FIFTH EDITION

REVISED

EMERGENCY CARE AND TRANSPORTATION

OF THE
SICK AND
INJURED

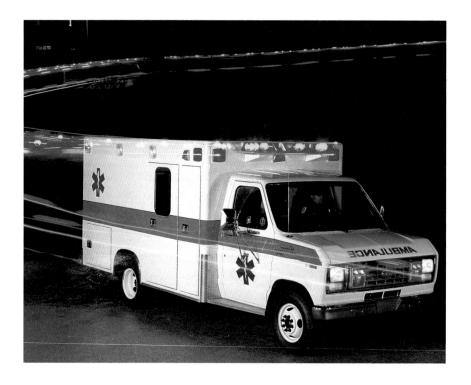

FIFTH EDITION

REVISED

EMERGENCY CARE AND TRANSPORTATION

OF THE
SICK AND
INJURED

JAMES D. HECKMAN, MD
CHAIRMAN, EDITORIAL BOARD

AMERICAN
ACADEMY OF
ORTHOPAEDIC
SURGEONS

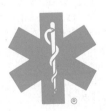
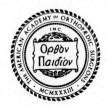

CREDITS

. . . .

Executive Director: Thomas C. Nelson
Deputy Executive Director: Fred V. Featherstone, MD
Director, Division of Education: Mark W. Wieting
Director, Department of Publications: Marilyn L. Fox, PhD
Production Manager: Loraine Edwalds
Senior Editor: Lynne Roby Shindoll
Production Editor: Kathy M. Brouillette
Editorial Assistants: Kathryn M. O'Brien, Susan Baim

Book design and art production: Image House, Inc.
Editor: Lynn Brown
Cover design: Image House, Inc.
Photography: Susan V. Steinkamp
Martin Simon

Emergency Care and Transportation of the Sick and Injured
Fifth Edition © 1991, Fourth Edition © 1987, Third Edition
© 1981, Second Edition © 1977, First Edition © 1971

ISBN 0-89203-049-6

Library of Congress Catalog Card Number 91-075604

Published and distributed by: American Academy of
Orthopaedic Surgeons

10 9 8 7 6 5

CONTENTS

. . . .

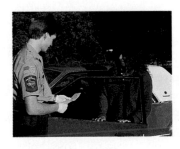
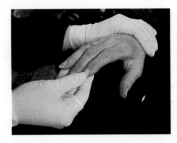

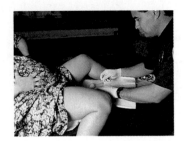
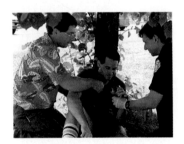
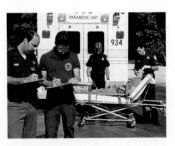
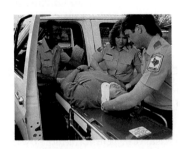
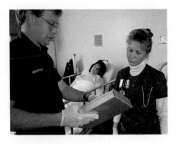

SECTION

12

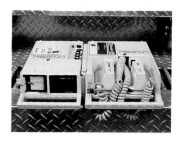

BOARD OF EDITORS

. . . .

DEDICATION

. . . .

This textbook is dedicated to the men and women
engaged in emergency medical services
whose unselfish devotion has improved, without
measure, the quality and effectiveness of prehospital
care.

CONTRIBUTORS

. . . .

Many individuals have contributed to the content of the fifth and previous editions of this textbook. It is impossible to list everyone, but the Board of Editors wishes especially to thank the following for their substantial contributions in recent years.

Cecil Arnold
Washington, DC
William Auchterlonie, EMT-PI/C
Wichita, Kansas
Mark D. Baker, EMT
Wichita, Kansas
George Berry, RPAC
New Hyde Park, New York
Marvin Birnbaum, MD, PhD
Madison, Wisconsin
Keith D. Bjork, MD
San Antonio, Texas
Dave Boersema, EMT-P
Crete, Illinois
Willis E. Brown, Jr., MD
San Antonio, Texas
Bruce D. Browner, MD
Houston, Texas
William E. Butler, BS, NREMT-P
San Antonio, Texas
Alexander M. Butman, EMSI, REMT-P
Akron, Ohio
R. Donovan Butter, DO
San Antonio, Texas
C. Robert Clark, MD
Lookout Mountain, Tennessee
Ewell A. Clarke, MD
San Antonio, Texas
Jo Ann Cobble, MA, NREMT-P, RN
Jacksonville, Arkansas
Nancy Colley, BSE, EMT
Riverside, Missouri

Richard O. Cummins, MD, MPH, MSc
Seattle, Washington
Ronald D'Acchioli
Santa Monica, California
Lorraine J. Day, MD
San Francisco, California
Robert DiLibero, JD
Boston, Massachusetts
Donna C. Dowd, MD
San Antonio, Texas
Carol L. Dunetz, MD
Lake Success, New York
Richard G. Dunford, MS
Seattle, Washington
Kurt Edelmann, NREMT-P
Park Ridge, Illinois
Mickey Stewart Eisenberg, MD
Seattle, Washington
Michael F. French, NREMT-A
Kirksville, Missouri
Charles E. Garoni, BA, EMT-P
San Antonio, Texas
Charles B. Gillespie, MD
Albany, Georgia
John C. Goll, EMT-P
Indianapolis, Indiana
James Gosselin, EMT-I
New Britain, Connecticut
Judith R. Graves, RN, MA
Seattle, Washington
John F. Gwin, MD
Fort Worth, Texas
Henry Alan Hooper, MD
Camarillo, California
Walter A. Hoyt, Jr., MD
Akron, Ohio
Raymond E. Humiston, EMT-P
Southbury, Connecticut
Diana Jansen, RN, CCRN, EMT-P
Madison, Wisconsin
Jerald J. Jansen, EMT-A
Madison, Wisconsin
George L. Johnson, EMT
Albany, New York

Lou Jordan, PA
Baltimore, Maryland
Richard L. Judd, PhD, NREMT-A
New Britain, Connecticut
Glen Kane, MD
Venice, California
Nancy D. Kellogg, MD
San Antonio, Texas
J.G. Kendrick, MD
Wichita, Kansas
William Koenig, MD
Pasadena, California
Russell Kulp
Braintree, Massachusetts
Cynthia C. Kurdi
San Antonio, Texas
Denny Kurogi, NREMT-A, EMT I/C
Overland Park, Kansas
Alexander Lampone, MD
Pacific Palisades, California
W.H. Leonard
Phoenix, Arizona
John H. Littlefield, PhD
San Antonio, Texas
Donald MacLachlan, MD
Calgary, Alberta, Canada
Brian D. Mahoney, MD
Minneapolis, Minnesota
Dennis Mauk, EMT-P
Wichita, Kansas
Newton C. McCollough, MD
Tubac, Arizona
William F. McManus, MD
Fort Sam Houston, Texas
Norman E. McSwain, MD
New Orleans, Louisiana
Kathleen K. Mechler, RN
San Antonio, Texas
Jean Worsing Merry, DDS
Minneapolis, Minnesota
T.A. Don Michael, MD
Bakersfield, California
William J. Mills, Jr., MD
Anchorage, Alaska

TECHNICAL CONSULTATION

REVIEWERS

. . . .

Linda M. Abrahamson, EMT-P
  EMS Instructor/Coordinator
  BroMenn Healthcare
  Normal, Illinois
Ben E. Blankenship, NREMT-A I/C
  Captain, Training Division
  North Little Rock Fire Department
  North Little Rock, Arkansas
Nancy Bryan, NREMT-A
  BLS Training Coordinator
  Wisconsin Division of Health, EMS Section
  Madison, Wisconsin
Kenneth E. Cole, Jr.
  Director, Bureau of Emergency Medical Services
  Missouri Department of Health
  Jefferson City, Missouri
Robert A. Franklin, Jr., NREMT-P
  Virginia EMT-Instructor
  Regional Training Coordinator
  Western Virginia Regional EMS Council
  Salem, Virginia
Alice (Twink) Gorgen, BSN, NRPM
  Paramedic Nurse Coordinator
  PreHospital Education Program, Creighton
  University
  Omaha, Nebraska
George L. Johnson, EMT
  Chairman ASTM Committee F30.02 on
  EMS Personnel Education and Training
  Albany, New York
W.H. Leonard
  Executive Vice President
  Az Star Center for Safety and Risk Management
  Phoenix, Arizona
Fred R. Matthes, EMT Instructor Coordinator
  Program Director, Public Safety Services
  Great Oaks JVSD
  Cincinnati, Ohio

Jeffrey T. Mitchell, PhD
  Clinical Associate Professor of Emergency
  Health Services
  University of Maryland (UMBC)
  Baltimore, Maryland
Lawrence D. Newell, EdD, NREMT-P
  Senior Associate, Development Health and Safety
  American National Red Cross
  Washington, DC
Daniel S. Shannon, EMT-P
  EMS Training Section
  Los Angeles City Fire Department
  Los Angeles, California
D. Terry Shorr, BS, NREMT-P
  Training Director
  West Virginia Office of EMS
  Charleston, West Virginia
Mark Stevens
  Director of Training
  Buck Medical Services
  Portland, Oregon
Mary Ann Talley, RN, BSN, MPA, EMT-B
  Program Director/Chairman
  Department of EMS Education
  University of South Alabama
  Mobile, Alabama
Tom Vines, EMT-D
  Editor
  Response Magazine
  Red Lodge, Montana
Jason White, BA, EMT-P
  State Training Coordinator
  Missouri Department of Health
  Jefferson City, Missouri
Robert L. Zickler, MS, ED
  Deputy Chief
  Indianapolis Fire Department
  Indianapolis, Indiana

FOREWORD

. . . .

In 1971, when the American Academy of Orthopaedic Surgeons published the first edition of *Emergency Care and Transportation of the Sick and Injured*, no one predicted that 20 years later we would be publishing our fifth edition. Nor would they have predicted that the field of emergency medical services would have come so far.

What in 1971 was a loosely organized group of undertrained, underequipped, and understaffed ambulance drivers has become a highly professional group of prehospital care providers. Emergency medical technicians and paramedics are essential elements in the continuum of care. The Academy, probably best known in the field as "AAOS," is proud to have been there at the beginning, and to have contributed along the way. But the real tribute should go to those in the field who have taught others, the instructors who have shared their knowledge and their hearts with the thousands of people who have come into the field at the ground level, who have taken the EMT-A training course.

The Academy has been committed to keeping up with the rapid rate of change in the EMS field, with new editions of "the Orange Book" in 1977, 1981, 1987, and now 1992. Along the way, with successive reprintings of the book, we have tried to refine concepts and add the most current information on such rapidly changing topics as infectious diseases and trauma care. This is our continuing commitment to the people who use this book.

It is not an easy effort. The Editorial Board for the fifth edition spent many long hours on this project—on airplanes, in hotel meeting rooms, and at their desks at home—writing and refining the text and the illustrations for this edition.

In addition, many other contributors and reviewers from all corners of the EMS world have given us the benefit of their knowledge and experience and have been an integral part of the development of this new edition. We cannot thank them enough for the assistance they gave us.

James D. Heckman, MD, chairman of the Editorial Board, was at the helm of this 20th anniversary edition of *Emergency Care and Transportation of the Sick and Injured*. He also headed the editorial boards of the third and fourth editions. He is chairman of the department and professor of orthopaedics, University of Texas Health Science Center in San Antonio. Ronald E. Rosenthal, MD, of New Hyde Park, New York, Robert A. Worsing, Jr., MD, of Kansas City, Missouri, and Arthur S. McFee, MD, of San Antonio have served the editorial boards of previous editions; Dr. McFee, in fact, served on the editorial board of the first edition. New members of the Editorial Board are Ralph J. DiLibero, MD, of Palos Verdes Estates, California, and Donald J. Gordon, MD, PhD, of San Antonio, who have brought new perspectives to the task.

On behalf of the Board of Directors of the American Academy of Orthopaedic Surgeons and all of the fellows of the Academy, it is my pleasure to congratulate the Board of Editors for producing this magnificent new edition of one of the most important books in health care publishing.

Augusto Sarmiento, MD
President
American Academy
of Orthopaedic Surgeons

PREFACE

· ·

The American Academy of Orthopaedic Surgeons is pleased to present this fifth edition of a textbook designed to provide current, accurate, and reliable information to the basic EMT student. Five years have elapsed since the publication of the fourth edition in this extremely dynamic field; many changes have occurred that advanced the quality of prehospital care. This new edition reflects these current concepts and draws from an increasingly large scientific base to provide evaluation and treatment plans in a logical and informed way.

As with previous editions of this text, the information has been collected from many sources. Numerous experts have been called upon to contribute to all stages of the project. Truly, this textbook is a consensus of the experts in the field, and the long list of contributors and reviewers presented here is a demonstration of the Academy's interest in providing the most useful information derived from the widest possible range of EMS experience.

The most current and correct information has been distilled from these many sources to provide a consistent and medically accurate textbook. Where controversy exists regarding the best approach to a specific emergency problem, the alternative methods are presented, or a synthesis of those methods designed to provide a practical and useful approach is described.

With each revision of this text, critiques of the previous editions are sought, carefully considered, and addressed. Because of the constantly changing nature of the emergency care field, the Editorial Board will continue to respect and respond to any criticism of this edition to assure continued currentness and appropriateness of its contents. The advances in textbook publication techniques will allow us to revise this fifth edition with each new printing, thus providing a more contemporary and accurate reflection of the current thinking of the leaders in prehospital care.

The specific changes in this edition most notably reflect the significantly increased emphasis on personal safety for the EMT in the field. Each section strongly emphasizes the importance of self-protection so that the EMT avoids self-injury and accidental infection. A new chapter, Chapter 3, is devoted entirely to EMT safety. The rapid advances in treatment of sudden cardiac arrest with automated external defibrillation have demanded that instruction in this modality be included in the text as a standard component of prehospital care education. At a meeting of 15 nationally recognized experts in the management of musculoskeletal trauma in January of 1990, the prehospital care of musculoskeletal injuries was reviewed in depth and chapters in this fifth edition accurately reflect the consensus of those deliberations. All of the principles outlined in the management of injuries are based on the principles of Prehospital Trauma Life Support as developed by the Committee on Trauma of the American College of Surgeons.

Many technical improvements have been made in this edition to enhance the student's ability to comprehend and retain the critical basic information. The quality and technical accuracy of the illustrations have been substantially improved. The Editorial Board has worked extremely hard to make the text as readable as possible, yet preserve the highly accurate and critical medical content that has been the hallmark of previous editions. Key words and goals have been created for each chapter to guide the student in learning the material. Finally, the accompanying workbook has been substantially rewritten, with questions that emphasize information essential for effective performance in the field.

This edition could not have been successfully completed without the extraordinary voluntary efforts of the members of the Board of Editors, who have devoted innumerable hours to this task. I express my sincere appreciation to each member for his outstanding contribution. The Editorial Board has had excellent administrative support and technical assistance from the publications staff of the American Academy of Orthopaedic Surgeons, and I would specifically like to thank Mr. Mark Wieting and his staff for their invaluable support. In particular, I would like to recognize Sally Jessee for getting the project off the ground, Kathy Brouillette for keeping track of it all, Katy Kohl and Susan Baim for word processing and proofreading, Loraine Edwalds for turning the raw materials into the finished product, and to Lynne Roby Shindoll for managing the workbook and related projects. Especially, I would like to thank Marilyn Fox, PhD, for overseeing all staff activities and for giving so much of herself to the project.

Special thanks must be extended to Stuart Paterson of Image House, Inc. for the design and art production of the book. The new photography in this edition is the work of Susan Steinkamp and Martin Simon. The consistency of the text is largely due to the excellent work of Lynn Brown, the medical copy editor.

Personally, I wish to thank Charles A. Rockwood, Jr., MD for his continuing encouragement, guidance, and support during the entire project; the Board of Directors of the American Academy of Orthopaedic Surgeons for their confidence, encouragement, and continuing support; Juanita Hammerstrom and Colleen Mann for their tolerance and extremely efficient editorial and secretarial skills; and finally to my family Susan, Coleman, and Betsy for their continuing love, support, and patient understanding during my many years of involvement with this project.

James D. Heckman, MD
San Antonio, Texas
1991

THE EMT CODE OF ETHICS

Professional status as an Emergency Medical Technician and Emergency Medical Technician-Paramedic is maintained and enriched by the willingness of the individual practitioner to accept and fulfill obligations to society, other medical professionals, and the profession of Emergency Medical Technician. As an Emergency Medical Technician at the basic level or an Emergency Medical Technician-Paramedic, I solemnly pledge myself to the following code of professional ethics:

A fundamental responsibility of the Emergency Medical Technician is to conserve life, to alleviate suffering, to promote health, to do no harm, and to encourage the quality and equal availability of emergency medical care.

The Emergency Medical Technician provides services based on human need, with respect for human dignity, unrestricted by consideration of nationality, race, creed, color, or status.

The Emergency Medical Technician does not use professional knowledge and skills in any enterprise detrimental to the public well being.

The Emergency Medical Technician respects and holds in confidence all information of a confidential nature obtained in the course of professional work unless required by law to divulge such information.

The Emergency Medical Technician, as a citizen, understands and upholds the law and performs the duties of citizenship; as a professional, the Emergency Medical Technician has the never-ending responsibility to work with concerned citizens and other health care professionals in promoting a high standard of emergency medical care to all people.

The Emergency Medical Technician shall maintain professional competence and demonstrate concern for the competence of other members of the Emergency Medical Services health care team.

An Emergency Medical Technician assumes responsibility in defining and upholding standards of professional practice and education.

The Emergency Medical Technician assumes responsibility for individual professional actions and judgment, both in dependent and independent emergency functions, and knows and upholds the laws which affect the practice of the Emergency Medical Technician.

An Emergency Medical Technician has the responsibility to be aware of and participate in matters of legislation affecting the Emergency Medical Technician and the Emergency Medical Services System.

The Emergency Medical Technician adheres to standards of personal ethics which reflect credit upon the profession.

Emergency Medical Technicians, or groups of Emergency Medical Technicians, who advertise professional services, do so in conformity with the dignity of the profession.

The Emergency Medical Technician has an obligation to protect the public by not delegating to a person less qualified, any service which requires the professional competence of an Emergency Medical Technician.

The Emergency Medical Technician will work harmoniously with and sustain confidence in Emergency Medical Technician associates, the nurse, the physician, and other members of the Emergency Medical Services health care team.

The Emergency Medical Technician refuses to participate in unethical procedures, and assumes the responsibility to expose incompetence or unethical conduct of others to the appropriate authority in a proper and professional manner.

*The National Association
of Emergency Medical Technicians*

THE EMT OATH

Be it pledged as an Emergency Medical Technician, I will honor the physical and judicial laws of God and man. I will follow that regimen which, according to my ability and judgment, I consider for the benefit of patients and abstain from whatever is deleterious and mischievous, nor shall I suggest any such counsel. Into whatever homes I enter, I will go into them for the benefit of only the sick and injured, never revealing what I see or hear in the lives of men unless required by law.

I shall also share my medical knowledge with those who may benefit from what I have learned. I will serve unselfishly and continuously in order to help make a better world for all mankind.

While I continue to keep this oath unviolated, may it be granted to me to enjoy life, and the practice of the art, respected by all men, in all times. Should I trespass or violate this oath, may the reverse be my lot. So help me God.

Adopted by The National Association of Emergency Medical Technicians, 1978

SECTION 1

INTRODUCTION

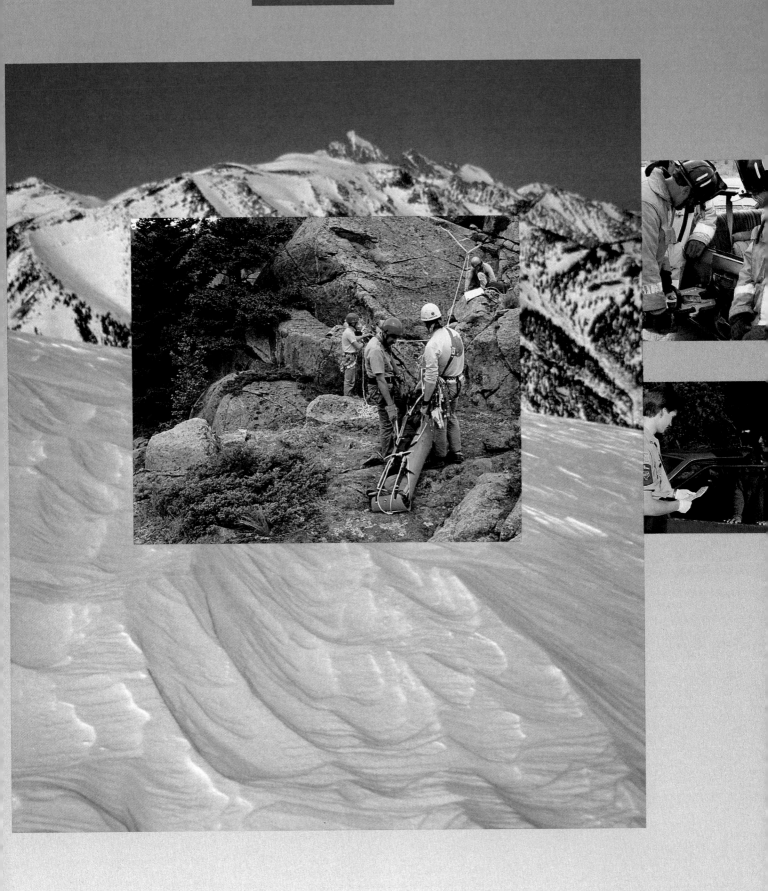

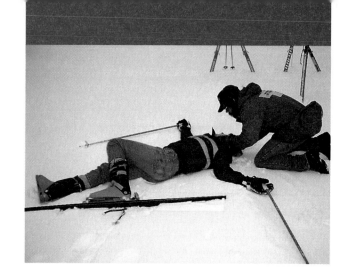

CHAPTER 1

ORIENTATION

KEY TERMS

basic life support (BLS) Simple emergency lifesaving procedures which can aid a person in respiratory or circulatory failure.

cardiopulmonary resuscitation (CPR) The artificial establishment of circulation of the blood and movement of air into and out of the lungs in a pulseless, nonbreathing patient.

Critical Incident Stress Debriefing (CISD) A program designed to help emergency medical personnel cope with psychological reactions to stressful job-related incidents.

emergency medical services (EMS) The combined efforts of several professionals and agencies to provide prehospital emergency care to the sick and injured.

emergency medical technician (EMT) A member of a prehospital emergency medical system who is trained to provide basic life support.

first responder The first person present at the scene of sudden illness or injury.

paramedic A trained professional EMT who provides sophisticated advanced life support in the field.

SURVIVE study technique Composed of the following techniques: *s*kim, *u*nderline, *r*ead, *v*erbalize, *i*ntegrate, *v*ary, and *e*valuate.

OVERVIEW

Emergency care of the sick and injured was inadequate in many areas of the United States until public attention brought needed reforms that were begun in the 1970s. These reforms resulted in the development of effective emergency medical services (EMS) systems staffed by well-trained emergency medical technicians (EMTs). This process continues today. And so, too, do we continue our role, with the fifth edition of *Emergency Care and Transportation of the Sick and Injured.*

As with the previous editions, the major portion of this text is devoted to instruction in the actual care of patients with specific emergency medical problems, from initial assessment through transportation to a medical facility. The book's content and objectives conform to the EMT National Standard Curriculum developed by the U.S. Department of Transportation in 1984. The theme that runs throughout the text is that in learning to give proper emergency care efficiently, you must be constantly mindful that the instructions contained in the various chapters are combined with the goal of saving lives. You must learn to avoid or reduce complications that might prolong recovery or cause permanent physical impairment. And last but not least, you must learn to combine effec-

tive interpersonal relationships with medical knowledge, skills, and practice.

Chapter 1 begins with a short history of how EMS systems came into being. The chapter then introduces the EMT. The roles and responsibilities of EMTs, their relationship with prehospital and hospital personnel, the emotional stress associated with the job, the importance of personal safety, and the training and certification needed by EMTs are covered. The last section of Chapter 1 explains more about the fifth edition of *Emergency Care and Transportation of the Sick and Injured* and about the "lifesaving" study technique we recommend called "SURVIVE."

GOALS

The goals of Chapter 1 are to
- identify the components of a functioning EMS system.
- get to know what is required of an EMT—roles and responsibilities, relationships with prehospital and hospital personnel, emotional strength, personal safety, and training and licensure standards.
- become familiar with the "SURVIVE" study technique.

THE EMERGENCY MEDICAL SERVICES (EMS) SYSTEM

For years there has been a wide gap between what is possible and what in fact has been delivered in emergency medical care. The knowledge and equipment necessary to develop an **emergency medical services (EMS)** sys-

tem existed long before such services became available to the public. In reality, EMS as we know it today had its beginnings 25 years ago in 1966. In that year, the Committees on Trauma and Shock of the National Academy of Sciences National Research Council jointly published "Accidental Death and Disability: The Neglected Disease of Modern Society." This report brought public attention to the inadequate emergency medical care being provided to the sick and injured in many areas of the country.

Two federal agencies initiated reform measures. The National Highway Traffic Safety Administration of the Department of Transportation (DOT), through the Highway Safety Act of 1966, and the Department of Health, Education, and Welfare (DHEW), through the Emergency Medical Services Act of 1973, created funding sources to develop improved prehospital emergency care. Thousands of dedicated individuals, assisted by a number of professional organizations and guided by regulatory input from various levels of government, organized and established local EMS systems in the early 1970s.

In the 1980s, practitioners took a hard look at what was done in the 70s, and the focus changed from establishing EMS systems to developing educational programs to provide consistent levels of quality care to the sick and injured. The programs included additional classroom training and "hands-on" skills sessions, as well as programs for certification, continuing education, and mandatory retraining. Despite the improvements in prehospital care, a great deal remained to be done. The gap between available services and the people who needed them was narrowing but still existed in many areas of the country. Likewise, the gap between what was theoretically feasible and what was realistically available also narrowed.

In the 1990s we have reached an era in which the value of the emergency medical technician (EMT) will truly be defined through scientific research. The responsibilities placed upon EMTs is increasing and will continue to expand. The level of care provided by basic EMTs will significantly increase for many reasons. Currently, 50 percent of the population of the United States is served by **paramedics** who provide sophisticated advanced life support in the field. That level of service, however, is costly and requires significant run volume to ensure skills maintenance. The 50 percent figure represents nearly total saturation of those areas that can both at once afford and utilize advanced life support in the prehospital setting, a situation that is unlikely to change greatly over the next several years. The greater need for well-trained EMTs in those areas not served by paramedics will likely fuel a move toward "training up" the existing and future EMTs to fill the gap.

The 1990s are also a time when advances in technology will become increasingly available. We will see the advent of several "high tech" products that will allow the basic EMT to perform certain "paramedic skills" with a safety factor that once required extensive training. The safety and efficiency of devices such as the automatic defibrillator make it possible for the basic EMT to provide sophisticated lifesaving care. This decade is an exciting and demanding time for the EMT.

The EMS system is made up of various components that work together to provide the sick and injured with the best possible emergency medical care in the shortest possible time. The EMS system represents the combined efforts of the first responder, the EMT with basic life-support skills, the EMT-intermediate or EMT-paramedic with advanced life-support skills, emergency department personnel, physicians, allied health personnel, hospital administration, EMS system administration, and the overseeing governmental agencies.

The way an EMS system functions varies widely, depending on the geographic area and population served. Regardless of whether it is in a rural area, a large city, or a vast metropolitan complex, the EMS system requires the following 14 essential elements:

1. An advisory council on emergency medical service.
2. Physician-directed medical control, including quality control review.
3. EMT training programs, including continuing education programs.
4. Instructor training programs.
5. A communications system, including system access.
6. Dispatch center(s).
7. Ambulance service(s).
8. EMT and emergency department personnel rapport and trust.
9. Reports and records.

10. Ongoing system evaluation with quality assurance, risk management, and outcome study programs.
11. Disaster plans.
12. Public information and education programs.
13. Categorized hospital emergency capabilities.
14. Funding.

THE EMERGENCY MEDICAL TECHNICIAN (EMT)

The cornerstone of the EMS system is the **emergency medical technician (EMT).** EMTs have the greatest opportunity of perhaps any group in society to relieve suffering and to reduce injury severity and death at the scene of an accidental injury or sudden illness and during transportation to a medical facility. To become a valued member of the prehospital emergency medical care team, you need the following:

1. Proper training and experience.
2. Ready availability of the proper equipment and supplies.
3. A properly designed vehicle to meet the needs of the sick and injured.
4. Treatment protocols and guidelines.
5. Radio communication with emergency department personnel.
6. Ready availability of physician-directed medical control.

Roles and Responsibilities of the EMT

You have to earn the respect and recognition of the community in which you live and work. You must be viewed as a responsible member of the emergency medical care team. To these ends, your attitude and conduct must at all times be professional and reflect a sincere dedication to serve humanity. Your moral and ethical standards must be of the highest order. You must take pride in your personal appearance, as well as in your technical knowledge and skills used to render care to the sick and injured.

Such knowledge and skills, however, must be continually expanded and updated. To this end, you must take responsibility for your learning and continuing education. You must strive for excellence in job performance, with full recognition of your personal limitations. You must accept and benefit from constructive criticism and advice.

EMTs are expected to perform under pressure with composure and self-confidence. Emotions have to be controlled and suppressed through self-discipline. The abnormal or exaggerated actions of patients and families under stress need to be handled with understanding and sympathy. These are the qualities of responsible leadership, which you must provide to ensure the health, survival, safety, comfort, and confidence of your patients from the time you arrive on the scene until you transfer patient care to other medical professionals.

No matter how severe the circumstances, you have a moral obligation to provide the best emergency medical care possible until relieved by a physician or other qualified person at the scene or at the hospital. Your primary responsibilities to the patient are to:

- Protect yourself and the patient from further harm.
- Carefully assess and evaluate all signs and symptoms.
- Give prompt and efficient medical care.
- Provide safe and efficient transportation.
- Arrange the orderly transfer of patient care at the receiving medical facility.
- Communicate with all parties and agencies involved.

In addition to the patient care responsibilities, EMTs have additional responsibilities, including maintaining control at the scene, gaining access to and disentangling patients, keeping accurate records, and operating and maintaining the emergency vehicle and its equipment and supplies. Last, but just as important, you have a responsibility to yourself and others at the scene to perform your duties with due regard for your own safety as well as the safety of those around you.

Prehospital Care Personnel and the EMT

In the structure of emergency medical service systems throughout the country, there are recognized differences among basic first-aid training, a DOT first responder training course, and a DOT-approved EMT training course. Basic first-aid and the slightly more advanced first responder training programs incorporate basic life-sustaining measures that members of the general public should learn in order to recognize the many hazards encountered during their daily activities.

Ideally, basic first-aid training should begin at the fifth-grade level. All EMTs should actively participate as instructors in these community training programs. This training should be made available to as many citizens as possible, but especially to those individuals who through their jobs or recreational interests are likely to encounter situations that might require the use of emergency medical techniques. First-aid and first responder training should be under the direction of and taught in part by knowledgeable physicians.

Professional emergency medical care, on the other hand, is administered at the scene of an accident or illness and during transport to a medical facility by highly trained EMTs. These individuals might be volunteers, employees of a commercial ambulance service, or members of a municipal ambulance operation.

The first responder plays an important role in the EMS system. The **first responder** is the first medically trained person to arrive at the scene of sudden illness or injury (Figure 1–1). The care given by a first responder is essential because it is given first. That first person could be a fire fighter, police officer, safety engineer, occupational health or school nurse, coach or trainer, lifeguard, youth leader, or one of many other professionals in public places.

These individuals should be trained to the level of the First Responder Curriculum, which has been developed by the Department of Transportation. This training includes **cardiopulmonary resuscitation (CPR).** First responders may have little or no equipment, and in reality they need none to sustain life until a trained EMT arrives on the scene. First responders can assess the injury or illness, provide air to the lungs, blood to the brain, and control bleeding. In other words, they can provide **basic life support (BLS).**

Just as it is essential for the first responder to do enough for the patient, it is essential for the first responder not to try to do too much. One of the greatest mistakes the general public and first responders make is to remove the injured victim from a vehicle or accident scene. Many additional injuries, including permanent paralysis, have been caused by such well-intentioned, but potentially dangerous, actions. At

FIGURE 1–1

The first responder is the first person present at the scene of sudden illness or injury. By using their hands, lungs, mouth, and brain, first responders can sustain life until a trained EMT or other professional emergency medical personnel arrive.

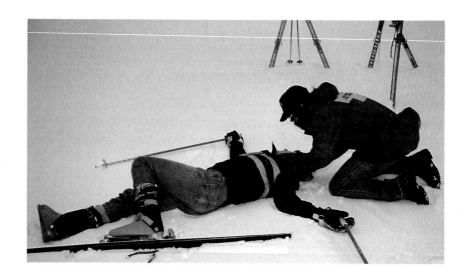

the scene of an injury, an unwarranted fear of fire or lack of training is frequently the cause for such intervention.

A first responder should attempt to gain access to the patient if possible and provide necessary, life-sustaining CPR, control accessible bleeding using pressure, comfort the patient, and await your arrival. Only if the patient's position prevents necessary life-sustaining care or if some circumstances exist that pose an immediate threat to the life of the patient or first responder—for example, fire or imminent collapse of a structure—should the first responder attempt to move the patient before you arrive with appropriate equipment.

On arrival, you should assume responsibility immediately but tactfully. Assess the quality and effectiveness of the care rendered by the first responders and ask the first responders to continue assistance as needed. Give credit for what was done and diplomatically suggest improvements for subsequent care, keeping in mind that the scene of an accident is not the place to be openly critical of the skills or techniques of a first responder. The training of first responders is a vital link in the EMT chain. Especially in rural areas, the training of first responders is one of the weakest elements of EMS systems. Therefore, you must be actively involved not only in promoting such training programs for the general public and first responders, but also in the instruction process. In addition, you must promote the continuing education and evaluation process for first responders and other EMTs. It is possible that the next life the first responder saves might very well be your own.

You may come in contact with two additional groups of prehospital emergency medical care personnel: the EMT-paramedic and the EMT-intermediate. The EMT-paramedic (EMT-P) has completed an extensive course of training in advanced life support, including intravenous therapy, pharmacology, cardiac monitoring, and defibrillation; advanced airway maintenance, including intubation; and other advanced assessment and treatment skills. Some states have established an intermediate level of training between the basic EMT and the EMT-

paramedic. The EMT-intermediate (EMT-I) has training in specific aspects of advanced life support (ALS). This training is generally limited to a very specific area, such as intravenous therapy, cardiac defibrillation, or advanced airway management. Whenever an EMT-I or EMT-P arrives on the scene, you should give a brief account of the situation, transfer the responsibility for patient care, and stand by to assist as requested.

Hospital Personnel and the EMT

There is no better way for you to understand how prehospital care influences full recovery or aids in reducing permanent physical impairment than to observe the continuation of emergency medical care by the staff of the emergency department. How much is learned depends on your sincerity of purpose; eagerness for self-improvement in knowledge, techniques, and skills; and willingness to accept advice and constructive feedback. An EMT with these attributes can enjoy a close working relationship with the hospital staff (Figure 1–2). It is for this reason that in-hospital observation programs are built into the EMT training program.

Although legal restrictions or local and hospital rules may prevent you from participating actively in all procedures in the emergency department, much can be learned through direct observation, instruction, demonstration, and assisting to the extent permitted. As an observer, you will become familiar with hospital equipment and its use, the functions of staff members, and the policies and procedures in all emergency areas of the hospital. In addition, you will keep abreast of advances in emergency care as well as in the use of new equipment. The experience gained from participation serves to emphasize the importance and benefits of proper initial emergency care and efficient transportation, as well as the consequences of delay, inadequate care, or poor judgment.

Rarely is a physician present at the scene of an accident or at the onset of unexpected illness to give on-the-spot directions to the EMT.

FIGURE 1–2

One of the best ways for an EMT to understand how important prehospital emergency care is in aiding full recovery and reducing permanent impairment is to observe the continuation of medical care in the hospital emergency department.

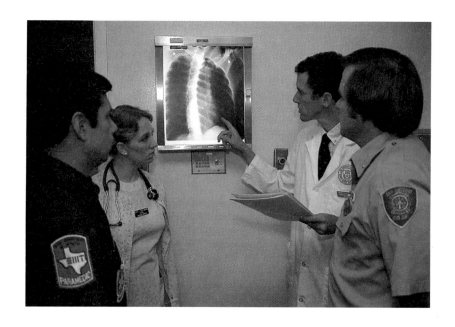

Consultation and advice are usually given over the radio through established medical control procedures. In addition to acting as an instructor for the medical subjects taught in this book, the emergency department physician can effectively train you in the emergency department by demonstrating assessment and treatment techniques on actual patients.

With such instruction, you become more comfortable using medical terminology, become better able to interpret the signs and symptoms of injury and disease, and develop needed patient management skills. At the same time, the physician becomes familiar with your capabilities and develops a degree of trust in your skills so there will be no hesitation in allowing you to proceed with patient care protocols if and when radio communication fails. Such prior face-to-face communication improves radio communication between you and the physician.

The people who staff the emergency departments of most hospitals are eager and willing to help improve the skills and efficiency of EMTs, not only during the initial phase of training but throughout their careers. A close rapport among all involved in providing emergency medical care not only ensures optimal patient care but also affords you and emergency department staffs the opportunity to discuss your mutual problems, benefit from each other's experiences, and better fulfill your respective roles as members of the emergency medical care team.

THE EMS SYSTEM MEDICAL DIRECTOR

The EMS system medical director plays an *extremely* important role in the delivery of prehospital emergency medical care. The medical director authorizes or delegates the privilege to perform medical acts to the field EMT. As prehospital medical care activities come under increasing scrutiny, it is increasingly important for the emergency medical service to have a medical director who takes an active role in supervising and supporting the activities of the field EMT.

It is the medical director's responsibility to coordinate and ensure the provision of appropriate and consistent prehospital emergency medical care. The medical director is expected to provide for on-line and off-line medical direction, commonly called medical control. On-line medical control is delivered by a physician or registered nurse who is authorized by the medical director to communicate medical orders directly to field EMTs in person, by radio, or by telephone.

Off-line medical control is delivered by standing orders or standard medical operating procedures (SMOPs) that are written down, authorized, and delegated in writing by the medical director and followed by field personnel in the absence of direct on-line medical control. The medical director is also responsible for ensuring appropriate EMT education and continuing training, providing a system of quality assurance and risk management for the EMS system, providing liaison with the medical community, and ensuring that appropriate standards are met by EMS personnel.

The medical director is the primary supporter of the field EMT, because it is through his or her medical authority that the EMT provides medical care. It is up to the medical director to coordinate the interaction of the EMT with all levels of health care professionals. Medical problems, including possible liability and infectious disease exposures, need to be immediately brought to the attention of the medical director for resolution.

Most states have an EMS law which requires that an EMS system providing advanced life support (ALS) services have a licensed physician as the system medical director. The state EMS law usually defines the duties and responsibilities of the medical director.

The medical director is in a unique position to supervise and provide assistance to you, because the director understands and supervises your day to day operations. All EMS systems should have a medical director who sets the standard of care and provides mentorship, apprenticeship, and role-modeling for the practice of prehospital emergency medicine.

PREPARATION FOR BECOMING AN EMT

Emotional Stress and the EMT

You need great willpower to remain calm and perform effectively when confronted with horrifying events, life-threatening illness, or injury. The kind of self-control you need to respond effectively to the suffering of others can only be developed through proper training, through gaining experience in dealing with all degrees of physical and mental distress, and especially through an unswerving dedication to serve humanity. At times, even the most experienced physician or combat-hardened medic may find it difficult to overcome personal reactions and proceed without hesitation to release patients from life-endangering situations, administer life-support measures to the mutilated, or recover the remains of those mangled in highway accidents, aircraft disasters, or explosions. You must learn to face these situations calmly and to act responsibly as a member of the emergency medical care team. You must also realize that the feelings that must be kept under control are normal feelings. They are experienced by everyone who has to deal with such situations, and they contribute to the emotional stress of an EMT's job.

There may arise an occasion when a disaster situation is so horrible that you are paralyzed and unable to respond. Do not be ashamed of such feelings, which affect approximately 20 percent of all people who respond to such events. If you feel overwhelmed, step back and call for help. Sometimes, simply knowing that additional help is on the way can free your inhibitions and enable you to respond to the situation. You should also be alert to see that your fellow EMTs are under control and not frozen or acting inappropriately in the face of a major disaster.

After a stressful run or a disaster, there is an emotional letdown. This phase is often overlooked, but often in the long run it is more important to deal with than the initial contact response. **Critical Incident Stress Debriefing (CISD)** is designed to deal with this emotional letdown phase. Never be ashamed to report your feelings, because such debriefing can be vital to your emotional well-being and should not be dismissed as trivial or nonessential.

A high percentage of the patients you treat will be rational and cooperative. Their concerns will generally be relieved by calm and efficient care and a simple explanation of what you are doing and why. Often you will realize that a given condition is not a true medical emergency, but for the patient it might seem to be truly serious. Neither by action nor word should you fail to take the patient's concern seriously. This means being extremely careful about what is said at the scene. During periods of great stress, words that seem immaterial or are uttered in jest might become fixed in the patient's mind and cause untold harm. Conversations at the scene must be appropriate. Statements such as "Everything will be all right" or "There is nothing to worry about" are inappropriate. A person who is trapped in a wrecked car, hurting from head to foot and worrying about the condition of a loved one or about the payments on the car, knows very well that all is not well. What will reassure the patient is that a trained EMT is present. You must explain briefly the emergency actions to be taken and discuss to which medical facility the patient wishes to be transported.

When you are unsure whether a true medical emergency exists, it is always best to transport the patient to a hospital for evaluation by a physician who then may decide to dismiss the patient; you do not have that option. For both ethical and medicolegal reasons, a physician must examine all patients transported by you and judge the degree of medical need of every "emergency" patient. You must also realize that the most subtle of symptoms may be early signs of catastrophe and that symptoms of many illnesses may be similar to those of alcohol and drug abuse or withdrawal, hysteria, or other conditions. You must not only accept the patient's complaints at face value but also provide appropriate care for the injury or illness reported until you are able to transfer the care of the patient to a hospital or physician. Local medical director protocols will direct your actions in these uncertain situations.

A patient's reaction to acute injury or illness may be influenced by certain personality traits. Some people may be highly emotional and demonstrative over what may seem to be a minor problem, whereas others show little or no emotion, even in the face of serious injury or illness. Many factors, such as social and economic background, dependence on others, level of maturity, fear of medical personnel, senility, mental disorders, alcoholism, drug addiction, reaction to medication, nutritional status, and chronic disease, may influence how a patient reacts.

Although you cannot be expected to know the underlying causes that might trigger unusual emotional responses, a quick, calm appraisal of the actions of the patient and of relatives and bystanders will help you to gain the confidence and cooperation of all concerned. Courtesy, calmness, proper tone of voice, sincere concern, and efficient action during the examination and treatment will go far to relieve anxiety, fear, and insecurity. Calm reassurance rather than abrupt dismissal, chiding, or accusation will inspire confidence and gain cooperation. Compassion is a notable attribute, but you must be careful that it does not overrule reason. For example, a screaming toddler with no obvious life-threatening injuries, yet covered with another victim's blood, can appeal to your compassion and attention, while an unconscious, nonbreathing adult nearby dies from lack of care.

Patients must be given the opportunity to express their fears and concerns, many of which may easily be relieved on the spot. The usual concerns are for the safety or well-being of others involved in the accident and for the damage or loss of personal property. Your response must be discreet and diplomatic, giving reassurance when appropriate. If possible, you should wait until an experienced person such as a minister or emergency department nurse can tell the patient of the death or critical injury of a loved one so that the psychological support the person may need is available.

Some patients, especially children and the confused or aged, may be terrified or feel rejected when separated from family members. Other patients may not want family members to share their stress or witness their disability or pain. The extent to which relatives participate in patient care, including whether they go with the patient to the hospital, must be decided on the basis of the best interests of the patient. It is usually best if parents go with their children and if relatives accompany confused, elderly patients.

The religious customs or needs of the patient must also be respected. Many people have strong convictions against the administration of drugs and blood and blood products. Some people will cling to religious medals or amulets, especially if an attempt is made to remove them. Others will express a strong desire for religious counsel, baptism, or last rites if death is imminent at the scene. You must try to accommodate these requests.

In the case of death, the body of the deceased must be handled with respect and dignity. It must be exposed as little as possible. You must be aware of local restrictions about moving the body or changing its position, especially if there is a possibility of a criminal investigation. Even under these circumstances, CPR and appropriate treatment must be instituted unless there are obvious signs of death, such as rigor mortis, decapitation, or other massive injuries not compatible with life.

The care of the handicapped patient presents special problems. This is particularly true of the deaf, the deaf-mute, and the blind. The hearing impaired patient who does not have a functioning hearing aid will have difficulty in understanding verbal questions about symptoms. The deaf-mute will be able to respond only with sign language or in writing. Unless pertinent information is needed at the scene, obvious problems should be treated. The patient can be reassured with efficient action and brief written notes. Detailed questioning may be delayed until the patient is transferred to a medical facility where relatives or others may act as interpreters.

Similar problems will occur with patients who do not speak English. In communities with large non-English-speaking populations, you will find it helpful to carry a card with frequently used medical words and their translations (Figure 1–3).

The blind patient, of course, will be able to talk with you, but you must be careful to explain what is occurring, the actions to be taken, and your qualifications to perform these actions. Although the majority of blind people are very self-reliant, they behave like any other patient when disoriented and confused. Such situations can be avoided by keeping them fully informed.

Personal Safety of the EMT

Chapter 3 of this text describes personal safety in detail, and it is emphasized throughout this text. The personal safety of all those involved in an emergency situation is very important—so

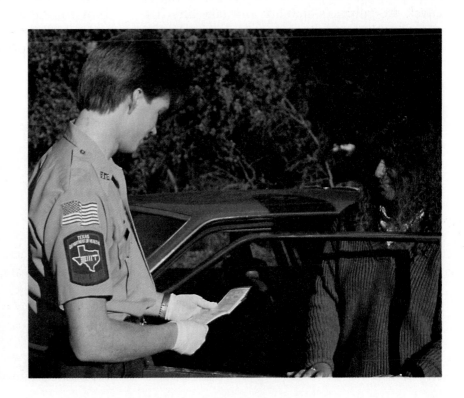

FIGURE 1–3

Language translation cards list frequently used medical words and their translations into English. EMTs who work in communities with large non-English-speaking populations should carry these cards.

important, in fact, that the steps you take to preserve personal safety must become automatic. A second accident at the scene or an injury to you compounds the problems, delays emergency medical care for the patients, increases the burden on the remaining EMTs, and may result in unnecessary fatalities.

Perhaps the easiest and most effective way in which you can protect yourself is by using seat belts and shoulder harnesses. When riding in a vehicle, you should wear belt devices at all times unless patient care makes it impossible. Many EMS units have instituted mandatory seat belt policies for the driver at all times, for all EMTs during transit to the scene, and for anyone riding with a patient.

The scene of an accident must be well marked, because a second accident often results in damage to the ambulance and injury to the EMTs. If the police have not already done so, proper warning devices should be placed at a sufficient distance from the scene to alert motorists coming from both directions. The ambulance should be parked at a safe, yet convenient, distance from the scene; the exact location will be determined by factors discussed later in the text. Before you make any attempt to access patients trapped in vehicles, check the vehicle's stability and take any necessary measures required to secure it. A vehicle's stability should not be determined by

pushing or rocking, because this may be all that is needed to overturn the vehicle or send it crashing into a ditch.

Your risk of injury when working at the scene of a wreck can be greatly reduced by wearing protective clothing. For example, a firefighter's helmet or hard hat, turnout gear, goggles or face shield, and leather gloves are all designed to decrease the risk of injury from broken glass or jagged metal during disentanglement of the patient (Figure 1–4).

To work effectively at night, you must have plenty of light. Poor lighting increases the risk of further injury to both you and the patient and results in poor emergency medical care for the patient. Proper lighting is included in the equipment requirements for ambulances. Reflective emblems or clothing help make you more visible at night and decrease your risk of injury (Figure 1–5).

You should never enter an unstable accident scene. Fires, poisonous gas, downed electrical wires, or hazardous materials require preliminary action by other public safety personnel. Unstable situations also include civil disturbances such as shootings, brawls, hostage situations, and riots. You must recognize hazardous situations and call for additional specialized assistance to stabilize the scene before you enter and render care; failure to do so may seriously jeopardize your personal safety. You

FIGURE 1–4

Wearing protective clothing, including a helmet or hard hat, turnout gear, goggles or a face shield, and leather gloves, will greatly reduce your risk of injury.

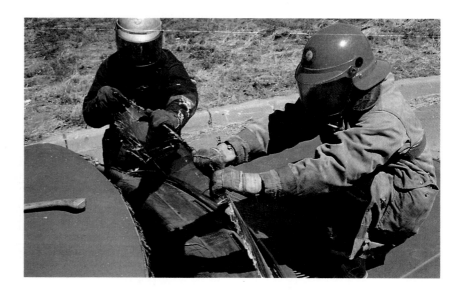

should rely on the advice of police or other public safety officials for the appropriate protective measures to take under these circumstances. Again, the general rule is that you should not enter an unsecured or unstable incident scene.

Finally, infection is another real and common hazard that will confront you. Universal infectious disease precautions must be taken in every instance where an exposure to body fluids is a possibility.

EMT Training

Emergency medical technology is an exciting field of study. Few areas offer more direct application of theory and skills. Everything that is taught in an EMT class will be important when it comes to saving lives and lessening human suffering. Emergency medical technology combines theoretical information, practical skills, and common sense. Becoming an effective EMT means mastering the information in this textbook, becoming competent in the technical skills taught in laboratory sessions, and using your common sense. You must also possess a great deal of compassion and understanding.

The Department of Transportation's Emergency Medical Technician-Ambulance: National Standard Curriculum specifies that training consist of a minimum of 110 hours; most EMT courses run from 110 to 140 hours. During your training program, you will develop the capabilities necessary to carry out your required responsibilities. The training may be divided into three main categories. The first and most important category is the care of life-threatening conditions. For such situations, you must learn to:

1. Establish and maintain an open airway.
2. Provide adequate pulmonary ventilation.
3. Perform cardiopulmonary resuscitation.
4. Control accessible bleeding.
5. Treat shock.
6. Care for cases of poisoning.

The second category of training covers conditions that, although not life-threatening, must be cared for before the patient is transported to a medical facility. To handle these situations, you must learn to:

1. Dress and bandage wounds.
2. Splint fractures and dislocations.
3. Deliver a baby.
4. Care for newborn infants, including premature infants.
5. Cope with the psychologic stresses on patients, families, colleagues, and yourself.

FIGURE 1–5

Adequate lighting is essential for providing emergency care. Poor lighting increases the risk of further injury to both you and the patient. Reflective emblems on clothing also make you more visible at night.

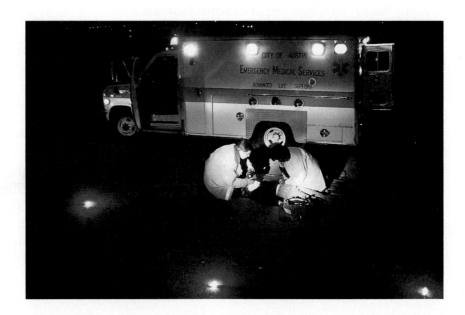

The third training category covers important nonmedical requirements. You must develop competence in the following areas:

1. Verbal and written communications skills.
2. Defensive and emergency driving skills.
3. Maintenance and use of supplies and equipment.
4. Proper extrication techniques and equipment.
5. Avoiding or coping with medicolegal problems.

Licensure, Certification, and Continuing Education for the EMT

Licensure, certification, recertification, and continuing education policies and procedures vary from state to state, although efforts are being made to establish a national standard. It is important for each EMT to understand and conform to the local requirements. EMT training is not a one-time effort. To maintain, update, and broaden needed knowledge and skills, you must continue to study. This responsibility for continuing educational effort exists whether you are affiliated with a full-time paid ambulance service or a rural volunteer rescue squad. In fact, rural volunteers probably have a greater need for continuing education, because they do not have as many opportunities to refresh their knowledge and skills in actual patient-handling situations.

Four major national organizations that are concerned with the education, licensure, and certification of EMTs are the National Council of State EMS Training Coordinators, Inc., the National Registry of Emergency Medical Technicians, the International Society of Fire Service Instructors, and the National Association of Emergency Medical Technicians.

The National Council of State EMS Training Coordinators, Inc. The purpose of the National Council of State EMS Training Coordinators is to promote the training of EMS personnel based on sound educational principles and current medical knowledge and practice. The council seeks acceptance of a standardized national EMT training curriculum, certification/recertification policies and procedures, and the reciprocity of certification from state to state. Public recognition and trust of the EMT as a health care professional is a major goal of the council. Forty-seven states are represented on the council, in addition to numerous liaison appointees from professional organizations that are involved in prehospital care.

The National Registry of Emergency Medical Technicians The National Registry of EMTs is the recognized national agency for certifying EMTs and documenting their level of competence according to recommended standards. The goals of the Registry are to promote and improve the delivery of emergency medical services by:

■ Assisting in the development and evaluation of educational programs to train EMTs.
■ Establishing qualifications for eligibility in applying for certification.
■ Preparing and conducting examinations designed to ensure the competence of EMTs.
■ Establishing a system of recertification every two years.
■ Establishing procedures for revocation of certification for cause.
■ Maintaining a national directory of registered EMTs.

The Registry also develops guidelines and programs to help registered EMTs raise their level of competence, thereby ensuring the provision of improved emergency medical services. Finally, the Registry will do any and all things necessary or desirable for the attainment of these goals.

The three levels of national certification available through the National Registry are basic (EMT-ambulance and EMT-nonambulance), intermediate (EMT-intermediate), and advanced (EMT-paramedic). The shoulder patch of the National Registry of EMTs has been copyrighted, and rockers (patches) attesting to the EMT's level of competence are available (Figure 1–6).

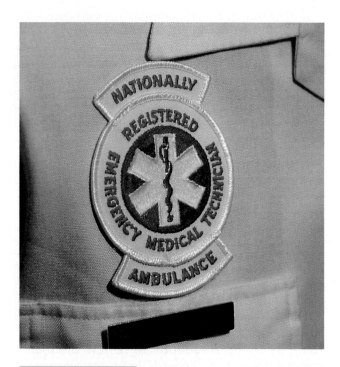

FIGURE 1–6

Rockers are small patches that are positioned below the National Registry patch. They indicate an EMT's level of competence and any specialized training.

The International Society of Fire Service Instructors The International Society of Fire Service Instructors has approximately 6,000 members in all 50 states and 10 foreign countries. Its EMS section is designed to meet the training and education needs of persons providing emergency medical services training. The society serves as a communication link for its members through newsletters, meetings, and other clearinghouse activities.

The National Association of Emergency Medical Technicians The National Association of Emergency Medical Technicians (NAEMT) was formed in 1975 by a representative group of nationally registered EMTs from existing state EMT organizations, national EMS leaders, and the National Registry of EMTs to serve the needs of EMTs throughout the country. The association has a membership in excess of 4,000 in 26 affiliated EMT associations. It sponsors continuing education programs on a national, regional, and local level. It provides a total of 15 other membership programs and services. The association's goals are to promote the professional status of the EMT, encourage the constant upgrading of the education and abilities of the EMT, and strive for a national standard of recognition for the skills and abilities of the EMT.

USING *EMERGENCY CARE AND TRANSPORTATION OF THE SICK AND INJURED,* 5TH ED.

This may be the first time you have been a student in several years, or this course may be part of your ongoing educational process. Whatever group you fall into, the editors have strived to ease your learning tasks. The content and objectives of this textbook conform to the EMT National Standard Curriculum developed by the United States Department of Transportation in 1984. The format of each chapter has been modified from previous editions to enhance student retention of the information presented. Each chapter begins with an overview of the topic to be covered and a list of educational goals that outline the core material. Key words are highlighted and defined at the start of each chapter. Other important new words are printed in italic and defined in the Glossary. Often a simple definition of these words follows their introduction in the text. Should you have forgotten the meaning of these new words or key terms when they are used in later chapters, check the Glossary at the end of the textbook. The end of each chapter contains a few thought-provoking questions under the heading "You Are the EMT." They should help you apply the principles within the chapter to the types of situations you will encounter as an EMT.

The student workbook is divided into sections that correspond to the chapters in the text. Each section contains questions on the material covered in the chapter. The questions are multiple-choice, fill-in-the-blank, true-false, or label the diagram. Answering the questions will help you retain the material that you have just studied. The end of each section in the workbook contains a series of multiple-choice questions. In addition to helping you review the material that you have just covered, these questions will also provide you with some practice in the testing format used in the written portion of most licensure and certification examinations.

To assist you in successfully completing the EMT course you have undertaken, the **SURVIVE study technique** was developed. Its purpose is to help you gain and retain more from your reading assignments and workbook activities. Take a few minutes to review this "lifesaving" study technique.

S – Skim

Read the chapter overview and goals. Briefly skim the chapter. Look at all the headings, pictures, charts, and diagrams.

U – Underline

Underline or highlight any unfamiliar words or medical terms that you have been asked to define. Do not highlight long sentences or passages. The purpose of highlighting is to allow the quick location of key information within the text. Excessive highlighting defeats this purpose.

R – Read

Read the goals at the beginning of the chapter again. Read the workbook questions and any questions distributed by your instructor. This enables you to direct your reading toward the specific goals of the chapter. Now, read the chapter.

V – Verbalize

Answer the questions from the workbook and your instructor out loud. This technique will help you to remember in two ways. First, it turns a written stimulus into an auditory response. At the same time, it holds the answer in your brain long enough for it to be transferred to long-term memory.

I – Integrate

Integrate the new information with the information you have previously learned in the textbook as well as in your lab sessions. Using the information helps make it meaningful and is an excellent way to increase your memory retention.

V – Vary

Vary your activity. Take a break from your studies so the newly acquired information can "sink in." Stop frequently to review the material you have just covered.

E – Evaluate

Evaluate the newly presented information. Does it conflict with previously presented materials? Do the lecturers say the same thing as the textbook? Were all of your questions answered? If not, you need to get those questions cleared up as soon as possible.

One of the most important tasks for the EMT student is learning to study effectively. The SURVIVE format is intended to provide the structure needed to sharpen your study skills. The following additional study hints will not only help you survive but also EXCEL!

- Do not miss any classroom lectures or lab sessions.
- Take advantage of any extra study or practical lab sessions.
- Form a study group with classmates who are serious about doing well.
- If your class is offered at a college, especially a community college, find out if a learning resource center is available and take advantage of programs offered.

- Come to class with a positive attitude. Plan to do better than just getting by.
- Always act in a professional manner.
- Be good to yourself and show pride in your accomplishments by treating yourself to something special when you have achieved your goals.

After you have successfully completed your EMT course and passed your certification and/or Registry exams, remember that your learning process never ends. Eagerly pursue recertification and continuing educational opportunities as time permits.

YOU ARE THE EMT

1. Right now you have passed a first responder course. What additional skills must you acquire to become an EMT? An EMT-P?
2. You will receive much of your EMT training in the hospital emergency department. Besides having the opportunity to practice assessment and treatment techniques on actual patients, what other benefits will you derive from this kind of experience? What benefits can emergency department physicians derive from teaching you?
3. Perhaps the most important step you can take to preserve your personal safety is to wear a seat belt and shoulder harness. What other precautions should EMTs take when responding to an automobile accident?
4. Describe an unstable accident scene. How would you go about stabilizing the situation?

CHAPTER 2

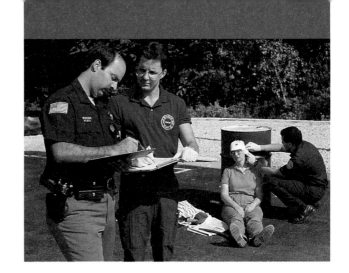

LEGAL
RESPONSIBILITIES

KEY TERMS

abandonment Failure of the EMT to continue emergency medical treatment.

actual consent Consent given by a person authorizing the EMT to provide care or transportation.

certification Formal notice of certain privileges and abilities after completion of certain training and testing.

duty to respond The responsibility of an ambulance service attached to a government agency to respond to calls within its jurisdiction. A commercial or volunteer service is not so obligated unless such care is advertised or is a requirement of its licensure.

immunity Exemptions granted by law to certain individuals or agencies freeing them from the burdens of compensating the injured or damaged individual.

implied consent Consent that is given by the fact that the individual voluntarily entered a situation.

informed consent Consent given by a person who understands the nature and extent of any procedure before agreeing to it and who has sufficient mental and physical capacity to make such a judgment.

licensure Formal permission to perform certain acts.

negligence Failure to perform an important or necessary technique or performance of such a technique in a careless or unskilled manner so as to cause further injury.

standard of care The manner in which an individual must act or behave when giving care.

OVERVIEW

An EMT involved in an emergency response situation may become involved in a variety of potential legal problems. One type of legal problem occurs when an individual is dissatisfied with the quality of emergency care rendered. Unskilled assessment or treatment performed by the EMT which worsens the patient's condition, or failure to protect the patient from further injury, may raise the question of negligence. And if negligence did occur, does the patient deserve a legal remedy or settlement? This type of potential legal problem is the focus of this chapter, as well as the concepts of consent and immunity.

Chapter 2 begins with a discussion of standard of care and how it is established—that is, whether standards are imposed by local custom, by law, or as a measure against professional or institutional standards. The chapter next explains the doctrine of negligence and the law of consent. The last part of the chapter discusses forms of immunity, duty to respond, and types of records and reports.

GOALS

The goals of Chapter 2 are to

- understand the basis of legal responsibility—the standard of care—and how standard of care can be established.
- become knowledgeable concerning the doctrine of negligence.
- become informed of the law of consent, including implied consent, consent to treat a minor, consent of the mentally ill, and the right to refuse treatment.
- identify the various forms of immunity granted by the law.
- distinguish between duty to respond and response on a volunteer basis.
- appreciate the importance of keeping accurate records and reports, especially regarding cases of child abuse , injuries during felonies, drug-related injuries, childbirth, crimes, and death.

STANDARD OF CARE

Regardless of the activity one is involved in, the law requires an individual to act or behave toward other individuals in a certain, definable way. Under given circumstances, the individual has a duty either to act or refrain from acting. Generally speaking, the individual must be concerned about the safety and welfare of other individuals when his or her behavior or activities have the potential for causing others injury or harm. The manner in which the individual must act or behave is called a **standard of care.**

Standard of care is established in many ways, among them being local custom, statutes, ordinances, administrative regulations, and case law. In addition, professional or institutional standards have a bearing on determining the adequacy of an EMT's conduct.

Standards Imposed by Local Custom

The conduct of an individual is to be judged in comparison with the conduct of other (hypothetical) persons of similar training and experience. For example, the conduct of an EMT employed by an ambulance service is to be judged in comparison with the expected conduct of EMTs from comparable ambulance services. Such standards are often based on locally accepted protocols. In the first place, you will not be held to the same standard of care as a physician or other more highly trained individuals. Further, your conduct must be judged in the light of the given emergency situation, taking into consideration the general confusion at the scene of the emergency, the needs of other patients, and the type of equipment available. Therefore, the prevailing custom of the community is an important element in determining the standard of emergency care required. Specifically, the standard of care is how a reasonably prudent person with similar training and experience would act under similar circumstances, with similar equipment, and in the same place.

Standards Imposed by Law

In addition to local customs, standards of emergency medical care may be imposed by statutes, ordinances, administrative regulation, or case law. In many jurisdictions, violating one of these standards is said to create *presumptive negligence*. Therefore, you must familiarize yourself with the particular legal standards that may exist in your state. In many states, this may take the form of published treatment protocols by a state agency.

Professional or Institutional Standards

In addition to the standards imposed by the force of law, professional or institutional standards may be admitted as evidence in determining the adequacy of an EMT's conduct. *Professional standards* include published recommendations of organizations and societies involved in emergency medical care. *Institutional standards* include specific rules and procedures of the ambulance service or organization to which the EMT is attached.

Two words of caution are important. First, you should familiarize yourself with the published standards of your organization. Second, an EMT who is involved in formulating standards for a particular agency should attempt to make the standards reasonable and realistic so that they do not impose an unreasonable burden on the EMTs. Optimum emergency medical care should be every EMT's goal, but it is not realistic to have institutional standards that *demand* optimum care.

In legal terms, the standard of care for an EMT may be stated as follows: "To perform as a reasonable, prudent, properly trained EMT would perform under the same or similar circumstances." A reasonably skillful, good faith effort to apply the information and skills that are presented in this book would generally meet the standard of care expected of a basic EMT.

THE DOCTRINE OF NEGLIGENCE

The legal doctrine of **negligence,** stated in its simplest terms, consists of three elements: duty, breach of that duty, and causation. Once called to the scene to render aid or assistance, the EMT has a duty to help the victim. The failure to do so, or the rendering of aid or assistance in a manner not consistent with the level of care that other similarly trained EMTs would render is a breach of duty. If that breach of duty is the causation of further injury, then the EMT has acted in a negligent manner and may be liable for the harm that results. All three elements—duty, breach of that duty, and causation of injury—must be present for the legal doctrine of negligence to be applicable.

Examples of potentially negligent conduct include the failure to render aid to a patient, the failure to perform an important or necessary technique, or the performance of a necessary technique in a manner not consistent with the skill with which other similarly trained EMTs would perform it.

When charged with negligent actions or behavior, the individual cannot be found liable before the facts of the case have been presented and weighed carefully. The performance of the individual must be weighed against the applicable standard of care. For an EMT, if the actions or performance of the EMT were those that might be expected of a reasonable, prudent, properly trained EMT operating in the same or similar circumstances, there would be no negligent action or behavior and, therefore, no liability. On the other hand, if the actions or performance of the EMT were reckless, careless, or lacking in skill, the standard of care would have been violated, and the EMT might be found negligent.

However, before the EMT can be found liable, it must be shown that the third element of negligence, causation of injury, has occurred. The requirement for proof of causation may be the major reason why very few lawsuits for negligence have been filed against EMTs. In most instances, EMTs are called to assist an individual who has a preexisting illness or injury. Because the illness or injury existed before the EMT arrived at the scene, the EMT cannot be held responsible for the preexisting condition. The EMT may, however, be held responsible for an aggravation or worsening of the condition that results from a violation of the standard of care.

It is important to recognize that the civil law of negligence is a system for evaluating an individual's behavior against a standard of behavior. If the behavior is found inappropriate, monetary compensation may be awarded. Regardless of the field of human activity, every individual has the right not to be subjected to undue harm. When the individual is subjected to undue harm and an injury or aggravation of a preexisting injury occurs, the person who caused that injury or aggravation is expected to compensate the injured individual.

Abandonment

Having begun to provide care, you must follow through with all necessary and appropriate treatment. You must continue to provide care until responsibility for patient care is transferred to another medical professional of an equal or higher level of skill, or until the patient is transferred to a medical facility. Failure to continue the treatment is referred to as **abandonment.** Abandonment is legally and ethically the most serious act an EMT can commit.

THE LAW OF CONSENT

Every experienced EMT has been confronted with the law of consent. It is a long-established legal right that an individual is entitled to be free from intentional touching or interference by another person without his or her consent.

Without consent, the intentional touching of an individual is said to constitute a technical battery. However, not every touching without consent results in possible exposure to legal action. People often enter situations in which a reasonable person could expect touching. For example, bumping in crowds at a sporting event does not result in legal action. Consent to such contact is implied from the fact that the individual voluntarily entered the situation. This type of **implied consent** is applicable to emergency situations. Just as a person voluntarily entering a crowd implies consent for bumping, emergency situations create an implication that the person consents to receive emergency medical care and to be transported to a medical facility.

In addition to implied consent, you will be frequently involved with another type of consent: **actual consent.** Actual consent occurs when the patient expressly authorizes you to provide care or transportation. Actual consent may take the form of words, a nod of agreement, or other expression of approval.

You should attempt to obtain actual consent whenever possible. At the same time, for consent to be binding, it should also be **informed consent.** Before granting informed consent, the patient must understand the nature and extent of any procedure and possible risks or complications. The patient should also have sufficient mental and physical capacity to make such a judgment.

Hospitals normally obtain a patient's consent by requiring a signature on a printed document. The signed document is useful as evidence that the patient was informed of what was to take place and willingly agreed to permit these activities. Most often, in field situations encountered by the EMT, obtaining written consent from the patient is not practical. Instead, oral consent will be obtained from the patient. Oral consent is valid and binding, although it may be difficult to prove unless a reliable witness can later be found.

Implied Consent

The law assumes that an individual who needs immediate emergency medical care to prevent death or significant physical impairment would consent to such care and transportation to a medical facility. However, this doctrine of implied consent is limited to true emergency situations. Generally, implied consent is appropriate when the patient is unconscious, delusional, or otherwise physically incapable of giving informed consent. In these cases, as well as in those where prompt action is necessary to prevent death or serious physical impairment, you may proceed with the required care and transportation without obtaining consent.

When the patient is unable to express consent but another responsible person or relative is present, it is advisable to obtain permission from that person or relative to proceed with care. The law in most instances recognizes the right of a spouse, close relative, or next of kin to give consent for injured persons unable to consent for themselves.

Consent to Treat Minors

The law recognizes that a minor may not have the wisdom, maturity, or judgment to give valid consent for emergency medical care. Therefore, the authority to consent for the minor is given to the parents or individuals who are so close to the minor as to be treated as the equivalent of parents. Despite this rule, the consent given by a minor may in some cases be valid, depending on the age and maturity of the individual. For example, the consent of a 17-year-old is more likely to be valid than that of a 4-year-old. Many states have enacted laws that permit minors to give a binding consent to receive medical care. The laws of many states also allow emancipated, married, or pregnant minors to be treated as adults for the purposes of consenting to medical treatment.

The laws and principles related to consent of minors merely determine who has the right to consent—not whether consent is needed. If a true emergency exists, the consent to treat the minor is implied. However, the consent of the parents should be obtained as soon as possible.

Consent of the Mentally Ill

A mentally incompetent person is not capable of giving an informed consent to receive medical treatment. However, unless the individual has been legally judged incompetent, there may be a question as to his or her capabilities. When a legal determination of incompetence has occurred, another individual, such as a guardian or conservator, usually possesses the right to consent on behalf of the patient.

In many field situations, you will encounter patients who may appear confused or in mental distress. These symptoms should be considered in deciding whether the patient can give a knowing or informed consent to medical treatment. When a true emergency situation exists, the doctrine of implied consent applies.

The Right to Refuse Treatment

Mentally competent adults have the right to refuse treatment. Injured or ill people who refuse treatment or transportation present EMTs with a dilemma: Do they care for such people against their will and risk being accused of battery, or do they leave them alone and risk a worsening of the condition and being accused of negligence or abandonment? Just as the consent to receive treatment must be informed, the refusal of treatment or transportation must also be informed. That means that if the refusing patient is delusional or confused, the EMT cannot assume that the refusal of treatment is a knowing refusal. On the other hand, competent adults who for religious reasons refuse specific kinds of treatment generally have a legal right to refuse such treatment.

When an individual refuses treatment, you must try to determine whether the individual's mental condition is impaired. When in doubt, it is always best to assume that there is mental impairment and to proceed with treatment. When compared to the decision to abandon a patient and having that patient's condition worsen, the decision to provide treatment is defensible from both legal and medical points of view.

A special situation occurs when a parent refuses to permit treatment of an ill or injured child. The EMT has an obligation to consider the emotional impact of the emergency on the parent's judgment. In this and virtually all cases of refusal to receive treatment, you usually can resolve the situation through patience and calm persuasion. When refusal is adamant, however, and no amount of persuasion can resolve the situation, it is essential that the refusing individual, guardian, conservator, or parent of the patient be asked to sign an official release form that acknowledges refusal. This form should be witnessed and stored with the run report and the medical incident report that are compiled by the ambulance personnel. It is advisable to include a comment about the refusal on the medical incident report and on the run report forms as well. In those instances in which the individual also refuses to sign the refusal form, the circumstances of the incident and the refusal should be thoroughly documented and the record stored for future reference.

The requirement for consent and the problem of refusing patients are related. Emergency medical care may be rendered only with the consent of the patient, and a mentally competent adult has the right to refuse treatment. These matters become more complex in cases involving minors or in cases where the patient appears to be delusional or confused. You should try to err on the side of rendering treatment rather than withholding it. Failure to render treatment to an individual invites much greater exposure to legal liability than rendering treatment to an individual who has failed to give consent or who expresses a refusal to be treated or transported. In most instances, the law is on the side of emergency medical care personnel. Also, in most cases, the problem of a refusing patient can best be resolved by the persuasive skills of the EMT in the field.

FORMS OF IMMUNITY

As stated earlier, the civil law of negligence is intended to provide legal remedies to persons who suffer injury or damage as a result of the negligent actions or behavior of another. Throughout the history of law, however, there have been limited situations where the law has granted **immunity** from the burdens of compensating the injured or damaged individual. Most of the forms of immunity have been based on the special status of the individual to whom the immunities applies.

For example, in English common law, the doctrine of *sovereign immunity* meant, in essence, that the king could do no wrong. Under this doctrine, injured or damaged individuals were deprived of a remedy when their injury or damage was caused by the negligence of the king or other member of the royal family. The resulting injustice eventually caused the doctrine to be abandoned.

Later, the doctrine of *governmental immunity* was adopted throughout the United States. Under this rule, government agencies were held to be immune from the legal consequences of their actions. Persons injured or damaged by the negligent actions, behaviors, or omissions of a government agency or its employees were deprived of a remedy. Injustice commonly resulted from this form of immunity, and it has been substantially eroded in recent years. In fact, more than half of the states have abandoned the doctrine of governmental immunity.

Some states, in balancing the needs of victims to recover for the negligent acts of their employees and the concern that employees might not otherwise act on behalf of the public for fear of the legal consequences, have adopted a limited form of governmental immunity. Massachusetts, for example, has abolished governmental immunity and adopted a statute similar to a federal law known as the Federal Tort Claims Act. Under this statute, the state or the appropriate municipality or governmental district is now responsible for the negligent conduct of its employees when the conduct occurs in the scope of their employment. Recovery under the statute is limited, however, to $100,000.

A relatively new form of immunity exists today. Adopted by statute in virtually all states, this new immunity seeks to protect citizens and other non-certified emergency medical care workers from legal liability. These *"Good Samaritan" laws* attempt to ensure that someone who voluntarily helps an injured or suddenly ill person at the scene is not legally liable for errors or omissions in rendering good faith emergency care. Most of these statutes do not provide immunity for gross negligence or willful and wanton misconduct that results in an injury.

Another group of laws, currently in effect in every state, seeks to grant immunity from liability to official emergency medical care providers, such as EMTs. The provisions of these laws vary widely from state to state. Massachusetts General Law c.111C, §14 provides in part:

> No emergency medical technician certified under the provisions of this chapter . . . who in the performance of his duties and in good faith renders emergency first aid or transportation to an injured person or to a person incapacitated by illness shall be personally in any way liable as a result of rendering such aid or as a result of transporting such person to a hospital or other safe place . . .

As with the "Good Samaritan" laws, most do not provide immunity when injury or damage is caused by gross negligence or willful and wanton misconduct. For example, Maryland provides limited immunity for ambulance and rescue personnel under the provisions of Maryland Ann. Code, art. 43, §149a:

> The members of volunteer ambulance and rescue squads shall not be liable for damages . . . except for gross negligence. . . . In order to be eligible . . . a person must have completed a basic and an advanced Red Cross or equivalent course or instruction in first aid. . . .

In considering immunities, you should recognize that any immunity granted to one individual has the potential for creating injustice to another. Making one person unaccountable for his or her negligence can mean that an individual injured by that negligence may have no legal recourse. Generally throughout the history of law, efforts to grant immunity to individuals with special standing or status have been relatively short-lived.

The current trend toward providing immunity to citizens and emergency care personnel has not been thoroughly tested by the courts, largely because few legal conflicts arise from emergency medical care and transportation in the field. Most legal scholars agree that the immunities granted by the various state laws are not absolute by any means. Furthermore, in order to determine whether an immunity applies in a particular case, it would be necessary to initiate a lawsuit and evaluate the relevant evidence and testimony. Although the immunity laws may provide some protection, it is clear that much better protection is provided by rendering top-quality emergency medical care.

EMERGENCY MEDICAL TECHNICIAN STATUTES

Most states have adopted specific statutes that grant special privileges to EMTs. These statutes frequently authorize the performance of certain specified medical procedures. Many also grant a partial immunity to the EMT and the physicians and nurses who give emergency instructions to EMTs, EMT-intermediates, or EMT-paramedics via radio or other forms of communication. A typical statute follows:

> No physician . . . and no nurse . . . and no hospital shall be liable in a suit for damages as a result of acts or omissions related to advice, consultation, or orders given in good faith to ambulance operators and attendants . . . who are qualified under section six, and are acting on behalf of an ambulance service duly licensed under section three, by radio, telephone, or other remote means of communica-

tion under emergency conditions and prior to arrival of the patient at the hospital, clinic, office, or other health facility from which the emergency communication to the ambulance operator or attendant is made; nor shall any said ambulance operator or attendant be liable in a suit for damages as a result of his said acts or omissions based upon said advice, consultation or orders by remote communication, if the said acts or omissions were made in good faith.Massachusetts General Laws c.111C, §13.

Exemptions from the Medical Practices Act

Nearly every state exempts emergency medical care from the licensure requirements of the Medical Practices Act for nonmedical personnel. Because many emergency medical care procedures may be construed to be the performance of a medical act, the EMT is protected in those situations. Such exemption is, however, not all-inclusive, because there are specific licensure or certification requirements for EMTs in all states. A state's requirement for specific licensure or certification of the EMT affects the exemption from the Medical Practices Act.

The Effect of Licensure or Certification

By definition, **licensure** is formal permission to perform certain acts. **Certification** is formal notice of certain privileges and abilities after the completion of certain training and testing. In states that require licensure or certification by a specified state agency, these requirements frequently are interpreted as necessary conditions to the rendering of emergency medical care on a regular or continuing basis. Furthermore, the possession of a license or certificate obligates the individual to conform to the standard of care of other licensed or certified emergency medical care personnel. In states that might not require licensure or certification, individuals rendering emergency medical care on a regular or continuing basis may nonetheless be held to the same standard of care expected of certified EMTs.

DUTY TO RESPOND

The primary distinction between an ambulance service attached to a government agency and one that is volunteer or commercial lies in the **duty to respond.** A municipal ambulance service, being part of a governmental service, may have a duty to respond to a call within its jurisdiction, whereas a commercial or volunteer service may not be so obligated unless such care is advertised or is a requirement of its licensure. However, once a response has been made by any type of ambulance service, the principles of duty to act and the standards of care are equally applicable to both types of emergency personnel.

RECORDS AND REPORTS

Society through its government has formulated a policy to protect its people by health regulations and statutes. Because certain individuals are in a position to observe and gather information about diseases, injuries, and emergency events, an obligation to compile such information and report it to certain agencies may be imposed. Even where there is no such requirement, it is advisable for you to compile a complete and accurate record of all incidents when you come in contact with sick or injured individuals. Most medical and legal experts believe that a complete and accurate record of an emergency medical incident is an important safeguard against legal complications. The absence of a record, or a substantially incomplete record, may mean that you have to testify to the events, your findings, and your actions relying on memory alone. Reliance on one's memory can prove to be wholly inadequate and embarrassing in the face of aggressive cross-examination.

Two rules of thumb relating to your reports and records should be followed. Typically applied in the courtroom setting, the first rule suggests that if an action or procedure is not recorded on the written report, it was not done. The second rule of thumb generally suggests that an incomplete or untidy report is evidence of incomplete or inexpert emergency medical care. Both of these potentially dangerous presumptions can be avoided by compiling and maintaining accurate reports and records of all events and patients.

Special Reporting Requirements

Child Abuse All states and the District of Columbia have enacted laws to protect abused children, and some have added other protected groups such as the elderly and "at-risk adults." Most states have a reporting obligation for certain individuals, whose definition may range from "physician" to "any person." You must be aware of the requirements of law in your state. Such statutes frequently grant immunity from liability for libel, slander, or defamation of character to the person obligated to report, even if the reports are subsequently shown to be unfounded, if the reports are made in good faith.

Injury During the Commission of a Felony Many states have laws requiring the reporting of any injury likely to have occurred during the commission of a criminal act or other specific injuries, such as gunshot or knife wounds or poisonings. Again, you must be familiar with the legal requirements of your state.

Drug-Related Injuries In some instances, drug-related injuries must be reported. These requirements may affect the EMT. However, it should be stressed that the United States Supreme Court has held that drug addiction, as opposed to drug possession or sale, is an illness and not a crime. Hence, an injury as a result of a drug overdose may not be within the definition of an injury resulting from a felonious act.

Some states, by statute, specifically establish confidentiality and excuse certain specified individuals from reporting drug cases, either to a government agency or a minor's parents, if, in the discretion of those individuals, withholding reporting is necessary for the proper treatment of the patient. Once again, you must be familiar with the legal requirements of your state.

Childbirth Many states require that anyone in attendance at a live birth in any place other than a licensed medical facility report the birth. As before, you must be familiar with state requirements.

Other Reporting Requirements

Other reporting requirements may include attempted suicides, dog bites, certain communicable diseases, assaults, and rapes.

Scene of a Crime

If there is evidence at an emergency scene that a crime may have been committed, you must notify the dispatcher immediately so that proper authorities can be informed. Provided that there is no active criminal activity occurring at the scene that renders the scene hazardous or unstable, such circumstances should not deter you from providing necessary emergency medical care to the patient and transporting the patient to the hospital, if necessary, before the authorities arrive. While emergency medical care is being provided, you must be careful not to disturb the scene of the crime any more than absolutely necessary. Notes and drawings should be made of the position of the patient and of the presence and position of any weapon or other objects that may be valuable to the investigating officers. You should confer periodically with local authorities and be aware of their wishes as to any actions you should take at the scene of the crime. It is best if these guidelines can be established by protocol.

The Deceased

In most states, EMTs do not have the authority to pronounce an individual dead. If there is any chance that life exists or that the patient can be resuscitated, you must make every effort to preserve that life at the scene and during transport to medical facilities. At times, however, death is obvious; rigor mortis has set in, decapitation has occurred, the body is consumed by fire, or there is a massive head injury with parts missing. In such instances, there is no urgent reason to move the body. The only immediate action required of you is to cover the body and prevent its disturbance. Local rules and protocols from the medical examiner or coroner will determine your ultimate action in these instances.

Occasionally an EMT will respond to a call for assistance because a patient has died from some disease and the family members present decide that they do not wish any resuscitative efforts to be made, but no written documentation to that effect has been initiated. This places the EMT in a very difficult position and one that will be occurring more frequently with the development of terminal nursing home placements, hospices, and home health programs. Generally speaking, in order to be valid, such "do not resuscitate" orders must meet the following requirements:

- Clearly state the patient's medical problem(s).
- Be signed by the patient or legal guardian.
- Be signed by one or more physicians.
- Be dated in the preceding 12 months.

Even in the presence of such an order, however, you are still obligated to provide supportive (oxygen, pain relief) and comfort measures whenever possible. Each ambulance service, in consultation with its medical director and legal counsel, must develop a protocol to follow in such circumstances.

CONCLUSION

It must be emphasized that only general legal principles have been discussed here, because state laws differ widely. Even though medico-legal responsibilities must be taken seriously, they should not intimidate you and prevent you from doing your job. In very few cases has liability been imposed on EMTs because of their

conduct. The liability for not performing is at least as great as the liability for performing improperly. The best legal defense is proper training, continuing education, skillful rendering of required emergency care, and careful written documentation.

YOU ARE THE EMT

1. Before you can be accused of negligence, what has to be proved?
2. Your patient, a middle-aged man, is unconscious and requires oxygen. You begin treatment, based on implied consent. What does that mean? A few minutes later his wife arrives. What kind of consent will you seek from her?
3. You have responded to a bicycle accident in which a 14-year-old boy appears to have suffered a severe concussion. You realize he should be transported to the hospital for X rays and examination by a doctor. He refuses to go and will not tell you his name. He says he's OK and will get in terrible trouble if his parents find out he was skipping school. What will you do?
4. You are a certified EMT. How does certification differ from licensure?

CHAPTER 3

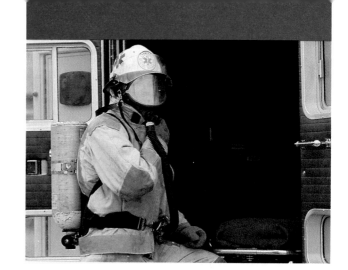

SELF PROTECTION/ PERSONAL SAFETY

. . . .

KEY TERMS

. . . .

decontamination (de"kon-tam-ĭ-na'shun) The orderly process by which radiation or chemical hazards can be removed from clothing, equipment, vehicles, and personnel.

frostbite Damage to tissues as the result of exposure to low environmental temperatures.

hemoglobin (he'mo-glo"bin) The oxygen-carrying pigment of the red blood cells.

hydration (hi-dra'shun) The act of combining or causing to combine with water.

hyperthermia (hi"per-ther'me-ah) A condition in which the internal body temperature increases above normal after prolonged exposure to heat.

hypothermia (hi"po-ther'me-ah) A condition in which the internal body temperature falls below 95 degrees F after prolonged exposure to freezing or near-freezing temperatures.

hypovolemia (hi"po-vo-le'me-ah) A decrease in the volume of circulating blood or other body fluids.

hypoxia (hi-pok'se-ah) A deficiency of oxygen reaching the tissues of the body.

pathogen Any disease-producing microorganism.

universal precautions Protective measures developed by the Centers for Disease Control (CDC) for use when dealing with objects that might accidentally puncture the skin of the health care worker.

OVERVIEW

The personal safety of all EMTs is vital to EMS operations. As a part of training, you will learn to recognize hazards and how to protect yourself from them. These hazards vary greatly, ranging from personal neglect to environmental and man-made threats to your safety as you perform your duties. As an EMT you make many daily decisions. Are you equipped to handle the current emergency? If not, what are your options? What is the best approach? When is it appropriate to think of yourself? The material in Chapter 3 is presented to help you answer these questions and others like them. The chapter begins with a discussion of factors that make up your personal well-being. Descriptions of common hazards and recommended protective measures are then discussed in detail.

GOALS

The goals of Chapter 3 are to
- understand the importance of nutrition and physical fitness for the EMT.
- know the role of protective clothing and equipment.
- understand the hazards associated with fires, fuel systems, and flares.
- understand the common water and ice hazards.
- understand the dangers of electricity, the terrain, and falling objects.
- understand the dangers of confined spaces.
- understand the hazards encountered in civil disturbances.

PERSONAL WELL-BEING

The personal well-being of the EMT is of primary importance to effective EMS operations. Your effectiveness and efficiency in performing your duties depend on your ability to stay in shape and to avoid the risk of personal injury. To accomplish these goals, you need to be in good physical condition. You need to develop an awareness of the potential hazards present in rescue and patient care and learn how to avoid or prevent personal injury or illness.

To perform efficiently, the human body must have adequate nutrition. Food is the fuel that makes the body run. The physical exertion and physical stress that are a part of your job require a high energy output. If you do not have a ready source of fuel, your performance may be less than satisfactory, endangering you, your patient, and your co-workers. Therefore it is important for you to learn about and follow the rules of good nutrition.

Simple sugars, contained in candy and soft drinks, are the foods most quickly absorbed and converted to fuel by the body. But sugars also stimulate the body's production of insulin, which reduces blood sugar levels. For some people, eating a lot of sugar can actually result in lower energy levels. Be aware that the body's need for sugar and its reaction to it vary from person to person.

More complex carbohydrates rank next to simple sugars in their ability to produce energy; however, some carbohydrates take hours to be converted into usable body fuel. On the other hand, complex carbohydrates such as pasta, rice, and vegetables, are among the safest, most reliable sources for long-term energy production.

Fats are also easily converted to energy, but overuse of foods containing high levels of fat can lead to obesity, cardiac disease, and other long-term health problems. The proteins in meat, fish, chicken, beans, and cheese take several hours to convert to energy.

Carry an individual supply of high-energy food to help you maintain your energy levels. Try eating several small meals throughout the day to keep your energy resources at constant high levels. Remember, however, that overeating may reduce your physical and mental performance. After a large meal, blood required for the digestive process is not available for other activities.

Your physical well-being also depends on maintaining an adequate fluid intake. **Hydration** is important for proper functioning of the human body. Fluids can be easily replenished by drinking any nonalcoholic, noncaffeinated fluid. Water is generally available, and it is absorbed by the body faster than any other fluid. Avoid fluids that contain high sugar levels. They can actually slow the rate of fluid absorption by the body and cause abdominal discomfort as well. One indicator of adequate hydration is frequent urination. Infrequent urination or urine that has a deep yellow color is an indication of dehydration. Keep your fluid intake at a level that maintains adequate hydration.

Finally, a regular program of exercise will enhance the benefits of maintaining good nutrition and adequate hydration. When you are in good physical condition, the stresses of your job can be more easily handled. A regular program of aerobic exercise will increase your strength and endurance.

PROTECTION FROM INFECTION

An immunization program should be in place in your EMS system to ensure that all rescue personnel stay up-to-date on their vaccinations. The minimum inoculations that should be kept current include tetanus, mumps, measles, rubella, and hepatitis.

The Centers for Disease Control (CDC) and the Occupational Safety and Health Administration (OSHA) have developed requirements for protection from blood-borne **pathogens** (disease-causing agents) such as the hepatitis and human immunodeficiency viruses. All EMS and rescue personnel need to study these regulations. Whenever there is a possibility of exposure to blood or other body fluids, you must wear gloves, eye protection, and a gown or other protective clothing. The **universal precautions** for protection against infection are described in detail in Chapter 35.

PROTECTIVE CLOTHING AND EQUIPMENT

Protective clothing and other gear appropriate for the task at hand play an important role in your personal safety. You need to become familiar with the protective equipment available to you. Then you will be able to select the proper clothing and gear for the job and know how to adapt or change items as the situation and environment change. Remember, too, that the clothing and other gear you need for protection are safe only when they are in good condition. It is your responsibility to consider these items unsafe and unusable until you have inspected them thoroughly, even if you must make the inspection your first priority at an emergency site.

Protection Against the Weather

A layered system of clothing is much better protection from the cold than a single thick cover. Layers offer more flexibility, allowing you to add or remove a layer to control your body temperature. Cold weather protection should consist of at least three layers:

1. A thin, inner layer next to the skin (sometimes called the transport layer) should wick moisture away from the skin to keep the wearer dry and warm. Underwear made from polypropylene or polyester material works well for the transport layer.
2. A thermal layer of bulkier material that acts as insulation should come next. Tradition-

ally, wool has been the material of choice for warmth, but it is rapidly being replaced by other materials, such as polyester pile.

3. The best outer layer is one made of material capable of resisting chilling winds and precipitation. The two top layers should have zippers to aid in venting body heat should you become too warm (Figure 3–1).

The type of material used in clothing determines how well the clothing protects the wearer from the weather. Cotton is one material that should be avoided when chilling from wetness is a possibility, because cotton tends to absorb moisture. For example, when a person wears cotton trousers and walks through wet grass, the cotton wicks the moisture from the grass up the pant legs, chilling the wearer in cold weather. Because cotton does absorb moisture and pulls heat away from the body, it is a good material for warm, dry environments.

Plastic-coated nylon can provide the waterproof protection needed for the outer layer of cold weather protective clothing, but it can also hold in body heat and perspiration, making the wearer as wet inside as out. Newer, less airtight materials have been designed to allow perspiration and some heat to escape while the material retains its water resistance. Avoid flammable or meltable synthetic material anytime there is any possibility of fire.

Clothing worn for rescue must be appropriate for the activity involved and the environmental conditions in which the activity will take place. The typical bunker gear worn for fire fighting, for example, is usually too restrictive for working on a patient in a confined space.

Temperature extremes can be a threat in any environment where the climate is not controlled. The human body works well within a narrow body core temperature range of around 98.6 degrees F (37.0 degrees C). Our bodies can maintain this optimal body temperature for a fairly long period of time regardless of the temperature extremes produced by weather or other environmental conditions. However, prolonged exposure can produce changes in body temperature. A difference of only a few degrees from the normal body temperature affects an individual's ability to think and act. As the body temperature continues to move away from the normal range, either up or down, there will be increasing loss of function and eventually unconsciousness may occur. Unless this trend is interrupted, death may

FIGURE 3–1

The proper cold weather protection consists of three layers: a thin inner transport layer, a thermal layer, and an outer protective layer.

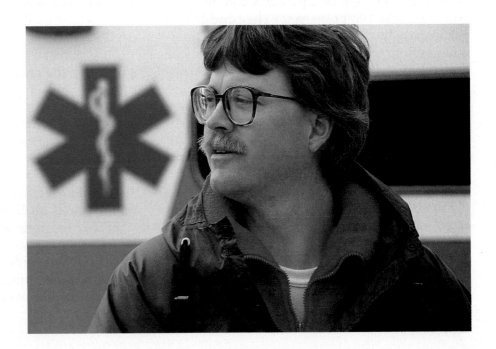

follow. You must continually monitor yourself, your squad, and your patients for dangerous temperature changes. Further, you must provide as much protection against temperature extremes as possible as a preventative measure.

Exposure to heat that increases body temperature above normal is known as **hyperthermia.** Heat exhaustion is the first indication that the body is being overheated. It develops when the body loses excessive water and minerals through perspiration. Mild **hypovolemic** shock results from this loss of body fluids. To prevent heat exhaustion, shield yourself from the sun and other heat sources, maintain an adequate fluid intake, and reduce excessive perspiration by removing excess layers of clothing.

Untreated heat exhaustion may progress to heat stroke. Heat stroke is a serious illness that results when the body is subjected to more heat than it can handle. The body's sweating mechanism becomes overwhelmed, and heat stroke victims do not perspire. They have hot, dry, flushed skin. Heat stroke is a life-threatening emergency. If untreated, it will result in death. To avoid hyperthermia, you must wear proper clothing, vent heat away from your body, use shelter to protect yourself from heat sources such as the sun, and consume adequate amounts of fluid.

Exposure to cold may result in a potentially dangerous lowering of the body's core temperature known as **hypothermia.** The condition is particularly hazardous because the central nervous system does not function well at lower than normal body temperature. Mental processes are affected, reducing a person's ability to care for himself. Because hypothermia may come on slowly, in a very subtle way, you may not realize it is happening to you. If the cooling process is not reversed, death can result. Protection from hypothermia includes adequate clothing, shelter, and nutrition.

Frostbite is the freezing of body tissue. The areas most susceptible to freezing are the feet (particularly the toes), and the hands (especially the fingers). Portions of the face, such as the ears and the nose, can also be frostbitten. Frostbite frequently develops because of exposure to chilling winds or water. It often results

from inadequate footwear or hand covering. Frostbite can also develop very quickly from contact with cold metal on equipment or vehicles or from contact with cooled liquids, such as gasoline, that have spilled.

Another factor contributing to frostbite is a lowered body temperature. As the body cools, circulation to the extremities is reduced to conserve warmth for the body's core: the brain, heart, and lungs. Anyone with impaired circulation because of a medical condition such as hypothermia or an injury to an extremity is particularly susceptible to frostbite. Especially at lower temperatures, winds increase chilling (Table 3–1). If there is a combination of low temperature and high wind, you must protect yourself and your patients from the dangers of wind chill. Take particular precautions to protect exposed flesh from frostbite.

Protection of Specific Body Areas

Head Helmets should be worn by all rescue personnel, but they are mandatory if you are working in a fall zone (an area where you are most likely to encounter falling objects). The helmet should provide top and side impact protection and have a secure chin strap. Objects frequently fall one after another. If the helmet has an inadequate chin strap, the first falling object may knock it off, leaving the head unprotected as the remaining objects fall (Figure 3–2).

Most construction-type helmets are not well suited for the rescue environment. They offer minimal impact protection and have inadequate chin straps. Modern fire helmets do offer impact protection, but the projecting brim at the back of the neck may get in your way in a rescue situation. Helmets that have been certified by the Union of International Alpine Associations (UIAA) offer the kind of protection required for high-angle specialized rescue.

In cold weather, a good bit of body heat can be lost by not wearing a head covering. An insulated hat made from wool or a synthetic material can be pulled down over the face and the base of the skull to reduce heat loss in extremely cold weather (Figure 3–3).

TABLE 3–1   Wind Chill Chart

Temperature (F°)	Wind Speed (mph)							
	5	10	15	20	25	30	35	40
35	32	22	16	12	8	6	4	3
30	27	16	9	4	1	−2	−4	−5
25	22	10	2	−3	−7	−10	−12	−13
20	16	3	−5	−10	−15	−18	−20	−21
15	11	−3	−11	−17	−22	−25	−27	−29
10	6	−9	−18	−24	−29	−33	−35	−37
5	0	−15	−25	−31	−36	−41	−43	−45
0	−5	−22	−31	−39	−44	−49	−52	−53
−5	−10	−27	−38	−46	−51	−56	−58	−60
−10	−15	−34	−45	−53	−59	−64	−67	−69
−15	−21	−40	−51	−60	−66	−71	−74	−76
−20	−26	−46	−58	−67	−74	−79	−82	−84
−25	−31	−52	−65	−74	−81	−86	−89	−92
−30	−36	−58	−72	−81	−88	−93	−97	−100
−35	−42	−64	−78	−88	−96	−101	−105	−107
−40	−47	−71	−85	−95	−103	−109	−113	−115

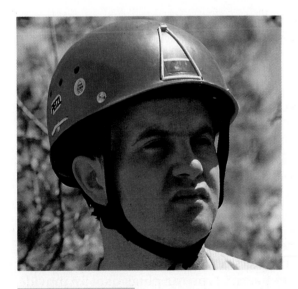

FIGURE 3–2

Rescuers working in a fall zone must wear helmets that offer both top and side impact protection and that have a secure chin strap.

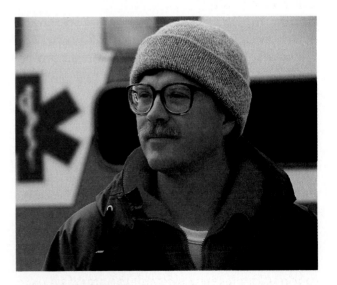

FIGURE 3–3

In cold weather, body heat is lost quickly from an uncovered head. An insulated hat will conserve body heat.

Feet Footgear should protect the feet, be water resistant, fit well, and be flexible so you can walk long distances comfortably. If much of your activity will be outdoors, select boots that cover and protect the ankles, keeping out stones, debris, and snow. In colder weather, your footwear must also protect you from the cold. Leather remains one of the best materials for footwear; however, certain synthetics, such as Goretex, are also very good. The soles must provide traction. Lug-type soles may grip well in snow, but they become very slippery when caked with mud.

The fit of boots and shoes is extremely important, because a minor annoyance can develop into a disabling injury. Excessive slipping of your feet inside the footgear will cause painful blisters. However, there should be enough space inside your boots or shoes to allow your toes to wiggle. Socks keep the feet warm and provide some cushioning for the impact of walking. In cold weather, two pairs of socks are generally preferable to one thick pair. A thin sock next to the foot helps to wick perspiration away to a thicker, outer sock keeping your feet warmer, drier, and generally more comfortable. When you purchase new shoes or boots, keep these points in mind.

Hands In many EMS operations you must protect your hands and wrists from injury. You will need gloves that provide maximum protection from heat, cold, and cuts while allowing the dexterity you need to use rescue tools and perform patient care duties. Anytime there is a possibility that you may be exposed to blood or other body fluids, you must wear rubber gloves to avoid direct contact with these fluids.

Eyes The human eye is very fragile, and permanent loss of sight can occur from very minor injuries. You need to protect your eyes from blood and other body fluids, foreign objects, plants, insects, and debris from extrication. Goggles or a face shield should be used whenever there is a risk of getting something in your eyes (Figure 3–4).

In snow or white sand, particularly at higher altitudes, eyes need the protection from ultraviolet (UV) exposure that can be provided by

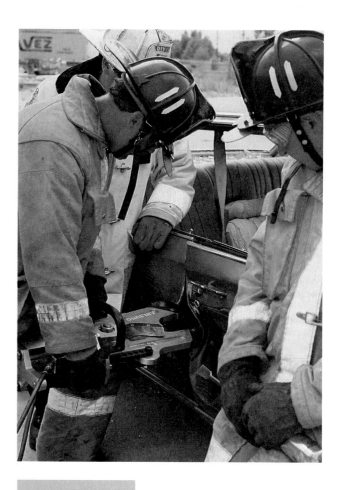

FIGURE 3–4

Eye protection, such as goggles, must be adaptable to the weather and physical demands of the rescue operation.

glasses or goggles designed for that purpose. In addition, eyewear must be adaptable to the weather and the physical demands of the task at hand. Clear vision must be maintained at all times.

Ears Long-term exposure to loud noises can cause permanent hearing loss. When working around equipment with high noise levels, such as helicopters and some extrication tools, soft foam industrial-type ear plugs usually provide adequate protection.

Skin Your skin needs protection against sunburn while you are working outdoors. It might be considered simply an annoyance, but sunburn is a first-degree thermal burn. In reflective areas such as sand, water, and snow, the risk of sunburn is increased. Protect your skin by applying a sunscreen with an appropriate rating and remember that skin can be burned even on a cloudy day.

Light Sources

Many EMS operations occur at night and in places without electricity or adequate lighting. Often, you will need to provide your own light sources. Each rescuer should have more than one light available. Flashlights are good sources of light but, because they must be held by hand, the rescue and patient care may be hampered. Headlamps that clip to a helmet or are mounted on a headband are an excellent alternative. In addition, you should always carry spare batteries and bulbs for each light source.

HAZARDS

The varied settings in which EMS personnel must function will expose you to many hazards. In situations that pose a physical threat to your survival, you must first take the required protective measures or avoid the hazard completely.

Fire

Fire is frequently encountered by EMTs. You should have a basic understanding of the hazards associated with fire in order to be safe and effective in your work. There are four common hazards in a fire:

- smoke.
- oxygen deficiency.
- high ambient temperatures.
- toxic gases.

Smoke is made up of suspended particles of tar and carbon, which irritate the respiratory system on contact. Many smoke particles are trapped in the upper respiratory system, but many smaller particles enter the lungs. Some smoke particles not only irritate the airway but

may be deadly. Appropriate airway protection must be worn at all times.

All fires consume oxygen. Particularly in a closed space, such as a room, the fire may consume most of the available oxygen, making breathing difficult for anyone in the closed space.

Thermal burns and damage to the respiratory system can result from the high ambient temperatures in a fire. Breathing air heated above 120 degrees F can damage the tissues of the respiratory tract.

There are a number of toxic gases present in a typical building fire. They include carbon monoxide, phosgene, nitrogen oxides, hydrogen cyanide, hydrogen chloride, and carbon dioxide.

Carbon monoxide is a colorless and odorless gas that is present in every fire. This gas is responsible for more fire deaths each year than any other by-product of combustion. Carbon monoxide combines with the **hemoglobin** in your *red blood cells* about 200 times more rapidly than oxygen does, blocking the ability of the hemoglobin to transport oxygen to your body tissues. Table 3–2 shows the toxic effects of carbon monoxide.

Phosgene is a colorless gas with the odor of musty hay. In small amounts, it causes eye and throat irritation. When phosgene is inhaled, it decomposes into hydrochloric acid, which burns the lungs.

Hydrogen cyanide is a colorless gas with a noticeable almond odor. It blocks the exchange of oxygen and carbon dioxide in the lungs. Symptoms of exposure include gasping, muscle spasms, increased heart rate, and sudden collapse.

Carbon dioxide is colorless and odorless, and exposure causes increased respirations, dizziness, and sweating. Breathing concentrations of carbon dioxide above 10 to 12 percent may cause death within a few minutes.

Hydrogen chloride is also a colorless gas with a strong, pungent odor. It can cause severe irritation to the respiratory tract and the eyes. It may also lead to an irregular heart rhythm. Inhalation may result in chemical burns of the upper respiratory tract.

TABLE 3–2	Toxic Effects of Carbon Monoxide

Percent Carbon Monoxide in Air	Symptoms
.01	No symptoms—No apparent illness
.02	Mild headache—Few other symptoms
.04	Headache following 1–2 hours
.08	Headache following 45 minutes, nausea/vomiting, unconscious following 2 hours
.16	Headache following 20 minutes, nausea/vomiting, unconscious following 45 minutes
.32	Headache following 5–10 minutes, nausea/vomiting, unconscious following 30 minutes
.64	Headache, ataxia following 1–2 minutes, unconscious following 10–15 minutes
1.28	Immediately unconscious, death following 1–3 minutes

Carbon Monoxide parts per million (ppm)

Adapted with permission from the International Fire Service Training Association, Oklahoma State University, Stillwater, Oklahoma.

Nitrogen oxides decompose into nitric oxide and nitric acid that are reddish-brown in color. Exposure may cause severe lung damage and death by suffocation.

Proper protective equipment such as a *self-contained breathing apparatus (SCBA)* must be worn by all rescuers to protect from these toxic gases (Figure 3–5).

Hazards in Structural Fires

EMS personnel should never enter a fire scene unless they are trained and appropriately equipped. An uncontrolled fire is a very dynamic situation; significant changes can occur rapidly. You must be aware of these potential hazards in any burning area: flashover, backdraft, and building collapse.

Temperatures in a free-burning fire can exceed 1,500 degrees F. Most of the combustible material in a building will burn at temperatures ranging from 400 to 1,400 degrees F. These combustibles are preheated to ignition temperature by the open fire situation. When all of the combustible items within a fire zone ignite sud-

denly, *flashover* (a violent reaction similar to an explosion) occurs. Anyone exposed to a flashover without protective clothing and equipment will probably die. Rescuers with protective equipment in place are still at risk for severe injury or death during a flashover, because even the best firefighting apparel cannot withstand these excessively high temperatures.

In a smoldering fire, burning is incomplete because of a lack of oxygen. Adding air to the smoldering process rekindles the flame and creates ideal conditions for a *backdraft*, an explosion of gases emitted in the smoldering phase of the fire as the gases are mixed with additional oxygen. The following are signs of an impending backdraft:

- Little, if any, fire visible outside of the building.
- Hot exterior doors and windows.
- Grayish-yellow puffs of smoke coming from the building.
- Air or smoke forcefully reentering the burning building.

■ Audible sounds such as whistling or moaning coming from the burning structure.

Your first priority as an EMT is the treatment of your patients. However, you should never let this priority override common sense. Should you hurriedly open a door or break a window in a burning structure where conditions are right, you may supply the fresh oxygen necessary for a backdraft to occur, further complicating your rescue effort.

Properly done, vertical ventilation allows the heated gases from a smoldering fire to escape in a controlled manner. Enter a burning building with extreme caution after ventilation. Always stand to the side when opening doors and windows. Have proper respiratory equipment, "envelope protection," and a backup water supply in place and ready for use.

Finally, there is always a potential for collapse of structural parts during and following a building fire. Frequently, there are no warning signs, and your hasty entry into a burning structure may result in serious injury and possible death. Once inside the burning building, you are subject to an uncontrolled, hostile environment. Fires are not selective about their victims. You must be extremely cautious when-

ever you are in or near a structure that is burning or in which a fire has just been extinguished. Always defer to trained fire-fighting personnel when rescue decisions must be made at the scene of any fire.

Fuels and Fuel Systems

The fuel and the fuel systems of vehicles involved in accidents present a hazard to you and your patients. Although the risk of a vehicle fire is less than 0.05 percent, any fuel may ignite under the right conditions. If there is a known fuel leak or if people are trapped in the vehicle, you must arrange for adequate fire protection. This means that at least one charged 1½ inch diameter hose line is staffed and ready for operation before beginning the rescue.

You must use respiratory protection as well as thermal protection if there is or has been a fire in the accident vehicle. The smoke from vehicular fires contains many toxic by-products. The use of full protective gear at an accident scene can reduce the risk to rescue personnel.

FIGURE 3–5

Self-contained breathing apparatus (SCBA) is essential equipment whenever you are in or near a fire scene.

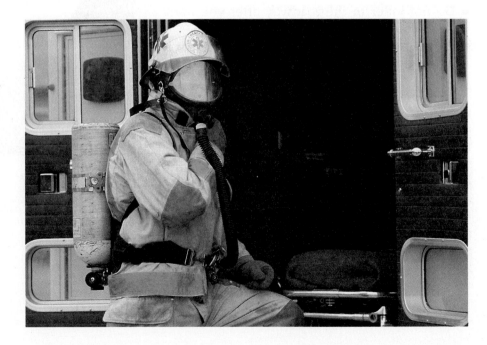

Flares

Flares are considered essential tools by some EMS personnel. They are used to warn oncoming traffic of a hazard and to route traffic. In the hands of a careless or inexperienced user, flares can be extremely dangerous. They are very hot and only burn for a limited period of time—10 to 60 minutes, depending on the wind. Flares are most dangerous during the lighting process. The following general safety guidelines when working with flares will decrease your chance of injury:

- Do not set flares near flammable materials such as gasoline spills, open flames, or dry brush.
- Extend flares toward oncoming traffic, at least 15 to 20 feet apart.
- Arrange flare patterns to direct traffic away from the scene yet keep traffic moving.
- Stack several flares together so that as one burns out, another will ignite.
- Put end caps on the nonburning ends of the flares to keep them upright.
- To avoid burns, do not hold onto or wave flares.
- Let flares burn out rather than risk splatter trying to extinguish them.
- Face downwind to light flares. This will lessen the danger of burns or inhalation of toxic fumes.
- Do not loiter in the roadway after you light flares.
- If the road is two-way and has only two lanes, place flares in both directions.

Water and Ice Hazards

There are many different kinds of water hazards that you may encounter. You should be aware of the types of water rescue you might have to perform in your locale and the hazards you could be called upon to face in those situations. For example, rising water can cover and conceal objects such as trees, bridges, and buildings that could hamper search and rescue activities by snagging or entangling equipment and personnel. In an ocean environment, currents and tides may prove hazardous because they may obstruct access to beaches near dunes and cliffs. Currents and tides also may flood rescue attempts around marine structures and docks, especially near low tide marks. In coastal regions, local tide charts are necessary decision-making tools for EMS operations. Undertows can be vicious and forceful. If you get caught in an undertow, do not fight the force of the current until you are too tired to make it to shore. Rather, relax and swim at an angle across the current.

You can avoid problems by understanding the forces that direct water flow. Special training in river operations may enhance your competency and safety in moving water. Knee-deep, flowing water may throw a wading person off balance in rivers and streams. A flow as slow as five miles per hour can pin you or your patients under water.

You must also avoid *strainers*, obstructions that allow water to flow through, yet trap objects such as boats or people. The pressures generated by water flowing around, over, or through a strainer such as a partially or completely submerged tree branch (Figure 3–6)

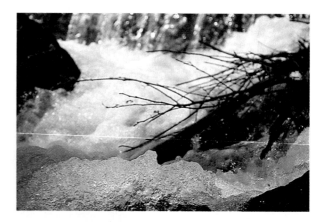

FIGURE 3–6

Strainers are obstructions in a moving stream that allow current to flow through yet may trap boats or people.

FIGURE 3–7

Low head dams can create dangerous hydraulics which may trap people in a backwash. The trapped victims often succumb to fatigue, hypothermia, and drowning.

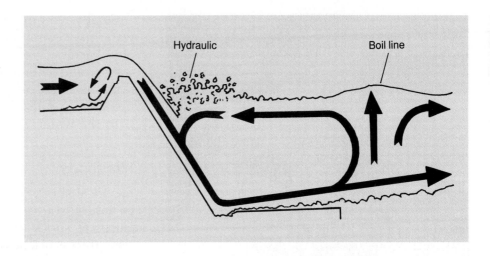

Hydraulic   Boil line

FIGURE 3–8

When floating in cold water, conserve body heat by using a body position that will reduce the escape of heat. (A) If alone, use the HELP position. (B) With other people, huddle together.

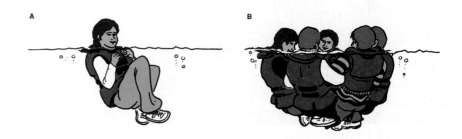

A   B

may cause major blunt trauma. The pressure of the flowing water may pin boats and bodies against the strainer. Approach strainers cautiously to avoid being caught.

Some alterations in natural water flow, such as low head dams, are man-made. They create hydraulics (powerful water movements or currents) that can trap people. These dams range in height from 6 inches to 10 feet. They frequently show a boil line downstream caused by the dangerous flow of water (Figure 3–7). The boil line is the result of some of the spillway flow backwashing upstream toward the dam. Anyone caught in the backwash will be pushed back toward the dam face, and be submerged by water rushing over the spillway. Then the current moves the victim downstream, along the river bottom, back into the boil line where the backwash will recapture the surfacing victim and begin the cycle again.

Those who are trapped often succumb to fatigue, hypothermia, or drowning. They also sustain injuries from impact with debris caught in the water with them.

In addition, the temperature of the water may cause problems. Hypothermia occurs rapidly in cold water. In fact, water draws body heat away 25 times faster than does air of the same temperature. You and the victim are at risk of developing hypothermia. To conserve heat, adopt the heat escape lessening posture (HELP), or huddle together with other people (Figure 3–8). Warm water (above 70 degrees F) can also be a problem, because it increases fatigue of both the victim and the rescuer.

All personnel involved in operations on or near the water must wear an approved personal flotation device (PFD). Several types of PFDs are available. Type I or Type II PFDs are preferred for water rescue work (Figure 3–9).

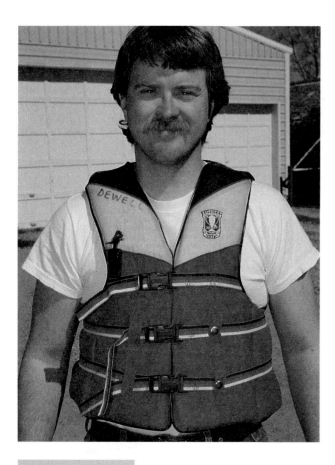

FIGURE 3–9

All personnel involved in a water rescue must wear a personal flotation device.

You should clean and inspect your PFDs regularly as part of your equipment maintenance program.

Never attempt a swimming rescue unless you are trained to do so, are experienced, and have the proper backup and equipment. Use shore-based rescue techniques, because they are safer and more effective. Ideally, a backup should be on hand to assist if the primary rescuer gets into trouble. The backup may also assist in treatment or evacuation of the patient.

Unless properly trained and equipped for cold water immersion, you should never attempt a rescue over ice. Instead use shore-based techniques. Try to direct the victim into self-rescue by having him grab a thrown rescue line. Do not use human chains that place additional stress on the irregular ice, inviting further breakup.

Finally, you must be aware that any body of water may contain hazardous materials including bacteria, parasites, sewage, industrial waste, and chemical spills. Appropriate precautions must be taken and **decontamination** procedures must be carried out after contact with the water.

Electricity

Electrical shock can be produced by man-made or natural sources. No matter what the source, electrical shock requires an evaluation of the risks to the rescuers and to the patient before aid can be rendered. The rescuers' level of skill is the most important factor affecting the outcome when dealing with the victim of an electrical accident.

The severity of man-made electrical emergencies varies greatly and depends on the current involved. Your local power company can assist with in-service education, providing training to evaluate the risks in electrical emergencies. They can also teach you how to deal with electric lines once the risks have been established. EMS personnel *should not* attempt to deal with downed electric lines except to establish a danger zone around the downed wires.

Dealing with power lines is beyond the scope of most EMS personnel. Energized power lines, particularly those carrying high voltage, behave in unpredictable ways. Using the equipment that is necessary to deal adequately with electrical emergencies requires in-depth training. The equipment also has specific storage needs and requires careful cleaning. Deposits of dirt or other contaminants can make this safety equipment useless or dangerous.

At the scene of a motor vehicle accident, above ground and below-grade power lines or feeds may both become electrical hazards. Disrupted overhead wires are usually a visible hazard; however, many EMS personnel become too casual about electrical hazards because visible sparks are not always present in charged wires. The area around downed power lines is always a danger zone, and it extends well beyond the normal accident scene. The utility poles that supported the broken lines should be used as landmarks for establishing the perimeter of the danger zone, which must become a restricted area for all emergency personnel, equipment, and vehicles.

In situations where man-made electrical hazards are present, you should use a helmet with chin strap and face shield. The shell of the helmet should be constructed of a certified electrical nonconductor. The chin strap should not stretch and should fasten securely so that the helmet stays in place if you are knocked down or a power line hits your head. You should be able to lock the face shield on the helmet to protect your face and eyes from power lines and/or flying sparks.

A bunker jacket provides minimal electrical protection, but it can protect you from heat, fire, possible flashovers, and flying sparks. The front opening of the jacket should be fastened and the jacket worn with the collar up and closed in front to protect your neck and upper chest. Proper fit is important so you can move freely.

Lightning is a complex natural phenomenon. It can be fatal to assume that "lightning never strikes in the same place twice." If the right conditions remain, a repeat strike in the same area can occur.

Lightning is a threat in two ways: by a direct hit and through ground current. After the lightning bolt strikes, the current drains along the earth following the most conductive pathway. To avoid being injured by this ground current, stay away from drainage ditches, moist areas, small depressions, and wet ropes. If you are in the open and a thunderstorm approaches, move down from ridge lines and peaks as soon as possible. Rescue operations may need to be suspended until the storm has passed. There are warning signs that occur just before a strike. As your surroundings become charged, you may feel a slight tingling sensation on your skin or your hair may even stand on end. In this situation, a strike may be imminent. Move immediately to the lowest possible area.

If you are caught in the open, try to present the smallest possible target for a direct hit or for ground current. To keep from being hit by the initial strike, stay away from projections from the ground such as a single tree. Drop all equipment, particularly metal objects that project above your body. Avoid fences and other metal objects, because they can transmit current from the initial strike over a long distance. A low crouch is a good protective position to take, because it exposes only your feet to the ground current whereas sitting on the ground exposes both the feet and buttocks. Place an object made of nonconductive material, such as a pack or sleeping bag, under your feet. Get inside a motor vehicle, if possible, because they provide good protection from lightning.

Terrain

In many rescue situations, the location of the incident and the surrounding terrain may become major obstacles and pose potential hazards for EMS personnel. The accident site may be remote; the only approach may be on foot. Equipment and supplies may have to be carried in, creating a major test of endurance.

During rescue operations, if there is a possibility that you or your patient might fall, preventive measures must be taken. When there is the potential for a fall, the situation is called *exposure*. Wherever there is exposure, you and your patient must be protected. One of your first actions at a scene with exposure should be to place a barrier line to prevent access to all dangerous areas. The restricted access should apply to EMS personnel as well as onlookers. In addition, you should establish safety lines and anchor them securely. Anyone who must work near the danger must wear appropriate safety equipment. A designated safety officer should oversee operations involving exposure to ensure that safety rules are followed.

A *belay* (safety rope) should be used anytime you or your patient are at risk of falling. When attached to a person on a litter, the belay can be used to control a fall. In most cases, the belay rope is controlled by a second person, the belayer. A patient on a litter must always be belayed where there is exposure during rescue, such as during lowering or raising of the litter

(Figure 3–10). Your need for a belay will depend on the particular situation, but anytime you feel the need, a belay should always be provided.

Any surface, natural or man-made, that creates the possibility of a fall or loss of control is an unstable surface. The surface can be natural or man-made. Natural unstable surfaces include creek beds, river rocks, cave surfaces, animal wastes, rotting vegetation, loose gravel, and ice. Some examples of man-made unstable surfaces are chemical spills; auto accident debris; chemical reaction vessels; tank cars; large metal, plastic, or glass surfaces; animal processing factories; cooling systems; and coal slurry or grain storage facilities. You must be aware of the potential for a mishap on unstable surfaces to protect you and your patients. Slips, falls, and collapse of the unstable surface can all result in injury.

When you plan for stable access to a patient or patients, remember that the overall safety of you and your patient is the primary consideration. If you lack training in this area, have trained and properly equipped rescue personnel bring the patient to you. Qualified rescuers always develop an escape plan first and have adequate standby equipment (ladder trucks, ropes, or boats) and a backup crew, dressed in the appropriate gear, ready to take action. Whenever there is the possibility of a fall, collapse, or serious slide, the rescuers and the patient(s) should wear a harness that is attached to a lifeline secured by a bombproof anchor.

Heavy, cleated hiking boots or structural firefighting boots work well when you must walk over very rough and unstable surfaces. However, that type of footwear can be very slippery on smooth, wet or frozen surfaces, such as the inside of glass or stainless steel tanks. A good pair of heavy-duty *crampons*, spiked metal plates that attach to boots or shoes, provide traction on ice, mud, stainless steel chemical tanks, mold or moss-covered rocks, or other hard surfaces that have a slippery covering. *Never* use any steel-cleated shoes or crampons on flammable liquids, however; the metal could cause sparks that might result in a flash fire.

Soft, rubber-soled shoes such as tennis shoes provide traction on some smooth surfaces. Remember that part of the purpose of footwear is foot protection, so soft tennis shoes are not appropriate in a situation where a foot injury is likely to occur.

FIGURE 3–10

When there is any risk of a litter sliding downslope during a carry, a safety or belay rope should be attached to the litter to support it.

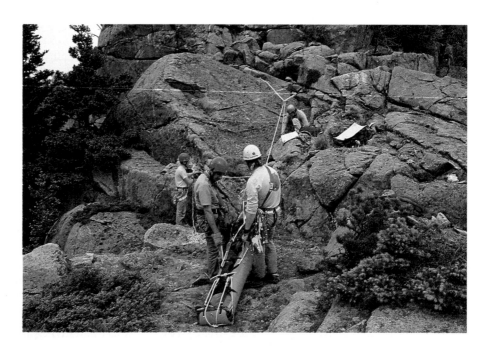

Another method to improve foot traction is to remove or alter the slippery surface as much as possible. Mud, oil, firefighting foam, and other substances can be washed down with a fire hose. Bulky material can be shoveled and hauled away to remove it from the area around a patient. Sodium chloride (table salt) or potassium chloride (road salt) can be sprinkled on a thin layer of ice that has covered a hard surface. However, chemical melting will not work well when temperatures have fallen below 10 degrees F. Other granules that work well in providing traction on ice are poultry grit and sand. Certain chemicals have been designed to absorb a tremendous amount of moisture from a slippery area, but these agents must be used by trained personnel.

When an unstable surface does not have the underlying strength necessary to support the weight of emergency personnel or the combination of personnel, equipment, and patient(s), place or build a covering around the scene of the accident or evacuation site. This will enable you to be lifted over the top of the unstable surface. On very loose materials, such as coal slurry or grain, place a large steel barrel over the top of the patient. This will protect the patient from further engulfment and will help stabilize the surrounding area until the material can be removed enough to gain access.

Stored grain can develop a surface crust when left standing for several months. As the grain shifts underneath, the crust may remain intact above an open space. If you stand on the crust, you could break through and become covered by the grain. Manure ponds and some chemical tanks may also have a crust form on top of the liquid beneath. Should you need to gain access to a patient across such a surface, it is best to use a boat or similar flotation device regardless of how strong the crust appears to be.

Dilapidated structures of rotting wood or rusting steel can be too unstable for walking or working. If the structure appears too flimsy to walk on, use an alternate means of patient access, such as a fire department's aerial apparatus or a rope system. Where the structure seems reasonably sound but the flooring appears unsafe, cover the old surface with plywood or lay a ladder on the floor to spread and support your weight.

Assume that any questionable, untested surface is hazardous. Never stand unsupported on top of any pile of grain, coal, pea gravel, or similar granular item. Always attach a lifeline to all rescuers and all patients on unstable surfaces as soon as possible. A lifeline may be used to locate the person tied to it in the event of secondary collapse.

Falling and Flying Objects

In any high-angle environment (buildings, caves, and mountain sides, for example), falling objects such as tools or rocks can become hazards. A *fall zone* is defined as the area where you are most likely to encounter falling objects. In back country, high-angle, or high-altitude areas, fall zones include gullies, washes, and runs. To reduce the risk of falling objects, you should immediately establish control of the area above the rescue site and banish any unauthorized and unnecessary persons from the scene. Travel up and down a slope or the side of a building often requires rappel/ascent lines or safety lines. These ropes may dislodge objects. Therefore, whenever possible, rescue ropes should be rigged off to the side of the patient and rescuers. If there is any danger of objects falling into the area, the patient must be protected with a backboard or other hard shield. Before accessing the patient in a fall zone, you should identify an escape route. The escape route does not necessarily have to be completely out of the danger area, but it should be away from the fall zone.

When strapped in a litter or stretcher, the patient is unable to ward off or avoid falling objects, brush or tree limbs, and other objects. Patients on litters must be protected with goggles, face shields, or litter shields (Figure 3–11).

When objects do fall, an easily understood alert must be given quickly. In a high-angle environment, standard words are used to warn others in the area of falling objects. When anything hard (e.g.: rock, hardware) falls, the warning word is *rock*. If the falling object is soft, such as a rope, webbing, or clothing, then the warning word is *rope.* The warning should be shouted by the person who first sees the object. The warning must be loud and distinct so that everyone hears and understands. If you are in the fall zone when you hear a warning, resist the natural reaction to look up, because the object could strike you in the face. Shield yourself and your patient as much as you can. Assume a position that will allow your helmet to protect you against the falling object and make your body as small a target as possible.

If the rescue situation is such that objects could fall on the rescue site without being seen, a safety observer should be stationed to watch and warn of any danger. If EMS personnel need to pass through an area that is prone to falling objects, scouts can "clean" the area by deliberately dislodging the dangerous objects before the personnel enter the area.

Flying objects are also a hazard, particularly when you are using power extrication equipment. Metal fragments can become dislodged; objects can be thrown by a hydraulic spreader. When flying objects are a possibility, you should take protective measures similar to those recommended for falling objects.

Confined Spaces

Confined spaces present a major potential hazard to EMS personnel. A confined space is any space not intended for continuous occupancy, with little or no ventilation, and limited entrance and exit. Confined spaces include but are not limited to water and waste removal pipes and systems, wells, caves, grain storage facilities, reaction vessels, ventilation and/or other duct work systems, liquid storage tanks, tank cars, ship holds, and utility vaults. A confined space is not necessarily a small space. The greatest potential hazards to EMS personnel involve limited entrance or exit and limited ventilation. A large grain elevator is a good example of a confined space although many people could fit within its walls. The elevator is not intended for continuous occupancy. It probably has little, if any, ventilation. Furthermore, it is difficult to get in and out of.

Many times a confined space may look safe. Even experienced EMS personnel can overlook the potential dangers, concentrating on the treatment of the patient. A tragic situation can be compounded when colleagues attempt to save a team member and also become victims of

FIGURE 3–11

Litter shields can help protect the patient from falling objects.

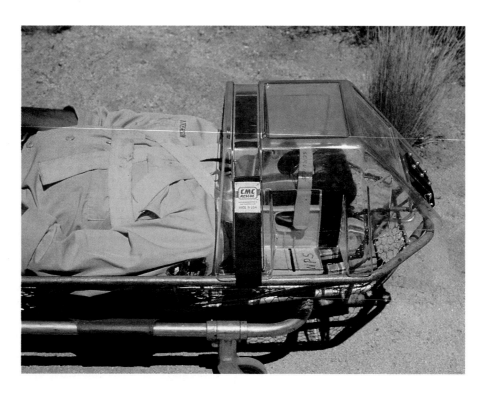

a dangerous confined space. *Never* enter any confined space unless it has been determined to be absolutely safe for entry. Entry and patient stabilization should be attempted only when you have had the appropriate training, have the proper equipment at hand, and have rendered the environment as safe as possible.

There are three groups of hazards in confined spaces: atmospheric, physical, and psychological. Atmospheric hazards are determined by the shape and makeup of the area, the amount of ventilation, and the presence of hazardous gases. Physical hazards include fire and hazardous materials, mechanical entrapment, electrical exposure, or product engulfment. Psychological hazards are the fears or anxieties that may be in your mind, which can profoundly affect your performance and the outcome of the rescue.

Normal air contains approximately 21 percent oxygen, 78 percent nitrogen, and 1 percent of other gases. Humans cannot function normally in an atmosphere that varies much from these percentages. Any atmosphere that has less than 19.5 percent oxygen must be considered immediately dangerous to life and health. You may fail to appreciate the effects of an oxygen-poor atmosphere, particularly when concentrating on patient care or rescue. The effects of **hypoxia** (low oxygen levels) vary, but typically an individual so affected will become excited, agitated, or confused. There are reported instances of people just sitting down and laughing in an oxygen poor environment. Agitation might make you rush to escape the area, only increasing your body's oxygen demand. On the other hand, disorientation, weakness, and lethargy could keep you from making any attempt at self-rescue from a low-oxygen atmosphere.

In a confined space, oxygen can be consumed by many sources. In some settings, natural, rotting vegetation consumes oxygen. The presence of rodents or other animals could also reduce the supply. In most incidents, however, methane, hydrogen sulfide, or other gases produced by decaying matter displace the oxygen. Hydrogen sulfide is heavier than air. It displaces oxygen from the low spaces in confined areas, causing death by suffocation.

Around factories, chemical plants, and construction sites, oxygen can be removed by chemical reactions. Freshly poured concrete consumes a tremendous amount of oxygen. Special care should be taken when you work around freshly poured, enclosed concrete structures.

In grain bins and silos, the atmosphere may be highly saturated with grain dust. Large tanks and manufacturing vessels may contain flammable vapors. Both grain dust and chemical vapors can explode when exposed to a single spark.

Atmospheric hazards encountered in confined spaces should be handled in two steps. First, the atmosphere must be tested with an acceptable testing device by someone familiar with this equipment. The most important readings indicate a potential immediate danger to life and health (IDLH) atmosphere: abnormal oxygen content or the presence of toxic and/or flammable gases and vapors. Second, ventilate the confined space thoroughly. Often the ventilation system built into the structure can be used. However, make sure the patient will not be injured if you start the ventilating system and ensure that air circulation will not introduce fire or explosion hazards or create a toxic atmosphere. Ventilation should be performed by trained experts.

Again, entry into a confined space with dangerous atmospheric conditions is extremely hazardous for EMS personnel. You must be properly equipped and have trained and practiced with competent instructors before you should consider any rescue attempt.

If you are not trained in the proper entry techniques, have trained personnel bring the patient to you for treatment.

The physical hazards of confined spaces include the potential for entrapment, electrocution, drowning, burns from steam, scalds from liquids, falls, and crush injuries. In addition, mechanical, electrical, or product transfer devices, such as augers, may endanger you or your patient.

Psychological stress is a challenging part of operations in confined spaces. A high level of anxiety can occur when you enter a tight enclosure with limited escape options, under emergency conditions and in the presence of electrical hazards, hazardous materials, and little or no breathable air. However, training and experience can prepare you to assist others safely in confined areas.

Your safety must always come first. You must answer yes to these three questions before contemplating a confined space entry:

- Am I absolutely sure that this area is safe?
- Do I have access to specialized equipment to work in this confined space?
- Am I trained in and do I feel comfortable with confined space entry and rescue?

If you answer "No" to any of the above questions, do not attempt the rescue.

Civil Disturbances

Civil disturbances (riots, strikes that become violent, and large gatherings of hostile or potentially hostile people) create many hazards for EMS personnel. Your safety and the safety of those with whom you work in civil disturbances are of primary concern. Several agencies will respond to these disturbances, and it is important to know who is in command and will be issuing orders.

If the incident is likely to become violent, you should wear protective clothing. Helmets with face shields, body armor (bulletproof vests), boots, and gas masks may be necessary because you could be the target for everything from dirt clods to bullets or tear gas.

Several types of body armor are currently being used by police agencies. They range from extremely light and flexible to heavy and bulky. The lighter vests do not stop large caliber bullets but offer more flexibility and are preferred by most law enforcement personnel. Lighter vests are commonly worn under a uniform shirt or jacket; the larger and heavier vests are worn on the outside.

Currently two types of gas masks are being used by police agencies and the military (Figure 3–12). The Grasshopper is popular because it is small and easy to store. However, it limits visibility and, after long periods of using it, causes a claustrophobic feeling. The M-17 gas mask is larger and easier to put on, and has large eye ports to increase visibility.

Exposure to tear gas destroys lung tissue. High concentrations of tear gas can also displace oxygen in a confined area and cause suffocation. Tear gas is actually a fine powder. The particles settle until movement scatters them or until they are removed by decontami-

FIGURE 3–12

The two types of gas masks used by police agencies and the military are the M-17 (left) and the Grasshopper (right).

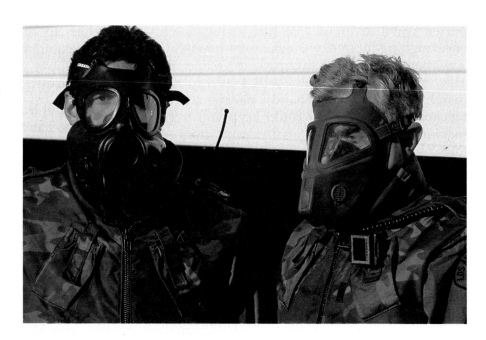

nation procedures. You can avoid exposure to tear gas by protecting your face with a gas mask, covering your arms and legs with tightly woven or knit material, and using proper footwear and gloves.

Once inside an area contaminated by tear gas, you should not move any items unless necessary. Fire service personnel can assist you with ventilation fans for air movement. After the incident, all exposed equipment and clothing must be thoroughly washed with soap and water for decontamination. A patient's skin, hair, and clothing can contain gas particles that may cause irritation when disturbed. Be aware that you can also be exposed to tear gas when you treat people who have been exposed, and you should take the same protective measures then as you would for primary exposure.

CONCLUSION

In summary, your personal safety is of utmost importance. You must thoroughly understand the risks of each environment you enter. You must have adequate protection from the dangers before you enter the scene, and you must seek help from trained personnel to create the safest environment for you and your patient(s).

Whenever you are in doubt about your safety, do not put yourself at risk and seek more expert and experienced assistance.

YOU ARE THE EMT

1. Choose appropriate clothing and gear for a rescue operation.
2. Select methods of protecting yourself from personal hazards.
3. Describe ways to avoid injury and protect patients in rescue operations involving fire.
4. Describe the tools and techniques of water and ice rescue.
5. Describe how to protect the patient from environmental threats in a high-angle environment during litter transport.

SECTION 2

PATIENT
ASSESSMENT

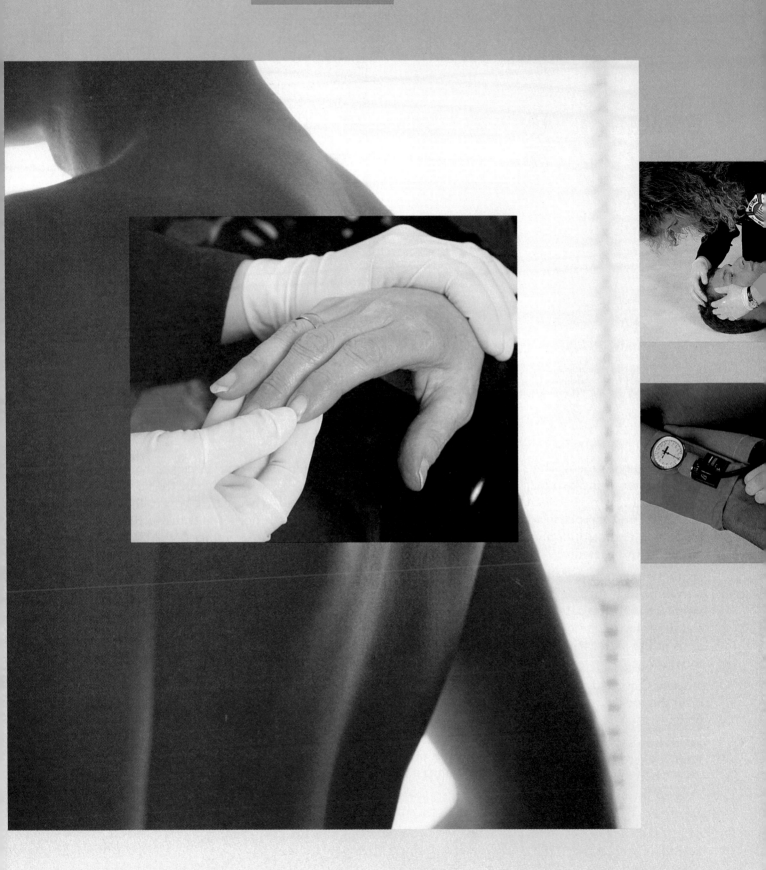

CHAPTER 4

GENERAL AND TOPOGRAPHIC ANATOMY

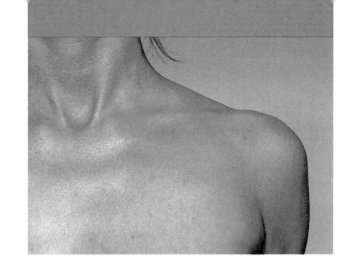

KEY TERMS

abdomen (ab-do′men) The more inferior of the two major body cavities, lying between the thorax and the pelvis and containing the major organs of digestion and excretion.

anatomic position (an″ah-tom′ik po-zish′un) A point of reference with the patient standing, facing the examiner, arms at the sides, with palms forward.

anterior Situated in front of or in the forward part of the body.

arterial pressure points Points where an artery passes over a bony prominence or lies close to the skin.

deep Pertaining to or situated inside the body and away from the skin.

distal (dis′tal) Farther from any point of reference; opposed to proximal.

inferior (in fēr′e-or) Referring to the lower portion of an organ or other structure.

lateral Away from the midline of the body or a structure.

medial (me′de-al) Pertaining to the middle; closer to the midline of the body or a structure.

midline The median line or median plane of the body.

pelvis A closed bony ring, consisting of the sacrum and two pelvic bones, that connects the trunk to the lower extremities.

posterior (pos-tēr′e-or) The back or dorsal surface of the body.

proximal (prok′sĭ-mal) Nearest; closer to any point of reference; opposed to distal.

superficial Pertaining to or situated near the surface.

superior (soo-pe′re-or) Situated above or directed upward.

thorax (tho′raks) The chest; the upper part of the trunk between the neck and the abdomen.

A working knowledge of human anatomy is essential for all medical personnel, including EMTs. Even though you are not expected to diagnose every injury or illness, you can aid emergency department personnel by conveying correct information using medical terminology. Such information is gathered after examination of a patient at the scene of an accident or sudden illness.

Topographic anatomy refers to how the superficial landmarks on the surface of the body are used as guides to locate the internal structures that lie beneath them. The language of topographic anatomy refers to the names of the principal regions of the body and the way the locations of these regions are described in relationship to one another.

Chapter 4 begins by defining the terms used to describe topographic anatomy when the body is in the anatomic position. The chapter then describes the topographic features of the seven major regions of the body. The last section of the chapter discusses arterial pulse points, or where on the body the major arteries can be palpated.

GOALS
. . . .

The goals of Chapter 4 are to
- define the common terms used in topographic anatomy.
- describe the major topographic features of the head, neck, thorax, shoulder girdle, upper extremity, abdomen, pelvis, and lower extremity.
- identify the major arterial pulse points.

. . . .

THE LANGUAGE OF TOPOGRAPHIC ANATOMY
. . . .

The surface of the body has many definite, visible features that serve as guides or landmarks to structures that lie beneath them. These external features, or topography, give form to the general anatomy of the body. Knowledge and awareness of the superficial landmarks of the body—its topographic anatomy—are vital to the accurate assessment of the sick or injured patient. This knowledge is also crucial to enable you to describe important patient findings to other medical personnel.

Visual inspection of the body is the simplest step in the primary and secondary surveys. Knowledge of topographic anatomy enables you to quickly spot abnormal findings. Because so much information regarding the extent of an injury or illness can be obtained through inspection, the importance of critical visual inspection of the patient cannot be overemphasized. In fact, many important facts about a patient's injury or disease might be missed because of inadequate visual inspection.

All medical personnel must be familiar with the language of topographic anatomy. The use of the proper terms will ensure that correct information is transmitted with the least possible confusion. The terms used to describe the topographic anatomy are applied to the body when it is in the **anatomic position**. This is a position of reference with the patient standing, facing the examiner, arms at the sides, with palms forward (Figure 4–1). When the terms *right* and *left* are used, they refer to the patient's

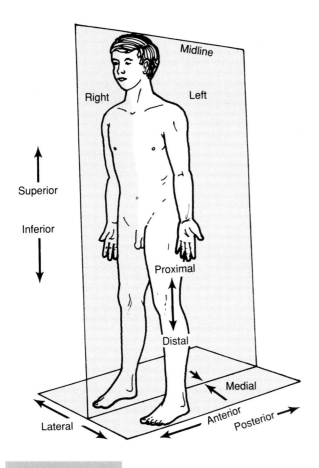

FIGURE 4–1

The terms used to describe the topographic anatomy are applied to the body in its anatomic position—that is, standing erect, facing the examiner, palms forward.

right and left. The principal regions of the body are the head, neck, thorax (chest), abdomen, and extremities (arms and legs).

The front surface of the body, facing the examiner, is the **anterior** surface. The surface of the patient away from the examiner is the **posterior** surface. An imaginary vertical line drawn from the midforehead through the nose and the *umbilicus* (navel) to the floor is termed the **midline** of the body. This imaginary line divides the body into two halves that are mirror images of each other. Parts of the body that lie at some distance from the midline are termed **lateral** structures. Parts that lie closer to the midline are termed **medial** structures. For example, we speak of the medial (inner) and

lateral (outer) aspects of the knee or the eye. The **superior** portion of the body, or any body part, is that portion nearer the head, whereas a portion nearer the feet is the **inferior** portion. We also use these terms to describe the relationship of one structure to another. For example, the nose is superior to the mouth and inferior to the forehead.

The terms *proximal* and *distal* are used to describe the relationship of any two structures on a limb. **Proximal** describes structures that are closer to the trunk. **Distal** describes structures that are nearer to the free end of the extremity. For example, the elbow is distal to the shoulder yet proximal to the wrist and hand. The term **superficial** means closer to or on the skin while the term **deep** means further inside the body and away from the skin. Many times these two terms are used to describe the extent or severity of an injury as well.

You should be familiar with all of these terms and be able to use them to describe the location of an injury or other physical findings. These terms are summarized in Table 4–1. When you use these terms properly, any other health care personnel examining the patient will know immediately where to look and what to expect. Visual inspection of the body should be sys-

TABLE 4–1	Topographic Anatomical Terms
Head	**Meaning**
Anterior	Front
Posterior	Back
Midline	Line drawn through nose and umbilicus
Medial	Closer to midline
Lateral	Farther from midline
Deep	Farther inside the body, away from the skin
Superficial	Closer to or on the skin
Superior	Closer to the head, higher
Inferior	Farther from the head, lower
Proximal	Closer to trunk
Distal	Farther away from trunk

tematic, thorough, and performed in exactly the same sequence for all patients. You should develop a specific examination routine so that you will not overlook a significant but perhaps subtle sign of injury or disease.

Whenever possible, the injured part should be compared to the corresponding uninjured part on the opposite side of the body. Although body structure varies significantly from individual to individual, the mirror image opposite side usually provides an excellent reference point for comparison (Figure 4–2).

THE HEAD

The head is divided into two parts: the cranium and the face. The cranium or skull contains the brain, which connects to the spinal cord through a large opening at the base of the skull (the *foramen magnum*). The most posterior portion of the cranium is called the *occiput*. On each side of the cranium, the lateral portions are called the temples or *temporal* regions. Between the temporal regions and the occiput lie the *parietal* regions. The forehead is called the *frontal* region. Just anterior to the ear, in the temporal region, one can feel the pulse of the superficial temporal artery. The thick skin covering the cranium and usually bearing hair is called the *scalp.*

The face is composed of the eyes, ears, nose, mouth, cheeks, and jowls. Six bones—the *nasal* bone, the two *maxillae* (upper jawbones), the two *zygomas* (cheekbones), and the *mandible* (jawbone)—are the major bones of the face.

The *orbit* of the eye is composed of the lower edge of the frontal bone of the skull, the zygoma, the maxilla, and the nasal bone. The bony orbit protects the eye from injury. By viewing the face from the side (Figure 4–3, right), one can observe the eyeball recessed in the orbit. Only the proximal one-third of the nose—the *bridge*—is formed by bone. The remaining two-thirds of the nose is composed of cartilage. Unlike the nose, the exposed portion of the ear is composed entirely of cartilage that is covered by skin. The visible part of the ear is called the *pinna*. The earlobes are the fleshy portions at the bottom of each ear. The *tragus* is a small rounded fleshy bulge immediately anterior to the ear canal. The superficial temporal artery can be palpated just anterior to the tragus. About one inch posterior to the external opening of the ear is a prominent bony mass at the base of the skull called the *mastoid process.*

The mandible forms the jaw and chin. Motion of the mandible occurs at a joint (the *temporomandibular joint*), which lies just in front of the ear on either side of the face. Below the ear and anterior to the mastoid process, the *angle of the mandible* is easily palpated.

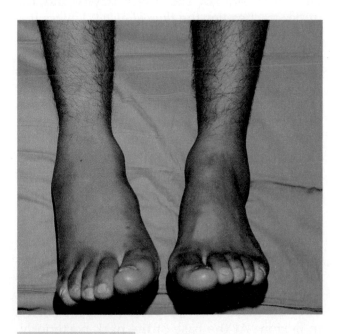

FIGURE 4–2

An injured, swollen right ankle is compared with the uninjured left ankle.

THE NECK

The neck contains many important structures. It is supported by the *cervical spine*, or the first seven vertebrae in the spinal column (C_1 through C_7). The *spinal cord* exits from the foramen magnum and lies within the spinal canal formed by the vertebrae. The upper part

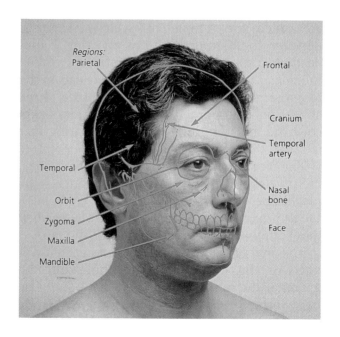

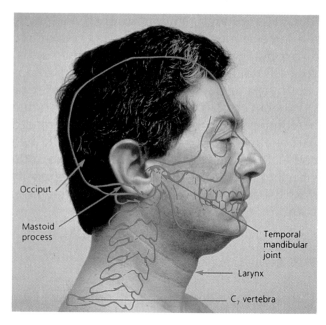

FIGURE 4-3

(Left) The major topographic features of the head.
(Right) The lateral view of the head and neck.

of the *esophagus* and the *trachea* (windpipe) lie deep in the midline of the neck. The carotid arteries may be found on either side of the trachea, along with the jugular veins and several nerves (Figure 4–4).

Several useful landmarks can be palpated and seen in the neck. The most obvious is the firm prominence in the center of the anterior surface commonly known as the "Adam's apple." Specifically, this prominence is the upper part of the *larynx*, the *thyroid cartilage*. It is more prominent in men than in women. The other portion of the larynx is the *cricoid cartilage*, a firm ridge of cartilage inferior to the thyroid cartilage, which is somewhat more difficult to palpate. Between the thyroid cartilage and the cricoid cartilage in the midline of the neck is a soft depression, the *cricothyroid membrane*. This is a thin sheet of connective tissue (*fascia*) that joins the two cartilages. The cricothyroid membrane is covered at this point only by skin.

Inferior to the larynx, several additional firm ridges are palpable in the anterior midline. These ridges are the cartilage rings of the trachea. The trachea connects the larynx with the main air passages of the lungs (the *bronchi*). On either side of the lower larynx and the upper trachea lies the *thyroid gland*. Unless it is enlarged, this gland is usually not palpable.

Pulsations of the carotid arteries are easily palpable in a groove 1 to 2 centimeters lateral to the larynx. Lying immediately adjacent to these arteries, but not palpable, are the internal jugular veins and several important nerves. Lateral to these vessels and nerves lie the *sternocleidomastoid muscles*. These muscles originate from the mastoid process of the cranium and insert into the medial border of each collarbone and the sternum (breastbone) at the base of the neck.

A series of bony prominences lie posteriorly, in the midline of the neck. They are the spines of the *cervical vertebrae*. The lower cervical spines are more prominent than the upper ones. They are more easily palpable when the neck is in flexion. At the base of the neck posteriorly, the most prominent spine is the seventh cervical vertebra (see Figure 4–3, right).

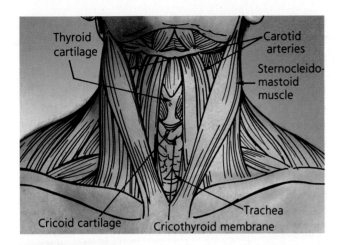

FIGURE 4-4

Anterior view of the neck.

THE THORAX

The **thorax** (chest) is the cavity that contains the heart, lungs, esophagus, and the great vessels (the aorta and two venae cavae). It is formed by the 12 *thoracic vertebrae* (T$_1$ through T$_{12}$)and their 12 pairs of ribs. The *clavicle* (collarbone) overlies its upper boundaries in front and articulates with the *scapula* (shoulder blade), which lies in the muscular tissue of the thoracic wall posteriorly (Figure 4–5). The lower boundary of the thorax is the *diaphragm*, which separates the thorax from the abdomen.

The dimensions of the thorax are defined by the *bony rib cage* and its attachments. Anteriorly, in the midline of the chest is the *sternum* (breastbone). The superior border of the sternum forms the easily palpable *jugular notch*. There are three components of the sternum: the manubrium, the body, and the xiphoid process. The upper quarter of the sternum is called the *manubrium*. The body comprises the rest of the sternum except for a narrow, cartilaginous tip inferiorly, which is called the *xiphoid process*. The junction of the manubrium and the body forms a very prominent ridge on the sternum, called the *angle of Louis*. The angle of Louis lies at the level where the second rib is attached to the sternum; it provides a constant and reliable bony landmark on the anterior chest wall.

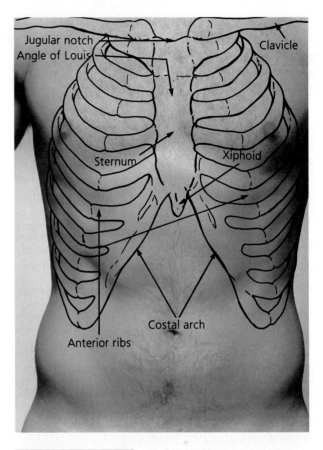

FIGURE 4-5

Anterior aspect of the thorax demonstrating the bony landmarks.

In the midline of the upper back, the spines of the 12 thoracic vertebrae can be palpated. Twelve *ribs* on each side form small joints with their respective thoracic vertebrae and extend around to the front to create the walls of the *thoracic cage*. The upper five ribs connect to the sternum through a short bridge of cartilage. The sixth through tenth ribs insert into the costal arch. The *costal arch* is a bridge of cartilage that connects the ends of the sixth through tenth ribs with the lower portion of the sternum. The eleventh and twelfth ribs are called *floating ribs*, because they do not attach to the sternum through the costal arch. The costal arch is easily palpable and represents the boundary between the lower border of the thorax and the upper border of the abdomen.

On the posterior chest wall the scapulae overlie the thoracic wall and are surrounded by large muscles (Figure 4–6). When the patient is standing or sitting erect, the two scapulae should lie at approximately the same level, with their inferior tips at about the level of the seventh thoracic vertebra. In the lower part of the thorax on each side an angle called the *costovertebral angle* is formed by the junction of the spine and the tenth rib. The kidneys lie deep to (beneath) the back muscles in the costovertebral angle.

The diaphragm is a muscular dome that forms the undersurface of the thorax, separating the chest from the abdominal cavity. Ante-riorly it attaches to the costal arch, and posteriorly it attaches to the *lumbar vertebrae*. The diaphragm cannot be seen or palpated.

Within the thoracic cage (Figure 4–7), the largest structures are the heart and lungs. The *heart* lies immediately under the sternum. It extends from the second to the sixth ribs anteriorly and from the fifth to the eighth thoracic vertebrae posteriorly. The lower border of the heart extends into the left side of the chest. Diseased hearts may be larger or smaller.

The major blood vessels that travel to and from the heart also lie in the chest cavity. On the right side of the spinal column, the *superior* and *inferior venae cavae* carry blood to the heart.

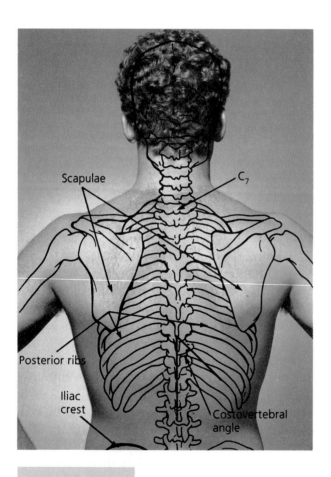

FIGURE 4–6

The topographic anatomy of the posterior view of the thorax. Major bony landmarks are also shown.

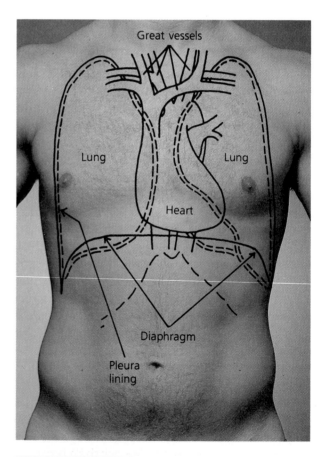

FIGURE 4–7

Anterior aspect of the thorax showing the relative positions of the major thoracic organs beneath the surface.

Just beneath the manubrium of the sternum, the *arch of the aorta* and the *pulmonary artery* exit the heart. The arch of the aorta passes to the left and lies along the left side of the spinal column as it descends into the abdomen. The esophagus lies behind the great vessels and directly on the anterior aspect of the spinal column as it passes through the chest into the abdominal cavity.

All space within the chest not occupied by the heart, great vessels, and esophagus is occupied by the *lungs*. Anteriorly, the lungs extend down to the surface of the diaphragm at the level of the xiphoid process. Posteriorly, the lungs extend farther inferiorly to the surface of the diaphragm at the level of the twelfth thoracic vertebra.

The major palpable landmarks in the chest are obviously the ribs. Most of them can be easily felt except for the first, which is hidden under and behind the clavicle. Both clavicles and the sternum can be easily palpated. The jugular notch is the top portion of the sternum. The angle of Louis is readily palpable in the upper portion of the sternum at the level of the space between the second and third ribs (the second intercostal space). Inferiorly, the costal arch is readily palpable on both sides of the anterior chest wall. In the midline, the tip of the xiphoid process is a tender and easily palpated landmark.

THE ABDOMEN

The **abdomen** is the second major body cavity. It contains the major organs of digestion and excretion. The diaphragm separates the thorax from the abdomen. Anteriorly and posteriorly, thick muscular abdominal walls create the boundaries of this space. Inferiorly, the abdomen is arbitrarily separated from the pelvis by an imaginary plane that extends from the *symphysis pubis* (also called the *pubic symphysis*) through the *sacrum*. Many organs lie in both the abdomen and the pelvis depending on the posture of the patient.

The simplest and most common method of describing the portions of the abdomen is by quadrants. In this system the abdomen is divided into four equal parts by two imaginary lines that intersect at right angles at the umbilicus. On the anterior abdominal wall the quadrants thus formed are right upper, right lower, left upper, and left lower (Figure 4–8). The terms *right* and *left* refer to the patient's right and left and not the observer's. Pain or injury in a given quadrant usually arises from or involves the organs that lie in that quadrant. This simple means of designation will allow you to identify injured or diseased organs that require emergency attention.

In the right upper quadrant (RUQ), the major organs are the *liver, gallbladder*, and a portion of the *colon* (Figure 4–9). Most of the liver lies in this quadrant almost entirely under the protection of the eighth to twelfth ribs. The liver fills the entire anteroposterior depth of the abdomen in this quadrant. Thus, injuries in this area are frequently associated with injuries of the liver. Tenderness without injury in the RUQ usually is a result of gallbladder disease.

In the left upper quadrant (LUQ), the principal organs are the *stomach*, the *spleen*, and a portion of the colon. The spleen is almost

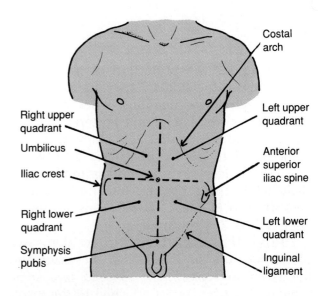

FIGURE 4–8

In the abdomen, quadrants are the easiest system for identifying areas. Major bony landmarks are also shown.

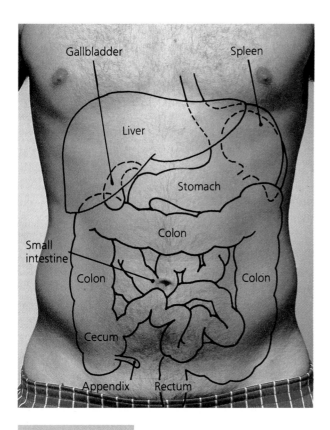

FIGURE 4–9

Anterior view of the abdomen showing the position of the major abdominal organs.

entirely under the protection of the left rib cage, whereas the stomach may sag well down into the left lower quadrant when full. The spleen lies in the lateral and posterior portion of this quadrant, under the diaphragm and immediately in front of the ninth to eleventh ribs. The spleen is frequently injured, especially when these ribs are fractured. Tenderness or pain in the LUQ following an injury often points to a ruptured spleen.

The right lower quadrant (RLQ) contains two portions of the large intestine: the *cecum* and the ascending colon. The *appendix* is a small tubular structure that is attached to the lower border of the cecum. Appendicitis is the most frequent cause of tenderness and pain in this region. In the left lower quadrant (LLQ) lie the descending and the sigmoid portions of the colon.

Several organs lie in more than one quadrant. The *small intestine,* for instance, occupies the central part of the abdomen around the umbilicus, and parts of it lie in all four quadrants. The *pancreas* lies just behind the abdominal cavity on the posterior abdominal wall in both upper quadrants. The *large intestine* also traverses the abdomen, beginning in the right lower quadrant and ending in the left lower quadrant as it passes through all four quadrants. The *urinary bladder* lies just behind the pubic symphysis in the middle of the abdomen and, therefore, lies in both lower quadrants and also in the pelvis.

The *kidneys* lie behind the abdominal cavity. They are termed *retroperitoneal* organs. They are above the level of the umbilicus, extending from the eleventh rib to the third lumbar vertebra on each side. They are approximately 5 inches long and lie just in front of the costovertebral angle (Figure 4–6).

The chief topographic landmarks in the abdomen are the costal arch, the umbilicus, the anterior superior iliac spines, the iliac crest, and the pubic symphysis. The costal arch, as noted earlier, is the fused cartilages of the sixth through the tenth ribs. It forms the superior arching boundary of the abdomen. The umbilicus, a constant structure, is in the same horizontal plane as the fourth lumbar vertebra and the superior edge of the iliac crest, the rim of the pelvic bone. The *anterior superior iliac spines* are the hard bony prominences at the front on each side of the lower abdomen just below the plane of the umbilicus (Figure 4–8). In the midline in the lowermost portion of the abdomen is another hard bony prominence, the pubic symphysis. Between the lateral edge of the pubic symphysis and the anterior superior spine on each side you can palpate the tough *inguinal ligament,* which stretches between these two structures. Below the ligament lie the femoral vessels.

Posteriorly, one does not usually refer to abdominal quadrants. The posterior portion of the iliac crest can be palpated, as can the spines of the five lumbar vertebrae (L_1 through L_5) in the midline. The lowermost rib on either side forms the costovertebral angle with the spines of the vertebrae.

THE PELVIS

The **pelvis** is a closed bony ring that consists of three bones: the sacrum and the two pelvic bones. Much like the skull, each pelvic bone is formed by the fusion of three separate bones. These three bones are called the *ilium,* the *ischium,* and the *pubis* (Figure 4–10). The pelvic cavity is bounded superiorly by an imaginary plane that runs from the symphysis pubis to the top of the sacrum. Its lateral walls are formed by the inner borders of the pelvic bone, and its inferior boundary is the *pelvic outlet,* a layer of muscles with openings for the gastrointestinal tract (the *rectum*), the female reproductive system (the *vagina*), and the urinary tract (the *urethra*). The pelvis contains the final portions of the gastrointestinal tract (the *rectosigmoid colon*), the female reproductive organs, and the urinary bladder.

The prominent anterior bony landmarks of the pelvis are the symphysis pubis in the midline and the anterior superior iliac spines. The inguinal ligament attaches to these two bony prominences and can be palpated in thin persons. Just distal to the midpoint of the inguinal ligament, the femoral artery can be palpated as it enters the thigh. From the anterior superior iliac spine, the ilium extends laterally and posteriorly to form the rim of the pelvis. This bony ridge is called the *iliac crest.*

Posteriorly, the pelvis has a flattened appearance, and in the middle third, the firm bony sacrum can be palpated. Just lateral to the sacrum on either side is a joint with the iliac portion of the pelvic bone (the *sacroiliac joint*). In the sitting position, a bony prominence is easily felt below the middle of each buttock. These prominences are the *ischial tuberosities.* The *sciatic nerve*—the major nerve to the lower extremity—lies just lateral to the tuberosity as it enters the thigh.

THE LOWER EXTREMITIES

The three major portions of the lower extremity are the thigh, the leg, and the foot. The joint

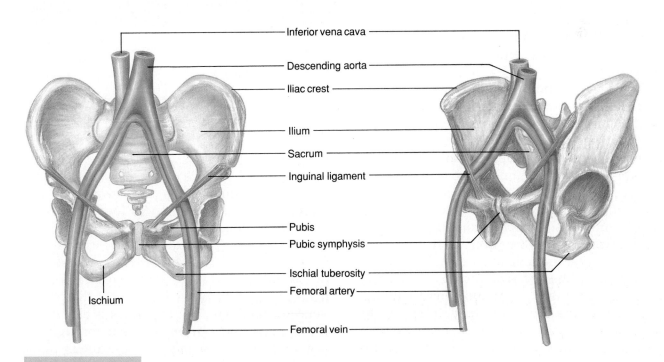

Inferior vena cava
Descending aorta
Iliac crest
Ilium
Sacrum
Inguinal ligament
Pubis
Pubic symphysis
Ischial tuberosity
Femoral artery
Femoral vein
Ischium

FIGURE 4–10   The pelvis, a very strong, closed bony ring, is composed of several separate elements and bears the sockets for the hip joints. The inguinal ligament lies just above the femoral vessels and helps protect them.

between the thigh and pelvis is called the *hip*. The joint between the thigh and the leg is the *knee joint,* and the joint between the leg and the foot is the *ankle joint.*

On the lateral side of the thigh just below the hip joint is a bony prominence called the *greater trochanter* (Figure 4–11). On examination, the position of this prominence should always be compared with that on the opposite side as a guide to fracture or dislocation of the hip.

The *femur,* the longest and strongest bone in the body, is the supporting bone of the thigh. It is surrounded by large muscles, and thus proximally, the only part of the femur that can be palpated is the greater trochanter. Near the knee, the medial and lateral *femoral condyles* can be palpated. Anteriorly, the large muscle of the thigh is called the *quadriceps;* the *hamstring muscles* lie posteriorly.

The *patella* (kneecap) is a specialized bone that lies within the tendon of the quadriceps muscle. It provides protection for the anterior aspect of the knee joint. The patella normally glides smoothly in a groove on the anterior surface of the femur. This groove lies between the rounded condyles that make up the distal end of the femur. Thus the knee joint is composed of the femoral condyles superiorly, the patella anteriorly, and the upper end of the tibia distally.

The leg is that portion of the lower extremity that extends from the knee joint to the ankle joint (Figure 4–12). The bones of the leg are the *tibia* (shin bone) and the *fibula.* The entire length of the tibia can be palpated on the anterior surface of the leg just under the skin.

The fibula lies on the lateral side of the leg. The rounded head of the fibula (the fibular head) can be easily palpated on the lateral side of the knee when the knee is flexed to 90 degrees. Lying immediately below the head of the fibula is the *peroneal nerve.* This nerve controls movement at the ankle and supplies sensation to the top of the foot. Injury to the fibula in this region or excessive pressure from a splint may cause permanent paralysis of this nerve.

The ankle joint is formed by the prominent distal ends of the tibia and the fibula. The end of the tibia forms the *medial malleolus,* and the

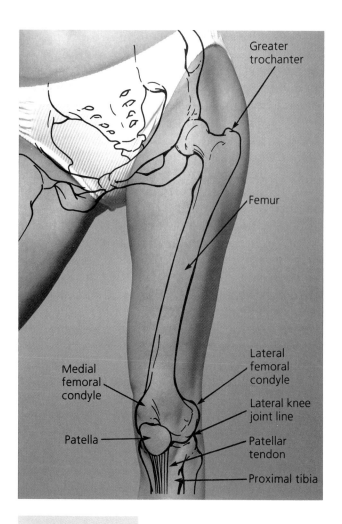

FIGURE 4–11

The major bony landmark in the upper portion of the lower extremity is the greater trochanter of the femur.

end of the fibula forms the *lateral malleolus.* These two bony prominences form the socket of the ankle joint. Both are usually visible and easily palpated. The two malleoli form a socket for the *talus,* or ankle bone. The undersurface of the talus has an articular surface for the *calcaneus* (heel bone), which forms the prominence of the heel. The calcaneus is also called the *os calcis* and can be palpated through the skin of the heel. The talus and calcaneus, along with five other bones, make up the rear portion of the foot. These seven bones are called tarsal bones. Five *metatarsal bones* form the substance of the foot. The five toes are formed by fourteen

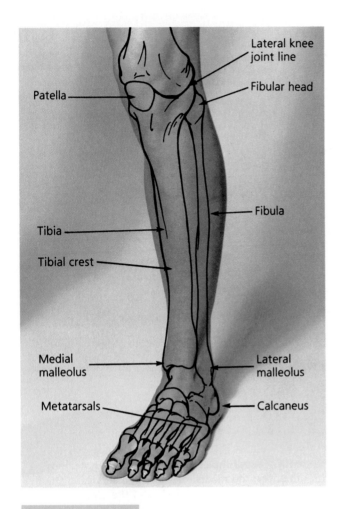

Patella

Lateral knee joint line

Fibular head

Fibula

Tibia

Tibial crest

Medial malleolus

Lateral malleolus

Metatarsals

Calcaneus

FIGURE 4–12

Anterolateral view of the leg and foot with the bony prominences labeled.

THE SHOULDER GIRDLE

The *shoulder girdle* is composed of the clavicle anteriorly, the scapula posteriorly, and the upper end of the *humerus* laterally. The clavicle, or collarbone, is firmly attached medially to the upper part of the sternum at the *sternoclavicular joint* (Figure 4–13). The clavicle is palpable throughout its entire length from the sternum to its attachment to the scapula. The *acromion process* of the scapula makes up the rounded lateral border of the shoulder girdle and forms a joint with the lateral end of the clavicle, the *acromioclavicular joint*, also called the *A/C joint*.

The scapula is a large, broad flat bone that overlies the posterior wall of the thorax and is surrounded by large muscles. Because of the presence of the muscles, only small portions of this bone are palpable. The acromion process can be palpated around the lateral edge of the shoulder girdle. It continues on as the spine of the scapula across the back (see Figure 4–6). The rounded appearance of the shoulder girdle is produced by the head of the humerus, the upper end of the arm bone, that articulates with a part of the scapula to form the true shoulder joint.

phalanges (singular form is phalanx): two in the great toe and three in each of the smaller toes.

Inspection of the lower extremity will identify injury in many instances. You should always compare the injured limb to the opposite, uninjured one. Any difference in the shape or appearance of the injured limb should make you suspicious of injury. Palpation of the bony landmarks (greater trochanter, femoral condyles, patella, fibular head, tibia, malleoli, calcaneus and metatarsal heads) should be included in any secondary survey of the injured limb to identify points to localized tenderness.

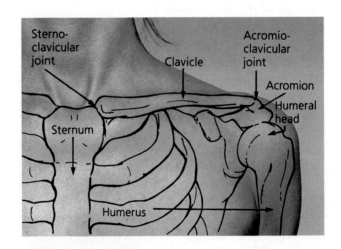

Sterno-clavicular joint

Clavicle

Acromio-clavicular joint

Acromion

Humeral head

Sternum

Humerus

FIGURE 4–13

The rounded prominence of the shoulder girdle laterally is created by the humeral head, covered by muscle.

THE UPPER EXTREMITY

The upper extremity extends from the shoulder girdle to the fingertips. It is composed of the arm, elbow, forearm, wrist, hand, and fingers. The arm extends from the shoulder to the elbow. The supporting bone of the arm is the humerus. Just like the thigh, there are few bony landmarks in the arm because it is covered by large muscles—the *biceps muscle* in the front and the *triceps muscle* in the back. Near the elbow joint, the medial and lateral *humeral condyles* form the medial and lateral borders of the upper portion of the elbow joint. These bony prominences are easily palpable when the elbow is flexed (Figure 4–14). The elbow is the joint between the distal end of the humerus and the two forearm bones, the ulna and the radius. The *olecranon process* of the ulna forms the point of the elbow, posteriorly.

The forearm is composed of two bones, the *ulna* and the *radius*. The ulna is larger in the proximal forearm, and the radius is larger in the distal forearm. The olecranon process of the ulna forms most of the elbow joint. The entire *ulna shaft* from the tip of the olecranon process distally can be palpated, because it lies just under the skin on the posterior surface of the forearm. The radius is covered by muscles and cannot be palpated except in the lower third of the forearm, where it enlarges to form a major portion of the wrist joint. Just as the two bones of the leg form a socket for the ankle joint, there are bony prominences on the ends of the radius and ulna to form the socket for the wrist joint. Here they are called *styloid processes*. Both the *radial styloid* and the *ulnar styloid* are easily palpable. The radial styloid is on the thumb side of the wrist, and the ulnar styloid is on the little finger side. Simultaneous palpation of these two processes will reveal that the radial styloid process usually lies about one centimeter distal to that of the ulna.

There are eight bones, called *carpal bones*, in the wrist. At the base of each finger lies a *metacarpal bone*. The metacarpals form the substance of the palm. The thumb has two phalanges, and each of the fingers has three phalanges (Figure 4–15).

As in the lower extremity, careful inspection of the upper extremity, especially when compared to the opposite limb, will often reveal an

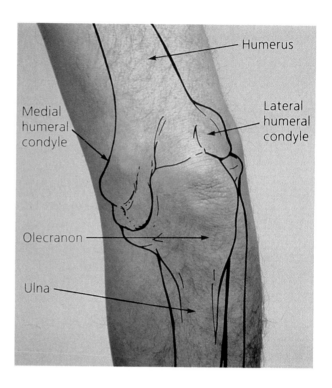

FIGURE 4–14

Posterior view of the elbow showing the three bony prominences: the medial and lateral condyles of the humerus and the olecranon process of the ulna.

abnormality. Palpation of the bony landmarks (clavicle, acromion process, humeral condyles, olecranon process, ulnar shaft, styloid processes, metacarpals, and phalanges) will identify points of local tenderness following injury.

ARTERIAL PULSE POINTS

An artery can be palpated wherever it passes over a bony prominence or lies close to the skin. At these points the arterial pulse can be taken. These points have been called **arterial pressure points** because in the past it was believed that compression at one of these points would help control hemorrhage distal to it. Although the theory behind this principle is sound, applying pressure over any single artery will rarely completely stop circulation distal to that point because there is always more than one artery supplying blood to an injury site. Therefore, local pressure on the wound is the best method for control of

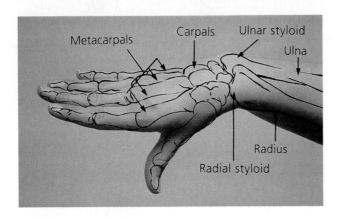

FIGURE 4–15

Dorsal view of the forearm, wrist, and hand.

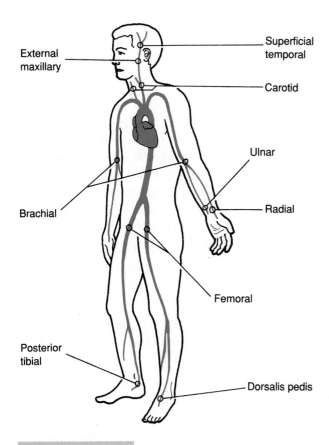

FIGURE 4–16

Major arterial pulse points.

hemorrhage. Pressure on the arterial pulse points can be used on occasion to supplement the control of rapid, severe bleeding.

Major arterial pulse points are shown in Figure 4–16. Palpation at these points enables

you to ascertain the presence of cardiac activity. In addition, following injury, decrease or absence of the pulse may indicate damage to the artery proximal to the pulse point.

Anterior to the upper portion of the ear, just over the temporomandibular joint, lies the *superficial temporal artery.* Anterior to the angle of the mandible on the inner surface of the lower jaw, the *external maxillary artery* can be palpated. It contributes much of the blood supply to the face. The *carotid arteries* may be palpated anteriorly in the neck just lateral to the larynx. On the inner surface of the arm, about 5 centimeters above the elbow, the *brachial artery* can be palpated. Arterial pulsations may be felt in both the *radial* and *ulnar arteries* at the wrist just proximal to the styloid processes. The *femoral artery* may be palpated as it passes beneath the inguinal ligament in the groin. Just posterior to the medial malleolus is the *posterior tibial artery.* On the anterior surface of the foot between the first and second metatarsals is the *dorsalis pedis artery.* This artery is not always present. When it is present, its pulsations may be felt easily.

YOU ARE THE EMT

1. The costovertebral angle is formed by the spine and tenth rib. What organs lie deep to the back muscles in the costovertebral angle?
2. Name three abdominal organs that lie in more than one quadrant and identify the quadrants they share.
3. The lungs take up a good portion of the thorax. What other structures lie in the thorax? What organ separates the thorax from the abdomen?
4. With severe trauma to the ankle, which three bones could be fractured?

CHAPTER 5

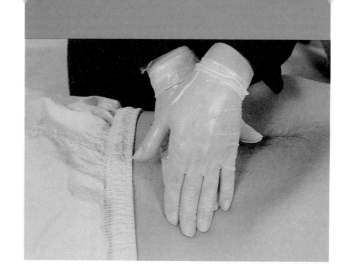

PATIENT ASSESSMENT

KEY TERMS

auscultation (aws"kul-ta'shun) Listening to sounds within the organs, usually with a stethoscope; a method of taking a patient's blood pressure.

blood pressure The pressure of the blood against the walls of the arteries.

chief complaint The first words out of a patient's mouth in response to a general question such as "What's wrong?" or "What happened?"

level of consciousness The degree of alertness or awareness of the patient.

palpation (pal-pa'shun) Examination by touch.

primary survey The process of finding and treating the most life-threatening emergencies first.

pulse The expansion and contraction of an artery, consistent with the beat of the heart, which may be felt with a finger.

secondary survey The final step in the assessment process in which the EMT carefully examines the patient from head to toe, looking for wounds and deformities and observing whether the patient feels pain or sensation.

sign A condition that the EMT observes, such as bleeding or a contusion.

symptom Something the patient tells the EMT, such as "I feel dizzy."

OVERVIEW

The most important function of the emergency medical technician is to identify and treat any life-threatening conditions first and then to assess the patient carefully for other complaints or findings that may require emergency treatment or transportation to a hospital. The importance of this function is stressed repeatedly because failure to perform patient assessment correctly will result in improper patient care and possibly permanent impairment or even death.

Chapter 5 begins by distinguishing between signs and symptoms. Then 10 basic diagnostic signs are described. The second half of Chapter 5 explains how patient assessment is carried out using these diagnostic signs. The sequence of assessment and treatment priorities is especially important, and thus the order in which topics are presented is significant.

GOALS

The goals of Chapter 5 are to
- distinguish between signs and symptoms.
- describe the four vital signs (pulse, respiration, blood pressure, and temperature) and six other diagnostic signs (skin color, capillary refill, pupil size and response to light, level of consciousness, ability to move, and reaction to pain).
- understand the sequence of assessment and treatment priorities, including the first assessment, arrival at the scene, the primary survey, the chief complaint, vital signs, history of present illness, and the secondary survey.

THE SETTING OF PATIENT ASSESSMENT

This chapter concentrates on the techniques of patient assessment and common findings to look for in assessing the patient. A general and customary emergency medical method of proceeding is presented. You must consider the nature of the situation in which you find the patient. The situation will sometimes modify the time spent on any one aspect of assessment but never negates the need to try to accomplish all aspects of assessment presented in this chapter.

The patient who is the victim of trauma is handled somewhat differently than the patient who has a primary medical complaint. The emphasis in trauma patient care is to minimize the time spent at the scene (to remain there only long enough to manage treatable life- and/or limb-threatening situations and stabilizing injuries to minimize worsening of those injuries). Patients with medical complaints must be assessed thoroughly and receive initial stabilizing treatment at the scene. Patients who are in shock or are unconscious are managed differently from patients who are talking and have stable vital signs. In all cases, the condition of the airway, breathing, and circulation will govern the depth of patient assessment and treatment of the sick or injured patient in the field. Always give priority to emergency care of the airway, breathing, and circulation to ensure life and limb saving treatment.

After discussing some of the more important diagnostic signs, a general method of examination will be presented, illustrated, and discussed. Before you can tailor your assessment to trauma versus medical problems, or to serious life-threatening versus less urgent problems, you must have a thorough understanding of the basic patient assessment method. This method begins with important diagnostic signs and associated symptoms.

SIGNS AND SYMPTOMS

The words *sign* and *symptom* are often used incorrectly, even by experienced medical personnel. A **symptom** is something that the patient tells you, such as, "My arm hurts," or "I feel dizzy," or "I can't breathe," or "I feel like I'm gonna die." A **sign** is something that you observe in a patient, such as deformity or bleeding in a fractured arm or the patient's blood pressure or wheezing in a patient struggling to breathe. Because they are actually observed by you, signs are considered to be more reliable than symptoms (Figure 5–1). Both signs and symptoms must be noted and relayed to higher-level emergency care personnel when you transport the patient.

DIAGNOSTIC SIGNS

To observe important diagnostic signs, you must have the proper tools, the most important of these being your eyes, ears, and hands. Above all, you must have the ability to use these "tools" calmly in a stressful environment. An EMT who panics at the scene will be unable to perform a proper assessment or set the right priorities for treatment. Other tools that are useful are a penlight, a wrist watch with a second hand, a stethoscope, and a blood pressure cuff. The stethoscope is easily misused — the earpieces should be placed *facing forward* into the ears (Figure 5–2).

Patient assessment requires you to look **(inspect),** listen **(auscultate),** and/or feel **(palpate)** for four vital signs (pulse, respiration, blood pressure, and temperature) and six other diag-

nostic signs (skin color, capillary refill, pupil size and response to light, level of consciousness, ability to move, and reaction to pain).

Pulse

The **pulse** is the pressure wave that is felt as the heart contracts and propels a volume of blood through the arteries. It is a useful indication of the condition of the heart, the blood vessels, and the blood itself. You measure the pulse by palpating an artery at a pulse point, which is where an artery lies close to the surface of the

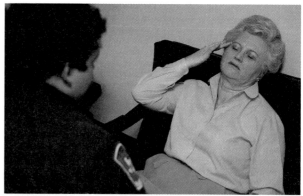

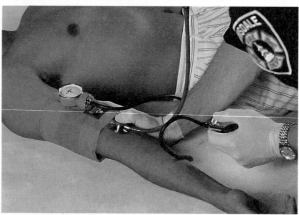

FIGURE 5–1

A *symptom* is a complaint that the patient relates to you. At the top, the patient is telling the EMT that she feels dizzy (a symptom). A *sign* is something you observe. At the bottom, the EMT is taking the patient's blood pressure (a sign). Both symptoms and signs should be recorded.

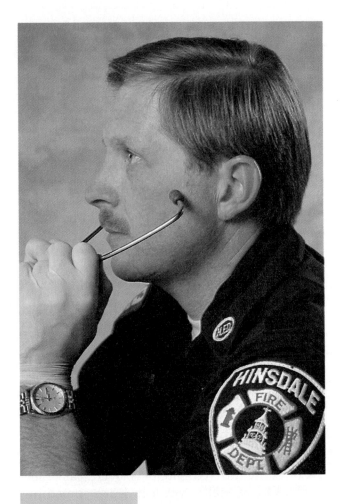

FIGURE 5-2

The ear pieces of a stethoscope should be placed facing forward in the ears.

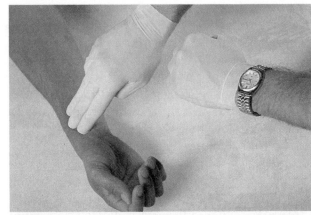

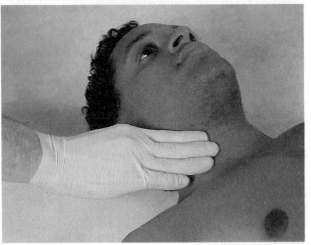

FIGURE 5-3

Palpation of the radial pulse at the wrist (top) and of the carotid pulse in the neck (bottom).

skin. Although the pulse can be palpated at any of the pulse points described in Chapter 4, the most common place to palpate for the pulse is in the wrist, along the path of the radial artery (Figure 5-3, top).

If the pulse cannot be palpated at either wrist, you should attempt to find it in the neck along the path of the carotid artery (Figure 5-3, bottom). The carotid pulse is more prominent than the radial pulse and it is easier to feel in an emergency situation particularly when the blood pressure is low. The carotid pulse is found in the neck under the anterior edge of the sternocleidomastoid muscle. When palpat-

ing the carotid pulse, you should first make sure that the patient is in a lying or sitting position. Never try to feel both carotid pulses at the same time because excessive pressure on the two arteries might cut off circulation to the brain.

"Taking a pulse" consists of an assessment of the rate, strength, and regularity of the pulse. The normal pulse rate is the number of beats per minute and is a reflection of the heart rate. The average adult's pulse rate ranges from 60 to 100 beats per minute. In a child, the normal rate is 80 to 100 beats per minute. In toddlers it is 100 to 120 beats per minute and in newborn infants, normal rates range from 120 to 140 beats per minute. The pulse rate is usually obtained by counting the number of beats that occur over a 15 second period and multiplying that number by 4. However, if the rate is found to be slower than 70 or is irregular, the rate should be counted for a full minute to more accurately measure the pulse rate.

The pulse volume is a rough indicator of the strength of the heart's contractions. After palpating the pulse in many patients, you will develop a sense of the pulse volume. A rapid, "thready," weak pulse can indicate shock from loss of blood. A "bounding" pulse can be present in fright or with high blood pressure. If the pulse is absent, it may mean that the artery being palpated is blocked from disease or injury or that the heart is weak or has stopped beating.

The third important characteristic of the pulse is the regularity of its rhythm. The pulse should have a regular frequency of beats. The absence of beats ("skipped beats") or irregularity of beats (palpitations) usually signals a heart rhythm problem.

The pulse is an instantaneous indicator of the condition of the patient and should be taken *and recorded* (rate, volume, and regularity) frequently during any emergency encounter. The frequency of recording the pulse and other vital signs should be governed by local medical director protocol. Pulse is one of the vital signs that you can monitor continuously in most emergency situations, including the back of a moving ambulance. For the conscious patient, the hands-on contact with the radial pulse by the caring EMT is a very reassuring gesture that has a medically useful function as well.

Respirations

Normal breathing occurs easily, without pain, noise, or effort. The rate of respirations can vary widely and is usually between 12 and 20 breaths per minute. Interestingly, well-trained athletes at rest may breathe only 6 to 8 times per minute. Normal respirations are not unusually shallow or deep. You should begin a record of the rate and character of respirations when you first see a patient, and observe and record any changes that occur.

Rapid, shallow respirations are frequently associated with shock. Very deep and rapid respirations in an unconscious patient with head trauma are ominous signs of severe injury. Deep, gasping, labored, and noisy breathing may indicate partial airway obstruction, respiratory failure, or chronic lung disease. With respiratory depression or respiratory arrest, there will be little or no movement of the chest and abdomen and little or no airflow felt or heard at the nose and mouth. A choking patient can be identified by the inability to cough or talk and the instinctive, nearly universal, gesture of clutching the throat that characterizes the choking victim (Figure 5–4).

Sputum is matter that is expectorated (coughed) from the lungs. Injury to the chest may cause the patient to cough up blood or frothy (foamlike) sputum. Heart failure can also cause the production of a frothy pink sputum. Patients with pneumonia and bronchitis may cough up thick sputum of various colors. You should note the volume, color, and other characteristics of any sputum that is produced.

Coughing up red blood is a critical emergency. Occasionally, you can learn something

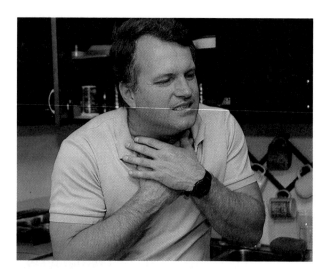

FIGURE 5–4

Nearly every choking person will grasp the throat.

about the patient by smelling the patient's breath. For example, the breath of patients with severe diabetic acidosis often gives off a sweet or fruity odor. Obviously, the intoxicated patient may smell of alcohol. However, you must not be misled by the smell of alcohol into thinking that the patient is "just drunk" when a more serious condition might exist. Any particularly obvious odor of the breath should be noted, recorded, and reported.

Blood Pressure

Blood pressure is the pressure of the circulating blood against the walls of the arteries. In an uninjured, healthy person, the arterial system is a closed system attached to a pump (the heart) and completely filled with blood. Changes in the blood pressure may indicate changes in the blood volume, capacity of the vessels to contain the blood, or ability of the heart to pump the blood. Changes in the blood pressure can occur rapidly but usually not as rapidly as pulse changes occur. This is because the body attempts to maintain a normal blood flow to critical organs by first increasing the pulse rate. Thus, a falling blood pressure is a late and ominous sign in injury or disease.

Blood pressure can fall markedly after severe bleeding, following a heart attack, or in other states of shock. Low blood pressure means there is insufficient pressure in the arterial system to supply blood to all the organs of the body. As a consequence, organs may be severely damaged. The causes of low blood pressure must be identified promptly and treated aggressively. The treatment of low blood pressure that is caused by severe bleeding requires emergency control of the source of such bleeding.

If the blood pressure is abnormally high, damage to or rupture of the vessels in the arterial circuit may occur. It is equally important that the cause of elevated blood pressure be found and treated. The treatment of elevated blood pressure is complex and may require hospitalization.

Blood pressure can change rapidly during transport of a patient to the hospital. It is important that emergency department person-

nel be notified of the status of your patient's blood pressure as early as possible in the course of the prehospital evaluation and also be made aware of any changes before arrival at the hospital. Therefore, during the course of emergency medical care, you should check and record the blood pressure at frequent intervals, along with the time it was taken.

Blood pressure is recorded at systolic and diastolic levels. Systolic pressure is the level present in the artery at the moment the heart contracts. Diastolic pressure is the level present during relaxation of the heart. Systolic pressure is the maximum pressure to which the arteries are subjected, and diastolic pressure represents the minimum amount of pressure that is always present in the arteries. With most diseases or injuries, these pressures change in a parallel fashion—in other words, both rise or both fall. Three exceptions to this rule occur: brain injury, cardiac tamponade, and tension pneumothorax. Brain injury, at times, causes a rise in the systolic pressure with a stable or falling diastolic pressure. A fall in systolic pressure, accompanied by a rising diastolic pressure, occurs in cardiac tamponade and in tension pneumothorax. In cardiac tamponade, blood fills the sac around the heart impeding its filling and pumping. In tension pneumothorax, air under abnormal pressure in the chest obstructs the filling of the right heart thereby limiting its output. Both conditions cause the systolic and diastolic pressures to approach each other; this condition is called a narrow pulse pressure.

Blood pressure is measured by one of two methods or a combination of the two. Both methods require the use of a blood pressure cuff, called a sphygmomanometer (Figure 5–5). It is important to select a cuff that is the appropriate size for the patient. The sphygmomanometer has a rubber bladder inside of it; this bladder should be long enough to encircle the patient's arm completely. The width of the bladder should be at least 20 percent greater than the diameter of the arm (Figure 5–6a). Narrow cuffs are made for taking children's blood pressure, and extra-wide cuffs are made for obese adults (Figure 5–6b). Cuffs that are too small may give falsely high readings, and

A

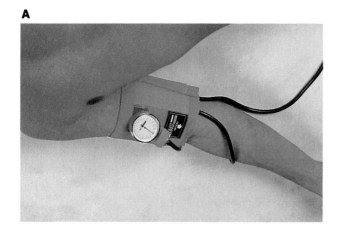

B

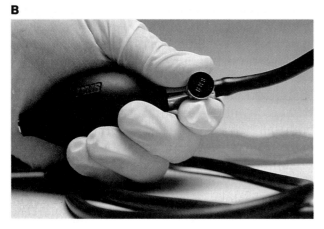

A

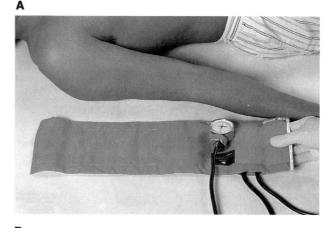

B

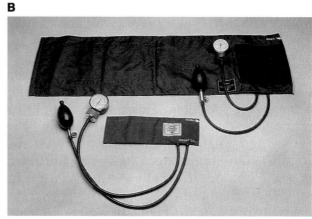

FIGURE 5–5

(A) A blood pressure cuff, or sphygmomanometer. (B) The EMT's thumb and index finger operate the knob that controls the release of air from the cuff, while the rest of the hand inflates the cuff using the bulb.

FIGURE 5–6

(A) It is important to use the right size cuff—one that is at least 20 percent wider than the diameter of the arm. (B) A pediatric cuff and an extra large cuff are shown.

cuffs that are too large may give falsely low readings. The blood pressure may also be taken in the thigh, using the extra large cuff.

Wrap the cuff snugly around the patient's upper arm, with the lower edge of the cuff about 1 inch above the inside of the patient's elbow (Figure 5–7). The center of the inflatable bladder, usually marked with an arrow on the cuff, should cover the patient's brachial artery along the medial aspect of the lower arm at the elbow.

You should first take the blood pressure by palpation. This is done by finding the patient's radial pulse. Then, with the other hand, inflate the blood pressure cuff until the pulse is no longer felt and then for another 30 millimeters of mercury (mm Hg) on the gauge of the blood pressure cuff. Deflate the cuff slowly until the pulse returns (Figure 5–8). The reading on the gauge when the pulse returns is the patient's systolic blood pressure, by palpation. Because the blood pressure determined by palpation is less accurate than if determined by auscultation, it should be recorded with the word "palpation" written beside it. Only the systolic pressure can be measured using the palpation method.

Then you should take the blood pressure by auscultation. Reinflate the cuff to the same point as before—about 30 mm Hg above the

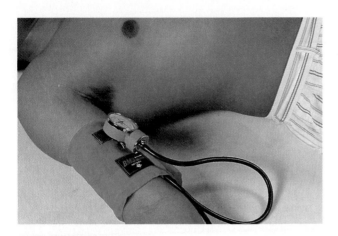

FIGURE 5–7

The cuff is wrapped securely around the arm about 1 inch above the elbow.

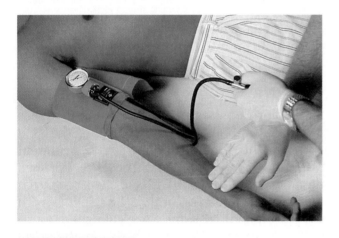

FIGURE 5–8

The pressure is first taken by palpation.

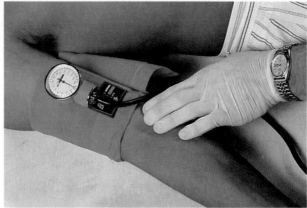

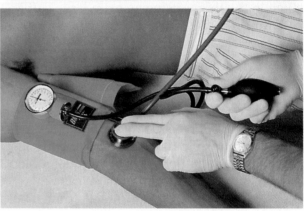

FIGURE 5–9

The brachial pulse (top) is palpated to determine where the stethoscope will be placed. The stethoscope (bottom) is placed over the brachial artery and the blood pressure is taken by auscultation.

systolic blood pressure as determined by palpation—and place the stethoscope in the patient's *antecubital fossa,* located at the anterior aspect of the elbow over the brachial artery (Figure 5–9). Gradually deflate the cuff while you listen for the sound of the pulse "tapping" in the artery. Record the sound first heard as the systolic pressure. Continue to deflate the cuff until the "tapping" sounds disappear. The

pressure at which the sounds disappear is the second reading, or the diastolic pressure. Record the blood pressure in the form systolic/diastolic; for example, 120/80 mm Hg. Also record the position of the patient (sitting, standing, or lying) and the extremity in which the pressure is taken.

Blood pressure levels vary with age and sex. One useful rule of thumb for estimating the normal systolic pressure in the male is to add 100 to the age of the patient, up to the level of 150 mm Hg. Normal diastolic pressure in the male ranges between 65 and 90 mm Hg. Both pressures are about 10 mm Hg lower in the female. Sounds at the elbow are, at times, impossible to hear in a moving ambulance, and often you must rely on measuring the blood pressure by palpation during transport. Occasionally, the blood pressure sounds do not disappear as you decrease the cuff pressure. This indicates continued turbulence in the artery after the pressure of the cuff has been released. The pressure is then reported as the systolic pressure and "all the way down"; for example, "120 over all the way down."

Only rarely can the upper extremities not be used to determine blood pressure. In such circumstances, the blood pressure may be taken in the thigh, using an extra large cuff and palpating for the pulse in the posterior tibial artery.

Temperature

Normal body temperature is 98.6 degrees Fahrenheit (37.0 degrees Centigrade). The skin is largely responsible for regulation of body temperature, by radiation of heat from skin blood vessels and the evaporation of sweat.

Changes in temperature result from illness or injury. A cool, clammy (damp) skin is indicative of a general response of the sympathetic nervous system to an insult, such as blood loss (shock) or heat exhaustion. As a result of nervous stimulation, sweat glands are hyperactive and skin blood vessels contract, resulting in cold, pale, wet, or clammy skin. These signs are often the first indication of shock or severe pain. Exposure to cold will produce a cool, dry skin. Dry, hot skin may be caused by fever or by exposure to excessive heat, as in heat stroke.

A patient's temperature is usually taken by mouth, with the bulb of the thermometer placed beneath the tongue. The thermometer should be left in place with the patient's mouth closed for 3 minutes. In a child or an uncooperative patient, the thermometer can be placed in the axilla (armpit), keeping the patient's arm at the side. Axillary temperatures are notoriously inaccurate, take a long time to register (10 minutes), and should be used only as a last resort. Rectal temperature is very accurate and is usually taken, if necessary, in the emergency department. The rectal temperature is routinely one-half to one degree above oral temperature

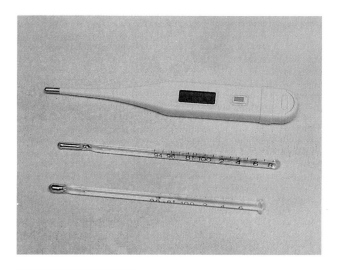

FIGURE 5–10

A digital (top), oral (middle), and a rectal (bottom) thermometer.

and is taken with a rectal thermometer left in place for 1 minute (Figure 5–10).

Skin Color

Skin color depends primarily on the presence of circulating blood in the vessels of the skin and on the amount and kind of pigment present in the skin. The presence of such pigment may hide skin color changes that result from illness or injury. In patients with deeply pigmented skin, color changes may be apparent in the fingernail beds, in the *sclera* (the "whites") of the eye, or the membranes inside the mouth. In lightly pigmented patients where changes are seen more easily, the skin colors of medical importance are red, white, and blue.

A red color may be present with high blood pressure, fever, late stages of carbon monoxide poisoning, alcohol intoxication, and heat stroke. The patient who has severe high blood pressure may sometimes be plethoric (dark, reddish-purple skin color due to filling of all visible blood vessels). The patient who has carbon monoxide poisoning is usually cherry red, as is the heat stroke patient (Figure 5–11).

A pale, white, ashen, or grayish skin is indicative of insufficient circulation and is seen

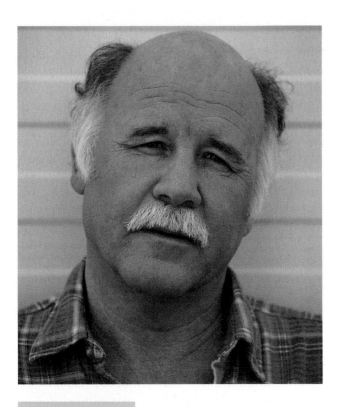

Red skin color may indicate high blood pressure, heat stroke, or carbon monoxide poisoning.

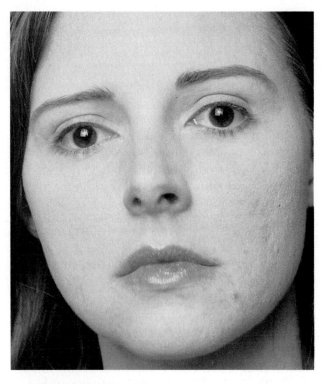

Pale skin color may indicate insufficient circulation.

in patients who are in shock, in certain stages of fright, or suffering from cold exposure. In these circumstances, there is literally not enough blood circulating in the skin (Figure 5–12).

A bluish color, *cyanosis,* results from poor oxygenation of the circulating blood. Blood is blue when it is oxygen poor and red when fully saturated with oxygen. Thus, cyanotic blood in the vessels makes them blue. Cyanosis always indicates a significant lack of oxygen and demands rapid correction of the underlying respiratory problems. Cyanosis is usually first seen in the fingertips and the lips (Figure 5–13).

Chronic illness may also produce color changes such as the jaundice (yellow color) seen in liver disease (see Chapter 34). In this condition, bile pigments that are normally present in the liver and the gastrointestinal tract are deposited in the patient's skin. Pa-

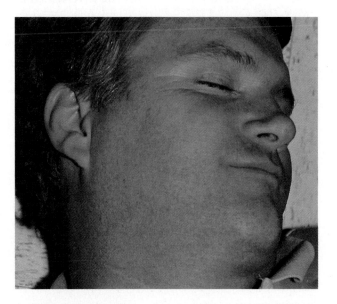

Blue skin color is characteristic of the lack of oxygen in the blood.

tients with the dangerous infection hepatitis are often jaundiced. The presence of jaundice should alert you to exercise appropriate infectious disease precautions, such as wearing gloves.

Assessment of the patient's color can lead to an immediate decision about the need for treatment. Oxygen may be necessary, arrest of bleeding may be required, or full resuscitation may be indicated. Sometimes a glance at the patient is all you need to identify treatment priorities.

Capillary Refill

Capillary refill is the ability of the circulatory system to restore blood to the capillary blood vessels after it has been squeezed out by the examiner. Customarily, the capillary bed under the fingernails is the most reliably tested area. Capillary refill should be both prompt and pink—that is, the normal pink color underneath the nail bed should return within 2 seconds after gentle compression is released. It may be delayed or completely absent. This test is not valid if the returning color is blue, because this may indicate that the capillaries are refilling from the veins, rather than with fresh, oxygenated blood from the arteries (Figure 5–14).

Pupil Size and Response to Light

The pupils of the normal eye are regular in outline and usually of the same size. Changes and variation in size of one or both pupils are important signs in emergency medical care. In a small percentage of normal persons, *anisocoria* (unequal pupil size) is found. Anisocoria (Figure 5–15) may be the result of a birth abnormality, dilation of the pupil with eyedrops, or a previous eye injury. The incidence of this phenomenon is so rare, however, that in the injured and unconscious patient, variation in pupil size is regarded as a reliable sign of possible brain damage.

Constricted pupils (Figure 5–16) are often present in a narcotic drug addict or a patient with a central nervous system disease. Variation in the size of the two pupils is seen in patients with head injuries or strokes. Dilated pupils (Figure 5–17) indicate a relaxed or unconscious state. Such dilation of the pupils usually occurs rapidly (within 30 seconds) after cardiac arrest. Head injury or previous drug use, however, may cause the pupils to remain constricted, even in patients with cardiac arrest.

Ordinarily, the pupils constrict equally and promptly when a bright light shines into either eye. This is a normal protective reaction of the eye (Figure 5–18). Failure of the pupils to

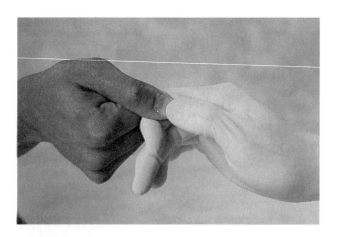

FIGURE 5–14

One important method of assessing the circulation is by observing the capillary refill.

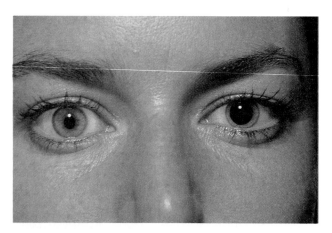

FIGURE 5–15

Variation of pupil size may indicate head injury or stroke.

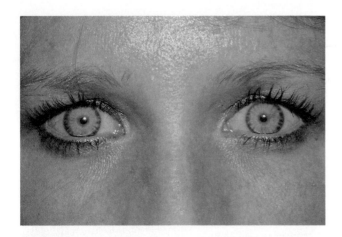

FIGURE 5–16

Constricted pupils in a dark environment may indicate drug usage or central nervous system disease.

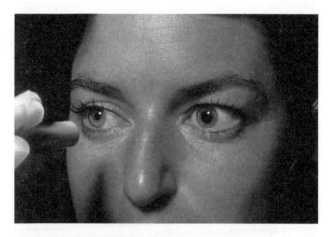

FIGURE 5–18

Normally, the pupil should constrict when light is shined into it.

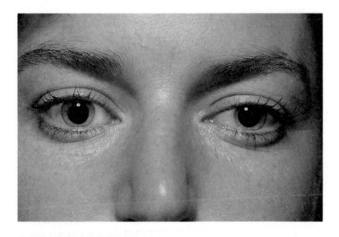

FIGURE 5–17

Dilated pupils in a bright environment or when being examined with a penlight may indicate a relaxed or unconscious state.

constrict when a light shines into the eye occurs in disease, poisoning, drug overdose, and injury. In death, the pupils are widely dilated and fail to respond to light.

The state of the pupils, especially any progressive change, is a rapid reflection of central nervous system injury or disease. Note all such changes. Report, and record them early in your examination of all patients.

Level of Consciousness

Normally a person is alert (awake), oriented (appropriately able to describe the time and place and his or her identity), and responsive to vocal and physical stimuli. Any change from that state indicates illness or injury. Recording such a change is extremely important in emergency medical care. Such changes may vary from mild confusion in an alcoholic or mental patient to deep coma in a poisoned person or a patient with a head injury. The patient's **level of consciousness** is probably the single most reliable sign in assessing the status of the central nervous system (Figure 5–19).

It is extremely important for you to note the level of consciousness of a patient early in the course of evaluation. All subsequent changes must also be noted, recorded, and reported. Progressive deterioration in the level of consciousness or increasing difficulty in rousing a patient are signs that indicate an urgent need for prompt attention at the hospital. This is especially true with a patient who is unconscious following an injury, then rouses and seems normal for a period of time (lucid interval), but suddenly becomes unconscious again. Such a patient is probably experiencing bleeding inside the skull and is in need of immediate surgery.

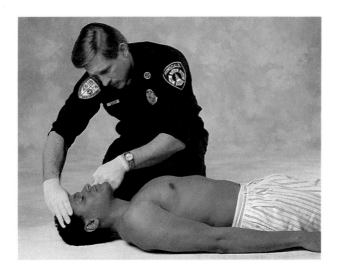

FIGURE 5–19

Increasing difficulty in rousing a patient indicates a
need for urgent attention at the hospital. This EMT is
protecting the patient's cervical spine with his right
hand while trying to rouse the patient with his left.

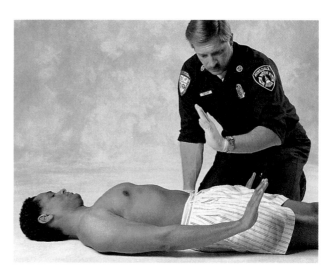

FIGURE 5–20

Inability to move the arms or legs can be a sign of spinal cord injury.

A specific place on the ambulance form
should be reserved for a neurological checklist
to record the reactive changes of the patient
and the specific time at which the observation
was made.

Ability to Move

Paralysis is the inability of a conscious patient
to move. It may occur as a result of illness or
injury. *Hemiplegia* (paralysis of one side of the
body) may occur as a result of bleeding or
blood-clot formation within the brain (a *stroke*).
Certain drugs, if used over long periods of
time, may also cause paralysis.

Inability to move the legs or arms after an
injury indicates damage to the spinal cord until
proven otherwise. Inability to move the legs
while the arms remain normal indicates a
spinal cord injury below the neck level. Paralysis is a particularly important sign, and its
presence and the time of onset must be recorded (Figure 5–20).

Reaction to Pain

Reaction by vocal response or body movement
to a painful physical stimulus is a normal
protective function of the body. Because the
patient is not screaming or clutching "where it
hurts" does not prove the absence of significant
injury. Changes in the normal reaction to pain
may result from loss of sensation following an
injury or illness. You should test the patient's
reaction to pain by gently pinching the skin.
Avoid extreme force or pressure (Figure 5–21).
Paralysis is usually accompanied by loss of
sensation in the affected extremities. Occasionally, however, movement is retained, and the
patient complains only of numbness or tingling
in the extremities. It is important for you to
recognize this fact as a sign of probable injury
of the spinal cord so that mishandling does not
aggravate the condition.

Severe pain in an extremity with loss of skin
sensation may be the result of blockage of the
main artery of the extremity. In such a case, the

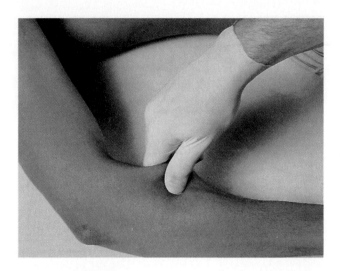

FIGURE 5–21

Use a gentle pinch to test the patient's reaction to pain.

patient lacks a pulse in the extremity. The ability to move the extremity is usually retained, although it is often held immobile because of pain.

Frequently, patients suffering from hysteria, shock, or excessive drug or alcohol use may feel no pain from an injury for several hours. This loss of pain sensation is not accompanied by paralysis, and the patient may continue to try to use the injured limb.

USE OF THE DIAGNOSTIC SIGNS

The alert EMT, using eyes, ears, hands, and a few simple instruments, can obtain a great deal of information about the patient by assessing the vital and diagnostic signs just listed. The four vital signs (pulse, respiration, blood pressure, and temperature) can be used to identify most critically ill patients. The diagnostic signs provide many clues as to the cause of the patient's injury or illness and help to assess the severity of the problem. Accurate assessment of the diagnostic signs is essential for proper patient management. Periodic reassessment of

the pertinent diagnostic signs at least every 10 to 15 minutes will allow you to determine whether the patient's condition is improving or deteriorating. Consult your local medical director's protocol for the required frequency of reexamination. It is essential for all observations to be recorded with the time each observation is made. A written record of the patient's course is valuable information for the emergency department personnel.

ASSESSMENT AND TREATMENT PRIORITIES

The rest of this chapter addresses the sequence of assessment and treatment that you should undertake for every patient. The highest priorities (the ABCs) must, of course, be addressed first, both in terms of assessment and treatment, before you proceed to less important priorities. The following procedures should be carried out in the order in which they are presented.

The First Assessment

The first assessment of the patient is not performed by an emergency medical technician in the field; rather, it is performed by the dispatcher who first receives the call. The dispatcher should obtain important information from the caller and relay this information to you. The minimum information obtained should consist of the patient's age, sex, and major apparent problem. Dispatch should also learn whether the patient is breathing and is conscious. Your EMS system medical director should dictate what additional information is essential and monitor the information actually transmitted to field personnel as a quality assurance measure. In the field, you should use this information to prepare mentally for the type of emergency to be encountered and to determine what equipment will be needed. The function of the dispatcher is extremely important and is covered in detail in Chapter 50 (Figure 5–22).

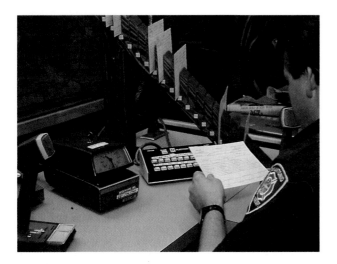

The EMS dispatcher provides the EMT in the field with important information.

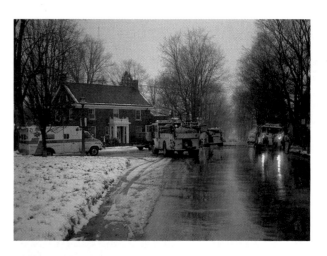

The initial assessment of the environment is an important source of information.

Arrival at the Scene

As you arrive at the scene, begin to assess the patient and the environment even before you get out of the ambulance. The presence of police cars may indicate the possibility of violence or trauma. A call originating from a restaurant may indicate that a person is choking. A patient who is lying outside on a cold or rainy day could be suffering from exposure to the elements. Any circumstances that relate to the event should always be mentally recorded because they may provide clues to the nature of the patient's problem or condition.

It is especially important for you to assess the scene for possible personal danger or danger to uninvolved bystanders (Figure 5–23). It is foolhardy and contrary to care standards for any EMT to enter a dangerous scene without taking self-protective measures. For example, when called to the scene of a shooting, you must wait for clearance from police officers at the scene before approaching the patient. And if you arrive before the police, waiting for them is still the best policy. Until the police have secured the area, you should keep bystanders from accidentally approaching the scene. Never become part of the problem.

When the patient has been injured, as in a motor vehicle accident, note the mechanism of injury as well. Is the windshield cracked or the steering wheel bent? Has the car rolled over? Was the patient thrown from the vehicle? Knowledge about the mechanism of injury will guide the thoughtful EMT to certain specific injuries and patterns of injury (see Chapter 13). Record and report this information.

To avoid further injuries, the safety of the patient should be considered next. For example, if a patient has suffered a heart attack while crossing a busy street, it may be necessary to divert the flow of traffic before you start to work on the patient. Or, in this situation, move the patient quickly to a safer place before or as the necessary assessment and treatment begin. As you approach the scene, you will notice many obvious findings at once—for example, bleeding, unconsciousness, or extreme agitation. Any obvious findings such as these should be noted, but they should not distract you from proceeding with a further orderly assessment of the patient.

You must also, at this point, be able to identify patients who are obviously dead at the scene. *Lividity* is the bluish red discoloration caused by blood pooling in the dependent parts of the body and is seen 15 to 30 minutes after death (Figure 5–24). Several hours later, *rigor mortis* will be noted by the resistance felt from the patient's body when an attempt is made to move it. Rigor mortis is best seen by trying to straighten a flexed extremity. Decomposition, incineration, and decapitation are other obvious signs of death. When they are present, resuscitation attempts should not be made.

The Primary Survey

The purpose of the **primary survey** is to help you find and treat the most life-threatening emergencies first. This is accomplished by assessing and stabilizing the following systems in this order of importance:

1. Airway.
2. Breathing.
3. Circulation.
4. Disability.

To assess the status of these four conditions in a seemingly unconscious patient, begin by attempting to rouse the patient (Figure 5–25). If the patient cannot be roused, assess the breathing (Figure 5–26), then circulation, and,

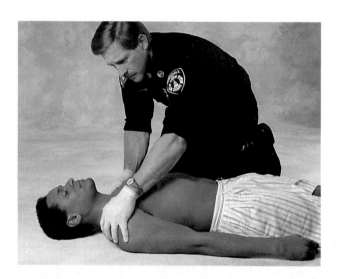

FIGURE 5–25

Assess airway, breathing and circulation in the seemingly unconscious person by first attempting to rouse the patient.

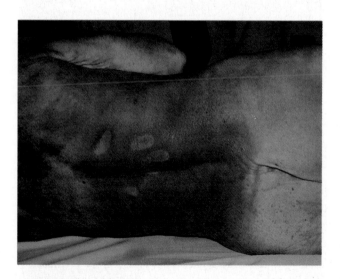

FIGURE 5–24

Dependent lividity, an obvious sign of death, is caused by blood settling to the lower parts of the body. This body was found in a supine position, with the lividity seen as purple discoloration of the back, except in those areas of firm contact with the ground (white areas across back at scapulae and buttocks).

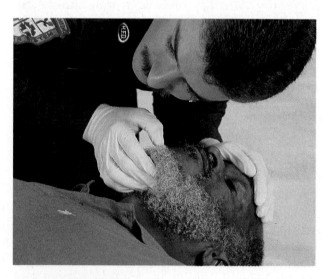

FIGURE 5–26

If the patient cannot be roused, "look, listen, and feel" for breathing.

if necessary, begin resuscitation as described in Chapters 7 and 9. If the patient is conscious or is unconscious but breathing, continue the assessment of airway, breathing, circulation, and disability with the following steps, which can be done in nearly one motion.

l. Place your face squarely in front of the patient's face while grasping the patient's wrist nearest to your hand.
2. Ask the patient, "Are you okay?" while you take the pulse (Figure 5–27). Observe the patient's response carefully and continue assessment of the following four critical factors:

Airway In assessing the airway, ask yourself the obvious: Is the patient breathing? Does the patient have an adequate airway? If the patient does not appear to be breathing or has an inadequate airway, start airway management immediately (see Chapter 7).

Breathing In determining whether the patient is having difficulty breathing, you should notice the character of the respirations—are they shallow or deep? Does the patient appear to be choking? Is the patient cyanotic, suggesting poor oxygenation? If the patient appears to have any difficulty breathing, you should immediately begin support of the patient's breathing, as described in Chapter 7 (Figure 5–28).

Circulation The next step is to check the circulation. Using one hand, you can assess the rate and quality of the radial pulse. If the radial pulse is absent, you should palpate for the carotid pulse in the neck or, if the patient is alert, the radial pulse in the other wrist. If the pulse is absent in both wrists and in the neck, give immediate circulatory support. Full cardiopulmonary resuscitation (CPR) should be carried out, as described in Chapter 9.

If the pulse is present, next assess the patient's skin color, temperature, and moisture. While looking at the patient's face, you should note color changes and excessive sweating.

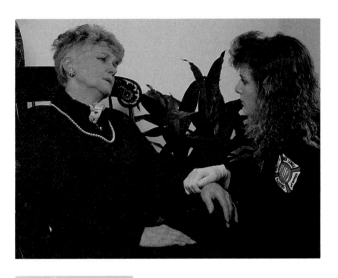

FIGURE 5–27

Squarely face the patient and ask "Are you okay?" while examining the patient's face and neck for signs of distress.

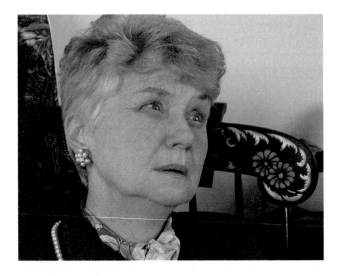

FIGURE 5–28

Examine the face and neck of the patient for the patient's overall level of distress, for difficulty in breathing, for cyanosis around the mouth, for distended neck veins, and for level of consciousness. Abnormal findings in these areas would indicate immediate administration of oxygen and possible ventilatory support.

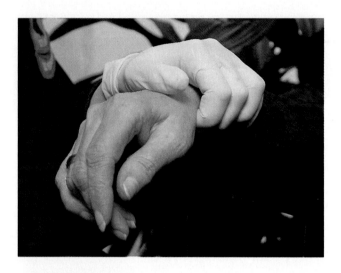

FIGURE 5-29

First, note the warmth, moisture, and color of the extremity. Then, assess the radial pulse for rate and quality. If you cannot obtain the radial pulse, check the other wrist. If both radial pulses are absent, check the carotid pulse and begin immediate circulatory support, if indicated.

While you take the pulse, palpate the skin and identify abnormalities in skin temperature and moisture (Figure 5-29).

After assessing the patient's pulse, skin temperature, and color, you should further assess the circulation by squeezing one of the patient's fingernails to check capillary refill (Figure 5-30). Find and quickly control any sources of external bleeding, as described in Chapter 11. In cases of significant trauma, remove all of the patient's clothing and find all sources of bleeding to complete your assessment of the circulation. If the trauma patient has signs of diminished circulation, examine the chest, abdomen, and thighs, because they may reveal evidence of internal bleeding. In certain circumstances, a pneumatic antishock garment should be used to support the circulation (see Chapter 11).

Disability Once you have assessed the airway, breathing, and circulation, move on to

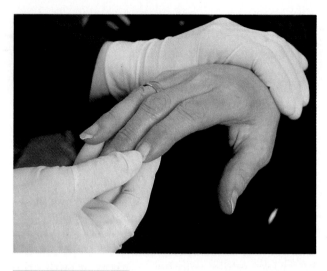

FIGURE 5-30

As a final check of the patient's circulatory status, assess the capillary refill.

assess the patient's level of consciousness. The patient's neurological status is assessed by noting the quality of the patient's response to the question, "Are you okay?" and by noting whether the patient's extremities move spontaneously. The patient's level of consciousness or "mental status" can be described using one of the following four terms:

- *Alert.* The patient's eyes open spontaneously and questions are answered in a clear manner. The patient knows and can correctly tell you the date, the location, and his or her own name. If the patient knows these facts, the patient is said to be "alert and oriented."
- *Responsive to verbal stimulus.* The patient's eyes do not open spontaneously, and the patient may not be oriented to time, place, and person but does respond in some meaningful way when spoken to.
- *Responsive to pain.* The patient does not respond to verbal stimuli but moves or cries out in response to a painful stimulus. This response is tested by gently, but firmly, pinching the patient's skin. An appropriate

response is withdrawal from this painful stimulus. If the patient has a paralyzed extremity, this examination is not valid in that extremity. Extremely painful stimuli should never be applied to the patient.

■ *Unresponsiveness.* The patient does not respond to the painful stimulus.

These four terms describing the patient's mental status are referred to as the *AVPU scale.*

If the patient has been injured and is unconscious, complains of pain in the head or neck, or is having difficulty moving any extremity, or if the mechanism of injury suggests significant trauma, all assessment and treatment should be done while another person guards the stability of the cervical spine. Injuries to the cervical spine caused by rough handling of the patient can produce immediate paralysis and death.

If the patient is unconscious or unable to respond, the patient's clothes, wallet, wrist, and neck should be checked for an emergency medical identification card or tag (Figure 5–31). These usually bear warning of any serious medical problem. Except for the desire to obtain information of medical importance that can be found in wallet cards, there is no reason for you to search the patient. If police are present, it is best that any search be done by them or in their presence and so recorded.

The primary assessment up to this point has been concerned with identifying life-threatening conditions. This concern must be uppermost in your mind. When you identify an abnormality in airway, breathing, or circulation, institute treatment as the abnormality is assessed and the deficit corrected to ensure adequate performance of the patient's vital functions. The airway, breathing, and circulation must be stabilized as a first priority, and they must be continuously supported until the patient is delivered to the emergency department. In assessing and transporting the injured patient, you must always remember to protect the spine from further injury.

Only after adequate performance of the patient's vital functions has been ensured should you proceed with further evaluation of the patient's problem. In rare instances, when the patient is critically ill or injured, the neces-

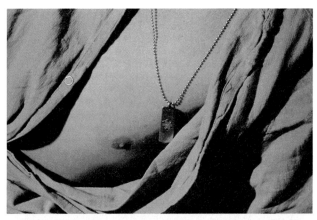

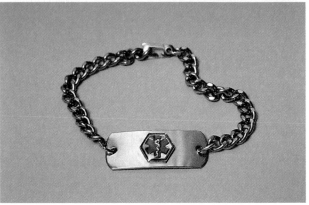

FIGURE 5–31

Emergency medical identification cards or tags may alert you that the patient has a known, life-threatening condition.

sity for resuscitation and immediate transport may mean that no further assessment is done.

The Chief Complaint

Until now, you have been concerned primarily with signs, or those conditions that can actually be observed. When asking the patient "Are you okay?" you have been concerned with the response only in terms of its quality. That is, the response was not assessed for content—only for an indication of the patient's ability to breathe and respond to a verbal stimulus. Now you must address the patient's symptoms.

Usually the first words out of the patient's mouth in response to a general question such as "What's wrong?" or "What happened?" are called the **chief complaint** (Figure 5–32). Despite what you have already observed, do not jump to any conclusions about what is troubling the patient. Now is the time to listen. It is important to understand the patient's problems in the patient's own terms.

Generally, the chief complaint is recorded in a few of the patient's own words, along with the duration of the symptoms: "I fell and hurt my arm two hours ago." "I have had pain in my chest since last night." If the patient is not capable of giving a chief complaint, it should be elicited from a family member or bystander (Figure 5–33). The informant's relationship to the patient should be indicated on the ambulance form. For example, Wife: "He passed out and stopped breathing five minutes ago."

Vital Signs

The vital signs (pulse, respirations, blood pressure, and, if indicated, temperature) should be determined at this point in your assessment of the patient. Generally, one EMT can do this while the other takes the history of present illness, as described next (Figure 5–34).

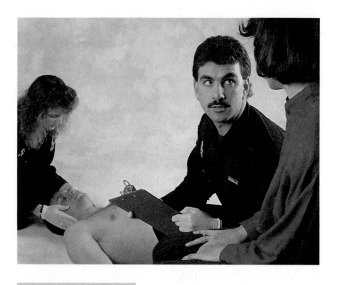

FIGURE 5–33

If the patient is unresponsive, obtain the chief complaint and any other pertinent history from bystanders.

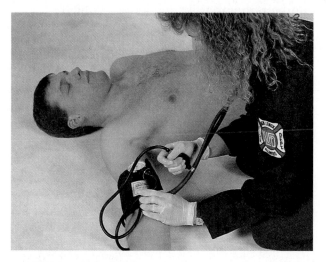

FIGURE 5–34

Determining the patient's vital signs is part of the patient assessment.

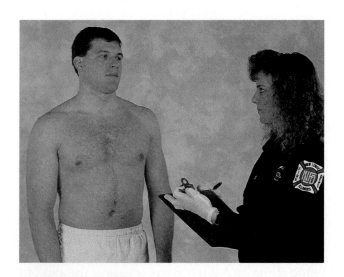

FIGURE 5–32

The patient's initial response to the question "What's wrong?" is the *chief complaint.*

History of Present Illness

If time permits, it is valuable to learn the events leading up to the current episode. To obtain this information, ask the patient or an informed bystander questions that shed light on the patient's current problem as it relates to the patient's overall medical state. It is important for you to know about any major medical problems such as diabetes or heart disease, the medications the patient takes, any allergies the patient may have, when the patient last ate or drank, and the events that led up to the current illness or injury. This information can be easily remembered through the use of the word "AMPLE":

A Allergies
M Medications
P Previous illness
L Last meal or drink
E Events preceding the illness or injury

One of the most common chief complaints is pain. Pain can, and will, be described in many different ways. It is important to question the patient about the nature and extent of the pain that is present. The questions relating to pain can be remember by the letters PQRST:

P *Provoke.* What causes the pain? What makes the pain worse? What makes the pain better?
Q *Quality.* What does the pain feel like? Sharp? Dull? Burning? Stabbing? Crushing?
R *Radiation.* Does the pain travel from one area to another? For example, does the patient's chest pain seem to go up into his or her jaw?
S *Severity.* Does the patient think the pain is mild, moderate, or severe?
T *Time.* Is the pain constant or intermittent? Has the pain occurred before? When did it start? Does it change in severity (get better, then worse)?

With trauma patients, you must record the mechanism of injury, because it may give a clue to significant hidden injuries. Patients who have been in automobile wrecks should also be asked about the path of their vehicle before and after impact, their position inside the car, and which parts of their body were struck during the impact. Certainly, if the patient has been thrown from the vehicle or if the vehicle has rolled over, this information should be indicated on the patient's record. Often this information can be indicated by diagram (Figure 5–35).

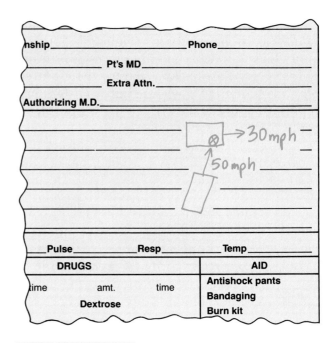

FIGURE 5–35

The mechanism of injury after an automobile accident can be easily illustrated with simple drawings. This diagram represents the patient as the passenger (indicated by the X) in a car that was going 30 miles per hour and was struck on the passenger's side by another vehicle traveling at 50 miles per hour. The circle around the symbol for the patient indicates that he was wearing his seat belt.

Secondary Survey (Head-to-Toe Examination)

The final step in the assessment process is examining the patient carefully from head to toe, looking for wounds and deformities, and observing whether the patient feels pain and has sensation. This head-to-toe examination is called the **secondary survey.** If the patient has been found to have life-threatening injuries during the primary survey, the necessity for immediate resuscitation and transport may mean that the secondary survey cannot be done. You should explain to the patient what is being done and why. By reassuring the patient throughout the examination, you can establish rapport and ensure better cooperation. The secondary survey is represented pictorially in Figures 5–36 through 5–77.

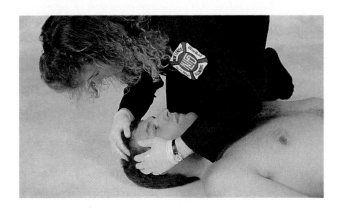

FIGURE 5–36

Look for lacerations or bruises of the scalp.

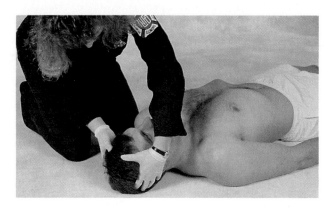

FIGURE 5–37

Note any tenderness, depressions of the skull, and deformities. Take care not to press firmly over areas of skull depression.

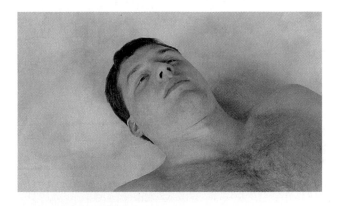

FIGURE 5–38

Note lacerations, bruises, and deformities of the face.

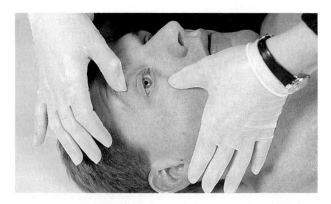

FIGURE 5–39

Inspect the eyes and lids in more detail.

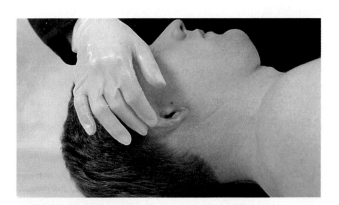

FIGURE 5–40

Pull the patient's ear forward to search for bruising of the mastoid process. Mastoid bruising is characteristic of a basilar skull fracture. See Chapter 20.

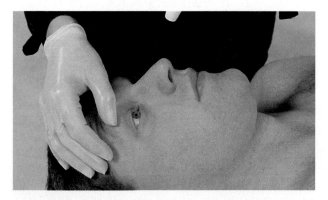

FIGURE 5–41

Examine the eyes for redness and for contact lenses, and assess the pupils.

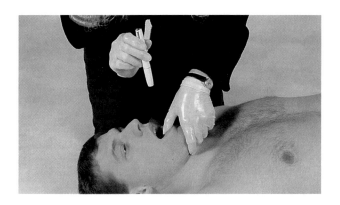

FIGURE 5–42

Examine the nose for drainage or bleeding, and examine the mouth for cyanosis, foreign bodies (including loose teeth or dentures), bleeding, lacerations, or deformities.

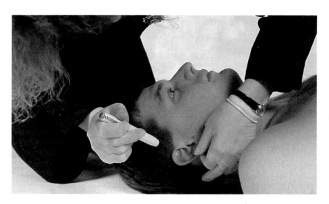

FIGURE 5–43

Use the penlight to look for drainage or blood in the ears.

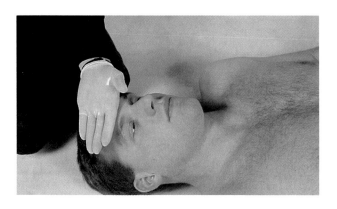

FIGURE 5–44

Feel the forehead for temperature and moisture.

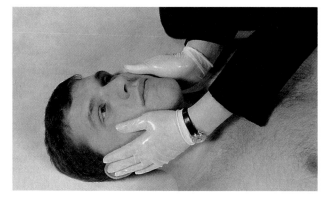

FIGURE 5–45

Palpate the zygomas (bones forming the lateral wall of the orbit of the eye) for tenderness or instability.

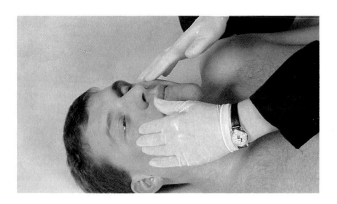

FIGURE 5–46

Palpate the maxillae (cheek bones).

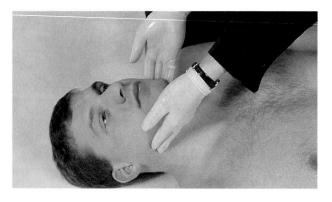

FIGURE 5–47

Palpate the mandible (jawbone).

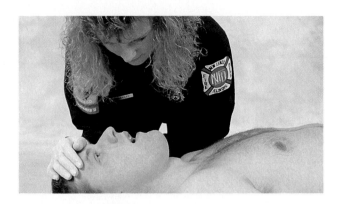

FIGURE 5–48

Check for unusual odors on the patient's breath.

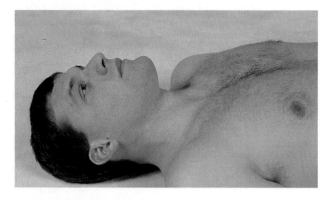

FIGURE 5–49

Look for distended neck veins, lacerations, bruises, and deformity. Distended neck veins are not necessarily significant when the patient is lying down. Veins that are distended when the patient is sitting upright, however, may indicate cardiac or other thoracic problems.

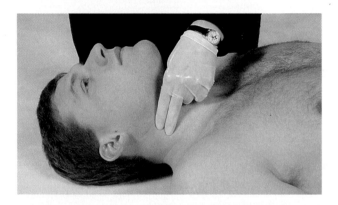

FIGURE 5–50

If the neck veins are distended, it may be significant to note that they refill from below after you have expressed all the blood with your examining hand.

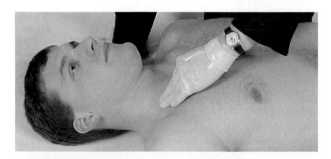

FIGURE 5–51

Note the trachea. It should be in the midline at the suprasternal notch. Deviation of the trachea may indicate pneumothorax.

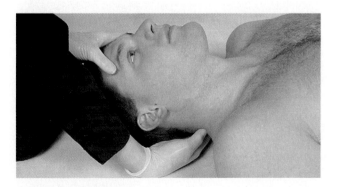

FIGURE 5–52

Palpate the cervical spine gently for deformity or tenderness.

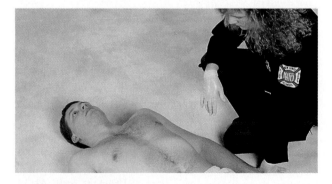

FIGURE 5–53

Look carefully for signs of injury before laying hands on the patient's trunk. Movement of the chest with respiration is also important to observe.

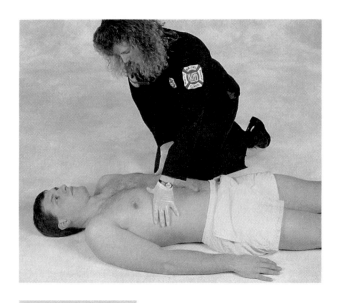

FIGURE 5–54

Gently press on the ribs to elicit tenderness. Avoid pressing over obvious bruises or fractures. Also note the presence of subcutaneous emphysema, a crackling sensation caused by air bubbles trapped in tissues beneath the skin.

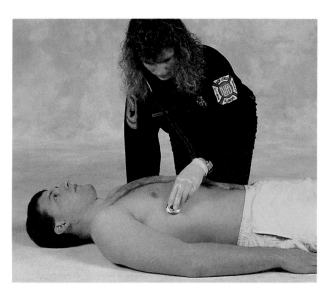

FIGURE 5–55

Listen at the nipple level in the mid-axillary line to compare the equality of the breath sounds on the two sides of the chest.

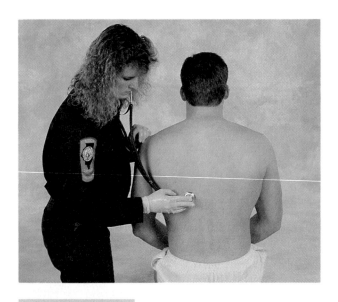

FIGURE 5–56

Examine the breath sounds from the back as well. Although the patient is shown here in the sitting position, you can usually perform this examination when the patient is in the supine position. Comparison of the two sides is helpful in determining if an abnormality exists.

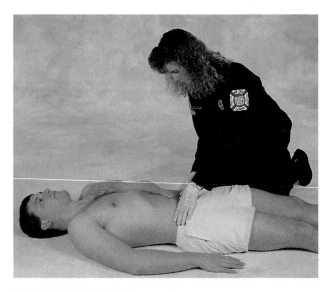

FIGURE 5–57

Look to see if the patient's abdomen is distended and examine for wounds, bruises, or other obvious signs of injury. If the patient has sustained trauma to the genital area, this should also be examined.

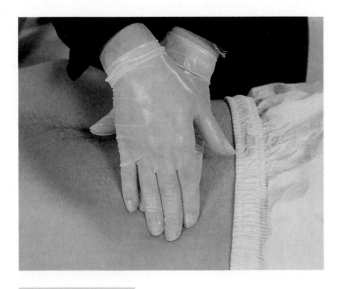

FIGURE 5–58

Press gently on the abdomen and note any tenderness. If the muscles of the patient's abdomen are unusually tense, this finding is called "rigidity" and is extremely significant.

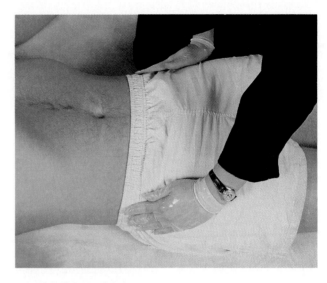

FIGURE 5–59

Compress the pelvis from the sides to determine whether it is tender.

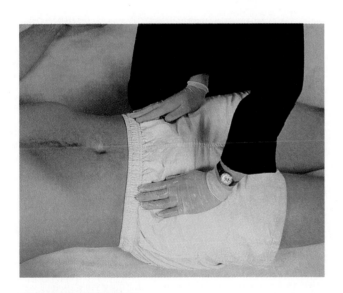

FIGURE 5–60

Press the patient's iliac crests to elicit signs of instability, tenderness, or crepitus.

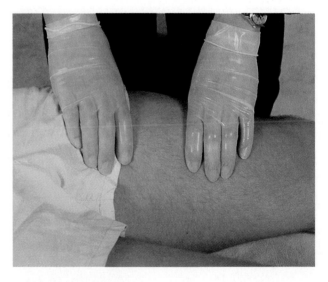

FIGURE 5–61

Inspect the lower extremities for lacerations, bruises, edema, or deformity. Then, palpate for tenderness, except over obvious fracture sites.

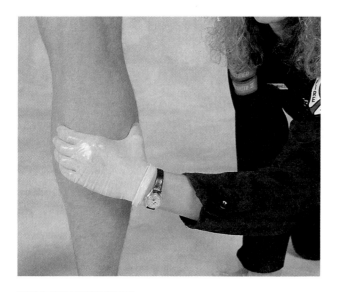

FIGURE 5–62

Tenderness elicited by squeezing the calves may indicate clots in the legs that may travel through the circulation to the lungs, where they can be fatal. Perform this examination gently and, if it is positive, do not repeat it, because the examination itself may dislodge clots.

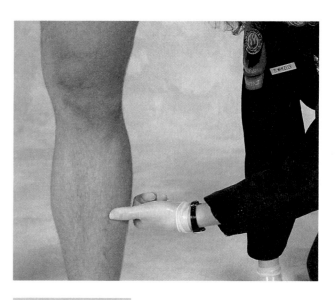

FIGURE 5–63

Press against the front of the shin to determine the presence of pretibial edema (swelling). When the swelling is extreme, the imprint of the examining finger will remain even after your finger is removed; this is called "pitting edema."

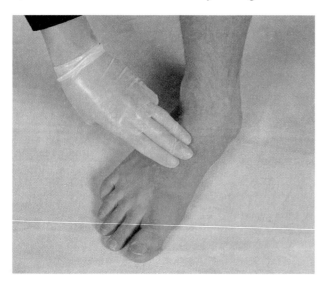

FIGURE 5–64

Check the dorsalis pedis pulse in each foot.

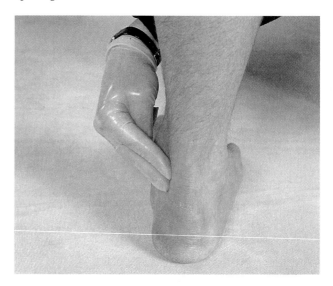

FIGURE 5–65

Examine the posterior tibial pulse on the medial side of each ankle.

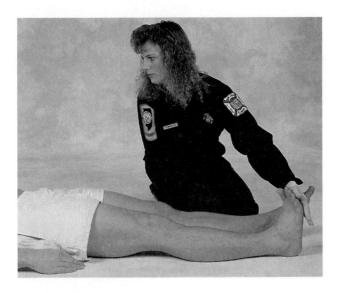

FIGURE 5-66

Test strength of the foot by having the patient press the foot against your hand. Compare this to the opposite side. Note the presence of sensation and movement.

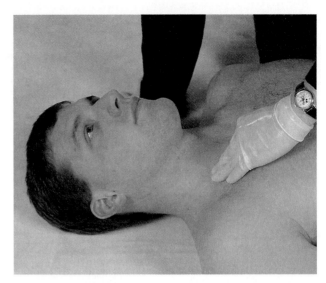

FIGURE 5-67

Include inspection and palpation of the clavicles when you check the upper extremities.

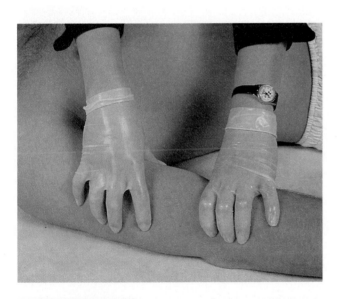

FIGURE 5-68

Squeeze the extremities to reveal any hidden fracture by eliciting tenderness.

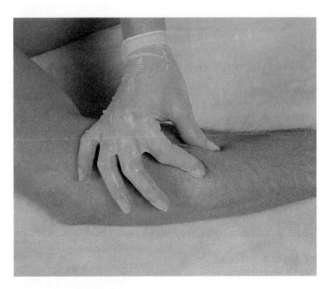

FIGURE 5-69

Use gentle pinching to test reaction to pain. This need not be done if the patient is able to identify the sensation of light touch in the extremities.

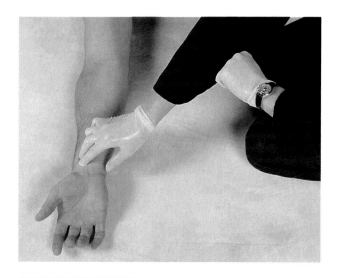

FIGURE 5–70

Check the pulses in each upper extremity.

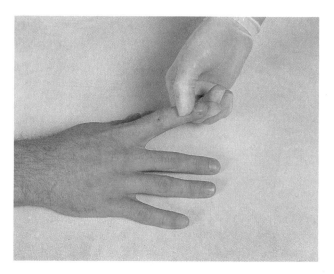

FIGURE 5–71

Test the patient's sensation of light touch by gently stroking the palmar surface of the tip of the index finger.

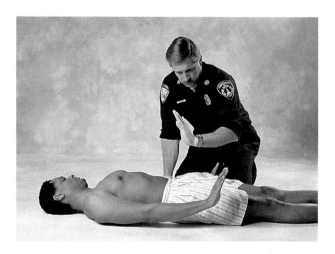

FIGURE 5–72

Test the patient's ability to move the hand. Ask the patient to open and close the fist as an additional means of testing neurological function. This is also a test of the patient's ability to follow commands.

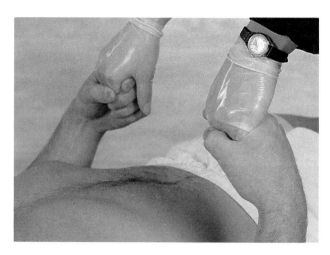

FIGURE 5–73

Comparing the patient's grip strength on the two sides is useful for determining the presence of weakness.

FIGURE 5–74

If you suspect spinal cord injury, carefully log-roll the patient to inspect the back.

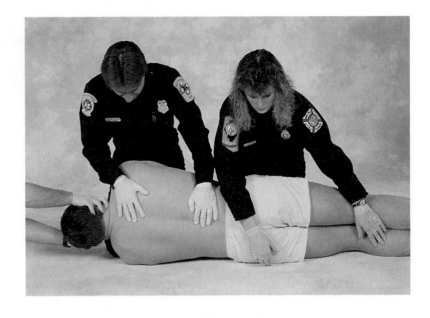

FIGURE 5–75

Carefully palpate the cervical spine for tenderness or deformity.

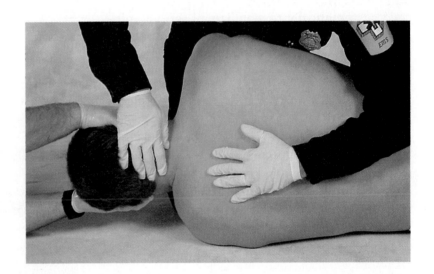

FIGURE 5–76

Likewise, examine the thoracic spine for possible injury.

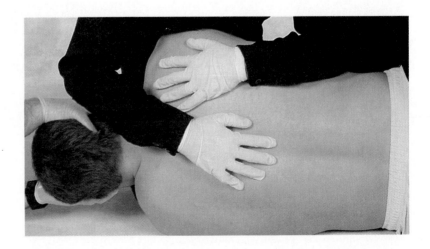

FIGURE 5–77

Similarly examine the lumbar spine.

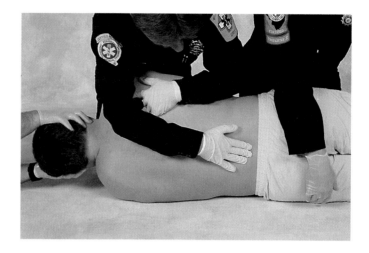

Once the secondary survey is completed, you will have compiled a mental list of all the patient's serious disorders. Then you can proceed systematically to stabilize all serious injuries while you continue to ensure adequacy of the patient's vital functions through periodic monitoring of the vital signs. Finally, you should make a careful recording of all findings and treatments. Repeat assessments should also be documented. The progression of vital signs and neurological status is especially important to hospital personnel and should be carefully recorded (Figure 5–78). Care is not complete until the case is completely recorded.

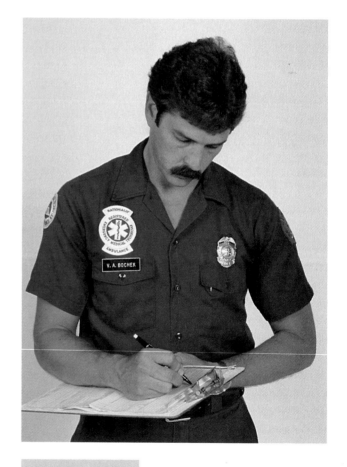

FIGURE 5–78

Document, document, document! A famous lawyer once said, "If it isn't written down, you didn't do it."

YOU ARE THE EMT

1. The patient tells you she has been vomiting all day and is worried because now she is vomiting blood. She began to have stomach pains the night before. Her temperature is 101 degrees F, and she is dizzy when she walks. She has a fierce headache. Her pulse is rapid and her blood pressure is 120/85. Which of these are signs and which are symptoms?

2. Your patient is a 50-year-old man. His blood pressure is 150/95. Which number is the diastolic pressure? The systolic? Is this blood pressure in the normal range? Why or why not?

3. You have taken the patient's pulse, respiration, and blood pressure. What is the fourth vital sign? Name four diagnostic signs.

4. Why is it so important to assess the level of consciousness? Describe the AVPU scale.

SECTION 3

CARDIOPULMONARY RESUSCITATION

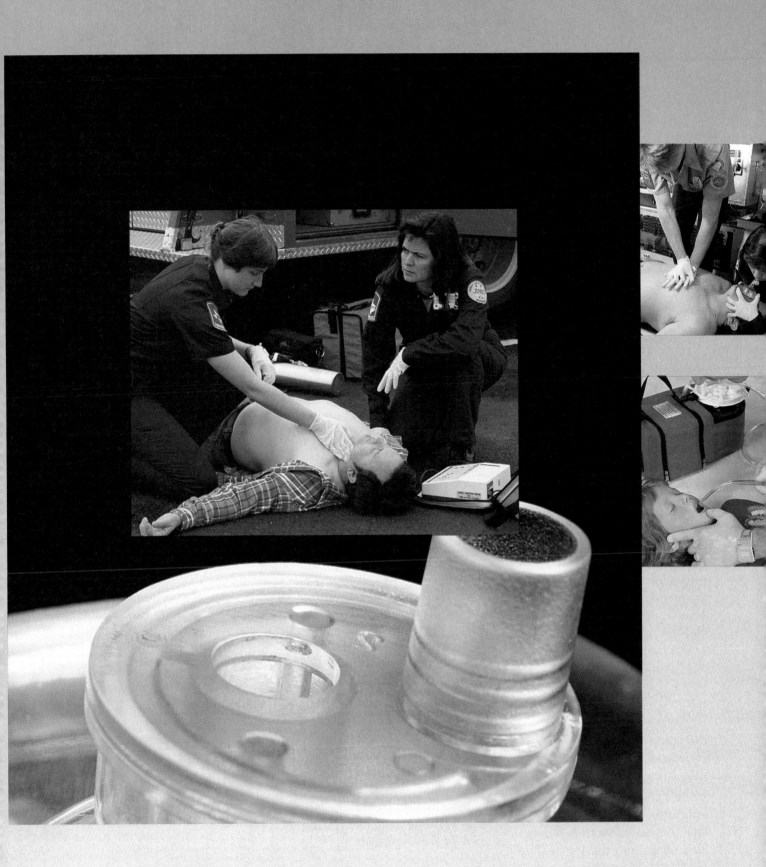

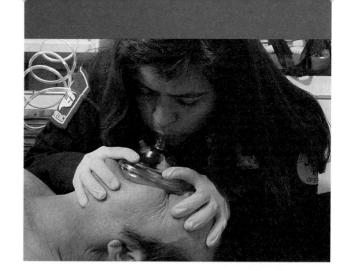

CHAPTER 6

THE RESPIRATORY SYSTEM

KEY TERMS

alveoli (al-ve′o-li) The air sacs of the lungs where the exchange of oxygen and carbon dioxide takes place.

anoxic (ah-nok′sik) Characterized by a total lack of oxygen.

diaphragm (di′ah-fram) A muscular dome that forms the undersurface of the thorax, separating the chest from the abdominal cavity. Contraction of the diaphragm (and the chest wall muscles) brings air into the lungs. Relaxation allows air to be expelled from the lungs.

diffusion (dĭ-fu′zhun) The spontaneous movement of molecules or particles in solution.

epiglottis (ep″ĭ-glot′is) A thin, leaf-shaped valve that allows air to pass into the trachea but prevents food or liquid from entering.

larynx (lar′inks) Voice box; a structure composed of thyroid cartilage on the top and cricoid cartilage on the bottom. It guards the entrance to the trachea and functions secondarily as the organ of voice.

mediastinum (me″de-as-ti′num) The space between the lungs in which lie the heart, the great vessels, the esophagus, the trachea and major bronchi, and many nerves.

metabolism (mĕ-tab′o-lizm) The sum of all the physical and chemical processes by which living organized substances are produced and maintained, and also the transformation by which energy is made available for the uses of the organism.

pleura (ploor′ah) The serous membrane covering the lungs and lining the thoracic cavity, completely enclosing a potential space known as the pleural space.

pleural space (ploor′al spās) The potential space between the parietal pleura and the visceral pleura. It is described as "potential" because under normal conditions the lungs fill this space.

pleurisy (ploor′ĭ-se) Inflammation of the pleura.

thorax (tho′raks) The chest; the upper part of the trunk between the neck and the abdomen.

trachea (tra′ke-ah) The windpipe; the main trunk for air passing to and from the lungs.

OVERVIEW

. . . .

The respiratory system consists of the body's structures that contribute to respiration, or breathing. The function of the respiratory system is to provide the body with oxygen and eliminate carbon dioxide. The exchange of oxygen and carbon dioxide takes place in the lungs and in the tissues. It is a complicated process that occurs automatically unless the airways or the lungs become diseased or damaged. In order to provide the lifesaving treatment required when a patient is not breathing effectively, you must be able to locate the structures of the respiratory system and understand their functions.

Chapter 6 begins with a description of the breathing process, including the exchange of oxygen and carbon dioxide that takes place. The airways and lungs are also described in this section. The chapter next discusses the mechanics of breathing and the role of the diaphragm and intercostal muscles. The last section of Chapter 6 explains how breathing is controlled by the brain and is stimulated by the level of carbon dioxide present in the arterial blood.

GOALS

. . . .

The goals of Chapter 6 are to
- describe the breathing process, including the exchange of oxygen and carbon dioxide and the role of the airways and lungs.
- understand the mechanics of breathing, or how the diaphragm and intercostal muscles contract and relax during inspiration and expiration.
- realize that breathing is controlled by the brain's response to levels of carbon dioxide and oxygen present in the arterial blood.

. . . .

THE BREATHING PROCESS

. . . .

The **thorax,** or chest, is the more superior (upper) of the two major body cavities. It is bounded by the rib cage anteriorly, superiorly, and posteriorly, and by the diaphragm inferiorly. The clavicles pass anterior to its uppermost portion. The thorax contains the lungs—one in each half, or *hemithorax.* Between the lungs, in a space called the **mediastinum,** lie the heart, the great arteries and veins, the esophagus, the trachea and major bronchi, and many nerves (Figure 6–1).

The *respiratory system* consists of all the structures of the body that contribute to normal respiration, or the process of breathing. It includes the nose, mouth, throat, larynx, tra-chea, and bronchi, which are all air passages or airways. The system also includes the lungs, where oxygen (O_2) is passed into the blood and where carbon dioxide (CO_2) is removed from the blood to be exhaled. Finally, the respiratory system includes the diaphragm, the muscles of the chest wall, and the accessory muscles of breathing, which permit normal respiratory movement (Figure 6–2).

In this text, the term *airway* usually refers to the upper airway or the passage above the **larynx** (voice box). "Clearing the airway" means removing obstructing material or tissue from the nose, mouth, or throat (Figure 6–3). "Maintaining the airway" means to keep the airway open to permit the unhindered flow of gases in and out. The lower airway includes the

FIGURE 6–1

The important anatomic structures of the chest cavity.

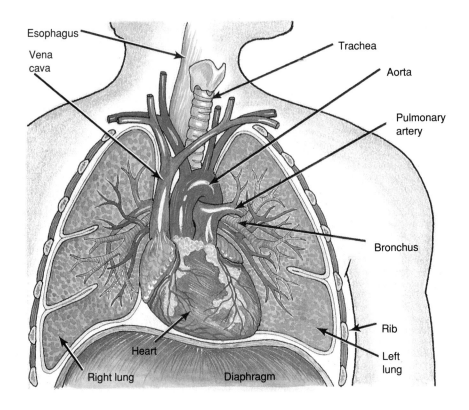

Esophagus
Vena cava
Trachea
Aorta
Pulmonary artery
Bronchus
Rib
Left lung
Heart
Right lung
Diaphragm

FIGURE 6–2

The respiratory system includes airways, lungs, and muscles. Some passages—the mouth and pharynx—are shared with the digestive system.

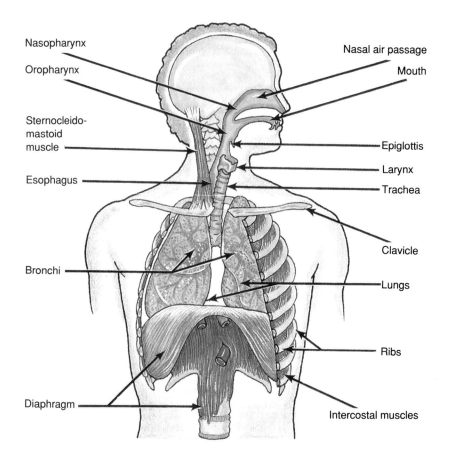

Nasopharynx
Oropharynx
Sternocleidomastoid muscle
Esophagus
Bronchi
Diaphragm
Nasal air passage
Mouth
Epiglottis
Larynx
Trachea
Clavicle
Lungs
Ribs
Intercostal muscles

FIGURE 6–3

The upper airway includes the air passages above the larynx, or the nose, mouth, and throat. The lower airway includes the larynx, trachea, major bronchi, and other air passages within the lungs.

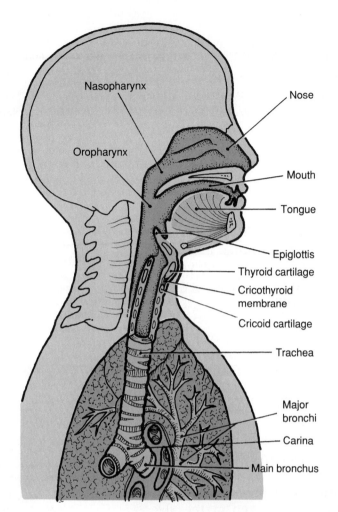

Nasopharynx

Nose

Oropharynx

Mouth

Tongue

Epiglottis

Thyroid cartilage

Cricothyroid membrane

Cricoid cartilage

Trachea

Major bronchi

Carina

Main bronchus

larynx, the trachea, the major bronchi, and other air passages within the lungs.

The Exchange of Oxygen and Carbon Dioxide

All living cells of the body are engaged in a series of chemical processes by which the energy needed to maintain life is extracted from nutrients. The name given to the sum of these processes is **metabolism**. In the process of metabolism, each cell combines nutrients and oxygen and produces energy and waste products (primarily water and carbon dioxide).

This basic metabolic chemical reaction occurs in all cells:

$$C_6H_{12}O_6 \;+\; 6O_2 \;\rightarrow\; 6CO_2 \;+\; 6H_2O \;+\; \text{Energy}$$
(Glucose) (Oxygen) (Carbon (Water)
Dioxide)

Cells not able to participate in metabolic processes are dead or dying.

Each living cell in the body requires a regular supply of oxygen; some cells are more dependent on a constant oxygen supply than others. Cells in the heart may be damaged if the oxygen supply is interrupted for more than a few seconds. Cells in the brain and nervous system may die after 4 to 6 minutes without oxygen. These cells can never be replaced, and permanent changes result from the **anoxic** (without oxygen) damage. Other cells in the body are not as vitally dependent on a constant oxygen supply. They can withstand short periods without oxygen and still survive. The respiratory system, which delivers oxygen to the lungs and allows the exhaust of carbon dioxide, is thus a very important part of the body. Normally, the air that we breathe contains 21 percent oxygen and 78 percent nitrogen. Small amounts of other gases make up the final 1 percent.

Blood that has passed through the body has given up oxygen to the tissues and absorbed carbon dioxide produced by cellular metabolism. Deoxygenated venous blood is collected in the right atrium of the heart and is pumped into the lungs by the right ventricle. In the lungs, it passes into a fine network of *pulmonary capillaries,* which are in close contact with the **alveoli** (air sacs) of the lungs. These air sacs receive the carbon dioxide that diffuses out of the blood. The alveoli also provide a ready supply of oxygen from the atmosphere to be absorbed by the blood in the pulmonary capillaries surrounding them. The reoxygenated blood now flows from the lungs into the left atrium. It then passes into the left ventricle, where it is pumped to the body to again carry oxygen to the body's cells.

The capillaries in the lungs are located in the walls of the alveoli. The walls of the capillaries and the alveoli are extremely thin. Air in the alveoli and blood in the capillaries are thus separated only by two very thin layers of tissue. Oxygen and carbon dioxide can diffuse rapidly across these thin membrane layers between the alveoli and capillaries. It is well known that molecules move from a region of higher concentration to a region of lower concentration through the process of **diffusion.** Because there is more oxygen in the alveoli than in the blood, oxygen moves from the alveoli into the blood. There is more carbon dioxide in the blood than in the inhaled air, so carbon dioxide diffuses from the blood into the alveoli. Figure 6–4 shows the exchange of gases and nutrients in tissues and of gases in the lung.

Not all inhaled oxygen is extracted by the blood as it passes through the body. Exhaled air contains 16 percent oxygen and 3 to 5 percent carbon dioxide. The remainder is nitrogen. This 16 percent concentration of oxygen is sufficient to support artificial ventilation. That is, even though you "exhale" breaths of air in mouth-to-mouth resuscitation, the patient still receives the 16 percent concentration of oxygen contained in each exhaled breath.

The Airways

The upper airway includes the nose, mouth, and throat. The nose and mouth lead to the

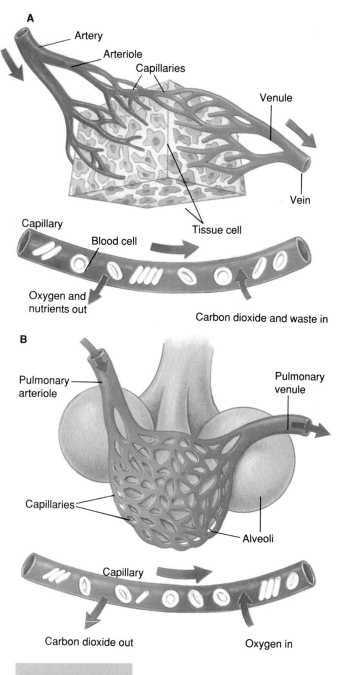

FIGURE 6–4

The exchange of oxygen and carbon dioxide in respiration. (A) Oxygen (O_2) passes from the blood through capillaries to tissue cells. In the reverse process, carbon dioxide (CO_2) passes from tissue cells through capillaries to the blood. (B) In the lung, oxygen is picked up by the blood and carbon dioxide is given off.

pharynx (throat). At the bottom of the pharynx are two passageways: the *esophagus* behind and the **trachea** (windpipe) in front. Food and liquids enter the pharynx and pass into the esophagus, which carries them to the stomach. Air and other gases enter the trachea and go to the lungs (Figure 6–3).

Protecting the opening of the trachea is a thin, leaf-shaped valve called the **epiglottis** (Figure 6–3). This valve allows air to pass into the trachea but obstructs food or liquid from entering the airway under normal circumstances. Air moves past the epiglottis into the larynx and the trachea.

The first part of the lower airway is the larynx, which consists of a rather complicated arrangement of tiny bones, cartilage, muscles, and the two *vocal cords*. The larynx is unable to tolerate any foreign solid or liquid material. A violent episode of coughing and spasm of the vocal cords will result from contact with solids or liquids. The *Adam's apple*, or *thyroid cartilage*, prominent in the neck, is the anterior portion of the larynx. Tiny muscles open and close the vocal cords and control tension on them. Sounds are created as air is forced past the vocal cords, making them vibrate. These vibrations make the sound. The pitch of the sound changes as the cords open and close. You can feel these vibrations if you place your fingers lightly on the larynx as you speak or sing. The vibrations of air are shaped by the tongue and muscles of the mouth to form understandable sounds.

Immediately inferior to the thyroid cartilage is the palpable *cricoid cartilage*. Between these two prominences lies the *cricothyroid membrane*, which can be felt as a depression in the midline of the neck just inferior to the thyroid cartilage (Figure 6–3). Below the cricoid cartilage is the trachea. The trachea is approximately 5 inches long and is a semirigid, enclosed air tube made up of rings of cartilage that are incomplete posteriorly. This enables food to pass through the esophagus, which lies right behind the trachea. The cartilaginous rings keep the trachea from collapsing when air is moved in and out of the lungs. The trachea ends at the *carina* by dividing into smaller tubes, the right and left *main bronchi*, which enter each lung. Each main bronchus immediately branches within the lung into smaller and smaller airways. Within the right lung, three major bronchi are formed;

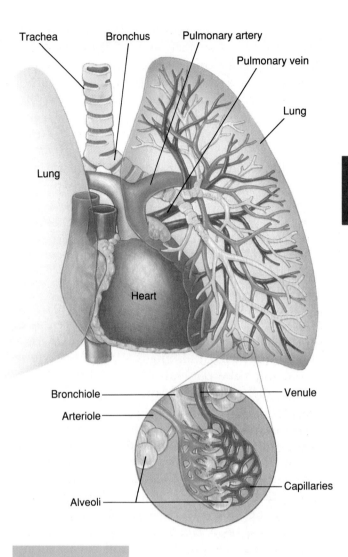

FIGURE 6–5

Within the lung, millions of air sacs (alveoli) lie at the ends of the air passages. Several alveoli are shown in the enlargement of a small area of the lung. Pulmonary capillaries are in very close contact with the alveolar wall.

within the left, there are only two. Each of these supply one lobe of the lung.

There are two *lungs*, one on each side of the thoracic cage (Figures 6–1 and 6–2). The lungs are suspended within the thoracic cage by the trachea, by the arteries and veins that run to and from the heart, and by the pulmonary ligaments. Within each lung, the main bronchi subdivide until they end in very fine airways called *bronchioles*. The bronchioles end in millions of tiny alveoli in each lung (Figure 6–5).

Healthy lungs contain about 700 million alveoli. The combined surface area of these alveoli is equal to about one-fourth that of a basketball court. The exchange of oxygen and carbon dioxide occurs within these alveoli.

The Lungs

The lungs hang freely within the chest cavity. They have no intrinsic capacity for expansion or contraction themselves because they have no muscle: there is, however, a very definite mechanism to ensure that they follow the motion of the chest wall and expand or contract with it. Covering each lung is a layer of very smooth, glistening tissue called **pleura** (Figure 6–6). Another layer of pleura lines the inside of the chest cavity. The two layers are called *parietal pleura* (lining the chest wall) and visceral pleura (covering the lungs).

Between the parietal pleura and the visceral pleura is the **pleural space,** which is not a space in the usual sense because normally these layers are in close contact everywhere. In fact, the layers are sealed tightly against one another by a thin film of fluid. When the chest wall expands, the lung is pulled with it and made to expand by the force exerted through these closely applied pleural surfaces. The pleural space is thus a potential one. Normally the pleural space is quite small and contains only the thin film of plural fluid as each lung entirely fills its chest cavity.

The potential space between the pleural surfaces can enlarge when the pleural surfaces are separated by blood from a lacerated chest wall or lung, or by air from a torn lung or a hole in the chest wall. If the surfaces are separated, the mechanism for normal expansion of the lungs is lost. If enough blood or air collects, the lung can be compressed to the extent that it cannot expand at all during inhalation, and insufficient oxygen is taken in to maintain life. Patients with this type of injury may die from lack of oxygen.

The smooth, lubricated pleural surfaces allow the lungs to move freely within the chest when one is breathing. If the pleural surfaces are injured or become diseased, they no longer have a friction-free, lubricated surface. Then, as

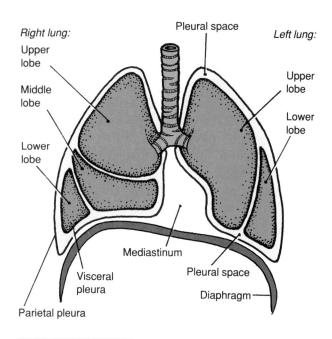

FIGURE 6–6

The pleura lining the chest wall and covering the lungs is an essential part of the breathing mechanism. The pleural space is not an actual space until blood or air leaks into it, causing the pleural surfaces to separate.

the lungs move in breathing, the surfaces rub together, causing friction and pain. This condition is called **pleurisy**.

THE MECHANICS OF BREATHING

Because the lungs contain no muscle tissue and cannot themselves move, expansion and contraction must be provided by other tissues. Movement of the thorax and diaphragm permits air to enter the lungs through the trachea and into the alveoli. The thoracic cage is a semirigid muscular and bony frame enclosed by skin. Contraction of the diaphragm and the intercostal and accessory muscles of breathing causes the thoracic cage to expand in three dimensions: anteroposterior, transverse, and inferiosuperior. Their attachments through the pleural surfaces enable the lungs to follow the chest wall motion exactly.

The **diaphragm** is one of the specialized muscles of the body. The diaphragm receives innervation from the *phrenic nerve,* which leaves the cervical spine between the third, fourth, and fifth cervical vertebrae. It is skeletal muscle in that it is attached to the costal arch and the vertebrae (Figure 6–7). It is *striated* (marked by streaks or lines under the microscope), like all other skeletal muscle. It is voluntary muscle in that one can take a deep breath, cough, or override breathing at will. However, unlike other skeletal or voluntary muscle, the diaphragm performs an automatic function. Breathing continues while we sleep and at all other times. The function and control of breathing can be overridden by conscious will; and people can temporarily breathe faster, slower, or hold their breath. However, these variations in breathing pattern cannot be continued indefinitely. Ultimately, when the concentration of carbon dioxide is close to being disturbed, automatic regulation of breathing resumes. Thus, although the diaphragm looks like voluntary skeletal muscle and is attached to the skeleton, it behaves, for the most part, like involuntary muscle.

The chest cage can be compared to a bell jar in which the lungs are suspended. The base is the movable diaphragm. The ribs maintain the shape of the chest. The only opening into the chest is the trachea. Air moves in through the trachea, to and from the interior of the lungs, to fill and empty the alveoli (Figure 6–8). When the diaphragm and chest wall muscles contract, the volume that the chest can hold is increased, causing a slight vacuum. Normally, the pressure within the chest cavity is slightly less than atmospheric pressure.

Contracting the diaphragm and intercostal muscles enlarges the thorax, causing intrathoracic pressure to decline still further. This respiratory motion of *inspiration* (inhaling) and chest expansion causes the higher air pressure outside to drive air in through the trachea, filling the lungs (Figure 6–8a). When the air pressure outside equals the air pressure inside, air stops moving. Any gas will move from a higher to a lower pressure area until the pressures are equal. When equalization occurs, movement of air ceases and inspiration stops. When the diaphragm and intercostal muscles relax during *expiration* (exhaling) and chest contraction, pressure inside the thorax becomes higher than that outside, and air is expelled (Figure 6–8b).

The active muscular part of breathing is inspiration. During inspiration, the diaphragm and intercostal muscles contract. When the diaphragm contracts, it moves downward and enlarges the thoracic cavity from top to bottom. When the intercostal muscles contract, they raise the ribs upward and outward. These actions combine to enlarge the chest cavity in all dimensions. Pressure within the cavity falls, and air rushes into the lungs. Take a deep breath to see how the chest increases in size with inspiration.

During expiration, the diaphragm and the intercostal muscles relax. As they relax, all

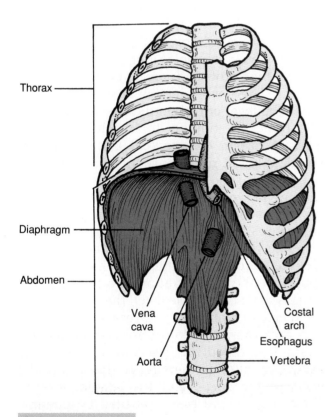

FIGURE 6–7

The dome-shaped diaphragm divides the thorax from the abdomen. It is pierced by the great vessels and the esophagus.

A Inhalation and chest expansion

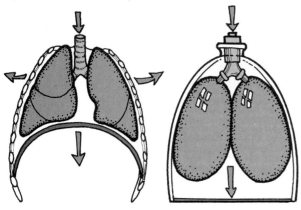

B Exhalation and chest contraction

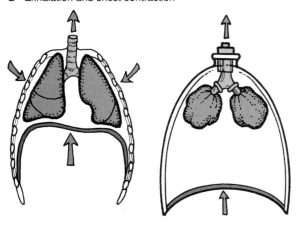

FIGURE 6-8

Inspiration and expiration can be visualized through the use of a bell jar containing balloons and closed at the end by a diaphragm. (A) When the diaphragm is depressed, pressure in the jar decreases and the balloons fill. (B) When the diaphragm is elevated, pressure increases in the jar and the balloons empty. Movement of the diaphragm causes movement of air in and out of the balloons, as in the lungs.

dimensions of the chest cavity decrease. When the volume of the chest cavity decreases, air in the lungs is compressed into a smaller space. Pressure is increased, and air is pushed out through the trachea.

The actual decrease in the size of the chest cavity after relaxation is accomplished largely by the action of elastic tissue in the lung which stretches during inspiration and recoils after relaxation of the muscular chest wall. In this situation, the chest wall, because of the pleural surface adhesion, follows the elastic recoil of the lung. There is also an inherent tendency for the chest wall (ribs and muscles) to assume a normal resting position, which aids in expiration. Unlike inspiration, expiration does not normally require muscular effort. It represents relaxation of effort and the assumption of a normal resting position.

Remember that there is only one normal opening into the chest cavity: the trachea. Although air may readily pass into the chest cavity if there is any other opening, it will not proceed to the interior of the lung or to the alveoli; rather it comes to lie in the pleural space, compressing the lung.

THE CONTROL OF BREATHING

The brain controls breathing. The center for this respiratory control is in the brain stem, one of the best-protected areas of the nervous system. The nerves in this area monitor and sense the level of carbon dioxide in the blood. The principal stimulus for respiration is the level of carbon dioxide (CO_2) in the arterial blood. When it rises above a certain level, the brain stem sends nerve impulses down the phrenic nerve and the nerves of the thoracic spine to cause the diaphragm and the intercostal muscles to contract, increasing the respiratory rate. The higher the level of carbon dioxide, the stronger the impulses to cause breathing. Once the concentration of carbon dioxide returns to an acceptable level, the strength and frequency of respiration decreases.

A backup system to control respiration also exists. It is called the *hypoxic drive*. There are oxygen-monitoring nerves in the brain, the walls of the aorta, and the carotid arteries. These sensors are easily satisfied by minimal levels of oxygen in the arterial blood. Thus, this hypoxic drive is much less sensitive and less powerful than the carbon dioxide sensors in the brain stem.

If the arterial levels of carbon dioxide or oxygen become abnormal, the brain automatically controls respiration. For these reasons, you cannot hold your breath indefinitely or breathe rapidly and deeply indefinitely. There are direct nervous connections from the brain to the lung and the muscles of respiration through which this control is exerted. Control of respiration by arterial carbon dioxide concentration is so sensitive that normally it adjusts with each breath.

If the carbon dioxide level rises above a certain level, the brain stem's carbon dioxide sensors become sluggish and poorly responsive to carbon dioxide levels in the arterial blood. This condition is called *carbon dioxide narcosis*. It occurs in some patients with a condition called *chronic obstructive pulmonary disease (COPD)*. Such patients are said to "retain CO_2." These patients become very dependent on their backup hypoxic drive to automatically control respiration. Extreme care must be taken when treating patients with COPD (see Chapter 31).

YOU ARE THE EMT

1. Where are the pulmonary capillaries located? What is their function?
2. Everyone knows that you inhale oxygen and exhale carbon dioxide. Why is it, then, that mouth-to-mouth resuscitation can revive a patient when the rescuer is "exhaling" into the patient's lungs?
3. What is pleurisy?
4. What stimulates a person to breathe?

CHAPTER 7

BASIC LIFE SUPPORT: AIRWAY AND VENTILATION

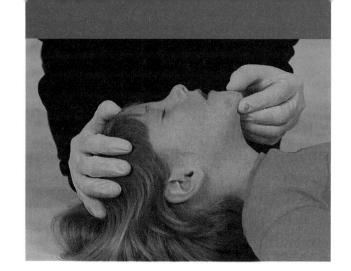

KEY TERMS

abdominal thrust maneuver A method of dislodging food or other material from the throat of a choking victim. Also referred to as the Heimlich maneuver.

advanced life support (ALS) Emergency lifesaving procedures performed by trained professionals, including the use of advanced procedures such as cardiac monitoring, defibrillation, intravenous drugs and advanced airway management devices, and drug infusion.

anoxia (ah-nok'se-ah) A lack of oxygen.

artificial circulation A means of providing circulation by external chest compression.

artificial ventilation Opening the airway and restoring breathing by mouth-to-mouth or mouth-to-nose ventilation and by the use of mechanical devices.

basic life support (BLS) Simple emergency lifesaving procedures which can aid a person in respiratory or circulatory failure.

cardiopulmonary resuscitation (CPR) The artificial establishment of circulation of the blood and movement of air into and out of the lungs in a pulseless, nonbreathing patient.

lividity (lĭ-vid'ĭ-te) Discoloration of dependent body parts, by the gravitation of the blood.

recovery position Position used for a patient who is not a trauma victim prior to transport to facilitate spontaneous breathing.

stridor (stri'dor) A harsh, high-pitched respiratory sound such as the inspiratory sound often heard in acute laryngeal obstruction.

OVERVIEW

Basic life support (BLS) is a series of emergency lifesaving procedure that is carried out in order to treat respiratory arrest, cardiac arrest, or both. Commonly known as cardiopulmonary resuscitation (CPR), it is a method of providing artificial ventilation and circulation. CPR depends for its effectiveness on prompt recognition of respiratory and/or cardiac arrest and the immediate start of treatment. You are expected to be able to recognize cardiac or respiratory arrest without difficulty and to quickly institute proper basic life support measures.

Several methods exist for opening the airway and providing artificial ventilation. Each has specific applications for conscious or unconscious patients, with or without head or spinal injury. Similarly, specific techniques must be used for removing foreign bodies that obstruct the airway. Again, all steps must be carried out as quickly and carefully as possible. Time is critical.

Chapter 7 begins with a discussion of basic life support—why it is lifesaving, how it came to be introduced, and the role of the EMT in instituting it. The chapter next describes the methods of opening the airway in adults, providing artificial ventilation in adults, and relieving foreign body obstruction in adults. The last section adapts all of these techniques of basic ventilatory support to infants and children. American Heart Association BLS skills sheets are included.

GOALS

The goals of Chapter 7 are to
- understand the need for basic life support, the urgency surrounding its rapid application, your responsibilities in beginning and terminating CPR, and the proper way to position a patient to receive basic life support.
- describe the four techniques for opening the airway in adults.
- learn how to perform mouth-to-mouth, mouth-to-nose, and mouth-to-stoma ventilation in adults and how to relieve gastric distension that sometimes occurs with artificial ventilation.
- learn how to distinguish foreign body obstruction from other conditions that cause respiratory failure and become familiar with the techniques for dislodging foreign objects that are obstructing the airway.
- know how to adapt basic ventilatory support procedures to infants and children.
- be aware of infectious disease issues related to rescue breathing.

GENERAL CONSIDERATIONS

Oxygen, present in the atmosphere at a concentration of about 21 percent, is essential to sustain life in all tissues and cells. The heart develops dangerous *arrhythmias* (irregular beats) within seconds after being deprived of oxygen. The brain undergoes potentially irreversible damage after the absence of oxygen in as little as 4 minutes (Figure 7–1).

The delivery of oxygen from the atmosphere to individual body cells of all types requires two

FIGURE 7-1

Time is critical. If the brain is deprived of oxygen for 4 to 6 minutes, brain damage is likely to occur. After 6 minutes without oxygen, brain damage is extremely likely.

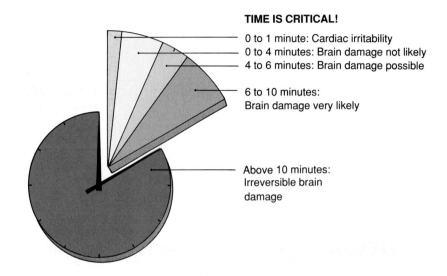

TIME IS CRITICAL!

0 to 1 minute: Cardiac irritability
0 to 4 minutes: Brain damage not likely
4 to 6 minutes: Brain damage possible
6 to 10 minutes:
Brain damage very likely

Above 10 minutes:
Irreversible brain
damage

necessary actions: breathing and circulation. Breathing means moving air from the atmosphere into and out of the lungs. Oxygen can then pass from the pulmonary *alveoli* to the capillaries to oxygenate the blood as it passes through the lungs. At the same time, carbon dioxide, produced by cells in the normal course of metabolism, moves from the blood into the alveoli and is exhaled. The blood, enriched with oxygen, is circulated to every part of the body by the pumping action of the heart. Any profound disturbance of the airway, breathing, or circulation can promptly produce disturbed heart function, brain damage, or death.

Basic life support (BLS) is a series of emergency lifesaving procedures to treat failure of the respiratory or cardiovascular systems. It is prompt treatment without the use of complex mechanical equipment that must be started as soon as possible after respiratory or cardiac arrest has occurred. The principles of basic life support were introduced in 1960. The specific techniques for life support have been reviewed and revised as necessary at national conferences on **cardiopulmonary resuscitation (CPR)** and *emergency cardiac care (ECC)* held every five to six years. These recommendations are published periodically in the *Journal of the American Medical Association*. The most recent gathering was the "1992 National Conference on Standards and Guidelines for Cardiopulmonary Resuscitation and Emergency Cardiac Care." Recommendations in this text follow those that were adopted at this conference with changes

later promulgated by the American Heart Association.

One of the most important findings in the evaluation of effectiveness of BLS measures has dealt with EMTs themselves. It has been noted that EMT competence in giving BLS is good immediately after training. However, it declines rapidly thereafter unless the EMT receives periodic retraining or is required to use the skills frequently. Techniques not regularly used tend to be performed poorly. Without regular usage, there are indications that basic skills must be practiced under close supervision every 90 days. The EMT must understand the urgent need to institute basic life support promptly and the absolute necessity for its being carried out properly. Retraining and maintenance of skills are absolutely necessary for effective performance of these lifesaving techniques.

As can be seen in Figure 7–2, prompt basic life support is indicated for:

A Airway (obstruction)
B Breathing (respiratory arrest)
C Circulation (cardiac arrest, or severe bleeding)

Basic life support is not the same as **advanced life support (ALS)**, which involves advanced procedures such as cardiac monitoring, administering intravenous fluids, medications, and the use of advanced airway management devices. Basic life support, on the other hand, can be provided by one EMT alone or

Airway **Breathing** **Circulation**

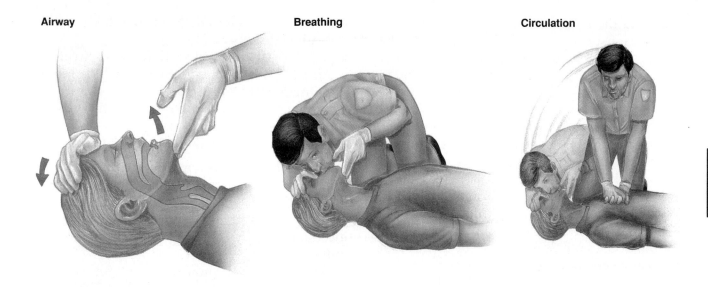

FIGURE 7–2 The ABC steps of cardiopulmonary resuscitation. Airway, Breathing, and Circulation are the essential components of basic life support.

two together. It can also be provided by alert and well-trained bystanders and first responders at the scene. It is the first line of treatment for respiratory or cardiac arrest. The correct application of BLS can maintain life until ALS can be delivered. In some instances (such as foreign body choking, drowning, or lightning injuries), BLS instituted early enough may be all that a patient needs to be resuscitated prior to transport to an appropriate medical facility.

Urgency in Instituting BLS

There must be a maximum sense of urgency in instituting basic life support. The outstanding advantage of cardiopulmonary resuscitation is that it permits the earliest possible treatment of airway obstruction, respiratory arrest, or cardiac arrest without the initial need for specialized equipment or material. Ideally, only seconds should elapse between the recognition of the need for BLS and the start of treatment. The inadequacy or absence of breathing or circulation must be determined promptly to allow the timely start of proper resuscitative procedures.

If breathing alone is inadequate or absent,

opening the airway with or without **artificial ventilation** may be all that is necessary. Frequently, clearing the airway alone will allow resumption of normal respiration. If there is no evidence of effective heart function, **artificial circulation** must be instituted in combination with artificial ventilation. If breathing ceases before the heart stops, enough oxygen will be available in the lungs to maintain life for several minutes. When cardiac arrest occurs first, delivery of oxygenated blood to the heart and brain ceases immediately. Permanent brain damage may occur when it is without oxygen for 4 to 6 minutes. After 6 minutes without oxygen, some brain damage is almost certain. Therefore, speed is essential in determining the need for beginning basic life support.

Primary Assessment

Because of the urgent need to start BLS, a prompt primary assessment, as described in Chapter 5, must be performed on all patients. The primary assessment is specifically designed to evaluate the adequacy of the airway, the quality of breathing, the quality of circulation, and the level of consciousness. The level of consciousness will be a good guide to the extent of BLS required by the patient. For example, the patient who is alert and oriented will not require BLS, whereas patients who are not fully conscious frequently do require at least some degree of basic life support. Not all unconscious patients require all components of basic life support, but all patients who are in need of BLS are unconscious.

For the unconscious patient in need of CPR, try to discover the cause of unconsciousness. Specifically, you must determine whether the unconscious state was caused by a head or cervical spine injury. In those injury cases, care must be taken during CPR to protect the spinal cord from injury. The presence of a head or spinal injury should not keep you from starting BLS. It simply indicates that BLS must be carried out within certain specific physical limits and with extra care to protect and maintain the spine to limit further possible damage. If there is even a remote possibility of neck trauma, appropriate precautions must be taken during the initial ABCs.

When the rescuer is alone, activating EMS is the highest priority after establishing unresponsiveness or the need for adult CPR; this may be called the "call first" rule. EMS should be activated before beginning CPR and the primary survey. If two rescuers are present, one should activate EMS, and the other should begin single-rescuer CPR.

Beginning and Terminating Basic Life Support

It is the responsibility of the EMT to institute basic life support in virtually all patients who have sustained a cardiopulmonary arrest. Only two general exceptions exist to this general rule. First, CPR should not be administered if obvious signs of irreversible biological death are present.

Obvious signs of biological death are known as dead on arrival (DOA) criteria. Two of these criteria are absence of the pulse and absence of respiration. Along with pulselessness and apnea, one of the following signs must also be present:

- *Rigor mortis*—stiffening of the body after death.
- *Livor mortis*—dependent **lividity.** A discoloration of the skin due to pooling of blood (see Figure 5–24).
- Putrefaction or decomposition of the body.
- Separation or obvious destruction of major body organs (such as the brain or heart).

Rigor mortis and livor mortis (lividity) evolve during a variable time after irreversible biological death. In severe injuries, decapitation, incineration, and other conditions obviously incompatible with life are also reasons not to initiate CPR.

Second, CPR is not indicated for certain persons in cardiopulmonary arrest who are known to have been in the terminal stage of an incurable disease. In this situation, CPR serves only to prolong the death of the patient. These individuals should have a living will available or certain other legal documents to inform you that CPR should not be started. You must be very familiar with local protocols and standards in your system before being called to treat terminally ill patients. Some EMS systems have computer annotations of patients preregistered with the system indicating the amount and extent of treatment desired at the time of the terminal event.

In all other circumstances, CPR is given to any individual who has sustained a partial or complete cardiopulmonary arrest. Even if a substantial amount of time has passed since the patient's collapse, it is impossible to know when the last instant of effective perfusion with oxygenated blood occurred. Extrinsic factors, such as the temperature of the environment, or intrinsic factors, such as the hardiness of the patient's tissues and organs, may affect the patient's ability to survive. Therefore, CPR should be instituted promptly in virtually all patients who have sustained a partial or complete cardiopulmonary arrest. Most legal advisers recommend that when there is any doubt, you should always err on the side of rendering too much care rather than too little. Thus, always start CPR if any doubt exists.

When resuscitation is started in the absence of a physician, it must be continued until one of the following events occurs:

S The patient *starts* breathing and has a pulse.

T The patient is *transferred* to a higher medical authority in accordance with accepted practice.

O You are *out of strength* or too fatigued to continue.

P A *physician* present assumes responsibility for the patient.

It is *not* your responsibility to terminate CPR unless you can no longer physically provide the support. In general, this decision to terminate CPR will not have to be made by you, because resuscitation should always be continued until the patient's care is transferred to a physician at the emergency department. In some systems, the medical director or a duly designated medical control physician may elect to order the cessation of CPR based on clinical factors.

In all instances, there should exist in each EMS system clearly delineated standing orders to provide you with guidance for starting and stopping CPR. Both the legal and medical communities should be in general accord with the written protocols. The information should be widely disseminated throughout the medical community to enable physicians to educate their patients when to call and when not to call EMS. Compliance with these protocols should be closely administered and reviewed by the EMS medical director.

Positioning the Patient

For cardiopulmonary resuscitation to be effective, the patient must be horizontal (lying down), supine (face up), and on a firm surface with enough clear space around the patient to allow two rescuers to perform CPR (Figure 7–3a). Optimal airway management and artificial ventilation require that the patient be supine. It is imperative to place the patient in a supine position as soon as possible. If the patient is crumpled up or lying face down, repositioning will be necessary. The few seconds spent in positioning the patient properly will greatly improve the delivery of CPR.

The **recovery position** is used in a patient who is not a trauma victim prior to transport in order to facilitate breathing. The patient is rolled onto his or her right or left side so that the head, shoulders, and torso move simultaneously without twisting. The patient's hands are placed under the cheek (Figure 7–3b). This

A

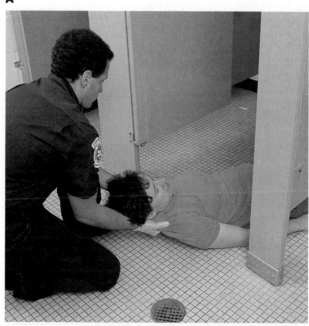

FIGURE 7–3

(A) It may be necessary to move the patient from a confined space. (B) The recovery position is used where spontaneous respirations are present prior to transport.

B

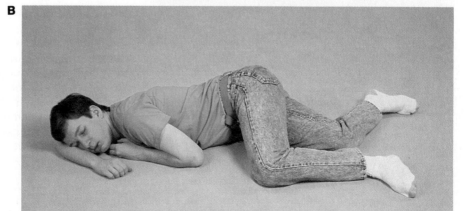

A

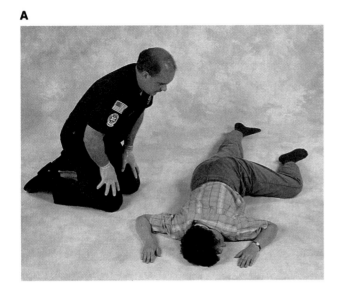

B

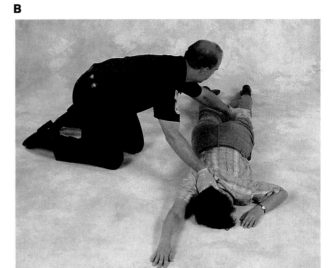

C

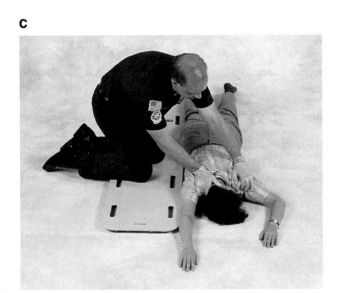

D

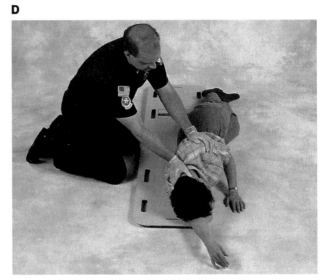

E

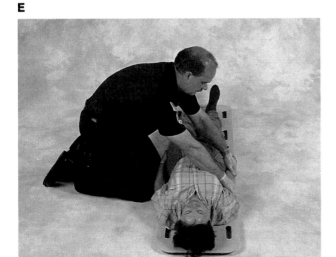

FIGURE 7–4

You should roll the patient into a supine position following these steps: (A) Kneel about 18 inches away from the patient's shoulder. (B) Bring the patient's nearer arm above the head and straighten patient's legs. (C) Place one of your hands behind the patient's head and neck and the other hand on the distant shoulder. (D) Roll the patient toward you by pulling the shoulder. (E) Once the patient is flat, bring the extended arm back to the side. When possible, two people should perform this maneuver with an injured person to ensure protection of the spine.

position is used to facilitate spontaneous breathing and allows for excretions, such as vomitus, to spontaneously drain out of the mouth. The recovery position is also used after the restoration of spontaneous respiration by initial resuscitation measures.

Considerable caution is necessary when a neck or back injury is suspected. The patient must be rolled as a single unit, including head, neck, and back.

For proper positioning, kneel beside the patient, but not in bodily contact. You must be sufficiently far away so that when rolled toward you, the patient does not come to rest in your lap (Figure 7–4a). Then rapidly straighten the patient's legs and move the nearer arm above the head (Figure 7–4b). Next, place one hand behind the back of the head and neck of the patient and the other on the distant shoulder (Figure 7–4c). The patient can then be turned toward you by pulling on the distant shoulder with the head and neck controlled so that they turn with the rest of the torso as a unit (Figure 7–4d). In this way, the head and neck remain in the same vertical plane as the back. Aggravation of any spinal injury is minimized. When the patient is flat on his or her back, bring the patient's farther arm back to the side (Figure 7–4e). When it is possible, the patient should be rolled onto a long spine board, which will provide support during transport and emergency department care. Once the patient is properly positioned, the adequacy of airway, breathing, and circulation should be reassessed and basic life support started if necessary.

In the situation where the patient has not been subject to spinal or head trauma and is noted to be breathing, placing the patient in the recovery position is appropriate.

OPENING THE AIRWAY IN ADULTS

Immediate opening of the airway is the most important factor in successful cardiopulmonary resuscitation. Without an open airway, artificial ventilation will not succeed. Far and away, the most common cause of airway obstruction in the unconscious patient is relaxation of the muscles of the throat and tongue. The airway is

obstructed by its own tissues, which tend to fall back into the throat to create the block (Figure 7–5). Dentures, blood clots, vomitus, mucus, food, or other foreign bodies may also cause obstruction. Obstruction of the airway from an aspirated foreign body is discussed later in this chapter. A variety of maneuvers exist to establish a patent airway when it is obstructed by relaxation of the muscles of the throat and tongue.

Head-Tilt/Chin-Lift Maneuver

Opening the airway to relieve an obstruction caused by relaxation of the tongue often can be accomplished easily and quickly by tilting the patient's head backward (Figure 7–6). This procedure is known as the *head-tilt maneuver*. Sometimes this simple maneuver is all that is required to cause the patient to resume breathing spontaneously. For the head tilt to be performed, the patient must be lying supine. Kneeling close beside the patient, place a hand on the patient's forehead and apply firm backward pressure with your palm, moving the patient's head as far back as possible. This extension of the neck will move the tongue forward, away from the posterior pharynx,

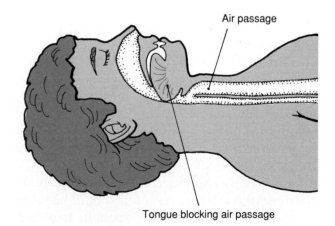

Air passage

Tongue blocking air passage

FIGURE 7–5

Muscular relaxation in the unconscious individual may allow the tongue to fall back into the airway and obstruct it.

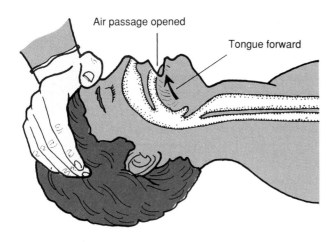

Air passage opened

Tongue forward

FIGURE 7-6

The head-tilt maneuver. The airway is opened by extending the neck with firm pressure applied to the forehead. The maneuver causes an anterior motion of the tongue to raise it from the posterior pharyngeal wall.

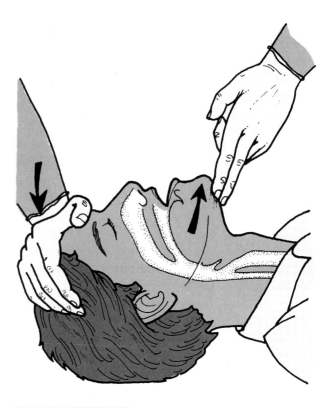

FIGURE 7-7

The head-tilt/chin-lift maneuver. While the head is tilted backward with one hand, the fingers of the other hand lift the chin forward, as indicated by the arrows.

clearing the airway. It will also straighten out the airway. An effective head tilt may be difficult to obtain with only one hand on the forehead. In this instance, the other hand can be used to apply a chin lift. The head tilt is the initial and often the most important general step in opening the airway.

Having achieved the head tilt, you can open the airway further with the *head-tilt/chin-lift maneuver*. You must be familiar with the chin-lift technique and be able to perform it well. Neither the head-tilt maneuver nor the head-tilt/chin-lift maneuver should be used in cases of trauma. The tips of the fingers of the hand not on the forehead are placed under the bony part of the chin. The chin is lifted forward, bringing the entire lower jaw with it, and helping to tilt the head back (Figure 7–7). The fingers must not compress the soft tissue under the chin, thereby obstructing the airway. The forehead hand continues to maintain the backward tilt of the head. The chin should be lifted so that the teeth are nearly brought together; however, you should avoid closing the mouth completely.

If the patient has loose dentures, they can be held in position with the chin lift, making obstruction by the lips less likely. If artificial ventilation is needed, a mouth-to-mouth seal is much more easily achieved when dentures are in place. If dentures cannot be managed in place, they should be removed. If a mask is utilized, most rescuers find that a mask-to-mouth seal is more easily accomplished if the dentures are removed.

Jaw-Thrust Maneuver

The two methods just described are effective for opening the airway for most patients. In some instances, however, forward movement of the lower jaw—the *jaw-thrust maneuver*—may be required. The jaw thrust is a triple maneuver in which you place your fingers behind the angles of the patient's lower jaw and then:

1. Forcefully move the jaw forward.
2. Tilt the head backward without significantly extending the cervical spine.
3. Use your thumbs to pull the patient's lower lip down, to allow breathing through the mouth as well as the nose.

The jaw thrust is performed best with you kneeling above the patient's head (Figure 7–8). When a cervical spine injury is suspected, this simple maneuver can be modified to keep the head in a neutral position while you thrust the jaw forward and open the mouth as described. Only a deeply unconscious patient will tolerate this maneuver. The resuscitation mask can be used easily with both hands doing the jaw thrust while at the same time you seal the mask around the mouth. When you perform mouth-to-nose ventilation with the jaw thrust maneuver, seal the patient's mouth with your cheek and do not retract the patient's lips. The nose may also be sealed with your thumbs using a modified jaw-thrust technique. In this maneuver, the index and long fingers are used to thrust the jaw anteriorly while the thumbs compress the patient's nose (Figure 7–9).

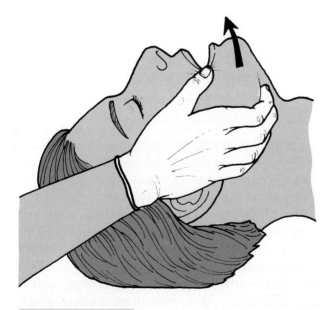

FIGURE 7–8

In the jaw-thrust maneuver, place your fingers behind the angle of the patient's jaw and forcefully bring it forward.

ARTIFICIAL VENTILATION IN ADULTS

Once the airway has been opened by one of the techniques just described, the patient may start to breathe spontaneously. To assess whether breathing has returned, place an ear about one inch above the nose and mouth of the patient and listen carefully for sounds of breathing (Figure 7–10). Your head should be turned to observe the patient's chest and abdomen. If you can feel and hear movement of air and can see the patient's chest and abdomen move with each breath, breathing has returned. Feeling and hearing the actual movement of air are far more important than seeing body movements. With airway obstruction, it is possible that there will be no air movement, even though the chest and abdomen rise and fall considerably with the patient's frantic attempts to breathe. In addition, observing chest and abdominal movement often is difficult with a fully clothed patient. Finally, there may be very little or no perceptible chest movement, even with normal breathing, particularly in some patients with chronic lung disease. When, using this "look, listen, and feel" technique, you discover that there is no movement of air, artificial ventilation must be started promptly.

In respiratory arrest, death results from **anoxia** (a lack of oxygen) combined with the accumulation of an excess of carbon dioxide. These changes cannot be corrected without good ventilation to get rid of carbon dioxide and provide oxygen. Adequate ventilation requires inspiration lasting 1½ to 2 seconds. Ventilations must be given slowly and deliberately. This gentle and slow method of ventilating the patient is done to keep from forcing air into the stomach.

Although no equipment is needed to ventilate a nonbreathing patient, to avoid any risk of disease transmission a resuscitation mask should be used. Once the need is identified, rescue breathing should be started immediately and should continue along with efforts to support the circulation and correct cardiac problems. Rescue breathing, whether mouth-to-mouth, mouth-to-nose, or mouth-to-stoma, will deliver exhaled gas from the rescuer. This

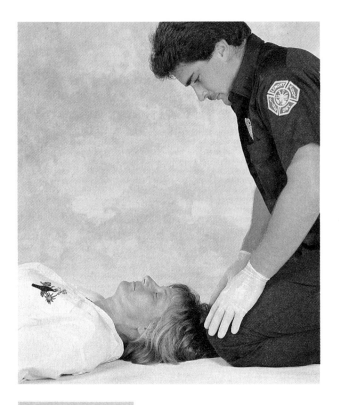

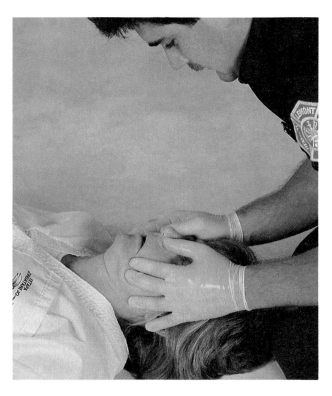

FIGURE 7–9   The modified jaw-thrust maneuver. Use the index and
long fingers to thrust the jaw forward while you compress the patient's nose with your thumbs.

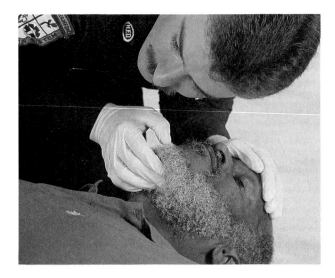

FIGURE 7–10

Respiration is determined by feeling the movement of
air on the cheek, by hearing it, and by seeing the chest
and abdomen move with each breath.

gas contains 16 percent oxygen, a level more
than sufficient to maintain the patient's life.

Mouth-to-Mouth Ventilation

To perform *mouth-to-mouth ventilation*, open the
airway with the head-tilt/chin-lift maneuver.
While you continue to exert pressure on the
forehead to maintain the backward tilt of the
head, pinch the patient's nostrils together
using the thumb and index finger of this hand
(Figure 7–11a). With this technique, the thumb
of the hand lifting the chin can be used to
depress the lower lip to help keep the mouth
open during mouth-to-mouth ventilation. Then
open the patient's mouth widely, take a deep
breath, make a tight seal with your mouth
around the patient's mouth, and exhale into it
(Figure 7–11b). Then remove your mouth and
allow the patient to exhale passively, turning
slightly to watch for movement of the patient's

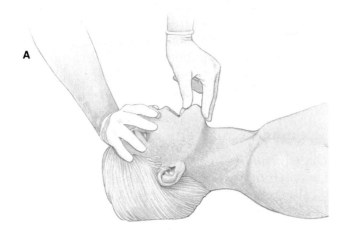

A

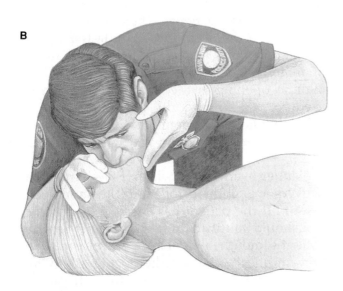

B

FIGURE 7–11

Mouth-to-mouth ventilation. (A) Seal off the patient's nose, and (B) after encircling the patient's open mouth with your own, exhale deeply into it.

chest. Breaths are given slowly each lasting 1½ to 2 seconds.

Adequate ventilation is ensured if, with every breath, you:

1. See the patient's chest rise and fall.
2. Feel the resistance of the patient's lungs as they expand.
3. Hear and feel the air escape during exhalation.

When you give mouth-to-mouth ventilation and use the jaw-thrust maneuver to maintain an open airway, you must move to the patient's side, keep the patient's mouth open with both thumbs, and seal the nose by placing your cheek against the patient's nostrils.

Mouth-to-Nose Ventilation

In some cases, *mouth-to-nose ventilation* is more effective than mouth-to-mouth ventilation. It is a good alternative to mouth-to-mouth ventilation. Mouth-to-nose ventilation is recommended when:

1. It is impossible to open the patient's mouth.
2. It is impossible to ventilate a patient through the mouth because of severe facial injuries.
3. It is difficult to achieve a tight seal around the mouth because the patient has no teeth.
4. You prefer the nasal route for some other reason.

For the mouth-to-nose technique, keep the patient's head tilted back with one hand on the forehead and use the other hand to lift the patient's lower jaw (Figure 7–12). This maneu-

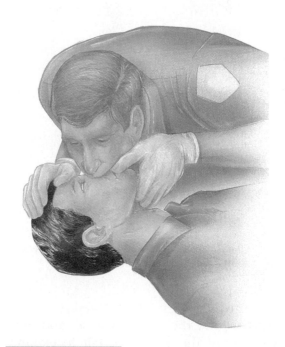

FIGURE 7–12

Mouth-to-nose ventilation using the chin-lift maneuver.

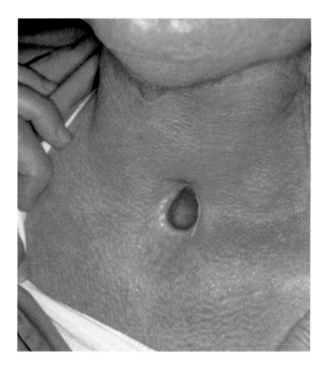

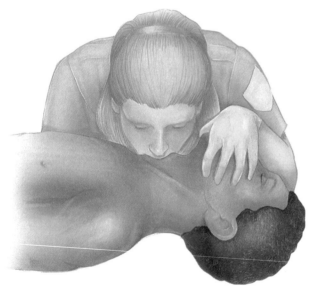

FIGURE 7–13

(Top) A tracheal stoma lies in the midline of the neck. (Bottom) Mouth-to-stoma ventilation.

ver seals the lips. Then take a deep breath, seal your lips around the patient's nose, and blow in slowly until the lungs are felt to expand. Then remove your mouth and allow the patient to exhale passively. You can see the chest fall when the patient exhales. It may be necessary to open the patient's mouth or separate the

patient's lips to allow air to escape during exhalation. As stated previously, when you use the jaw thrust to maintain the airway, use your cheek to seal the patient's mouth and do not use your thumbs to retract the lower lip when you give mouth-to-nose ventilation.

Mouth-to-Stoma Ventilation

Direct *mouth-to-stoma ventilation* must be used for patients who have had a *laryngectomy* (surgical removal of the larynx). These patients have a permanent *tracheal stoma* (an opening in the neck that connects the trachea directly to the skin). It may be seen as an opening at the center, at the front and the base of the neck. In many of these patients, there will be other openings in the neck, according to the type of operation done. Any opening other than the midline tracheal stoma should be ignored. The midline opening is the only one that can be used to put air into the patient's lungs. In general, other neck openings will lie to one side or the other, but not in the midline (Figure 7–13).

Neither head-tilt/chin-lift nor jaw-thrust maneuvers are required for mouth-to-stoma ventilation. If the patient has a tube in the stoma, you should ventilate through the tube. Seal the patient's mouth and nose with one hand to prevent a leak of air up the trachea when you ventilate through a tracheal tube or stoma. Release the seal of the patient's mouth and nose for exhalation. This allows the air to exhale through the upper airway.

Gastric Distension

Artificial ventilation frequently causes *gastric distension* (the stomach becomes filled with air). It happens most often in children, but it is also common in adults. It is most likely to appear when excessive pressures are used for ventilation or when the airway is obstructed. Slight gastric distension may be disregarded. Marked inflation of the stomach is dangerous because it causes regurgitation of gastric contents during CPR. Abdominal distension can also reduce the lung volume by elevating the diaphragm.

Gastric distension has been found by investigators to occur when high ventilatory pressures are used or when several rapid breaths are administered quickly in succession. Slower, periodic air flow at lower pressures is more effective in ventilating the lungs.

Acute, massive gastric distension that interferes with adequate ventilation must be relieved promptly. Frequently, this can be done by exerting moderate pressure on the patient's abdomen between the umbilicus and the rib cage with the flat of the hand after positioning the patient on his or her side. You must be alert to the fact that regurgitation will include air, gastric juice, and food. Aspiration of the gastric contents into the lungs must be prevented during this maneuver. The patient's entire body should be turned, preferably to the left side, and a suction device should be used promptly to remove any regurgitated material.

FOREIGN BODY AIRWAY OBSTRUCTION IN ADULTS

There can be several causes of airway obstruction: muscular relaxation in an unconscious patient; vomited or regurgitated stomach contents; blood clot, bone fragments, or damaged tissue after an injury; dentures; or foreign bodies. The maneuvers to open the obstructed airway that has been caused by muscle relaxation have been discussed. Loose dentures and large pieces of vomited food, mucus, or blood clots should be swept forward and out of the mouth with your gloved index finger. Once it becomes available, suctioning should be used to maintain a clear airway. On occasion, a large foreign body will be aspirated and block the upper airway.

Recognition of Foreign Body Obstruction

Sudden airway obstruction by a foreign body in an adult usually occurs during a meal. In a child, it occurs during mealtime or at play (choking on small objects placed into the mouth).

Early recognition of airway obstruction is the key to successful management. You must learn to differentiate between airway obstruction caused by a foreign body and that resulting from respiratory failure or arrest, such as fainting, stroke, or acute myocardial infarction.

You may be faced with two situations in which upper airway obstruction is present: The patient may be conscious when discovered and become unconscious, or the patient may be unconscious when discovered.

Conscious Patient Sudden upper airway obstruction is usually recognized when the patient who is eating or has just finished eating is suddenly unable to speak or cough, grasps the throat, develops cyanosis, and demonstrates exaggerated efforts to breathe (see Figure 5–4). Air movement is either absent or not detectable. Initially, the patient will remain conscious and be able to indicate quite clearly the nature of the problem for a short period of time. A standard simple question such as "are you choking?" will frequently be answered by the patient nodding "yes." Doubt about the obstruction is then removed. If the obstruction is not removed in a short period of time, oxygen in the lungs will be used up, and unconsciousness and death will follow.

Unconscious Patient When a patient is discovered unconscious, the cause is initially unknown. The unconsciousness may have been caused by airway obstruction, cardiac or cardiopulmonary arrest, or a number of other problems. Any patient found unconscious must be managed as a patient with cardiopulmonary arrest. The obstructed airway must be dealt with when discovered. The obstruction should be suspected in the unconscious patient when the standard airway maneuvers and ventilation efforts do not result in effective ventilation of the patient's lungs. If, after opening the airway, resistance to blowing into the patient's lungs is encountered or pressure builds up in your mouth, it may be assumed that some degree of obstruction is present and steps must be taken to relieve the obstruction.

Maneuvers to Relieve Upper Airway Obstruction

Two manual maneuvers are recommended for relieving foreign body airway obstruction: (1) abdominal thrusts (the Heimlich maneuver), and (2) finger sweeps and manual removal of the object.

Abdominal Thrust Maneuver The **abdominal thrust maneuver,** commonly referred to as the Heimlich maneuver is the preferred initial treatment to dislodge an aspirated foreign body in adults and children. The abdominal thrust maneuver is the most effective method of dislodging and forcing an obstructing object from the airway. Residual air, which is always present in the lungs, is compressed upward and used to expel the object.

A series of five abdominal thrusts is applied until the obstructing body is dislodged. With the patient sitting or standing, follow these steps:

1. Stand behind the patient, with your arms wrapped around the patient's waist.
2. Grasp one fist with the other hand and place the thumb side of the fist against the patient's abdomen, just above the umbilicus and well below the xiphoid.
3. Press your fist into the patient's abdomen with a quick inward and upward thrust (Figure 7–14).
4. Repeat the thrusts until the object is expelled from the airway, or the patient becomes unconscious.

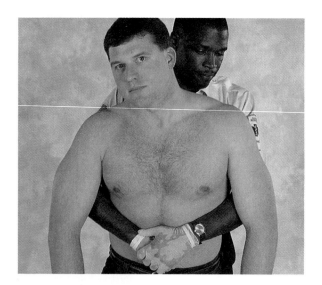

FIGURE 7–14

Proper positioning of the hands for applying abdominal thrusts in an adult who is standing or sitting.

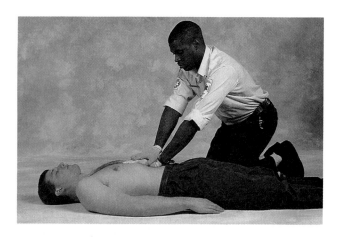

FIGURE 7–15

Proper positioning of the hands for applying abdominal thrusts in the supine patient.

With the patient supine, modify the technique as follows:

1. Position the patient supine and kneel close to the patient's hips or straddle either the hips or legs of the patient.
2. Place the heel of one hand against the patient's abdomen well below the xiphoid process and above the umbilicus; place the second hand on top of the first.
3. Press the hand into the patient's abdomen with a quick inward and upward thrust and repeat five times (Figure 7–15).

This maneuver can be accomplished safely in all adults and children with good results. Pregnancy and obesity do not contraindicate its use; however, the chest thrust is recommended for patients in advanced stages of pregnancy, or for the markedly obese and for children less than one year of age.

Manual Removal of a Foreign Body If at any time the foreign body causing an airway obstruction appears in the mouth, or is believed to be in the mouth, it should be removed cautiously with your gloved fingers. Abdominal thrusts may dislodge the foreign body but not expel it. Use either a cross-finger technique or a tongue-jaw lift combined with a finger probe to remove the foreign material.

A

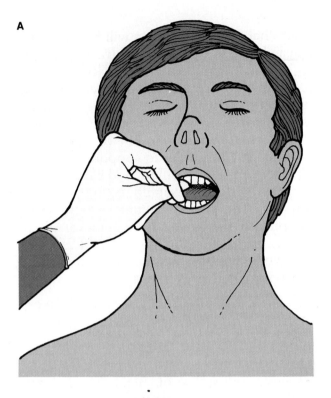

B

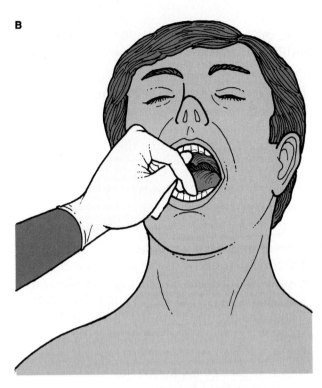

C

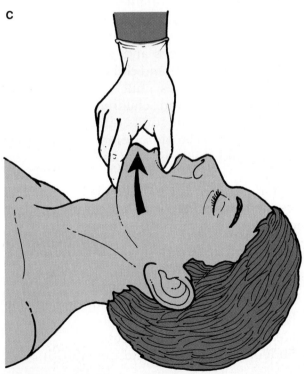

D

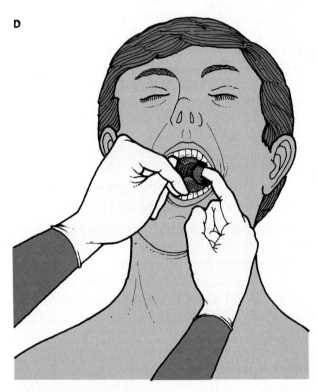

FIGURE 7–16   Manual removal of a foreign body. (A) Using the cross-finger technique, brace the thumb and index finger on the patient's teeth and (B) force the jaws apart. (C) Using the tongue-jaw-lift maneuver, lift the tongue and jaw to open the mouth and to help visualize the foreign body. (D) A finger probe is used to sweep the foreign body out of the mouth.

The *cross-finger technique* for opening the mouth includes these steps:

1. Cross your thumb under your index finger.
2. Brace your thumb and index finger against the patient's lower and upper teeth, respectively (Figure 7–16a).
3. Use your fingers to force the patient's jaws open (Figure 7–16b).

The *tongue-jaw-lift maneuver* for opening the mouth includes these steps:

1. Keep the head in the neutral position.
2. Open the patient's mouth by grasping both the tongue and the lower jaw between your thumb and fingers and lifting them forward (Figure 7–16c). This action will help pull the tongue back away from the throat and away from the foreign body that may be lodged there.

Finger probes to remove foreign bodies include these steps:

1. Hold the patient's mouth open by using either the cross-finger or tongue-jaw-lift technique.
2. Use the index finger of your opposite hand as a hook to sweep down inside the patient's cheek to the base of the tongue (Figure 7–16d).
3. Dislodge any impacted foreign body up into the mouth.
4. When the foreign body comes up within reach, grasp it and carefully remove it.

Take care when you use finger probes not to push the dislodged foreign body farther back into the airway. For this reason, finger sweeps are not advised in infants or small children. Instead, the advice is to seize the foreign object under direct visualization with the index finger and thumb.

Partial Airway Obstruction On occasion, a partial airway obstruction will be present. The patient will be able to exchange some air but will still have some degree of respiratory distress. Breathing is noisy and the patient may be coughing. Great care must be taken with this patient to prevent a partial airway obstruction from becoming a complete airway obstruction.

Abdominal thrusts generally will be ineffective in dislodging the partially obstructing object, and manual manipulation is dangerous because the object could be forced farther down the airway and completely obstruct it. In the case of a partial airway obstruction, the airway maneuvers (head-tilt/chin-lift or jaw-thrust) should be used in order to support the airway in its most efficient position, and supplemental 100 percent oxygen should be administered promptly. The patient should be transported promptly to the hospital for removal of the partially obstructing foreign body. Of course, if air movement stops completely, an immediate Heimlich maneuver is indicated.

BASIC VENTILATORY SUPPORT IN INFANTS AND CHILDREN

The basic principles of BLS are the same whether the patient is an infant, child, or adult. The differences in BLS for the infant and child relate to the different underlying causes of emergencies in infants and children and the smaller size of infants and children. In the great majority of instances, full cardiopulmonary arrest in infants and children results from respiratory arrest. In adults cardiac arrest usually occurs first. The causes of respiratory arrest in infants and children are numerous. If uncorrected, respiratory arrest will lead to cardiac arrest and death. Some of the major crises that necessitate resuscitation in infants and children include:

- Aspiration of foreign bodies into the airway: peanuts, candy, small toys.
- Poisonings and drug overdose.
- Airway infections, such as croup and epiglottitis.
- Near drowning or electrocution.
- Sudden infant death syndrome (SIDS).

For this reason, in single-rescuer CPR of children and infants, 1 full minute of CPR actions are to be delivered before EMS is activated.

For the purposes of BLS, anyone under 1 year of age is considered an *infant*. A *child* is between the ages of 1 and 8 years. Above 8 years of age, techniques used for adults can generally be applied. These definitions are to be considered guidelines only. The fact is that variations do occur among infants and children in size relative to age. Small children may well be treated best as infants, and large ones as adults.

Opening the Airway

In children and infants, attention first must be directed by you, or any first responder, to clearing the airway and to providing proper ventilation. If the child is breathing or struggling to breathe, the EMS system should be activated first to speed the patient's delivery to an ALS facility. In many instances, opening the airway and adequate rescue breathing are all that is needed for effective resuscitation.

After the primary assessment, you will have established whether the infant or child is unresponsive, is in acute respiratory distress, or is cyanotic. The next step is to secure an open airway. In children (1 through 8 years of age), the preferred technique is the chin-lift maneuver (Figure 7–17). The head-tilt technique, because of the suppleness of the child's neck, may result in excessive extension of the neck that itself can produce obstruction. In general, it is best to maintain the child's neck in a neutral position and to use the chin lift to open the airway.

The jaw-thrust maneuver without head tilt may be used as an alternative technique to open the child's airway and is the preferred method when neck injury is suspected. It should be performed in the same manner as for an adult.

As soon as the airway is opened, the adequacy of breathing should be assessed. Place your ear over the patient's mouth and nose and look toward the chest and abdomen. The patient is breathing if you:

- See the chest and abdomen rise and fall.
- Feel the air move from the mouth and nose.
- Hear air move during exhalation.

Artificial Ventilation

If the patient is not breathing or has cyanosis, rescue breathing must be started for 1 minute before activating the EMS system. If more than one rescuer is initially present, EMS should be called by one rescuer, while another rescuer begins CPR on the child. Children who are experiencing respiratory distress and are struggling to breathe will assume a position to optimize the patency of their airway. They should be able to stay in that position as long as their partial airway obstruction does not become a complete airway obstruction. For infants, the preferred technique of artificial ventilation is *mouth-to-nose-and-mouth ventilation*. You must cover both the mouth and the nose with your mouth and make a seal. If the child is large enough so that a tight seal cannot be made over both mouth and nose together, mouth-to-mouth ventilation is performed as in the adult.

Once an airtight seal has been established, two 1 to 1½ second gentle breaths are delivered. The initial breaths serve as a means of checking for airway obstruction as well as expanding the lungs. The lungs of a child, and especially an infant, are much smaller than those of an adult. Therefore, the volume of air

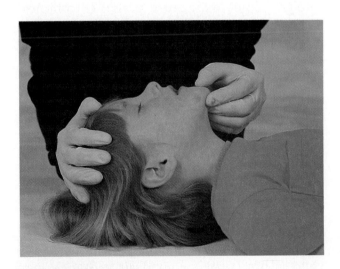

FIGURE 7–17

The chin-lift technique is used to open the airway in the infant or child. The tips of one or more fingers lift the lower jaw forward while the other hand maintains the head in a neutral position.

needed for effective ventilation will be less than in an adult and should be limited to the amount needed to cause the chest to rise. On the other hand, the smaller air passages of the child provide a greater resistance to airflow, and therefore the ventilatory pressure needed to inflate the lungs will probably be greater than anticipated. As soon as you see the chest rise and fall, the correct amount of force is being used.

Ventilatory rates for infants and children under conditions of resuscitation should be more rapid than for adults. Newborn infants should be ventilated once every 3 seconds or 20 times per minute; children and older infants should be ventilated once every 4 seconds or 15 times per minute. These rates will require appropriate pauses in cardiac compression if it is being given.

If air enters freely with the initial breaths and the chest rises, you can assume that the airway is clear. You can then proceed to check the pulse. If air does not enter freely, the airway must be checked for obstruction. The maneuvers (repositioning, chin-lift or jaw-thrust) to open the airway should be repeated, and if air still does not enter freely, an obstruction must be suspected. The airway must be cleared.

Gastric Distension

Artificial ventilation can cause stomach distension, especially if high ventilatory pressures are used. Massive distension can interfere with artificial ventilation by elevating the diaphragm, decreasing lung volume, and posing a threat of gastric regurgitation. Gastric distension can be minimized by limiting ventilation volumes to the point at which the chest rises and by using slow, 1 to 1½ second breaths. Attempts at relieving gastric distension by pressure on the abdomen should be made when you recognize the condition and before the abdomen is so tense that ventilation is ineffective. To relieve gastric distension turn the infant's entire body to the left side, head down, and applying firm manual pressure to the abdomen. The danger of aspiration of stomach contents into the lungs is such that pressure maneuvers should be done when you

are prepared to suction regurgitated material out of the throat promptly.

Foreign Body Airway Obstruction

As has been pointed out, primary airway obstruction is a common problem in infants and children. Airway obstruction is usually caused by a foreign body or an infection, such as *croup* or *epiglottitis,* resulting in swelling and narrowing of the airway. Distinguishing between a foreign body and an infectious cause is important. With infection, the steps for dislodging a foreign body will not be helpful, can be dangerous, and will cause a delay in transporting the child to the hospital.

The signs of croup or epiglottitis develop in a child who has been ill with a fever, has a barking cough, and develops progressive airway obstruction. The patient should be given humidified and warmed oxygen and transported promptly to the hospital. This child will require treatment for the infectious disease causing airway obstruction.

A previously healthy child who, while eating, playing with small toys, or crawling about the house, has sudden difficulty breathing has probably aspirated a foreign body. As in adults, foreign bodies may cause partial or complete airway obstruction. With a partial airway obstruction, air exchange can be either good or poor. With good air exchange, the patient can cough forcefully, although there may be wheezing between coughs. As long as good air exchange continues (the patient can breathe, cough, or talk), you should not interfere with the patient's attempts to expel the foreign body. Oxygen should be given, and the child should be transported promptly to the hospital. The emergency department personnel should be notified of the problem and the expected time of arrival.

Poor air exchange may be present when the child is first seen, or good air exchange may progress to poor air exchange. Poor air exchange is characterized by an ineffective cough, **stridor** (high pitched noises while inhaling), increased respiratory difficulty, and, especially, cyanosis. When available, oxygen should be given to the patient with poor air exchange.

When oxygen is unavailable or oxygen administration does not convert poor air exchange into good air exchange, partial obstruction with poor air exchange must be managed as a complete obstruction.

Relief of a complete foreign body obstruction in children is achieved with the use of the Heimlich maneuver. Five thrusts should be delivered to the unconscious child, until the foreign body is expelled. If the foreign body is not expelled, the mouth should be opened, and if the foreign body is visualized, the jaw and tongue lifted forward, and a finger sweep of the mouth performed to remove the object. In the rare instance when the foreign body cannot be retrieved, mouth-to-mouth ventilation should be attempted while the patient is transported rapidly to the hospital.

The actual technique for delivering the abdominal thrust may vary with the size of the child. Ordinarily, it will be convenient to administer it with the child supine. In the older child (over 8 years old) the technique with the patient erect may be similar to that for adults.

Some concern exists that the abdominal thrust might injure the liver of an infant. For this reason, you should deliver a series of five quick back blows and then a series of five chest thrusts when you clear an infant's airway that has become obstructed by a foreign body.

To deliver chest thrusts or back blows to an infant, place one hand on the infant's back and neck and the other supporting the chest, jaws, and face. The infant thus is sandwiched between your hands and arms. While you continue to provide support for the head and neck, the infant is placed with the head lower than the trunk. Five back blows can then be delivered in rapid succession between the shoulder blades (Figure 7–18a). External chest compressions are subsequently done by turning the child face up with the head slightly lower than the trunk, and doing five chest thrusts on the sternum in the same fashion as for cardiac

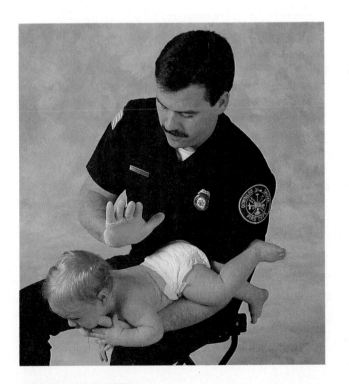
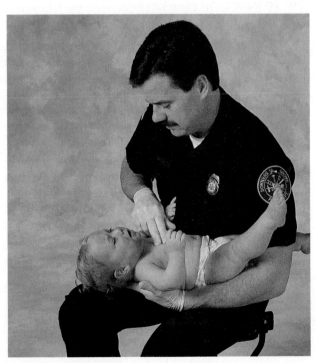

FIGURE 7–18 (A) The proper position for delivering back blows to relieve airway obstruction in the infant. (B) After giving five back blows, turn the infant over and give five chest compressions.

Skill Performance Sheet Adult Foreign-Body Airway Obstruction — Conscious

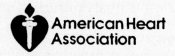

American Heart Association

Student Name _____ Date _____

Performance Guidelines	Performed
1. Ask "Are you choking?"	
2. Give abdominal thrusts (chest thrusts for pregnant or obese victim).	
3. Repeat thrusts until effective or victim becomes unconscious.	
Adult Foreign-Body Airway Obstruction — Victim Becomes Unconscious	
4. Activate the EMS system.	
5. Perform a tongue-jaw lift followed by a finger sweep to remove the object.	
6. Open airway and try to ventilate; if still obstructed, reposition head and try to ventilate again.	
7. Give up to 5 abdominal thrusts.	
8. Repeat steps 5 through 7 until effective.*	

*If victim is breathing or resumes effective breathing, place in recovery position.

Comments _____

_____

_____

Instructor _____

Circle one: Complete   Needs more practice

FIGURE 7–19 Management of a foreign body obstructed airway in a conscious adult.

Reproduced with permission. Basic Life Support Heartsaver Guide, 1993. Copyright ©
American Heart Association.

Skill Performance Sheet
Adult Foreign-Body Airway Obstruction — Unconscious

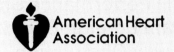

American Heart Association

Student Name _____ Date _____

Performance Guidelines	Performed
1. Establish unresponsiveness. Activate the EMS system.	
2. Open airway and try to ventilate; if still obstructed, reposition head and try to ventilate again.	
3. Give up to 5 abdominal thrusts.	
4. Perform a tongue-jaw lift followed by a finger sweep to remove the object.	
5. Repeat steps 2 through 4 until effective.*	

*If victim is breathing or resumes effective breathing, place in recovery position.

Comments _____

_____

_____

Instructor _____

Circle one: Complete   Needs more practice

FIGURE 7–20   Management of a foreign body obstructed airway in an unconscious adult.

Reproduced with permission. Basic Life Support Heartsaver Guide, *1993. Copyright ©* American Heart Association.

Skill Performance Sheet Infant Foreign-Body Airway Obstruction — Unconscious

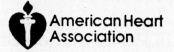
American Heart Association

Student Name _____ Date _____

Performance Guidelines	Performed
1. Establish unresponsiveness. If second rescuer is available, have him or her activate the EMS system.	
2. Open airway and try to ventilate; if still obstructed, reposition head and try to ventilate again.	
3. Give up to 5 back blows and 5 chest thrusts.	
4. Perform a tongue-jaw lift, and if you see the object, perform a finger sweep to remove it.	
5. Repeat steps 2 through 4 until effective.*	
6. If airway obstruction is not relieved after about 1 minute, activate the EMS system.	

*If victim is breathing or resumes effective breathing, place in recovery position.

Comments _____

_____

_____

Instructor _____

Circle one: Complete   Needs more practice

FIGURE 7–21   Management of a foreign body obstructed airway in an unconscious infant.

Reproduced with permission. Basic Life Support Heartsaver Guide, *1993. Copyright ©*
American Heart Association.

resuscitation except at a slightly faster rate (Figure 7–18b). You must be careful as you use the technique of placing your hands surrounding the infant not to compress the upper abdomen and damage the liver as you do the chest thrusts.

Blind finger sweeps done prior to attempting to dislodge the foreign body by back blows or thrusts should be avoided in infants and children, because the foreign body can easily be pushed farther back in the throat and cause further obstruction. In the unconscious pediatric patient, immediately after the chest or abdominal thrusts, the tongue and the lower jaw are lifted forward and the mouth opened. This maneuver is done by placing the thumb in the patient's mouth, over the tongue, with the fingers wrapped around the lower jaw. If the foreign body is seen, it can be removed with a finger sweep of the other hand.

If the patient has not started breathing after these maneuvers, the airway should again be opened and another attempt made to deliver artificial ventilation. If the chest does not rise, reposition the head and attempt ventilation again. If the chest still does not rise, obstruction persists. The preceding techniques should be repeated in an attempt to relieve the obstruction.

The 1993 American Heart Association standard skills sheets are presented in summary to specify steps in initial airway management (Figures 7–19 to 7–21).

YOU ARE THE EMT

1. When should you start BLS? When should you not start BLS?
2. You have started BLS on an unconscious patient in cardiac arrest. Under what circumstances should you discontinue it?
3. What is the difference between cardiac arrest and respiratory arrest? Which occurs more frequently in children? Why?
4. You have been called to treat a 2-year-old who is having trouble breathing. The mother thinks her daughter may have choked on a penny. What are your management steps?

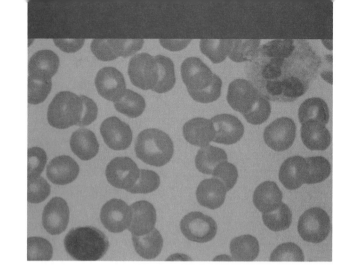

CHAPTER 8

THE CIRCULATORY SYSTEM

aorta (a-or′tah) The major artery leaving the left side of the heart, that carries freshly oxygenated blood to the body.

artery A tubular vessel that carries blood from the heart to the body tissues.

atrium (a′tre-um) Either of the two upper chambers of the heart.

blood pressure The pressure of the blood against the walls of the arteries.

cardiac muscle The muscle of the heart.

diastole (di-as′to-le) The dilatation, or resting period, of the heart, especially of the ventricles.

heart A hollow muscular organ that receives blood from the veins and propels it into the arteries.

heart rate (pulse) The wave of pressure that is created by the heart contracting and forcing blood out the left ventricle and into the major arteries.

inferior vena cava (in-fēr′e-or ve′nah ka′vah) One of the two largest veins in the body that carries blood from the lower extremities and the pelvic and abdominal organs into the heart.

myocardium (mi″o-kar′de-um) The heart muscle.

perfusion (per-fu′zhun) The process whereby blood enters an organ or tissue through its arteries and leaves through the veins providing tissue with nourishment and removing wastes.

superior vena cava (soo-pe′re-or ve′nah ka′vah) One of the two largest veins in the body that carries blood from the upper extremities, head, neck, and chest into the heart.

systole (sis′to-le) The contraction, or working period, of the heart, especially that of the ventricles.

vein A tubular vessel that carries blood from the capillaries and venules into the right atrium of the heart.

ventricle (ven′trĭ-k′l) Either of the two lower chambers of the heart.

venule (ven′ūl) A small vein into which blood passes from the capillaries.

The circulatory system is what keeps the "human machine" running. It delivers oxygen and nutrients to the brain and to the cells of all of the body tissues. It takes away cellular wastes and carbon dioxide. It works as a closed circuit—blood is continuously pumped by the heart from the left ventricle through the aorta; into the arteries, the arterioles, the capillaries, the venules, the veins; and back into the heart. It is a long route, but in only one minute the body's entire blood volume of 5 to 6 liters has circulated through all these vessels.

Problems occur whenever something interferes with this complicated circulation system. Illness such as heart attack or stroke or injuries in which vessels are lacerated can be of life-threatening proportions within minutes because the human machine will not run if the blood cannot deliver oxygen and glucose to the brain.

Chapter 8 begins with an explanation of how blood circulates in the body. It then describes the elements that make up the circulatory system. These include blood, the heart, arteries, and veins. The last section is about pulse and blood pressure, both of which relate to how blood is pumped through the circulatory system.

GOALS

. . . .

The goals of Chapter 8 are to
- learn how blood circulates in the body.
- describe the components of the circulatory system—blood, the heart, the arteries, and the veins.
- become familiar with pulse and blood pressure and understand how loss of blood pressure can bring on shock.

. . . .

HOW BLOOD CIRCULATES
. . . .

The *circulatory (cardiovascular) system* is a complex arrangement of connected tubes that include arteries, arterioles, capillaries, venules, and veins. At the center of the system, and providing its driving force, is the heart. Blood circulates throughout the entire body under pressure generated by the two sides of the heart. The *systemic circulation,* sometimes called the greater circulation, carries oxygenated blood from the left ventricle of the heart throughout the body and back to the right atrium of the heart. The *pulmonary circulation,* sometimes

called the lesser circulation, carries deoxygenated blood from the right ventricle through the lungs and back to the left atrium. In the greater circuit, as blood passes through the tissues and organs it gives up oxygen and nutrients and absorbs cellular wastes and carbon dioxide. The cellular wastes are eliminated in passages through the liver and the kidneys. In the lesser circuit, as blood passes through the lungs it gives up carbon dioxide and absorbs oxygen.

Oxygenated blood flows out from the left ventricle of the heart through the aorta to pass to the body in general (Figure 8–1). It leaves

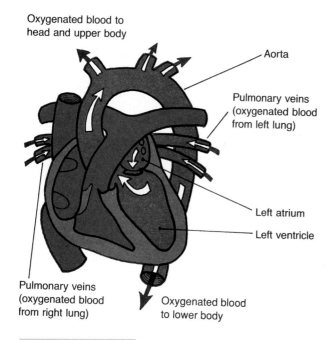

FIGURE 8–1

The left-sided, or higher-pressure, pump of the heart circulates oxygenated blood to all parts of the body.

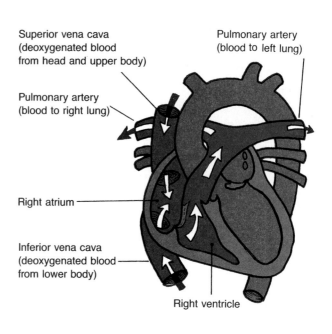

FIGURE 8–2

The right-sided, or lower-pressure, pump of the heart circulates blood from the body to the lungs.

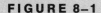

the aorta through **arteries.** The arteries gradually become smaller, and at the *arterioles* (smallest arteries), the blood finally passes into the *capillaries.* Arterioles, like all arteries, contain a muscle layer in their walls; this vessel type regulates the blood flow into the capillaries. Capillaries are small, thin-walled vessels in which individual red blood cells and plasma can make close contact with the individual cells of the body. The blood then empties into small veins **(venules),** which unite and become larger the closer they get to the heart. Veins deliver blood to the right atrium of the heart at the junction of the superior and inferior venae cavae (Figure 8–2). The blood then passes to the right ventricle, where it is pumped to the lungs. The blood passes through the pulmonary arteries, arterioles, capillaries, venules, veins, large pulmonary veins, left atrium, and finally flows into the left ventricle, where it is again circulated to the body.

The circulatory system is entirely closed, with capillaries connecting arterioles and venules. There are two circuits in the body. The

circuit in the lungs reoxygenates the blood and allows carbon dioxide to leave the blood. The circuit in the body delivers oxygenated blood to the tissues and also picks up carbon dioxide and other waste products of cellular activity. The capillaries are the fine-channel network where these exchanges take place. The life of the organism as a whole depends on the life of each cell within it. Capillary perfusion of tissues, the process whereby oxygen and nutrients are brought to every cell and waste and carbon dioxide are removed, is the key to continuous healthy existence.

Perfusion must be very clearly understood. It means that blood is entering an organ or tissue through its arteries and leaving through the veins. It also implies that nutrients and oxygen are successfully delivered to all body cells and that the waste products of cellular activity are picked up and transported to the lungs, liver and kidneys to be eliminated. To do so, the blood must pass through the appropriate capillary bed and provide tissue nourishment and waste removal. Thus, adequate perfusion means the provision of adequate oxygen and nutrition for each cell in the body. It also means adequate removal of waste and carbon dioxide. Perfusion of an organ can fail because of local vessel injury, shock, heart failure, or a number of more complex causes. With inadequate perfuson, cells and tissues die.

COMPONENTS OF THE CIRCULATORY SYSTEM

Blood

Blood is a complex, thick, red fluid composed of *plasma*, red blood cells called *erythrocytes*, white blood cells called *leukocytes*, and *platelets* (Figure 8–3.) Plasma is a sticky, yellow fluid that carries the blood cells and nutrients. It also transports cellular waste material to the organs of excretion. It contains most of the compounds needed to produce a blood clot. The iron-containing hemoglobin molecules in red blood cells (RBCs) give color to the blood and carry oxygen. White cells play a role in the body's immune defense mechanisms against infection. Platelets are tiny, disc-shaped elements that are much smaller than the cells; they are essential in the initial formation of a blood clot, the mechanism that stops bleeding.

Blood under pressure will gush or spurt intermittently from an artery and is bright red. From a vein, it will flow in a steady stream and is dark bluish-red. From capillaries, it will ooze at many tiny individual points. Clotting normally takes from 6 to 10 minutes.

The Heart

The **heart** is a hollow muscular organ approximately the size of an adult's clenched fist. A wall called the *septum* divides the heart down the middle into right and left sides. Each side of the heart is divided again into an upper chamber **(atrium)** and a lower chamber **(ventricle).**

The heart works as two paired pumps. The right side of the heart receives blood from the veins of the body. The blood enters from the venae cavae into the right atrium, then fills the

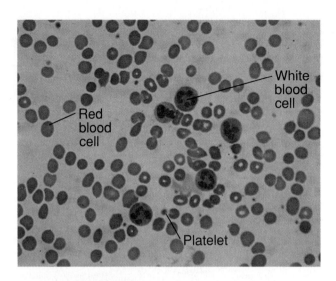

Red blood cell
White blood cell
Platelet

FIGURE 8–3

The microscopic appearance of the three major elements of the blood: red blood cells, white blood cells, and platelets.

right ventricle passing through a valve that closes to prevent backflow after the right atrial muscle contracts. Contraction of the right ventricle causes blood to flow into the pulmonary artery and the pulmonary circulation (Figure 8–2).

The left side receives oxygenated blood from the lungs through the pulmonary veins into the left atrium where it passes through a valve into the left ventricle. Contraction of this most muscular of the pumping chambers pumps the blood into the aorta and then to the arteries of the body (Figure 8–1).

The exit of each of the four heart chambers is governed by a one-way valve. The valves prevent the backflow of blood and keep it moving through the circulatory system in the proper direction. When a valve controlling the filling of a heart chamber is open, the other valve allowing it to empty is shut and vice versa. Normally, blood moves in only one direction through the entire system.

When a ventricle (lower chamber) contracts, the valve to the artery opens, and the valve between the ventricle and atrium (upper chamber) closes. Blood is forced from the ventricle out into the pulmonary artery or aorta. At the end of contraction, the ventricle relaxes. Back pressure causes the valve to the artery to close, and the entry valve to the ventricle opens as the ventricle relaxes. Blood then flows from the atrium into the ventricle. When the ventricle is stimulated to contract, the cycle is repeated.

The complete cycle that a blood cell makes in the circulatory system is shown in Figure 8–4.

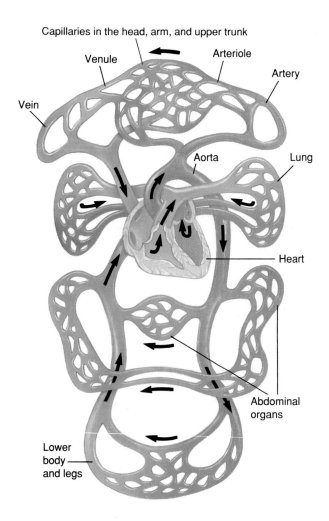

FIGURE 8–4

A schematic representation of the circulatory system, including the heart, arteries, veins, and interconnecting capillaries. The capillaries, the smallest vessels, connect arterioles with venules. In the capillaries an exchange of nutrients and waste products occurs between tissues and blood. In the lung an exchange of gases takes place between blood and air in the alveoli.

In the normal adult, the heartbeat may range from 50 to 180 beats per minute, depending on the level of activity. A very well-conditioned athlete may have a normal resting **heart rate (pulse)** of 50 to 60 beats per minute. During vigorous physical activity, the heart rate may rise normally to as fast as 180 beats per minute. The "usual" adult resting heart rate is between 60 and 100 beats per minute. At each beat, 70 to 80 milliliters of blood are ejected from the adult heart. In one minute, the entire blood volume of 5 to 6 liters is circulated through all the vessels.

The heart is made of a unique, adapted tissue called **cardiac muscle** or **myocardium.** It is actually two paired pumps with the one on the left being more muscular. The heart must function as a muscle continuously from birth to death and has developed special adaptations to meet the needs of this continuous function. It can tolerate a serious interruption of its own blood supply for only a very few seconds before the signs of a heart attack develop. Thus, its blood supply is as rich and well distributed as possible. It receives the first blood distribution from the aorta (Figure 8–5). The two main coronary arteries have their openings immediately above the aortic valve at the beginning of the aorta where the pressures are highest.

The heart is an *involuntary muscle*. As such, it is under the control of the *autonomic nervous system*. However, it has its own intrinsic regulatory system and will continue functioning even if its central nervous system control is lost. It is distinct from skeletal or smooth muscle both in its microscopic appearance and its requirement for a continuous supply of oxygen and nutrients.

The Arteries

The **aorta** is the major artery leaving the left side of the heart. It carries freshly oxygenated blood to the body. This blood vessel is found just in front of the spine in the chest and abdominal cavities. The aorta has many branches that supply the heart, head, neck, arms, and abdominal and thoracic organs before it ends in the lower abdomen. It divides at the level of the umbilicus into the two common *iliac arteries* that lead to the lower extremities (Figure 8–6a). All of the aorta's branches ultimately become arterioles leading into the body's capillary network.

In the body there are billions of cells and billions of capillaries. Capillary vessels are fine end divisions of the arterial system that allow contact between cells of the body tissues and the plasma and the red blood cells. At this level, each individual cell of the body lives. Oxygen and other nutrients pass from blood cells and plasma in the capillaries to the individual tissue cells through the very thin wall of the capillary (Figure 8–7a). Carbon dioxide and other metabolic waste products pass in a reverse direction from the tissue cells to the blood to be carried away. Blood in arteries is characteristically bright red, because its hemoglobin is rich in oxygen. Blood in the veins is dark bluish red, because it has passed through a capillary bed and given up its oxygen to the cells. Capillaries connect directly at one end with the flow regulating arterioles and at the other with the venules.

The Veins

Blood from the capillary system returns to the heart through the veins. Capillaries empty into small venules that join to form the **veins**. The larger veins of the entire body ultimately join to form two major vessels, the **superior vena cava** and **inferior vena cava** (Figure 8–6b). Blood returning from the head, neck, shoulders, and upper extremities passes through the superior vena cava. Blood from the abdomen, pelvis, and lower extremities passes through the inferior vena cava. The superior and inferior venae cavae join at the right atrium of the heart. The right ventricle receives blood from the right atrium and pumps it through the pulmonary arteries into the lungs.

FIGURE 8–5

The coronary arteries are the first branches of the aorta. They provide a rich supply of blood to the cardiac muscle.

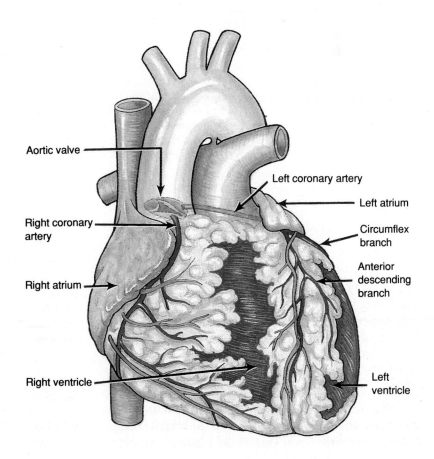

Aortic valve

Right coronary artery

Right atrium

Right ventricle

Left coronary artery

Left atrium

Circumflex branch

Anterior descending branch

Left ventricle

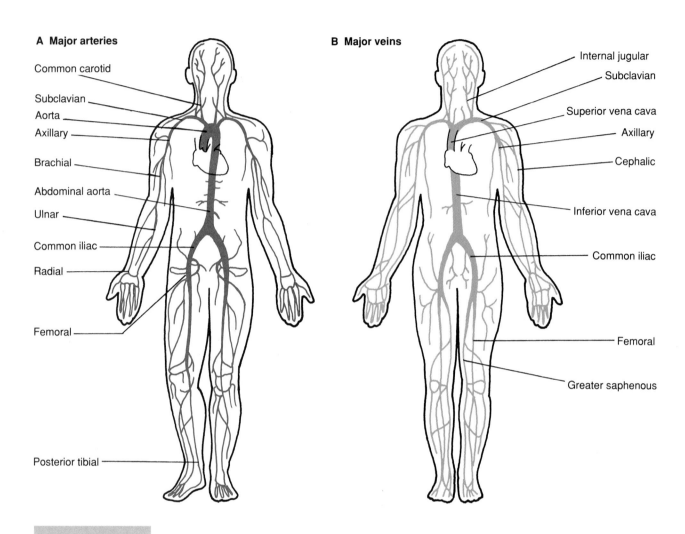

A Major arteries

- Common carotid
- Subclavian
- Aorta
- Axillary
- Brachial
- Abdominal aorta
- Ulnar
- Common iliac
- Radial
- Femoral
- Posterior tibial

B Major veins

- Internal jugular
- Subclavian
- Superior vena cava
- Axillary
- Cephalic
- Inferior vena cava
- Common iliac
- Femoral
- Greater saphenous

FIGURE 8–6   (A) The major arteries of the body distribute oxygenated blood from the heart to the principal organs or regions of the body. The name of each artery corresponds to the organ or region served. (B) The major veins are named to correspond to the regions of the body they drain. Blood is returned by these veins to the heart, which pumps it through the lungs for oxygenation.

Circulation in the Lungs

The general plan of circulation through the lungs is essentially the same as that in the rest of the body. Blood vessels from the right side of the heart branch and rebranch, finally forming capillaries. The *pulmonary capillaries* lie close to the *alveoli* (air sacs) of the lungs. The exchange of oxygen and carbon dioxide between air in the lung and blood in the capillaries is rapid (Figure 8–7b). Oxygen from the air in the alveoli diffuses to the red blood cell's hemoglobin molecules turning the cell a bright red. Carbon dioxide from the blood plasma rapidly

diffuses into the alveoli. The oxygenated blood from the lungs enters the four *pulmonary veins* that unite at the left atrium. It then passes to the left ventricle and is pumped to the body again.

PULSE AND BLOOD PRESSURE
· ·

The Pulse

The *pulse*, which is palpated most easily at the neck, wrist, or groin, is created by the forceful

A

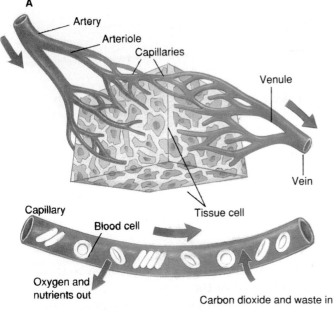

B

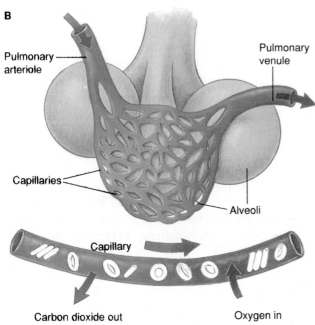

FIGURE 8–7

The exchange of oxygen and carbon dioxide between blood in vessels and tissue cells. The capillary is no larger than a single blood cell. (A) Oxygen (O_2) passes from the blood through capillaries to tissue cells. In the reverse process, carbon dioxide (CO_2) passes from tissue cells through capillaries to the blood. (B) In the lung, O_2 is picked up by the blood and CO_2 is given off.

pumping of blood out the left ventricle and into the major arteries. It is present throughout the entire arterial system. It can be felt most easily where the larger arteries are near the skin. The *carotid artery pulse* can be felt at the upper portion of the neck; the *radial artery pulse* is felt at the wrist, at the base of the thumb; the *femoral artery pulse* is felt in the groin. The pulse rate is the same as the heart rate. The usual adult resting pulse can range from 60 to 100 beats per minute, and in infants and children, it is normally slightly higher (see Table 8–1).

Blood Pressure

Blood pressure is the pressure that the blood exerts against the walls of the arteries as it passes through them. When the cardiac muscle of the left ventricle contracts, it pumps blood from the ventricle into the aorta. This muscular contraction phase is called **systole.** When the muscle of the ventricle relaxes, the ventricle fills with blood. This phase is called **diastole.** The pulsed forceful ejection of blood from the left ventricle of the heart into the aorta is transmitted through the arteries as a pulsatile pressure wave. This pressure wave keeps the blood moving through the body. The high and low points of the wave can be measured with a *sphygmomanometer* (blood pressure cuff) and are expressed numerically in millimeters of mercury (mm Hg). The high point is called the systolic blood pressure (measured as the heart muscle is contracting). The low point is called the diastolic blood pressure (measured when the heart muscle is in its relaxation phase).

Normal adult arterial blood pressure is usually 120/80 mm Hg. In infants and children it is less (see Table 8–1). Normal systolic blood pressure in children ranges from 90 to 110 mm Hg; in infants it ranges from 50 to 90 mm Hg. The diastolic blood pressure normally ranges between 60 and 80 mm Hg in children. Because diastolic pressure is the level to which arteries are subjected constantly, it is regarded as very important in patients with hypertension. Sustained high diastolic blood pressure is more significant for patients than an intermittent high systolic reading.

Both the wave and the flow of blood can be stopped by applying pressure on an artery.

	Premature Infant	Term Infant	1 Year	3 Years	6 Years	10 Years	14 Years
Table 8-1 Pulse Rate, Systolic Blood Pressure and Respiratory Rate, by Age							
Pulse Rate	140	140	130	80	80	75	75
Systolic Blood Pressure	50-60	70	90±30	100±25	100±15	110±20	115±20
Respiratory Rate	50-60	40-60	22-30	20-26	20-24	18-22	14-20

Applied pressure must exceed the pressure of the blood that flows through the artery. Several factors control *arterial pressure.* They include the blood volume itself, the state of the arteries and arterioles (whether they are dilated or constricted), the capacity of the heart muscle to contract normally, and the normal elasticity of the arteries.

Pressure of blood in the veins (*venous pressure*) is much less than that in the arteries. This low pressure aids in the return of blood to the heart. If the venous pressure falls below normal, insufficient blood is returned to the heart, and a failure in the circulatory system occurs. Two factors control the venous pressure: blood volume (the amount of blood within the circulatory system) and vascular volume (the capacity of the veins).

The average adult has approximately 6 liters of blood in the vascular system. Children have less—2 to 3 liters—depending on their age and size; infants have only about 300 milliliters. The loss of an amount of blood that may be negligible for an adult could be fatal for a baby.

In all healthy people, the circulatory system is automatically adjusted and readjusted constantly so that 100 percent of the capacity of the arteries, veins, and capillaries holds just 100 percent of the blood at that moment. Never are all the vessels fully dilated or constricted (Figure 8-8). The size of arteries and veins is controlled by the nervous system, according to the amount of blood available and many other factors to keep blood pressure normal at all times. Under the condition of normal pressure, with a system that can hold just 100 percent of

the blood available, all parts of the system will be perfused all of the time.

Loss of normal blood pressure is an indication that the blood is no longer circulating efficiently to every organ in the body. There are many reasons for loss of blood pressure. The result in each case is the same: organs, tissues, and cells are no longer adequately perfused or supplied with oxygen and food, and wastes can accumulate. Under these conditions, cells, tissues, and whole organs may die. The state of inadequate perfusion, when it involves the entire body, is called *shock.*

When a patient loses a small amount of blood, the arteries, veins, and heart automatically adjust to the smaller new volume. The adjustment occurs in an effort to maintain adequate pressure throughout the circulatory system and thereby maintain circulation for every organ. The adjustment occurs very rapidly after the loss, usually within minutes. Specifically, the vessels contract to provide a smaller bed for the reduced volume of blood to fill. And the heart pumps more rapidly to circulate the remaining blood more efficiently. As the blood pressure falls, the pulse increases to attempt to keep the cardiac output constant at 5 to 6 liters per minute. If the loss of blood is too great, the adjustment fails and the patient goes into shock.

The change in the size of arteries and veins is brought about by muscles in their walls under the continuous control of the autonomic nervous system. These muscles can contract or relax in response to changes in blood volume, heat, cold, fright, an injury, or an infection.

The contraction or relaxation of the muscle causes a change in the diameter of the artery or vein. These muscles do not act as pumps; they only change the diameter of the vessels and hence their volume. If the muscles of the arteries and veins contract, the vessel diameters decrease; the system therefore holds less fluid. If these muscles relax, then the vessels dilate and the system can hold a larger volume of blood. Massive dilation of the vessels can produce a system too large for the normal volume of blood available. Once again, shock occurs, and all organs, because they are poorly perfused, are at risk. Figure 8–8 is a schematic representation of some of these relationships.

Finally, shock can also be a signal that the muscle of the heart is incapable of pumping sufficiently to maintain circulation. This condition is seen in the patient with a *myocardial infarction* (heart attack) from direct damage of the muscle itself. The topic of shock is more fully discussed in Chapter 12.

A Normal system (6 liters)

Blood reservoir

Blood vessels

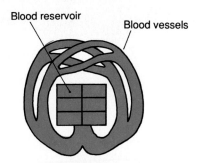

B Constricted system (shock)

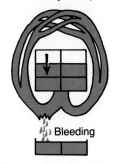

Bleeding

C Dilated system (shock)

Inadequate blood supply

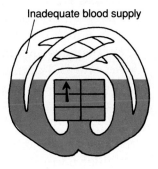

FIGURE 8–8

A schematic representation of the volume of blood in the body under varying circumstances. (A) The normal blood volume in an adult is 6 liters. (B) When bleeding occurs, the blood volume in the veins and arteries decreases, and the blood vessels constrict. If severe bleeding causes the volume of blood in circulation to be reduced rapidly, the patient may go into shock. (C) If the walls of the blood vessels become relaxed, the peripheral vascular system enlarges to hold more blood, thereby reducing the amount of blood in circulation as effectively as if bleeding to the outside of the body had occurred. Therefore, shock can be produced in a patient without any loss of blood from the body.

YOU ARE THE EMT

1. Where does the systemic circulation carry oxygenated blood? Where does the pulmonary circulation carry oxygenated blood?
2. What is capillary perfusion? Why is it so important?
3. What is the difference between venous pressure and arterial pressure? What two factors control venous pressure?
4. Does shock occur when the arteries and veins contract or dilate? Explain.
5. Name the only major artery in the body that normally carries unoxygenated blood.

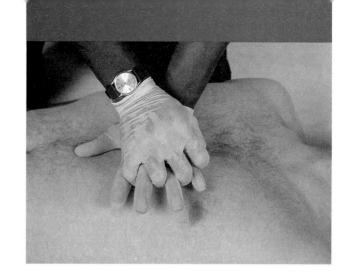

CHAPTER 9

BASIC LIFE SUPPORT: ARTIFICIAL CIRCULATION

KEY TERMS

acute myocardial infarction (ah-kūt' mi"o-kar'de-al in-fark'shun) Heart attack; specifically, death of the heart muscle from obstruction of its blood flow.

arrhythmia (ah-rith'me-ah) An irregular or abnormal heart rhythm.

asystole (ah-sis'to-le) Complete absence of heart activity.

automated external defibrillator (AED) Equipment that analyzes the electrical activity of the patient's heart and, under the right conditions, delivers an electrical charge to restore the heartbeat.

cardiac arrest A sudden ceasing of heart function.

cardiopulmonary resuscitation (CPR) The artificial establishment of circulation of the blood and movement of air into and out of the lungs in a pulseless, nonbreathing patient.

electrocardiogram (ECG or EKG (e-lek"tro-kar'de-o-gram") A recording of the electrical current that flows through the heart. The results are displayed on a paper strip or a display screen or (usually) both.

ischemic (is-kem'ik) Lacking oxygen.

pulseless electrical activity (PEA) The form of cardiac arrest in which the electrocardiogram displays an adequate heart rate and rhythm, but the heart is incapable of generating a palpable pulse and blood pressure in the circulation.

ventricular fibrillation (ventrik'u-lar fi-brĭ-la'shun) A continuous, uncoordinated quivering of the cardiac muscle.

ventricular tachycardia (ventrik'u-lar tak"e-kar'de-ah) A very rapid heart rate.

OVERVIEW

The patient is in cardiac arrest. Time is critical. Only minutes separate life and death. Before CPR training was taught in schools and communities, death usually won out. Now, however, more and more people know how to perform cardiopulmonary resuscitation and take advantage of those few life-and-death minutes. Thus you are apt to arrive at the scene and find someone has already begun CPR on a cardiac arrest patient. You must then evaluate the patient, assess the technique, and assist the rescuer, without ever interrupting the stride. Or, you may arrive and discover there is no assistance available. In this situation, you must use the few precious minutes that are available to institute one-rescuer CPR. In any cardiac arrest emergency, your role is critical.

Chapter 9 begins by defining cardiac arrest and naming its major causes. The chapter next focuses on the techniques of providing artificial circulation to adults, including external chest compression with a single rescuer, with the entry of a second rescuer, and with two rescuers. Also discussed are the modifications necessary when artificial circulation is ad-

ministered to infants and children. American Heart Association skills sheets are included.

Chapter 9 concludes with a discussion of the primary cause— ventricular fibrillation—of cardiac arrest and defibrillation, its best treatment. The current rationales and use of automated external defibrillation are fully described and discussed.

GOALS

The goals of Chapter 9 are to
- define cardiac arrest and identify its causes.
- become knowledgeable in the techniques of administering artificial circulation to adults.
- recognize the adjustments that have to be made when you provide artificial circulation to children or infants.
- become familiar with the rationale and use of automated external defibrillators.

CARDIAC ARREST

Cardiac arrest is the failure of the heart to generate an effective and perceptible blood flow. In cardiac arrest, pulses are not palpable, even in the major vessels (the carotid and femoral arteries). Effective blood flow does not exist. Cardiac arrest does not mean that the heart is without any muscular or electrical activity. Indeed, the heart can consume a great

deal of energy during cardiac arrest and demonstrate much muscular activity. However, uncoordinated or excessively rapid beating does not produce effective blood flow. Indeed, in situations in which muscular activity remains but is uncoordinated and produces no blood flow, the heart continues to consume energy while cut off from perfusion itself. The consumption of energy will ultimately cause more damage to the heart tissue, in part because of the accumulation of waste products. The four major causes of cardiac arrest are ventricular tachycardia, ventricular fibrillation, electromechanical dissociation, and asystole.

Ventricular tachycardia (rapid ventricular rate) is an **arrhythmia** (abnormal heart rhythm) in which the ventricles of the heart beat so fast that there is not enough time for the pumping chambers to fill adequately between beats. The ventricular contraction rate commonly ranges between 140 and 250 beats per minute. When ventricular tachycardia persists, effective body and heart perfusion declines. The heart becomes more **ischemic** (lacking oxygen), wastes build up, and ventricular fibrillation usually ensues. In ventricular tachycardia, the **electrocardiogram (ECG or EKG)** tracing shows recognizable waves. These waves disappear as this arrhythmia degenerates into fibrillation.

In **ventricular fibrillation,** the major pumping chambers of the heart undergo continuous and chaotic uncoordinated muscular quivering (fibrillation). This is the most common arrhythmia occurring in up to 70 percent of all cardiac arrests. No effective blood flow comes out of the heart, because the ventricles do not contract. This state may occur because of loss of blood supply to the heart muscle or an electrical malfunction of the heart's intrinsic electrical coordination system. This is usually a result of coronary artery disease. Because the heart itself is not perfused, no oxygen and nutrients reach it to support the muscular activity. In the absence of oxygen, the muscle contractions rapidly deplete the heart of its own energy stores and produce waste products that further weaken the heart muscle. If this arrhythmia is not terminated by immediate electrical countershock, the heart muscle will continue to lose energy and stop beating completely.

Pulseless electrical activity (PEA) is that form of cardiac arrest in which the EKG displays an apparently adequate heart rate and rhythm, but no palpable pulse or blood pressure is detectable. Pulseless electrical activity is usually caused by a variety of disorders: hypoxia, massive blood loss, cardiac tamponade, tension pneumothorax, acute pulmonary embolism, anaphylactic shock, acidosis, or a se-

vere heart attack. Obviously, in these cases it is necessary to identify the most likely cause of the pulseless electrical activity and proceed rapidly with attempts to correct it. Meanwhile, because the heart is not beating effectively, it is necessary to institute **cardiopulmonary resuscitation (CPR).**

The conditions leading to pulseless electrical activity often progress rapidly. They must be treated promptly. These considerations underscore the need for prompt treatment of the underlying cause and for *absolutely prompt* restoration of circulation. Rapid CPR is mandatory to restore adequate perfusion and oxygenation of the heart so that it can continue to function while proper definitive care is directed at the cause of the arrest.

In **asystole,** the heart is essentially without any electrical or detectable muscular activity. It is not beating. No pulses are felt. There is no electrical activity to record on an electrocardiogram. This stage is the final point to which all other cardiac arrest states may come without appropriate intervention. It certainly is the state found when someone is ultimately, irreversibly dead.

In ventricular fibrillation, pulseless electrical activity, and asystole, the institution of CPR is not sufficient by itself to resuscitate and maintain the patient. Advanced procedures and drugs are often needed. Rapid and safe patient transport is also needed. Therefore, the American Heart Association's 1992 guidelines recommend that the rescuer activate EMS even before beginning initial rescue breathing or a primary survey in unconscious adult patients.

ARTIFICIAL CIRCULATION IN ADULTS

Disturbances of the regular electrical rhythm and activity of the heart may prevent adequate cardiac muscular contraction and result in the failure of the heart to generate blood flow and produce a pulse. Any significant damage of the heart muscle itself from **acute myocardial infarction** or various cardiac muscle diseases may render the heart unable to contract properly. The absence of a strong, palpable central pulse, such as the carotid or femoral, indicates no blood flow and hence the presence of cardiac arrest.

Assessment of Circulation

Unconsciousness is always present in cardiac arrest states lasting more than 10 seconds, because the brain is not being properly perfused. After determining the patient's level of consciousness, calling for help, turning the patient if necessary, opening the airway, assessing the patient's respiratory status, and starting artificial ventilation, you must assess the circulation. Cardiac arrest is determined by the absence of a palpable pulse in a large artery, usually the carotid. The carotid artery is palpated in the neck. It is found most easily by locating the *larynx (Adam's apple)* at the front of the neck and then sliding two fingers toward one side. The pulse is felt in the groove between the larynx and the *sternocleidomastoid muscle*, with the pulp of the index and long

fingers held side by side (Figure 9–1). Light pressure is sufficient to palpate the pulse. Excessive pressure must not be applied because it can obstruct the carotid circulation, dislodge blood clots, or produce marked reflex slowing of heart activity.

Another conveniently felt large artery near the skin is the femoral artery in the groin. When pulses are not palpable, you can confirm the absence of heart activity by listening over the left chest using your ear or a stethoscope.

When the patient has been positioned for artificial ventilation, the hand on the forehead that has been maintaining backward head tilt is left in position to maintain the airway. The other hand is used to locate the carotid pulse. If the pulse is present but breathing is absent, you should perform rescue breathing as described in Chapter 7 until adequate breathing resumes. If the pulse is absent, begin *external*

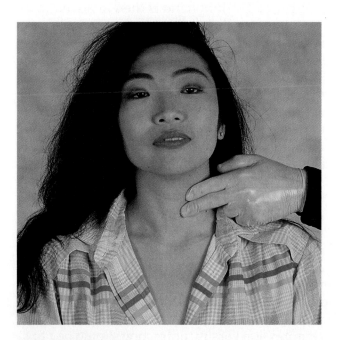

FIGURE 9–1

The carotid pulse is felt in the groove between the larynx and the sternocleidomastoid muscle.

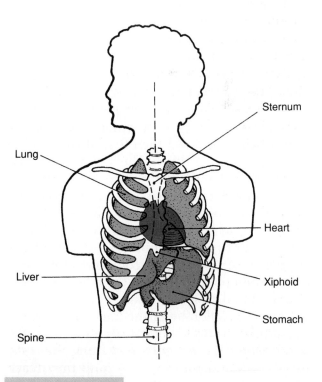

FIGURE 9–2

The heart lies slightly to the left of the middle of the chest between the sternum and the spine, with the lungs on either side and with the liver and stomach below.

chest compressions, which adds artificial circulation to the already initiated artificial ventilation.

External Chest Compression

The heart lies slightly to the left of the middle of the chest between the sternum and the spine (Figure 9–2). Rhythmic pressure and relaxation applied to the lower half of the sternum is believed to compress the heart between it and the spine and produce an artificial circulation.

In any patient with cardiac arrest, the cardiac output resulting from external chest compression, even flawlessly performed, is only about one-quarter to one-third of normal. For this flow rate to be achieved, the patient must be on a firm, flat surface. It may be the ground, the floor, or a spine board on an ambulance litter. The patient who is in bed must be placed rapidly on the floor. This step is quicker than looking for some type of firm support and minimizes the delay in starting cardiac compression. External chest compression must always be accompanied by artificial ventilation.

With a Single Rescuer If you are working alone, first activate the EMS system, and then position the adult patient properly. Then kneel close to the patient's side, with one knee at the level of the head and the other at the level of the upper chest. Place the heel of one hand on the lower half of the body of the sternum. Take great care *not* to place the hand on either the xiphoid process, which extends downward over the upper abdomen and liver, or beside the sternum onto the ribs or costal cartilages (Figure 9–3). The former could result in lacerated abdominal organs, and the latter results in fractured and dislocated ribs.

Correct positioning of the hands is achieved by sliding the index and long fingers of the hand nearer the patient's feet along the *costal margin* (edge of the rib cage) until they reach the xiphoid notch in the center of the chest (Figure 9–4a). The long finger is pushed as high as possible into the notch, and the index finger is then laid on the lower portion of the sternum with the two fingers touching (Figure 9–4b). The heel of the other hand is then placed on the lower half of the sternum (Figure

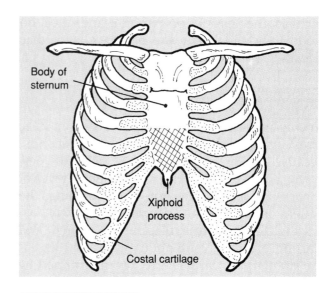

FIGURE 9–3

The xiphoid process is at the lower tip of the sternum and extends downward over the upper abdomen. The shaded area of the sternum is compressed.

9–4c) so that it touches the index finger of the first hand. The first hand is then removed from the notch in the center of the rib cage and applied over and parallel to the hand now resting on the patient's lower sternum (Figure 9–4d). *Only the heel of one hand is in contact with the lower half of the sternum.* The technique may be improved or made more comfortable if the fingers of your lower hand are interlocked with the fingers of your upper hand and pulled slightly away from the chest wall.

Exert pressure vertically downward through both arms to depress the adult sternum 1½ to 2 inches. A rocking motion, rising gently upward, allows pressure to be delivered vertically down from your shoulders while your elbows are kept straight (Figure 9–5). Vertical downward pressure produces a compression that must be followed immediately by an equal period of relaxation. The ratio of time devoted to compression versus contraction should be 1 to 1.

The actual motions must be smooth, rhythmic, and uninterrupted. Short, jabbing compression strokes are ineffective in producing artificial blood flow. The heel of your hand should not be removed from the chest during

A

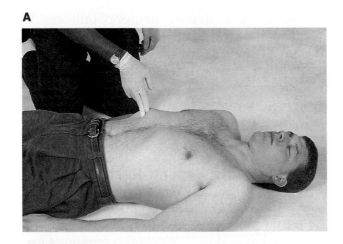

B

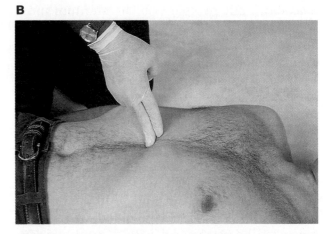

C

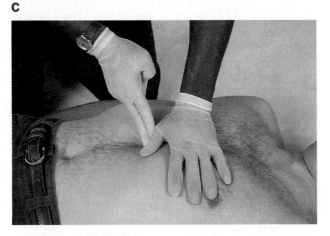

D

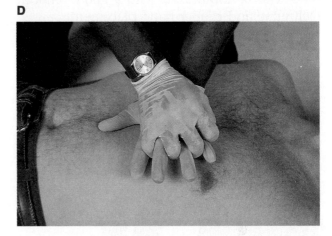

FIGURE 9–4

The correct hand position for chest compression: (A) Slide your index finger and your long finger nearest the patient's feet along the center of the patient's rib cage to the notch in the center of the chest. (B) Push the long finger high into the notch, and lay the index finger on the lower portion of the sternum. (C) Then place the heel of the second hand on the lower half of the sternum, touching the index finger of your first hand. (D) Remove your first hand from the notch and place it over and parallel to the hand on the sternum.

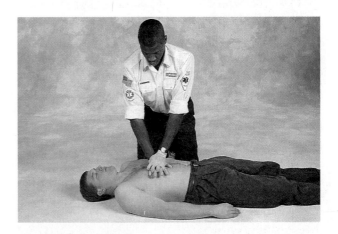

FIGURE 9–5

External chest compression is produced by vertical downward pressure through both extended arms to depress the adult sternum 1½ to 2 inches.

relaxation, but pressure on the sternum must be completely released so it can return to its normal resting position between compressions. Compression and relaxation must be rhythmic. Your hand must not bounce or come away from the patient's chest during compression (Figure 9–6). Considerable attention must be given to the actual technique of compression because, even well done, it carries some risk. Complications of cardiac compression have included fractured ribs, lacerated liver, ruptured spleen, or fracture of the sternum. Although these injuries cannot be entirely avoided, their occurrence can be minimized with a good, smooth technique and proper hand placement.

When alone, you must pause to give artificial ventilation. Then cardiac compressions must be resumed at a rate of 80 to 100 per minute. After every 15 cardiac compressions, you should deliver 2 ventilations (ratio 15:2). The 15 compressions are delivered in approximately 10 seconds. Two full ventilations are delivered in the next 4 to 5 seconds using at least 1½ to 2 seconds for each inspiration. A check for the return of spontaneous carotid pulsations (pulse check) should be done after the first minute of CPR and then at least every 5 minutes thereafter (Figure 9–7).

With Entry of a Second Rescuer When a second EMT becomes available after single-EMT CPR has been started and is in progress, the recommended procedure for entry into the resuscitation is simple. Without stopping CPR, the original EMT announces clearly that everything is ready for a switch to two-person CPR.

The logical point of entrance is after a sequence of 15 compressions and 2 breaths. The second EMT begins by initially assuming responsibility for chest compressions. This starts after a CPR assessment, a pulse check, and a ventilation.

The second rescuer feels for the patient's carotid or femoral pulse as the first rescuer finishes a sequence of 15 compressions. This CPR assessment includes evaluating the CPR pulse wave generated by the first rescuer's compressions, the rescuer's hand positioning, the patient's color, the patient's position, and the overall effectiveness of the CPR. While the first rescuer delivers two respirations and then feels for a spontaneous carotid pulse for 5 seconds, the second rescuer should position his or her hands in the proper sternal location and prepare to deliver chest compressions. If the first rescuer finds no pulse, he or she should deliver a single respiration over a 1½ to 2 second interval, and command, "Continue CPR," whereupon the second rescuer begins a series of five chest compressions.

The ratio with two rescuers is *five* compressions to *one* 1½ to 2 second rescue breath. Pulse checks should be approximately 5 seconds in duration and should be conducted after the first minute of CPR and then every 5 minutes thereafter. The ideal time to switch positions is when these pulse checks occur.

When EMTs are switching positions, then follow the same sequence. It is accomplished following a ventilation, a five second check for

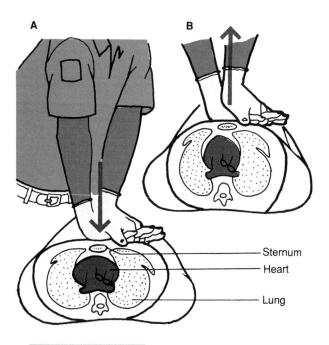

A   B

Sternum
Heart
Lung

FIGURE 9–6

(A) Compression and relaxation should be rhythmic and of equal duration. The heel of the hand should not be removed from the sternum. (B) Pressure on the sternum must be released so it can return to its normal resting position between compressions.

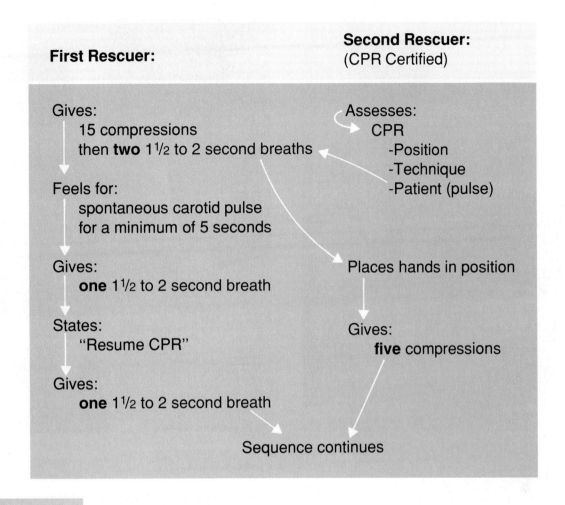

First Rescuer:

Gives:
    15 compressions
    then **two** 1½ to 2 second breaths

Feels for:
    spontaneous carotid pulse
    for a minimum of 5 seconds

Gives:
    one 1½ to 2 second breath

States:
    "Resume CPR"

Gives:
    one 1½ to 2 second breath

Second Rescuer:
(CPR Certified)

Assesses:
    CPR
    -Position
    -Technique
    -Patient (pulse)

Places hands in position

Gives:
    five compressions

Sequence continues

FIGURE 9–7   A suggested sequence for two-rescuer CPR.

a spontaneous carotid pulse, and yet another slow 1½ to 2 second ventilation by the new respirator while the other rescuer establishes his or her hand position on the sternum. Compressions start with the command, "Resume CPR."

Professional rescuers (rescue squad members, EMTs, medical and paramedical professionals) should be proficient in both one- and two-rescuer techniques. Two-rescuer CPR provides an opportunity for a coordinated effort that is less fatiguing and more effective. The two-rescuer technique allows better treatment of the patient and should be used whenever possible.

When two EMTs arrive to treat one patient, both must act promptly. One rescuer goes to the head of the patient and performs a primary

survey, while the second EMT gets in position to give chest compressions. The EMT at the head checks for absence of breathing and pulse by performing the "look, listen, and feel" procedure while feeling for the carotid pulse with one hand. If both breathing and pulse are absent, the EMT at the head gives two rescue breaths and CPR is begun.

Two-EMT CPR should be performed with the EMTs on opposite sides of the patient (Figure 9–8). They can easily switch positions when necessary without significant interruption in the ventilation-compression sequence. To switch, the EMT who is providing ventilation, after giving a breath, moves into position to begin cardiac compression. The EMT performing compression, after the fifth compression, moves to the patient's head and checks

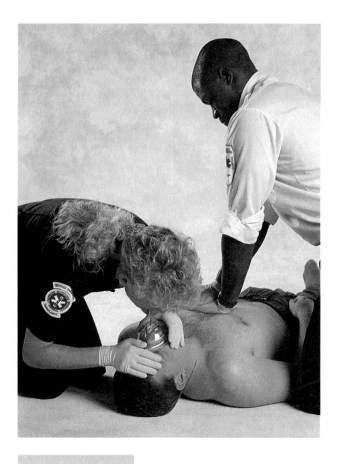

FIGURE 9–8

When two EMTs perform CPR, one is on each side of
the patient. Here, one EMT performs mouth-to-mask
ventilation while the other delivers external chest
compression.

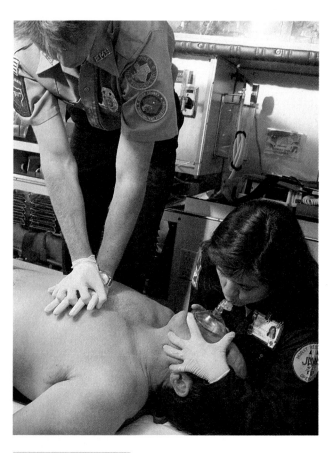

FIGURE 9–9

In an ambulance, two EMTs perform CPR from the
same side of the patient.

the pulse for 3 to 5 seconds. If no pulse is felt,
the EMT at the head ventilates the patient and
states, "No pulse; continue CPR."

When performing CPR on a litter in an
ambulance, both EMTs must work from the
same side of the patient (Figure 9–9). They can
switch positions using the following technique:
The EMT ventilating the patient rapidly moves
behind the EMT doing chest compressions and
assumes that role. The other EMT moves to the
head of the patient to check the pulse and
continue ventilation.

Effectiveness of CPR

It is appropriate to monitor the effectiveness
of cardiopulmonary resuscitation. The carotid
pulse must be palpated periodically for 3 to 5

seconds during CPR to check the effectiveness
of chest compression or the return of a spontaneous, effective heartbeat. Palpation should be
done after the first minute of CPR and every 5
minutes thereafter.

Pulse checks are performed by the EMT
doing the ventilation, particularly just before
switching positions during CPR. Pupils are
often assessed for responsiveness. Pupillary
reaction to light is generally considered a good
sign. However, normal pupillary reactions may
be altered in the elderly by eye operations. The
reactions are also drastically changed by the
use of medications and the presence of heightened levels of adrenalin. Return of normal skin
color or the resolution of cyanosis may also be
a positive sign.

The carotid pulse must be palpated periodically during CPR to check the effectiveness of chest compression or the return of a spontaneous, effective heartbeat.

There is ongoing research in measuring the possible efficacy of new techniques to improve CPR blood flow. These include pneumatic vest CPR, interposed abdominal compression CPR, and active compression-decompression CPR. The American Heart Association believes that more scientific proof is needed before they can present new techniques and change CPR guidelines.

CPR Interruption

Basic CPR should not be interrupted for more than 5 seconds, except when it is absolutely necessary to move a patient or in conditions where it is impossible to continue effective resuscitation. When a patient has to be moved up or down stairs, it is best to perform CPR at the head or foot of the stairs, then interrupt at a given signal and move quickly to the next level, where effective activity can be resumed. Interruptions should be held to as short a time as possible. The patient should not be moved until all transportation arrangements are set and you are ready and have sufficient assistance to provide uninterrupted CPR during transport.

Without advanced life support (monitoring, an intravenous line, cardiac medications, and defibrillation), basic life support will rarely be sufficient for patient survival, regardless of how well it is performed. If advanced life support modalities cannot be brought to the scene, the patient must be moved promptly to the hospital. Two-person CPR should be continued during transport to the hospital. CPR is an important "holding action," providing minimal circulation and ventilation until the patient can receive definitive care for the condition that caused the cardiopulmonary arrest.

CPR may be stopped in certain circumstances. When a physician or higher medical authority assumes responsibility for the patient, orders to "Stop CPR" may be appropriately observed; local protocols should govern these situations. When advanced life support procedures are to be performed, CPR may have to be briefly interrupted. When you become exhausted and are without the capability to transport the patient to a medical facility, as would occur in a wilderness or rural setting, CPR may have to be halted. When the patient regains pulse and respirations, CPR is, of course, discontinued.

ARTIFICIAL CIRCULATION IN INFANTS AND CHILDREN

The basic principles of CPR are the same whether the patient is an infant, child, or adult. The differences in performing CPR on an infant and child relate to the different underlying causes of emergencies in infants and children and the need for techniques that apply to variations in size.

In the majority of instances, cardiopulmonary arrest in infants and children begins with a respiratory arrest. Children consume oxygen two to three times as rapidly as do adults. Secondary cardiac arrest results from hypoxia and myocardial ischemia. Therefore, you must direct your major initial attention to the airway and ventilation. In many cases restoration of an open airway and adequate ventilation of the lungs is all that is needed for resuscitation.

For the purposes of CPR, anyone under 1 year of age is considered to be an infant. A child is classified as being between the ages of 1 and 8 years. Above 8 years, techniques for adults can generally be applied. Ninety pounds is often used as a weight guideline to separate children from adults. Variations can occur frequently among infants and children in size relative to age.

Assessment of Circulation

Once the airway and ventilation have been assessed and problems corrected as needed, you can focus on the circulation. As in the adult, this routine begins with a check for a palpable pulse. As in the adult, too, absence of a palpable major pulse defines the need for external chest compression to circulate the blood.

The pulse in a child can be felt over the carotid artery in a manner similar to that described for the adult. Palpating this pulse in an infant may present a problem. Unfortunately, the very short and, at times, fat neck of an infant makes the carotid pulse difficult to palpate. In infants, the brachial artery should be palpated to assess the quality of the patient's pulse.

The brachial artery is located on the inner side of the arm, midway between the elbow and shoulder (Figure 9–10). Place your thumb on the outer surface of the arm between the elbow and shoulder. Then position the tips of your index and long fingers to press lightly toward the bone, on the medial side of the biceps, to palpate the pulse.

External Chest Compression

It is in the technique of external chest compression that differences among infants, children, and adults become most apparent. The differences are related to the small size of the chest, the faster heart rate of the infant and the child, and the relative fragility of the surrounding organs.

Position of the Heart As the chest grows, the proportion of space occupied by the heart diminishes. The heart in the infant or child is situated at approximately the same level as in adults. If an imaginary line is drawn between the nipples, the proper area for compression lies one finger's breadth below this line on the sternum. Place your index finger just below the line as it crosses the sternum. The adjacent long finger identifies the most superior point for compression (Figure 9–11).

Using the same technique as described for the adult, locate the xiphoid notch in the center of the chest with your long finger. The area just under your index finger is then the appropriate place for compression. The sternum of the child is only 6 to 7 cm long. The thickness of two fingers of an adult EMT is 3 to 4 cm. Two fingers will easily cover the lower half of the sternum.

Chest Size The chest of an infant or child is smaller and more pliable than that of an adult. Two hands are not necessary for effective compression. In an infant, two fingers are adequate. With your fingers on the lower sternum, depress it ½ to 1 inch. As with adults, the patient must be on a hard surface for optimal results.

With a child, more force may need to be exerted, but the use of two or three fingers is usually adequate. If the child is large enough so that the sternum will not easily compress with

Checking the brachial pulse in an infant. This major pulse is located on the inner aspect of the upper arm, midway between elbow and shoulder. The tips of the index and middle finger are used to locate and palpate the brachial pulse.

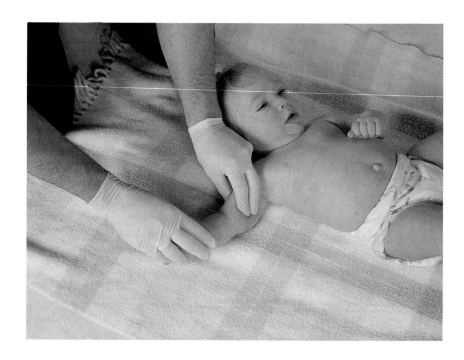

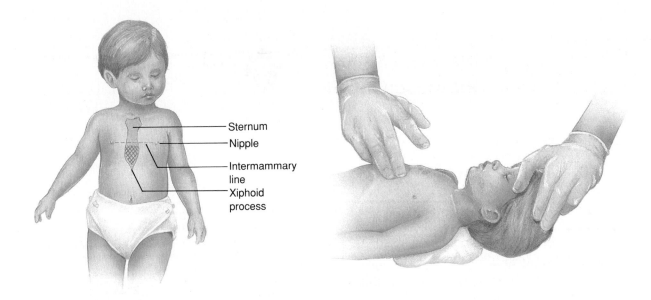

Sternum
Nipple
Intermammary line
Xiphoid process

FIGURE 9–11   The proper area for cardiac compression in a child is in the midline, one finger's breadth below the intermammary line.

three fingers, use the heel of one hand. The hand closest to the head should remain on the child's forehead during compressions. The hand performing compressions may remain on the chest during the ventilation cycle. If the chest does not rise, remove the compression hand and perform the head-tilt/chin-lift maneuver. Return the compression hand to the chest. Relocating the exact position of the sternum is not necessary. Place only the heel of your hand on the sternum; keep your fingers off the chest. If the patient is large enough to require the heel of the hand, the depth of compression should be 1 to 1½ inches.

Heart Rate Because of the faster heart rate in infants and children, the compression rate must also be faster. For infants and children, the minimum compression rate is 100 per minute.

Fragility of Organs Especially in infants, the liver is relatively large, immediately under the right diaphragm, and very fragile. The spleen on the left is much smaller and much less fragile than in adults. Each, however, may be injured by carelessly applied CPR. The fingers you will use for compression must be placed in the midline of the chest.

External chest compression on a child must be coordinated with ventilation, as in the adult. The rate of compression to ventilation is 5:1 for both single-EMT and dual-EMT rescue. When you are the only EMT present, after each fifth compression you open the airway and ventilate the patient once. If two EMTs are present, the ventilation is given during a pause after the fifth compression. For infants, one ventilation (1 to 1½ seconds per breath) should be given after every fifth compression. For infants, only one-person CPR is usually practiced in the field, although two-person CPR is certainly possible in highly favorable settings.

AMERICAN HEART ASSOCIATION GUIDELINES

On the following pages you will find the 1993 American Heart Association standard skill sheets for one- and two-rescuer CPR on adults, and one-rescuer CPR for children and infants. Also, the American Red Cross publishes skill sheets that are almost identical to those of the AHA. Consult your local protocols and state agencies for guidelines that may differ from the examples enclosed (Figures 9–12 through 9–15).

Skill Performance Sheet
Adult One-Rescuer CPR

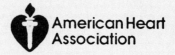

American Heart Association

Student Name _____ Date _____

Performance Guidelines	Performed
1. Establish unresponsiveness. Activate the EMS system.	
2. Open airway (head tilt–chin lift or jaw thrust). Check breathing (look, listen, feel).*	
3. Give 2 slow breaths (1½ to 2 seconds per breath), watch chest rise, allow for exhalation between breaths.	
4. Check carotid pulse. If breathing is absent but pulse is present, provide rescue breathing (1 breath every 5 seconds, about 12 breaths per minute).	
5. If no pulse, give cycles of 15 chest compressions (rate, 80 to 100 compressions per minute) followed by 2 slow breaths.	
6. After 4 cycles of 15:2 (about 1 minute), check pulse.* If no pulse, continue 15:2 cycle beginning with chest compressions.	

*If victim is breathing or resumes effective breathing, place in recovery position.

Comments _____

_____

_____

Instructor _____

Circle one: Complete   Needs more practice

FIGURE 9–12   Adult one-rescuer CPR performance sheet.

Reproduced with permission. Basic Life Support Heartsaver Guide, *1993. Copyright ©
American Heart Association.*

Skill Performance Sheet
Adult Two-Rescuer CPR

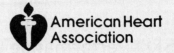

American Heart Association

Student Name _____ Date _____

Performance Guidelines	Performed
1. Establish unresponsiveness. EMS system has been activated.	
RESCUER 1	
2. Open airway (head tilt–chin lift or jaw thrust). Check breathing (look, listen, feel).*	
3. Give 2 slow breaths (1½ to 2 seconds per breath), watch chest rise, allow for exhalation between breaths.	
4. Check carotid pulse.	
RESCUER 2	
5. If no pulse, give cycles of 5 chest compressions (rate, 80 to 100 compressions per minute) followed by 1 slow breath by Rescuer 1.	
6. After 1 minute of rescue support, check pulse.* If no pulse, continue 5:1 cycles.	

*If victim is breathing or resumes effective breathing, place in recovery position.

Comments _____

_____

_____

Instructor _____

Circle one: Complete   Needs more practice

FIGURE 9–13   Adult two-rescuer CPR performance sheet.

*Reproduced with permission. Basic Life Support Heartsaver Guide, 1993. Copyright ©
American Heart Association.*

Skill Performance Sheet
Child One-Rescuer CPR

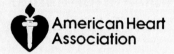 American Heart Association

Student Name _____ Date _____

Performance Guidelines	Performed
1. Establish unresponsiveness. If second rescuer is available, have him or her activate the EMS system.	
2. Open airway (head tilt–chin lift or jaw thrust). Check breathing (look, listen, feel).*	
3. Give 2 slow breaths (1 to 1½ seconds per breath), watch chest rise, allow for exhalation between breaths.	
4. Check carotid pulse. If breathing is absent but pulse is present, provide rescue breathing (1 breath every 3 seconds, about 20 breaths per minute).	
5. If no pulse, give 5 chest compressions (100 compressions per minute), open airway with chin lift, and provide 1 slow breath. Repeat this cycle.	
6. After about 1 minute of rescue support, check pulse.* If rescuer is alone, activate the EMS system. If no pulse, continue 5:1 cycles.	

*If victim is breathing or resumes effective breathing, place in recovery position.

Comments _____

_____

_____

Instructor _____

Circle one: Complete   Needs more practice

FIGURE 9–14   Child one-rescuer CPR performance sheet.

Reproduced with permission. Basic Life Support Heartsaver Guide, 1993. Copyright © American Heart Association.

Skill Performance Sheet
Infant One-Rescuer CPR

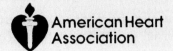

American Heart Association

Student Name _____ Date _____

Performance Guidelines	Performed
1. Establish unresponsiveness. If second rescuer is available, have him or her activate the EMS system.	
2. Open airway (head tilt–chin lift or jaw thrust). Check breathing (look, listen, feel).*	
3. Give 2 slow breaths (1 to 1½ seconds per breath), watch chest rise, allow for exhalation between breaths.	
4. Check brachial pulse. If breathing is absent but pulse is present, provide rescue breathing (1 breath every 3 seconds, about 20 breaths per minute).	
5. If no pulse, give cycles of 5 chest compressions (rate, at least 100 compressions per minute) followed by 1 slow breath.	
6. After about 1 minute of rescue support, check pulse.* If rescuer is alone, activate the EMS system. If no pulse, continue 5:1 cycles.	

*If victim is breathing or resumes effective breathing, place in recovery position.

Comments _____

_____

_____

Instructor _____

Circle one: Complete   Needs more practice

FIGURE 9–15   Infant one-rescuer CPR performance sheet.

*Reproduced with permission. Basic Life Support Heartsaver Guide, 1993. Copyright ©
American Heart Association.*

AUTOMATED EXTERNAL DEFIBRILLATION

In an ever-increasing number of communities, automated external defibrillators are becoming standard equipment on basic life support rescue vehicles. In areas that had no advanced life support capabilities but where early defibrillation was instituted, survival rates from cardiac arrest quadrupled. The American Heart Association and the International Association of Fire Chiefs have endorsed the delivery of early defibrillation at the basic EMT and CPR level as a standard of care. This final section presents the rationale for this technique, a brief description of the available equipment, the American Heart Association's recommended method of application and coordination with basic and advanced life support, and possible problems which may occur.

Ventricular fibrillation is best treated with defibrillation, the application of a sufficient amount of electrical energy directed across the heart to stop the heart from fibrillating. If defibrillation is successful, the heart begins beating on its own, with a rhythm that allows it to successfully perfuse the body. Automated external defibrillation is the use of a highly sophisticated device designed to permit the safe and reliable delivery of this lifesaving therapy by basic life support (BLS) rescuers. The difference between this automated method of delivering lifesaving therapy and *manual* defibrillation (discussed in Supplement C) lies in the fact that the AED computer program analyzes the electrical and mechanical activity of the patient's heart. Manual defibrillation, on the other hand, requires that the EMT be proficient in ECG rhythm analysis and be able to judge when defibrillation is or is not required.

Defibrillation was previously reserved for EMT-paramedic level or higher levels of emergency care personnel, but now automatic external defibrillation (AED) is often performed by BLS rescue personnel. The technology has been shown to be safe and sound. The protocols have become standardized. Its use is easy to learn and maintain. Most of all, it has been shown to increase substantially the percentage of lives saved.

The 1992 American Heart Association National Conference on Cardiopulmonary Resuscitation and Emergency Cardiac Care strongly endorsed the principle of early defibrillation. This principle states that "all personnel whose jobs require that they perform basic CPR be trained to operate and be permitted to use defibrillators, particularly automated external defibrillators (AEDs)." This guideline is intended to include all first-responding BLS trained in-hospital or out-of-hospital emergency personnel. Early defibrillation has become the standard of care for patients with either prehospital or in-hospital cardiac arrest, except in sparsely populated and remote settings. Thus, early defibrillation is a critical link in the chain of survival, following early access and early CPR and preceding early advanced cardiac life support (ACLS).

Rationale for Early Defibrillation

The most frequent abnormal rhythm following sudden cardiac arrest is ventricular fibrillation. More than 385,000 people in the United States experience sudden death from cardiovascular disease each year. In areas without advanced EMS systems, only 5 percent of those experiencing sudden cardiac arrest survive to be admitted to the hospital. In areas where the EMS system is strong, up to 70 percent of people with ventricular fibrillation who have a cardiopulmonary arrest in the prehospital setting reach the hospital with a spontaneous pulse and blood pressure.

Sixty-five percent of deaths from acute myocardial infarctions are due to ventricular fibrillation and occur within the first hour of the attack. If basic life support begins within 4 minutes and defibrillation occurs within 8 minutes of the cardiac arrest, it has been shown that 40 percent of these patients will live to be discharged from the hospital.

The chances of successful defibrillation decrease as the delay to defibrillation increases. After 10 minutes without CPR and without defibrillation, fewer than 1 in 250 have been resuscitated. Effective artificial circulation and ventilation has been shown to extend the ability of the heart to survive for longer times in fibrillation. However, CPR alone cannot reinstitute normal rhythm for hearts in ventricular fibrillation. Ventricular fibrillation decays to asystole as the heart becomes ischemic. The most effective treatment for ventricular fibrillation is electrical defibrillation as early as possible after cardiac arrest. The major determinant of survival is "time to defibrillation."

Types of Automated External Defibrillators

An **automated external defibrillator (AED)** is a device which, when hooked up to a patient, can enable you to deliver an appropriate defibrillatory shock to the heart. To do so, the AED must sense the electrical and mechanical changes of the heart and analyze these inputs using an internal computer. It will assess whether a patient is in ventricular fibrillation or pulseless ventricular tachycardia. If the patient

has one of these conditions, the AED will charge its capacitors to a preset level to deliver a defibrillatory countershock. During the use of the AED, CPR and all other patient contact must cease (Figure 9–16).

Automated external defibrillators currently in use are transportable and durable and have a means of recording the patient's electromechanical cardiac condition and the actions taken at the scene. This record is necessary to facilitate quality assurance and medical control by your system's medical director. A semi-automatic or "shock-advisory" AED (Figure 9–17) analyzes the patient's condition. When appropriate, this AED charges its capacitor, but it will not deliver the shock until the operator presses a shock button. An automatic AED, on the other hand, proceeds to deliver an appropriate shock after the operator hooks it up and initiates the machine's rhythm analysis mode without further intervention by the operator.

Exhaustive testing and years of practical experience have made the presently available AED models very reliable. Their main errors

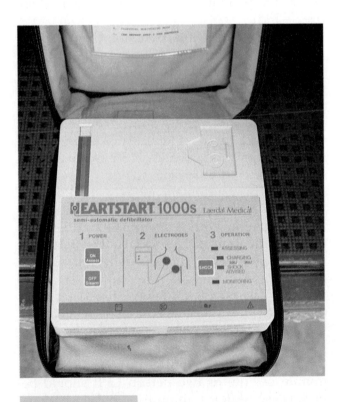

FIGURE 9–16

Automated external defibrillator (AED).

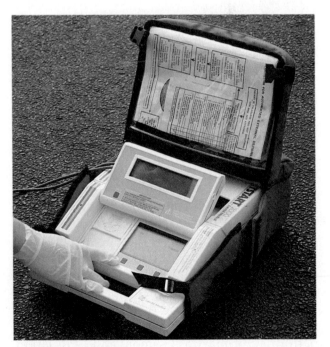

FIGURE 9–17

A semiautomatic AED.

occur when the operator fails to recognize subtle varieties of ventricular fibrillation or tachycardia. AEDs have not shocked a patient who was not in need of defibrillation; they are specifically programmed to prevent this from happening. AEDs have not been fooled by patient seizures, by agonal respirations, by movement of the patient, or by artifactual signals. Although no inappropriate shocks have been reported during the past 10 years, an AED should *only* be placed on a patient and switched on if the patient is assessed to be in cardiac arrest and all patient movement, CPR, and/or transport has ceased.

AEDs are programmed to check for radio transmissions, 60-cycle interference, loose electrodes, pacemakers, patient movements, continued heartbeat, and poor electrode contact. They take multiple samples or "looks" at the patient's heart rhythm. Each analysis lasts just a few seconds. Several of these analyses must confirm the presence of ventricular fibrillation or fast ventricular tachycardia for the AED to charge its capacitors and permit the delivery of a defibrillatory current.

AED Operations

All AEDs operate by completing a relatively simple process that starts when you attach the device to the patient and turn it on. The AED starts to analyze the patient's rhythm. If indicated, the machine then delivers an appropriate shock. Various models have differing features and controls. You must become thoroughly familiar with the specific model you are using. This information will be taught to you in a skills oriented training program. Maintain your skills through continuing practice.

A minimum of two persons are required in an AED rescue team. One member begins CPR while the other operates the AED. The AED operator should govern the initial management of the cardiopulmonary arrest patient.

After the patient has been moved to a flat surface with plenty of working room, one EMT performs a primary assessment and CPR. Upon verification of an arrest, the AED operator places the AED near the patient's ear (Figure 9–18a).

Next, the machine is turned on (Figure 9–18b). This activates the voice and ECG tape or solid state recorder and permits the machine to record the operator's statements as well as the patient's cardiac rhythm. Identifying data and patient history should be stated loudly and clearly by the operator as he or she removes the adhesive pads from their sealed envelopes and attaches them to the AED's cables.

The patient's chest should be bared and dried, if sweaty. If excessive hair is present, a prep razor is used to clear a small area for the placement of the defibrillator pads (Figure 9–18c). One pad is placed on the upper right chest and one on the lower left chest, just to the left of the heart's apex. If the patient has a pacemaker implanted, the pads should be placed 4 to 6 inches away from the battery pack of the pacemaker. The left lead is often color-coded red, and the right lead colored white, which you can remember with "White to the right, red over the heart."

Once the AED is turned on and the pads affixed to the patient, the operator should inform all present not to touch the patient by saying, "Clear the patient," or "Everybody clear" (Figure 9–18d).

On most AEDs, the operator checks to be sure that no one is touching the patient, then presses the analyze button (Figure 9–18e). The device takes from 5 to 15 seconds to analyze the patient's rhythm. If a treatable rhythm is present, the AED emits an audible tone that rises in pitch as the defibrillator charges, its screen (if present) advises, "Shock advised," and a voice synthesizer states, "Shock advised." A fully automatic model would deliver the shock at this point, and the patient would be seen to jerk. With semiautomatic AEDs, the operator must press the shock control button at this point. After the shock is delivered, CPR is not restarted. The analyze button is again pressed. The goal is to deliver three shocks as quickly as the machine advises that mode of therapy.

After the third shock, the patient is assessed for the presence of a pulse. If none is found, 1 minute of one- or two-person CPR should be performed. After 1 minute, a pulse check is performed and the patient is "cleared." The AED's analyze button is again pushed. Again, if treatable rhythms are present, three stacked

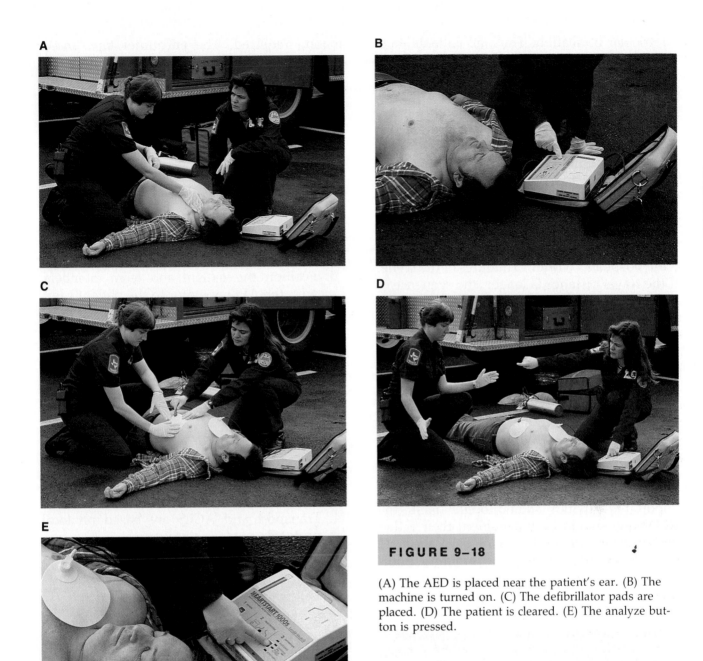

A

B

C

D

E

FIGURE 9–18

(A) The AED is placed near the patient's ear. (B) The machine is turned on. (C) The defibrillator pads are placed. (D) The patient is cleared. (E) The analyze button is pressed.

shocks are delivered without any intervening contact with the patient. After this basic sequence, local protocol and the availability of advanced life support services will govern further patient rescue activities.

Up to 92 percent of patients who are success-fully defibrillated respond to the first two countershocks. After a successful response, the patient usually requires ventilatory support and the administration of 100 percent oxygen. You must be aware that up to 25 percent of patients who are defibrillated will go back into ventricular fibrillation. Thus, all patients must be closely monitored and the AED operation repeated if the patient again arrests.

When advanced life support services arrive, the AED operation should be smoothly incorporated into existing defibrillation protocols. The AED team should be allowed to deliver the first three countershocks while the advanced life support team prepares for intravenous and endotracheal therapy. In systems without advanced life support services, transport is recommended following two sets of three stacked countershocks, with CPR being given en route if the hospital is within 15 minutes of the scene. If the travel distance is longer, the sequence of three stacked shocks with an intervening minute of CPR are continued until an effective pulse returns or local protocol dictates that no further shocks be given. This instance should be governed by the protocols of the local medical director.

The AED can be left attached to the patient (Figure 9–19) during ambulance transport to monitor the cardiac rhythm, but it should not be placed in the analyze mode because the vehicle motion will interfere with its operation.

After each field defibrillation effort, two very important activities should occur. First, the AED crew should fully document their activities for future reference. The medical director's protocols will dictate the basic minimum infor-

mation required. The encounter tape and/or memory module should be transmitted with the written documentation to the medical director for review. Second, the treatment of each arrest should be critiqued as outlined by policies and procedures of your medical director.

The steps in automated defibrillation are:

1. At the beginning of each shift, check all equipment and batteries, and designate an operator.
2. En route to the scene, anticipate AED use.
3. At the scene, find and assess the patient.
4. Institute CPR.
5. Position the patient and team members, with the AED operator to the patient's left.
6. When the primary assessment shows no pulse, the decision to use AED occurs.
7. Turn on machine. Attach pads to cables and then to patient.
8. Cease all contact with patient.
9. Press the analyze button.
10. Announce patient data and team data.
11. Shock if indicated, 3 times.
12. Do a pulse check, 1 minute of CPR, then another pulse check.
13. Repeat AED analysis and repeat shock if indicated, 3 times.
14. Transport and ACLS are based on local protocol.

Precautions, Energy, Age and Weight Guidelines

The energy sequence usually programmed into the AED for the three stepped shocks is 200 Joules-200 Joules-360 Joules. Your local medical director may choose to alter the second energy level to 300 Joules. All shocks after the third shock should be at the 360-Joule energy level. When ventricular fibrillation returns after successful defibrillation, it is recommended that the initial energy level be the same as the last successful countershock.

Defibrillation should not be attempted when anyone is in contact with the patient, when the patient is lying in a pool of water, when there are explosive vapors around, or when the patient is hypothermic.

Cardiac arrest in the pediatric age group is not usually caused by ventricular fibrillation.

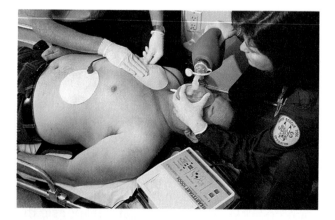

FIGURE 9–19

The AED can be left attached during transport.

Automated Defibrillators: Operator's Shift Checklist

Date _____ Shift _____ Location _____

Mfr/Model No. _____ Serial No. or Facility ID No. _____

At the beginning of each shift, inspect the unit. Indicate whether all requirements have been met. Note any corrective actions taken. Sign the form.

	OK as Found	Corrective Action/ Remarks
1. Defibrillator Unit Clean, no spills, clear of objects on top, casing intact		

2. Cables/Connectors
   a. Inspect for cracks, broken wire, or damage
   b. Connectors engage securely and are not damaged*		

3. Supplies
   a. Two sets of pads in sealed packages, within expiration date*
   b. Hand towel
   c. Scissors
   d. Razor
   e. Alcohol wipes*
   f. Monitoring electrodes*
   g. Spare charged battery*
   h. Adequate ECG paper*
   i. Manual override module, key, or card*
   j. Cassette tape, memory module, and/or event card plus spares*		

4. Power Supply
   a. Battery-powered units
     (1) Verify fully charged battery in place
     (2) Spare charged battery available
     (3) Follow appropriate battery rotation schedule per manufacturer's recommendations
   b. AC/battery backup units
     (1) Plugged into live outlet to maintain battery charge
     (2) Test on battery power and reconnect to line power		

5. Indicators*/ECG Display
   a. Remove cassette tape, memory module, and/or event card*
   b. Power-on display
   c. Self-test OK
   d. Monitor display functional*
   e. "Service" message display off*
   f. Battery charging; low battery light off*
   g. Correct time displayed; set with dispatch center		

6. ECG Recorder*
   a. Adequate ECG paper
   b. Recorder prints		

7. Charge/Display Cycle
   a. Disconnect AC plug—battery backup units*
   b. Attach to simulator
   c. Detects, charges, and delivers shock for VF
   d. Responds correctly to nonshockable rhythms
   e. Manual override functional*
   f. Detach from simulator
   g. Replace cassette tape, module, and/or memory card*		

8. Pacemaker*
   a. Pacer output cable intact
   b. Pacer pads present (set of two)
   c. Inspect per manufacturer's operational guidelines		

Major Problem(s) Identified (Out of Service)		

*Applicable only if the unit has this supply or capability

FIGURE 9–20   AED daily checklist.
Reproduced with permission. Textbook of Advanced Cardiac Life Support, *1994. Copyright © American Heart Association.*

Defibrillation in the pediatric age group should not take priority over airway clearance and maintenance. Priority should be given to rescue breathing. AEDs should not be used on patients younger than 12 years old or weighing less than 90 pounds.

The most common sources of problems in all defibrillator programs are two: human and machine. Although the initial training on the AED takes less than 8 hours, it must be refreshed at 90-day intervals to maintain peak skill levels. Lack of familiarity with the equipment or treatment protocols is a cause of treatment delay. It is recommended that the AED be checked each shift to be sure that it functions properly. Battery failure is a common defibrillator problem. A fully charged spare battery should always be carried with the AED. A daily maintenance sheet as shown in Figure 9–20 should be kept. Proper AED maintenance is critical and is described further in Supplement C.

Summary of AED Operation

The following points regarding AED operation merit emphasis:

- Always perform the basic ABCs before attaching the AED.
- Once the AED is attached and activated, CPR ceases until analysis is performed and no shock is advised or three shocks are delivered.
- Always shock in sets of three.
- Anytime the chest is touched after the first assessment, it should be to perform CPR for 1 minute.
- Continue to shock until the "no shock indicated" message is received unless the patient is being transported to a hospital within 15 minutes of the arrest location.
- Advanced life support personnel arriving on the scene have scene authority.
- Once the patient regains a spontaneous pulse, close supportive care is mandatory, especially ventilatory support.

YOU ARE THE EMT

1. How does ventricular fibrillation differ from ventricular tachycardia? Why are both called arrhythmias?

2. You have been told that the patient you are about to treat is in cardiac arrest. How will you confirm this report?

3. Why must external chest compression be accompanied by artificial ventilation?

4. You and your partner have been performing two-EMT CPR on a patient for 10 minutes. How do you monitor the effectiveness of your efforts?

5. Explain why all contact with the patient ceases when the AED is being used on a patient in cardiac arrest. Outline the AED protocol.

CHAPTER 10

VENTILATION EQUIPMENT AND OXYGEN THERAPY

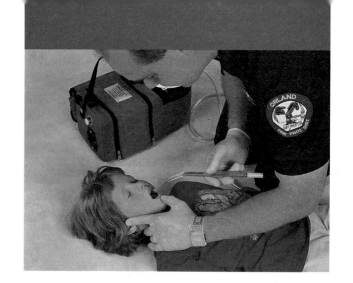

KEY TERMS

barrier device A protective item, such as gloves or a mask, that provides a relatively effective barrier to patient secretions and limits intimate patient contact during basic life support or mouth-to-mouth resuscitation.

cannula (kan'u-lah) A tube for insertion into a duct or cavity.

cerebrovascular accident (ser"ĕ-bro-vas'ku-lar ak'sĭ-dent) (stroke) A sudden lessening or loss of consciousness, sensation, and voluntary movement caused by rupture or obstruction of an artery in the brain.

chronic obstructive pulmonary disease (COPD) A slow process of dilation and disruption of the airways and alveoli, caused by chronic bronchial obstruction.

cyanosis (si"ah-no'sis) Blue color of the skin resulting from poor oxygenation of the circulating blood.

emphysema (em"fĭ-se'mah) Disease of the lungs in which there is extreme dilation and eventual destruction of pulmonary alveoli, with poor exchange of oxygen and carbon dioxide. Also called chronic obstructive pulmonary disease (COPD).

flowmeter A flow regulator attached to the pressure regulator on emergency medical equipment. It permits the regulated release of gas measured in liters per minute.

humidification (hu-mid"ĭ-fĭ-kay'shun) Process of adding moisture during artificial ventilation to prevent pure oxygen from drying the patient's mucous membrane surfaces.

hypoxia (hi-pok'se-ah) A deficiency of oxygen reaching the tissues of the body.

myocardial infarction Heart attack; damage or death of an area of the heart muscle.

nasopharyngeal airway (na" zo-fah-rin'je-al ār'wa) An artificial airway placed in the nasal cavity.

oropharyngeal airway (o"ro-fah-rin'je-al ār'wa) An artificial airway positioned in the mouth to prevent blockage of the upper airway by the tongue.

pocket mask Mask with an oxygen inlet that allows you to ventilate the patient with air from your own lungs while at the same time supplying supplemental oxygen.

pulmonary edema (pul'mo-ner"e ĕ-de'mah) Fluid building up in the lungs, a result of congestive heart failure.

suctioning The use of negative air pressure to remove materials from the airway.

Venturi mask A breathing unit that provides a specific concentration of oxygen through a delivery tube connected to a face mask.

Although basic life support for a patient with respiratory or cardiac arrest may be carried out without any mechanical aids, common practice at the EMT level now requires the routine use of certain ventilatory adjuncts to care for the respiratory needs of the sick or injured patient. You should take every advantage of this equipment as it becomes available to assist in the provision of prehospital ventilatory care. You should be thoroughly familiar with exactly how to provide oxygen-enriched air to all types of patients.

The various means of providing oxygen and regulating the delivery to patients who require supplementary oxygen are standard in the United States. Several precautionary systems exist to ensure that patients do not receive wrong gases by error. Of course, it is imperative that you become skilled in the use of all artificial ventilation equipment, because incorrect or inefficient use could cause a patient's condition to worsen.

Chapter 10 begins with a definition of hypoxia (oxygen deficiency) and its effects on the body. Then the ways of delivering supplemental oxygen are described. Suctioning devices for keeping the airway clear of mucus or vomitus are discussed next. The last sections cover when to use oxygen, its possible hazards, its storage, and equipment for its delivery.

GOALS

The goals of Chapter 10 are to
- define hypoxia and understand why sick or injured patients usually need supplemental oxygen.
- learn how to use the various artificial ventilation devices.
- become familiar with suctioning devices and their use.
- recognize when supplemental oxygen is needed.
- identify the hazards of supplemental oxygen.
- learn how to handle oxygen in compressed gas cylinders, recognize the different types of regulators, and know when to replace a cylinder.
- become knowledgeable about the equipment available for oxygen delivery.

BARRIER DEVICES

Many devices on the market today provide a relatively effective barrier to patient secretions and limit intimate patient contact during basic life support mouth-to-mouth resuscitation. Some of these **barrier devices** are shown in Figure 10–1. These breathing devices all feature a plastic barrier placed on the patient's face and a one-way valve to prevent backflow of secretions and gases. It is a good idea for all rescuers to carry these devices on all runs. They are good infection control barriers and provide a measure of confidence to the BLS rescuer and thus reduce the reluctance to perform mouth-to-mouth rescue breathing on a stranger.

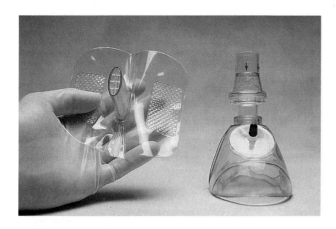

FIGURE 10–1

Barrier devices can be used to protect the rescuers from the patient's secretions.

THE NEED FOR SUPPLEMENTAL OXYGEN

The atmosphere contains more oxygen than we need to maintain proper function of our vital organs: heart, lungs, and brain. Oxygen is present in the air at a concentration of about 21 percent. We inhale air containing 21 percent oxygen, extract about one-fourth of it, and exhale air containing 16 percent oxygen. Thus, during mouth-to-mouth ventilation, 16 percent oxygen is delivered to the patient. This concentration is sufficient to oxygenate the blood passing through the lungs and provide enough oxygen to sustain life. Because external chest compression produces at best an effective cardiac output of only 33 percent of normal, only a limited amount of oxygen can be delivered to the body's vital organs. The combination of a low inspired oxygen concentration and a markedly reduced cardiac output leaves the patient *hypoxic* (oxygen deficient) even with the best artificial ventilation and cardiac compression techniques.

Hypoxia causes vital tissues to deteriorate rapidly. Injured tissues have an even greater need for oxygen than do healthy tissues. Therefore, the use of supplemental oxygen as early as possible will increase the patient's chances for recovery. Oxygen should be delivered at 100 percent concentration to any patient who has sustained a cardiopulmonary arrest. Any patient who has sustained any injury is likely to benefit from supplemental oxygen. Oxygen should never be withheld from any sick or injured patient.

ARTIFICIAL VENTILATION EQUIPMENT

During cardiopulmonary arrest, circulation and ventilation are both absent. Artificial ventilation using a high oxygen concentration must have an oxygen source and an effective method of delivery.

Pocket Mask with an Oxygen Inlet

A **pocket mask** with an oxygen inlet has been designed to provide supplemental oxygen during mouth-to-mouth ventilation (Figure 10–2). Other models of this device come with a one-way valve that attaches between your mouth and the mask. Extension tubes may also facilitate ventilation of the patient. The use of this valved mask is recommended for all EMTs performing basic life support. The mask allows you to ventilate the patient with air from your own lungs while at the same time supplying supplemental oxygen. The actual artificial

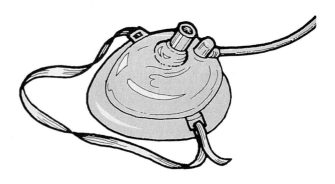

FIGURE 10–2

A pocket mask with a chimney can be used for mouth-to-mask ventilation. An inlet port for supplemental oxygen is shown.

breathing is done by you, but significant oxygen enrichment of inspired air is possible. The mouth-to-mask system frees both of your hands to aid in keeping the airway open and provide a better seal between the mask and the face. The one-way valve prevents backflow of oral secretions from the patient to the rescuer.

The mask, triangular in shape, has a narrow angle at the apex that is placed across the bridge of the nose. The base of the mask is placed in the groove between the lower lip and the chin. Rising from the center of the dome of the mask is a chimney with a 15 millimeter connector. You should follow these steps when using the pocket mask during mouth-to-mask ventilation:

1. Stand or kneel at the patient's head and open the airway with a head-tilt maneuver.
2. Connect the one-way valve to the face mask. Place the mask on the patient's face with the apex over the bridge of the nose and the base in the groove between the lower lip and chin.
3. Grasp the patient's mandible with the index, long, and ring fingers of each hand (the ring finger being on the ramus behind the angle) and place your thumbs on the dome of the mask. Maintain an airtight seal by applying firm pressure between the thumbs and the fingers (Figure 10–3a).
4. Keep the airway open by the upward and forward pull of the fingers on the mandible.
5. Take a deep breath and exhale through the open port of the one-way valve atop the chimney (Figure 10–3b).
6. Remove your mouth and observe the patient's chest collapsing during passive exhalation (Figure 10–3c). The timing of each breath is the same as that described for the standard mouth-to-mouth technique of artificial ventilation (Chapter 7).

The oxygen concentration of air delivered to the patient can be increased by the addition of the gas through the oxygen inlet valve. Any oxygen delivered to the patient is diluted with your exhaled breath. For example, 10 liters of oxygen per minute running to the mask will provide the patient with inspired air at approximately 50 percent oxygen concentration; 15

A

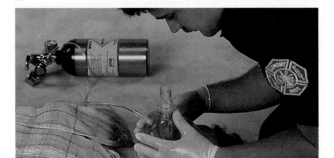

B

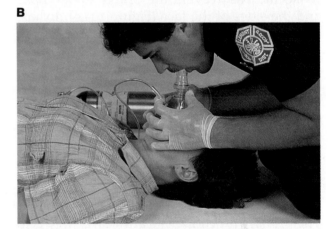

C

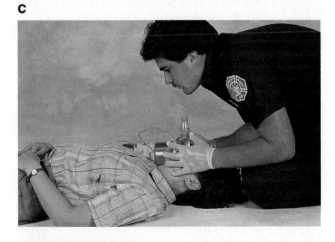

FIGURE 10–3

The steps in mouth-to-mask ventilation using a pocket mask: (A) Seal the mask to the face using both hands. The apex of the mask is over the bridge of the nose, and the base is between the lips and chin.
(B) Exhale into the chimney of the mask.
(C) During expiration, you must see the chest fall and feel the motion of exhaled air on your cheek.

liters per minute will provide inspired air at approximately 55 percent oxygen.

Provided that oxygen is being given and an airway can be maintained, this system also works well for the patient who is breathing spontaneously and does not require full ventilatory assistance but does require supplemental oxygen. The mask has an elastic strap for use with those patients who can breathe spontaneously.

The pocket mask may also be used for an infant. In this case the mask is turned around, and the apex is placed under the infant's chin while the base covers the bridge of the nose and the sides of the face (Figure 10–4). Exhale small breaths of air into the open port of the chimney, giving one breath over 1½ seconds. You must feel the resistance of the child's lungs as air is breathed in and must hear and feel the exhaled air move out. The rise and fall of the chest with each cycle should also be observed. Supplemental oxygen can be given in the same manner as described above for adults.

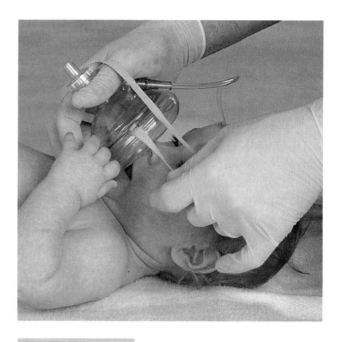

FIGURE 10–4

For an infant, the pocket mask is reversed, and the base is placed over the nose.

Artificial Airways

The primary function of an artificial airway is to prevent obstruction of the upper airway by the tongue and allow passage of air and oxygen to the lungs.

Oropharyngeal Airways An **oropharyngeal airway** keeps the tongue from occluding the upper airway, thus allowing the passage of respiratory gases and facilitating suctioning. The device is positioned in the mouth with the curvature of the airway following the contour of the tongue. The flange should rest against the lips; the other end opens into the pharynx. This airway has an opening down the center or along either side to permit the free passage of air or oxygen and to allow easy access for suctioning. An oropharyngeal airway should be inserted only in an unconscious patient or a patient without a gag reflex. If introduced into a conscious or semiconscious patient with an intact gag reflex, it could cause vomiting or *spasm* of the vocal cords. If incorrectly placed, instead of maintaining the airway the device can displace the tongue backward into the pharynx and actually produce airway obstruction. The technique for insertion of an oropharyngeal airway includes these steps:

1. Select the proper sized airway by measuring from the ear lobe to the corner of the mouth on the side of the face (Figure 10–5).
2. Open the patient's mouth with one hand using the cross-finger technique as described in Chapter 7.
3. Holding the airway device upside down in the other hand, insert it into the patient's mouth, rotating it through 180 degrees until the flange comes to rest on the patient's lips or teeth. In this position, the airway will hold the tongue forward. Moistening the airway with a small amount of water will ease introduction (Figure 10–6).

An alternate way of placing the airway involves opening the mouth, depressing the tongue with two or three stacked tongue blades, and sliding the airway into

FIGURE 10–5

The proper size of airway is as long as the distance between the ear lobe and the corner of the mouth.

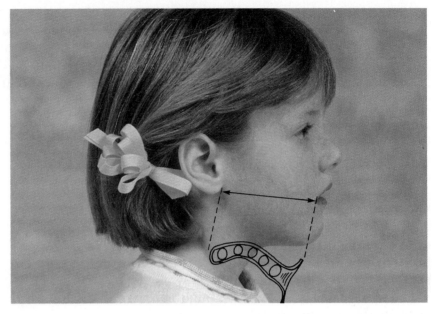

A

FIGURE 10–6

The oropharyngeal airway is rotated 180 degrees as it is inserted. (A) Using the cross-finger technique, the patient's mouth is opened. (B) The airway is then inserted until the flange rests on the lips or teeth.

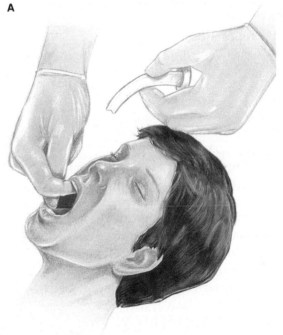

B

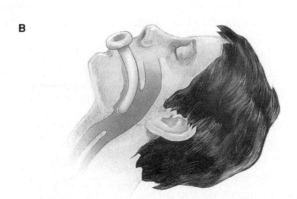

place either directly or sideways with a 90-degree rotation as the tongue is pressed forward and away from the roof of the mouth. Lifting the mandible away from the upper jaw will also facilitate the placement.

Take care to avoid injuring the *hard palate* when you insert the oropharyngeal airway. Rough insertion can cause bleeding, which may aggravate airway problems and may even cause vomiting.

The airway of an unconscious patient who is breathing spontaneously can be maintained with greater ease if an oropharyngeal airway is in place rather than with the constant use of the head-tilt or other maneuvers. The oropharyngeal airway should be used promptly for an unconscious patient who is breathing spontaneously. In the patient who is suspected of having a spinal injury, the oropharyngeal airway is a safe and effective means of keeping the airway open.

Nasopharyngeal Airways A conscious patient who is not able to maintain a natural airway may benefit from the use of a **nasopharyngeal airway.** A semiconscious or seizing patient may also benefit from this type of airway. This adjunct is usually well tolerated and is not as likely as the oropharyngeal airway to stimulate vomiting. A disadvantage is that it is usually not large enough in diameter, however, to allow passage of a standard suction tip or large suction catheter. Also, airway positioning techniques to ensure an open airway may still need to be applied with this type of airway.

Length sizing is accomplished by measuring from the tip of the nose to the ear lobe.

A nasopharyngeal airway is positioned in one nostril with its curvature following the curve of the floor of the nose. The flange, or trumpet-like flare, rests against the nostril while the other end opens into the posterior pharynx. The airway must be well coated with a water-soluble lubricant before it is inserted. Take care to select the patient's nostril large enough to accommodate the airway. In almost everyone, one nostril is larger than the other. Once the proper nostril is selected, the airway

device is inserted gently, without force, through the nostril until the flange rests against the skin (Figure 10–7). If an obstruction is met as the airway is introduced, the airway should be removed and inserted into the other nostril. It is not uncommon to cause slight bleeding even when this airway device is inserted properly. It should never be forced into place.

A

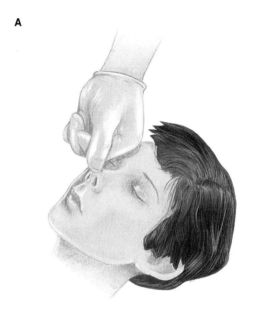

B

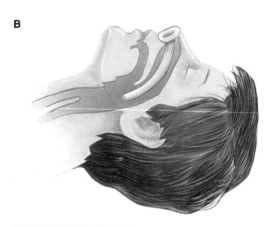

FIGURE 10–7

A nasopharyngeal airway can help to maintain an open airway in a conscious patient. (A) During insertion, its curvature should follow the curve of the floor of the nose. (B) Once in place, the flange should lie against the flare of the nostril so that the other end will lie in the pharynx.

Exercise caution when you consider the use of the nasopharyngeal airway in the patient with severe head or facial trauma because it may accidentally penetrate into the cranium. Consult your local medical director for guidance in this area.

The Bag-Valve-Mask System

The *bag-valve-mask system* should be used when it is desirable to deliver greater than 50 percent oxygen concentrations to the patient who is not breathing spontaneously or to assist respirations in a patient with severe respiratory failure. Both mouth-to-mouth and mouth-to-mask ventilation techniques can provide large volumes of inspired air—up to 4 liters per breath. In contrast, the bag-valve-mask system can deliver only as much gas as can be squeezed out of the bag by hand, which is usually about 1 liter. A volume of 10 to 15 mL/kg should be delivered over 2 seconds. Using the mouth-to-mouth technique, the concentration of oxygen delivered is only 16 percent, and the mouth-to-mask technique at best will provide only 50 to 55 percent oxygen. At the same oxygen flow rate (10 liters per minute), the bag-valve-mask system with an oxygen reservoir attached is capable of delivering air with more than 90 percent oxygen (Figure 10–8).

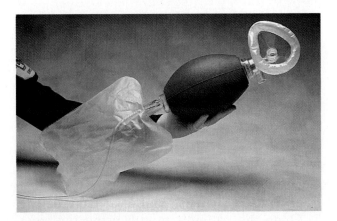

FIGURE 10–8

A bag-valve-mask system with all its component parts. Note the oxygen supply, oxygen reservoir, and resuscitation bag, in addition to the mask.

Patients deemed to be in severe respiratory distress are those whose minute volume is inadequate. The minute volume is that volume of air cycled through the alveoli in 1 minute. For practical purposes in the prehospital care arena, those patients whose respiratory rate falls below 12 breaths per minute or is greater than 24 breaths per minute are deemed to have inadequate respirations. Fast and shallow breathing can be as dangerous as a very slow breathing rate. Rapid, shallow breathing moves mostly dead space air, air in the larger airways only, whereas air in the alveoli is not exchanged adequately to provide fresh oxygen and flush out carbon dioxide waste gas.

The technique for using the bag-valve-mask system includes these steps:

1. Position yourself at the patient's head and maintain the patient's neck in extension.
2. Insert an oropharyngeal airway to maintain an open airway.
3. To achieve the best fit, you must select the correct mask size: the adult size for adults, a children's size for the smaller face, or one of three infant sizes (including a "premie" size for very tiny patients).
4. Place the triangular mask over the patient's face with the apex over the bridge of the nose and the base in the groove between the lower lip and the chin.
5. If the mask has an inflatable collar, blow it up before use to obtain a better fit and seal to the face.
6. Hold the mask in position by placing the little, ring, and long fingers on the mandible. The little finger is on the ramus, and the ring and long fingers are on the body of the mandible; be careful to avoid grabbing the fleshy part of the neck. Hold your index finger over the lower portion of the mask while securing the upper portion of the mask with your thumb; this is known as the "C-clamp." Firm pressure between the fingers on the mandible and the finger and thumb on the mask maintains the seal while the mandible is pulled forward to help maintain an open airway (Figure 10–9).
7. With the mask firmly applied to the patient's face and the neck maintained in extension

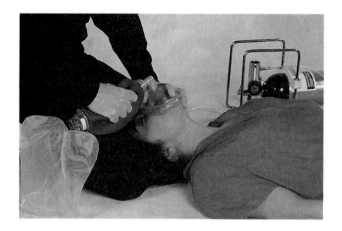

FIGURE 10–9

The mask of the bag-valve-mask system is held firmly against the patient's face. Three fingers are on the mandible, and the thumb holds the upper part of the mask.

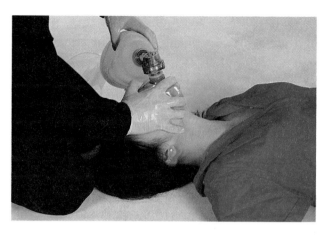

FIGURE 10–10

The bag-valve-mask system with an oxygen reservoir. Its limitations in terms of volume of oxygen delivered are apparent, because it can deliver only the volume that one hand can displace.

with one hand, use your other hand to compress the bag in a rhythmic manner once every 5 seconds (Figure 10–10). Proper ventilation must be evident by the symmetrical rise and fall of the chest.

8. Whenever possible, two rescuers should provide bag-valve-mask ventilation. It is very difficult to maintain a proper seal between the mask and face using just one hand. If two people are available, one should secure the mask to the face with *two* hands while the second squeezes the bag.

When this system is used with external chest compression, ventilation should be given during pauses in compression: one after every fifth or two after every fifteenth compression. At least 1½ to 2 seconds should be allowed for each ventilation.

You should adopt the following sequence in artificial ventilation when using a bag-valve-mask system with an airway:

1. Open the oxygen tank to the oxygen regulator and check that the pressure in the tank is adequate.
2. Connect the plastic oxygen line to the flowmeter nipple and connect the other end to the bag-valve-mask unit with the reservoir in place (Figure 10–11).

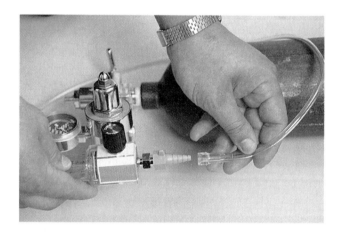

FIGURE 10–11

Connections of the bag-valve-mask with reservoir and oxygen tank flowmeter.

3. Open the regulator knob to the flowmeter to deliver 10 liters of oxygen per minute.
4. Select the correct size of mask for the patient and attach the mask to the valve on the bag.
5. Open the patient's mouth using the cross-finger technique and insert an oropharyngeal airway.
6. With one hand, maintain the face mask seal and neck extension.

7. With the other hand, ventilate the patient by squeezing the bag. Some EMTs compress the bag against their knee to facilitate more complete emptying of the bag. This is not usually necessary, because the minute volume may be increased by giving a higher number of ventilations per minute.
8. Check to be sure lung expansion is occurring by observing the symmetrical rise and fall of the chest during the respiratory cycle.

SUCTIONING DEVICES

Portable and fixed suctioning equipment is essential for resuscitation. The portable **suction** unit must provide a vacuum pressure and flow adequate for effective pharyngeal suction. The unit should be fitted with wide bore, thick-walled, non-kinking tubing and rigid, plastic, pharyngeal suction tips (tonsil tips). A non-breakable collection bottle and a supply of water for rinsing the tips should be available. The fixed suction unit should generate an airflow of more than 30 liters per minute and a vacuum of more than 300 mm of mercury when the tubing is clamped. The suction yoke, collection bottle, water for rinsing, and the suction tube should be readily accessible at the patient's head.

Plastic pharyngeal suction tips are best for suctioning the pharynx. They are large bore and do not collapse. A curved contour allows easy and rapid placement of the tip in the pharynx. They should be used with the greatest caution in conscious or semiconscious patients because of the hazard of inducing vomiting. Suction equipment should be cleaned and decontaminated after each use.

Hand-operated suction devices with disposable chambers are reliable and relatively inexpensive (Figure 10–12).

When using metered suction devices, follow these steps:

1. Inspect the unit for proper assembly of all its parts; switch on the suction; clamp the tubing and note if the pressure dial registers more than 300 mm of mercury.

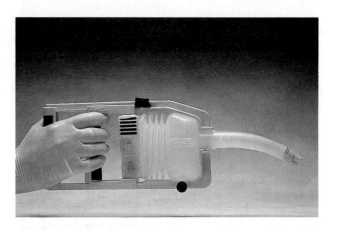

FIGURE 10–12

A hand operated manual suction device.

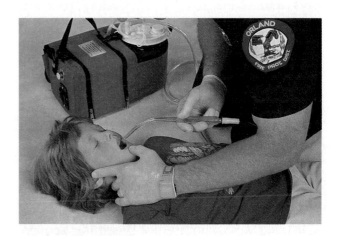

FIGURE 10–13

After opening the mouth with the cross-finger technique, insert the suction tip until the pharynx is reached.

2. Attach the pharyngeal suction tip to the tubing.
3. Open the patient's mouth with the cross-finger technique.
4. Insert the suction tip with its convex side along the roof of the mouth until the pharynx is reached (Figure 10–13).
5. After the tip is in place, release the clamp on the tube and suction as you withdraw the

suction tip from the pharynx and mouth.

6. Never suction for more than 15 seconds at one time, because suctioning removes oxygen from the airway very effectively.
7. Suctioning may be repeated only after the patient has been ventilated and reoxygenated.

WHEN TO USE SUPPLEMENTAL OXYGEN

As noted earlier, hypoxia is a condition in which there is a deficiency of oxygen reaching the cells of the body. It is extremely dangerous, and if it persists, death will occur. Some tissues and organs, especially the heart, the central nervous system, lungs, adrenal glands, kidneys and liver, require a virtually constant supply of oxygen to function normally. Regardless of how well the mechanics of artificial ventilation are performed, unless supplemental oxygen is used, recovery from hypoxia will be slow and often incomplete. Therefore, it is essential that you know the specific indications for the use of oxygen and the various modes of its storage and delivery.

Patients Requiring Oxygen Therapy

Oxygen should be given to two major groups of patients: those who are not breathing spontaneously and those who can breathe but who are unable to move a sufficient amount of air with each breath to ensure adequate oxygen delivery to the lungs. Those in the first group will rapidly develop hypoxia of the vital organs, especially the brain and heart. Death occurs within a matter of minutes if systemic hypoxia is not reversed. Patients in the second group (with an insufficient minute volume) will show varying signs of hypoxia, which may include apprehension, the use of accessory muscles, *dyspnea, tachypnea,* **cyanosis,** and even chest pain. The onset and the degree of tissue damage will depend on the degree of respiratory inadequacy. These patients have poor air exchange and require oxygen and varying degrees of ventilatory support.

Conditions Causing Hypoxia

The early signs of hypoxia are *tachycardia* (heart rate equal to or greater than 100 beats per minute), nervousness, irritability, apprehension, and fear. Conscious patients will complain of shortness of breath and may not be able to talk in complete sentences due to breathlessness. Cyanosis is a later finding. The best time to give oxygen is before any symptoms are noted and whenever you suspect tissue damage of any kind. Certainly oxygen must be supplied before severe damage occurs to the brain, heart, kidneys, and other essential organs. The following are some conditions that are commonly associated with hypoxia:

1. **Myocardial infarction** (heart attack). Hypoxia from myocardial infarction is associated with inadequate circulation of blood carrying oxygen to the tissues due to pump failure. There is usually no lung damage, airway obstruction, or poor air exchange in the lungs.
2. **Pulmonary edema.** Fluid accumulates within the lungs and markedly decreases the efficiency of the transfer of oxygen to the blood from the alveoli. Pulmonary edema may occur following a myocardial infarction.
3. *Acute drug overdose.* Respirations in patients who have taken an overdose of a drug may be very depressed. Infrequent, shallow breaths do not provide a sufficient amount of oxygen.
4. *Smoke and toxic inhalation exposure.* Damage of the lungs resulting from inhalation of smoke and products of combustion. Such damage produces local pulmonary edema and destroys lung tissue. In this situation, gas exchange in the lungs is markedly impaired. In addition, carbon monoxide, a product of combustion, will interfere with the oxygen-carrying capacity of the blood.
5. **Cerebrovascular accident** (stroke). The cause of hypoxia in a patient who has suffered a stroke is poor control of respiration and heart rhythms by the brain. Both the rate and depth of breathing may be severely decreased and cardiac output may be decreased.

6. *Chest injury.* Hypoxia results because of pain and damage to the chest and underlying lung tissue. Pain prevents full chest wall expansion; lung damage prevents efficient gas exchange.

7. *Shock.* Shock often occurs as a result of injuries in which much blood is lost. Oxygen is carried by the red blood cells' hemoglobin and with a significant loss of blood, not enough oxygen may be provided to the tissues to sustain them.

8. **Chronic obstructive pulmonary disease (COPD)(emphysema).** Long-standing chronic irritation of the lungs and air passages (smoking or inhaling toxic fumes) produces direct alveolar damage and increasingly poor gas exchange.

All patients who are hypoxic, from whatever cause, should be treated with supplemental oxygen. The method of oxygen delivery will vary, depending on the cause and the severity of the hypoxia.

HAZARDS OF SUPPLEMENTAL OXYGEN

General Considerations

Oxygen does not burn or explode; however, it does support combustion. The more oxygen there is around, the faster the combustion progresses. A small spark can become a flame in an oxygen-enriched atmosphere. For example, a glowing cigarette can burst into flames. Therefore, any possible source of fire must be kept away from the area while oxygen is in use. Adequate ventilation of the area where oxygen is administered should always be provided, especially in industrial settings where hazardous materials may be present and where sparks are easily generated. Keep this warning in mind at all times.

Patient Considerations

Normally, increasing levels of carbon dioxide in the blood are sensed by the respiratory center in the brain, stimulating the primary drive for breathing. However, when the CO_2 level in the blood rises beyond a certain point these brain cells are "poisoned" and no longer provide the stimulus to breathe. Severe chronic obstructive pulmonary disease causes this condition. Approximately 3 percent of patients with COPD do not have an effective CO_2 stimulus to breathe. These patients are called "CO_2 retainers." For these patients, a low blood oxygen level becomes the primary (and only) stimulus to breathe. This is called the *hypoxic drive*, or secondary drive. Giving oxygen to this set of COPD patients may eliminate this stimulus to breathe and cause a decrease in ventilation to the point that breathing ceases altogether. Inspired oxygen concentrations greater than 25 to 30 percent must be given with caution in these patients, and you must be prepared at all times to provide assisted or artificial ventilation for these patients.

Oxygen should *never* be withheld from any patient whose cells may benefit from it, even if ventilation must be assisted to provide adequate gas exchange.

It is important to remember that keeping oxygen levels low should never be a consideration in the setting of respiratory arrest or cardiopulmonary arrest. These patients are dying. Nothing should be done to make their situation worse. These patients need as much oxygen as possible.

Oxygen given in high doses for prolonged periods of time can be toxic. Pulmonary oxygen toxicity, however, in adults and children, only occurs after the lungs have been exposed for several days to an inspired oxygen concentration in excess of 50 percent and usually delivered at higher than normal pressures. The short-term delivery of high concentrations of oxygen does not cause lung damage, and this is not a valid reason to withhold it in the prehospital setting.

The management of cardiorespiratory arrest in the newborn requires the use of high oxygen concentration for two reasons. First, most newborns who suffer arrest do so because of respiratory insufficiency. Second, even when performed well, external chest compression only partially restores cardiac output. Oxygen will cause no harm to children and infants in the emergency and prehospital setting. Any problems that arise from oxygen toxicity will only occur after more than 24 hours of 100 percent oxygen administration. Therefore, during resuscitation the principles of oxygen administration are identical for adult, child, and neonate: All should be given oxygen in any arrest situation.

SOURCES OF SUPPLEMENTAL OXYGEN
· ·

Compressed Gas Cylinders

In locations other than hospitals and similar facilities, oxygen is usually supplied as a com-

pressed gas in green seamless steel or aluminum cylinders, available in various sizes. The two most frequently used in emergency medical care are the D (or super D) (Figure 10–14) and M cylinders (Figure 10–15). The D (or super D) cylinder can be carried from the vehicle to the patient and the M tank is used on board ambulances as a main supply tank. When filled with oxygen at a pressure between 2,000 and 2,400 pounds per square inch (PSI), the D size contains 620 liters, and the M size, 3,000 liters of oxygen.

Cylinders of D size or smaller have outlet valves designed to accept pressure-reducing

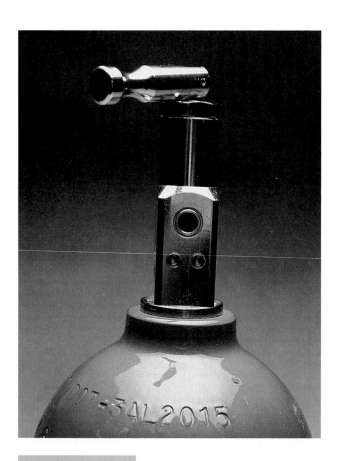

FIGURE 10–14

A size D cylinder.

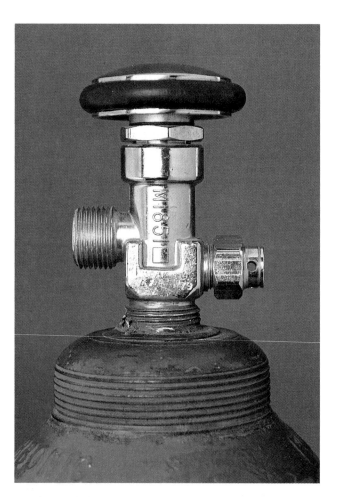

FIGURE 10–15

A size M oxygen cylinder has a valve with the threaded-connector gas outlet of the American Standard Safety System.

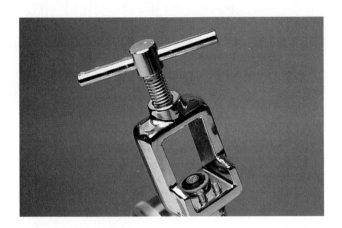

A yoke connector is used with small oxygen cylinders.

gauges of the yoke type (Figure 10–16). To prevent attachment of a pressure regulator for a different gas to an oxygen cylinder, the yoke contains a pin-indexing safety attachment system (Figure 10–17). The system comprises a series of pins on the yoke that must be matched with the holes on the valve stem attachment of the gas cylinder. The arrangement of the pins and holes varies for different gases according to accepted national standards. Each cylinder of a specific gas has a given pattern and a given number of pins. When two or more different gases are being used, one cannot, for example, attach a cylinder of nitrous oxide to an oxygen regulator by mistake because the nitrous oxide cylinder will not fit. For oxygen, there are two pins and two matching holes. Ideally, the connections should be greaseless and dirt-free.

Cylinders larger than D size are equipped with threaded gas outlet valves. The inside and outside thread sizes of these outlets vary according to the medical gas contained in the cylinder. Therefore, the gas cylinder will not accept a regulator valve unless it is properly threaded to fit that regulator. This safety system for large cylinders is known as the American Standard System (Figure 10–18). The purpose of these safety devices is to prevent the accidental attachment of a regulator to a wrong supply tank (for example, to nitrous oxide or carbon dioxide instead of to oxygen).

Compressed gas cylinders must be handled carefully, because their contents are under pressure. Regulators must be firmly attached to the cylinders before they are transported. A loose regulator or perforation of the tank can cause it to become a deadly missile. The cylinder should not be handled by the neck assembly alone. Safe use and respect for the potential destructive properties of compressed gas cylinders must be emphasized.

Regulators

Pressure Regulators The pressure of gas in an oxygen cylinder is too high to be useful medically. Pressure regulators must be attached to medical gas cylinders to reduce the pressure to the useful range of 40 to 70 pounds per square inch (PSI). Most pressure regulators

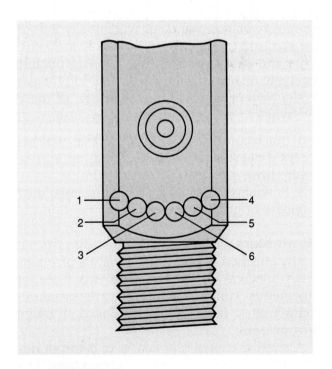

The locations of the pin-indexing safety system holes in a cylinder valve face. Various pairs constitute indexes for different gases.

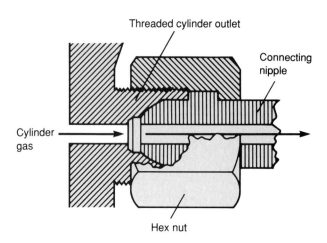

FIGURE 10-18

The typical American Standard connection is used to attach a reducing valve to a large high-pressure cylinder.

in medical use today reduce the pressure in a single stage, although multistage regulators do exist. A two-stage regulator will initially reduce the pressure to 700 PSI and then to 40 to 70 PSI. After the pressure is reduced to a workable level, the final attachment for delivering the gas to the patient is usually through one of these two ways:

- A quick-connect female fitting that will accept a quick-connect male plug from a pressure hose or ventilator or resuscitator.
- A flowmeter that will permit the regulated release of gas measured in liters per minute.

Flowmeters Flowmeters are usually permanently attached to pressure regulators on emergency medical equipment. The two types of **flowmeters** commonly in use are pressure-compensated flowmeters and Bourdon gauge flowmeters.

A *pressure-compensated flowmeter* incorporates a float ball within a tapered calibrated tube. The float rises or falls according to the gas flow within the tube. The flow of gas is controlled by a needle valve located downstream from the float ball. This type of flowmeter is affected by gravity and must always be maintained in an

upright position for an accurate flow reading (Figure 10–19).

The Bourdon gauge flowmeter is very common in emergency medical use, because it is not affected by gravity and can be used in any position. It is actually a pressure gauge calibrated to record flow rate (Figure 10–20). The major disadvantage of this flowmeter is that it does not compensate for back pressure and will usually record a higher flow rate when any obstruction to gas flow is encountered downstream.

Humidification Oxygen from a cylinder source is extremely dry. For all practical purposes, it is completely free from water vapor. Therefore, to prevent the drying of the patient's mucous membrane surfaces, **humidification** is an important consideration in oxygen administration (Figure 10–21). Excessive drying of the mucous membranes of the nose, mouth, and lungs can interfere with respiration. This is especially important when you are treating asthma and bronchitis, in which mucus plugging of the airway may be an important factor. Humidification systems, because they contain water, can easily become contaminated and serve as a reservoir for infection. Therefore, if used on an ambulance, they must be kept clean and

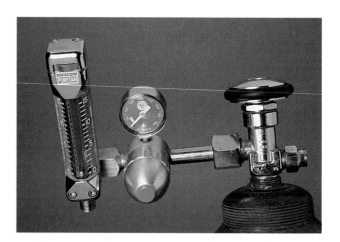

FIGURE 10-19

A pressure-compensated flowmeter attached to a large gas cylinder via a threaded connection allows a regulated flow from 0 to 15 liters of oxygen per minute.

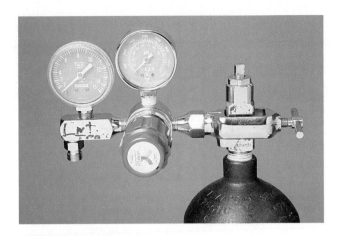

FIGURE 10-20

A Bourdon gauge flowmeter attached to a small gas cylinder via a yoke attachment allows a regulated flow from 0 to 15 liters of oxygen per minute.

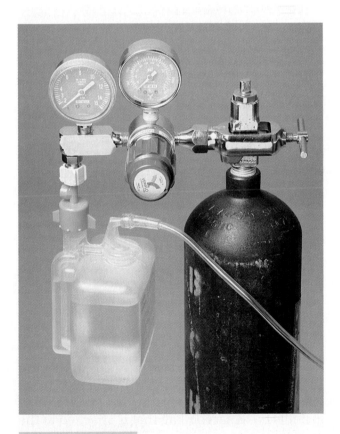

FIGURE 10-21

An evaporative oxygen humidifier is attached to a Bourdon gauge flowmeter/pressure regulator. Humidification prevents excessive drying of the mucous membranes of the nose, mouth, and lungs.

changed frequently. Single-use and disposable humidification devices are preferred. They should be filled with water at the time they are to be used, not prior to use.

Replacement of Oxygen Cylinders

Several methods are available for calculating how long an oxygen cylinder can be used before its contents are depleted. It should be emphasized that you must always make arrangements to switch to a fresh cylinder before the one in use becomes completely empty. Normally, a cylinder is replaced at a certain level (usually 200 PSI) above the 0 PSI reading on the pressure gauge. This level is called the *safe residual*. Knowing the current pressure reading, the current flow in liters per minute, and the safe residual, you can calculate how much useful life remains in any cylinder. One way of calculating the remaining duration of flow in the cylinder after it has been partially used is shown in Table 10–1.

EQUIPMENT FOR OXYGEN DELIVERY

Nasal Cannula

With a nasal **cannula** (Figure 10–22), oxygen is administered to the patient through two small tubular prongs that fit into the patient's nostrils. If the flowmeter is set for 6 to 7 liters per minute, it is possible to obtain inspired oxygen concentrations ranging from 35 to 50 percent. Because the nasal cannula delivers dry gas directly into the nostrils, humidification is necessary to prevent discomfort and possible damage to the nasal mucosa. This is especially important when long transport time is anticipated. A patient who is a mouth breather or who has a nasal obstruction derives little or no benefit from this type of oxygen administration.

Simple Face Mask

Simple *face masks* (Figure 10–23) contain a small bore inlet port and an elastic strap to secure the mask and for a snug fit. Perforations on either side allow the escape of excess gases, especially

TABLE 10–1	Calculating the Duration of Cylinder Flow (in Minutes)					
Formula			Factors in Various Oxygen Cylinders	Safe Residual Pressure	Example	Solution
$\dfrac{\left(\begin{array}{c}\text{Gauge pressure}\\ -\text{ Safe residual}\end{array}\right) \times \text{Factor}}{\begin{array}{c}\text{Flowrate}\\ \text{(liter flow per minute)}\end{array}}$	$\begin{array}{c}= \text{Duration}\\ \text{of flow}\\ \text{(in minutes)}\end{array}$		D 0.16 E 0.28 G 2.41 H 3.14 K 3.14 M 1.56	200 psi	M cylinder, gauge pressure at 1,200 psi, safe residual is 200 psi, flowmeter set for 5 liters per minute.	$\dfrac{\left(\begin{array}{c}1{,}200\\ -\ 200\end{array}\right) \times 1.56}{5} = \dfrac{1{,}560}{5} =$ 312 minutes (or 5 hours, 12 min)

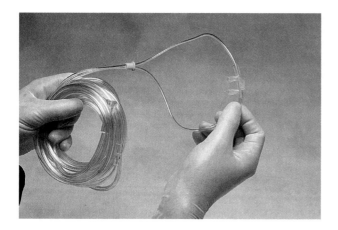

FIGURE 10–22

Nasal cannula used to administer oxygen in concentrations of 35 to 50 percent.

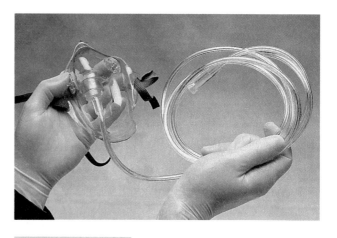

FIGURE 10–23

A simple face mask.

during exhalation. Different sizes of face masks are available, including infant and pediatric. All types of masks are fitted to the face in the same manner—the apex across the bridge of the nose and the base between the lower lip and chin. Face masks designed for infants should be designed to provide a tight seal and have a low dead space. (A newborn's should have less than 5 mL.) With a flow rate of 8 to 10 liters per minute, inspired oxygen concentrations of 35 to 60 percent can be attained. As with the nasal cannula, humidification should be provided.

Mask with Reservoir Bag

In the *mask and reservoir bag system* (Figure 10–24a), the mask is similar to the face mask just described. However, in this system, oxygen fills the reservoir bag that is attached to the mask by a one-way valve. This system is called a *non-rebreathing mask* because the exhaled gas escapes through flapper valve ports at the cheek areas of the mask. The valve also prevents rebreathing of the exhaled gases as the gas in the reservoir flows into the mask during inhalation. With a good seal and 100 percent

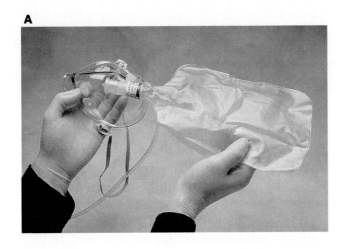

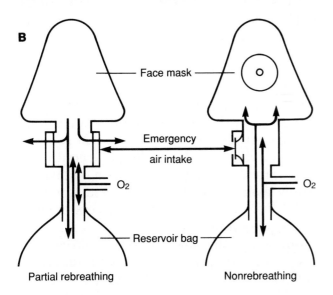

FIGURE 10-24

(A) A non-rebreathing mask with reservoir bag. (B) Removal of flapper valves converts it to a partial rebreathing mask.

oxygen supplied to its intake, it is capable of providing 95 percent inspired oxygen to the patient.

Removal of the flapper valves on the mask converts this system to a "partial rebreathing mask" and reservoir (Figure 10-24b). These valves may be removed to provide for proper fit and when necessary to handle large exhalation volumes. Oxygen concentrations of greater than 60 percent in inspired air can be obtained with this partial rebreathing system.

In both of the systems using a reservoir bag, the oxygen flow should be set at whatever flow

rate will prevent the use of more than ⅔ of the bag volume during inhalation. With infants and children, obviously a smaller bag will be needed, because the volume inhaled each time is less. As with the other systems, humidification is necessary when prolonged administration is anticipated.

Venturi Masks

A **Venturi mask** is a breathing unit that provides a specific concentration of oxygen through a delivery tube connected to a standard face mask (Figure 10-25). Before the oxygen delivery tube reaches the mask, it passes through an air entrainment device that mixes air and oxygen and specifically regulates the concentration of delivered oxygen and also the total volume of gas delivered to the patient per unit of time. Venturi masks are usually designed to deliver inspired oxygen concentrations of 24, 28, 35, or 40 percent. However, the stated concentrations are not highly accurate. The major advantage of this system is a high volume of inspired air with gradually increasing and controlled concentrations of oxygen. Venturi masks are commonly used for patients with COPD. Humidification is a consideration when a long transport time is anticipated; local protocols should be consulted when you provide humidification with Venturi masks.

Bag-Valve-Mask Resuscitators

All types of bag-valve-mask resuscitators have these common components (Figure 10-26):

- A transparent self-inflating, deflatable bag.
- A valve that incorporates the exhalation port, the oxygen inflow, a means of connection between the face mask and the bag, and attachment for the transparent reservoir bag or tube.
- A face mask that should also be transparent.

The total amount of gas contained within the bag of an adult resuscitator is 1,200 to 1,600 cubic centimeters (cc). The pediatric bag contains approximately 500 to 700 cc, and the infant bag holds 150 to 240 cc. The majority of the bag-valve-mask resuscitators on the market today are available with modifications or acces-

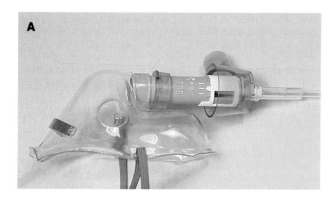

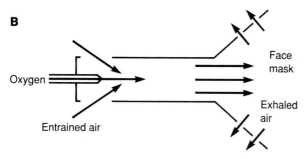

FIGURE 10–25

(A) A typical Venturi mask. (B) Diagrammatic representation of the functions of the Venturi mask. As oxygen is delivered, a certain amount of room air is also entrained with each inhalation, providing a given oxygen concentration. The amount of room air taken in is dependent on the size of the ports through which the air passes.

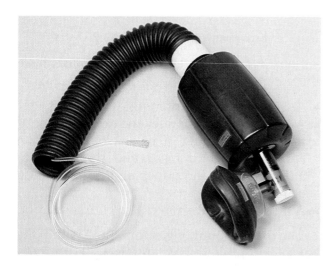

FIGURE 10–26

A bag-valve-mask resuscitator with modification for administration of a high concentration of oxygen.

sories to permit the delivery of oxygen concentrations approaching 100 percent. Without these modifications, it is difficult to achieve concentrations above 50 percent.

The oxygen inlet of a bag-valve-mask resuscitator is attached to the flowmeter nipple of the oxygen cylinder by the small bore tube. These units may be used to assist the respiration of patients who are breathing spontaneously but are not ventilating adequately. These are patients with a respiratory rate less than 8 or greater than 26 breaths per minute or patients who clearly demonstrate respiratory distress. When using the unit to assist respirations, you should deflate the bag simultaneously with the patient's inspiratory effort and ultimately attempt to achieve a more normal rate and depth of respiration. The function of the unit is under your manual control. Considerable practice must be performed on ventilation manikins before using a bag-valve-mask resuscitator on a real patient.

Bag-valve-mask resuscitators specially designed for neonatal resuscitation should be readily available to EMTs expected to deliver babies, because more than 12 percent of births will require some sort of resuscitation. These self-inflating bags and reservoirs have an intake valve at one end to allow rapid reinflation and blow by oxygen. Ensure that the bag will deliver oxygen passively through the mask. Some bag-valve-mask resuscitators are equipped with a "pop-off" valve at 30 to 35 cm H_2O. The neonate may require higher pressures for its initial breaths; therefore, a bypass to this pop-off valve may be desirable. The fit of the face mask is important, and those with cushioned rims are recommended as most effective.

Oxygen-Powered Mechanical Ventilation Devices

There are two basic types of oxygen-powered mechanical ventilation devices: automatic and manual. The most common of these devices are intermittent positive-pressure breathing (IPPB) resuscitators, demand-valve resuscitators (Figure 10–27), and resuscitator inhalators. Conventional, pressure-cycled, automatic resuscitators should not be used by EMTs for artificial

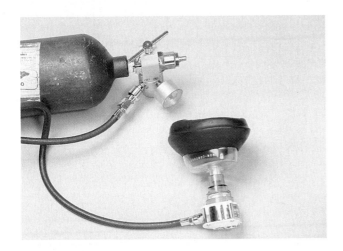

FIGURE 10–27

A demand-valve resuscitator with high-pressure hose and quick-connect fitting.

ventilation, especially in conjunction with external chest compression. External chest compression prematurely triggers termination of the inflation cycle of these devices, and inadequate ventilation results.

Federal specifications require that resuscitators used in ambulances be manually controlled (timed cycle). Manually controlled resuscitators have high instantaneous flow rates that allow them to be used for artificial ventilation alone, as well as in conjunction with external chest compression. The majority of these units will function as inhalators for patients who are breathing spontaneously but require oxygen.

Manually controlled oxygen-powered resuscitators should do the following:

- Provide flow rates of 40 to 50 liters per minute and an inspiratory pressure safety release valve that opens at approximately 35 to 50 cm of water. (You must be alert for gastric distension as a result of such a high flow rate).
- Provide 100 percent oxygen.
- Operate satisfactorily under varying environmental conditions.
- Have a prefitted lever arm manual control so that both of your hands can remain on the mask to provide an airtight seal while supporting and tilting the patient's head and keeping the jaw elevated.

The amount of pressure necessary to ventilate a patient adequately will vary according to the size of the patient, the patient's lung volume, and the condition of the lungs. A patient with stiff, diseased lungs or chronic obstructive pulmonary disease will require a greater pressure to receive a given volume than would be necessary for a patient with normal lungs.

The problem you will face in using these resuscitators, just as with the bag-valve-mask units, is the airtight fit between the patient's face and mask. Practice and strict adherence to proper technique will minimize this problem.

Significant concern exists about the inherent danger in the use of oxygen-powered mechanical ventilation devices, especially because they are widely available. These devices should not be used on children or infants. Their usefulness makes it necessary to include them in this discussion, but the need for proper training is vital if you are to use them correctly. Local medical protocols should be observed carefully when you use these devices.

YOU ARE THE EMT

1. What are the major advantages of mouth-to-mask ventilation compared with mouth-to-mouth ventilation?
2. The patient is unconscious and needs an artificial airway. Will you insert an oropharyngeal airway device or a nasopharyngeal airway device? Why?
3. What is hypoxia? What are the early signs of hypoxia? The later signs? How can it be reversed?
4. What may occur if oxygen in concentrations greater than 25 to 30 percent is administered to patients with chronic obstructive pulmonary disease?

SECTION 4

BLEEDING AND SHOCK

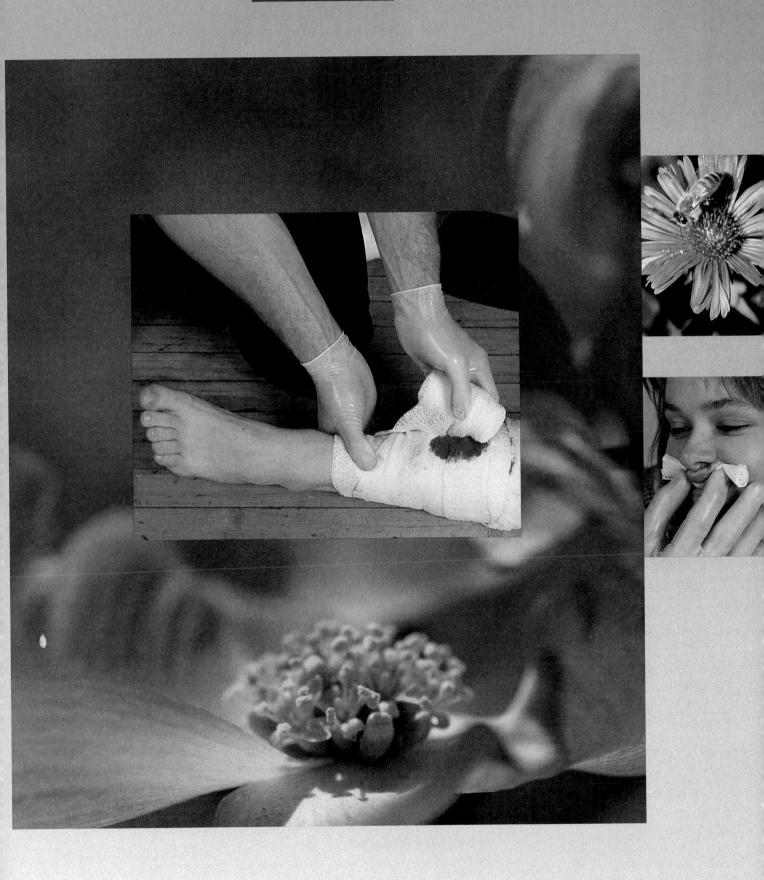

CHAPTER 11

THE CONTROL OF BLEEDING

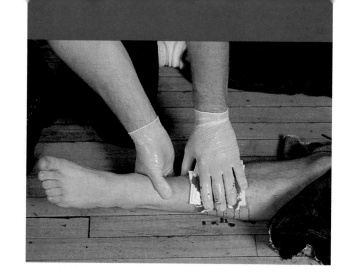

KEY TERMS

artery (ar'ter-e) A vessel through which blood passes away from the heart to the various parts of the body.

capillary (kap'ĭ-lar"e) Any one of the minute blood vessels that connect the arterioles and venules.

coagulation (ko-ag"u-la'shun) The process of blood clot formation; blood clotting.

collateral circulation (kŏ-lat'er-al ser"ku-la'shun) The ability of secondary blood vessels to replace or compensate for circulation lost by a damaged or blocked vessel.

ecchymosis (ek"ĭ-mo'sis) A small area of bleeding in the skin or mucous membrane; a bruise or "black and blue" mark.

epistaxis (ep"ĭ-stak'sis) Nosebleed; a hemorrhage from the nose.

hematemesis (hem"ah-tem'ĕ-sis) The vomiting of blood.

hematoma (hem"ah-to'mah) A collection of blood contained within the body in tissue or in a cavity, occasionally palpable as a discrete mass.

hematuria (hem"ah-tu're-ah) The discharge of blood in the urine.

hemophilia (he"mo-fil'e-ah) An inherited tendency to abnormal bleeding caused by a deficiency of clotting factors.

hemoptysis (he-mop'tĭ-sis) The expectoration of blood or blood-tinged sputum; the coughing up of blood.

hemorrhage (hem'or-ij) Bleeding.

occlude (ŏ-klood') To close or block.

pulse The expansion and contraction of an artery, consistent with the beat of the heart, which may be felt with a finger.

shock A condition of acute peripheral circulatory failure, causing inadequate and progressively failing tissue perfusion.

tourniquet (toor'nĭ-ket) An instrument for the compression of a blood vessel for the purpose of controlling the flow of blood.

vein A tubular vessel that carries blood from the capillaries and venules into the right atrium of the heart.

OVERVIEW

Unquestionably, bleeding is a major emergency problem. You must recognize its existence—obvious when the bleeding is external but not so obvious when it is internal—assess its seriousness, and know how to control it effectively. Several methods exist for controlling obvious external bleeding; they offer varying degrees of success. When patients have internal bleeding, recognition of its existence and prompt transportation are paramount because you have very limited means to control it.

Chapter 11 first discusses the significance of bleeding and includes a comment concerning the patient with hemophilia. External bleeding and the common methods of controlling it are described, as are some of the lesser used means. The last section of Chapter 11 discusses internal bleeding and includes a number of definitions. The focus for internal bleeding is on its seriousness, because of the difficulty of controlling this type of blood loss in the field. A final word concerning EMT safety is included.

GOALS

The objectives of Chapter 11 are to

- understand the significance of bleeding, both external and internal.
- be familiar with the term hemophilia and the significance of this disease for the patient who has it and is injured.
- know how to control external bleeding using direct pressure and elevation, an air pressure splint, or a simple splint.
- know the indications for using the less common methods of controlling external bleeding: proximal arterial pressure, pneumatic counterpressure devices, or tourniquets.
- know the drawbacks of each method of controlling bleeding and how it affects the use of that method to control hemorrhage.
- know how to manage the patient with epistaxis.
- recognize the signs and symptoms of internal bleeding and know the principles of treating patients with suspected internal bleeding.

THE SIGNIFICANCE OF BLEEDING

Bleeding and **hemorrhage** mean the same thing—namely, that blood is escaping from arteries, **capillary** vessels, or veins. Bleeding may be external and obvious or internal and hidden. In either case, it is dangerous. Hemorrhage initially causes weakness and, ultimately, if uncontrolled, **shock** and death. The average adult body contains 6 liters of blood. The acute loss of over 10 percent of that circulating blood volume (in an adult, 600 ml; in a child, 200 to 300 ml) cannot be compensated by the body and will cause shock. In an infant, the loss of as little as 25 or 30 ml (1 ounce) of blood can cause shock. These figures for bleeding represent maximum tolerable losses in otherwise healthy people. In some instances, blood loss can be very rapid and the resultant shock can be severe. Blood loss in any situation is an extremely serious problem that demands first priority attention for treatment after the airway is cleared and breathing is stabilized.

Blood is transported within the circulatory system through blood vessels. Injuries and some diseases can disrupt vessels and cause bleeding. Characteristically, blood from an open **artery** is bright red and spurts, under pressure, in time with the **pulse** (the beat of the heart). Blood from an open **vein** is much darker and flows steadily, under much less pressure, without the spurt. Bleeding from damaged capillary vessels is a continuous, slow, steady ooze (Figure 11–1).

The rapidity of bleeding is very important. The average adult may comfortably lose a unit (500 ml) of blood donated in a blood center over 15 to 20 minutes. While the blood is being withdrawn, the normal individual can adapt fairly rapidly to the decrease in blood volume quite well. If larger amounts are lost (more than 10 percent of the volume), especially if the loss is rapid, the patient may develop hypovolemic shock and may even die. In these circumstances, the blood loss has been so large or so fast that the body cannot compensate well. In general, a normal human being cannot compensate well for an acute blood loss greater than 10 percent of the total circulating volume.

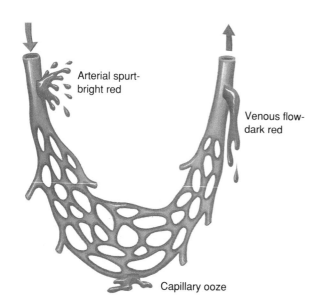

FIGURE 11–1

A capillary loop connecting an arteriole and a venule is shown in this schematic drawing. Bleeding on the arterial side is bright red and spurting; from the venous side it is dark red, or reddish-blue, with a steady flow. Bleeding from the capillaries themselves is a slow, steady ooze.

In this situation, *acute* means a loss of volume taking place over 10 minutes or less.

EXTERNAL BLEEDING

External bleeding is hemorrhage that can be seen coming from a wound. Examples of external hemorrhage are bleeding from open fractures, bleeding from open wounds, and nosebleeds.

In most instances, bleeding stops spontaneously after 6 to 10 minutes, because the intrinsic defense mechanisms that arrest bleeding are very effective. When a cut occurs, for example, blood at first gushes from the cut vessels. Then the completely cut ends of the vessel narrow to reduce the hemorrhage. A clot forms at the cut ends of these vessels. This process is called **coagulation.** Bleeding stops as the clot increases in size and plugs the hole. Bleeding will *never stop* without the formation of a clot, unless the entire blood supply to the injured vessel is cut off. Ultimately, clotting is the mechanism that arrests blood flow from vessels of every size.

Direct contact with the various body tissues and their juices is the common mechanism that activates the clotting factors in blood. When exposed to these tissues and fluids, blood clots rapidly to seal the injured portions of any damaged vessel. Normally, blood within an artery or vein is protected from direct contact with body tissue or tissue juice by the vessel wall and therefore does not clot unless the vessel is injured.

A number of medications interfere with normal clotting. This interfering action is called anticoagulation. Aspirin is one that is very commonly used. Most individuals use aspirin for headaches or mild joint or muscle problems. They have no knowledge at all that it is also an effective anticoagulant. Medications are frequently prescribed to anticoagulate the blood for a number of reasons. It is, therefore, helpful to know whether a bleeding patient is taking any anticoagulant drug and the schedule of its dose. Commonly used anticoagulant drugs are aspirin, Persantine®, dicumarol, Coumadin®, and heparin.

A very small portion of the population may lack one or some of the different substances that cause clotting. These patients have **hemophilia.** There are several forms of this problem; most are congenital, some are severe, and almost all result in a significant increased capacity to bleed because blood does not clot. For hemophiliacs, all injuries, no matter how trivial, are potentially serious. Sometimes, bleeding may occur spontaneously in hemophilia. The identification of an injured patient as a hemophiliac is important and requires immediate transportation to the emergency department.

In some patients who have undergone a severe injury, the damaged blood vessels may be so large that clots cannot **occlude** (block) them. Sometimes only a portion of the vessel wall may be cut, preventing the wall from retracting or constricting. In these cases bleeding will continue unless stopped by external means. Blood loss may, occasionally, be so rapid that, if one waits for the bleeding to stop spontaneously, the patient may die before normal protective processes such as clotting can be effective. It is absolutely imperative for you to know how to control external bleeding. After securing an airway and being certain that the injured patient can breathe, you must always address the second matter for immediate concern—the control of hemorrhage.

Controlling External Bleeding

The control of external bleeding is often very simple. Almost all instances of external bleeding can be controlled by applying direct local pressure at the bleeding site. Pressure stops the physical flow of blood and permits normal blood coagulation to occur.

Six ways exist to control visible external bleeding. For practical considerations, there are three recommended common means that are used frequently and three less recommended, or less frequently used, methods. The three recommended means are

- Direct local pressure and extremity elevation.
- Splinting.
- Air pressure splinting.

The less commonly used means are

- Proximal arterial pressure.
- Pneumatic air pressure devices.
- Tourniquets.

Recommended Methods to Control Bleeding

Local Pressure and Elevation Direct pressure may be exerted over the wound by a finger or hand or by the application of a pressure dressing. This method is, by far, the most effective way to control local external hemorrhage. Bleeding is nearly always stopped when pressure is applied directly over the wound (Figure 11–2a). Initially, pressure may be applied with the finger or hand, but a sterile gauze pressure dressing is preferred; 4 × 4 or 4 × 8 sterile gauze pads should be used for small wounds and a sterile universal dressing for larger wounds. Once bleeding is controlled using local manual pressure over sterile pads, compression can be maintained by wrapping the entire wound circumferentially and firmly with a sterile, roller, self-adhering bandage. The entire sterile compressive dressing should be covered above and below the wound by the roller bandage, stretched sufficiently tight to control the hemorrhage (Figure 11–2b). If sterile pads are not immediately available, a handkerchief, a sanitary napkin, a clean cloth, or a gloved hand can be used to apply pressure.

Do not remove the dressing until the patient has been evaluated by the physician at the emergency department. Bleeding that continues after the dressing is in place usually means that not enough pressure has been applied to the wound. In such instances, apply additional manual pressure through the dressing; then add additional gauze pads over the first dressing and secure them both with a second roller bandage applied more tightly. Almost always when the pressure of the dressing exceeds arterial pressure, the bleeding will stop.

Elevation of a bleeding extremity is also important. Elevation by as little as 10 inches often stops venous bleeding. Elevation of the bleeding part should be combined with local pressure whenever possible (Figure 11–2c).

A

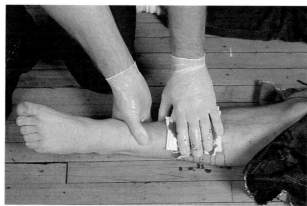

B

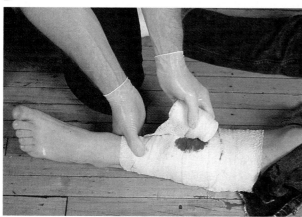

C

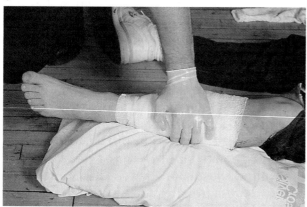

FIGURE 11–2

Methods of controlling external hemorrhage. (A) The best and most effective way to control external hemorrhage is the application of local pressure. (B) Maintain compression by wrapping a sterile roller bandage over the entire compressive dressing. (C) Elevation of a bleeding extremity is extremely efficient especially in controlling venous bleeding.

Splints Much bleeding from injured extremities occurs because muscles and other tissues are cut by the sharp ends of broken bones. As long as a fracture has not been stabilized, motion of the bone ends will cause continued injury to partially clotted vessels. Achieving stability of a major fracture is a principal priority in ensuring prompt control of bleeding. Often, the application of a simple splint to a fractured extremity will allow prompt control of the hemorrhage associated with the injury (Figure 11–3). The principles of applying splints are given in Chapter 16.

Pressure Splints Many ambulances throughout the United States carry *air pressure splints* (Figure 11–4). Air splints can control severe soft tissue hemorrhage when massive or complex lacerations of soft tissue have occurred. An

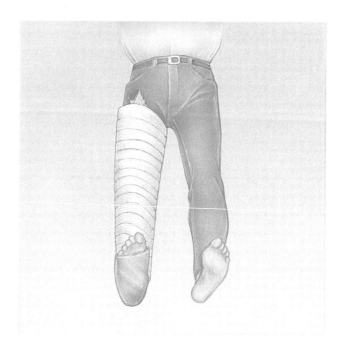

FIGURE 11–3

Often the application of a simple splint will allow control of severe soft tissue bleeding associated with a fracture. Limb stability is an absolute necessity in these cases.

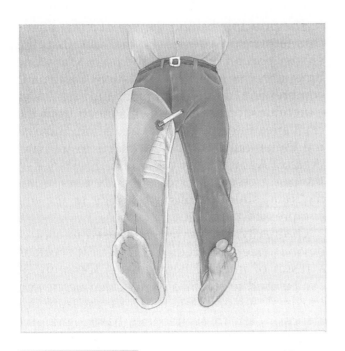

FIGURE 11–4

Air pressure splints can be applied around an extremity to control bleeding. Numerous sizes and designs exist. The inflated splint supplies pressure to the wound and splints the limb.

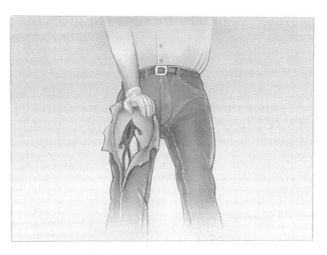

FIGURE 11–5

Proximal arterial pressure may aid in control of bleeding, but it is rarely totally effective alone in controlling hemorrhage.

air splint acts like a pressure bandage applied to the entire extremity rather than to a localized area. It can be used as an effective, much larger, local pressure dressing. At the same time, effective splinting of a coexisting fracture can be accomplished. The use of such a splint solely for the pressure control of hemorrhage is entirely appropriate in the patient with only extensive soft tissue lacerations and no fracture. For fractures, the use of air pressure splints is described in Chapter 16.

Less Commonly Used Methods to Control Bleeding

Proximal Arterial Pressure When pressure dressings are not available or when direct pressure with reinforced dressings does not control wound bleeding, proximal arterial pres-

sure control can sometimes be used to arrest bleeding (Figure 11–5). Pulse points, also known as pressure points, for all the major arteries are described in Chapter 4. To use proximal arterial pressure well, you must be thoroughly familiar with the location of these pulse points. Only rarely does proximal compression of a major feeding artery completely arrest hemorrhage from a more distal wound, because usually the wound is supplied by more than one major artery. Thus, this technique can aid temporarily to some degree in the control of severe hemorrhage if it is predominantly from one major vessel, but it should not be the primary or the sole method of bleeding control. It can be used to supplement direct pressure. When bleeding continues from a wound when compression is used directly over the wound, putting additional pressure over a proximal pulse point may slow the bleeding.

Pneumatic Counterpressure Device Frequently, hemorrhage is a severe or fatal complication of fractures of the pelvis or the proximal femur. Bleeding may not be observed externally in these patients because the blood collects behind the peritoneum and in the tissues around both hips. A pneumatic counterpressure device (pneumatic trousers, air pressure pants, pneumatic antishock garment, or MAST trousers) can be used in the treatment of hypovolemic shock from such injuries and from certain other causes (Figure 11–6). The device may be effective in a few very specific instances:

- For controlling significant internal bleeding into the tissues from a fractured pelvis or from fractures of the proximal femurs.
- For helping to counteract the shock from significant internal bleeding.
- For stabilizing fractures of the pelvis and proximal femurs.
- For supporting the systolic blood pressure when it falls below 100 mm Hg following trauma when a source of bleeding is not evident.

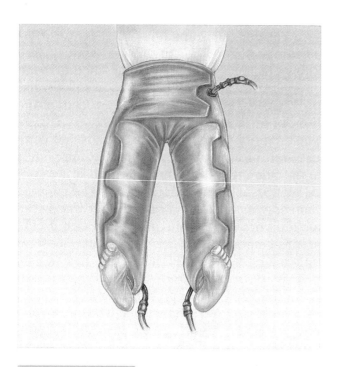

The pneumatic counterpressure device has few, very specific uses in treating bleeding.

The principle behind the use of a pneumatic counterpressure device is the fact that the greater portion of blood in the body at any one time is in the capillary circulation. Systematic compression of the abdomen and the lower extremities forces much of this blood from the capillaries into the central circulation, increasing the amount of blood available to the vital organs. Additionally, peripheral resistance in the compressed areas of the body rises, automatically shunting blood centrally to the uncompressed parts.

Ordinarily, the device is *not* used to control obvious external bleeding but to treat shock as a result of internal hemorrhage. Certainly, it can be used to stabilize complicated pelvic and proximal femoral fractures. In the rare instances when these fractures have significant external bleeding, the device also provides some soft tissue compression. It is not, in the main, a device to be used for bleeding control. Its uses are

- To counteract hypovolemic shock from a number of causes.
- To help stabilize the pelvis, hip joints, and upper femurs in cases of severe and complex fractures.

Do not use the pneumatic counterpressure device when the following conditions exist:

- Pregnancy.
- Chronic pulmonary edema secondary to long-standing heart disease.
- Acute cardiac failure.

More relative contraindications to the use of these devices include

- Penetrating chest injuries.
- Groin injuries.
- Major head injuries.
- Relatively short anticipated transport times.

In these situations, the use of this device may worsen or complicate the patient's condition. The device should not remain inflated for more than 2 hours or the time needed to transport a patient to the hospital. If prolonged use is absolutely necessary, inform medical control.

Major complications can arise from the use of the pneumatic counterpressure device. The most common of them is severe hypovolemic shock caused by unsupervised, uncontrolled, or too rapid deflation of the device in the emergency department. This situation usually is not your direct concern, because you rarely participate in this segment of the patient's care. You do, however, apply the device and you should be aware of problems that can arise in removing it. Emergency department personnel must be prepared to administer large volumes of intravenous fluid and blood to restore adequate blood volume *before* the device is deflated. Failure to do so may cause the patient to develop hypovolemic shock as the device is deflated.

Recently, there have been reports of muscle tissue death caused by excess pressure within the garment when it remains inflated for prolonged periods of time. The medical literature also reports several inappropriate uses of pneumatic counterpressure devices. Use it only as just indicated because of its potential for serious complications.

Several research studies have failed to identify a positive effect on patient care with the pneumatic counterpressure device. It has not yet, in general, been identified as a lifesaver for patients that would otherwise be lost.

There is general agreement, however, that the garment can stabilize major pelvic and femoral fractures. It can also support the blood pressure to a degree in instances of hypovolemic shock. You must remember, however, that emergency support of blood pressure is achieved at the cost of high and sometimes lethal tissue pressures in the lower extremities and abdomen. It is also achieved at the cost of delaying transport and more definitive care to apply the garment.

If you remember that the device is not an aid to control bleeding but one to help in managing shock and that many serious problems have been identified with its use, you are likely to use·it only when it is absolutely needed. The foregoing indications and contraindications are fairly stringent and enable you to apply this device when it can help. Local medical directors should prescribe indications and contraindications for its use.

In applying the device, the best results can be obtained by its careful inflation, in increments, with constant monitoring of the patient's blood pressure. As a general rule, pressure in the garment should be gradually increased in the legs of the garment before the abdominal portion is inflated. Do not increase pressure beyond that needed to produce the return of an adequate (greater than 100 mm Hg) systolic blood pressure. Avoid extremity pressures in the garment above 40 mm Hg, because they will damage tissue locally. If a garment has no pressure gauges, monitor the distal neurovascular status of the limbs to which it is applied. Pulses, sensation, and motion should not disappear. The effectiveness of this mode of treatment is measured by the return of blood pressure toward normal and by stabilization of vital signs. Remember that the pressure gauges on a pneumatic antishock garment are used to measure the air pressure in the device itself and have no bearing whatsoever on the patient's blood pressure. Thus, you should monitor and record the blood pressure, and its changes, at least every 5 minutes before, during, and after application.

While considerable work has been done to investigate whether the use of pneumatic counterpressure devices increase carotid artery blood flow during cardiopulmonary resuscitation, there still are no data demonstrating improved outcome from cardiac arrest with their use. Hence, these devices are not currently recommended for routine CPR in the treatment of cardiac arrest.

Whenever air pressure splints or pneumatic counterpressure devices are used and it is necessary to transport the patient either in a helicopter or in areas where temperature or pressure changes may be marked, you must remember that the volume of the air within the device changes with changes in external temperature and air pressure. In helicopters and in unpressurized airplanes, external pressure drops with increasing height, and the air in the splint expands. Accordingly, a splint or pressure garment will become much tighter aloft than it was when applied on the ground. Similarly, cold makes air within the device contract. If an emergency situation requires the application of such a device in areas of low temperature, the pressure within the splint or garment must be adjusted as the patient enters a warm room or transporting vehicle. The air in the garment or splint will expand with warmth, and it will again tighten.

You must inform the emergency department personnel about the patient's blood pressure, when the device was applied, and the results observed after its application. You must also note and record the time the device was applied and inflated. Removal of a pneumatic counterpressure device is done only in the hospital with gradual deflation, after the administration of appropriate intravenous solutions and with careful supervision. It is never done outside the emergency department or operating room. The technique of applying the pneumatic counterpressure device is illustrated in Figure 11–7.

Tourniquet Tourniquets are considered as a *final resort* in the control of bleeding for the following reasons:

- Their use is rarely necessary.
- Their use is not generally beneficial or effective.
- Their use often produces more problems than benefits.
- The absolute indications for their use are very few.

Tourniquets, improperly applied, can crush tissue beneath them and cause permanent damage to nerves, muscles, and blood vessels. Thus, they often make an extremity injury worse. Left on for a long time, a tourniquet causes *gangrene* (death) of all tissues distal to it. Use of a tourniquet is not indicated in wounds of the trunk, or for those distal to the elbow or knee. Tourniquets are frequently used in the operating room when it is convenient to keep an extremity bloodless for the completion of a surgical procedure. In these circumstances, control of the tourniquet is strict and the limb is monitored consistently. The types of injuries

for which they may be effective are limited, and the problems they cause are frequent. For these reasons, the current feeling is that tourniquets should virtually *never* be used to control bleeding in an emergency situation.

Nevertheless, a properly applied tourniquet may be lifesaving for a person whose bleeding from a major extremity vessel cannot be controlled in any other way. Specifically, the tourniquet is useful for the patient who has severe bleeding from a traumatic partial or complete amputation or when local pressure supplemented by proximal pressure point control fails to arrest major arterial hemorrhage in an injured extremity.

If a tourniquet must be used, to avoid problems it should be applied in the following very specific manner (Figure 11–8).

1. Fold a triangular bandage until it is 3 to 4 inches wide and 6 to 8 layers thick.
2. Wrap this long, 4-inch-wide bandage twice around the extremity, at a point proximal to the bleeding but as far distal on the extremity as possible (Figure 11–8a).
3. Tie one knot in the bandage. Place a stick or rod on top of the knot and tie the ends of the bandage over the stick in a square knot (Figure 11–8b).
4. Use the stick as a handle and twist to tighten the tourniquet until the bleeding has stopped (Figure 11–8c). Once the bleeding has ceased, make no more turns with the stick. Secure it in place and make the wrapping neat and smooth (Figure 11–8d). The technique of using a rod passed through a bandage to achieve pressure is called the *"Spanish Windlass."* This technique is also occasionally used for the application of traction in the treatment of fractures.

A blood pressure cuff can serve as a very effective tourniquet (Figure 11–9). Apply the cuff proximal to the bleeding point and inflate it to a pressure just in excess of that required to arrest the bleeding. Leave the cuff inflated.

Observe the following precautions when you use a tourniquet:

- Use as wide a bandage as possible and be sure that it is tightened securely. If possible,

A

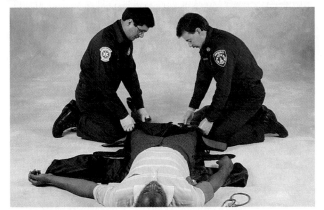

B

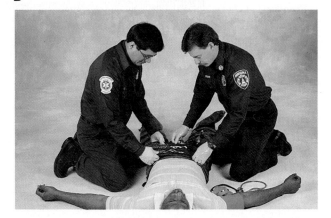

C

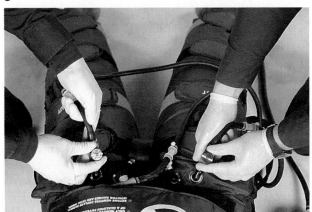

D

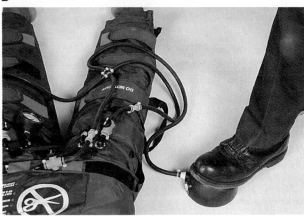

E

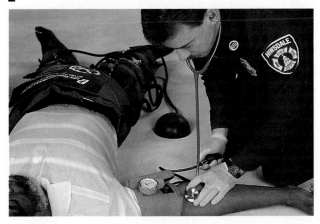

FIGURE 11–7

The application of a pneumatic counterpressure device. In effect, the unit is a large air splint for the lower half of the body. It can be used to provide stability for severe pelvic fractures. (A) Apply trousers to rib cage level. (B) Enclose both legs and abdomen and close velcro straps over zippers. (C) Open stopcocks. (D) Inflate with foot pump. (E) Check blood pressure and close stopcocks when systolic pressure reaches 100 mm Hg. Continue to monitor the patient's vital signs during transport.

use wide padding under the tourniquet to protect tissues.
- Never use wire, rope, a belt, or any other material that is narrow or will cut into the skin.

- Do not loosen the tourniquet once it has been applied. It will be loosened in the emergency department once measures have been taken to control the expected bleeding.
- Never cover a tourniquet with a bandage. Leave it open and in full view.

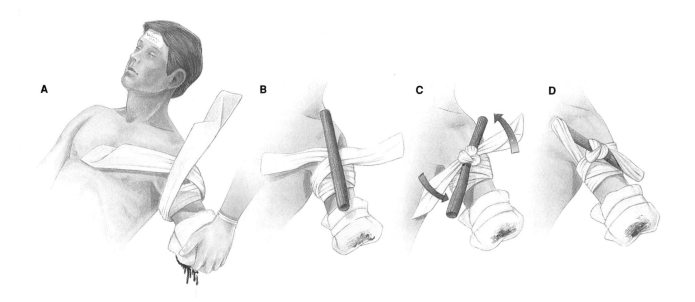

A   B   C   D

FIGURE 11–8 Steps in the application of a tourniquet. (A) Wrap a 4-inch bandage twice around the limb, just above the bleeding site. (B) Tie a single knot and place a stick on top of it. (C) Tie a square knot over the stick and then twist the stick until the bleeding stops. (D) Secure the stick so that it will not unwind.

FIGURE 11–9 A blood pressure cuff can serve as a very effective tourniquet.

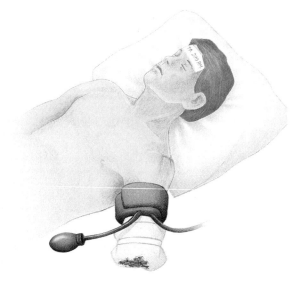

■ Always signify that the patient has had a tourniquet applied by writing "TK" and the time of tourniquet application on a piece of adhesive tape securely fastened to the patient's forehead (Figures 11–8a and 11–9). The phrase to use is "time applied" with the correct hour and minute. Record this infor-

mation on the ambulance run report form and notify the emergency department personnel on arrival that a tourniquet is in place.

■ Never place a tourniquet below the knee or elbow. In these more distal areas in the extremities, nerves lie close to the skin and may be injured by the compression. Furthermore, rarely, if ever, will you encounter bleeding distal to the knee or elbow that requires tourniquet control.

■ If you use a blood pressure cuff, continuously monitor the gauge to be sure that the pressure in the cuff is not being lost gradually. It may be necessary to clamp the tube leading from cuff to the inflating bulb to prevent loss of pressure.

Although you can control bleeding very efficiently with tourniquets, their use is *not recommended*, because

■ They are often improperly applied.
■ Most often the situations in which they might be effective do not produce much bleeding.
■ Tissue damage in the long run has exceeded patient benefit.

EPISTAXIS

Epistaxis (nosebleed) is a common emergency. The amount of blood that a person can lose in a nosebleed may occasionally be enough to cause shock. The blood seen actually coming from the nose may represent only a small amount of the total loss, because much may pass down the throat into the stomach as the patient swallows. A person who swallows a large amount of blood may become nauseated and may vomit. In this situation, sometimes a mistaken diagnosis of bleeding from the stomach may be made. Epistaxis can be caused by the following conditions:

■ A fractured skull.
■ Facial injuries, including those caused by a direct blow to the nose.
■ Sinusitis, infections, nosedrop use and abuse, dried or cracked nasal mucosa, or other abnormalities of the inside of the nose.
■ High blood pressure.
■ Bleeding diseases.

Bleeding from the nose or ears following a head injury may indicate that a skull fracture is present. Such bleeding is difficult to control, and excessive pressure at the fracture site may increase pressure on the brain as the blood leaking through the ear and the nose now

collects within the head. Treat bleeding from the nose caused by a skull fracture with a dry sterile local dressing and only moderate compression; avoid excessive pressure.

Nosebleeds resulting from all other causes should be initially treated at the scene. The following techniques are usually successful in stopping most nosebleeds (Figure 11–10):

1. Apply pressure by pinching the nostrils together or by placing a rolled 4 × 4 gauze bandage between the upper lip and the gum and pressing against it with your fingers. The patient can sometimes apply enough pressure to stop the bleeding by stretching the upper lip tightly against the rolled bandage and pushing it up into and against the nose (Figures 11–10a and b).
2. Keep the patient in a sitting position with the head tilted forward whenever possible so that blood will not trickle down the back of the throat or be aspirated into the lungs.
3. Keep the patient quiet. This rule is particularly important if the patient suffers from high blood pressure or is anxious. Anxiety tends to increase the blood pressure, and the nosebleed may worsen.
4. Apply ice over the nose. Local cooling treatment is helpful in controlling hemorrhage (Figure 11–10c).
5. Spend time to achieve control; most often, failure is related to releasing the pressure too soon; 15 minutes usually is adequate to allow time for good clot formation.

You must understand that the person with a prolonged nosebleed or one who is subject to frequent nosebleeds should be taken promptly to the hospital to be seen by a physician.

Most nosebleeds usually arise from an injury of the mucous membrane covering the nasal septum, which is anterior in the nose. Accordingly, the local measures just listed are frequently successful in stopping nosebleeds. A few nosebleeds, however, arise posteriorly, in the nasopharynx. This type of epistaxis cannot be stopped by these normal emergency methods. Such a nosebleed may require the application of a nasopharyngeal pack, which must be done in the hospital by the doctor. Transport any patient with a nosebleed that does not

A

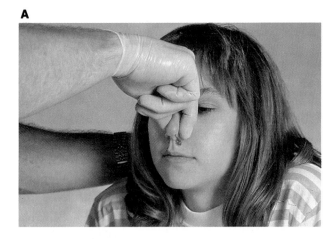

B

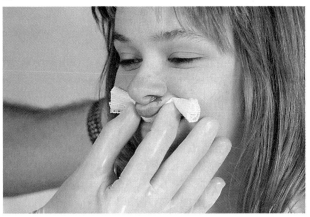

C

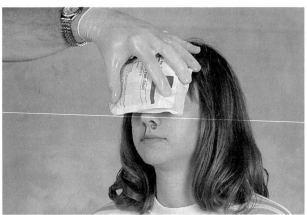

FIGURE 11–10

Methods of controlling epistaxis are shown. (A) To apply pressure, pinch the nostrils together or (B) place a rolled 4 × 4 gauze bandage between the upper lip and the gum. Keep the patient quiet and in a sitting position with the head tilted forward. (C) Apply ice over the nose.

respond to the measures listed to the hospital for treatment to avoid the development of hypovolemic shock.

INTERNAL BLEEDING

Signs and Symptoms of Internal Hemorrhage

Although not usually evident, internal bleeding can be very serious, and the patient with severe internal hemorrhage may develop hypovolemic shock before you realize the extent of blood loss. Bleeding, however slight, from any body opening is serious, because it usually indicates an internal source of hemorrhage that may not be readily seen or reached for control. Bleeding from the mouth or rectum or blood in the urine may indicate serious internal injury or disease. Nonmenstrual bleeding from the vagina is always significant.

Probably the most common evidence of internal bleeding is a bruise (contusion). It indicates hemorrhage into the soft tissues and may be seen after a slight or severe injury. The following are some other examples of internal hemorrhage:

- Bleeding from a peptic, gastric or duodenal ulcer, usually manifested as vomited blood or dark, tarry stools.
- Bleeding from a closed fracture of any bone, usually seen as bruising and swelling about the fracture site.
- Bleeding from a lacerated spleen or liver within the abdomen; usually, there is no evident sign of bleeding; you must suspect this problem with bruises over the lower chest, or with fractured ribs.

Signs that may point to internal bleeding and that are not evident at the body surface are those indicating the development of hypovolemic shock:

- The patient's pulse becomes weak and rapid ("thready").
- The patient's skin becomes cold and moist ("clammy").

- The eyes are dull; the pupils may be slightly dilated and slow to respond to light.
- The blood pressure falls; this event occurs *late* in the course of blood loss and means the patient can no longer compensate well.
- The patient is usually thirsty and almost invariably anxious, with a feeling of impending doom.
- The patient may feel nauseated and may vomit.

A person with a bleeding stomach ulcer may lose a large amount of blood internally very quickly. Fractured ribs may result in severe internal hemorrhage both into the chest cavity and into the soft tissues of the chest wall. Occasionally, with problems such as these, the patient vomits blood from the stomach or coughs up bright red blood from an injured lung. Vomited blood may be bright red, dark red, or look like coffee grounds suspended in gastric juice *(coffee grounds vomitus)*.

A person who has suffered a severe blunt abdominal injury with a laceration of the liver or spleen may lose a considerable quantity of blood within the abdominal cavity without any evident external sign of bleeding. Ordinarily, in addition to the signs and symptoms of shock, this patient develops a tender abdomen that progressively distends. Additionally, such patients sometimes complain of pain in the shoulder on the side of the injury. A patient with a liver injury may complain of right shoulder pain while one with an injured spleen may report left shoulder pain. Such referred pain, when there is no obvious shoulder injury, should make you suspect internal abdominal bleeding.

A person with a fracture of the shaft of the femur can easily lose a liter of blood or more into the soft tissues of the thigh with little or no immediate external indication of such blood loss. Local swelling is usually seen with closed fractures of major bones, largely as a result of an accumulation of blood around the ends of the fractured bone. Often the only signs of such bleeding are swelling of the tissue about the fracture site and local bruising.

Control of Internal Bleeding

The control of internal bleeding depends on the site of the hemorrhage. There is nothing you can do, in the field, to control internal hemorrhage within the body cavities or from the major organs. The likelihood of such bleeding must be suspected on the basis of the injuries sustained; it is confirmed by observing the vital signs. Immediate transportation to the emergency department is required for the injured patient whom you suspect has internal bleeding. Usually, an urgent operation or complex equipment is needed to control internal hemorrhage.

Following are some specific terms indicating acute internal bleeding from a variety of diseases and injuries:

- **Hematemesis** (the vomiting of bright red blood).
- **Hemoptysis** (the coughing up of bright red blood).
- *Melena* (the passage of dark black stools with the consistency of tar and a characteristic foul odor; it represents digested blood).
- *Hematochezia* (the passage of bright red blood from the rectum).
- *Coffee grounds vomitus* (the vomiting of coffee-ground-like material from the stomach; it represents semidigested blood).
- **Hematuria** (the passage of blood in the urine).
- **Ecchymosis** (a black and blue discoloration of the skin caused by bleeding; a bruise).
- **Hematoma** (a "blood tumor," a mass of blood accumulated in the soft tissues beneath the skin).

All patients with these findings are at risk; some may be in dangerous situations. These patients may continue to bleed; or, if they have stopped, they may bleed again massively at any moment. Transport all patients suspected of having internal bleeding promptly to the hospital for evaluation and treatment. Diagnosis of the exact cause of bleeding is frequently facilitated if the doctor can see the patient while the bleeding is active.

Usually you can control internal bleeding into the extremities quite well on the scene in a number of ways. Simple splinting of an injured or fractured extremity may allow control. In most cases, single-extremity air splints will effectively control bleeding. Only on rare occasions is the use of a pneumatic counterpressure device required. Tourniquets should not be used to control closed, internal, soft tissue bleeding.

Internal bleeding within the abdomen and thorax cannot be controlled in the field. The most serious complication of internal bleeding in these cavities, hypovolemic shock, can be treated to some degree by use of the pneumatic counterpressure device. This equipment does not treat the cause of the problem and may unnecessarily delay transport to the hospital.

The principles of treating any patient with suspected internal bleeding in the field are these:

1. Monitor and record the vital signs at least every 10 minutes (especially pulse, respiratory rate, and palpable systolic pressure).
2. Give oxygen. As blood is lost, the tissues of the body are deprived of their needed oxygen supplies. Administration of oxygen may be lifesaving.
3. Control all obvious external bleeding.
4. Treat obvious internal soft tissue bleeding in an extremity by applying a splint or an air pressure splint.
5. Treat severe uncontrolled hypovolemic shock with a pneumatic counterpressure device.
6. Anticipate that the patient will vomit; give nothing by mouth (not even small sips of water) and keep the patient supine, preferably on one side.
7. Elevate the patient's feet 6 to 12 inches to increase the return of the blood to the vital organs.
8. Transport the patient as expeditiously as possible to the emergency department.

EMT SAFETY

More than in any other situation, you are exposed to potentially infective body fluids when you must handle the patient who is actually bleeding. In these situations, barriers between you and the patient are absolutely necessary. Gloves, goggles, and masks are all required by the OSHA and by CDC guidelines. Any EMT with an open sore, cut, scratch, or ulcer that can be exposed to the patient must be especially careful. The risk of airborne infection is as slight as with any other routine, non-coughing patient; you must be careful here of direct contact with body fluids. Attention to barriers and frequent good hand washing and disinfection after every run is complete are important and will be generally successful in providing you adequate protection.

YOU ARE THE EMT

1. One of the ways that external bleeding can be controlled is to apply direct pressure to the wound using a finger, hand, or pressure dressing. Describe two other common ways you can control external hemorrhage. What are the most effective means of controlling external bleeding?

2. Why aren't tourniquets used very often to control bleeding? Under what type of circumstances are they useful?

3. How do pneumatic counterpressure devices work to control bleeding? What must be done before these devices are deflated to prevent hypovolemic shock in the patient?

4. What is the difference between hematemesis and hemoptysis? Between ecchymosis and hematoma? What do these four terms have in common?

5. You are called to treat a patient with epistaxis. How would you approach the treatment of this problem? If methods fail and the patient continues to bleed, what is your next step?

6. A patient has sustained a "twisted ankle" in a fall. He tells you that he has hemophilia. The ankle does not look very swollen 20 minutes after the injury. It is mildly tender. What do you do?

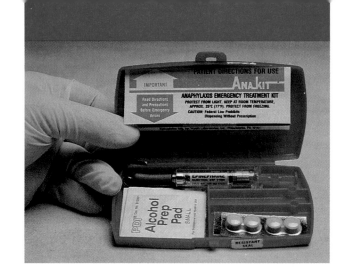

CHAPTER 12

SHOCK

KEY TERMS

anaphylaxis (an"ah-fĭ-lak'sis) An unusual or exaggerated allergic reaction of the organism to foreign protein or other substances.

autonomic nervous system (aw"to-nom'ik ner'vus sis'tem) That part of the nervous system that regulates functions, such as digestion and sweating, that are not controlled by a voluntary act of conscious will.

cyanosis (si"ah-no'sis) Blue color of the skin resulting from poor oxygenation of the circulating blood.

dehydration (de"hi-dra'shun) Loss of water from the tissues of the body.

dyspnea (disp'ne-ah) Difficulty in breathing.

edema (ĕ-de'mah) The presence of abnormally large amounts of fluid in the extracellular tissue spaces of the body, causing swelling of the affected area.

hypothermia (hi"po-ther'me-ah) A condition in which the internal body temperature falls below 95 degrees F after prolonged exposure to freezing or near-freezing temperatures.

perfusion (per-fu'zhun) The process whereby blood enters an organ or tissue through its arteries and leaves through the veins, providing tissue with nourishment and removing wastes.

shock A condition of acute peripheral circulatory failure causing inadequate and progressively failing perfusion of tissue.

sphincter muscle (sfingk'ter mus'el) Circular muscles that encircle a duct, tube, or opening in such a way that their contraction constricts the opening.

OVERVIEW

Shock has a variety of meanings. For example, it is used to denote the receiving of any amount of electrical current by an individual; it is also used to describe the psychological reaction to bad news, fright, or other emotional stress. In this chapter, shock describes a state of collapse and failure of the cardiovascular system. When that happens, blood circulation slows and eventually ceases. After even a few minutes without blood flow, the cells of certain organs, particularly the brain and heart, die. If the conditions causing shock are not promptly treated, death soon follows.

Shock is caused by a number of different factors, including blood loss, dilation of blood vessels, and failure of the heart to pump effectively. It can also be associated with respiratory failure and acute allergic reactions. You will frequently encounter shock, because it so often accompanies the events, such as heart attacks and automobile accidents, to which you must respond. Therefore, it is imperative that you be able to anticipate and recognize shock, treat it, and, hopefully, reverse it to save a life.

Chapter 12 begins with a description of the cardiovascular system and an explanation of perfusion. The lack of adequate tissue perfusion is shock. The three major physiologic causes of shock are described, together with a wider variety of specific clinical situations. The chapter next discusses the signs and symptoms of shock. The last section describes the general treatment for shock, including appropriate measures for treating each of the clinical situations seen. Specific measures for counteracting major allergic reactions causing shock are discussed and illustrated.

GOALS

The goals of Chapter 12 are to

- understand the basic physiology of circulation and tissue perfusion and the causes of shock.
- identify the three specific physiological processes responsible for the various clinical presentations of shock.
- recognize the signs and symptoms common to all types of shock.
- know the basic treatment for shock and the treatments for the specific, clinical pictures seen with shock.

CIRCULATION AND THE CAUSES OF SHOCK

The cardiovascular system circulates blood to all of the cells and tissues in the body. Through this system, oxygen and nutrients are brought to each cell, and metabolic waste products are removed from them. Certain parts of the body, such as the brain, the spinal cord, and the heart, require a constant flow of blood to live. These organs cannot tolerate the arrest of blood flow for more than a few minutes or their cells will die. Furthermore, these tissues do not have the ability to generate new cells. Once cells in these organs die they are replaced only by scar tissue. Permanent loss of function or, if enough cells die, death of the patient will result.

The Cardiovascular System

The cardiovascular system can be described as consisting of two parts: a container and its contents. The container consists of the *heart* and its system of blood vessels: arteries, veins, innumerable small arterioles and venules, and capillaries. They are the tubes that extend to every cell in the body.

In this system, capillary vessels nourish and carry oxygen to the individual cells of the body. Through these tiny tubes, just the size of a red blood cell, oxygen and nutrients are carried to tissue or organ cells, and waste and carbon dioxide are removed.

In the arteries and at the arterial ends of the capillaries, the vessels have distinct circular muscular walls. They can constrict and dilate automatically under the control of the **autonomic nervous system.** Whether the small capillary vessels that pass between individual cells and link arterioles with venules receive any blood at all is controlled by these **sphincter muscles.** When they are open, blood passes into the capillaries to be in close proximity to each cell of that tissue. When they are closed, there is no capillary flow. The opening (dilation) and the closing (constriction) of these arteriolar sphincters are entirely automatic functions and under the control of the autonomic nervous system. Stimuli that cause the dilation and constriction of blood vessels include fright, heat, cold, the specific need for oxygen, and the need to dispose of metabolic waste. An individual cannot exert any voluntary control over this system. Never are all the vessels fully dilated or fully constricted at one time in a normal individual. Most tissues in the body require circulating blood intermittently during the day when they are active. Some tissues never rest and require a constant blood supply.

The second part of the cardiovascular system is the contents in the container: the blood. Normally, there is just enough blood to fill the system entirely; in an average adult, this amount is 6 liters. The heart, a muscular pump, circulates the blood through the system. Nor-

mally, in an adult, the heart pumps 6 liters of blood per minute through a system that can hold just 6 liters. Thus, every part of the system receives a regular supply of blood every minute.

Any condition under which the circulatory system fails to provide sufficient circulation to every part of the body to carry out its functions is called **shock.**

As mentioned previously, some certain tissues cannot live without a constant, high level of blood flow. The heart, the central nervous system (brain and spinal cord), the lungs, and the kidneys are tissues that must function continuously. Regardless of what happens, the functions of these organs must continue, and they require a constant blood supply to do so.

It is just as important to realize that not every part of the body, nor every part of every tissue, receives the same blood flow all the time. Certain tissues are used very heavily but only on an intermittent basis. For example, muscles are at rest during sleep but require a very large blood supply during exercise. The gastrointestinal tract requires a high flow of blood after a meal; but it can be deprived of a good deal of this flow without significant problems after digestion of that meal is completed. Blood is shunted (redirected) automatically by the autonomic nervous system from such organs as the skeletal muscles and the gastrointestinal tract in emergency situations to the heart, brain, lungs, and kidneys. The blood supply to all the various tissues and organs of the body is regulated by this nervous system on a moment-to-moment basis in response to various stimuli. The vascular system is dynamic and constantly changing, depending on the needs of each of the body parts.

Perfusion (the circulation of blood within an organ or tissue) occurs if blood is entering an organ or tissue through the arteries and leaving it through the veins in adequate amounts to meet its current needs (Figure 12–1). To reach the veins, the blood must pass through the arterioles, connecting capillaries, and venules. In doing so, the blood gives up

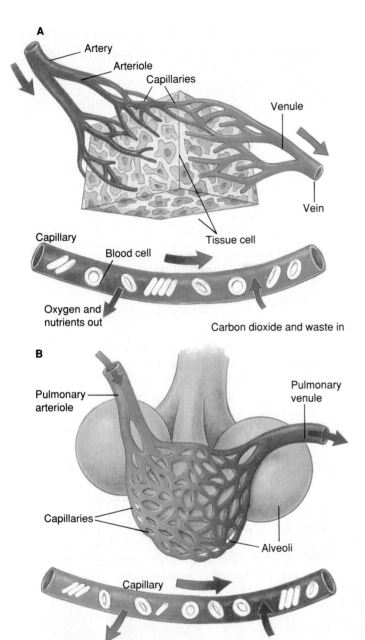

A

Artery
Arteriole
Capillaries
Venule
Vein
Capillary
Tissue cell
Blood cell
Oxygen and nutrients out
Carbon dioxide and waste in

B

Pulmonary arteriole
Pulmonary venule
Capillaries
Alveoli
Capillary
Carbon dioxide out
Oxygen in

FIGURE 12–1

The exchange of gas(es), nutrients, and wastes between capillary blood and tissue cells is shown schematically. The capillary vessel is no larger than a red cell. (A) Perfusion of blood through tissues is shown. Oxygen and nutrients pass from the capillary vessels to tissue cells; carbon dioxide and waste pass into the blood. (B) In the lung, capillary vessels surround an air sac (alveolus). Here the blood picks up oxygen and gives up carbon dioxide to be exhaled. Other waste products are processed by the liver or kidneys.

nutrients and oxygen to cells and picks up the waste from the organ or tissue that is being perfused. Blood must pass through this system fast enough so that each cell receives enough oxygen and nutrients and can get rid of wastes adequately. Perfusion of the whole body by blood keeps its component cells alive and healthy. The body depends on adequate, continuous perfusion of its organs and tissues by blood to bring food to them and to dispose of their metabolic waste products generated in the course of normal daily activity. In states of shock, perfusion of organs and tissues slows, falls below critical levels for cellular and tissue survival, and finally fails.

You must know which organs of the body are more susceptible than others to the lack of adequate perfusion. The heart requires *constant* perfusion or it will not function properly. The brain and the spinal cord (the central nervous system) cannot lack perfusion for more than 4 to 6 minutes without permanent damage to nerve cells. Permanent damage in the kidney results after inadequate perfusion for a period of 45 minutes. Skeletal muscle, if subjected to the loss of perfusion for more than 2 hours, will be permanently damaged. The gastrointestinal tract can exist with limited (but not absent) perfusion for a number of hours.

No part of the body can exist without adequate perfusion for an indefinite period of time. Permanent injury results when the organ systems that are most sensitive to the lack of perfusion are damaged. In order, these organs are heart, central nervous system, lung, and kidney. Each of the time periods listed for a safe length of time without perfusion assumes a normal body temperature. An organ or tissue that is considerably below normal body temperature (98.6 degrees F or 37.0 degrees C) is much more resistant to damage from lack of perfusion.

It is critical for you to understand the concept of perfusion, because it is the unifying element among the different types of shock. Of equal importance is understanding the varying susceptibility of tissues to the lack of perfusion.

Physiologic Causes of Shock

Shock has a number of separate causes; however, there are really only three ways by which shock can be caused in a living body. The following are the three basic causes of shock (Figure 12–2):

- *Pump failure:* The heart can be damaged by intrinsic muscular disease or injury, so that it fails to act properly as a pump. It does not generate sufficient energy to move blood through the system.
- *Relative hypovolemia:* The blood vessels constituting the container can dilate so that the blood within them, even though it is of normal volume, is insufficient to fill the system and provide efficient perfusion.
- *Hypovolemia:* Blood or plasma can be lost so that the volume of fluid contained within the vascular system is insufficient to perfuse all areas well each minute.

Whatever the cause of shock, damage occurs because perfusion of organs and tissues is insufficient. As soon as perfusion ceases or is impaired, tissues start to die. Regardless of the cause, the results of shock are all exactly the same. Insufficient perfusion of blood through the tissues of the body affects all local body processes. If the conditions causing shock are not promptly arrested and reversed, death soon follows.

Shock itself, however, cannot be seen. It is not a specific disease or injury. It is a physiologic state with specific manifestations. Its signs and symptoms include

- A rise in pulse.
- Agitation, anxiety, and a feeling of impending doom.
- Skin that is pale, ashen, cool, and moist.
- Air hunger (shortness of breath).
- Poor urinary output.
- Ultimately, a falling blood pressure.

You must learn to anticipate shock based on your assessment of each situation. The signs must trigger your response to treat imminent, severe cardiovascular collapse. In many critical situations, you must automatically expect shock—for example, after or accompanying massive external or internal bleeding, multiple severe fractures, an acute abdomen, spinal

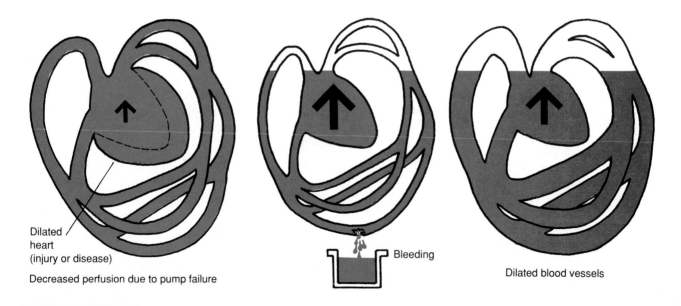

Dilated heart
(injury or disease)

Decreased perfusion due to pump failure

Bleeding

Dilated blood vessels

FIGURE 12–2

There are three basic causes of shock and impaired tissue perfusion: (left) pump failure due to heart disease or injury; (middle) decreased blood volume, usually a result of bleeding; and (right) dilation of blood vessels, making the container too large and decreasing the blood pressure.

injury, a severe infection, or a major heart attack. Whatever the cause, you must recognize the existence of shock promptly and immediately institute measures to counteract it.

TYPES OF SHOCK AND THEIR CAUSES

Shock may accompany many emergency situations. It is convenient to relate it to its basic physiologic cause since a more rational approach to its treatment can be made. There are both vascular and nonvascular causes of shock. The three major vascular causes of shock are

- Pump failure.
- Vessel failure (loss of muscle tone or damage of the vessels themselves).
- Content failure (loss of intravascular contents, blood or plasma).

The nonvascular causes of shock are respiratory insufficiency and anaphylaxis.

Vascular Causes of Shock

Pump Failure: Cardiogenic Shock *Cardiogenic shock* is caused by inadequate function of the heart. Circulation of blood throughout the vascular system requires the constant pumping action of a normal and vigorous heart muscle. Many diseases can cause destruction or inflammation of this muscle. Within certain limits, the heart can adapt to these problems. If too much muscular damage occurs, however, as sometimes happens after a heart attack, the heart no longer functions well.

The muscular contraction of the heart moves blood through the vessels at distinct pressures. A certain pressure is required to force the blood through the entire system. The heart must also beat enough times each minute so that the blood volume can be circulated throughout the system efficiently. To this end, the heart has its own electric system which initiates and regulates its beating. Disease or injury can damage or destroy this system causing irregular and uncoordinated beats.

Shock from cardiac origin develops when the heart muscle can no longer impart sufficient

pressure to circulate the blood to all organs. It can also occur when the regularity of the heartbeat is so disrupted that the volume of blood within the system can no longer be handled efficiently. Direct pump failure is the cause of shock in each of these situations, whether the muscular force is destroyed or the heartbeat itself is disrupted.

Vessel Failure: Neurogenic Shock Damage of the spinal cord, particularly at the upper cervical levels, may cause significant injury to that part of the nervous system that controls the size and muscular tone of the blood vessels. *Neurogenic shock* is usually the result. In this condition, the muscles in the walls of the blood vessels are deprived of the nerve supply that causes them to contract. Thus, all the vessels below the level of the spinal injury dilate widely and increase the size and capacity of the vascular system. The available 6 liters of blood can no longer fill the enlarged vascular system and failure rapidly follows. Even though no blood or fluid has been lost, perfusion of organs and tissues becomes inadequate, and shock occurs. In this condition, a radical change in the size of the vascular system has caused shock.

You must remember also that many other functions under the control of this part of the nervous system are also lost in this situation. The most important of them, in an acute injury setting, is that the patient loses the ability to control body temperature. Body temperature in the patient with neurogenic shock can rapidly fall to match that of the environment. In many situations, significant **hypothermia** (low body temperature) occurs, severely complicating the situation.

Psychogenic Shock *Psychogenic shock,* or fainting, is called *syncope* and is a sudden reaction of the nervous system that produces a temporary, generalized vascular dilation. The result is a temporary reduction of blood supply to the brain because the blood momentarily pools in dilated vessels in other parts of the body. When the blood supply to the brain is suddenly and sharply reduced, the brain ceases to function normally, and the patient faints.

Fear, bad news, sometimes good news, the sight of an injury or blood, the prospect of medical treatment, severe pain, and anxiety are among the many precipitating causes of psychogenic shock. A person who is not feeling well, is tired or worried, or is obliged to stand quietly in a stuffy room may be susceptible to fainting.

Once fainting has occurred, the patient collapses and becomes supine; circulation to the brain is promptly restored and the episode passes quickly. In this type of shock, your major concern is any injury sustained by the patient during the fainting spell, such as striking the head. The vascular cause of psychogenic shock is a sudden enlargement of the container so that perfusion, for the moment, becomes ineffective.

Content Failure: Hypovolemic Shock Following injury, shock is commonly a result of fluid or blood loss. This type of shock is called *hypovolemic* (low-volume) *shock*. When caused by blood loss, this type of shock is more specifically called *hemorrhagic shock*. External bleeding is common in patients who have suffered severe lacerations or fractures. Internal bleeding follows a variety of injuries or diseases: rupture of the liver or the spleen, lacerations of the great vessels within the abdomen or the chest, bleeding peptic ulcers, or tumors. Hypovolemic shock also occurs with severe thermal burns. In burns, a considerable amount of intravascular plasma (the colorless part of the blood) leaks from the circulatory system into the tissues that have been burned and that lie adjacent to the injury. Crushing injuries may also result in the loss of blood and plasma into the injured tissues from damaged blood vessels.

If **dehydration** (loss of body water) is present before the injury, the state of shock will be aggravated. In all these circumstances, the common factor is an insufficient volume of blood within the vascular system (the container) to provide adequate circulation to all the organs of the body, resulting in shock.

Metabolic Shock Occasionally, severe untreated illnesses may cause a state of *metabolic shock* because of profound fluid losses from vomiting, diarrhea, or excess urination. Disturbances of body fluid and chemical balance occur in uncontrolled diseases such as diabetes mellitus. These patients can become severely dehydrated and not have a sufficient volume of fluid within the vascular container to provide proper perfusion of tissues and organs. Patients who develop metabolic shock in the course of a chronic disease are desperately ill. They may have reached the end of their capacity to compensate for the problems of that particular disease. You may be called to transport such a patient whose disease has been sorely neglected. During transport this patient will require all available support measures.

Combined Vessel and Content Failure: Septic Shock In some patients who have severe bacterial infections, toxins (poisons) can be generated by the bacteria or by infected body tissues to produce a state called *septic shock*. In this condition, blood vessel walls are damaged and become leaky. They also lose the capacity to contract well. The shock state results from widespread dilation of vessels in addition to the loss of plasma through the injured vessel walls. This type of shock is a complex problem. There is an insufficient volume of fluid in the container because much of the blood has leaked out of the vascular system (hypovolemia). At the same time, there is a larger than normal blood vessel bed to contain the smaller than normal volume of intravascular fluid.

Septic shock almost always is seen as a complication of some very serious illness, injury, or operation. For it to develop, the patient must have a rather long-lasting and severe focus of infection or dead tissue. From time to time, you may be required to transport a patient in septic shock. You must be familiar with the term and its meaning for the patient. It is a serious problem.

Nonvascular Causes of Shock

There are two causes of shock that do not result from disturbances of the vascular system: respiratory insufficiency and anaphylaxis.

Respiratory Insufficiency A severe chest injury or obstruction of the airway may result in a patient's being unable to breathe adequately so that an insufficient amount of oxygen is inspired. Inadequate breathing capacity can produce shock as rapidly as the vascular causes. In these instances, shock is produced because an insufficient concentration of oxygen exists in the blood. The volume of blood, the volume of the vascular container, and the action of the heart may all be normal. The amount of oxygen carried in the blood is not sufficient to sustain the tissues adequately. Without oxygen the organs in the body cannot survive, and their cells promptly start to deteriorate.

Because this problem may develop in patients with airway obstruction or with diseased or injured lungs, the first step in adequate resuscitation is always securing an airway and the second is restoring respiration. Circulation of nonoxygenated blood will have no benefit at all for the patient.

Anaphylactic Shock *Anaphylactic shock (anaphylaxis)* occurs when an individual who has been sensitized to some substance by a previous contact with it reacts violently to a subsequent dose or contact. It is the most severe form of an allergic reaction. Because the first exposure did not cause an allergic reaction, do not be misled by a patient who reports prior contact with a suspected substance without incident. You should also remember that each subsequent exposure after sensitization tends to produce a progressively more severe reaction. Instances that most often cause allergic reactions fall into the following four groups:

- *Injection:* The injection of sera such as tetanus antitoxin or drugs such as penicillin may cause an immediate and severe allergic reaction.
- *Sting:* A sting is an injection of a specific venom. The sting of a honeybee, wasp, yellow jacket, or hornet can cause severe, immediate allergic reactions in those people who are allergic to the injected toxin. These reactions are similar in their rapidity to those seen with injected medicines.

- *Ingestion:* The eating of certain foods such as shellfish or the use of some medications or drugs such as oral penicillin can cause slower but equally severe reactions in anyone sensitive to the agents.
- *Inhalation:* The inhalation of dusts, pollens, or materials to which the patient is sensitive may similarly cause a rapid and severe allergic reaction.

Anaphylactic shock is a very complex and severe reaction. Anaphylactic reactions can develop in minutes or even seconds after contact with the substances to which the patient is allergic. Obvious reactions in the skin, respiratory system, and circulation result. The signs are not those usually associated with shock from other causes. The following evidences of an anaphylactic or allergic reaction are quite characteristic:

- *Skin:* There is flushing, itching, or burning of the skin, especially over the face and upper chest. *Urticaria* (hives) may spread over large areas of the body. **Edema** (swelling), especially of the face and tongue, may occur. Specific marked swelling of the lips may be seen. **Cyanosis** may become marked about the lips. The skin reactions may precede all others.
- *Respiratory System:* At first, the patient may sneeze or perceive an itch in the nasal passages. Then tightness in the chest develops, with an irritating, persistent dry cough. Wheezing and **dyspnea** (difficulty in breathing) then develop. Fluid and mucus are secreted into the bronchial passages and *alveoli* in reaction to the sensitizing agent and the patient tries to cough them up. Fluid is also secreted into the tissue of the lung. Bronchi constrict, and the movement of air into the lungs becomes increasingly difficult. Expiration, normally the passive and relaxed part of the breathing cycle, becomes forced and requires exertion. The fluid in the air passages and the constricted small bronchi cause the development of a characteristic wheeze as the patient works hard to exhale. Breathing rapidly becomes increasingly difficult and ultimately may cease.

- *Circulatory System:* The response of the peripheral vascular system is dilation. Ultimately, there will be a perceptible drop in blood pressure; the development of a weak, barely palpable pulse; pallor; and dizziness as the vascular system fails. Fainting and coma may follow.

With anaphylactic shock, there is no loss of blood, no vascular damage, and only a slight possibility of direct cardiac muscular injury; but there is vascular dilation. The body is rapidly deprived of needed oxygen by the respiratory system reaction. The combination of poor oxygenation and poor perfusion may easily prove fatal.

SIGNS AND SYMPTOMS OF SHOCK

Certain signs and symptoms are common to all types of shock, with the exception of anaphylactic shock, which presents its own special signs. The following signs and symptoms are common clinical indicators for all the other types of shock described in this chapter:

- Restlessness and anxiety may precede all other signs.
- A weak and rapid pulse ("thready" or difficult to feel) occurs rapidly.
- Cold and wet skin (commonly described as "clammy") reflects a major sympathetic nervous system response.
- Profuse sweating is common.
- Paleness, and later cyanosis, reflect decreasing oxygen delivery to tissues.
- Shallow, labored, rapid, or possibly irregular or gasping respirations (especially if a chest injury is associated with the development of shock) are common.
- Dull and lusterless eyes with dilated pupils occur as the process develops.
- Thirst may become intense.
- Nausea or vomiting usually reflect other injuries but may occur as shock develops.
- Gradual and steadily falling blood pressure is a common and *late* sign. (In general, although some people normally have a systolic blood pressure of only 90 to 100 mm Hg, it is best to assume that shock is developing in any adult whose systolic blood pressure in the field is 90 millimeters of mercury or lower.)
- Loss of or alterations in consciousness occur in cases of rapidly developing or severe shock.

You must remember that, although shock means the failure of the cardiovascular system to perfuse blood through organs and tissues at proper pressures and flow rates, blood pressure may be the last measurable parameter to change. Many mechanisms react automatically to help maintain blood pressure. When falling blood pressure is observed, shock is far along in its development. This late stage of shock (when the blood pressure is falling) has been described as *decompensated shock*. Prior to the time when the blood pressure starts to fall, the patient has been able to compensate. This earlier phase of shock is sometimes referred to as *compensated shock*.

TREATMENT OF SHOCK

Any patient who exhibits any of the signs or symptoms of shock must be vigorously treated as soon as the diagnosis is made. Recognizing the probable cause of shock is important so that treatment can be given logically. However, many specific principles of the initial treatment can be applied to all patients in shock. These initial principles are as follows:

1. First, secure and maintain an open airway and give oxygen as needed. Be certain the patient can breathe well. Assist or control respiration when appropriate. Give oxygen.
2. Control all obvious external bleeding by direct compression.
3. Elevate the lower extremities about 12 inches.
4. Prevent the loss of body heat by placing blankets under and over the patient. Do not, however, overload the patient with covers or attempt to warm the body unduly.
5. Splint fractures. Splinting will lessen bleeding from the injured site and minimize pain

and discomfort that can further aggravate shock.

6. Avoid rough and excessive handling.

7. In general, keep an injured patient supine. Remember, however, that some patients in shock after a severe heart attack or with lung disease cannot breathe as well when supine as when sitting up or in a semisitting position. With such a patient use the most comfortable position.

8. Accurately record the patient's pulse, blood pressure, and other vital signs. Maintain a record of them at 10-minute intervals until the patient is delivered to the emergency department.

9. Do not give the patient anything to eat or drink.

10. Plan the use of a *pneumatic counterpressure device* or pneumatic antishock garment (PASG) when it is indicated. The use of the device may help patients in shock from injuries of the pelvis or from intraabdominal bleeding. Occasionally, when the specific cause of shock is unknown, the device may also help. Any critically injured patient, any patient with a systolic blood pressure of less than 100 mg Hg, or any patient with a falling blood pressure or a rising pulse rate should be placed in an uninflated PASG prior to transport. This measure will facilitate rapid inflation should the patient's condition worsen en route to the hospital. The application, indications for its use, and hazards of this device are discussed in Chapter 11.

Lack of oxygen may rapidly cause shock; thus, it is important for you to observe the patient's breathing. Inadequate ventilation may be either the primary cause or a major contributing factor in shock. Respiratory difficulty may be the result of an easily removed obstruction in the throat, or it may require full ventilatory support. You must establish and maintain an open airway and be certain that breathing is adequate. Oxygen must be given to all patients in shock. A few assisted breaths using a ventilatory apparatus with added oxygen will substantially raise the patient's arterial blood oxygen concentration. If the cause of shock is hypovolemia, supplemental oxygen will permit the remaining blood to absorb and transmit a much higher than normal concentration of oxygen. This effect compensates to some degree for the actual loss of oxygen-carrying capacity with blood loss.

All obvious external bleeding must be controlled. It is best done with sterile gauze compresses placed over the bleeding sites and secured with local circumferential pressure dressings. Sufficient pressure must be applied to stop any bleeding. Elevating the lower extremities of the patient allows the blood in the legs to be returned to the heart more rapidly. It is a simple way, after severe hemorrhage, of supplying as much blood to the heart as possible. It is also a simple way of controlling venous bleeding in any part of the body that can be elevated. Do not attempt elevation if the patient has fractures of the legs until they are well splinted or the patient is on a spine board. Then elevate the foot of the board 6 to 10 inches.

Fractures must be splinted. Splinting, at this point, is not a definitive treatment for the fracture. It minimizes the amount of damage the broken ends of bone can do to adjacent soft tissue and decreases hemorrhage at the fracture site. In general, splinting makes it easier to move the patient and makes the patient much more comfortable. Some soft tissue injuries may very well be handled best by splinting and occasionally by the use of air splints for compression.

Although the loss of body heat should be prevented, you should not try to overwarm the patient. It is better for the patient to be slightly cool than too hot. The use of external heat sources such as hot water bottles or heating pads may harm the person in shock.

Do not give any liquids by mouth to the patient in shock. The rule is specifically, *nothing by mouth*, under any circumstances, regardless of the patient's urgent requests. Nothing should be given orally until the patient has been seen in the emergency department by the doctor. Alcoholic drinks (depressants) are never given to treat shock; stimulants such as coffee have little or no value in the treatment of shock. The intense thirst that frequently accompanies shock may be alleviated by allowing the patient to chew or suck on a moistened piece of gauze.

Table 12–1 lists the general supportive measures for the major types of shock. Not every measure is used for every type of shock. The appropriate measures for each type of shock are explained in greater detail in the following sections.

Pump Failure: Cardiogenic Shock

The patient in shock as a result of a heart attack specifically does not require a transfusion of blood, intravenous fluids, elevation of the legs, or a pneumatic counterpressure device. In this condition, shock results from the heart's inability to handle the volume of blood that the patient already has. The damaged heart muscle simply cannot generate the necessary power to pump the patient's blood through the circulatory system. If chronic obstructive pulmonary disease is associated with this condition, as is frequently the case, oxygenation of the blood passing through the lungs is impaired. Chronic lung disease will aggravate cardiogenic shock. This patient is often able to breathe better in a sitting position and may tell you so. This patient should be permitted to sit up during transport. Usually, these patients do not have any injury; but they have had and may still be having chest pains. The pulse commonly is irregular; and it may be weak. Blood pressure is low. Cyanosis is frequently present about the lips and underneath the fingernails. The patient may be anxious. Occasionally, patients who have had heart attacks vomit.

TABLE 12–1   General Measures to Treat Shock Based On Its Cause

	Identification					Treatment		
Major Cause Of Shock	Failure	Type Of Shock	Use Oxygen	Use Epinephrine	Elevate Legs	Pneumatic Antishock Garment	Position	Possible Other Injuries
Vascular	Pump	Cardiogenic	Yes	No	No	No	Sitting or semi-upright	No
Vascular	Vessels	Neurogenic	Yes	No	Yes	Maybe	Supine	Yes
Vascular	Vessels	Psychogenic	Maybe	No	No	No	Supine	Yes
Vascular	Contents	Hemorrhagic Hypovolemic	Yes	No	Yes	Maybe	Supine	Yes
Vascular	Contents	Metabolic	Yes	No	Yes	Maybe	Supine	No
Vascular	Contents and vessels	Septic	Yes	No	Yes	Maybe	Supine	No
Nonvascular	Respiratory system	—	Yes	No	No	No	Sitting or semi-sitting	Yes
Nonvascular	Respiratory system	Anaphylactic	Yes	Yes*	No	No	Sitting or semi-seated	Yes

*Use will depend on local protocol; consult your medical director.

Treat these patients by placing them in the position in which they can breathe most easily, by administering oxygen, by assisting ventilation when necessary, and by transporting them promptly to the emergency department. Reassurance and a calm demeanor are required in treating a patient after a heart attack.

Vessel Failure: Neurogenic Shock

Shock that accompanies spinal cord injury is best treated by a combination of all the known supportive measures. The patient who has suffered this kind of injury will ordinarily require hospitalization for a long time. Emergency treatment must be directed at obtaining and maintaining a proper airway, assisting impaired breathing as needed, conserving body heat with blankets, and providing the most effective circulation possible. The patient usually is not losing blood; but the capacity of his blood vessels has become significantly larger than the volume of blood they contain. In this specific instance, the pneumatic anti-shock garment may be useful.

This patient requires supplemental oxygen so that the blood may carry a greater than normal concentration of this gas. The patient must be kept as warm as possible, because the normal control of body temperature may well be lost with the injury. Prompt transportation to the hospital is mandatory.

Psychogenic Shock

Usually, a common fainting spell will pass very quickly. If the attack has caused the patient to fall, you must be alert for any injury sustained. The older patient is more likely to have sustained such an injury. In the absence of any injuries, the patient usually recovers consciousness within a few minutes. As soon as the patient has fallen, collapsed, or become supine, the blood supply to the brain improves and consciousness returns. If it does not or if the patient is confused after such a mishap, you must suspect a head injury, particularly if the patient has struck the head during the fainting spell. In such an instance, prompt transportation to the emergency department is necessary.

You must record your initial observations of the vital signs and level of consciousness. In addition, before transporting the patient try to learn from bystanders how long the patient had been unconscious.

Content Failure: Hypovolemic Shock

The emergency treatment of hypovolemic or hemorrhagic shock includes the control of all obvious external bleeding after you are sure that the patient can breathe properly. You must be aware that continued bleeding will result from the following:

- Failure to apply sufficient pressure to obvious external bleeding points.
- Failure to splint fractures properly.
- Failure to handle the injured patient gently.

Elevate the lower extremities by raising the legs from the hips 6 to 10 inches and keeping the knees straight. This maneuver increases blood flow to the heart from the lower body and may combat shock using the patient's own blood to the best advantage. Remember, however, that in a head-down position, the entire weight of the abdominal organs falls on the diaphragm. The patient may be unable to breathe easily in this position and may require some assistance with ventilation.

It is difficult to recognize internal hemorrhage. On occasion it can be identified when blood passes from the mouth or anus. Nothing can be done in the field to control internal bleeding. You must recognize the existence and severity of internal bleeding and provide vigorous general support. Be certain that the patient does not, in the instance of bleeding from the mouth, aspirate any vomitus into the lungs. Secure and maintain an airway and give respiratory support. Occasionally the application of a pneumatic antishock garment may help this patient. Because so little can be done to control the internal bleeding itself, you must transport the patient as rapidly as possible to the emergency department.

In some instances where hemorrhage is located about the pelvis, hips, or femurs; within the abdomen; or occasionally when it is suspected, but its location is unknown, a PASG may be helpful in treating shock. Its use is described in Chapter 11.

Ventilatory support must be part of the treatment for hypovolemic shock. It may include only assisted ventilation and the use of supplemental oxygen while the patient is being transported to the hospital. It may require full respiratory support. With too little circulating blood, additional oxygen may be lifesaving. The patient with hypovolemic shock must be taken as promptly as possible to the emergency department for definitive care.

Metabolic Shock

Metabolic shock is usually the result of an illness that has been present for a long time or has been extremely severe over a brief period. It is associated with unusual and excessive loss of fluid and electrolytes from vomiting, diarrhea, or urination. With inadequate food and fluid intake to cover the loss of body water, the patient will become severely dehydrated. This patient must be transported to the hospital as promptly as possible and again given all the support necessary, including oxygen, during transport. You should try to find out which contributory illnesses, such as diabetes or severe gastroenteritis, might be present.

Combined Vessel and Content Failure: Septic Shock

The proper treatment of septic shock requires complex hospital management. If this condition is suspected, transport the patient to the hospital as promptly as possible while giving all the general support available. The use of oxygen during transportation is advisable. Full ventilatory support may be necessary as well as elevation of the legs and keeping the patient warm with blankets.

Nonvascular Causes of Shock

Respiratory Insufficiency The proper emergency management of shock as a result of inadequate respiration involves the immediate securing and maintaining of an airway. Clear the mouth and throat down to the larynx of mucus, vomitus, foreign material, or anything obstructing the air passages. Provide manual ventilations using ventilatory aids or administer mouth-to-mouth resuscitation when necessary. Give supplemental oxygen. Prompt transportation to the emergency department is mandatory.

Anaphylactic Shock The only really effective treatment for a severe, acute, allergic reaction is immediate, subcutaneous, intramuscular, or intravenous injection of medication to combat the agent causing the reaction. In general, the intramuscular injection of 0.3 to 1.0 ml of 1:1000 *epinephrine* (0.3 mg) will alleviate the immediate signs and symptoms of these reactions. Often the patient may know of a specific sensitivity and may carry a kit containing epinephrine to combat the reaction (Figure 12–3). The patient should be assisted in using the epinephrine. If he or she cannot inject the medication, it may be necessary that you do so when local protocols in your system allow it. The injection may need to be repeated if the patient's signs and symptoms recur or worsen. Frequently, a drug that is a specific counteragent for the compound causing a reaction can be given. This specific treatment must be given by a doctor at a medical facility. Prompt transportation to the emergency department while you give all support possible is necessary.

In general, you will be principally concerned with supplying respiratory support and ventilatory assistance. You should also attempt to discover what caused the reaction—a drug, an insect bite or sting, or food—and how the agent was received—was it by mouth, by inhalation, or by injection (needle or sting)? The severity of such reactions can vary greatly. Symptoms may range from mild itching and burning of the skin to generalized edema, profound coma, and rapid death. Because it is often impossible to know at once how severe any reaction may become, you must undertake the most prompt transportation to the emergency department possible and be prepared to give all available supportive measures en route.

A

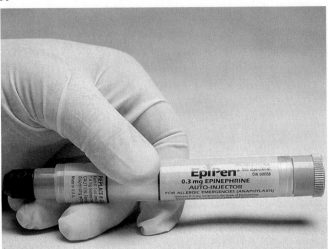

B

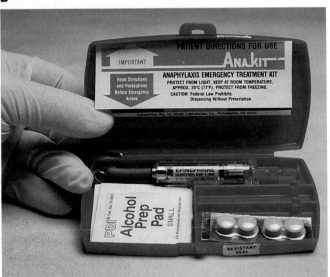

FIGURE 12–3

Two commercially available kits for the treatment of allergic emergencies (anaphylaxis) are shown. These items may not be available for use in every state. Consult with your local medical director regarding their use in your area. (A) The *Epi-Pen*® requires removal of the gray safety cap. Placing the black tip on the thigh and pushing hard will force the injector to function. A dose of 0.3 mg of epinephrine is given intramuscularly; it is contained in 0.3 ml of solution. (B) The *Ana-Kit*® contains a preloaded syringe with epinephrine and oral antihistaminic agents. When the needle is bared and the syringe barrel properly aligned, a dose of up to 0.3 mg of epinephrine in 0.3 ml of solution can be given intramuscularly. The syringe is calibrated to allow smaller doses. Tablets provide a longer-term allergic therapy.

SECTION 5

INJURIES

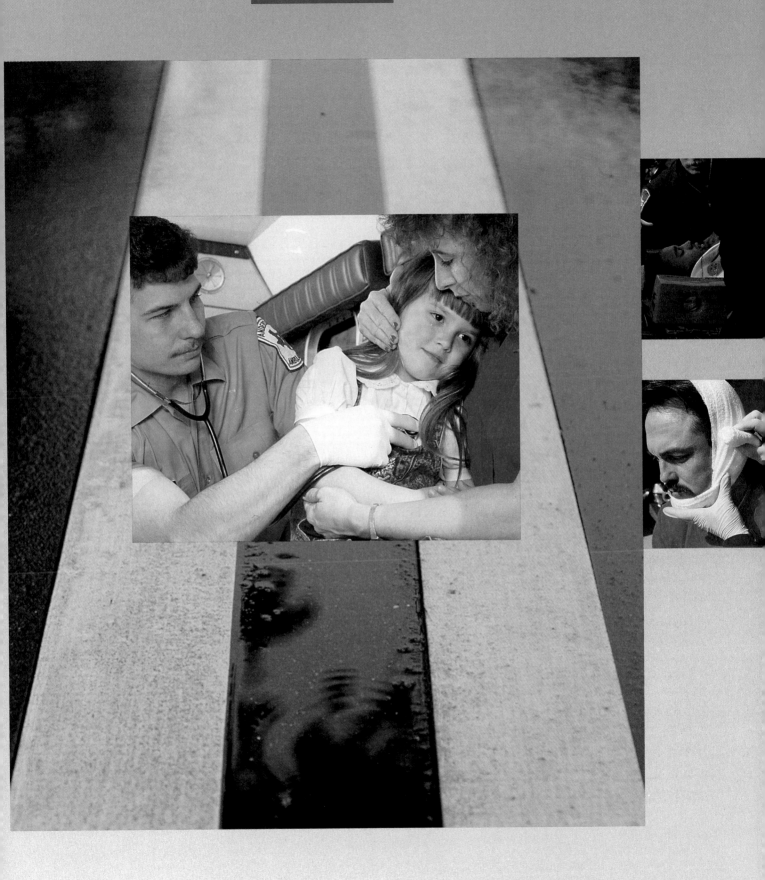

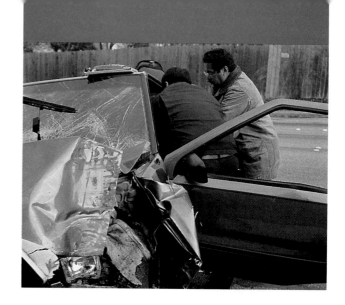

CHAPTER 13

INJURY

KEY TERMS

blunt injury Injury in which the force of impact is concentrated over a large area of contact; the force of impact does not break the skin but damages the tissues and organs below the skin.

deceleration (de-sel″er-a′shun) Reduction in speed.

ecchymosis (ek″ĭ-mo′sis) A small area of bleeding in the skin or mucous membrane; a bruise or "black and blue" mark.

edema (ĕ-de′mah) The presence of abnormally large amounts of fluid in the extra cellular tissue spaces of the body, causing swelling of the affected area.

fracture Any break in the continuity of a bone.

impaled object An object, such as a knife or splinter of wood or glass, that penetrates the skin and remains in the body.

kinetic energy (ki-net′ik en′er-je) Energy associated with motion.

open wound Injury caused by a penetrating object that breaks the skin or mucous membranes.

penetrating injury Injury in which the force of impact is concentrated on a small point of contact between the skin and the wounding implement, creating an open wound.

rupture (rup′chur) A break or tear of an organ or tissue.

trauma (traw′mah) A wound or injury.

Injuries are the leading cause of death and disability in the United States among children and young adults. Each year, one person in three sustains an injury that requires medical treatment, and more than 140,000 people die from injuries.

In fact, more Americans between the ages of 1 and 34 years die from injuries than from all other diseases combined. Trauma is the leading cause of death up to the age of 44 years, and it causes the loss of more working years of life than do cancer and heart disease combined. As can be seen from these statistics, you will be exposed frequently to patients with injury. Indeed, one out of every eight hospital beds is occupied by a patient who has sustained an injury. Proper prehospital evaluation and care can do much to minimize suffering, long-term disability, and death from trauma.

Chapter 13 begins by defining the mechanisms of injury—that is, how the different forms of energy cause injury to the body. The chapter next describes various patterns of injury and how these injury patterns are related to the environment in which you work. The last part of Chapter 13 discusses the principles of treatment of injuries—scene assessment, the primary survey, assessment of vital signs, stabilization of injuries prior to transport, and recognition of life-threatening signs and symptoms that require the patient's immediate transport for treatment.

GOALS

The goals of Chapter 13 are to
- define the mechanisms of injury.
- be familiar with the common types of injury patterns.
- understand the basic principles of the treatment of injury.

MECHANISMS OF INJURY

Injury results from sudden exposure of the body to energy. Energy cannot be created or destroyed; it only changes form. Some of energy's many forms are heat, electricity, and kinetic energy. **Kinetic energy** is energy in action that produces motion. The human body is frequently exposed to high levels of energy that cause permanent, sometimes fatal, damage to it. **Trauma,** another word for injury, is the term frequently used to describe the injury process.

The kinetic energy of an object in motion (such as a car) must be converted from speed into another form of energy when the motion stops. When the motion stops gradually (as when the brakes are applied), the kinetic energy is converted to heat (in the brakes). When the motion stops suddenly (as when the car strikes a wall), the energy of impact deforms the moving object, the object that is struck, or both (Figure 13–1). The human body's tolerance for sudden deformity is very limited. A gentle punch of the fist to the nose will cause the nose to deform temporarily and

important factor in this formula is the velocity of the object because the amount of kinetic energy increases dramatically as the object's velocity increases. In the following examples, doubling the speed of a 1000 pound car from 30 to 60 miles per hour increases its kinetic energy four times, whereas doubling its weight to 2000 pounds only doubles its kinetic energy:

$$\begin{aligned}
\text{Kinetic energy} &= M/2 \times V^2 \\
&= 1000/2 \times 30^2 \\
&= 500 \times 900 \\
&= 450{,}000
\end{aligned}$$

$$\begin{aligned}
\text{Kinetic energy} &= M/2 \times V^2 \\
&= 1000/2 \times \mathbf{60}^2 \\
&= 500 \times 3600 \\
&= 1{,}800{,}000
\end{aligned}$$

$$\begin{aligned}
\text{Kinetic energy} &= M/2 \times V^2 \\
&= \mathbf{2000}/2 \times 30^2 \\
&= 1000 \times 900 \\
&= 900{,}000
\end{aligned}$$

The velocity factor is especially significant when you consider the wounding potential of firearms. Although larger bullets cause more damage than smaller ones (with less mass), the more important variable is speed. As bullet speed increases, the amount of damage produced increases greatly. For this reason, gunshot wounds are separated into two basic categories: high velocity and low velocity. Bullets traveling at a muzzle velocity greater than 2,000 feet per second cause high-velocity injury. The type and amount of tissue damage is much greater than the damage produced in low-velocity bullet injuries (Figure 13–2). Because the extent of injury is so different between these two types of gunshot wounds, the surgical treatment for each is different. Therefore, it is essential for you to identify the type of firearm used and report this information to the emergency department personnel.

The type of injury that occurs from the impact of kinetic energy also depends on the specific tissue that is being deformed. Soft tissue such as the skin can stretch or deform to some degree and sustain only minor damage. With further deformity, however, soft tissues will be torn apart and permanently damaged. Firmer tissues, such as bone and certain organs

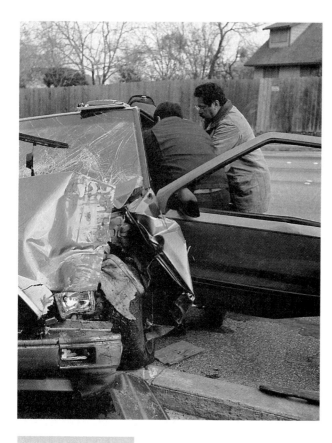

FIGURE 13–1

When the rapid motion of a vehicle suddenly stops, the kinetic energy is converted into deformity of the moving object.

absorb the energy of impact without permanent damage. A violent punch, however, will cause greater deformity of the tissues of the nose and result in permanent damage to them. The tissues will continue to deform until all of the kinetic energy is used up. Thus, tissue damage continues until all of the kinetic energy is spent. In high-energy injuries, several structures may be damaged at the same time.

The amount of kinetic energy that is present in a moving object is proportional to the mass (weight) of the object and to the square of its velocity (speed). The formula:

$$\text{Kinetic energy} = M/2 \times V^2$$
(where M = mass and V = velocity)

is used to calculate the kinetic energy of any object. It is this amount of energy that must be absorbed at the moment of impact. The more

that are contained within a firm capsule—for example, the liver and spleen—can resist or absorb small forces. When a large amount of energy is applied, however, these tissues deform and ultimately break apart, causing **fracture** (break in a bone) or **rupture** (break or tear in organs like the liver and spleen).

Some structures of the body are more susceptible to injury than others. The brain and the spinal cord are especially fragile and vulnerable to injury. They are protected from injury by the surrounding skull, the spinal column, and several layers of soft tissues. The eye is another susceptible structure that lies recessed in a bony socket of the skull. The anterior portion of the eye is still vulnerable to injury, and even small forces may cause serious and permanent damage (Figure 13–3).

Forces applied to the body are generally separated into two broad categories: penetrating and blunt. In **penetrating injury,** there is usually a very small point of contact between the skin and the wounding implement. The

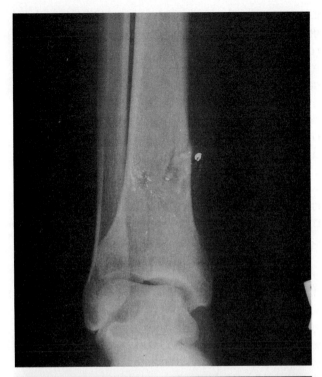

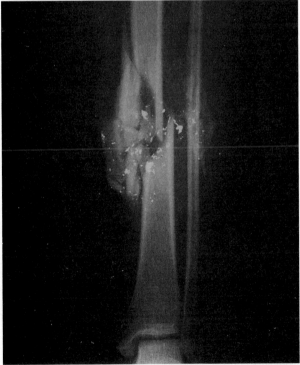

FIGURE 13–2

All gunshot wounds can inflict serious injury, but more injury is produced by high-velocity bullets. The X ray (top) shows a simple fracture of the tibia produced by a low-velocity bullet wound. A high-velocity bullet (bottom) has caused the tibia to shatter.

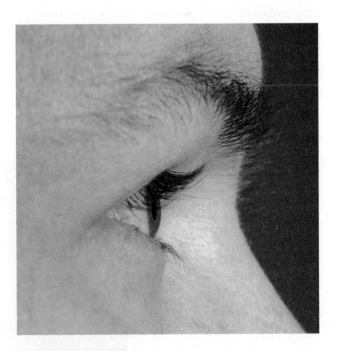

FIGURE 13–3

The eye is recessed in the skull to protect its fragile structures from injury; however, the front of the eye remains exposed and is quite vulnerable.

force of impact is concentrated on this small point, and the wounding object is driven through the skin to produce a *laceration* (cut). When the skin is cut by a penetrating object, the wound produced is called an **open wound.** The penetrating object may go only through the skin or it may pass entirely through the body and exit at some distant site. All structures in its path are vulnerable to injury. Occasionally, the object remains in the body. These are called **impaled objects.** Blood loss from the open wound and the potential for infection resulting from the damage to the protective covering of the skin may create serious problems for the patient.

In **blunt injury,** the area of contact between the object and the body is large enough so that skin penetration either does not occur or is only superficial. However, the force of impact is transmitted through the skin, and the deeper tissues are damaged. Often blood vessels below the skin are sheared from their attachments, producing bleeding under the skin and into the deeper body tissues. In addition, blunt trauma tends to cause hollow organs to rupture and solid organs to break apart (fracture or rupture).

Not all injury occurs from striking the body with a moving object. Significant injury can also occur when the body is in motion and strikes a fixed object. Sudden **deceleration** (decreased speed) occurs at the moment of impact, and both blunt and penetrating injury can result. In addition, specific deceleration injuries can occur because certain parts of the body come to a stop more rapidly than do others. For example, when the head strikes the dashboard in a car wreck, the skull quickly stops moving forward; however, the brain, which floats within the skull, continues to move forward until it strikes the inner surface of the skull. This "second impact" is often the cause of brain injury (Figure 13–4).

A similar phenomenon occurs with certain organs in the chest—the heart and aorta—and in the abdomen—the liver, small intestine, and spleen. Deceleration injury of the internal organs may be fatal, although the severity of such an injury may not be appreciated on initial examination because the outward signs of injury, such as laceration or bruising, may not be great.

The critical determinant of the degree of injury is the amount of kinetic energy that was absorbed at the moment of impact. The greater the force of impact, the greater the damage. You must realize the potential for severe and multiple injuries with all high-energy (high-

FIGURE 13–4

Sudden deceleration of the skull resulted in fatal brain injury when the brain continued its forward motion and struck the inside of the skull.

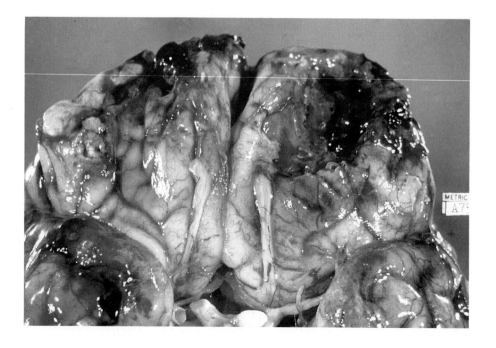

velocity) injuries. Car wrecks, certain gunshot wounds, and falls from heights are just a few examples of these high-energy injuries. It is imperative to identify high-energy injuries quickly. They often produce such severe injury that the patient's life can only be saved by rapid transportation to a trauma center.

Other mechanisms of bodily injury exist as well. *Crushing injury* implies the application of force to body tissue over relatively long periods of time as opposed to the very short time of blunt or penetrating trauma. In addition to causing some direct soft tissue damage, continued compression of the soft tissues during the crushing will cut off their circulation and produce further tissue destruction. For example, a person whose legs are trapped under a collapsed pile of rocks will continue to suffer tissue damage until the compressing rocks are removed.

Another form of compression injury can result from the tissue damage itself. Whenever tissues are injured, swelling occurs. The cells that are injured leak watery fluid **(edema fluid)** into the spaces between the cells, producing a local increase in size of the tissues. If swelling is excessive or occurs in a confined space such as the skull, the tissue pressure will increase to dangerous levels. The pressure of the edema fluid may become great enough to compress the tissue and cause further damage, particularly if the blood vessels become compressed, cutting off the flow of blood to the tissue. Excessive swelling often follows injury of the brain, the spinal cord, and the extremities.

There are many different mechanisms of injury, and several factors determine the extent and severity of the injury produced. The amount of kinetic energy absorbed, the degree of tissue deformity and displacement, and the particular tissue injured are three important variables that you must consider when evaluating each injury.

TYPES OF INJURY

You will come in contact with a wide spectrum of injury and must be prepared to deal with many different types of trauma. However, the frequency of exposure to specific types of injury will be directly related to the environment in which you work, because certain specific types of injury are more common in certain settings. For example, a great contrast is evident in the types of injuries commonly seen in urban and rural environments.

The EMT who works in a large city will respond to a great many injuries resulting from personal assaults with weapons such as knives and guns—injuries rarely seen in the rural environment. In addition, the urban EMT must be prepared to deal with patients injured in construction and industrial accidents. In contrast, in the rural setting the EMT will respond to a large number of agricultural accidents resulting from farm machinery accidents with augers, cornpickers, combines, and many other specialized pieces of farm equipment (Figure 13–5). Silos and grain elevators present special dangers to both the injured patient and to rescue personnel, especially first responders unfamiliar with the potential for such hazards.

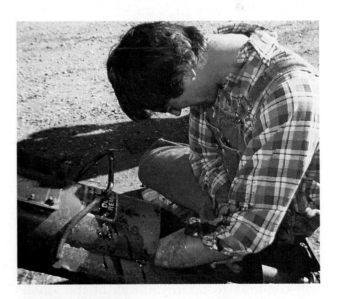

FIGURE 13–5

Certain injuries are unique to the environment in which they occur. For example, specialized farm equipment can cause unusual injuries and difficult extrication problems.

Other environments also present unique and unusual potentials for injury. EMTs who work near large bodies of water, particularly those used for recreational purposes, will respond to many different types of water-related injuries that range in severity from sunburn to drowning.

Because of the specialized nature of the injuries common to certain environments, it is essential for you to become familiar with the common types of injuries seen in your particular locale. Furthermore, you may have to develop specialized rescue and treatment skills to facilitate the management of environment-related injuries. For example, in rural areas, the EMT must become familiar with the specialized rescue and extrication techniques for injury situations caused by farm machinery. Books, courses, and other instructional materials are available to prepare you for this specialized type of work. As a general principle, all EMTs must become familiar with the injury patterns common in their area and be prepared to deal with them before training is completed.

INJURY COMBINATIONS

With certain mechanisms of injury, two or more specific injuries frequently occur together. Certain combinations of injuries are particularly seen in motor vehicle accidents. When you are aware that certain injuries frequently occur together, you can be on the lookout for them.

One example of a group of injuries that occur together is seen in a front-end collision, when the front seat passenger continues forward and strikes his or her knee against the dashboard (Figure 13–6). Obviously, a knee injury (patellar fracture or knee dislocation) can occur, but in addition the femur may fracture, and the hip may dislocate or the pelvis may fracture. Injury will continue to occur until all of the kinetic energy is used up.

If the driver of a car in a head-on collision goes up and over the steering wheel, injuries to the face, head, and perhaps spine can occur. In addition, the driver's chest and abdomen will strike the steering wheel causing injury to the

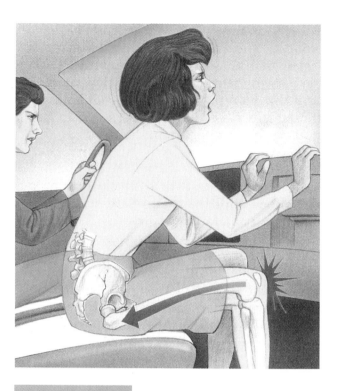

FIGURE 13–6

When the knee strikes the dashboard forcefully, the energy of impact can be transmitted to the hip, fracturing the pelvis or even dislocating the hip.

lungs, heart, great vessels, or abdominal organs. The more serious injury is usually the chest or abdominal injury, but because the face is bleeding all of your initial attention may be directed to it. If you realize that with this mechanism of injury serious chest or abdominal injuries may result, you will be better prepared to deal with them.

These are just two examples of commonly occurring combined injuries. Familiarity with the mechanism of injury will enhance your ability to identify such combinations and improve your assessment and diagnostic skills.

PRINCIPLES OF INJURY TREATMENT

Because you are so often called to evaluate and treat injuries, you must understand the basic principles of injury care. These principles have been developed and refined over the past 20 years as we have gained experience in the prehospital management of injured patients. The National Association of Emergency Medical Technicians, in cooperation with the Committee on Trauma of the American College of Surgeons, has organized these principles into courses called Pre-Hospital Trauma Life Support (PHTLS), Basic and Advanced. These courses provide an in-depth understanding of the management of injuries much as Basic and Advanced Cardiac Life Support courses do for cardiorespiratory problems.

The first step in trauma assessment as outlined by PHTLS is to evaluate the scene before you reach the patient. The three Ss make up this evaluation:

1. *Safety:* Evaluate all possible dangers. Make sure that none still exist for you or the injured person(s). Never become a victim yourself.
2. *Scene:* What was the mechanism of injury? What types of injuries should be expected? What severity of injury might be expected judging from the amount of kinetic energy expended?
3. *Situation:* How many people have been injured? What special circumstances need to be dealt with (crowds, weather, patient access)?

Once you reach the patient, you should complete a primary survey. As with other emergencies, evaluating an injured person begins with the primary survey of airway, breathing, and circulation. Clearing the airway, assuring adequate ventilation, and controlling hemorrhage must therefore be the top priorities in the care of any injured patient. Because head injury is common and because a change in the level of consciousness is often a sign of hypoxia or hypoperfusion of the brain, PHTLS recommends that a "D," disability, be added to the routine ABCs of the primary survey. The purpose of this step is to assess the patient's level of consciousness using the AVPU scale as described in Chapter 5.

The entire primary survey should be done quickly, within 15 seconds. As you approach the patient, look from head to toe for bleeding and to see if he or she is awake or unconscious, moving or still. When you reach the patient, grasp the wrist to check the radial pulse and at the same time ask "What happened?" The quality of the patient's response will tell a great deal about his or her level of consciousness, airway status, and ability to ventilate. Asking the responsive patient a second question "Where do you hurt?" will help you to localize the injuries. Any life-threatening problem that is identified in the primary survey must be stabilized immediately. You must pay particular attention to obtaining and maintaining an adequate airway and controlling hemorrhage right away.

The third step in the general management of a patient who has been injured is to assess the vital signs. Injury frequently results in bleeding, and significant bleeding will result in tachycardia and hypotension. Injuries of the head, neck, and chest can interfere with the normal mechanisms of breathing. Many other injuries may also affect the vital functions and alter the vital signs. Thus, an initial assessment of the vital signs must be carried out on all injured patients. The vital signs must then be monitored at least every 15 minutes until the patient reaches the hospital. More frequent observations are needed in the seriously injured patient who has unstable vital signs.

Rapid deterioration of one or more of the vital signs is seen frequently in the severely injured patient. Initially, many patients are able to compensate for blood loss or moderate respiratory insufficiency. During this early phase, the vital signs are maintained near normal levels. However, with significant injury the compensatory mechanisms eventually fail, and the vital signs and vital functions deteriorate rapidly. That is why it is essential for you to recheck the vital signs frequently in all injured patients in anticipation of the possibility of significant, rapid deterioration.

The 15-second global primary survey, combined with continued close monitoring of the vital signs in all injured patients, will help you to identify those who are critically injured. Although the critically injured represent only about 5 percent of all injured patients, their injuries are immediately life threatening and cannot be treated in the field. These include:

- A compromised airway that cannot be opened and maintained.
- Respiratory insufficiency.
- Hemorrhagic shock.
- Deteriorating neurological function.

These critically injured trauma patients usually have only 60 minutes ("The Golden Hour") from the time of injury to reach definitive surgical treatment. Therefore, you must recognize these patients quickly, spend little time in the field providing only essential life-saving care, and transport them rapidly to a hospital where the appropriate care can be given immediately. PHTLS recommends that your time at the scene with such patients should not exceed the "Golden Ten Minutes." Maintain the airway, ventilate the patient if necessary, give oxygen, control bleeding, protect the spine from further injury, rapidly package the patient on a long spine board, and transport the patient rapidly to an appropriate medical facility. Do not waste time in the field with these critically injured patients.

THE SECONDARY SURVEY
· ·

The remaining 95 percent of injured patients are not critically injured. They have isolated injuries that are not life threatening. After the completion of the primary survey (ABCD) and an assessment of the vital signs indicate that a critical injury is not present, the next phase of assessment of the injured patient is a complete secondary survey. A complete head-to-toe examination should be performed to identify all injury sites which will require stabilization prior to transport.

Pain and loss of function usually accompany injury. Any injured patient who complains of pain should be considered to have a significant injury deserving a thorough evaluation. Because injury also frequently results in a loss of function of a specific organ or body part—for example, difficulty in breathing, double vision, or inability to bend the elbow—any complaint of loss of function should result in a complete, in-hospital evaluation.

The absence of these complaints does not mean that the patient has not sustained a significant injury. Obviously, the unconscious injured patient will not complain at all. In addition, sometimes the pain of a severe injury will be so great that the patient does not realize that he or she has sustained another equally serious, yet less painful, injury. Therefore, a secondary survey of all injured persons must be carried out to identify these common signs of injury:

- Tenderness.
- Swelling.
- Ecchymosis.
- Deformity.
- Loss of function.

Gentle palpation of the trunk and extremities is designed to identify areas of tenderness following injury. Frequently, more than one injury site may be present. A careful examination will reveal all points of injury and enable you to set priorities for treatment.

Swelling, as described earlier, is a very common, nonspecific sign of injury. Damaged cells leak edema fluid very soon after injury. Massive swelling may occur as a result of damage to blood vessels and bleeding into the soft tissues. Thus, swelling is one of the earliest and most consistent signs of injury.

Ecchymosis (bruising or discoloration of the tissues) is caused by damage to blood vessels. Blood from the damaged vessels leaks into the area of injury and gives a blue or blue-black discoloration to the tissues.

When a force is applied to body tissues, they deform in an attempt to absorb the energy of impact. All tissues can deform to some degree without sustaining permanent damage. With excessive force, however, tissue damage and persistent deformity occur. Deformity is readily seen in many fractured limbs as well as in soft tissues, such as the skin, that have been stretched or torn beyond their limits.

The patient often complains of a loss of function of a specific body part, and you also may observe this loss. For example, impaired breathing following a chest injury can frequently be seen by the careful observer. Such observations are especially important for patients who for some reason are unable to express complaints about pain and loss of function.

With specific injuries, other specific symptoms and signs will be present. The subsequent chapters in this section detail these particular findings. A careful assessment of the patient's vital signs, symptoms, and physical signs will enable you to evaluate the patient's condition and set priorities for treatment. In general, after the airway, breathing, and circulation have been secured, isolated injuries should be stabilized and the patient transported to the hospital for definitive treatment. In most cases, stabilizing the injury in the field will allow the patient to be transported in an efficient yet safe manner.

Recently, several trauma scales have been developed to help in the field assessment of the severity of the injury and objectively identify those patients with injuries severe enough to require immediate and rapid transport to the hospital. The scales use the objective measurements of vital signs, level of consciousness, and specific sites and mechanisms of injury to give a severity of injury rating to the patient. The use of these trauma scales is discussed further in Chapter 46.

The following chapters in this section describe the specific injuries that you will encounter. The principles of evaluation and field stabilization are presented in detail for each of the areas of the body.

EMT SAFETY

In treating trauma patients, two major risks to your safety occur: personal injury from the dangerous or unstable environment and contamination from blood and other body fluids.

In any trauma situation, the scene must be stabilized before you access and treat the patients. For example, on the highway following a car accident, your first priority must be to protect yourself and others from the hazards of fire, spilled gasoline, moving traffic, and unstable vehicles. Immediately on arrival at the scene, you should consider any trauma situation unstable and potentially dangerous. Be cautious and ensure scene safety as a top priority so that you, other rescuers, and bystanders are not exposed to injury.

With all injured individuals, you must be alert to protect yourself from unnecessary contact with the blood or body fluids of the patient. You must be certain that all of the appropriate barriers exist between you and the patient. They include gloves, mask, goggles (if the patient is coughing violently), and protective clothing. You must use all of these aids and pay special attention to good hand-washing and vehicle cleaning once the run is completed. In general, a combination of all these procedures will be very effective protection against contamination from blood or other body fluids.

YOU ARE THE EMT

1. You are responding to a gunshot injury. Why is it important for you to know the approximate muzzle velocity of the weapon that inflicted the injury?
2. Explain how an accident or set of circumstances can simultaneously cause blunt injury and penetrating injury.
3. Your cousin works for a rural EMS, and you work for an urban EMS. You are having a "friendly argument" about who has the hardest job. What examples will you give of "difficult" city situations? What kind of situations do you think your cousin will describe? What problems do you both share?
4. What five common signs of injury should you look for during the secondary survey? Which of these signs can be detected in an unconscious person?
5. How do you identify the critically injured patient? Why is it essential to identify such a patient quickly?

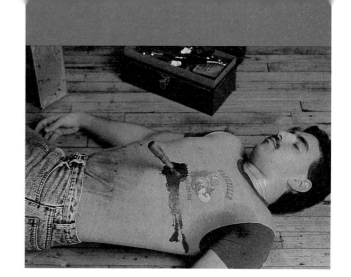

CHAPTER 14

SOFT TISSUE INJURY

KEY TERMS

abrasion (ah-bra'zhun) Loss of skin as a result of a body part being rubbed or scraped across a rough or hard surface.

avulsion (ah-vul'shun) An injury in which a piece of skin is either torn completely loose from all of its attachments or is left hanging as a flap.

contamination The presence of infective organisms on or in objects such as dressings, water, food, or on the patient's body.

contusion (kon-tu'zhun) A bruise.

dermis (der'mis) The inner layer of the skin, containing hair follicles, sweat glands, nerve endings, and blood vessels.

epidermis (ep"ĭ-der'mis) The outer layer of skin, which is made up of cells that are sealed together to form a watertight protective covering for the body.

hematoma (hem"ah-to'mah) A collection of blood contained within the body in tissue or in a cavity, occasionally palpable as a discrete mass.

laceration (las"er-a'shun) A cut that may leave a smooth or jagged wound through the skin, subcutaneous tissues, muscles, and associated nerves and blood vessels.

metabolism (mĕ-tab'o-lizm) A sum of all physical and chemical processes of living organisms; the process by which energy is made available for the uses of the organism.

mucous membrane (mu'kus mem'brān) The lining of body cavities and passages that communicate directly or indirectly with the environment outside the body.

subcutaneous tissue (sub"ku-ta'ne-us tish'u) Tissue, largely fat, that lies directly under the dermis and serves as an insulator of the body.

Injury to the soft tissues is quite common and understandably so—the skin acts as the first line of defense against external forces. Even though the skin is relatively tough, it is still quite susceptible to injury. Injuries to the soft tissues range from simple bruises and abrasions to serious lacerations and amputations. All wounds require bandaging. Therefore, you must become familiar with the specific techniques of applying dressings and bandages to various body parts. In all instances, the principles of controlling bleeding, preventing further contamination, and protecting the wound from further damage must be followed.

Chapter 14 begins with the anatomy and physiology of the skin, the largest single organ in the body. The chapter next describes the two types of soft tissue injuries—closed wounds and open wounds—and the treatment of each. The last section of Chapter 14 covers the general principles of applying dressings and bandages.

GOALS
. . . .

The goals of Chapter 14 are to

- understand the anatomy and physiology of the skin.
- describe the characteristics of closed and open soft tissue injuries and learn how to treat them.
- become familiar with the general principles of the application of dressings and bandages.

. . . .

ANATOMY AND PHYSIOLOGY OF THE SKIN
. . . .

The skin, the largest single organ in the body, serves three major functions:

1. To protect the body in the environment.
2. To regulate the temperature of the body.
3. To transmit information from the environment to the brain.

The protective functions of the skin are numerous. Over 70 percent of the body is composed of water. The water contains a delicate balance of chemical substances in solution. The skin is watertight and serves to keep this balanced internal solution intact. The skin also protects the body from the invasion of infectious organisms—bacteria, viruses, and fungi. These organisms are everywhere and are routinely found lying on the skin surface and deep in its grooves and glands; they never, however, penetrate through the skin. Germs cannot pass through the skin unless it is broken by injury; thus, the skin provides a constant protection against outside invaders.

The energy of the body is derived from **metabolism** (chemical reactions) that must take place within a very narrow temperature range. If the body temperature is too low, these reactions cannot proceed, metabolism ceases, and the body dies. If the temperature becomes too high, the rate of metabolism increases.

Dangerously high temperatures producing too high a metabolic rate can result in permanent tissue damage and death.

The major organ for regulation of body temperature is the skin. Blood vessels in the skin constrict when the body is in a cold environment and dilate when the body is in a warm environment. In a cold environment, constriction of the blood vessels shunts the blood away from the skin to decrease the amount of heat radiated from the body surface. When the outside environment is hot, the vessels in the skin dilate, the skin becomes flushed or red, and heat radiates from the body surface.

Also, in the hot environment, sweat is secreted to the skin surface from the sweat glands. Evaporation of the sweat requires energy. This energy, as body heat, is taken from the body during the evaporation process, which causes the body temperature to fall. Sweating alone will not reduce body temperature; evaporation of the sweat must also occur.

Information from the environment is carried to the brain through a rich supply of sensory nerves that originate in the skin. Nerve endings that lie in the skin are adapted to perceive and transmit information about heat, cold, external pressure, pain, and the position of the body in space. The skin thus recognizes any changes in the environment. The skin also reacts to pressure, pain, and pleasurable stimuli.

The skin is divided into two parts: the superficial epidermis, which is composed of several layers of cells, and the deeper dermis, which contains the specialized skin structures. Below the skin lies the subcutaneous layer of fat (Figure 14–1a). The cells of the **epidermis** are sealed to form a watertight protective covering for the body (Figure 14–1b).

The epidermis is actually composed of several layers of cells. At the base of the epidermis is the germinal layer, which continuously produces new cells that gradually rise to the surface. On the way to the surface these cells die and form the watertight covering. The epidermal cells are held together securely by an oily substance called sebum, which is secreted by the *sebaceous glands* of the dermis. The

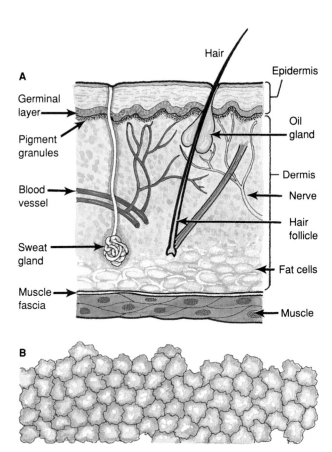

FIGURE 14–1

(A) The skin has two layers, the epidermis and the dermis. All of the major structures lie in the dermis. A layer of subcutaneous fat lies below the dermis. (B) Cells of the epidermis are fitted closely together on the skin surface to form a watertight protective layer.

outermost cells of the epidermis are constantly rubbed away and then replaced by new cells produced by the germinal layer. The deeper cells in the germinal layer also contain pigment granules that (along with the blood vessels lying in the dermis) produce skin color.

The epidermis varies in thickness in different areas of the body. On the soles of the feet, the back, and the scalp it is quite thick, but in some areas of the body the epidermis is only 2 or 3 cell layers in thickness. The watertight seal provided by the epidermis prevents the invasion of bacteria and other organisms.

The deeper part of skin, the **dermis,** is separated from the epidermis by the layer of germinal cells. Within the dermis lie many of the special structures of the skin: sweat glands, sebaceous (oil) glands, hair follicles, blood vessels, and specialized nerve endings.

Sweat glands produce sweat for cooling the body. The sweat is discharged onto the surface of the skin through small pores, or ducts, that pass through the epidermis onto the skin surface. The sebaceous glands produce sebum, the oily material that seals the surface epidermal cells. The sebaceous glands lie next to hair follicles and secrete sebum along the hair follicle to the skin surface. In addition to providing waterproofing for the skin, sebum keeps the skin supple so that it does not crack.

Hair follicles are the small organs that produce hair. There is one follicle for each hair connected with a sebaceous gland and also with a tiny muscle. The muscle serves to pull the hair into an erect position when the individual is cold or frightened. All hair grows continuously and is either cut off or worn away by clothing.

Blood vessels provide nutrients and oxygen to the skin. The blood vessels lie in the dermis. Small branches extend up to the germinal layer. There are no blood vessels in the epidermis. A complex array of nerve endings also lie in the dermis. These specialized nerve endings are sensitive to environmental stimuli: they respond to these stimuli and send impulses along the nerves to the brain.

Beneath the skin, immediately under the dermis and attached to it, lies the **subcutaneous tissue.** The subcutaneous tissue is largely composed of fat. The fat serves as an insulator for the body and as a reservoir to store energy. The amount of subcutaneous tissue varies greatly from individual to individual. Beneath the subcutaneous tissue lie the muscles and the skeleton.

The skin covers all of the external surface of the body. The various *orifices* (openings to the body)—including the mouth, nose, anus, and vagina—are not covered by skin. Orifices are lined with mucous membranes (Figure 14–2).

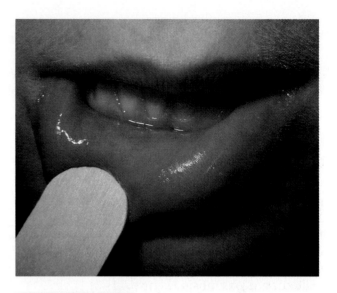

FIGURE 14–2

All body openings are lined with mucous membranes. Just like the skin, these membranes prevent the invasion of bacteria into the body. They secrete a watery mucus for lubrication and moisture.

Mucous membranes are quite similar to skin in that they provide a protective barrier against bacterial invasion. Mucous membranes differ from skin in that they secrete *mucus*, a watery substance that lubricates the openings. Thus, mucous membranes are moist whereas the skin is dry. A mucous membrane lines the entire gastrointestinal tract from the mouth to the anus.

SOFT TISSUE INJURIES

Because the soft tissues are the first line of defense against most injuries, they are often damaged. Soft tissue injuries or wounds are divided into two types: closed and open. A closed wound is one in which soft tissue damage occurs beneath the skin or mucous membrane surface, but the surface remains intact. An open wound is one in which there is a break in the surface of the skin or the mucous membrane.

Closed Soft Tissue Injuries

Contusions and Hematomas A blunt object that strikes the body will crush the tissue beneath the skin. This injury is called a **contusion** (a bruise). The epidermis remains intact. Damage beneath the epidermis will extend to varying depths, depending on the force of injury. In the dermis, cells are damaged and small blood vessels are usually torn. Varying amounts of edema fluid and blood leak into the damaged area. This leakage produces swelling and pain. As blood accumulates in the damaged area, a characteristic discoloration occurs. Usually, the discoloration is black or blue and is called an ecchymosis (Figure 14–3).

When large amounts of tissue are damaged beneath the outer layer of the skin, large blood vessels may tear and cause rapid bleeding. A pool of blood called a **hematoma** will collect within the damaged tissue. A hematoma occurs whenever a large blood vessel is damaged. The formation of a hematoma is not limited to soft tissue injuries; it can also occur following a fracture or when blood vessels to any organ in the body are damaged. When a large bone such as the femur or pelvis fractures, the hematoma that forms may contain more than a liter of blood.

Closed soft tissue injuries are characterized by a history of injury, pain at the site of injury, swelling beneath the skin, and ecchymosis. They may be mild or quite extensive.

Management of Closed Soft Tissue Injuries Small bruises require no special emergency medical care. With more extensive closed injuries, swelling and bleeding beneath the skin can be extensive and may even result in hypovolemic shock. You can control bleeding and swelling in the deep soft tissues to some degree by applying ice and local compression immediately following the injury. Ice or cold packs will cause the blood vessels to constrict, which will slow the bleeding. Firm manual compression over the area of injury will compress the blood vessels and also decrease bleeding. Immobilizing the soft tissue injury with a splint is another way to decrease bleeding. In addition, application of cold packs and

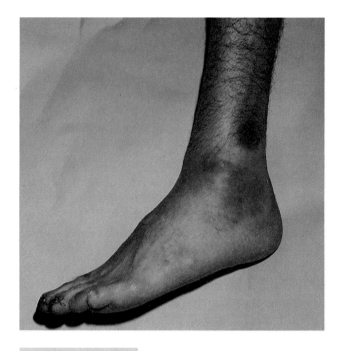

FIGURE 14–3

A closed soft tissue injury—a contusion—is characterized by swelling and ecchymosis.

splinting decreases the patient's pain. Elevating the injured part to a point just above the level of the patient's heart decreases the amount of swelling in the region. Therefore, when treating a patient with a closed soft tissue injury, you can think of ICES (ice, compression, elevation, and splinting) to remember the four steps in treatment.

Severe closed injuries can cause fracture or other injury to important deeper structures. At times it is difficult to estimate the degree of injury to the deeper structures. Therefore, all closed injuries should be treated with the immediate application of cold and then compression, elevation, and splinting, as discussed in Chapter 16.

Open Soft Tissue Wounds

Open soft tissue wounds differ from closed wounds in that the protective skin layer is damaged. This damage can result in more extensive bleeding. More importantly, however, once the protective skin layer has been

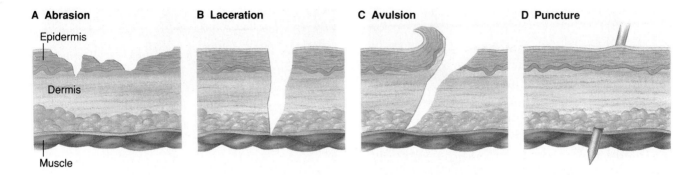

A Abrasion   **B Laceration**   **C Avulsion**   **D Puncture**

Epidermis

Dermis

Muscle

FIGURE 14–4   The four general types of open soft tissue injuries: (A) Abrasions involve variable depths of the dermis and epidermis. (B) Lacerations are cuts produced by sharp objects. (C) Avulsions raise flaps of tissue, usually along normal tissue planes. (D) Puncture wounds may penetrate to any depth.

violated, the wound becomes contaminated and may become infected. These two problems (bleeding and contamination) must be addressed in the treatment of open soft tissue wounds.

There are four types of open soft tissue wounds: abrasions, lacerations, avulsions, and puncture wounds (Figure 14–4).

Abrasion An **abrasion** is the loss of a portion of the epidermis and part of the dermis as a result of the skin being rubbed or scraped across a rough or hard surface. Blood may ooze from the injured capillary blood vessels in the dermis, but the abrasion usually does not penetrate completely through the dermis. Extremely painful, abrasions are known by a variety of common names, such as road rash, strawberry, and mat burn (Figure 14–5).

Laceration A **laceration** is a cut produced by a sharp object. The cutting object may leave a smooth or jagged wound through the skin and may penetrate into the subcutaneous tissue, the underlying muscles, and the nearby nerves and blood vessels (Figure 14–6).

Avulsion An **avulsion** is an injury in which a piece of skin is either torn completely loose from all of its attachments or is left hanging as a flap. Avulsed tissues ordinarily separate at

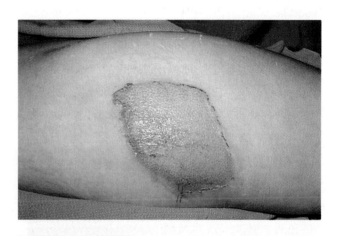

FIGURE 14–5

An abrasion of the skin. Blood is oozing from the damaged capillaries of the dermis.

normal anatomical planes, usually between the subcutaneous tissue and the muscle fascia. Usually there is significant bleeding from the bed of the wound. If the avulsed part remains attached only by a small pedicle of skin, the circulation to the flap may be in jeopardy (Figure 14–7).

Puncture Wound A puncture wound results from a stab with a knife, ice pick, splinter, or any other pointed object or from a bullet.

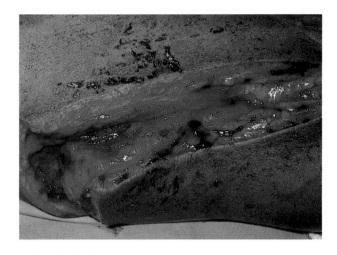

FIGURE 14–6

A laceration of the skin and subcutaneous tissue. The fascia covering the muscle is seen in the depths of the wounds.

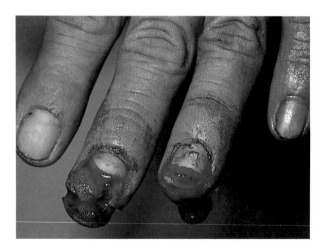

FIGURE 14–7

An avulsion attached only by a small pedicle of skin.

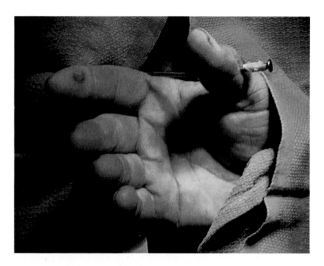

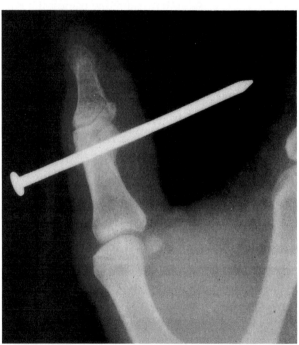

FIGURE 14–8

A puncture wound. Even though the entrance wound is small and the external bleeding is not severe, damage to the internal structures may be serious.

External bleeding from a puncture wound is usually not severe because the entrance wound is relatively small (Figure 14–8). However, the wounding object may injure structures deep within the body and cause rapid, fatal bleeding if the wound occurs in the chest or abdomen. Assessing the amount of damage sustained from a puncture wound is very difficult. *Perforating* (through and through) wounds, especially those in the extremities, may pass through the entire limb and exit on the opposite side. You should always look for and note an exit wound, especially in the case of gunshot injury. Stabbings and shootings often result in multiple puncture wounds. You must examine the victim of such assaults carefully to identify all of the wounds.

Management of Open Wounds Initially, it is imperative to assess the extent and severity of the soft tissue wound. A complete assessment can be accomplished only by removing any clothing that is covering the wound. Usually it is better to tear or cut the clothing away from the wound rather than attempt to remove it in a normal manner, because excessive motion of the injured part will cause pain and possibly additional tissue damage. As you cut or tear the clothing, remove it with minimal movement of the patient. What may seem an insignificant motion to you may cause excruciating pain for the patient. In addition, such motion may dislodge any blood clots that have formed at the injury site, allowing the wound to begin bleeding once again.

Once the wound is clear of any clothing, you can assess its severity and begin treatment. Three general steps govern the management of open soft tissue wounds:

1. Control bleeding.
2. Prevent further contamination.
3. Immobilize the part.

With open wounds, the amount of bleeding may be extensive and severe. The first priority in the emergency management of an open wound is to control the bleeding by applying a dry sterile compression dressing to the entire wound. Figure 14–9 summarizes steps in control of bleeding. Initially, apply pressure to the dressing with your gloved hand. Maintain continued pressure by firmly applying a roller bandage to the injured part. If bleeding continues or recurs, the original dressing should be left in place and a second dressing should be applied and secured with an additional roller bandage. Once the bleeding is controlled, the dressing is held in place with a splint.

All open wounds are contaminated and at risk for infection. **Contamination** occurs as soon as the protective covering of the skin or mucous membrane is broken. It is impossible to sterilize a wound in the prehospital setting. You can, however, prevent further contamina-tion of an open wound by applying a dry, sterile dressing. This will help keep foreign matter such as hair, clothing, and dirt out of the wound and decrease the risk of secondary infection. However, in the initial management of open wounds, do not try to remove material in the wound no matter how dirty it may be. Rubbing, brushing, or washing an open wound will only cause further bleeding. Cleansing of the wound is a procedure for the physician to carry out in the hospital.

Frequently, the control of bleeding from soft tissue wounds—whether or not they are asso-ciated with a fracture—is improved by splint-ing the extremity. Splinting can also help the patient feel more comfortable. In addition, splinting facilitates movement of the patient, minimizing further damage to an already in-jured arm or leg. Therefore, an initial step in the control of soft tissue bleeding is appropriate splinting to immobilize the injured part.

The following procedures list summarizes the treatment of open soft tissue injuries:

1. All wounds must be thoroughly inspected and then covered with a dry, sterile com-pression dressing to control bleeding and prevent further contamination.
2. Once bleeding is controlled by compression, the limb should be splinted to further con-trol bleeding, stabilize the injured part, minimize the patient's pain, and facilitate the patient's transport to the hospital.
3. As with closed soft tissue injuries, the injured part should be elevated to just above the level of the patient's heart to minimize swelling.

Management of Avulsion Injuries When a flap of skin has been partially avulsed, the circulation to the skin flap is jeopardized. The blood supply must come through the pedicle of the flap, which may be kinked if the flap is folded back on itself. If compression is applied to the flap in this abnormal position, the blood vessels may be compressed and further dimin-ish the blood supply to the flap. Fold back any partially avulsed flap of skin onto the wound so that it is aligned normally. Once you have replaced the flap into its bed, place a dry, sterile compression dressing over it (Figure 14–10).

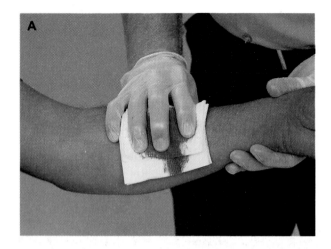
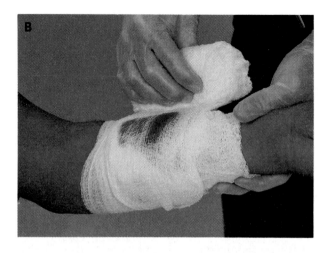
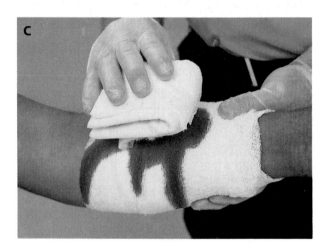
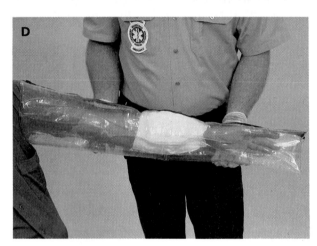

FIGURE 14–9 (A) Bleeding from an open wound is first controlled by manual pressure applied to a dry, sterile dressing. (B) The dressing can be held in place by a circular pressure bandage. (C) If bleeding continues, an additional layer of compression dressing should be applied to the first dressing. (D) A splint is used to hold the dressing in place.

If the avulsion is complete, so that piece of soft tissue has been amputated, the avulsed or amputated part should be collected and taken to the emergency department along with the patient. You may encounter persons who have had avulsion injuries of small or large pieces of skin or who have lost portions or all of an extremity. It is now often possible to replace or reimplant these totally avulsed tissues. Therefore, the avulsed part should be wrapped in sterile gauze and placed in a plastic bag. The

bag should be placed in a cool container. The tissue, however, should not be allowed to freeze (Figure 14–11).

Management of an Impaled Object Occasionally, following a puncture wound the impaled object (knife, splinter, or piece of glass) remains in the wound (Figure 14–12). In addition to controlling local bleeding, you must follow three rules in treating a patient who has an impaled object in a wound:

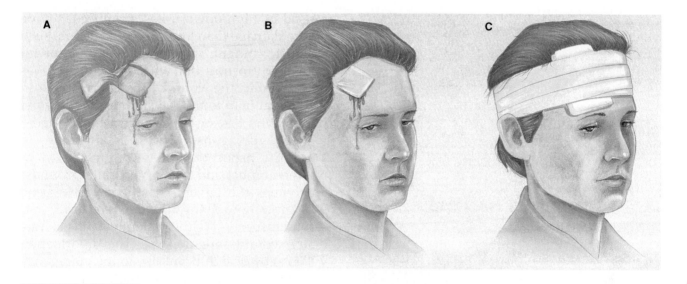

FIGURE 14–10 (A) An avulsed flap of skin may lose its blood supply if the pedicle attachment is kinked or twisted. (B) The flap should be carefully restored to a more normal position. (C) A compression dressing is then applied.

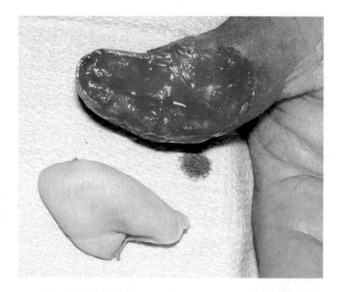

FIGURE 14–11

Amputated body parts should be saved, wrapped in a dry, sterile gauze, placed in a plastic bag, kept cool, and transported with the patient to the hospital.

1. Do not move or remove the object unless that object lies in the upper airway and obstructs the airway. In this circumstance, the need to restore the airway is of greater concern than the problems produced by removing the impaled object. Any motion may cause damage to nerves, blood vessels, or muscles lying close to the object. Try to stop any bleeding from the entrance wound by applying direct pressure but avoid exerting any force on the impaled object or on any tissue directly adjacent to its cutting edge.

2. Use a bulky dressing to stabilize the impaled object. Any motion of the impaled object will cause further soft tissue damage. The object should be incorporated within the dressing to minimize or eliminate its motion after the bandage is applied.

3. Transport the patient promptly to the emergency department with the object still in place. Ordinarily, the patient will need a surgical procedure to remove the object and to examine the tissues immediately surrounding it.

Occasionally, you will encounter very long impaled objects. Again, the impaled object should not be removed. Rather, the exposed portion should be cut off—that is, short-

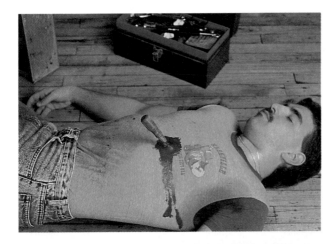

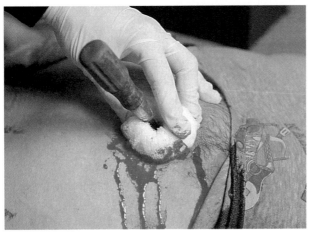

FIGURE 14-12

An impaled foreign object should be left in place and
secured with a stabilizing dressing.

ened—to facilitate transport of the patient.
Before the object is cut, however, it must be
secured to minimize any motion transmitted to
the patient. Such motion may cause further
internal damage and, most certainly, pain for
the patient.

Management of Gunshot Wounds Gunshot
wounds are a form of puncture wound that
have some unique characteristics that require
special prehospital care. The degree of damage
from a gunshot wound is directly proportional
to the square of the velocity of the bullet. Thus,
high-velocity gunshot wounds, such as those

caused by high power rifles, produce far more
severe damage than low-velocity wounds, such
as most handgun injuries. It is important for
you to try to find out what type of gun was
used to inflict the wound. This information can
be of great help to the physicians attending the
patient who has sustained a gunshot wound.

Frequently, gunshot wounds are multiple.
You must inspect the patient carefully to identify the number and sites of the bullet wounds.
Sometimes the patient or others at the scene
will know how many rounds were fired, and
careful inspection of the patient will reveal how
many wounds are present. This information
will also be of significant use to the emergency
department physicians in their care of the
patient.

Usually, the wound of entrance is smaller
than the wound of exit when a through-and-
through bullet wound occurs. Often the patient
will have a small entrance wound on the
anterior aspect of the body and a large exit
wound on the opposite side. You must look
carefully for the exit wound. Because of its size,
an exit wound may be bleeding excessively and
yet not be as readily apparent as the entrance
wound. In addition to being smaller in size, an
entrance wound that is sustained at close range
will have powder burns around its edges
(Figure 14–13).

Bear in mind that small-caliber bullets, due
to their small mass, can be deflected by bone or
dense organs within the body and end up at a
point well away from the entry site. Thus, a
bullet that enters the chest can strike a rib and
be deflected downward into the abdomen,
causing abdominal as well as chest injuries. For
this reason, it is important to do a complete
assessment looking for associated injuries, not
merely ones near the point of entry.

Careful recording of the circumstances of
injury, the status of the patient, and the
treatment given is most important with gunshot wounds, because most will involve litiga-
tion at some future date. You may be called by
the court to testify regarding conditions at the
scene and any treatment that was administered. Only a carefully written record will be of
use to you then.

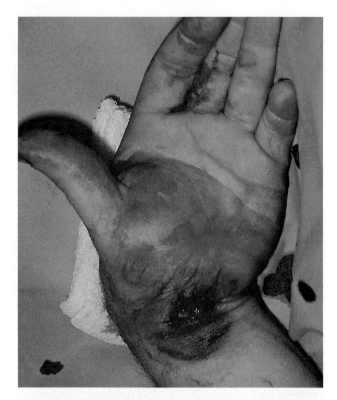

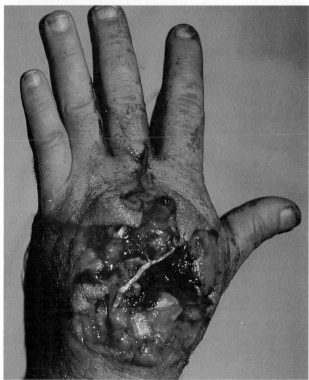

FIGURE 14–13

A close-range gunshot wound. Note the powder burns around the smaller entrance wound. Also note the large wound of exit.

APPLYING DRESSINGS AND BANDAGES

All wounds require bandaging. In most instances, splints will also be used to help control bleeding or provide firm support for the dressing. There are many different types of dressings and bandages, and you should be familiar with their functions and their proper application. Dressings and bandages have three major functions: to control bleeding, to protect a wound from further damage, and to prevent further contamination of the open wound.

Sterile Dressings

All ambulances must carry sterile dressings. Universal dressings, conventional 4″ x 4″ and 4″ x 8″ gauze pads, an assortment of small adhesive-type dressings, and soft self-adherent roller dressings will provide coverage for most wounds (Figure 14–14). A universal dressing is made of thick, absorbent material. It measures 9″ x 36″ and is packed folded into a compact size (Figure 14–15). These dressings are available commercially in sterilized packages. The universal dressing material can also be purchased

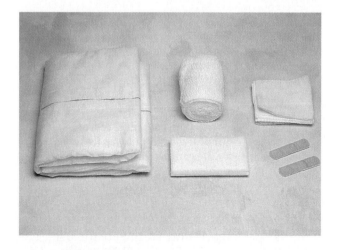

FIGURE 14–14

The standard types of dressings carried in an ambulance: universal dressings; conventional 4″ x 4″ and 4″ x 8″ gauze pads; small adhesive-type dressings; and soft self-adherent roller dressings.

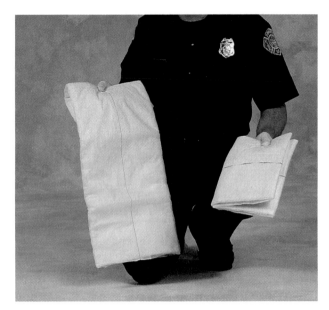

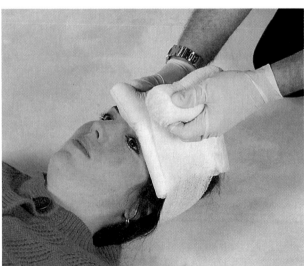

FIGURE 14–15

The universal dressing (top) can be folded to fit almost any large-size wound. It is held in place (bottom) by a self-adherent roller dressing.

in 20-yard rolls that can be cut into 3-foot lengths, packaged, and sterilized for use. The universal dressing provides ideal coverage for large open wounds, and the smaller gauze pads should be used for less extensive wounds. The universal dressing is also an efficient pad for rigid splints.

Bandages

Dressings must remain in place during transport. The stability of the dressing can be provided by soft roller bandages, rolls of gauze, triangular bandages, or adhesive tape. The self-adherent soft roller bandages are probably easiest to use. They are slightly elastic, which makes them easy to apply. The layers adhere somewhat to one another, and the end of the roll can be tucked back into a deeper layer to secure it in place. Adhesive tape holds small dressings in place and helps secure larger dressings. Some people, however, are allergic to adhesive tape; paper or plastic tape should be used for these patients.

Elastic bandages should not be used to secure dressings. With swelling, the elastic bandage may act as a tourniquet on an injured limb and cause further damage. Bandages should not interfere with circulation to the limb. You should always check a limb distal to a bandage after it is applied for signs of impaired circulation or loss of skin sensation.

Occlusive Dressings

An *occlusive dressing* prevents the passage of air and liquids. They are used for sucking chest wounds and abdominal eviscerations. A sucking chest wound must be sealed so that air does not pass through it. The wound can be occluded by Vaseline gauze or other impermeable dressings that will block the passage of air. Use a large enough dressing so that the dressing itself will not be sucked into the chest cavity. The dressing should be taped to the chest wall on three sides to keep it in place. One edge should be left untaped to allow for the escape of air (see Chapter 24).

Abdominal eviscerations must be kept moist. Occlusive dressings serve this purpose best. Exposed abdominal organs should be covered with a moistened universal dressing. The universal dressing is then covered with sterile aluminum foil that is taped to the abdomen. This dressing will keep the exposed abdominal contents moist and prevent further contamination (Figure 14–16).

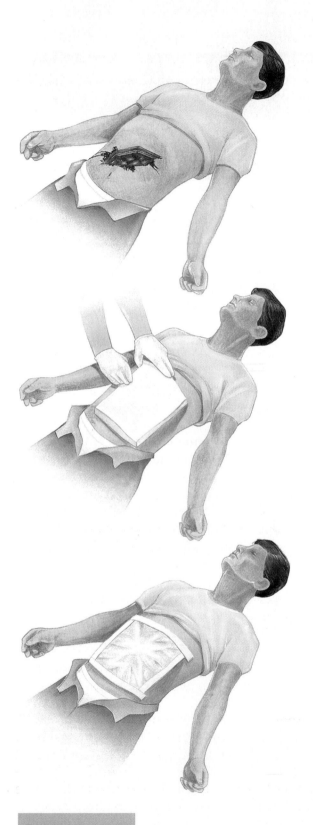

FIGURE 14–16

An abdominal evisceration is kept moist with a universal dressing soaked with sterile normal saline. The moistened dressing is sealed with aluminum foil securely taped on all sides to the skin of the abdomen.

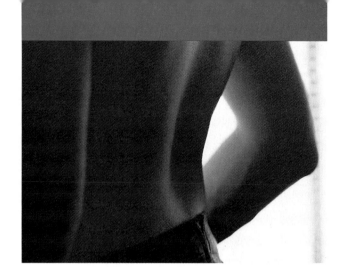

CHAPTER 15

THE MUSCULOSKELETAL SYSTEM

KEY TERMS

articular cartilage (ar-tik'u-lar kar'tĭ-lij) A thin layer of cartilage, covering the articular surface of bones in synovial joints.

joint The place where two bones come in contact.

ligament (lig'ah-ment) A band of fibrous tissue that connects bones to bones. It supports and strengthens a joint.

musculoskeletal (mus"ku-lo-skel'ĕ-tal) Pertaining to or composing the skeleton and the muscles, as the musculoskeletal system.

osteoporosis (os"te-o-po-ro'sis) Reduction in the amount of bone mass, leading to fractures after minimal trauma.

skeletal muscle (skel'ĕ-tal mus'el) Striated muscles that are attached to bones and usually cross at least one joint.

smooth muscle Nonstriated, involuntary muscle; it constitutes the bulk of the gastrointestinal tract and is present in nearly every organ to regulate automatic activity.

tendon (ten'dun) A tough, ropelike cord of fibrous tissue that attaches a skeletal muscle to a bone.

The human body is a well-designed system whose form, upright posture, and movement are provided by the musculoskeletal system. As its combination form suggests, the term musculoskeletal refers to the bones and voluntary muscles of the body. The musculoskeletal system also protects the vital internal organs of the body. It is susceptible to external forces, however, that can cause injury. And more than muscles and bones are at risk. The tendons that attach muscles to bones, the joints that form wherever two bones come into contact, and the ligaments that hold the bone ends of a joint together all are susceptible to injury.

As an EMT you are expected to understand the basic anatomy of the body's skeletal system. Although muscles are technically soft tissue, they are considered in this chapter because of their close anatomic and functional relationship to the skeleton. Chapter 15 thus begins with a description of the three basic types of muscles. The rest of the chapter focuses on the anatomy of the skeleton.

GOALS

The goals of Chapter 15 are to

- describe the three types of muscle found in the human body: skeletal muscle, smooth muscle, and cardiac muscle.
- be able to name and locate the major bones of the body.

MUSCLE

Muscles are a form of tissue that allows body movement. Although there are more than 600 muscles in the **musculoskeletal** system, they are generally divided into three types: skeletal, smooth, and cardiac.

Skeletal Muscle

Skeletal muscle, so named because it attaches to the bones of the skeleton, forms the major muscle mass of the body. It is also called *voluntary muscle,* because all skeletal muscle is under direct voluntary control of the brain and can be stimulated to contract or relax at will. Skeletal muscle is also called *striated muscle,* because when viewed under the microscope it has characteristic stripes (striations). All bodily movement results from skeletal muscle contraction or relaxation. Usually, a specific motion is the result of several muscles contracting and relaxing simultaneously.

All skeletal muscles are supplied with arteries, veins, and nerves (Figure 15–1). Arterial blood brings oxygen and nutrients to the muscle, and the veins carry away the waste products of muscular contraction (carbon dioxide and water). Muscles cannot function without this ongoing supply of oxygen and nutrients and removal of waste products. Muscle cramps result when insufficient oxygen or food is carried to the muscle or when acidic waste products accumulate and are not carried away.

Skeletal muscle is under the direct control of the nervous system and responds to a command from the brain to move a specific body part. Specific nerves pass directly from the brain to the spinal cord. There they connect with other nerves that exit from the spinal cord

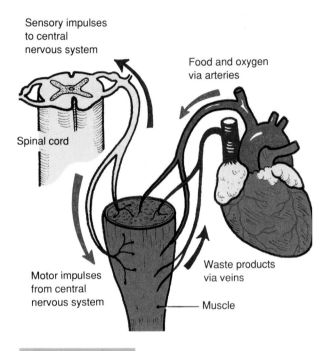

FIGURE 15-1

All skeletal muscles receive arterial blood carrying oxygen and nutrients. Waste products of muscle activity are removed by veins. Peripheral nerves, which extend from the spinal cord to each skeletal muscle, transmit electrical signals from the brain that cause the muscle to relax or contract.

and pass to each skeletal muscle. Electrical impulses are carried from the cells in the brain and spinal cord along the peripheral nerves to each muscle, signaling it to contract. When this normal nerve supply is lost through injury to the brain, spinal cord, or peripheral nerves, the voluntary control of the muscle is lost and the muscle becomes paralyzed.

Most skeletal muscles attach directly to bone by tough, ropelike cords of fibrous tissue called **tendons,** which continue the fascia that covers all skeletal muscles. The *fascia* is much like the skin of a sausage in that it encases the muscle tissue. At either end of the muscle the fascia extends beyond the muscle to attach to a bone. This *musculotendinous unit* crosses a joint and is responsible for the motion of that joint. The proximal point of attachment of the musculotendinous unit is its *origin*, and the distal

bony attachment is called the *insertion* of the muscle (Figure 15–2). When a muscle contracts, a line of force is created between the origin and the insertion, which pulls the points of origin and insertion closer together. This motion occurs at the joint between the two bones.

Smooth Muscle

Smooth muscle carries out much of the automatic work of the body; therefore, it is also called *involuntary muscle*. Smooth muscle is found in the walls of most tubular structures of the body, such as the gastrointestinal tract, the urinary system, the blood vessels, and the bronchi of the lungs. Contraction and relaxation of smooth muscle propels or controls the flow of the contents of these structures along their course. For example, the rhythmic contraction and relaxation of the smooth muscles of the wall of the intestine propel ingested food

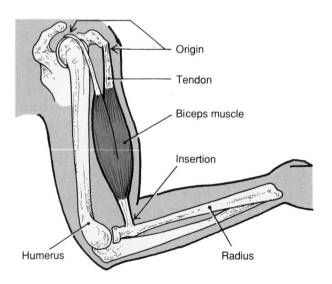

FIGURE 15-2

The biceps muscle causes the elbow to bend (flex) when it contracts. Note the points of tendon origin and insertion. As the muscle fibers contract and shorten, the origin and insertion are pulled closer together with motion occurring at the elbow joint.

through it, and smooth muscle in the walls of a blood vessel can alter the diameter of the vessel to control the amount of blood flowing through it (Figure 15–3).

Smooth muscle responds only to primitive stimuli such as stretching, heat, or the need to relieve waste. An individual cannot exert any voluntary control over this type of muscle. A more extensive description of smooth muscle function can be found in Chapter 25.

The Diaphragm

The *diaphragm* is unique because it has characteristics of both voluntary and involuntary muscle. Under the microscope it has striations like skeletal muscle. Also, it is attached to the costal arch and the lumbar vertebrae like other skeletal muscles. Thus, in many ways it looks like a voluntary muscle; however, we do not have complete voluntary control over its function. When we take a deep breath, the diaphragm flattens and its central part moves downward. This movement increases the vol-

ume of the chest cavity, allowing us to inhale air. When the diaphragm relaxes, its central part rises and air is exhaled. For the most part, breathing is automatic and continuous, so the diaphragm muscle should be thought of as an involuntary muscle. Automatic control of breathing can be overridden by the conscious person, and one can breathe faster or slower or hold one's breath for short periods of time. However, this voluntary control cannot continue indefinitely, and in the end automatic control resumes. Hence, although the diaphragm looks like voluntary skeletal muscle and is attached to the skeleton, it behaves like involuntary muscle most of the time.

Cardiac Muscle

The heart is a large muscle composed of a pair of pumps of unequal force—one of lower and one of higher pressure. The heart must function continuously from birth to death. It is an especially adapted involuntary muscle with a very rich blood supply and its own intrinsic regulatory system. Microscopically, it looks different from both skeletal and smooth muscle. *Cardiac muscle* can tolerate an interruption of its blood supply for only a few seconds. It requires a continuous supply of oxygen and glucose for normal function. Because of its special structure and function, cardiac muscle is placed in a separate category.

SKELETON

The skeleton is composed of about 206 bones. The skeleton functions to:

- Give form to the body.
- Allow bodily movement.
- Provide protection of vital, internal organs.
- Produce red blood cells.
- Serve as a reservoir for calcium, phosphorus, and other important body chemicals (Figure 15–4).

The skeleton is a framework for the attachment of muscles; it allows an erect posture against the pull of gravity and gives a constant and recognizable form to the body. Yet it is

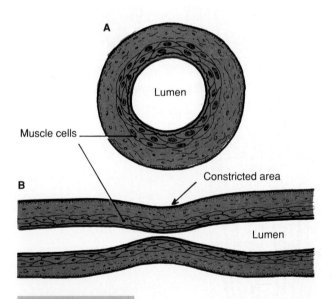

FIGURE 15–3

(A) Smooth muscle lines the walls of the tubular structures of the body. (B) Contraction of the muscles narrows the diameter of the structure, and relaxation allows the diameter to increase in size.

FIGURE 15–4

The human skeleton gives
form to the body, allows bodily
movement, protects internal
organs, produces red blood
cells, and stores calcium,
phosphorus, and other body
chemicals.

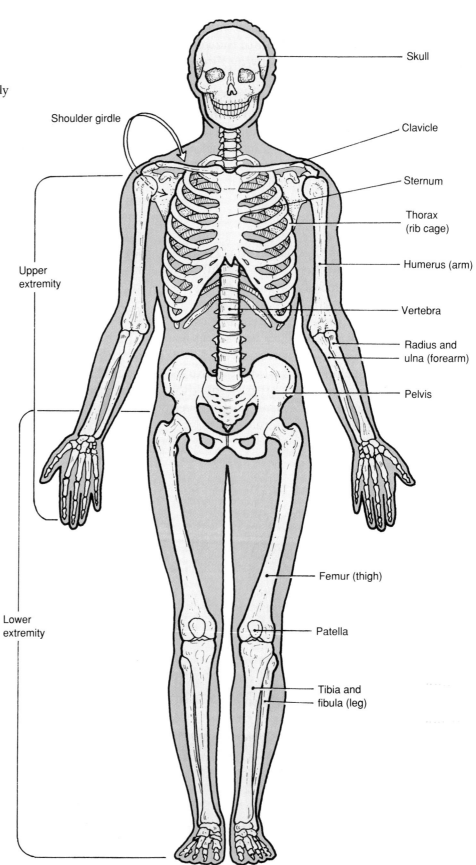

Shoulder girdle

Upper
extremity

Lower
extremity

Skull

Clavicle

Sternum

Thorax
(rib cage)

Humerus (arm)

Vertebra

Radius and
ulna (forearm)

Pelvis

Femur (thigh)

Patella

Tibia and
fibula (leg)

designed to allow motion of the body as well. The bones come in contact with one another at joints where controlled motion is accomplished by muscle action.

The skeleton also protects vital internal organs. The brain lies within the skull. The heart, lungs, and great vessels are protected by the thorax. Much of the liver and spleen is protected by the lowermost ribs. The spinal cord is contained within and protected by the bony spinal canal formed by the vertebrae.

The central portion of all bones is composed of bone marrow. *Bone marrow* produces red blood cells. These red blood cells have a short life-span of about 120 days. Thus, the bone must continuously supply new red blood cells to the circulation to ensure adequate transport of oxygen and carbon dioxide.

Each bone is composed of a protein framework that allows for its growth and remodeling. Calcium and phosphorus are deposited into this framework to make the bone hard and strong. Throughout the lifetime of the individual, calcium and phosphorus are constantly being deposited in bone and withdrawn from it under the control of a very complex metabolic system. Calcium must be maintained at a very specific concentration in the circulation for skeletal muscles to contract normally and for proper function of cardiac muscle.

Bone is just as much a living tissue as are muscle, skin, and other tissues. A rich blood supply constantly provides the oxygen and nutrients required by the bones. Each bone also has an extensive nerve supply. Thus, a fracture of bone produces severe pain from irritation of the nerves as well as significant bleeding from damage to the bone's blood vessels.

Although bones form the skeleton, not every bone is fully developed at birth. Bones must be rigid and unyielding to fulfill their structural support function, but they must also grow and adapt as we grow. As a rule, bone growth ends when a person reaches the late teens. Unless some abnormality is present, there is usually little outward skeletal change after this period.

Bones in young children are more flexible than in the adult and therefore are less likely to fracture. However, because children are so active, fractures still occur frequently. Bone

heals by forming new bone. It is the only tissue in the body that heals by forming more of itself. Other tissues in the body heal by forming scar tissue. Scar tissue, however, is not strong enough to function as bone should; therefore, bone has retained the ability to heal by forming more of itself.

As humans age, bone gradually becomes weaker due to a loss of calcium. This condition of gradual, progressive weakening of the bone is called **osteoporosis.** Osteoporosis is particularly common in women and is especially severe after menopause. Thus, elderly people, and in particular postmenopausal women, are more susceptible to fracture because of the weakened condition of the bone. Even trivial injuries may produce significant fractures in patients with osteoporosis (Figure 15–5).

Anatomy of a Bone

The various parts of a bone are designated by specific names depending on their shape and function. Many bones have a rounded end that allows joint rotation. This part is called the head. The region below the head is called the neck. The shaft is the long, straight cylindrical midportion of a bone. The *condyles* (called *malleoli* at the ankle and *styloid processes* at the wrist) are prominences at one or both ends of the bone that usually serve as points of ligament attachment. *Tuberosities* and *trochanters* are prominences of the bone where tendons insert (Figure 15–6).

The *epiphyseal plate* is a transverse cartilage plate near the end of a long bone of a child. It is responsible for the growth in length of the bone. Because it is made of cartilage, it can be seen on an X ray as a clear transverse line near the end of the child's bone (see also Figure 16–8).

Joints

Wherever two bones come in contact, a **joint** (articulation) is formed. Most joints allow motion—for example, the knee, hip, or elbow—whereas some bones fuse with one another at joints so that a solid, immobile, bony structure results. For instance, the skull is composed of

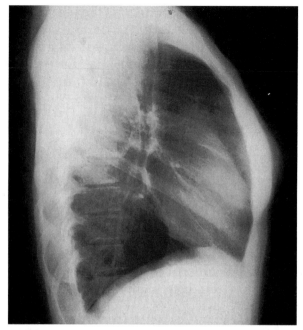

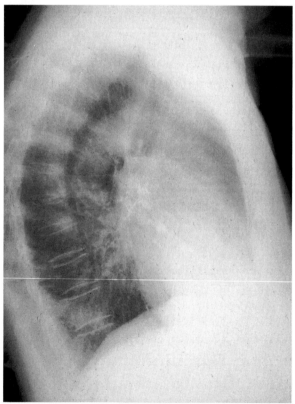

FIGURE 15–5

X ray of the spine of a healthy 25-year-old (top) and a 79-year-old with osteoporosis (bottom). Note the loss of bone density with age. Multiple fractures of the vertebrae have resulted in collapse of the spine and a "humpback" deformity.

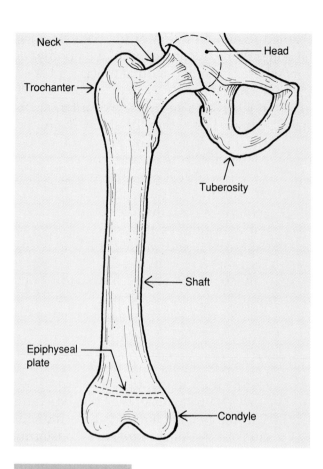

FIGURE 15–6

Specific regions of many bones have special names as indicated by the labels on this "typical bone."

several bones that fuse as the child grows. The infant, whose skull bones are not yet fused, has *fontanelles* (soft spots) between the bones. The fontanelles close as the bones fuse together when the child's skull reaches the adult size. Some joints have slight, limited motion. The bone ends are held together by fibrous tissue. Such a joint is called a *symphysis*.

A joint consists of the ends of the bones that make up the joint and the surrounding, connecting, and supporting tissue (Figure 15–7). Most joints in the body are named by combining the names of the two bones that form that joint. For example, the sternoclavicular joint is the articulation between the sternum and the clavicle.

In joints where motion occurs, the ends of bones that articulate with each other are cov-

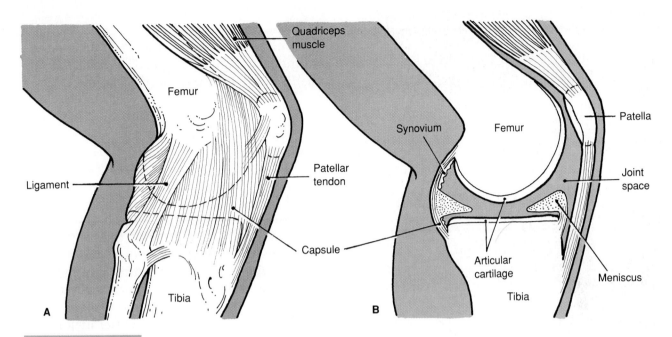

FIGURE 15-7

(A) The knee joint is stripped of the soft tissues that surround it to demonstrate its capsule and ligaments. (B) The knee is cut longitudinally to show the interior of the joint.

ered with a smooth, shiny surface called **articular cartilage.** Inside some joints, most notably the knee, cushions made of cartilage fill up spaces between the bones and aid in the gliding motion of the joint. Such a cushion is called a *meniscus,* or sometimes simply a cartilage. If injured and torn from its attachments, the meniscus can produce symptoms of locking or catching in the joint.

The bone ends of a joint are held together by a fibrous tissue *joint capsule.* At certain points around the circumference of the joint, the capsule is lax and thin so that motion can occur. In other areas it is quite thick and resists stretching or bending. These bands of tough, thick capsule are called **ligaments.** A joint such as the sacroiliac joint that is virtually surrounded by tough, thick ligaments will have little motion, whereas a joint such as the shoulder, with few ligaments, will be free to move in almost any direction (and will, as a result, be more prone to dislocation).

The degree of freedom of motion of a joint is determined by the extent to which the ligaments hold the bone ends together and also by the configuration of the bone ends themselves. The hip joint is a *ball-and-socket joint,* which allows rotation as well as bending (Figure 15-8). The finger joints and the knee are *hinge joints,* with motion restricted to one plane. They can only flex (bend) and extend (straighten). Rotation is not possible because of the shape of the joint surfaces and the strong restraining ligaments on both sides of the joint (Figure 15-9). Thus, although the amount of motion varies from joint to joint, all joints have a definite limit beyond which motion cannot occur. When a joint is forced beyond this limit, damage to some structure must occur: either the bones that form the joint will break, or the supporting capsule and ligaments will be disrupted.

The *synovium* (inner surface of the joint capsule) produces a fluid that nourishes and lubricates the articular cartilage. It is called synovial fluid. It is thick, almost oily, and clear yellow in color. Normally, only a few cubic centimeters of synovial fluid are present within a joint. With injury or disease, however, more fluid is produced to protect the joint, resulting

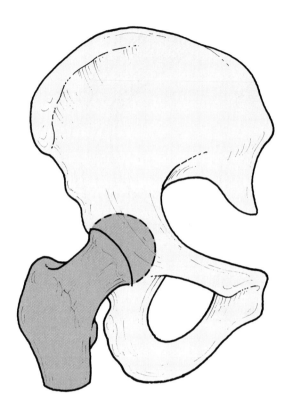

FIGURE 15-8

The hip joint is a typical ball-and-socket joint.

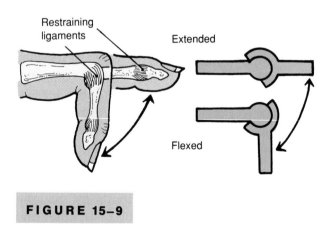

FIGURE 15-9

The finger joints are hinge joints, which allow motion in only one plane.

in swelling inside the capsule—for example, the so-called "water on the knee".

The Skull

The skull has two major divisions: the cranium and the face (Figure 15-10). The *cranium* (brain case) is composed of a number of thick bones that fuse together to form a shell that protects the brain. The face is also composed mostly of bones fused together to provide protection for important structures. For example, the *orbit* (eye socket) is composed of two facial bones, the maxilla and the zygoma, as well as the frontal bone of the cranium, to form a solid bony rim that protrudes around the eye to protect it. The *maxilla* contains the upper teeth and forms the *hard palate* (roof of the mouth). The *mandible,* (lower jaw) is the only movable facial bone having a joint (the *temporomandibular)* with the cranium just in front of each ear. The *nasal bone* is very short, as the majority of the nose is composed of flexible cartilage. The *mastoid process* of the cranium is a bony prominence behind the ear.

The Spinal Column

The *spinal column* is the central supporting structure of the body (Figure 15-11). It is composed of 33 bones, each called a *vertebra.*

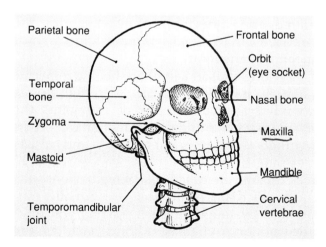

FIGURE 15-10

The skull includes the bones of the cranium, which are fused, and the facial bones. The mandible (lower jaw) is freely movable.

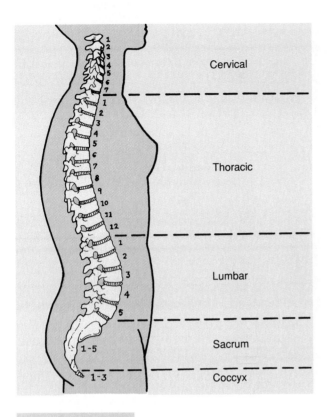

The spinal column consists of 33 vertebrae in 5 definite sections. The vertebrae protect the spinal cord.

with strong ligaments at the sacroiliac joints to form the *pelvic girdle.* The last three or four vertebrae form the *coccyx* (tailbone).

The skull rests on the first cervical vertebra and articulates with it. The *spinal cord* is an extension of the brain. It is composed of virtually all the nerves that carry messages between the brain and the rest of the body. It exits through a large hole (the *foramen magnum*) in the base of the skull and is contained within and protected by the vertebrae of the spinal column.

The front part of each vertebra consists of a round, solid block of bone, the *body.* The back part of each vertebra forms a *bony arch.* This series of arches from one vertebra to the next forms a tunnel that runs throughout the length of the spine and is called the *spinal canal.* The spinal canal encases and protects the spinal cord (Figure 15–12). Nerves branch from the spinal cord and exit from the spinal canal between each two vertebrae to form the motor and sensory nerves of the body (Figure 15–13).

From the top down, the spine is divided into these five sections:

- Cervical (neck).
- Thoracic or dorsal (upper part of the back).
- Lumbar (lower part of the back).
- Sacral (part of the pelvis).
- Coccygeal (coccyx or tailbone).

The vertebrae are named according to the section of the spine in which they lie and are numbered from top to bottom. The first seven vertebrae form the *cervical spine* (C_1 through C_7). The next 12 vertebrae make up the *thoracic* or *dorsal spine.* One pair of ribs articulates with each of these thoracic vertebrae. The next five vertebrae form the *lumbar spine,* or the lower back. The five sacral vertebrae are fused together to form one bone called the *sacrum.* The sacrum is joined to the iliac bones of the pelvis

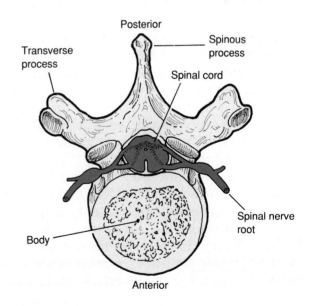

FIGURE 15–12

The top view of a thoracic vertebra showing the spinal canal protecting the spinal cord.

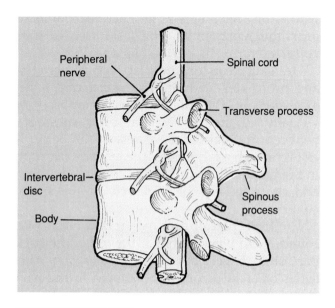

FIGURE 15–13

Between each two adjacent vertebrae, peripheral nerves exit the spinal canal. These nerves transmit information between the brain and specific parts of the body.

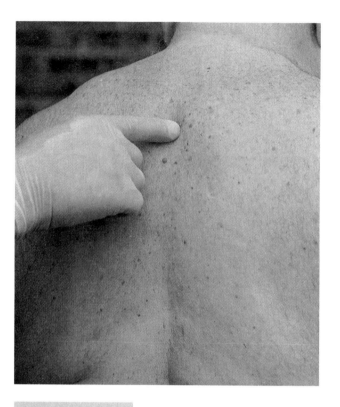

FIGURE 15–14

Even in the obese patient, it is usually possible to palpate the posterior spinous processes in the midline.

The vertebrae are connected by ligaments, and between each two vertebral bodies is a cushion, the *intervertebral disc*. These ligaments and discs allow some motion to occur between every two vertebrae, thus allowing the trunk to bend forward and back; however, they also act to limit motion of the vertebrae so that the spinal cord will not be injured. When a fracture of the spine occurs, protection of the spinal cord and its nerves may be lost. Until the fracture is stabilized, you must guard against injury to the spinal cord.

The spinal column itself is virtually surrounded by muscles; however, the *posterior spinous process* of each vertebra can be palpated, as it lies just under the skin in the midline of the back (Figure 15–14). The most prominent and most easily palpable spinous process is that of the seventh cervical vertebra at the base of the neck.

The Thorax

The *thorax* (rib cage) is made up of the ribs, the 12 thoracic vertebrae, and the *sternum* (breast bone) (Figure 15–15). There are 12 pairs of *ribs*, which are long, slender, curved bones. Each rib forms a joint with its respective thoracic vertebra and then curves around to form the rib cage. At the front of the rib cage, ribs 1 through 10 connect with the sternum through a bridge of cartilage. For the lower five ribs, this cartilaginous bridge is called the *costal arch*.

The sternum forms the middle part of the front of the thoracic cage. In the adult, this bone is approximately 7 inches long and 2 inches wide. The sternum has three parts: the *manubrium* (upper part), the *body*, and the *xiphoid process*. The junction of the manubrium and the body of the sternum is located at the level of the second ribs. Here there is a consistent bony prominence, the *angle of Louis*, that can be palpated on all patients. The xiphoid process of the sternum projects from the lower part of its body. It is made of cartilage and is very tender to palpation.

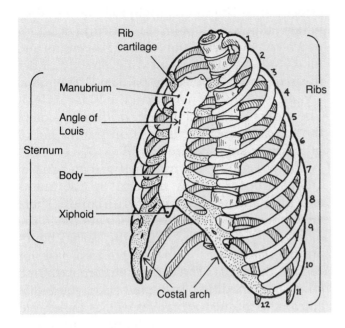

FIGURE 15-15

In the thoracic cage, 12 pairs of ribs articulate with the vertebrae in the spinal column through small joints. The first 10 pairs also articulate with the sternum or the costal arch in front, through a cartilaginous bridge.

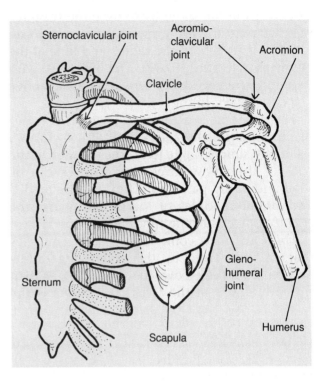

FIGURE 15-16

The shoulder girdle is composed of the clavicle, scapula, and proximal humerus.

The Upper Extremity

The proximal portion of the upper extremity is called the *shoulder girdle* (Figure 15–16). It consists of three bones: the clavicle, the scapula, and the humerus. The shoulder girdle serves as a base of attachment for the upper extremity to the trunk. The upper extremity can be moved through a wide range of motion, allowing the hand to be placed in almost any position. This motion occurs at three joints within the shoulder girdle: the *sternoclavicular joint*, the *acromioclavicular joint*, and the *glenohumeral joint*. Only slight motion occurs normally at the sternoclavicular and acromioclavicular joints. On the other hand, the ball-and-socket arrangement of the glenohumeral joint (the true shoulder joint) allows great freedom of motion in almost any direction.

The *clavicle* (collar bone) is a long, slender bone that lies just under the skin and serves as a support or prop for the upper extremity. Its medial end is attached by very strong ligaments to the manubrium of the sternum to form the sternoclavicular joint. Its lateral end forms a joint with the acromion process of the scapula to create the acromioclavicular joint.

The *scapula* (shoulder blade) is a large, flat, triangular bone interposed between the clavicle and the humerus and held against the back of the thorax by large muscles. It has two specially named regions that form joints with the clavicle and the humerus. The *acromion process*, anteriorly, forms part of the acromioclavicular joint, and the *glenoid fossa* is the recess for the articulation of the humeral head, forming the glenohumeral joint. The spine and medial border of the scapula can be seen and palpated posteriorly. The acromion process forms the rounded edge of the shoulder girdle and can be felt anteriorly as one walks a finger along the clavicle and across the acromioclavicular joint.

The head of the *humerus* is covered by muscles that form the rounded prominence of the shoulder girdle laterally. The humerus extends from the shoulder to form the supporting structure for the arm, and the distal end articulates with both the radius and ulna at the elbow joint (Figure 15–17). The humerus, with its long, straight shaft, serves as an effective lever for heavy lifting.

The humerus articulates with the two bones of the forearm, the *radius* and *ulna,* to form a relatively simple hinge joint, the elbow. On the back of the elbow three prominences can be seen and easily palpated. They are the medial and lateral condyles of the humerus and the *olecranon process* of the ulna (Figure 15–17).

The forearm is composed of many muscles that are supported by the underlying radius and ulna. At the elbow, the ulna is larger than the radius, but at the wrist, the radius is the larger bone. The radius rotates about the ulna, which allows the palm to be turned up or down. At the wrist, the ends of the radius and ulna (the styloid processes) lie directly under the skin and can be easily palpated. The radial styloid is slightly longer than the ulnar styloid. The radius lies on the lateral, or thumb, side of the forearm, and the ulna is on the medial or little finger side (Figure 15–18).

The wrist joint is a modified ball-and-socket articulation formed by the ends of the radius and ulna and several small wrist bones. There are eight bones in the wrist. They are called the *carpal bones.* Extending from the carpal bones are five *metacarpals,* which serve as a base for each of the digits. The carpometacarpal (thumb joint) is a modified ball-and-socket joint that allows the thumb to rotate as well as to flex and extend. The other joints in the hand are simple hinge joints. In the thumb, there are two bones beyond the metacarpal: the proximal and distal *phalanges* (singular, *phalanx*). The remaining four digits of the hand are named in order: the index, the long, the ring, and the little finger. Each of these contains three phalanges (Figure 15–19).

The Pelvis and Lower Extremity

The *pelvis* (Figure 15–20) is a bony ring that is formed posteriorly by the sacrum and antero-

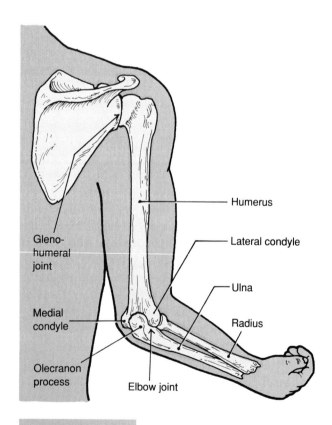

FIGURE 15–17

The arm is that portion of the upper extremity between the shoulder and the elbow joint. Three bony prominences can be seen at the elbow joint.

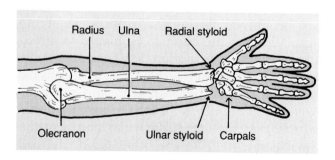

FIGURE 15–18

The forearm is made up of two bones, the radius and the ulna. The radius is larger distally and lies on the thumb side of the forearm. The ulna is larger proximally and lies on the little-finger side.

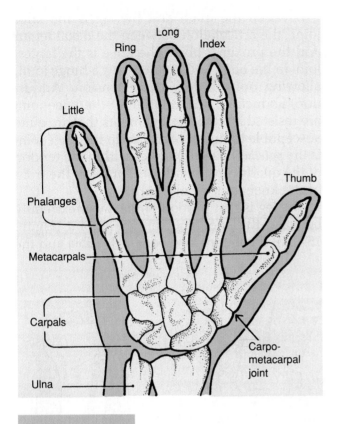

FIGURE 15–19

The bones of the wrist and hand. Note the proper name of each digit.

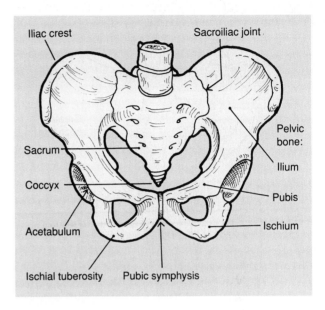

FIGURE 15–20

The pelvis is comprised of three bones: the sacrum and the two pelvic bones. The sacrum firmly articulates with the two pelvic bones posteriorly, and anteriorly the symphysis pubis joins the two pelvic bones.

laterally by the large winglike pelvic bones. Each pelvic bone is formed by the fusion of three separate bones, much as the skull is composed of several bones fused together. The three bones are the *ilium*, with its *iliac crest* laterally; the *ischium*, with its *ischial tuberosity* palpable in the buttock; and the *pubis*, palpable anteriorly.

The sacrum and the two pelvic bones articulate at three joints: the two posterior *sacroiliac joints* and the anterior, midline *symphysis pubis*. All three joints allow very little motion, as they are firmly held together by strong ligaments. Thus, the pelvic ring is strong and stable, because it is designed to support the body weight and protect the structures within the pelvic cavity (the bladder, the rectum, and the female reproductive organs). On the lateral side of each pelvic bone where the three

component bones join is the socket for the hip joint. This depression in which the femoral head fits very snugly is called the *acetabulum*.

The lower extremity consists of the thigh, the leg, and the foot (Figure 15–21). The *femur* (thigh bone) is the longest and one of the strongest bones in the body. The femoral head forms the hip joint with the acetabulum of the pelvis. This ball-and-socket joint allows flexion, extension, adduction (motion of the limb toward the midline), and abduction (motion of the limb away from the midline), and internal and external rotation of the entire lower extremity.

In the proximal lateral thigh, the prominence of the *greater trochanter* of the femur can be easily palpated. This prominence is sometimes called the "hip bone." The shaft of the femur is surrounded by large muscles (the quadriceps anteriorly and the hamstrings posteriorly). Just above the knee, the medial and lateral femoral condyles can be palpated.

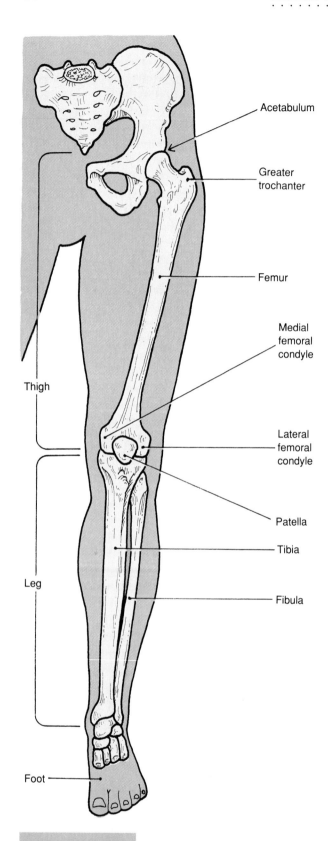

Between the thigh and the leg is the knee joint, the articulation between the distal femur and the proximal tibia. The knee is the largest joint in the body and is essentially a hinge joint, allowing only flexion and extension. Adduction, abduction, and rotation of the knee joint are resisted by complex ligaments that are quite susceptible to injury. Anterior to the knee joint is the *patella* (kneecap). It lies within the tendon of the quadriceps muscle and protects the front of the knee joint from injury.

The leg is that portion of the lower extremity between the knee and the ankle joint (Figure 15–22). It contains two bones: the tibia and the

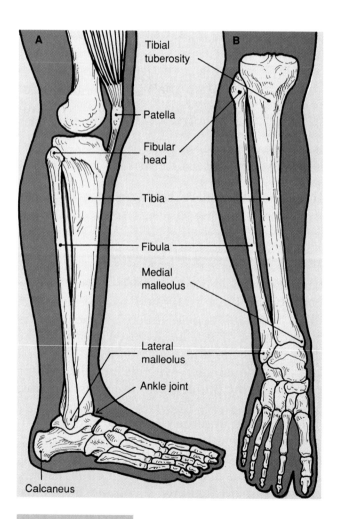

FIGURE 15–21

The femur is the single bone of the thigh. The leg is formed by the fibula and the tibia. The foot contains seven tarsal bones.

FIGURE 15–22

(A) A lateral view of the knee and leg showing the patella in the tendon of the quadriceps muscle. (B) An anterior view of the leg.

fibula. The *tibia* (shin bone) is the larger bone and lies in the anterior aspect of the leg. Its edge is just under the skin and is easily palpable from the tibial tuberosity (the insertion of the patellar tendon) to the medial malleolus at the ankle. The *fibula* lies laterally. Its head can be palpated on the lateral aspect of the knee joint, and its distal end forms the lateral malleolus of the ankle joint.

The ankle joint is a hinge joint that allows flexion and extension of the foot on the leg. The end of the tibia provides a smooth articular surface for the *talus* (ankle bone) (Figure 15–23). The talus is one of seven *tarsal bones*. The *calcaneus* (*os calcis*, or heel bone) is the other large tarsal bone. It forms the prominence of the heel. The *Achilles tendon* inserts into the back of the calcaneus. There are five *metatarsals* that articulate with the tarsal bones, and, as in the hand, each gives rise to its respective digit. The great toe has two phalanges, and the lesser four toes have three phalanges each, similar to the arrangement of the bones in the fingers.

YOU ARE THE EMT

1. Would you describe the biceps muscle as a smooth or skeletal muscle? Why? Which muscle looks like skeletal muscle but behaves like involuntary muscle?
2. You know that bones heal by forming new bone. Can this process still occur in an elderly person? Describe the condition called osteoporosis.
3. Your patient has "water on the knee." What is the medical explanation for this phenomenon?
4. What is the difference between hinge joints and ball-and-socket joints? Name two hinge joints and two ball-and-socket joints.

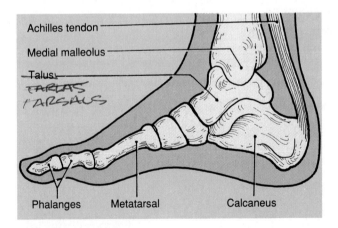

FIGURE 15–23

This view of the ankle and foot shows the articulation of the talus with the distal tibia. The talus and calcaneus are both tarsal bones.

FRACTURES, DISLOCATIONS, AND SPRAINS

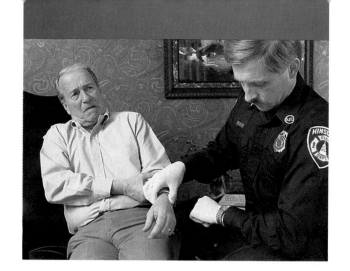

KEY TERMS

dislocation (dis"lo-ka'shun) The disruption of a joint such that the bone ends are no longer in contact.

displaced fracture A fracture that produces deformity of the limb.

fracture Any break in the continuity of a bone.

open fracture A fracture in which there is an external wound that communicates with the fracture site.

splint A rigid or flexible appliance used to keep in place and protect an injured part.

sprain A joint injury in which some of the supporting ligaments are damaged.

strain An overstretching or overexertion of a muscle.

traction The act of exerting a pulling force on a structure.

Musculoskeletal injuries are among the most common problems seen in emergency care work. You must check each injured patient for the possibility of fracture, dislocation, or sprain and be prepared to manage that injury properly. Effective emergency care of musculoskeletal injuries decreases immediate pain and reduces the possibility of shock and further nerve or vessel injury; it also improves the patient's chances for a rapid recovery and early return to normal activity.

Chapter 16 begins with a description of the types and causes of musculoskeletal injuries. It then discusses fractures, dislocations, and sprains. The chapter next describes the steps in the examination of musculoskeletal injuries. The last part of Chapter 16 focuses on the treatment of musculoskeletal injuries—specifically, the methods of splinting and transporting the injured patient.

GOALS

The goals of Chapter 16 are to
- describe the types and causes of musculoskeletal injuries.
- recognize the various types of fractures.
- recognize a dislocation.
- recognize a sprain.
- learn how to carry out an examination of an injured limb.
- learn how to treat a musculoskeletal injury, including the various methods of splinting and the proper way to transport a patient with an injured limb.

TYPES AND CAUSES OF MUSCULOSKELETAL INJURY

A **fracture,** known commonly as a broken bone, is any break in the continuity of a bone. The break may range in severity from a simple crack to severe shattering that produces multiple fracture fragments. The break can occur anywhere on the surface of the bone (Figure 16–1), even across the surface of the joint.

Dislocation means disruption of a joint so that the bone ends are no longer in contact. Such a disruption of the joint can happen only if the supporting ligaments and capsule of the joint tear, allowing the bone ends to separate completely from each other (Figure 16–2).

A fracture-dislocation is a twofold injury in which the joint is dislocated and a part of the bone near the joint also fractures (Figure 16–3).

A **sprain** is a joint injury in which the joint is partially, temporarily dislocated, and some of the supporting ligaments are either stretched or torn. Following the injury, the joint surfaces fall back into alignment so that immediately after the injury persistent displacement of the joint surfaces does not occur (Figure 16–4). Sprains vary in severity from mild to severe, depending on the amount of damage that has occurred to the supporting ligaments. A severe sprain often causes as much damage to the supporting ligaments and the joint capsule as does a complete dislocation.

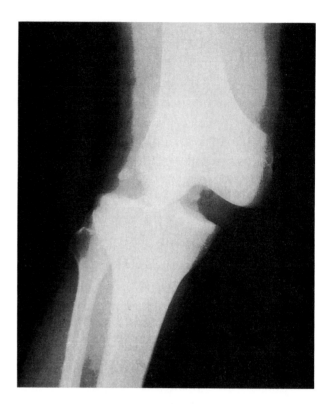

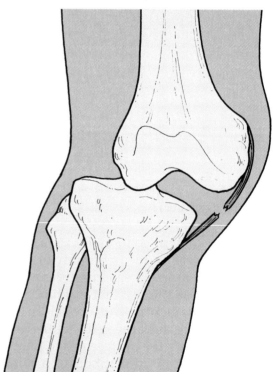

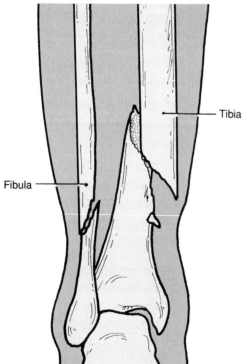

Tibia

Fibula

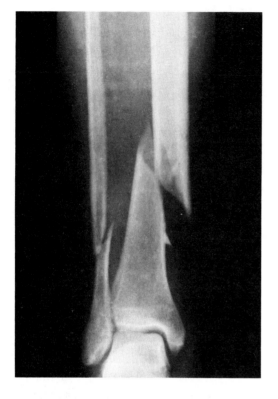

FIGURE   16–1

FIGURE   16–2

Fracture of the tibia and fibula. (Top) X ray appearance of fracture fragments; (bottom) line drawing of the fracture.

Dislocation of the knee joint. (Top) X ray appearance of the dislocated joint; (bottom) line drawing of the dislocation.

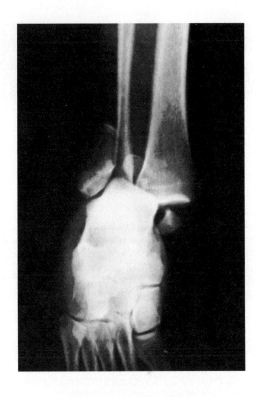

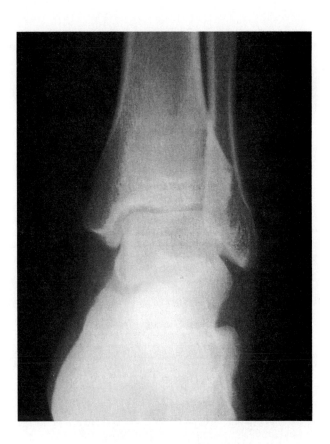

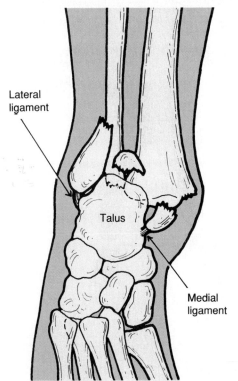

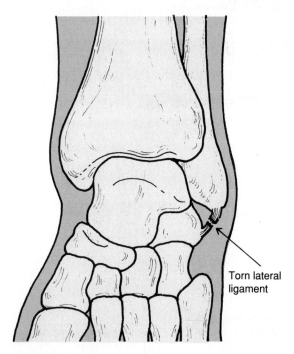

FIGURE 16–3

Fracture-dislocation of the ankle joint. (Top) X ray appearance of the talus dislocated from the distal tibia with fracture of both the medial and lateral malleoli; (bottom) line drawing of the fracture-dislocation.

FIGURE 16–4

An ankle sprain. (Top) X ray of the injured ankle appears normal because there is no injury of the bones. (Bottom) The line drawing, however, shows that the supporting ligament on the lateral side of the ankle has been torn.

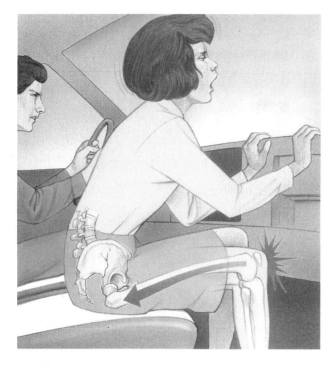
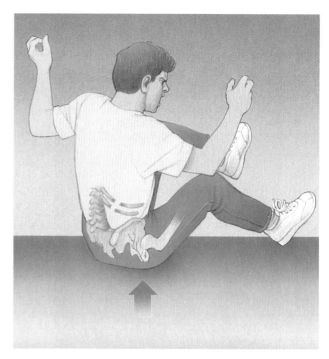
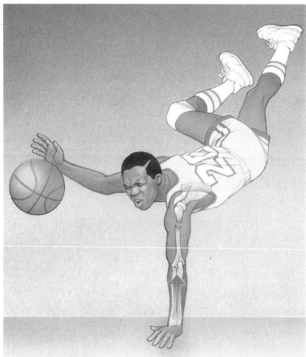
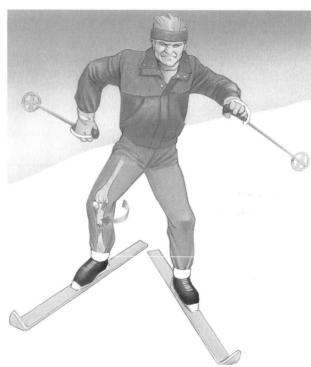

FIGURE 16–5   Various mechanisms of injury may produce fractures and dislocations.

A **strain** (muscle pull) is a stretching or tearing of a muscle. Unlike a sprain, no ligament or joint damage occurs. A strain is a muscle injury. The muscle fibers are partially pulled apart, producing pain and occasional swelling and ecchymosis of the local soft tissues.

Because musculoskeletal injuries occur so frequently, you must be able to evaluate them properly. Injury to the bones and joints is often associated with injury to the surrounding soft tissue (especially the adjacent nerves and arteries). In addition, other areas of the body at a distance from the fracture may sustain injury as well. Therefore, do not focus exclusively on a patient's obviously deformed arm or leg without first completing a primary assessment to ensure that associated and perhaps even more serious injuries are not overlooked.

Significant force is usually required to cause fractures or dislocations. The force may be applied to the limb in several ways. Direct blows, indirect forces, twisting forces, or high-energy injury all may cause significant musculoskeletal injury (Figure 16–5). A direct blow is a common cause of fracture. The fracture from a direct blow occurs at the point of impact. For example, the patella may be fractured when it strikes the dashboard in an automobile accident.

Indirect forces can also result in fracture or dislocation. In such instances, the force is applied to one part of the limb, and the site of injury is some distance away from the point of impact, usually proximal to it. The best example of an indirect force that causes a fracture is the wide range of fractures that occurs when an individual falls and lands on an outstretched hand. The patient may fracture the bones of the wrist, or forearm, the humerus, or even the clavicle. Indeed, this is the most common mechanism of fracture of the clavicle.

Twisting forces can also result in musculoskeletal injury. Such a force is a common cause of tibial fractures as well as knee and ankle ligament injuries. With this mechanism of injury, the foot is usually fixed to a point on the ground as the patient falls. Skiing injuries frequently occur this way, when the ski becomes caught and the skier falls, applying a twisting force to the lower extremity.

High-energy injury—as in automobile accidents, falls from heights, gunshot wounds, and injuries from other extreme forces—produces severe damage to the skeleton, its surrounding soft tissues, and the vital internal organs it is designed to protect. More than one bone in a limb may be fractured or dislocated, and multiple injuries to many parts of the body commonly occur following high-energy injury.

Not all fractures result from the application of a violent force, however. Some people have a localized destructive lesion of bone, such as a bone tumor, that so weakens the bone that only a slight force will cause it to break. A common generalized bone disease, *osteoporosis*, weakens the bone and causes it to be very susceptible to fracture with minimal force. Osteoporosis is common in elderly patients, particularly postmenopausal women. Minor falls, simple twisting injuries, or even contraction of the muscles can cause a bone to fracture in people who have osteoporosis. Thus, you must suspect the presence of a fracture in any older patient who has sustained even a mild injury.

FRACTURES

Fracture Classification

The most important factor to identify in the initial evaluation of a fracture, or any extremity injury, is the integrity of the overlying skin and soft tissues. Just as with soft tissue injuries, fractures are classified as open or closed.

An **open fracture** is any fracture in which the overlying skin has been damaged (Figure 16–6). Laceration of the skin can occur when sharp bone ends protrude through it or by a direct blow that lacerates the skin at the time of the fracture. The wound may vary in size from a small puncture wound to a gaping hole with much exposed bone and soft tissue. The bone may or may not be visible in the wound. Regardless of the extent and severity of the injury to the skin, any fracture in which the protective covering of skin has been damaged is considered to be an open fracture. In con-

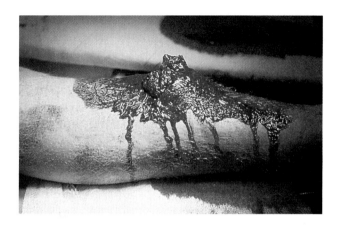

FIGURE 16–6

An open (compound) fracture with exposed bone. The fracture does not have to be visible to be classified as open.

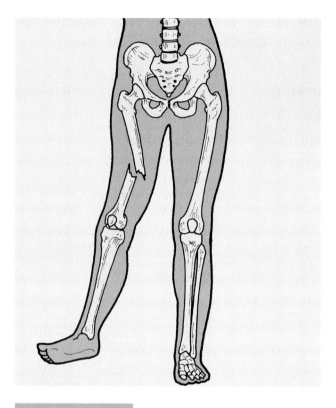

FIGURE 16–7

Fracture of the shaft of the right femur with angulation, shortening, and rotation of the limb below the fracture site.

trast, a closed fracture is one in which the skin has not been penetrated by the bone ends and no wound exists anywhere near the fracture site.

It is extremely important for you to determine whether the fracture is open or closed. Open fractures are much more serious than closed fractures for two reasons. First, greater blood loss occurs with open fractures than with closed fractures. Second, and more important, the bone is contaminated by being exposed to the outside environment, and the fracture site may become infected. An infected fracture sometimes causes serious life-long problems for the patient. For these reasons, all fractures should be described to emergency department

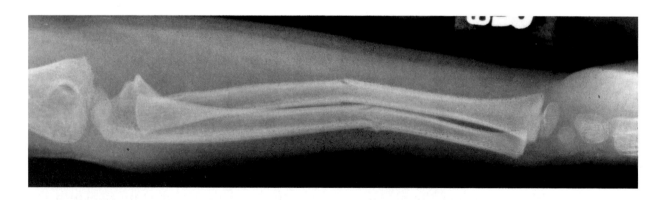

FIGURE 16–8

X ray of a greenstick fracture of the radius and ulna. These incomplete fractures occur only in children. Note the epiphysis at the distal end of the radius.

personnel as either open or closed so that the proper treatment can be undertaken on arrival at the hospital.

Fractures are also described by the degree of displacement of the fracture fragments. A **displaced fracture** produces deformity of the limb. The deformity is slight if the displacement is minimal, or it may be extreme if gross displacement of the fracture fragments has occurred. Many different deformities may occur. Angulation at the fracture site and rotation of the limb distal to the fracture site are common types of displacement. In addition, the limb may be shortened if the fracture fragments are displaced and their ends overlap (Figure 16–7).

The deformity associated with displaced fractures makes their diagnosis easy. It is much more difficult to diagnose nondisplaced fractures without the aid of X rays. Because there is no deformity, these fractures may be missed or thought to be only a bruise or a sprain. Use a high index of suspicion when you evaluate an injured person who complains of pain in the extremity. A patient exhibiting any one of the signs of fracture described later in this chapter must be considered to have a fracture, even if there is no deformity of the limb.

On occasion, special terms are used to describe particular types of fractures. Because these terms are used commonly by medical personnel, you should be familiar with their meaning:

■ *Greenstick fracture:* Occurs only in children and is an incomplete fracture that passes only partway through the shaft of a bone (Figure 16–8).
■ *Comminuted fracture:* One in which the bone is broken into more than two fragments (Figure 16–9).
■ *Pathologic fracture:* Occurs through weak or diseased bone, as in osteoporosis, and can be produced by a minimal force (Figure 16–10).
■ *Epiphyseal fracture:* Occurs in growing children. It is an injury to the growth plate of a long bone that may lead to an arrest of bone growth if not properly treated (Figure 16–11).

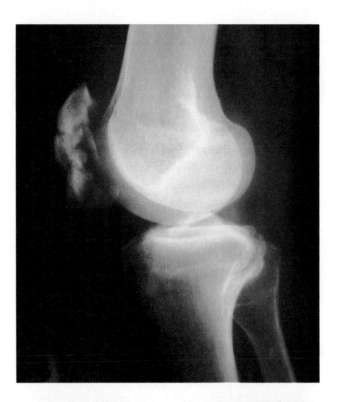

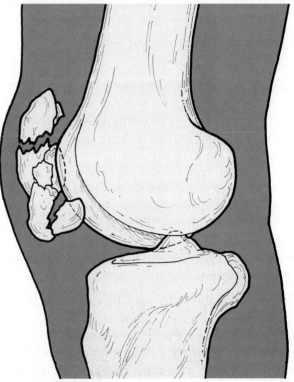

FIGURE 16–9

A comminuted fracture of the patella. (Top) X ray appearance of the patella; (bottom) line drawing of the comminuted fracture.

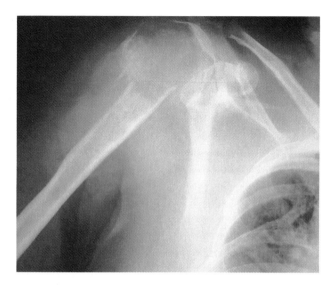

FIGURE 16–10

X ray of a pathologic fracture that has occurred through the upper end of the humerus weakened by a tumor.

Signs and Symptoms of Fractures

Any patient with a history of injury who complains of musculoskeletal pain must be suspected of having sustained a fracture. Although bone ends protruding through the skin or gross deformity of a limb make fracture recognition easy, many fractures—particularly nondisplaced fractures—are less obvious. You must know the following seven signs of fractures. All seven signs do not need to be present to make the diagnosis. The presence of any one of these signs should arouse suspicion of a fracture, and you should institute proper emergency treatment.

- *Deformity.* The limb may lie in an unnatural position, shortened, angulated, or rotated at a point where no joint exists. If you are uncertain whether a deformity exists, use the opposite limb as a mirror image for comparison. Always compare the injured limb with the uninjured opposite limb when you check for deformity (Figure 16–12).
- *Tenderness.* Tenderness is usually sharply localized at the site of the injury. This sensitive spot can be located by gently pal-

pating along the bone with the tip of one finger. This sign is called point tenderness and is the most reliable indication of an underlying fracture (Figure 16–13).

- *Guarding* (inability to use the extremity). A patient who has sustained a fracture or serious injury usually guards the injured part and will refuse to use it because motion causes increased pain. It is the patient's way of "splinting" the injured limb to minimize motion and pain. Although the inability to use a limb is a reliable sign of a significant injury, you must realize that the reverse is *not* true: The ability to use an extremity does not mean that a fracture does not exist. Occasionally, nondisplaced fractures are not very painful, and some patients may continue to use an injured limb even though a fracture is present. Such is the case particularly with

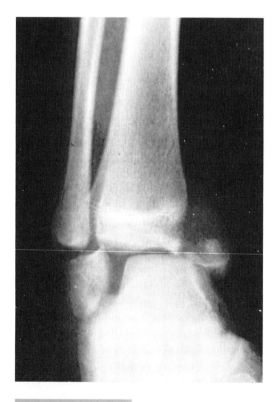

FIGURE 16–11

Epiphyseal (growth) plates are present in children near the ends of all long bones. X ray appearance of a displaced fracture through the epiphysis of the distal fibula.

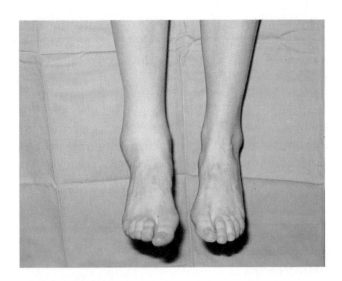

FIGURE 16–12

The EMT should always compare the injured limb with the uninjured limb when checking for deformity.

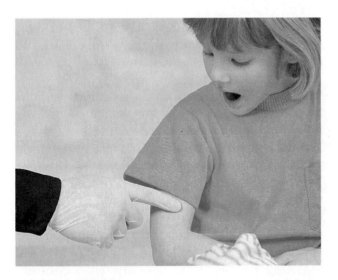

FIGURE 16–13

Point tenderness, the sensitive spot at the site of injury that can be located by gentle palpation along the bone with the tip of the EMT's finger, is the most reliable sign of an underlying fracture.

multiple fractures, where one injury is very painful and masks the pain of other fractures.

■ *Swelling and ecchymosis.* Fractures are virtually always associated with swelling and bruising of the surrounding soft tissues. These signs are also present following almost any injury and are not specific for fractures. However, rapid swelling occurring immediately after an injury usually indicates bleeding from the fracture site into the soft tissues from damaged blood vessels. Indeed, the swelling may be severe enough to mask the deformity of a limb produced by the broken bones. Generalized swelling of the limb also occurs as a result of fracture several hours after the injury.

■ *Exposed fragments.* An open fracture's bone ends may protrude through the skin or be seen in the depths of the wound itself, an obvious sign of fracture.

■ *Crepitus* (grating). A grating or grinding sensation called crepitus can be felt and sometimes even heard when the raw bone ends rub together.

■ *False motion.* Motion at a point in the limb where it usually does not occur is a positive indication of fracture. This is called false motion.

The first five signs listed are the only ones that need to be evaluated to diagnose a fracture in the field. Crepitus and false motion only appear when a limb is moved or manipulated. These conditions are, however, extremely painful to the patient, and the limb should not be manipulated to elicit these signs. Inspection of the limb with the clothing removed will allow you to see any deformity, swelling, ecchymosis, or exposed bone fragments. An unwillingness of the patient to use the injured limb indicates guarding and loss of function. Finally, palpation with one finger over the injured bone will elicit point tenderness. Any one of these signs is sufficient grounds to assume that a fracture is present.

DISLOCATIONS

With dislocation of a joint, injury to the supporting ligaments and capsule is so severe that the joint surfaces are completely displaced from one another. The bone ends lock in the displaced position, making any attempt at motion of the joint difficult as well as painful. Among the joints most susceptible to dislocation are the small joints of the fingers, the shoulder, the elbow, the hip, and the ankle. You may see the following signs and symptoms when a joint is dislocated:

- Marked deformity of the joint.
- Swelling in the region of the joint.
- Pain at the joint which is aggravated by any attempt at movement.
- Virtually complete loss of normal joint motion (a "locked" joint).
- Tenderness to palpation about the joint.

SPRAINS

A joint sprain occurs when a joint is twisted or stretched beyond its normal range of motion. As a result, some of the supporting capsule and ligaments are stretched or torn. Because it is an injury to a joint, a sprain should be considered to be a partial dislocation. The bone ends are not completely displaced from one another by the force of injury, so they can fall back into alignment when the force is released. Therefore, the severe deformity seen with a dislocated joint is not present with a sprain. Sprains vary in severity from a slight injury to severe disruption of the supporting ligaments and capsule. Although sprains most often occur in the knee and ankle, any joint may be sprained. The following are signs of sprain:

- *Tenderness.* Point tenderness can be elicited over the injured ligaments, just as point tenderness is found over a fracture site.
- *Swelling and ecchymosis.* A sprain usually tears blood vessels, producing swelling and ecchymosis at the point of ligament injury.
- *Inability to use the extremity.* Because of the pain of injury, the patient often cannot move or use the limb normally.

The signs of a sprain are the same as some of those for a fracture. Indeed, it is impossible at times to differentiate between a nondisplaced fracture and a sprain. The important point to remember is that although an injury may appear to be just a sprain, a fracture may be present as well. In the field, the working diagnosis whenever any one of the signs of fracture, dislocation, or sprain is present should be "injury to the limb." Even though you will often be able to make a more specific diagnosis of fracture, dislocation, or sprain, all extremity injuries require evaluation in the emergency department. *The basic principles of field management are the same for all three types of limb injury.*

EXAMINATION OF MUSCULOSKELETAL INJURIES

There are three essential steps in the examination of patients with musculoskeletal injuries:

1. Make a general assessment of the patient.
2. Examine the injured part.
3. Evaluate the distal neurovascular function.

You should conduct a general, primary assessment of the injured patient before you focus attention on an injured limb. Multiple injuries occur frequently, and the patient's general condition must be assessed and stabilized first. Bleeding from an extremity should be controlled as part of the primary stabilization, but further treatment of the extremities should await full stabilization of the patient's vital functions.

When the patient is critically injured and the vital functions cannot be stabilized in the field, rapid transportation to a trauma center is necessary. In this situation, extensive evaluation and splinting of limb injuries in the field only wastes valuable time. Secure this critically injured patient to a long spine board to rapidly immobilize the spine, pelvis, and extremities.

When no critical life-threatening injuries can be found and the patient's general condition has been stabilized, attention can be directed at evaluating the injured limb. During the secondary survey, inspection and palpation are used to identify musculoskeletal injuries. You should look at the injured limb and compare it with the opposite, uninjured side. Gently and carefully remove the patient's clothing so that a thorough inspection will reveal any of the following:

1. Open fracture or dislocation (and its accompanying risks of bleeding and contamination),
2. Deformity,
3. Swelling, and/or
4. Ecchymosis.

Then gently palpate the extremities and the spine to identify any areas of point tenderness—the best indicator of an underlying fracture, dislocation, or sprain.

Inspection and palpation will enable you to identify the presence of a significant limb injury in most instances. It is not important to differentiate fractures, dislocations, sprains, or simple contusions. The working diagnosis in most instances will be "injury to the limb." All limb injuries are treated in the same manner and therefore it is not critical to differentiate among the various types of extremity injuries.

If the patient has no signs of injury following inspection and palpation, ask the patient to move each limb carefully. With any significant musculoskeletal injury, movement of an injured part will be painful for the patient. The patient can usually localize the point of maximal discomfort. If even the slightest motion by the patient produces pain, no further motion should be attempted. This step should not be attempted when evaluating an injured person who complains of neck or back pain, because even the slightest motion may cause permanent damage to the spinal cord.

Once you have diagnosed an injury to the limb, it is essential to perform an evaluation of the distal neurovascular function. Many important vessels and nerves lie close to the bone, especially around the major joints. Therefore, any fracture or dislocation may have associated vessel or nerve injury. A neurovascular examination must be carried out initially and repeated every 15 minutes until the patient is hospitalized.

It is also imperative to recheck the neurovascular status after any manipulation of the limb (such as splinting). This reevaluation after a splint is applied is most important because

manipulations during splinting might have caused a bone fragment to press against or impale an important nerve or vessel. A pulseless limb will die if circulation is not restored, and you must give priority to such patients in the emergency care system. Perform the following neurovascular examination and record the results for each injured limb:

1. *Pulse.* Palpate the pulse distal to the point of injury. Palpate the radial pulse in the upper extremity and the posterior tibial pulse in the lower extremity (Figure 16–14).
2. *Capillary refill.* Note and record skin color, identifying any pallor or cyanosis. The cap-

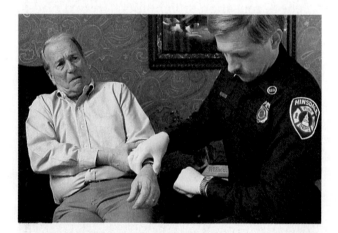

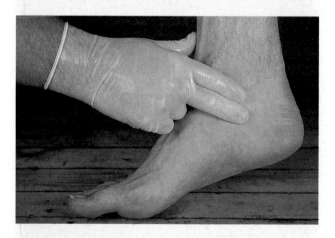

FIGURE 16–14

The first step in a neurovascular examination following a limb injury is to palpate the pulse distal to the injury: (Top) palpation of the radial pulse; (bottom) palpation of the posterior tibial pulse.

illary bed is best seen in the finger or toe underneath the nail. Firm pressure on the tip of the nail will cause the nailbed to blanch (turn white). On release of the pressure, the normal pink color should return to the nailbed by the time it takes to say "capillary filling." If a pink color does not return in this two-second interval, it is considered delayed and indicates impairment of circulation. The capillary refill should be pink and brisk (Figure 16–15).

3. *Sensation.* The patient's ability to sense light touch in the fingers or toes distal to a fracture site is a good indication that the nerve supply remains intact. In the hand, check sensation to light touch in two places: on the pulp of the index and the little fingers. In the foot, check the feeling on the pulp of the big toe and laterally on the dorsum of the foot (Figure 16–16).

4. *Motor function.* When the injury is proximal to the patient's hand or foot, make an estimate of muscular activity. If the injury involves the hand or foot itself, do not perform this test, because it will cause the

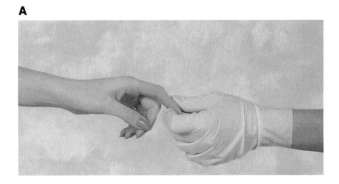

A

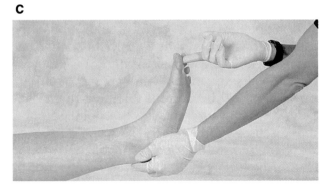

B

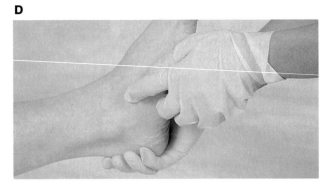

C

D

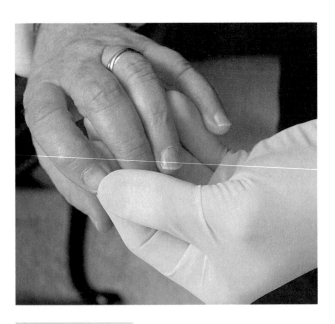

FIGURE 16–15

The second step in a neurovascular examination following a limb injury is to note and record skin color. Capillary refill (best seen in the nailbed) should be pink and brisk.

FIGURE 16–16

The third step in a neurovascular examination following a limb injury is to check sensation in four critical areas: (A) the pulp of the index fingertip; (B) the pulp of the little fingertip; (C) the pulp of the big toe; and (D) the dorsolateral aspect of the foot.

patient pain. The test can be done simply by having the patient open and close the fist for an upper extremity injury and wiggle the toes or move the foot up and down to test the motor function of the lower extremity

(Figure 16–17). Sometimes, an attempt at motion will produce pain at the injury site. If pain occurs, do not persist with this part of the examination.

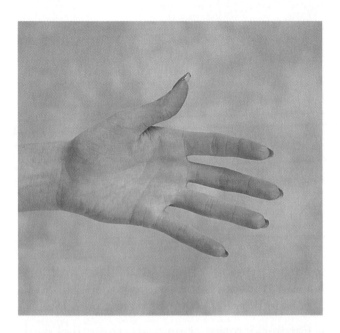

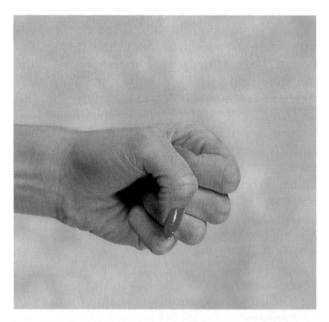

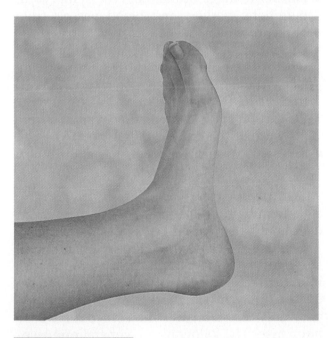

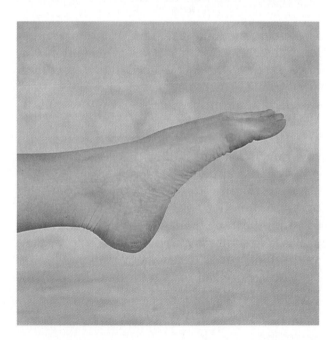

FIGURE 16–17 The fourth step in a neurovascular examination following a limb injury is to check motor function: (top) upper extremity motor function is tested by having the patient open and close the hand; (bottom) lower extremity motor function is tested by wiggling the toes or moving the entire foot up and down.

Taken together, these examination findings are often referred to as CMS (for circulation, motor and sensory functions). Thus, a patient with good pulses, capillary refill, motor responses, and sensations is said to have "good CMS" on examination.

In the unconscious patient, many of the steps just listed cannot be carried out because they require patient cooperation. After the primary assessment is completed and vital functions are stabilized, any limb deformity, swelling, ecchymosis, or false motion should be considered evidence of a limb injury and treated as such. Monitoring the distal pulses and capillary filling can be done in the unconscious patient, but assessing sensation and motor function cannot be done without the cooperation of the patient. In addition, you must always assume that *any unconscious, injured patient has a spinal fracture that will require spinal immobilization.*

TREATMENT OF MUSCULOSKELETAL INJURIES

The emergency management of fractures, dislocations, and sprains takes place after you have assessed and stabilized the injured patient's vital functions. Then, and only then, should attention be directed to the musculoskeletal injury.

All open wounds are managed initially by covering the entire wound with a dry, sterile dressing and applying local pressure to control bleeding (Figure 16–18). Once a sterile compression dressing has been applied to an open fracture, it can be managed in the same way as a closed fracture by applying an appropriate splint. Emergency department personnel must be notified of all wounds that have been dressed and splinted.

Splinting

All fractures, dislocations, and sprains should be splinted before the patient is moved unless the patient's life is in immediate danger. Splinting prevents motion of fracture fragments, a dislocated joint, or damaged soft tissues, thus

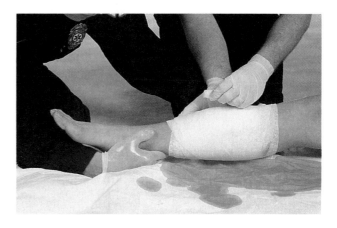

FIGURE 16–18

The first step in the management of any open extremity wound is the application of a dry sterile compression dressing.

reducing pain. Splinting also facilitates the transfer and transportation of the patient. In addition, splinting will help prevent the following:

- Further damage of muscles, the spinal cord, peripheral nerves, and blood vessels from broken bone ends.
- Laceration of the skin by broken bone ends. One of the primary indications for splinting is to prevent the conversion of a closed fracture to an open fracture.
- Restriction of distal blood flow resulting from pressure of the bone ends on blood vessels.
- Excessive bleeding of the tissues at the injury site.

Because splinting has so many advantages, all extremity injuries, regardless of their severity, should be splinted prior to transport.

A splint can be fashioned from any material. It is simply a device to prevent motion of the injured part. However, you should have an adequate supply of standard commercial splints, and only occasionally should you have to improvise. The following are general principles of splinting that all EMTs should know how to carry out:

1. In most situations, remove clothing from the area of any suspected fracture or dislocation to allow inspection of the limb for

open wounds, deformity, swelling, and ecchymosis.

2. Note and record the circulatory (pulse and capillary refill) and neurological (sensation and movement) status distal to the site of injury. Continue to monitor the neurovascular status until the patient reaches the hospital.

3. Cover all wounds with a dry sterile dressing before applying a splint. Notify the receiving hospital of all open wounds.

4. Do not move the patient before splinting extremity injuries unless there is an immediate hazard to the patient or yourself.

5. In a suspected fracture of the shaft of any bone, make sure the splint immobilizes the joint above and joint below the fracture.

6. With injuries in and around the joint, make sure the splint immobilizes the bone above and the bone below the injured joint.

7. Pad all rigid splints to prevent local pressure.

8. During application of the splint, use your hands to minimize movement of the limb and to support the injury site until the limb is completely splinted.

9. Align a limb severely deformed from a fracture of the shaft of a long bone with constant gentle manual traction so that it can be incorporated into a splint.

10. If you encounter resistance to limb alignment when you apply traction, splint the limb in the position of deformity.

11. Immobilize all suspected spine injuries in a neutral in-line position.

12. When in doubt, **splint.**

Principles 9 and 10 refer to the use of traction in managing musculoskeletal injury. **Traction** is the action of drawing or pulling on an object. Traction is the most effective way to realign a fracture of the shaft of a long bone so that the limb can be splinted more effectively. Excessive traction can be very harmful to an injured limb. When applied correctly, however, traction stabilizes the bone fragments and improves the overall alignment of the limb. You should not attempt to reduce (set) the fracture or force all the bone fragments back into anatomic alignment. This is the physician's responsibility. In

the field, the goals of traction are (1) to stabilize the fracture fragments to prevent excessive movement, and (2) to align the limb sufficiently to allow it to be placed in a splint.

The amount of pull required to accomplish these objectives varies, but rarely will it exceed 15 pounds. You should use the least amount of force necessary to achieve alignment of the limb. When you apply traction, grasp the foot or hand firmly so that once the traction pull is applied it will not be released until the limb is fully splinted. Discomfort to the patient will be minimized by having a second person support the injured limb under the site of the fracture.

The direction of traction pull is always along the long axis of the limb. Imagine where the normal, injured limb would lie and pull along the line of that normal, imaginary limb. The alignment of the deformed, injured limb will then approximate this posture as gentle traction is applied (Figure 16–19). Grasping the foot or hand and the initial pull of traction usually causes slight discomfort as the fragments move. This initial discomfort quickly subsides, and further gentle traction may then be applied. If the patient strongly resists the traction or if it causes more pain that persists, it must be stopped and the limb must be splinted in the deformed position.

Remember that many different materials can be used as splints if necessary. Even when no splinting materials are available, the arm can be bound to the chest wall and an injured leg can be splinted to the patient's uninjured leg to provide at least temporary stability. Although splints can be fabricated from many different materials, there are three basic types: rigid, formable, and traction splints.

Rigid Splints Rigid (nonformable) splints are made from firm material and are applied to the sides, front, and/or back of an injured extremity to prevent motion at the injury site. Common examples of rigid splints include padded board splints, molded plastic and metal splints, padded wire ladder splints, and folded cardboard splints (Figure 16–20). After assessing the distal neurovascular function, two EMTs following these steps are needed to apply rigid splints:

FIGURE 16–19

Apply gentle traction to the limb in a line parallel to the normal axis of the injured, deformed limb.

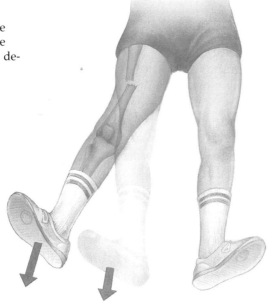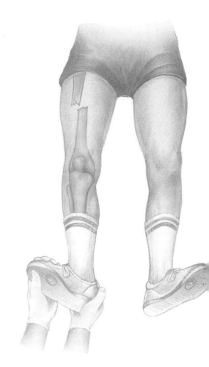

FIGURE 16–20

A rigid splint. Two EMTs are needed to apply a rigid splint.

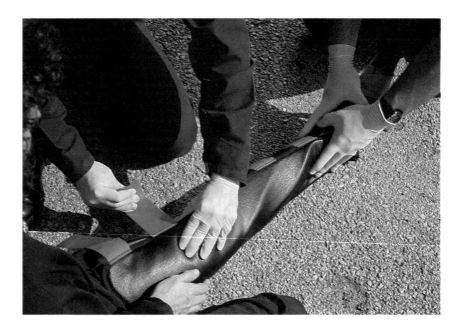

1. First EMT: Gently support the limb at the site of injury and apply gentle steady traction if necessary. Maintain this support until the splint is completely applied.
2. Second EMT: Place the rigid splint under or alongside the limb.
3. Place padding to ensure even pressure and even contact between the limb and the splint, paying particular attention to bony prominences.
4. Apply bindings to hold the splint securely to the limb.

5. Check and record the distal neurovascular function.

When severe limb deformities are present—as is the case with many dislocations—or when resistance or pain is encountered upon application of gentle traction to the fracture of a shaft of a long bone, the deformed limb must be splinted in the position of deformity. In this situation, splinting is accomplished by applying padded board splints to each side of the limb and securing them with soft roller bandages (Figures 17–18 and 18–13).

Formable Splints The most commonly used formable or soft splint is the precontoured, inflatable, clear plastic *air splint*. These splints are available in a variety of sizes and shapes, with or without a zipper that runs the length of the splint. After application, the splint is inflated by mouth—never with a pump. The air splint is comfortable for the patient, provides uniform contact, and has the added advantage of applying firm pressure to a bleeding wound. It is used to immobilize injuries below the elbow or below the knee.

The air splint has some disadvantages, particularly in cold weather areas. The zipper can stick, clog with dirt, or freeze. With significant temperature changes, the pressure of the air in the splint will vary, decreasing with cold and increasing in warm environments. Changes in pressure will also occur with changes in altitude—sometimes becoming a problem with helicopter transport of patients.

The method of applying an air splint depends on whether it has a zipper. With either type, first you cover all wounds with a dry, sterile dressing. If the splint has a zipper, hold the injured limb slightly off the ground with gentle traction and support under the site of injury. Place the open, deflated splint around the limb, zip it up, and inflate it by mouth (Figure 16–21).

If you use a nonzippered or partially zippered type of air splint, two EMTs should follow these steps:

1. First EMT: Place your arm through the splint. Once your hand is extended beyond

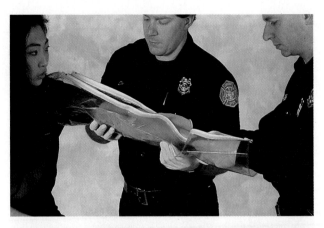

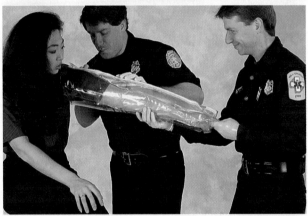

FIGURE 16–21

A zippered air splint. (Top) The deflated splint is first placed under the limb and zipped up. (Bottom) Then the EMT inflates the air splint by mouth.

the splint, grasp the hand or foot of the injured limb (Figure 16–22a).
2. Second EMT: Support the patient's injured limb until splinting is accomplished.
3. First EMT: Apply gentle traction to the hand or foot while sliding the splint onto the injured limb (Figure 16–22b). The hand or foot of the injured limb should always be included in the splint.
4. Inflate the splint by mouth (Figure 16–22c).
5. With either type of air splint, test the pressure in the splint after application. With proper inflation, you should be just able to compress the walls of the splint together with a firm pinch between the thumb and

A

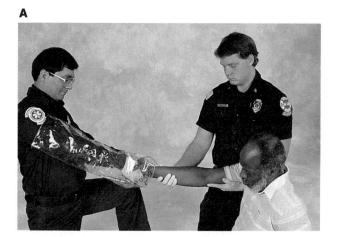

C

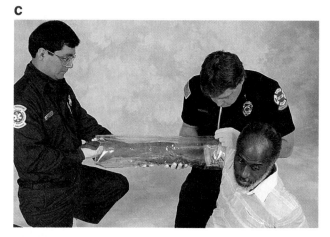

B

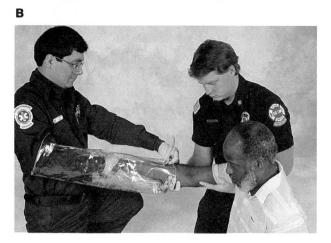

D

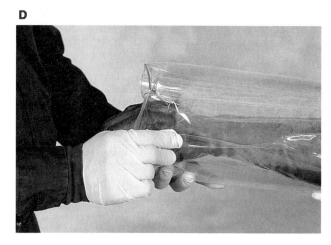

FIGURE 16–22   Steps in the proper application of a nonzipper air splint:
(A) the EMT places the splint on his arm; (B) he then
applies gentle traction to the hand while sliding the
splint in place; (C) the splint is inflated by mouth; (D)
proper inflation is checked by pinching the end of the
splint.

index finger near the edge of the splint
(Figure 16–22d).
6. As with any other splint, check and record
the distal neurovascular function after application and monitor it periodically until the
patient reaches the hospital.

Other soft splints such as pillow splints, the
SAM splints, and a sling and swathe are used
extensively and will be discussed in Chapters
17 and 18. The pneumatic antishock garment
should also be regarded as a formable splint to
immobilize pelvic fractures. Vacuum splints are
another type of formable splint. They can be

easily shaped, just like an air splint, to fit
around a deformed limb. Suction is then applied to a valve in the splint to remove the air
from inside. When the air is sucked out and the
valve is sealed, the vacuum splint becomes
rigid, conforming to the shape of the deformed
limb and immobilizing it (Figure 16–23).

Traction Splints Traction splints are used
primarily to secure fractures of the shaft of the
femur. Several different types of lower extremity traction splints are commercially available.
Each brand has its own unique method of
application. You must be thoroughly familiar

FIGURE 16–23

(A) The injured limb is carefully placed onto the vacuum splint. (B) The splint is then wrapped around the limb and the air removed to conform to the shape of the limb.

A

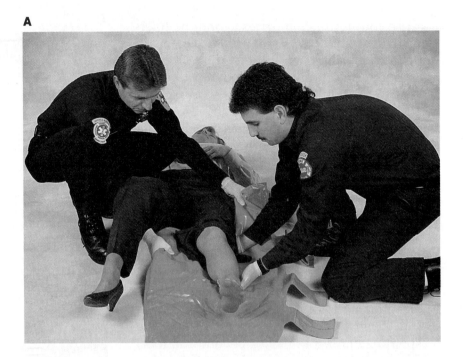

B

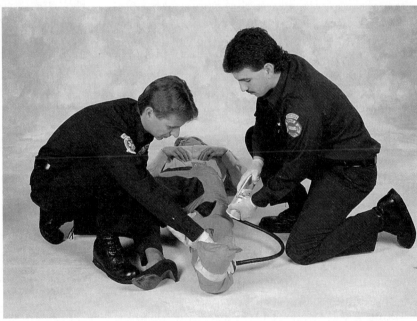

with and practiced in the technique of applying the particular splint being used. One of the more commonly used brands is the Hare Traction Splint. When traction is applied to the foot through the ankle hitch, a force is exerted by the upper end of the splint against the ischial tuberosity of the patient's pelvis. This force is called countertraction. The Hare splint must be seated well on the ischial tuberosity for effective countertraction. Because countertraction is essential to proper function of the splint, it is not suitable for use in the upper extremity because countertraction forces cannot be tolerated by the major nerves and blood vessels in the patient's axilla.

Proper application of a traction splint requires two well-trained EMTs working together. It is impossible for one person to apply this splint. Knowledge of the precise technique of application of the traction splint is extremely important. You should practice the steps until the sequence and necessary teamwork have become routine. Follow these eight steps (Figure 16–24):

1. Cut open the patient's trouser leg or otherwise expose the injured lower extremity so that you can see exactly what is being done.
2. Place the splint beside the patient's uninjured leg and adjust it to the proper length (the ring at the ischial tuberosity and the splint extending 12 inches beyond the foot) (Figure 16–24a). Open and adjust the four velcro support straps that should be positioned at the mid-thigh, above the knee, below the knee, and above the ankle.
3. First EMT: Manually support and stabilize the injured limb so that no motion will occur at the fracture site while the second EMT fastens the appropriately sized ankle hitch about the patient's ankle and foot (Figure 16–24b). Customarily, the shoe is removed from the patient's foot.
4. First EMT: Support the leg at the site of the suspected injury (Figure 16–24c) while the second EMT simultaneously applies gentle longitudinal traction manually to the ankle hitch and foot. Apply only enough traction to align the limb so that it will fit into the splint. Do not attempt to align the fracture fragments anatomically.
5. First EMT: Slide the splint into position under the patient's injured limb (Figure 16–24d), making certain that the ring is seated well on the ischial tuberosity. Pad the groin and gently apply the ischial strap (Figure 16–24e).
6. First EMT: While the traction is maintained, connect the loops of the ankle hitch to the end of the splint (Figure 16–24f). Then

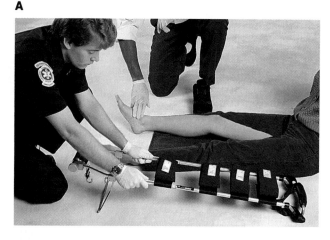

A

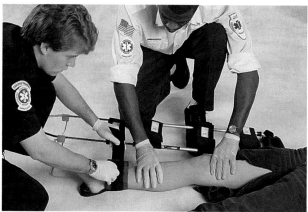

B

FIGURE 16–24

Proper sequence of steps used in the application of a traction splint to an injured lower extremity: (A) the EMT positions the splint against the patient's uninjured leg and adjusts it to the proper length; (B) the ankle hitch is fastened around the patient's ankle and foot; (C) the leg is supported at the site of suspected injury; (D) the EMT slides the splint into position under the patient's leg; (E) the groin area is padded, and the ischial strap is fastened; (F) the loops of the ankle hitch are connected to the end of the splint; (G) the support straps are fastened; (H) Place the splinted patient securely on a long spine board for transport.

apply gentle traction to the connecting strap between the ankle hitch and the splint, just strongly enough to maintain limb alignment. This splint comes with a ratchet

C ~ Never ⊗ THIS

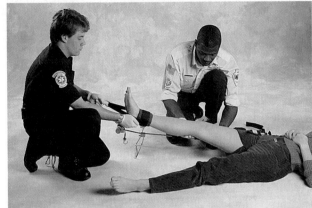

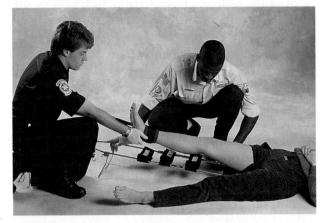

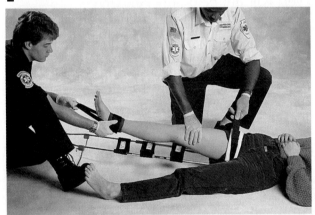

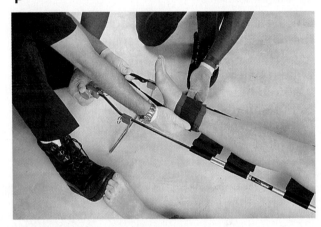

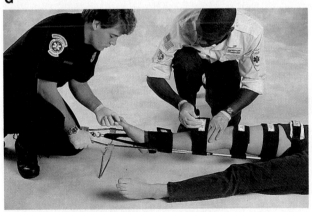

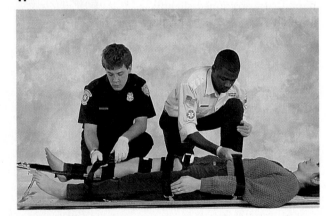

mechanism to tighten the strap. This mechanism can generate an excessive amount of force, which can overstretch the limb and further injure the patient.

7. Once proper traction has been applied,

fasten the support straps so that the limb is securely held in the splint (Figure 16–24g).

8. Place the splinted patient securely on a long spine board for transport to the emergency department (Figure 16-24h).

Because this traction splint immobilizes the limb by producing countertraction on the ischium and in the groin, use care to pad these areas well and especially to avoid excessive pressure on the external genitalia. Commercial padded ankle hitches are readily available and must be used rather than pieces of rope, cord, or tape. Such improvised hitches are painful and can obstruct circulation in the foot.

Another commonly used brand of traction splint is the Sager splint. Its method of application is presented in Chapter 18.

Transportation

Once an injured limb is adequately splinted, the patient is ready to be transferred to a litter and transported. The exact position of the patient will vary somewhat, depending on the type of injury. With most isolated upper extremity injuries, the patient will be most comfortable in a semiseated position rather than lying flat. Either position is acceptable. With lower extremity injuries, the patient should lie supine, with the limb elevated, about 6 inches to minimize swelling. In all cases, the injured part should be positioned slightly above the level of the heart (Figure 16–25). The injured limb should never be allowed to flop about or dangle off the edge of the litter.

Swelling can also be minimized to some degree by applying cold packs to the splinted injury site. Take care to avoid placing the cold packs directly on the skin or other exposed tissues. Placing a cold pack on top of an air splint or other thick, insulating material, however, will not be of any benefit.

Very few, if any, musculoskeletal injuries require excessively rapid ambulance transportation. Once dressed and splinted, the limb is stable and the patient can be transported in an orderly fashion. With the pulseless limb, a sense of urgency develops, and the patient must be given a higher priority in the transpor-

FIGURE 16–25

Transport the patient with the injured part positioned slightly above the level of the heart.

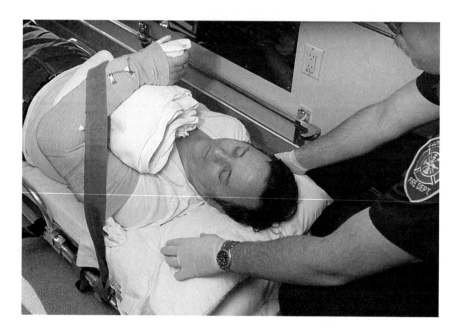

tation system. If the hospital is only a few minutes away, reckless speeding to the emergency department will make little or no difference to the patient's eventual outcome. If the treatment facility is an hour or more away, however, evacuation of the patient with a pulseless limb by helicopter or rapid ground transportation should be given high priority. In every instance of impaired circulation to the distal limb, medical control should be notified of the patient's problem so that proper steps can be taken once the patient arrives in the emergency department.

YOU ARE THE EMT

1. Which condition—an open or closed fracture—is more serious? Why?

2. A young boy has fallen out of a tree and is guarding his arm. What does that mean? What condition does guarding indicate?

3. A strain is a muscle injury. What kind of injury is a sprain? What are three signs of a sprain?

4. You are not sure whether your patient's ankle is sprained, dislocated, or broken. Why should you splint it? What kind of splint will you use?

SHOULDER AND UPPER EXTREMITY FRACTURES AND DISLOCATIONS

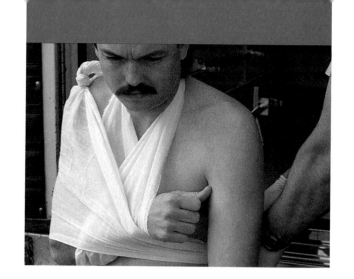

KEY TERMS

acromioclavicular joint (ah-kro"me-o-klah-vik'u-lar joint) Joint at the top of the shoulder, formed by bony projections of the scapula and clavicle.

clavicle (klav'ĭ-k'l) The collarbone. It is attached medially to the sternum and laterally to the scapula.

glenohumeral joint (gle"no-hu'mer-al joint) The true shoulder joint.

humerus (hu'mer-us) The supporting bone of the upper arm that articulates with the scapula to form the shoulder joint and with the ulna and radius to form the elbow joint.

radius (ra'de-us) The bone on the thumb side of the forearm.

scapula (skap'u-lah) The shoulder blade.

sling A triangular bandage or material that is tied around the neck and is used to support the weight of the injured upper extremity.

swathe (swäth) A bandage that passes around the chest to secure an injured arm to the chest.

ulna (ul'nah) The inner and larger bone of the forearm, on the side opposite the thumb.

OVERVIEW

Injuries to the upper extremity are quite common. Although many types of forces cause these injuries, one of the most frequent mechanisms is a fall on the outstretched hand. When people fall, they invariably extend their hands in a protective reflex to prevent injury to the head and face. The hands receive the weight of the body, and the stage is set for injury to occur anywhere between the hand and the clavicle. Persons of all ages are prone to upper extremity injuries, although certain injuries are more frequent in particular age groups.

Before you evaluate and splint any limb injury, always perform a primary assessment of the patient and stabilize any serious problems. Always follow the general principles of splinting, as listed in Chapter 16. Distal neurovascular function must be evaluated immediately and frequently monitored. Bleeding must be controlled, and all wounds must be protected from further contamination.

Chapter 17 first describes injuries to the clavicle and scapula. The next injuries covered are dislocation of the shoulder and fracture of the shaft of the humerus. Then elbow injuries are discussed. The last two sections of Chapter 17 cover fractures of the forearm and injuries to the wrist and hand.

GOALS

The goals of Chapter 17 are to

- identify and splint injuries to the clavicle, scapula, and proximal humerus.
- know how to recognize and immobilize a dislocation of the shoulder.
- learn how to splint and, if necessary, apply traction to realign humeral fracture fragments.
- appreciate the significance of elbow injuries.
- know how to splint injuries of the elbow.
- recognize fractures of the forearm and learn how to immobilize the injured arm.
- learn how to splint wrist and hand injuries using a bulky hand dressing.

INJURIES TO THE CLAVICLE AND SCAPULA

The **clavicle** (collarbone) is one of the most frequently fractured bones in the body. Fracture of the clavicle most commonly occurs in children, usually from a fall on the outstretched hand. Clavicle fractures are also seen in association with crushing injuries of the chest. A patient with a fracture of the clavicle will complain of pain in the shoulder girdle and will usually hold the injured arm against the chest wall, supporting the elbow or forearm with the opposite hand to "splint" the site of injury (Figure 17–1). Frequently, a younger child will complain of pain throughout the limb and express unwillingness to use any part of that limb. These complaints sometimes make it difficult to localize the point of injury. Generally, there is swelling and point tenderness over the clavicle. Occasionally the skin is tented over a fracture fragment because the clavicle lies just beneath the skin. The clavicle lies directly over the major arteries, veins, and

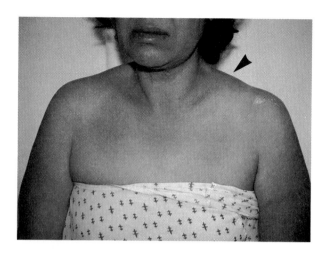

FIGURE 17–1

The clavicle is one of the most frequently fractured bones.

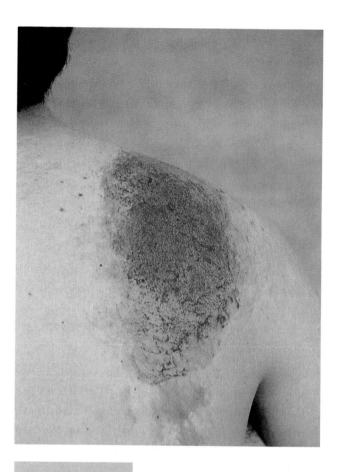

FIGURE 17–2

Contusions or abrasions over the scapular region may indicate a fracture. You must be aware of the high likelihood of respiratory problems found frequently with this injury.

nerves that supply the upper extremity. Thus, fractures of the clavicle may damage these important neurovascular structures.

Fractures of the **scapula** occur much less frequently, because this bone is well protected by many large muscles. Scapular fractures almost always occur following a violent blow to the back, directly over the scapula. Because the force required to break the scapula is so great and because the thoracic cage lies just beneath it, a patient suspected of having a scapular fracture must be evaluated very carefully. Respiratory insufficiency, secondary to rib fractures or other chest injuries, may exist. You must carefully assess such patients for signs of respiratory insufficiency. Administer oxygen and provide rapid transportation to the emergency department for the patient in severe respiratory distress. The signs of scapular fracture include abrasions, contusions, swelling, and tenderness about the scapula, as well as signs of respiratory difficulty (Figure 17–2). The patient will limit use of the arm because of pain at the fracture site.

The joint between the outer end of the clavicle and the acromion process of the scap-

ula is called the **acromioclavicular joint** (Figure 17–3). This joint is frequently dislocated, especially in football players. The injury is often called a shoulder separation or simply an A/C separation. Dislocations occur when the individual falls and lands on the point of the shoulder, driving the scapula distally away from the outer end of the clavicle. Pain, including point tenderness over the acromioclavicular joint, is usually accompanied by prominence of the distal end of the clavicle.

Fractures of the clavicle and scapula and acromioclavicular separations can all be splinted effectively with a sling and swathe. The principal effect of the **sling** is to support the weight of

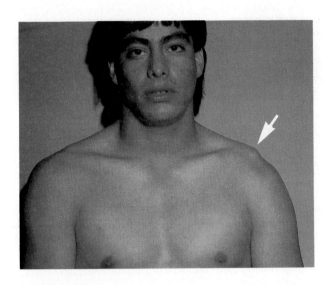

FIGURE 17–3

Acromioclavicular separation. Note the prominence of the dislocated outer end of the clavicle.

A

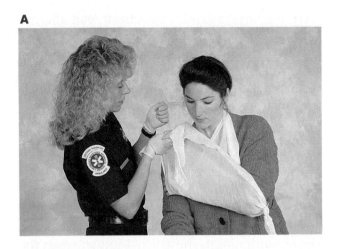

B

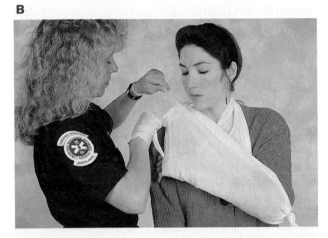

C

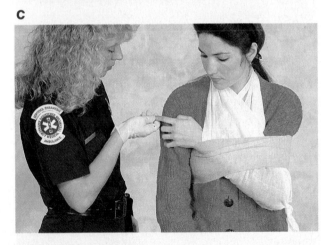

FIGURE 17–4

Splinting with a sling and swathe: (A) The sling should be applied so that the knot is tied to one side of the neck; (B) the sling should support the weight of the arm; (C) a swathe is used to bind the arm to the chest wall to prevent it from swinging freely.

the upper extremity and relieve the downward pull of gravity on the injury site. The triangular sling must apply gentle upward support to the *olecranon process* of the ulna to be effective. The knot of the sling should be tied to one side of the neck so that it does not press uncomfortably on the cervical spinous processes (Figure 17–4).

A sling alone, however, does not fully immobilize the shoulder region. A **swathe** must be added to bind the arm to the chest wall for adequate immobilization. The swathe should be tight enough to secure the limb to the chest wall to prevent it from swinging freely. However, the swathe should not be so tight as to compress the chest and compromise breathing. The hand should remain exposed so that you can perform neurovascular evaluations periodically after you have applied the splint.

Two slings can be combined to achieve effective splinting of these shoulder injuries also. Apply the first triangular sling just as for the sling and swathe. The second sling replaces the swathe. Tie a knot at the apex and apply this portion over the injured shoulder. Then, tie the two ends snugly around the chest to hold the arm against the chest wall (Figure 17–5).

When slings are not available, the injured limb can be splinted fairly effectively with a T-shirt by placing the shirt over the arm, as demonstrated in Figure 17–6. Commercially available shoulder immobilizers also provide adequate splinting for these injuries of the shoulder region (Figure 17–7).

DISLOCATION OF THE SHOULDER

The shoulder joint, the articulation between the humeral head and the glenoid fossa of the scapula (the **glenohumeral joint**), is the most commonly dislocated large joint in the body. Almost always, the humeral head dislocates anteriorly, coming to lie in front of the scapula. This anterior dislocation of the humeral head is caused by forceful abduction and external rotation of the arm. Shoulder dislocation is extremely painful, and the patient will resist any motion of the locked joint. The patient will try

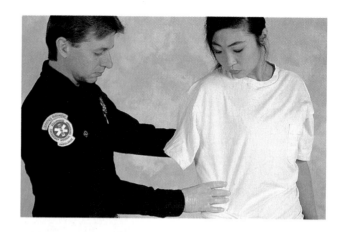

FIGURE 17–6

A T-shirt sling.

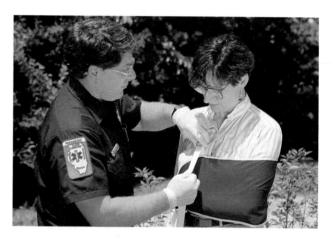

FIGURE 17–7

A commercially available "shoulder immobilizer" can also provide adequate support.

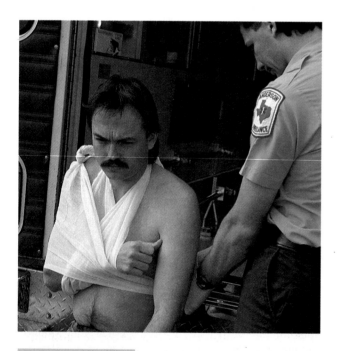

FIGURE 17–5

Two slings can be combined to achieve effective splinting.

to protect the injured shoulder by holding the dislocated arm with the opposite hand to "splint" it. On careful inspection from the front, you will be able to see that the normal rounded contour of the shoulder is not present when compared with the opposite side (Figure 17–8). Instead, the shoulder is squared off—flattened laterally. The humeral head can be seen protruding anteriorly, lying underneath

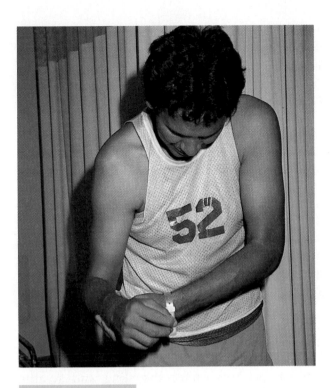

FIGURE 17–8

Anterior dislocation of the shoulder. The normal rounded contour of the shoulder is not present when compared with the opposite side, and there is a space between the elbow and the patient's chest wall.

the pectoralis muscle on the anterior chest wall. Frequently, there is numbness in the upper extremity because the head of the humerus is pressing on the major nerves in the *axilla* (armpit).

Dislocation of the shoulder disrupts many of the supporting ligaments on the anterior aspect of the shoulder joint. Often these ligaments do not heal well after the shoulder dislocation is reduced (put back in place). Therefore, some patients will have frequent, recurrent dislocations of this joint so that it will eventually require surgical repair. Much less force is required to dislocate a shoulder that previously has been dislocated, and many patients will have recurrent dislocations of the shoulder with trivial trauma. Simply raising one's hand to put on a T-shirt is all that may be necessary to allow the humeral head to slip out of place. You will see many patients who have primary

or recurrent dislocations of the shoulder joint. Never, however, should you attempt to reduce a dislocated shoulder. This maneuver should only be done in the hospital after X rays have been taken.

Immobilizing a shoulder dislocation is difficult, because the patient will hold his or her arm in a fixed position away from the chest wall. Any attempt to bring the arm in toward the chest will produce pain. The joint must be splinted in the position that is most comfortable for the patient. You can overcome the difficulty that this fixed position of the arm causes by gently placing a pillow or rolled blanket between the arm and the chest wall to fill up the space between them (Figure 17–9). Once the arm is stabilized against the pillow, the elbow can usually be flexed to 90 degrees without causing further pain for the patient. A sling can then be applied to the forearm and wrist to support its weight. The arm in the sling is secured to the pillow and chest with a swathe. The patient should be transported in a sitting or semiseated position.

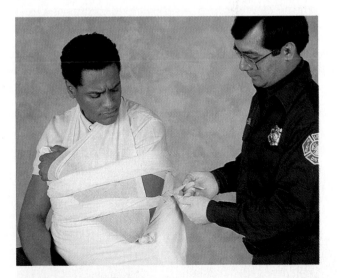

FIGURE 17–9

A dislocated shoulder must be splinted in the position of deformity with a pillow, sling, and swathe.

FRACTURE OF THE SHAFT OF THE HUMERUS

The shaft of the **humerus** is frequently broken. Two regions of this bone are prone to fracture. In the elderly, the proximal portion near the shoulder joint is frequently fractured as a result of a fall. Fracture near the midshaft occurs more frequently in the young adult, usually as a consequence of a more violent injury.

The proximal shaft fracture causes mild to moderate deformity of the upper arm. Frequently, deformity is masked by swelling and by the large muscles that surround this part of the arm (Figure 17–10). With fractures of the midshaft of this bone, there is usually gross angulation at the fracture site and marked instability of the fracture fragments (Figure 17–11).

Occasionally, because of the close proximity of the radial nerve to the humeral shaft (Figure 17–12), this nerve is lacerated, compressed, or trapped at the midshaft fracture site. When this nerve is injured, the patient cannot extend (dorsiflex) the wrist or fingers. The patient may also experience numbness on the dorsum of the hand. The weakness produces the characteristic "wristdrop" of a radial nerve palsy.

Fractures of the proximal humerus and all minimally displaced fractures of the shaft of this bone can be immobilized with a sling and swathe or a shoulder immobilizer. Use the chest wall as a splint and secure the injured arm to the chest wall, as you would with injuries about the shoulder girdle. You can place a short padded board splint on the lateral side of the arm under the sling and swathe to provide additional lateral support (Figure 17–13).

With a severely angulated fracture of the shaft of the humerus, you should apply traction to realign the fracture fragments prior to splinting them. Support the site of the fracture

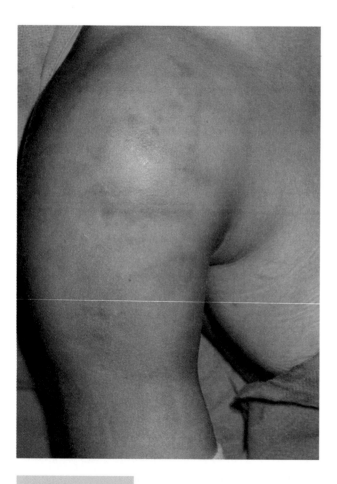

FIGURE 17–10

Fracture of the proximal end of the humerus is usually associated with significant soft tissue swelling at the fracture site.

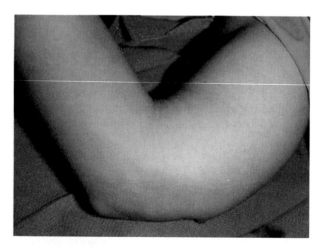

FIGURE 17–11

Fractures in the midshaft of the humerus are usually displaced, producing significant deformity of the arm.

with one hand and with the other hand grasp the two humeral condyles just above the elbow. Pulling gently in line with the normal axis of the limb will align the arm so that splinting can be accomplished more effectively (Figure 17–14). Once you achieve gross alignment of the limb, splint the arm with a sling and swathe, supplemented by a padded board splint on the lateral aspect of the arm. If the patient exhibits significant pain or resistance to gentle traction, splint the fracture in the deformed position with a padded wire ladder splint or a padded board splint and pillows to support the injured limb.

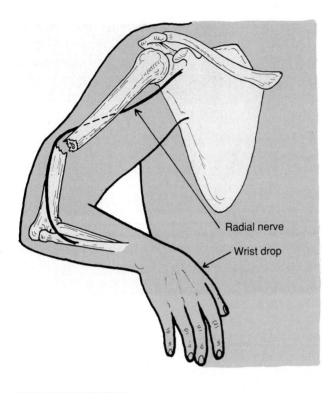

FIGURE 17–12

The radial nerve lies right against the shaft of the humerus and may be damaged or trapped in the fracture site.

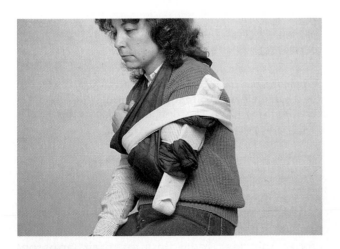

FIGURE 17–13

A sling and swathe, supplemented with a lateral padded board splint, provides good immobilization for humeral shaft fractures.

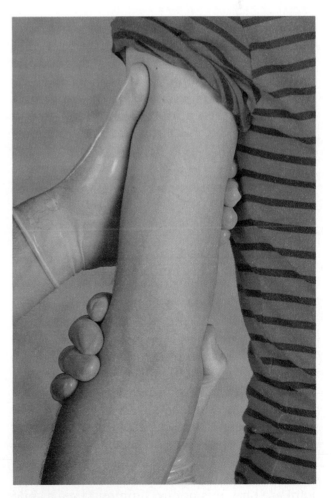

FIGURE 17–14

To align the severely deformed arm with a humeral shaft fracture, apply gentle traction to the humeral condyles, as is demonstrated on this normal subject.

ELBOW INJURIES

Fractures and dislocations occur commonly around the elbow. They are all considered here because they are difficult to distinguish from each other without the use of X rays. The clinical deformities produced are quite similar, and the emergency care is the same for all of these injuries. Nerve and vessel injuries occur quite commonly in this region and can be produced or worsened by inappropriate emergency care, particularly by excessive manipulation of the injured joint.

Types of Elbow Injuries

Fracture of the Distal Humerus Fracture of the distal end of the humerus is called a supracondylar fracture, because the fracture line lies just across the humerus above the level of the condyles (Figure 17–15). These fractures are commonly seen in children. Frequently, a significant rotation of the fracture fragments takes place and produces a deformity and exposes the bone surfaces to the nearby vessels and nerves (Figure 17–16). Nerve and vessel injury is common with this fracture. Swelling occurs rapidly and may be severe.

Dislocation of the Elbow This injury usually occurs in teenagers and young adults and is frequently an athletic injury. The ulna and radius, which both articulate with the distal humerus, are most commonly displaced posteriorly, making the olecranon process of the ulna much more prominent (Figure 17–17). The joint is locked with the forearm moderately flexed on the arm. Any attempt at motion of the elbow is very painful. As with a supracondylar fracture, there is swelling and the potential for significant vessel or nerve injury.

Elbow Joint Sprain Sprains of the elbow joint are rare. It is not uncommon to see a child who has sustained a mild or moderate elbow injury that could readily be dismissed as a simple sprain. Very frequently the "sprain" turns out to be a nondisplaced or minimally displaced fracture or a partial dislocation of this

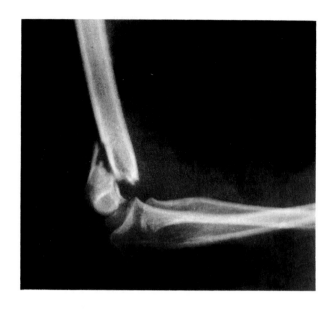

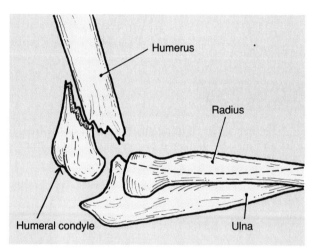

FIGURE 17–15

Supracondylar fracture of the humerus: (Top) X ray of the injured elbow; (Bottom) line drawing showing fracture line lying just across the humerus above the level of the condyles.

joint that requires prompt treatment to avoid problems later as the child grows. Thus, all elbow injuries, regardless of their apparent severity, require X ray evaluation in the emergency department.

Olecranon Fracture Fracture of the olecranon process of the ulna is usually the result of

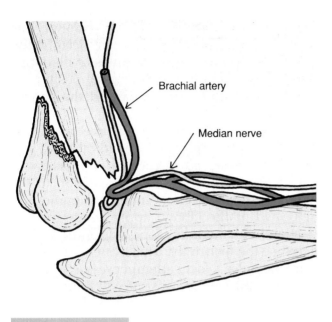

FIGURE 17–16

Note the close proximity of the brachial artery and median nerve to the fracture fragments in a supracondylar fracture.

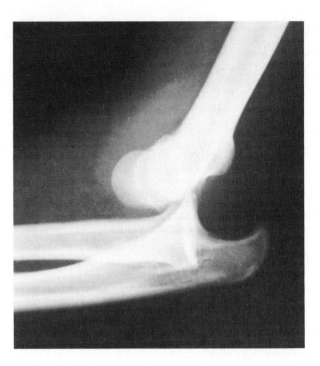

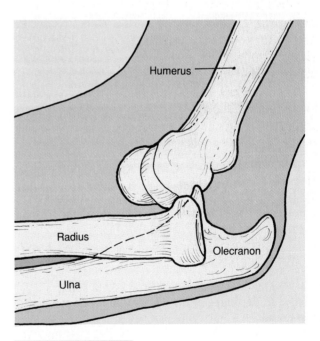

FIGURE 17–17

Dislocation of the elbow: (Top) X ray of the elbow; (Bottom) line drawing showing prominence of the olecranon process.

a direct blow. Thus, abrasions or lacerations are commonly present over this fracture site.

Care of Elbow Injuries

You must take all elbow injuries seriously and exercise caution in their emergency management. Perform a careful distal neurovascular evaluation on all patients with elbow injuries.

If strong pulses and good capillary filling are present when the patient is first evaluated, splint the fracture or dislocation in the position in which you found it. Two padded board splints, applied to each side of the limb and secured with soft roller bandages, usually provide adequate stability. The boards should extend from the shoulder joint to the wrist joint, immobilizing the entire bone above and below the injured joint (Figure 17–18). A padded wire ladder splint or a SAM splint can also be molded to the shape of the limb to splint it in the position found (Figure 17–19). You can add a wrist sling to support the weight of the

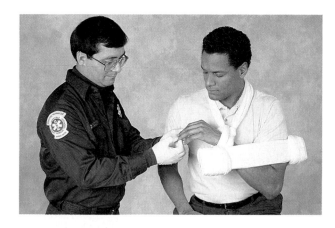

FIGURE 17–18

Two padded board splints adequately stabilize the injured elbow. A wrist sling further supports the weight of the arm.

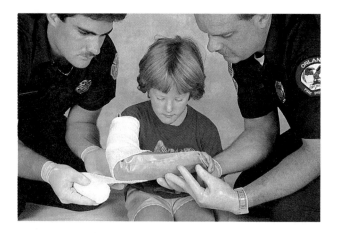

FIGURE 17–19

Use a padded wire ladder splint or a SAM splint molded to the shape of the limb to splint it in the position found.

arm and further support the limb with a pillow, if necessary.

If the patient's hand is cold, pale, or has a weak or absent pulse and poor capillary refill, you must assume that the vessels have been injured; a high priority must be given to this patient. Notify medical control immediately of

these findings because further care of this patient should be dictated by a physician. If the patient is within 10 to 15 minutes of definitive medical care, splint the limb in the position in which you found it and transport the patient promptly to the hospital.

If there will be a prolonged time before the patient can reach definitive medical care, you may be directed by medical control to try to realign the limb to improve circulation to the hand. If the pulseless limb is significantly deformed at the elbow, apply gentle manual traction in line with the long axis of the limb to decrease the deformity. This maneuver may restore the pulse. Never attempt excessive manipulation, however, because it will only worsen the vascular problem. If the pulse can be restored by gentle longitudinal traction, splint the limb in the position that allows the strongest pulse. If no pulse returns after one manipulation, splint the limb in the most comfortable position for the patient. Prompt transfer to the emergency department is required for all patients with impaired distal circulation.

FRACTURES OF THE FOREARM

Fractures of the shaft of the **radius** and the **ulna** are common in persons of all age groups but are seen particularly often in children. Usually both bones break at the same time when the injury is the result of a fall on the outstretched hand (Figure 17–20). An isolated fracture of the shaft of the ulna may occur as the result of a direct blow to it.

Fracture of the distal radius is especially common in the elderly, osteoporotic patient. In fact it is so common that it has a special name, Colles' fracture. It results from a fall on the outstretched hand that usually produces a characteristic "silver fork deformity," because the injured wrist assumes a curvature similar to the profile of a dinner fork (Figure 17–21). In children, a fracture similar in appearance occurs through the epiphyseal plate.

You can use a variety of splints to immobilize fractures of the forearm bones. A padded board,

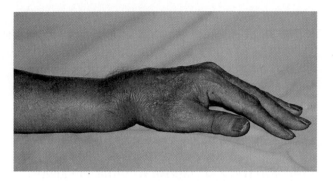

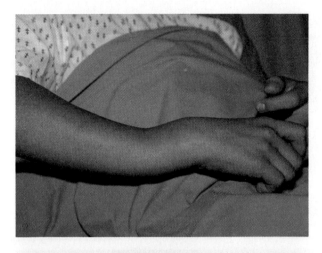

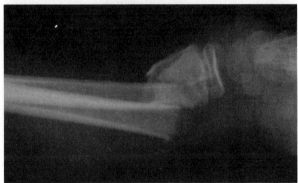

FIGURE 17–20

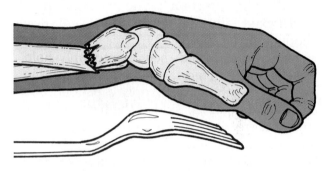

FIGURE 17–21

Fracture of the distal radius, also called a Colles' fracture, produces a characteristic silver fork deformity.

(Top) Fractures of both bones of the forearm occur in children as a result of a fall on the outstretched hand. (Bottom) X ray showing fractures of the shafts of the radius and ulna.

air, vacuum, or pillow splint are all effective. Immobilization of fractures of the shaft of these bones must include the elbow joint. Elbow joint splinting is not essential with fractures near the wrist, but the patient will be more comfortable if a sling or supporting pillow is added to the immobilization.

INJURIES TO THE WRIST AND HAND

Dislocation of the wrist is uncommon. It is usually associated with fracture of one or more of the carpal bones, producing a fracture-dislocation. Wrist sprains frequently occur.

Another common injury is an isolated, nondisplaced fracture of one of the carpal bones. As with other joint injuries, these wrist bone fractures cannot be diagnosed without X rays. Thus, all apparent wrist sprains must be splinted until they can be evaluated in the emergency department.

You will be called to treat a great variety of hand injuries. All can be potentially serious for the patient. Industrial, recreational, and home accidents commonly result in lacerations (with frequent underlying nerve, tendon, or vessel injury), burns, amputations, fractures, or dislocations. The very intricate function of the fingers and hand is so important that any injury, if inadequately or belatedly treated, may result in permanent deformity and disability. All injuries to the hand must be evaluated promptly by a physician so that proper care can be instituted. Even simple lacerations should be treated with respect (Figure 17–22). Dislocated finger joints should not be "popped" back into place. Any amputated parts should be brought with the patient to the hospital, following the procedures outlined in Chapter 14.

All hand and wrist injuries can be effectively splinted with a bulky hand dressing. First cover all wounds with a dry, sterile dressing. Then form the injured hand into what is called the "position of function": The wrist is slightly dorsiflexed and all finger joints are flexed moderately (Figure 17–23). This is the position in which one would most comfortably hold a baseball. Then place a soft roller bandage into the palm of the hand. Apply a padded board splint to the palmar side of the hand and wrist and secure it with a soft roller bandage throughout the length of the splint. Prop the splinted hand and wrist on a pillow or on the patient's chest during transportation to the hospital.

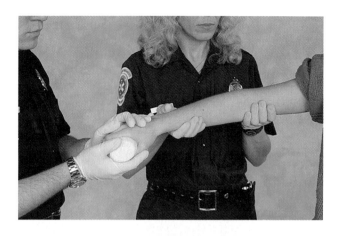

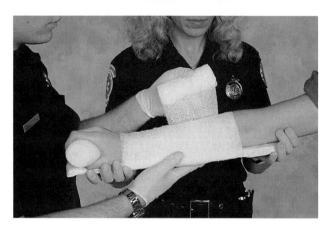

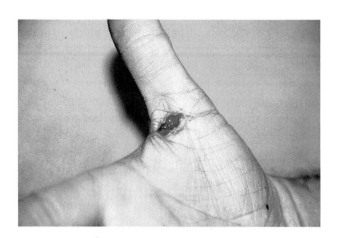

FIGURE 17–22

A small laceration to the base of the thumb that, upon surgical exploration, was found to have produced laceration of two tendons and nerves.

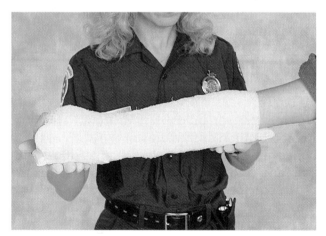

FIGURE 17–23

The injured hand is splinted in the "position of function"—the position that one would most comfortably hold a baseball.

YOU ARE THE EMT

1. What is the difference between a shoulder separation and dislocation of the shoulder? How would you treat each injury?

2. You suspect your patient has a humeral shaft fracture. After performing a careful neurovascular evaluation, you decide the limb does not need to be realigned before splinting. What findings contributed to this decision? What signs would have made you decide realignment was necessary?

3. What bone is involved in a Colles' fracture and produces a silver fork deformity? These fractures are more common in elderly people who suffer from what disease? How would you splint this injury?

4. Your patient is a young girl who fell off a deck about 12 feet off the ground. She has pain in her arm and is holding it to her chest with her other arm. What other injury should you suspect, and what will you look for to confirm your suspicions?

INJURIES OF THE PELVIS AND LOWER EXTREMITY

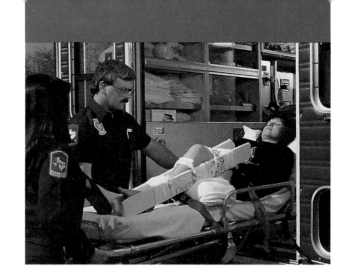

KEY TERMS

calcaneus (kal-ka′ne-us) The heel bone.

femur (fe′mur) The thigh bone; it extends from the pelvis to the knee and is the longest and largest bone in the body.

fibula (fib′u-lah) The outer and smaller of the two bones of the leg, extending from just below the knee and forming the lateral portion of the ankle joint.

hematuria (hem″ah-tu′re-ah) The discharge of blood in the urine.

ilium (il′e-um) One of three bones (ilium, ischium, and pubis) that fuse to form the pelvic bones.

patella (pah-tel′ah) The kneecap; a specialized bone that lies within the tendon of the quadriceps muscle.

retroperitoneal space (re″tro-per″ĭ to-ne′al spās) The space between the abdominal cavity and the posterior abdominal wall, containing the kidneys, certain large vessels and parts of the gastrointestinal tract.

sciatic nerve (si-at′ik nerv) The major nerve to the lower extremity.

symphysis pubis (sim′fĭ-sis pu′bis) The firm fibrocartilaginous joint between the two pubic bones.

tibia (tib′e-ah) The shin bone; the larger of the two bones of the leg.

OVERVIEW

The bones of the pelvis and lower extremity are large and strong because they are designed to bear weight. Injuries to these structures usually result from severe trauma, such as falls and automobile accidents. These injuries can range from a simple contusion to severe, multiple fractures that often result in permanent deformity and loss of function.

The general principles of splinting as outlined in Chapter 16 should be followed with injuries to the lower extremity, after, of course, you perform a general primary assessment of the patient. You must stabilize serious problems identified in the primary survey before you evaluate and splint the limb injury. You must also evaluate and monitor the distal neurovascular function frequently until the patient is delivered to the hospital.

Chapter 18 examines pelvic fractures, dislocation of the hip joint, fractures of the proximal femur, femoral shaft fractures, knee injuries, tibia and fibula fractures, ankle injuries, and foot injuries. The discussion of each of these injuries includes their signs and symptoms, how to evaluate them, and the best way to stabilize them.

GOALS

The goals of Chapter 18 are to

- identify and know how to stabilize injuries of the pelvis, including fractures of the pelvis and dislocation of the hip joint.
- learn how to evaluate and splint fractures of the proximal femur and the femoral shaft.
- become familiar with the evaluation and splinting of injuries about the knee.
- know the techniques of splinting fractures of the tibia, fibula, ankle, and foot.

INJURIES TO THE PELVIS

Fractures of the Pelvis

Fracture of the pelvis is commonly a result of direct compression in which the pelvis is literally crushed by a heavy impact. This injury is often seen after a fall from a height or a direct crushing blow to the pelvic region. Indirect forces can also produce injury of the pelvis—for example, in a car accident, the knee can strike the dashboard of the car, whereupon the impact of the force is transmitted along the **femur,** driving the femoral head into the pelvis and causing it to fracture (Figure 18–1). Not all pelvic fractures result from violent trauma. Even a simple fall can produce a fracture of the pelvis, especially among elderly people who have osteoporosis.

Fractures of the pelvis may be accompanied by severe blood loss. Large blood vessels lie adjacent to the pelvis and are easily torn or lacerated at the time of the fracture. A large amount of blood can drain from these lacerated vessels into the **retroperitoneal space,** an area that can hold several liters of blood. As a result, the patient may develop hypovolemic shock and even die from blood loss following a fracture of the pelvis.

Keeping in mind the possibility of shock associated with this fracture, you must take immediate steps to combat it, even if there is only minimal swelling or other external signs of bleeding. The extent of blood loss in a closed fracture of the pelvis may not be apparent because the bleeding occurs within the pelvic cavity into the retroperitoneal space. According to the principles of Prehospital Trauma Life Support, the critically injured patient with a

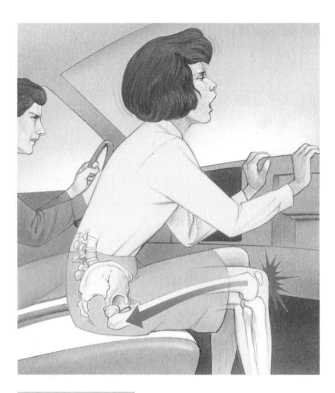

FIGURE 18-1

When the knee strikes the dashboard forcefully, the energy of impact can be transmitted to the hip, fracturing the pelvis or even dislocating the hip.

fracture of the pelvis should be transported immediately to an appropriate medical facility.

Open fractures of the pelvis are quite rare, because the pelvis is surrounded by heavy muscles. Occasionally, pelvic fracture fragments will lacerate the rectum or vagina and create an open fracture.

The urinary bladder is especially susceptible to injury following a fracture of the pelvis. Pelvic bone fragments may lacerate the bladder, or the force of impact at injury may cause the bladder to rupture. Thus, the important structures that the pelvis is designed to protect (the blood vessels, the bladder, the vagina, and the rectum) are all susceptible to injury once the protective pelvic ring has been broken.

You should suspect a fracture of the pelvis in any patient who has sustained a high-velocity injury. Frequently, such a patient complains of pain in the pelvic region or the lower abdomen. Because the area is covered by heavy muscles and other soft tissues, deformity of the pelvis

or swelling in the pelvic region is difficult to see. The best sign of fracture of the pelvis is tenderness on firm compression and palpation. Because of its ring-like structure, firm compression on the two iliac crests will produce pain at a fracture site at any point around the pelvic ring. First, place the palms of your hands over the lateral aspect of each iliac crest and apply firm inward pressure on the pelvic ring (Figure 18–2a). Then, with the patient lying supine, place each of your palms over the anterior aspect of each iliac crest and apply firm downward pressure (Figure 18–2b). In addition, firm palpation with the palm of the hand over the **symphysis pubis** will elicit tenderness if there is injury to the anterior portion of the pelvic ring (Figure 18–2c). If there has been injury to the bladder or the urethra, the patient will have lower abdominal tenderness and may have **hematuria** (blood in the urine) or a bloody discharge from the urethral opening.

Once you suspect a pelvic fracture, assess the patient's general condition carefully and monitor vital signs closely because of the high likelihood of developing hypovolemic shock. You can immobilize isolated fractures of the pelvis in stable patients with a long spine board or a scoop stretcher. Place a pneumatic anti-shock garment on the spine board or stretcher underneath the patient (Figure 18–3). During transport, elevate the foot of the immobilization device 6 to 12 inches. If the patient is in shock or develops signs of hypovolemic shock due to a severe pelvic fracture, supplement the immobilization with a pneumatic antishock garment (see Chapter 10). The device will provide adequate immobilization of the fracture and will also decrease the severity of the hypovolemic shock. Once the pneumatic anti-shock garment is applied, all of the rules governing its use (particularly the method of deflation and removal) must be followed. Such critically injured patients must be transported immediately to the hospital without any unnecessary delay.

Dislocation of the Hip Joint

The hip joint is a very stable ball-and-socket joint that dislocates only following significant injury. Virtually all dislocations of the hip are

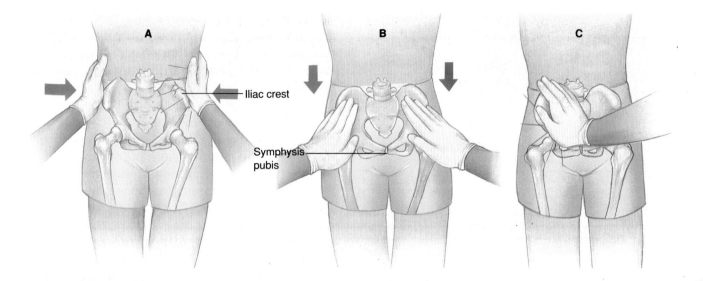

(A) To identify pelvic fracture tenderness, place your hands over the lateral aspect of each iliac crest and compress the pelvic ring. (B) Then, with the patient supine, place your palms over the anterior aspect of each iliac crest and apply firm downward pressure. (C) Finally, palpate firmly over the symphysis pubis with the palm of one hand.

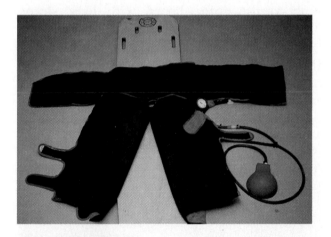

Any patient suspected of having a pelvic fracture should be placed on a spine board or stretcher with a pneumatic antishock garment in place. The garment can then be applied and inflated promptly should the patient develop signs of hypovolemic shock.

posterior. The femoral head is displaced posteriorly, coming to lie in the muscles of the buttock. Posterior dislocation of the hip most commonly occurs during automobile accidents, when a direct force is applied to the knee and the entire femur is driven posteriorly, dislocating the joint. Thus, you should suspect a hip dislocation in any patient in a car accident in which a contusion, laceration, or obvious fracture is present in the knee region.

Very rarely does the femoral head dislocate anteriorly. In this circumstance, the legs are suddenly and forcefully spread wide apart.

Posterior dislocation of the hip is frequently complicated by injury to the **sciatic nerve.** Located directly behind the joint, the sciatic nerve is the most important nerve in the lower extremity. It controls the activity of some of the muscles in the thigh and all of the muscles below the knee as well as all of the sensations in the leg and foot.

When the head of the femur is forced out of the acetabulum, it damages the sciatic nerve by pressing on it or stretching it (Figure 18–4). Partial or complete paralysis of this nerve can result from posterior dislocation of the hip. The patient with paralysis of the sciatic nerve will have decreased sensation in the leg and foot. In addition, there will frequently be weakness of the foot muscles, particularly those muscles that *dorsiflex*, or raise, the toes or the foot. This muscular weakness is commonly called a "foot drop" and is characteristic of damage to the sciatic nerve.

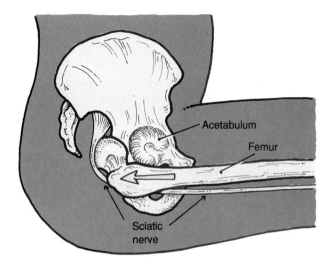

FIGURE 18-4

Posterior dislocation of the hip joint allows the head of the femur to press against the sciatic nerve, causing partial or complete paralysis of this nerve.

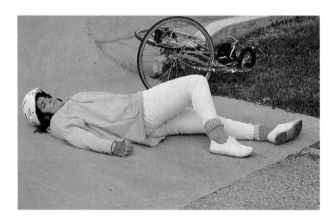

FIGURE 18-5

The usual position of a patient with a posterior dislocation of the hip: The hip joint is flexed and the thigh is rotated inward and adducted across the midline of the body.

A characteristic deformity occurs with posterior dislocation of the hip. The patient lies with the hip joint flexed (the knee drawn up toward the chest), and the thigh rotated inward and adducted across the midline of the body (Figure 18-5). The flexed thigh on the dislocated side lies across the midline of the body over the top of the thigh of the normal leg. With the rare anterior dislocation of the hip, the limb is in the opposite position—extended straight out, rotated outward, and pointing away from the midline of the body.

Because of the unique deformities associated with dislocation of the hip, inspection of the patient will usually lead you to the correct diagnosis. The patient will have severe pain in the hip, and any attempted motion of the joint will be met with great resistance. Palpation of the lateral and posterior aspects of the hip region will elicit tenderness, and in some thin individuals the femoral head can be palpated lying deep to the muscles of the buttock. Careful examination of sensation and motor function in the lower extremity may identify a sciatic nerve injury.

As with any other dislocated joint, you should make no attempt to reduce the dislocated hip in the field. Splint the dislocation in the position of deformity. Place the patient supine on a long spine board. Support the limb with pillows and rolled blankets, particularly under the flexed knee. Then secure the entire limb to the spine board with long straps. Stabilize the limb well enough to the spine board to eliminate all motion in the hip region (Figure 18-6).

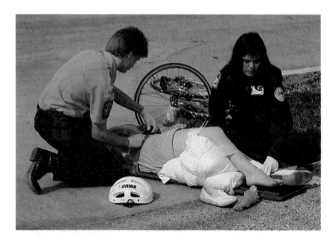

FIGURE 18-6

Posterior dislocation of the hip is splinted with the limb in the deformed position, supported with pillows and secured to the long spine board with straps.

INJURIES TO THE FEMUR

Fractures of the Proximal Femur

Some of the most common fractures are those of the upper (proximal) end of the femur. Over the years, these fractures have been called "hip fractures," even though the hip joint is rarely involved. The break goes through the neck of the femur, the intertrochanteric area, or across the proximal shaft of this bone. The fractures are then respectively called *femoral neck, intertrochanteric,* or *subtrochanteric fractures.* Fractures of the upper end of the femur occur in two distinctly different groups of patients—the elderly and young adults. Fractures of the hip most commonly occur in elderly persons (particularly women) with osteoporosis. Because of the brittleness of the osteoporotic bone, a simple fall sustained while standing or walking may result in fracture. On rare occasions fracture of the proximal end of the femur occurs in a younger individual with normal bone who sustains more severe trauma.

All patients with displaced fractures of the proximal femur displays a very characteristic deformity. They lie with the leg externally rotated, and the injured leg is usually shorter than the opposite uninjured limb (Figure 18–7). If the fracture is not displaced, this deformity is not present. Most patients with a hip fracture are unable to walk or move the leg because of pain. Usually the pain is in the hip region or along the inner aspect of the thigh. On occasion, however, the pain is referred to the knee, and it is not uncommon for an elderly person with a fracture of the hip to complain of knee pain after a fall. Because fractures of the proximal femur are so common, any elderly individual who has fallen and complains of pain in the hip or knee, even though there is no deformity, should be splinted and transported to the emergency department for X rays.

Palpation about the hip region will usually elicit tenderness in a patient with a fracture of the hip. You should apply gentle, manual pressure to the greater trochanter to elicit this tenderness (Figure 18–8).

The method of splinting the fractured hip will be determined by the age of the patient and the severity of the injury. Fractures of the hip that occur as a result of violent injury in young people are best immobilized with a traction splint or the combination of a pneumatic antishock garment and a spine board. The traction splint is applied in the same manner as for femoral shaft fractures. Special care should be taken to protect the injured region about the hip from excessive pressure from the ring of a Hare Traction Splint. In the seriously or multiply injured patient, the pneumatic antishock garment will provide effective immobilization of the pelvis and hip region when combined with a spine board. In addition, the pneumatic antishock garment will help control hemorrhage in the region.

In contrast to the violently injured patient, the elderly individual with an isolated hip fracture does not require a traction splint for

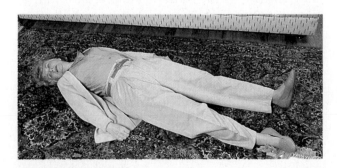

FIGURE 18–7

The patient with a displaced "fractured hip" will have shortening and external rotation of the injured limb.

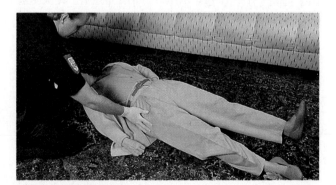

FIGURE 18–8

Palpation of the greater trochanter is usually painful in the patient with a "hip fracture."

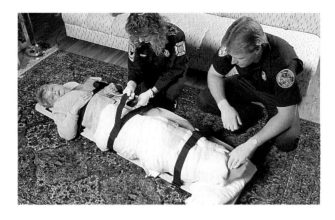

FIGURE 18-9

Splinting of most patients with a ''hip fracture'' can be accomplished with a spine board and pillows.

adequate immobilization. To effectively immobilize such a fracture, place the patient on a long spine board or a scoop stretcher using pillows or rolled blankets to support the injured limb in the deformed position. You should secure the injured limb carefully to the stretcher with long straps or cravats (Figure 18-9).

All patients with hip fractures may lose significant amounts of blood. Therefore, you should watch for shock in these patients and monitor the vital signs carefully.

Femoral Shaft Fractures

Fractures of the femur can occur in any part of the shaft, from the hip region to the femoral condyles just above the knee joint. Following fracture, the large muscles of the thigh go into spasm to ''splint'' the unstable limb. The muscle spasm frequently produces significant deformity of the limb, with severe angulation or rotation at the fracture site. Usually the limb shortens significantly as well. Often, fractures of the femoral shaft are open, and fragments of bone may protrude through the skin.

There is always a significant amount of blood loss following a fracture of the shaft of the femur. As much as 500 to 1,000 ml of blood can be lost with this fracture. With open fractures, the amount of blood loss may be even greater.

Thus, it is not unusual for a patient with a fracture of the femur to develop hypovolemic shock. You must be extremely careful in handling these patients, because any extra movement or fracture manipulation will increase the blood loss.

Because of the severe deformity that occurs with these fractures, bone fragments may penetrate or press on important nerves and vessels and produce significant damage. Careful evaluation of the distal neurovascular function is imperative in patients who have sustained a fracture of the shaft of the femur.

Remove the clothing from the limb of a patient suspected of having a fracture of the shaft of the femur so you can adequately inspect the injury site for any open wounds. Monitor the patient's vital signs closely and continually to identify the onset of hypovolemic shock. You must be prepared to transport the patient immediately in this situation.

If a wound is present, cover it with a dry, sterile compression dressing. If the foot or leg below the level of the fracture shows signs of impaired circulation (pale, cold, or pulseless), apply gentle longitudinal traction to the deformed limb. Apply the traction in line with the long axis of the limb, and gradually turn the leg from the deformed position to restore the limb's overall alignment. Frequently, restoring the limb to a more normal position restores or improves circulation to the foot. If there are no signs of the return of circulation after traction has been applied and realignment achieved, a serious vascular injury may have occurred, and the patient requires prompt medical treatment.

A fracture of the femoral shaft is best immobilized with a traction splint. In addition to knowing the precise sequence of steps to apply the splint properly, you must practice the splinting technique frequently to maintain the necessary skills. The technique for applying a Hare Traction Splint is described in Chapter 16. Another type of traction splint is called the Sager splint. You can apply it by yourself when necessary. It is lightweight and easily stored, applies a measurable amount of traction, and can be used with a pneumatic antishock garment. It should be applied using the following steps:

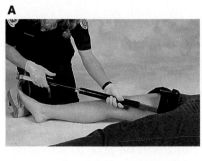

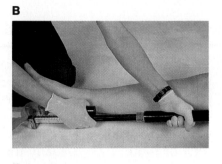

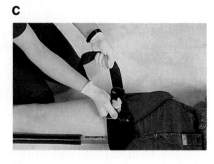

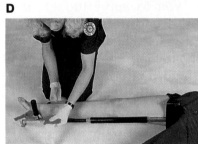

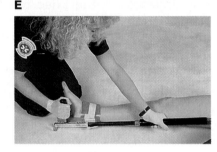

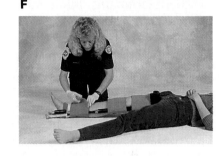

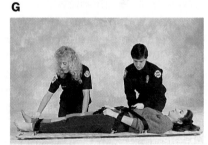

FIGURE 18–10

Application of a Sager splint for a femoral shaft fracture.

1. Before applying the splint, adjust the thigh strap so that it will lie anteriorly when secured in place (Figure 18–10a).
2. Get a rough estimate of the proper splint length by placing it alongside the injured limb so that the wheel is at the level of the heel (Figure 18–10b).
3. Arrange the ankle pads to fit the size of the patient's ankle.
4. Place the splint along the inner aspect of the limb and slide the thigh strap around the upper thigh so that the perineal cushion is snug against the groin and the ischial tuberosity. Tighten the thigh strap snugly (Figure 18–10c).
5. Secure the ankle harness tightly around the patient's ankle just above the malleoli (Figure 18–10d).
6. Snugly pull the cable ring up against the bottom of the foot.

7. Pull out the inner shaft of the splint to apply traction of approximately 10 percent of body weight (a maximum of 15 pounds) (Figure 18–10e).
8. Secure the limb to the splint using elasticized cravats (Figure 18–10f).
9. Secure the splinted patient to a long spine board (Figure 18–10g).

INJURIES ABOUT THE KNEE

Many different types of injuries can occur about the knee. Ligament injuries, for example, range from mild sprains to complete dislocation of the joint. The **patella** can also dislocate. In addition, all of the bony elements of the knee (the distal femur, the upper tibia, and the patella) can fracture. The knee is very vulnerable to injury, and injuries frequently occur in this region.

Injuries of the Knee Ligaments

The knee is especially prone to ligament injuries that may range in severity from mild sprains to complete disruption of one or more of the stabilizing ligaments. These injuries occur when abnormal bending or twisting forces are applied to the joint. They are commonly seen in both recreational and competitive athletes. The ligaments on the medial side of the knee are the ones most frequently injured. This injury usually results when the foot is fixed to the ground and the lateral aspect of the knee is struck by a heavy object such as when a football player is clipped or tackled from the side (Figure 18–11).

Usually the patient with a knee ligament injury will complain of pain in the joint and is unable to use the extremity normally. Examination will show swelling and occasionally ecchymosis, as well as point tenderness at the area of ligament injury.

You must splint all suspected knee ligament injuries. The splint must extend from the hip joint to the foot, immobilizing the bone above the injured joint (the femur) and the bone below (the tibia). A variety of splints can be used: a padded rigid long leg splint, or two padded board splints securely applied to the medial and lateral aspects of the limb. A long spine board, a pillow splint, and simply binding the injured limb to the opposite uninjured limb are also acceptable but less effective splinting techniques.

Usually the patient will be able to straighten the knee to allow you to apply the splint. If resistance or pain is encountered when you attempt to straighten the knee, splint it in the flexed position. Following the application of the splint, assess and monitor the distal neurovascular function until the patient reaches the hospital.

Dislocation of the Knee

Complete disruption of the ligaments supporting the knee may result in dislocation of the joint. When this happens, the proximal end of the tibia completely displaces from its articulation with the lower end of the femur, usually producing a significant deformity. Although substantial ligament damage always occurs with a knee dislocation, the immediate seriousness of this injury is not related to the ligament damage but to injury to the *popliteal artery*. Often, the popliteal artery is lacerated or compressed by the displaced tibia (Figure 18–

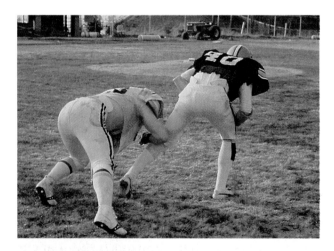

FIGURE 18–11

The knee joint is especially vulnerable to injury, particularly during athletics.

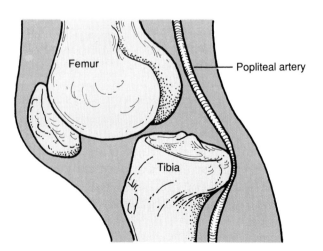

FIGURE 18–12

Dislocation of the knee frequently results in serious injury to the popliteal artery in the back of the knee.

12). When a dislocation of the knee is suspected because of gross deformity, severe pain, and an inability to move the joint, you must always check the distal circulation carefully before taking any other step. If the distal pulses are absent, notify medical control immediately because further steps in field stabilization must be directed by medical control.

If adequate distal pulses are present, a dislocated knee should be splinted in the position in which it is found, and the patient should be transported promptly to the hospital. Make no attempt to manipulate or straighten any severe knee injury when strong distal pulses are present. If the limb with good pulses is straight, apply standard rigid long leg splints to at least two sides of the limb to provide adequate immobilization (Figure 18–13). If the

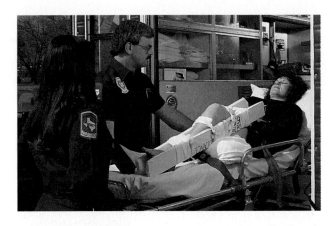

FIGURE 18–14

The flexed knee can be immobilized adequately by padded board splints applied securely to each side of the limb.

knee is bent and the foot has a good pulse, splint the joint in this position. Parallel padded board splints secured at the hip and ankle joint will provide a stable A-frame splinting configuration. Further support the limb with pillows and straps to a spine board or stretcher to eliminate any motion of the limb during transport (Figure 18–14).

On rare occasions, the medical control physician may request that you realign a deformed, pulseless limb in order to restore distal circulation. You should *only make one attempt* to realign the limb and thus reduce compression of the popliteal artery. Gently straighten the limb by applying gentle longitudinal traction in the axis of the limb. Monitor the posterior tibial pulse during the application of traction to determine whether the pulse returns. Splint the limb in the position in which the strongest pulse is felt. If traction significantly increases the patient's pain, make no further attempts to realign the limb. Once you apply manual traction, maintain it until the limb is fully splinted; otherwise, the limb will return to its deformed position.

If you are unable to restore the distal pulse, splint the limb in the position most comfortable for the patient; then transport the patient promptly to the hospital. Medical control should be notified of the status of the distal pulse so that arrangements can be made in advance to receive the patient.

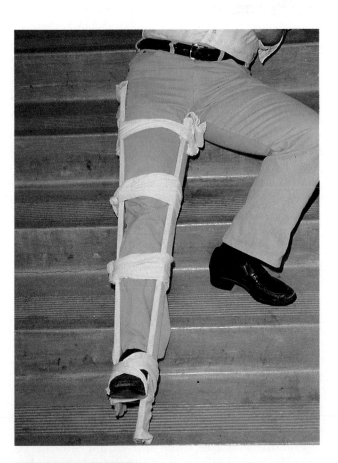

FIGURE 18–13

When the injured knee is straight, it should be splinted with padded board splints extending from the hip to the ankle.

Fractures about the Knee

Fractures about the knee may occur at the distal end of the femur, at the proximal end of the tibia, or in the patella. Nondisplaced or minimally displaced fractures are sometimes confused with a ligament injury because of their local tenderness and swelling. On the other hand, displaced fractures about the knee may produce significant deformity and be confused with a knee dislocation. When you suspect a fracture about the knee, manage it in a manner similar to the knee injuries just described. If there is an adequate distal pulse and no significant deformity, splint the limb with the knee straight. If there is significant deformity and an adequate pulse, splint the joint in the position of deformity. If the pulse is absent below the level of the injury, medical control should be notified immediately, and you should follow the instructions from medical control with regard to further management of this injury.

Dislocation of the Patella

The patella may be dislocated from its articulation with the front of the distal femur. This injury usually occurs in teenagers and young adults engaged in athletic activities. Some patients have recurrent dislocations of the patella in which only a minor twisting of the knee will produce the dislocation, just as occurs with recurrent dislocation of the shoulder. Usually the dislocated patella displaces to the lateral side, and the knee is held in a partially flexed position. The displacement of the patella produces a significant deformity (Figure 18–15).

The knee should be splinted in the position in which it is found, usually with the knee flexed to a moderate degree. Padded board splints applied to the medial and lateral aspects of the joint extending from the hip to the ankle provide adequate immobilization when combined with pillows to support the limb on the stretcher.

Occasionally, as the splint is being applied, the patella will return to its normal position spontaneously. When this occurs, immobilize the limb as for a knee ligament injury in a

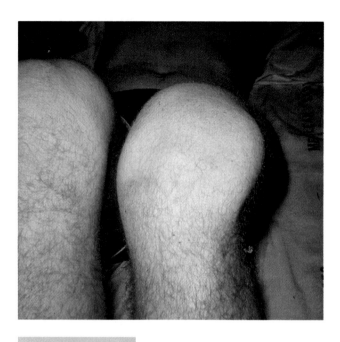

FIGURE 18–15

The typical appearance of a dislocated left patella, with the patella displaced laterally and the knee moderately flexed.

padded long leg splint. Even if the patella does return to its normal position, the patient needs to be evaluated in the emergency department. Any time a joint reduces spontaneously, you should report this occurrence to emergency department personnel so that they will know the severity of the injury.

INJURIES TO THE TIBIA AND FIBULA
. . . .

Fracture of the shaft of the **tibia** or the **fibula** may occur at any place between the knee joint and the ankle joint. Usually both bones fracture simultaneously. Because the tibia is located just beneath the skin, open fractures of this bone are quite common. These fractures may result in severe deformity, with significant angulation or rotation (Figure 18–16).

Fractures of the tibia and fibula should be immobilized with a padded, rigid long leg splint or an air splint that extends from the foot to the upper thigh. Alternatively, you can use a traction splint; however, constant traction is not usually necessary to maintain limb align-

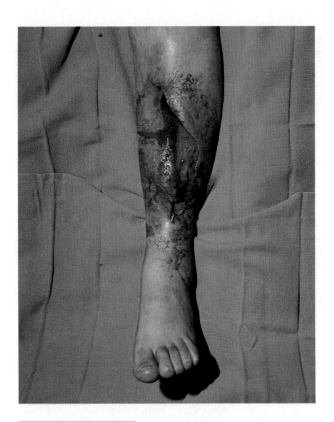

FIGURE 18–16

The typical appearance of an open fracture of the tibia and fibula.

ment with isolated tibial fractures. When both the tibia *and* femur in the same limb have been fractured, a properly applied traction splint will provide sufficient immobilization for both bones. As with most other fractures of the shaft of long bones, you should correct severe deformity prior to splinting by applying gentle longitudinal traction. The goal of applying traction is to achieve adequate alignment of the limb so that a standard splint can be applied. It is not necessary to replace the fracture fragments in their anatomic position.

Vascular injury is not uncommon with fractures of the tibia and fibula and is frequently due to the distorted position of the limb following injury. Realignment of the limb frequently corrects the impaired blood supply to the foot. If adequate circulation is not present or is not restored when the limb is realigned, transport the patient promptly to a hospital and notify the emergency department en route.

INJURIES TO THE ANKLE AND FOOT

Ankle Injuries

The ankle is one of the most commonly injured joints. Injuries occur in people of all ages and range in severity from a simple sprain that heals after a few days' rest to severe fracture-dislocations. As is true with other joints, it is sometimes difficult to distinguish nondisplaced ankle fractures from a simple sprain by clinical examination (Figure 18–17). Therefore, any ankle injury that produces pain, swelling, localized tenderness, or the inability to bear weight must be evaluated by a physician. The most frequent mechanism of ankle injury is twisting, which stretches or tears the supporting ligaments. A more extensive twisting force may produce fracture of one or both malleoli (Figure 18–18). When dislocation of the ankle occurs, it is usually associated with fractures of both malleoli.

The wide spectrum of injuries to the ankle should all be managed in the same way. Dress all open wounds, evaluate distal neurovascular function, correct any gross malalignment by applying gentle longitudinal traction to the heel, and apply a splint before the traction is released. Splinting can be accomplished with a

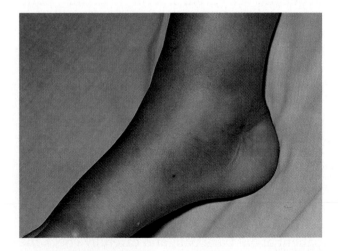

FIGURE 18–17

Swelling about the ankle is characteristic of both sprains and fractures.

FIGURE 18–18

(Left) X ray of an ankle fracture. (Right) Line drawing showing that both malleoli are broken.

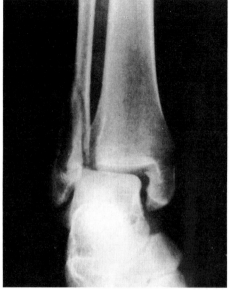
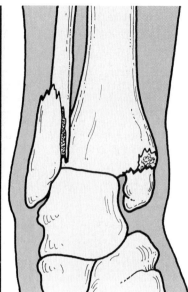

padded rigid splint, an air splint, or a pillow splint. The splint should include the entire foot and extend up the leg to the level of the knee joint.

Foot Injuries

Injuries of the foot can result in the fracture of one of the several tarsals, metatarsals, or phalanges of the toes. Toe fractures are especially common.

Of the tarsal bones, the **calcaneus** is the most frequently fractured. Fracture of this bone usually occurs when the patient falls or jumps from a height and lands directly on the heel(s). The force of injury causes the calcaneus to be compressed and produces immediate swelling and ecchymosis about the heel. If the force of impact is great enough, as from a fall from a roof or tree, additional fractures may occur as well.

Frequently, the force of injury is transmitted up the legs to the spine, producing a fracture of the lumbar spine (Figure 18–19). When a patient who has jumped or fallen from a height complains of heel pain, you must question the patient about back pain and carefully check the spine for tenderness or deformity.

Injuries of the foot are associated with significant swelling but rarely with gross deformity. Vascular injuries are uncommon. As in the

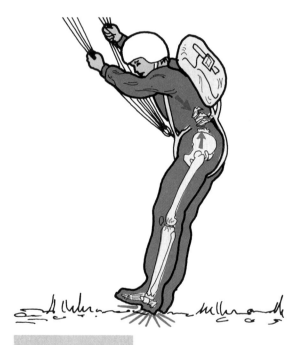

FIGURE 18–19

When a jumper lands on the heels, the energy is transmitted to the spine, producing spine injury as well as injury to the foot and ankle.

hand, lacerations about the ankle and foot may damage important underlying nerves and tendons. Puncture wounds of the foot occur frequently and may cause serious infection if not treated early. All of these injuries must be evaluated and treated by a physician.

To splint the foot, apply a rigid padded board splint, an air splint, or a pillow splint, all of which must immobilize the ankle joint as well as the foot (Figure 18–20). The toes should remain exposed for periodic neurovascular checks.

Slightly elevate the foot after splinting to minimize swelling. When the patient is lying on the stretcher, prop up the foot approximately 6 inches. All patients with lower extremity injuries should be transported supine to adequately elevate the limb. The foot and leg should never be allowed to dangle off the stretcher on the floor or ground.

Any patient who has fallen from a height and complains of heel pain should, in addition to having the foot splinted, be transported on a long spine board to immobilize any possible spinal injury (Figure 18–21).

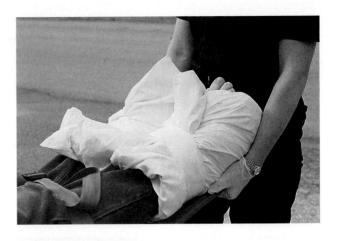

FIGURE 18–21

Any patient who has fallen from a height should be transported on a long spine board to immobilize any possible spine injury.

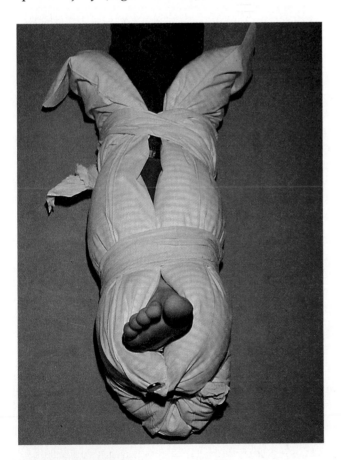

FIGURE 18–20

A pillow splint provides excellent immobilization of the foot with suspected fractures.

YOU ARE THE EMT

1. Your patient has a closed pelvic fracture. What internal organs could be injured? What are some of the signs of such injuries?
2. Why is hypovolemic shock likely to occur with pelvic and femoral injuries? What should you do once you determine the patient is in shock?
3. Your patient has a serious knee injury, but you are not sure whether his knee is dislocated or fractured. What are the signs of each? How should you prepare this patient for transport?
4. You have identified a posterior dislocation of the hip in a patient injured in an automobile accident. What signs led you to this diagnosis? What would anterior dislocation of the hip look like?

CHAPTER 19

THE NERVOUS SYSTEM

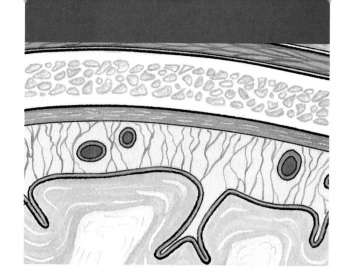

KEY TERMS

autonomic nervous system (aw"to-nom'ik ner'vus sis'tem) That part of the nervous system that regulates functions, such as digestion and sweating, that are not controlled by a voluntary act of conscious will.

brain stem Area of the brain between the spinal cord and cerebrum, surrounded by the cerebellum; controls functions necessary for life, such as respiration.

central nervous system The brain and spinal cord.

cerebrum (ser'ĕ-brum) The largest of the three subdivisions of the brain, sometimes called the "gray matter"; it is made up of several lobes that control movement, hearing, balance, speech, visual perception, emotions, and personality.

meninges (mĕ-nin'jēz) The three layers of tissue that envelop the brain and spinal cord: the dura mater, pia mater, and arachnoid.

motor nerves Nerves that transmit impulses to muscles, causing them to move.

peripheral nervous system (pĕ-rif'er-al ner'vus sis'tem) The part of the nervous system that consists of 31 pairs of spinal nerves and 12 pairs of cranial nerves. These peripheral nerves may be sensory nerves or motor nerves.

sensory nerves (sen'so-re nervz) Nerves that carry sensations of touch, taste, heat, cold, pain, or other modalities.

somatic nervous system (so-mat'ik ner'vus sis'tem) Part of the nervous system that regulates functions over which there is voluntary control.

spinal cord An extension of the brain, composed of virtually all the nerves carrying messages between the brain and the rest of the body. It lies inside of and is protected by the spinal canal.

The nervous system is a complex system of nerve cells that enables all parts of the human body to function. It is basically composed of the brain, the spinal cord, and several billion nerve fibers that carry information to and from all parts of the body. Because the nervous system is so vital, it is well protected. The brain lies beneath the skull, and the spinal cord lies inside the bony spinal canal. Despite its being well protected, the nervous system can be injured from serious impacts and blows. To make an accurate assessment of nervous system injuries, you must understand the anatomy of the nervous system and how it functions.

Chapter 19 first describes the anatomic and functional components of the nervous system. It then discusses its two basic anatomic divisions: the central nervous system and the peripheral nervous system. The chapter next presents the nervous system's two functional divisions: the somatic nervous system and the autonomic nervous system. The last part of the chapter describes how the nervous system is protected within the body.

GOALS

The goals of Chapter 19 are to

- understand the anatomic and functional components of the nervous system.
- describe the central and peripheral nervous systems.
- describe the somatic and autonomic nervous systems.
- identify the protective coverings of the nervous system.

ANATOMIC AND FUNCTIONAL COMPONENTS OF THE NERVOUS SYSTEM

Anatomically, the nervous system is divided into two parts: the central nervous system and the peripheral nervous system. The **central nervous system (CNS)** is made up of the brain and the spinal cord. From a practical point of view, the central nervous system can be considered the part of the nervous system that is covered and protected by bones. The brain is covered by the skull, and the spinal cord is covered by the spinal column. The major parts of most nerve cells (the nucleus and the cell body) lie within the central nervous system. Many of the cells in the central nervous system have long fibers that extend from the cell body out through openings in the bony covering to form a cable of nerve fibers that link the central nervous system to the various organs of the body. These cables of nerve fibers make up the **peripheral nervous system.** The two major types of nerves are sensory and motor nerve fibers. The **sensory nerves** carry information from the body to the central nervous system; the **motor nerves** carry information from the central nervous system to the muscles of the body.

The nervous system controls virtually all activities of the body, including those over which one has voluntary control (voluntary) and those over which one has no voluntary control (involuntary). The part of the nervous system that regulates activities over which there is voluntary control is called the **somatic nervous system.** Such activities include walking, talking, and writing. Many body functions occur without voluntary control. These activities are under the control of the autonomic, or involuntary, nervous system. The **autonomic nervous system** controls automatic body functions such as digestion, dilation and constriction of blood vessels, sweating, and all other involuntary actions necessary for basic bodily functions. Some of the cells that form the autonomic nervous system are inside the central nervous system, and others lie alongside the spinal column in the cervical and lumbar regions.

Thus, the nervous system as a whole can be divided *anatomically* into the central and peripheral nervous systems, and *functionally* into somatic (voluntary) and autonomic (involuntary) components.

CENTRAL AND PERIPHERAL NERVOUS SYSTEMS

Central Nervous System

The central nervous system is composed of the brain and the spinal cord.

The Brain

The *brain* is the controlling organ of the body. It is the center of consciousness. It is responsible for all our voluntary body activities, the perception of our surroundings, and the control of our reactions to the environment. In addition, the brain enables us to experience all the fine shadings of thought and feeling that make us individuals. The brain is subdivided into several areas, all of which have specific functions. Three major subdivisions of the brain are the cerebrum, the cerebellum, and the brain stem.

The largest part of the brain is the **cerebrum,** which is sometimes called the "gray matter." It makes up about three-fourths of the volume of the brain and is itself composed of several lobes—frontal, parietal, temporal, and occipi-

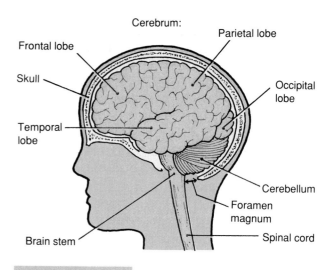

FIGURE 19–1

The brain lies well protected within the skull. Its major subdivisions are the cerebrum, cerebellum, and brain stem.

tal (Figure 19–1). The cerebrum on one side of the brain controls activities on the opposite side of the body. Each lobe of the cerebrum is responsible for a specific function. For example, one group of brain cells in the frontal lobe is responsible for the activity of all the voluntary muscles of the body. Brain cells in this area generate impulses that are sent along nerve fibers that extend from each cell into the spinal cord. Another area in the parietal lobe has cells that receive sensory impulses from the peripheral nerves of the body. Other parts of the cerebrum are responsible for other body functions. For instance, the occipital region, on the back of the cerebrum, receives visual impulses for the eyes, and other areas control hearing, balance, and speech. Still other parts of the cerebrum are responsible for emotions and other characteristics of an individual's personality.

Underneath the great mass of cerebral tissue lies the *cerebellum,* sometimes called the "little brain" (Figure 19–1). The major function of this area is to coordinate the various activities of the brain, particularly body movements. Without the cerebellum, very specialized muscular activities such as writing or sewing would be impossible.

The **brain stem** is so called because the brain appears to be sitting on this portion of the central nervous system as a plant sits on its stem. The brain stem is the most primitive part of the central nervous system. It lies deep within the cranium and is the best protected part of the central nervous system (Figure 19–1). The brain stem is the controlling center for virtually all body functions that are absolutely necessary for life. Cells in this part of the brain control cardiac, respiratory, and other basic body functions.

The brain has many other anatomic areas, all of which have specific and important functions. The brain receives a vast amount of information from the environment, sorts it all out, and directs the body to respond appropriately. Many of the responses involve voluntary muscle action; others are automatic and involuntary.

The Spinal Cord

The **spinal cord** is the other major portion of the central nervous system (Figure 19–2). Like the brain, the spinal cord contains nerve cell bodies, but the major portion of the spinal cord is made up of nerve fibers that extend from the cells of the brain. These nerve fibers transmit information to and from the brain. All the fibers join together just below the brain stem to form the spinal cord. The spinal cord exits through a large opening at the base of the skull called the *foramen magnum*. It is encased within the spinal canal down to the level of the second lumbar vertebra. The *spinal canal* is created by the vertebrae, stacked one on the other. Each vertebra surrounds the cord to form the bony spinal canal (see Figures 15–12 and 15–13).

The major function of the spinal cord is to transmit messages between the brain and the body. These messages are passed along the nerve fibers as electrical impulses, just as messages are passed along a telephone cable. The nerve fibers are arranged in specific bundles within the spinal cord to carry the messages from one specific area of the body to the brain and back.

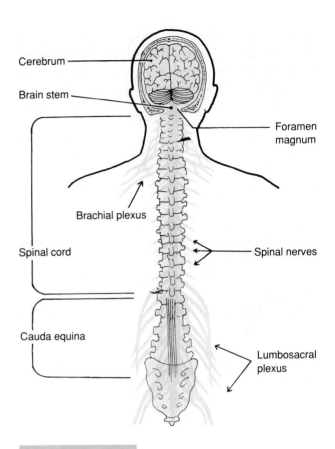

Cerebrum
Brain stem
Foramen magnum
Brachial plexus
Spinal cord
Spinal nerves
Cauda equina
Lumbosacral plexus

FIGURE 19–2

The spinal cord is the continuation of the brain stem. It exits the skull at the foramen magnum and extends down to the level of the second lumbar vertebra.

The Peripheral Nervous System

The peripheral nervous system is composed of 31 pairs of peripheral nerves called *spinal nerves* and 12 pairs called *cranial nerves*. At each vertebral level from the first cervical to the fifth sacral, on each side of the spinal cord, a spinal nerve exits the spinal cord and passes through an opening in the bony canal (Figure 19–3). This spinal nerve is composed of nerve fibers from nerve cells that originate within the spinal cord. The nerve fibers conduct sensory impulses from the skin and other organs to the spinal cord. They also conduct motor impulses from the spinal cord to the muscles that are present in that segment of the body. For example, between the seventh and eighth ribs the spinal nerve carries sensory fibers from the

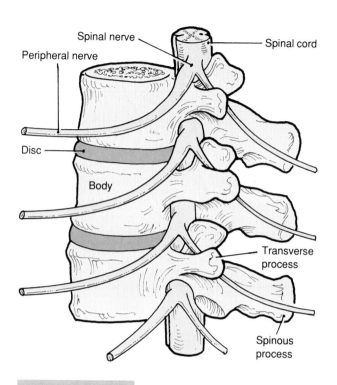

FIGURE 19-3

At each vertebral level, spinal nerves containing both motor and sensory fibers exit the spinal canal between each pair of vertebrae.

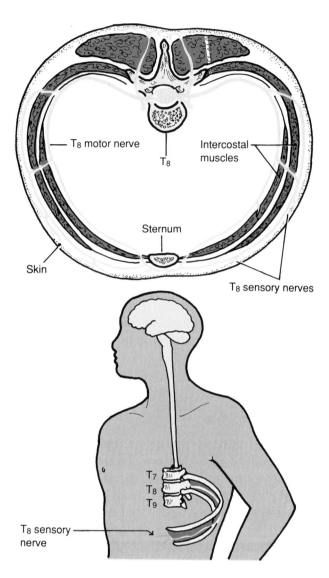

FIGURE 19-4

The T_8 peripheral nerve supplies motor nerve fibers to the intercostal muscles between the seventh and eighth ribs and sensory nerve fibers to the skin in this interspace.

skin between those two ribs and also has motor nerve fibers to innervate the intercostal muscle between the seventh and eighth ribs (Figure 19–4). This specific arrangement of nerve fibers becomes more complex and confusing in both the cervical and lumbar regions because of the large number of muscles in the arms and legs that must be supplied with nerve fibers. The spinal nerves combine to form complex nerve networks (*plexuses*) in these two areas—the *brachial plexus* for the upper extremity and the *lumbosacral plexus* for the lower extremity (Figure 19–2).

Cranial nerves are 12 pairs of peripheral nerves that exit the brain through holes in the skull. For the most part, they are very specialized nerves designed to provide specific functions in the head and face. For example, the facial (seventh cranial) nerves send motor impulses to many of the facial muscles.

There are three major categories of peripheral nerves: sensory nerves, motor nerves, and connecting nerves.

Sensory Nerves   Sensory nerves of the body are quite complex. There are many different types of sensory cells in the nervous system. One type forms the retina of the eye; others are responsible for the hearing and balancing mechanisms in the ear. Other sensory cells are located within the skin, muscles, joints, lungs, and other organs of the body. When a sensory cell is stimulated, it transmits its own special message to the brain. There are special sensory nerves to detect heat, cold, position, motion, pressure, pain, balance, light, taste, and smell, as well as other sensations. Specialized nerve endings are adapted for each cell so that it perceives only one type of sensation and it transmits only that message.

The sensory impulses constantly provide information to the brain about what the different parts of our body are doing in relation to our surroundings. Thus, the brain is continuously made aware of its surroundings. The cranial nerves supply sensations directly to the brain. Visual sensations (what we see) reach the brain directly by way of the *optic nerve* (the second cranial nerve) in each eye. The nerve endings for the optic nerve lie in the retina of the eye. The nerve endings are stimulated by light, and the impulses are carried along the nerve that passes through a hole in the back of the eye socket and carries impulses to the occipital portion of the brain.

When sensory nerve endings in the extremities are stimulated, the impulses are transmitted along a peripheral nerve to the spinal cord. The cell body of the peripheral nerve lies in the spinal cord. The impulse is then transmitted from that cell body to another nerve ending in the spinal cord. The impulse is then sent up the spinal cord to the sensory area in the parietal lobe of the brain, where the sensory information can be interpreted and acted on by the brain (Figure 19–5).

Motor Nerves Each muscle in the body has its own motor nerve. The cell body for each motor nerve lies in the spinal cord, and a fiber from the cell body extends as part of the peripheral nerve to its specific muscle. Electrical impulses produced by the cell body in the spinal cord are transmitted along the motor nerve to the muscle and cause it to contract. The cell body in the spinal cord is stimulated by an impulse produced in the motor strip of the cerebral cortex.

This impulse is transmitted along the spinal cord to the cell body of the motor nerve.

Connecting Nerves Within the brain and the spinal cord are cells with short fibers that connect the sensory nerves with the motor nerves. In the spinal cord they connect the sensory and motor nerves directly, bypassing the brain. These *connecting nerves* allow sensory and motor impulses to be transmitted from one nerve to another within the central nervous system.

FUNCTIONAL DIVISIONS OF THE NERVOUS SYSTEMS

The Somatic Nervous System

The somatic nervous system controls the voluntary activities of the body. Sensory information from the peripheral nerves is interpreted by the cerebral cortex of the brain. The brain then sends signals to voluntary muscles in response to these sensory stimuli. The somatic nervous system is responsible for almost all of the body's coordinated muscular activities such as walking, eating, and driving a car.

The Autonomic Nervous System

The autonomic nervous system is involuntary—the brain has no voluntary control over its activity. It is a very primitive system that controls the function of many of the body's vital organs. The autonomic nervous system is composed of two counterbalancing parts: the sympathetic nervous system and the parasympathetic nervous system. These two divisions have equal and opposite effects on the body's vital organs, increasing or decreasing their activity depending on basic bodily needs.

The Sympathetic Nervous System The cells of the *sympathetic nervous system* lie outside of the spinal canal in clusters on either side of the cervical and lumbar spine near the points where the spinal nerves exit the canal. The

FIGURE 19–5

A simplified schematic representation of the nerves in the central and peripheral nervous systems.

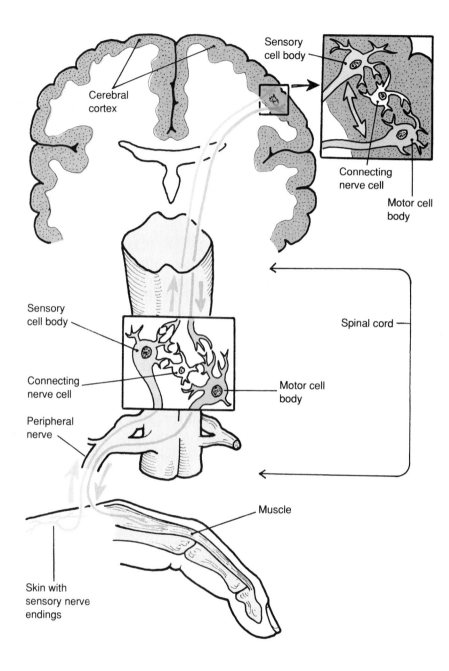

sympathetic nerves respond to stress and prepare the body to respond to threatening situations (the "fight or flight" phenomenon). Thus, the sympathetic nervous system causes blood vessels to constrict, stimulates sweating, increases the heart rate, causes the sphincter muscles to constrict, and prepares the body to respond to stress.

The Parasympathetic Nervous System In contrast, the *parasympathetic nervous system* acts in the opposite manner. The cells of the parasympathetic nervous system are found in the brain stem and also in the sacral area of the spinal cord. Its functions are opposite those of the sympathetic nervous system. The parasympathetic nervous system causes blood vessels to dilate, slows the heart rate, and relaxes muscle sphincters, among other effects.

Both divisions of the autonomic nervous system are equally effective. They tend to counterbalance one another so that stable and effective basic body functions can be maintained.

Activities of the Somatic and Autonomic Nervous Systems

The combined actions of the somatic and the autonomic nervous systems control all the body activities. The body responds either voluntarily or involuntarily to external stimuli. There are three basic categories of nervous system activity: voluntary, involuntary, and reflex.

Voluntary Activity The skeletal muscles are under voluntary control. A person can decide to move an arm or leg to accomplish a specific task. A conscious decision is made to perform this task. Sensory input will be used to determine the specific muscular activity. Driving a car is an example of voluntary activity of the nervous system. Sensory input from the eyes and ears and the general sensation of road bumps and vehicle speed are synthesized in the brain. This information dictates the specific muscular activity necessary to drive the car toward a specific objective, avoiding danger. This action is a series of willed or voluntary acts, each resulting from a separate, conscious decision.

Involuntary Activity Both the central nervous system and the autonomic nervous system control basic bodily functions independent of the thought process. For example, breathing is done automatically. Although, to a certain extent, we can breathe rapidly or hold our breath by conscious will, neither can be done indefinitely. A complex system of chemical controls takes over when a person approaches danger from excessive voluntary breathing control. The respiratory rate is controlled involuntarily until normal levels of oxygen and carbon dioxide are restored. This response is one of the most primitive functions of the brain and is present at every level of animal development. Similarly, heart rate, dilation and constriction of blood vessels, and the function of many other organs are controlled by involuntary activity of the central and autonomic nervous systems.

Reflex Activity The connecting nerves in the spinal cord complete a *reflex arc* between the sensory and motor nerves of the limbs. An irritating stimulus to the sensory nerve (such as heat) will be transmitted from the sensory nerve along the connecting nerve and directly to the motor nerve, causing it to be stimulated (Figure 19–6). The muscle responds promptly, withdrawing the limb from the irritating stimulus even before this information can be transmitted to the brain. The physician who taps on

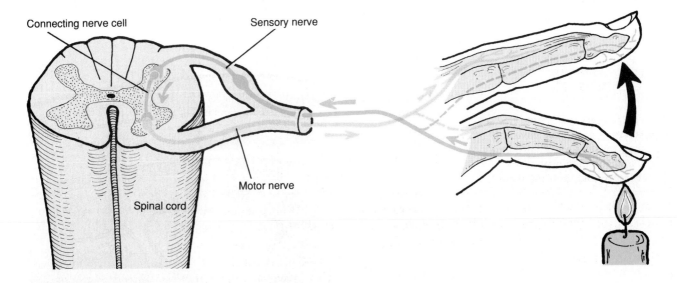

Connecting nerve cell

Sensory nerve

Motor nerve

Spinal cord

FIGURE 19–6   The reflex arc is a primitive response to irritating stimuli that allows prompt stimulation of the muscles to withdraw from the source of irritation.

the patellar tendon with a rubber hammer is testing to see whether the patient's reflex arc is intact.

PROTECTIVE COVERINGS OF THE NERVOUS SYSTEM

The cells of the brain and spinal cord are soft and easily injured. Once damaged, cells in the central nervous system cannot be regenerated or reproduced. Therefore, the body has developed an extensive protective covering for the central nervous system (Figure 19–7). The entire central nervous system is contained within this protective framework. The skull is covered by a thick layer of skin (the *scalp*) and underneath the skin by a layer of muscle fascia. The spinal canal is also surrounded by a thick layer of skin and muscles.

The skull and spinal canal are thick and withstand injury very well. The skull, in fact, has two layers—an inner table and an outer table—doubling the amount of bone protecting the brain. In addition to these layers of protective covering, the central nervous system is further protected by a set of special coverings called the **meninges**. The meninges are three layers of tissue that suspend the brain and the spinal cord within the skull and the spinal

canal. These layers are distinct. The outer one is a tough fibrous layer, much like leather, called the *dura mater*. The dura mater forms a sac to contain the central nervous system. The peripheral nerves exit through small openings in the dura.

The inner two layers of the meninges are much thinner than the dura mater. They are called the *arachnoid* and the *pia mater*. Blood vessels that nourish the brain and spinal cord lie in these layers. *Cerebrospinal fluid* is produced by and fills the spaces between the arachnoid and the pia mater. The brain and spinal cord essentially float in this cerebrospinal fluid. The fluid is an excellent shock absorber that buffers the central nervous system from injury.

All of these protective layers combine to isolate the central nervous system and protect it from injury. However, closed head injuries can result in serious problems caused in part by these firm protective coverings. Severe injury may cause bleeding of the vessels under the dura. The hematoma that develops (a *subdural hematoma*) will then compress the softer brain tissue. The increased pressure inside the confined space of the skull will require prompt surgical decompression to avoid permanent brain damage.

If the outer protective layers are damaged

FIGURE 19–7

The central nervous system has several layers of protective covering: the skin, muscles and their fascia, bone, and the meninges (dura mater, arachnoid, and pia mater).

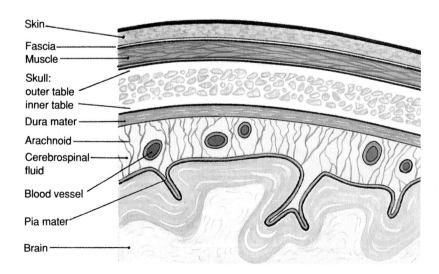

Skin
Fascia
Muscle
Skull:
outer table
inner table
Dura mater
Arachnoid
Cerebrospinal fluid
Blood vessel
Pia mater
Brain

(the skin, fascia, skull, and dura), cerebrospinal fluid may leak to the body surface. Such cerebrospinal fluid leaks most frequently occur from the nose and the ears. Cerebrospinal fluid is clear and watery. If a head injury patient has a "runny nose" or watery fluid draining from the ear or from an open skull fracture, you must assume that the watery fluid is cerebrospinal fluid.

YOU ARE THE EMT

1. The nervous system can be divided anatomically into what two divisions? Into what two parts is it divided functionally?
2. What are the three categories of peripheral nerves? Describe the function of each.
3. Which part of the nervous system causes blood vessels to constrict? Which part causes them to dilate? Are constriction and dilation voluntary or involuntary activities? Why?
4. How is the central nervous system protected from injury? What kinds of injuries do you think might endanger the central nervous system?

CHAPTER 20

HEAD INJURIES

amnesia (am-ne′ze-ah) Lack or loss of memory; inability to remember past experiences.

cerebral edema (ser′ĕ-bral ĕ-de′mah) Swelling of the brain.

cerebrospinal fluid (ser″ĕ-bro-spi′nal floo′id) Fluid that fills the spaces between the arachnoid and the pia mater. The brain and spinal cord essentially float in this fluid.

concussion (kon-kush′un) A temporary loss of some or all of the abilities of the brain to function without physical damage to the brain.

contusion (kon-tu′zhun) A bruise.

convulsion (con-vul′shun) A seizure.

epidural (ep″ĭ-du′ral) Superficial to the dura, deep to the skull.

Glasgow Coma Scale (glas′gōw ko′mah skāl) A rating system used to assess the patient's level of consciousness and the extent of loss of brain function.

intracerebral (in″trah-ser′ĕ-bral) Inside or within the brain.

intracranial (in″trah-kra′ne-al) Within the skull.

retrograde amnesia (ret′ro-grād am-ne′ze-ah) Inability to recall events that occurred before the actual onset of an event, such as a head injury.

All head injuries are potentially life-threatening. Over 70 percent of the injuries sustained in automobile accidents involve the head. In addition, a significant number of patients with head injuries also have sustained a neck injury with spinal cord damage or the potential for such damage.

The severity of head injuries can range from a trivial scalp laceration to fatal brain damage. Intracranial bleeding can produce rapid neurological deterioration and death. The patient's best chances for survival and recovery of normal function frequently depend on the quality of the initial care that is given and prompt transportation to a hospital capable of dealing with such injuries.

Chapter 20 first describes the various types of head injuries and the complications that can arise from these specific injuries. The chapter then describes the signs and symptoms that can occur with a head injury and the method of evaluating and monitoring these signs and symptoms in the head injury patient. Next, Chapter 20 describes the general principles of treatment of all head injury patients. It concludes with a discussion of some of the specific problems seen with head injury patients, describing the best way to manage these specific problems.

GOALS

The goals of Chapter 20 are to
- know the various patterns of injury that may affect the head.
- understand the common complications that occur following head injury.
- know how to assess the major and minor signs and symptoms of head injury.
- understand the importance of assessing and interpreting the patient's level of consciousness.
- understand the general principles of treatment of head injury.
- understand the methods needed to manage some of the specific consequences of head injury.

TYPES OF HEAD INJURY

Scalp Laceration

Scalp lacerations vary from minor to very extensive. Because the face and scalp both have an unusually rich blood supply, significant amounts of blood may be lost quickly, even from very small lacerations. On rare occasions, blood loss from a scalp laceration may be severe enough to cause hypovolemic shock, particularly in children. In the multiply injured patient, bleeding from scalp or facial lacerations will contribute to or accentuate hypovolemia. Because a scalp laceration results from a direct blow to the head, other, more serious deeper injuries are often present as well.

Skull Fracture

The main function of the skull is to protect the brain from injury. Fracture of the skull is an indication that a significant force has been exerted on the head. As with any other fracture, a skull fracture may be open or closed, depending on whether there is an overlying laceration of the scalp. The diagnosis of a skull fracture is usually made in the hospital by x-ray examination, but you may conclude that a fracture is present if the patient's head appears deformed. If there is a scalp laceration, there may be a visible crack in the skull in the depths of the laceration. Injuries from bullets or other penetrating weapons frequently result in fracture of the skull. Another sign of skull fracture seen occasionally is ecchymosis that develops under the eyes (a condition known as "raccoon eyes") or behind one ear over the mastoid process ("Battle's sign") (Figure 20–1).

Concussion

A blow to the head or face may cause concussion of the brain. There is no universal agreement on the appropriate definition of a concussion, but it is accepted that **concussion** represents a temporary loss of some or all of the abilities of the brain to function *without* actual physical damage having occurred to the brain. A concussion may result in a temporary abnormal function in any part of the brain. For example, the person who "sees stars" after being struck in the head has suffered a concussion that affects the occipital portion of the brain. A concussion may result in unconsciousness and even the inability to breathe for short periods of time. The patient may be confused or have **amnesia** (loss of memory). Occasionally the patient cannot remember events that occurred prior to the injury. This is called **retrograde amnesia.**

Usually, the concussion is of very short duration. In fact, it is often over by the time you arrive. Nevertheless, any patient who has sustained a head injury should be questioned for symptoms of a concussion. A patient who has not sustained a concussion should have a clear memory of the accident and should not complain of dizziness, weakness, visual changes, or any other symptoms that would indicate temporary loss of part or all of the brain's function.

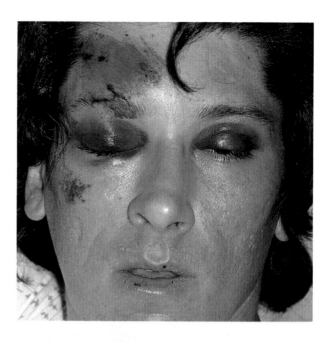

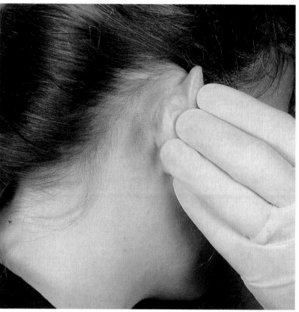

FIGURE 20–1

Signs of skull fracture: (top) bruising around the eyes; (bottom) bruising behind the ear over the mastoid process, or "Battle's sign."

Contusion

Just as with any other soft tissue in the body, the brain may sustain a **contusion,** or bruise, when the skull is struck. A contusion is a far more serious condition than a concussion, because physical injury to the brain tissue has occurred. As with contusions elsewhere, there is associated bleeding and swelling from injured blood vessels. Contusion of the brain may produce long-lasting, and perhaps permanent, damage to the brain tissue. A patient who has sustained a brain contusion may exhibit any or all of the signs of brain injury described later in this chapter.

Intracranial Bleeding

Laceration of a blood vessel inside the brain or of the meninges that cover the brain will produce an **intracranial** hematoma. The brain occupies nearly the entire space inside the skull. There is very little room for a hematoma that results from a laceration or a rupture of a blood vessel within the skull. An intracranial hematoma can be found in one of three areas (Figure 20–2):

■ Outside the dura and under the skull: an **epidural** hematoma.

■ Beneath the dura but outside the brain: a *subdural* hematoma.
■ Within the substance of the brain tissue itself: an **intracerebral** hematoma.

The bleeding that results from a lacerated or torn blood vessel within the skull will form a hematoma that compresses the brain tissue, causing loss of brain function. The hematoma may develop rapidly, as seen with an epidural hematoma, or may develop very slowly over several days, as may be seen with a subdural hematoma. The expanding hematoma will cause progressive loss of brain function and death if not treated promptly.

COMPLICATIONS OF HEAD INJURY

Cerebral Edema

Cerebral edema (swelling of the brain) is one of the most common and serious complications

---

FIGURE 20–2

Bleeding from injured blood vessels within the skull can produce a hematoma which compresses the brain tissue causing irreversible damage. The hematoma can be: (A) Subdural, (B) intracerebral, or (C) epidural.

A. SUBDURAL

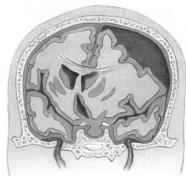

B. INTRACEREBRAL

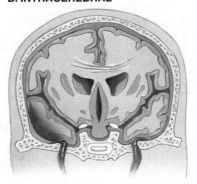

C. EPIDURAL

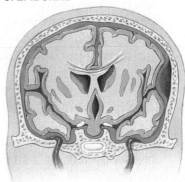

associated with any head injury. Just as any other injured tissue, the brain swells when it has been injured. Swelling within the closed space of the skull results in compression of the brain tissue and loss of brain function. Cerebral edema is aggravated by low oxygen levels in the blood and can be decreased or minimized by high blood oxygen levels. For these reasons, it is of primary importance in your treatment of the head injury patient (particularly the unconscious patient) to secure an adequate airway, ensure adequate ventilation, and provide high-flow supplemental oxygen. High-flow supplemental oxygen should always be administered to the head injury patient, because there is strong evidence that oxygen decreases cerebral edema in the acutely injured brain. You should not wait for the appearance of cyanosis or other obvious signs of hypoxia to diagnose low arterial oxygen levels in the head injury patient. Cyanosis is a very late finding in these patients, and many patients need oxygen and ventilatory support before cyanosis appears.

Convulsions

It is not uncommon for the head injury patient to have a **convulsion** or a seizure as a result of the injury. Direct injury to the brain or the accumulation of edema fluid within the skull compressing the brain tissue may result in convulsions. You must be prepared to manage convulsions in all patients who have sustained a head injury.

Vomiting

Head injury patients commonly vomit. The vomiting usually results from increased intracerebral pressure and it occurs very often, even after trivial head injuries. In all head injury patients you must be prepared to manage vomiting with particular attention to protecting the airway in these patients.

ASSESSMENT OF HEAD INJURY

The assessment of a patient with a head injury begins by having a high index of suspicion for such an injury when you arrive on the scene. The common causes of head injury (motor vehicle accidents, direct blows, falls from heights, assaults, and sports injuries) should alert you immediately to this possibility, and you should seek specific signs and symptoms of head injury during your patient assessment. During the assessment of all head injury patients, it is especially important to evaluate and monitor the patient's level of consciousness, paying particular attention to any changes that may occur.

Signs and Symptoms of Head Injury

All head injuries are potentially serious. Those that initially may seem trivial may end up being life-threatening, if not properly treated. Conversely, severe lacerations of the scalp or fractures of the skull may occur with little or no brain injury and produce minimal or no long-term problems. Specific major signs of head injury include the following:

- Laceration or contusion of the scalp.
- Visible fractures, or deformities of the skull.
- Ecchymosis about the eyes (raccoon eyes) or behind the ear over the mastoid process (Battle's sign). Both of these signs usually indicate a fracture of the base of the skull.
- **Cerebrospinal fluid** leakage from a scalp wound, the nose, or the ear indicating a fracture of the skull associated with a tear of the underlying dura. A tear of the dura combined with a fracture of the skull allows the watery, clear or pink cerebrospinal fluid to leak to the outside.
- Failure of the pupils to respond to light.
- Unequal pupil size.
- Loss of sensation and/or motor function.

The following less specific signs and symptoms may also be the result of a head injury:

- A period of unconsciousness.
- Amnesia (loss of memory).
- Retrograde amnesia (the inability to remember events prior to the injury).
- Confusion.
- Dizziness.
- Visual complaints.
- Combative or other abnormal behavior.

Any combination of these signs and symptoms may occur following a head injury. Following an injury, any patient who exhibits one or more of these signs or symptoms should be evaluated promptly in the emergency department.

Level of Consciousness

Once you have concluded that a head injury is present, it is imperative for you to assess and monitor the patient's level of consciousness. You should perform an initial, baseline evaluation using the AVPU scale and record the time of the initial observations. Reevaluations should be made and recorded on the ambulance street form every 10 minutes until the patient reaches the hospital. Any change in the level of consciousness (either improvement or deterioration) is the most important measurement any medical person can make in the head injury patient. Frequently, the level of consciousness fluctuates—improving, deteriorating, and then improving again with time. On other occasions there is a gradual, progressive deterioration in the patient's response to stimuli. Such deterioration usually indicates serious brain damage that may require prompt and vigorous surgical treatment.

The physicians taking care of the patient must know when loss of consciousness occurred. The baseline neurological evaluation that you performed in the field will be compared with the neurological evaluations obtained once the patient reaches the emergency department. The sooner you obtain this baseline evaluation, the more information physicians will have for planning an appropriate course of treatment. The level of consciousness of a patient, or any change in it, is the *single most important* observation that an EMT can make to assess the severity of brain injury.

The **Glasgow Coma Scale** is used by many hospitals and some EMS systems to assess the patient's level of consciousness and the extent of loss of brain function. It is a more detailed scale than the AVPU scale and may be the choice of your EMS system (see Figure 20–3).

When you report the patient's level of consciousness, it is important to use simple, easily understood terms such as "does not remember

GLASGOW COMA SCALE		
Eye Opening	Spontaneous	4
	To Voice	3
	To Pain	2
	None	1
Verbal Response	Oriented	5
	Confused	4
	Inappropriate Words	3
	Incomprehensible Words	2
	None	1
Motor Response	Obeys Command	6
	Localizes Pain	5
	Withdraws (pain)	4
	Flexion (pain)	3
	Extension (pain)	2
	None	1
Glasgow Coma Score Total		

TOTAL GLASGOW COMA SCALE POINTS	
14 - 15 = 5	
11 - 13 = 4	CONVERSION =
8 - 10 = 3	APPROXIMATELY
5 - 7 = 2	ONE-THIRD
3 - 4 = 1	TOTAL VALUE

FIGURE 20–3

The Glasgow Coma Scale. Note that the lower the score, the more severe is the extent of brain injury.

events immediately preceding injury" or "confused about time and date." Terms such as obtunded or dazed have different meanings to different people and thus should not be used in either written or verbal reports.

TREATMENT OF HEAD INJURIES

General Principles

Patients with head injuries often sustain injuries to the cervical spine. You should assume for all patients with head injuries that the cervical spine is unstable and carry out all treatments without undue movement of the neck until the spine can be appropriately splinted. When it is necessary to restore the airway, use the trauma jaw-thrust maneuver (Figure 20–4) or the trauma chin-lift maneuver (Figure 20–5). With both of these maneuvers, the cervical spine and head are stabilized manually in a neutral, in-line position to protect them from movement. In the patient with a head injury, never hyperextend the cervical spine to open the airway except in the mass casualty situation (see Chapter 46). Rather, the mandible should be moved forward to open the airway.

Bearing in mind the precaution to protect and stabilize the cervical spine at all times, you should treat the patient with a head injury following these general principles, designed to protect and maintain the critical functions of the central nervous system:

1. Establish an adequate airway: if necessary, begin and maintain ventilation; and always provide high-flow supplemental oxygen.
2. Control bleeding and provide adequate circulation to maintain cerebral perfusion (institute CPR, if necessary).
3. Assess the patient's baseline level of consciousness and continuously monitor it.

In addition, you must subsequently assess and treat other injuries, splint fractures, anticipate and deal with vomiting to prevent aspiration, be prepared for convulsions, and transport the patient promptly and with extreme care.

Airway Maintenance

While you remember the possibility of a cervical spine injury, your most important step in the treatment of patients with head injury, regardless of the severity, is to establish an adequate airway. Foreign bodies, secretions, and vomitus must be removed manually and by suction from the oropharynx. In the unconscious patient, the airway may be compromised by loss of voluntary control. If the tongue obstructs the airway, use the trauma jaw-thrust or the trauma chin-lift maneuver to overcome the obstruction.

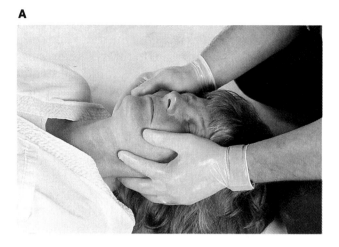

A

B

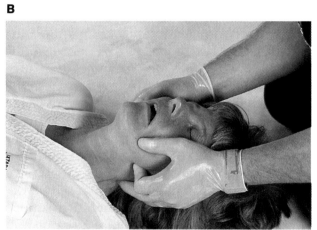

FIGURE 20–4

The trauma jaw-thrust maneuver. (A) Stabilize the patient's head and neck in a neutral in-line position. (B) Push the angle of the mandible anteriorly with the ring and little fingers of both hands.

Adequate ventilation is of equal importance. Ventilation will be inadequate if there has been damage to the respiratory control center of the brain, resulting in an ineffective rate or depth of breathing. Ventilation may also be limited by chest injuries or by paralysis of some or all of the muscles of respiration due to a spinal cord injury.

High-flow supplemental oxygen should always be given. It minimizes two problems: hypoxia (inadequate oxygenation) and cerebral edema. More than any other part of the body, the brain requires a constant, rich supply of

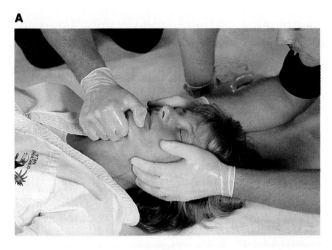

A

B

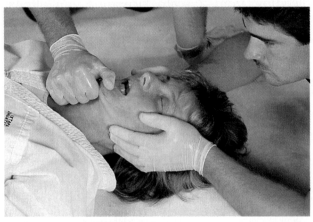

FIGURE 20–5

The trauma chin-lift maneuver. (A) One EMT stabilizes the patient's head and neck in a neutral in-line position while the second EMT grasps the chin between the thumb and the index and middle fingers. (B) While the first EMT keeps the head from moving, the second lifts the chin anteriorly to elevate the mandible and open the airway.

oxygen, and without it, severe brain damage or death may result in minutes. An injured brain is even less tolerant of hypoxia than is a normal brain. Studies have shown that the administration of supplemental oxygen can reduce brain hypoxia.

As discussed earlier, cerebral edema is another problem encountered in the patient who has a head injury. Just as other tissues swell when injured, so does the brain. There is little

extra space inside the skull. As the brain swells, the pressure inside the skull increases. This increased intracranial pressure reduces the blood flow to the brain and accentuates hypoxia. Hypoxia increases cerebral edema. The body attempts to overcome this "vicious cycle" by slowing the pulse, improving cardiac output, and raising the blood pressure. However, these compensatory mechanisms will fail at a certain point, and death will occur from uncontrolled, increased intracranial pressure, fed by the hypoxia. To a significant degree, ventilatory support and administering supplemental oxygen can limit this series of events. To be effective, these measures must be started as soon as possible. Do not wait until the patient becomes cyanotic. You must continue to ventilate and administer oxygen until the patient reaches the hospital.

Circulation

If the heart is not beating, providing airway maintenance, ventilation, and oxygen accomplishes nothing. You must initiate full CPR if cardiac arrest is present.

Furthermore, active blood loss accentuates hypoxia by reducing the available number of oxygen-carrying red blood cells. Continued blood loss must be controlled. Scalp lacerations, although they rarely alone cause shock (except in infants and children), are often associated with the loss of large volumes of blood. The blood loss accentuates hypoxia and, therefore, should be controlled. Bleeding inside the skull may elevate intracranial pressure to life-threatening levels, although the actual volume of blood lost inside the skull will be relatively small.

In the patient with a head injury, shock is usually due to hypovolemia caused by bleeding from other injuries. The occurrence of shock in such a patient, as in other trauma patients, indicates a critical situation. Such a patient must be transported immediately to a trauma center for treatment. Maintain the airway while you protect the patient's cervical spine, ensure adequate ventilation, administer 100 percent oxygen, control any obvious sites of bleeding with direct pressure, place the patient supine on a spine board, keep the patient warm, and transport the patient rapidly to the emergency department.

Cervical Spine Injury

Determining whether the patient has sustained a spine injury is often very difficult, even in a conscious patient with a head injury. There may be no neurological loss, and spine pain may not be appreciated because of shock, or the patient's attention may be directed to more painful injuries. The diagnosis is even more difficult in the unconscious patient. Because any manipulation of the unstable cervical spine may cause permanent and irreversible damage to the spinal cord, you must assume the presence of spinal injury in all patients who have sustained head injuries. Manual in-line immobilization may be replaced by a cervical collar and securing the patient to a long spine board, as described fully in Chapter 21.

Level of Consciousness

Once you have established the airway, controlled bleeding, ensured circulation, and stabilized the cervical spine, the next most important step in evaluating a patient with a head injury is to assess the level of consciousness. Use the AVPU scale or the Glasgow Coma Scale to assess the patient's initial baseline level of consciousness and record the time of this initial observation. Remember to reevaluate and document the patient's level of consciousness at least every 10 minutes until the patient reaches the hospital. Hospital medical staff will compare your baseline neurological evaluation with those done in the emergency department. With certain injuries, particularly certain types of intracerebral bleeding such as an epidural hematoma, the patient's level of consciousness will deteriorate rapidly. A patient with only moderate symptoms may suddenly lose consciousness or develop other signs indicating loss of brain function. Only with careful close observation will you be able to identify such changes and be able to respond effectively.

On occasions, particularly with some subdural hematomas, bleeding occurs slowly and the neurological changes appear only hours or days after a head injury. Therefore, whenever you assess a patient with an altered level of consciousness, specifically inquire about the possibility of a head injury in the hours or days preceding the onset of symptoms.

TREATMENT OF SPECIFIC HEAD INJURIES
· ·

Scalp Laceration

Bleeding from a scalp laceration can almost always be controlled by local manual pressure with a dry, sterile dressing applied directly over the wound. In some instances, you will have to apply firm compression for several minutes in order to control the bleeding from a scalp laceration. Sometimes triangular or square flap type lacerations of the scalp will occur. The flap of skin should be folded back down onto its bed before the compression dressing is applied. As with bleeding from other areas, you should not remove the dressing even if it becomes soaked with blood. In this case, apply a second dressing over the first one to reinforce it. Continue manual pressure until the bleeding is controlled. Once the bleeding is under control, secure the compression dressing in place with a soft, self-adhering circumferential roller bandage (Figure 20–6). If you suspect an underlying skull fracture do not apply excessive pressure to the open wound, as doing so may push fracture fragments into the brain.

Fractures

It is often difficult to diagnose a skull fracture in the field but, on occasion, bone fragments will be obvious in the depths of a scalp laceration. Treat all open fractures by applying a dry, sterile, gentle compression dressing to control bleeding. You should avoid excessive manual pressure to prevent displacement of any of the fracture fragments. Closed fractures of the skull and contusions of the scalp, which may have an underlying skull fracture, will need thor-

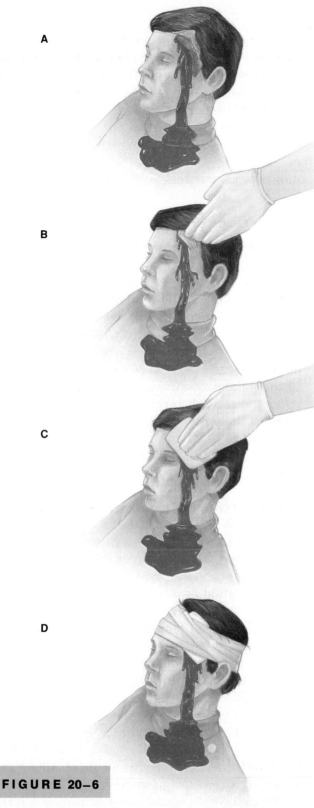

A

B

C

D

FIGURE 20-6

Scalp laceration. (A) Bleeding from a scalp laceration may be extensive; often, flap-type lacerations occur. (B) Replace the flap into its bed. (C) Apply compression with a dry, sterile bandage. (D) Once bleeding is controlled, the dressing can be secured with a soft roller bandage.

ough evaluation in the emergency department. Your attention should be directed to the airway, breathing, circulation, cervical spine, and level of consciousness. The patient should be well splinted on a spine board to prevent any further injury. Take care to avoid applying pressure to an area of the skull that may be fractured. This is particularly important in the occipital region, where prolonged pressure against the spine board may aggravate the problem. A foam rubber pad should be placed over any area of contusion or possible fracture of the skull to avoid excessive pressure on this region during transport.

Concussion

Usually a concussion lasts for only a short period of time and it may be over by the time you arrive at the scene. If the patient has any complaints consistent with a concussion, regardless of the patient's degree of recovery, observe and record the level of consciousness. Transport the patient to the hospital for close monitoring over the next several hours to ensure that progressive neurological symptoms do not develop.

Brain Contusion

Any patient who has sustained a brain contusion may exhibit any or all of the signs of brain injury. The contused brain will swell rapidly. The swelling causes increased intracranial pressure that may cause further brain damage. Therefore, the importance of adequate ventilation and the administration of oxygen cannot be overemphasized in the treatment of patients with this condition. High blood oxygen levels will decrease the amount of brain swelling and thus minimize the amount of brain damage that may occur. Monitor the patient's level of consciousness closely and transport the patient promptly to the hospital for expert neurological evaluation and care.

Intracranial Bleeding

Intracranial bleeding results in the formation of a hematoma. The patient with an expanding hematoma inside the skull often requires prompt surgical treatment to avoid permanent brain damage. When the bleeding occurs rapidly within the brain, the patient's neurological status may deteriorate within a matter of minutes. Any patient who develops rapidly progressive deterioration of the neurological signs following a head injury should be considered to have an intracranial hematoma that will require rapid evaluation and probably surgical treatment. Complete the same steps in treatment as for a cerebral contusion and transport the patient rapidly to the hospital.

Cerebrospinal Fluid Leakage

An indirect indication of a fracture of the skull is the appearance of clear or pink watery fluid dripping from the nose, from the ear, or from an open scalp wound. This cerebrospinal fluid can leak to the outside only if the dura and the skull have both been penetrated. When you see cerebrospinal fluid draining from the skull, make no attempt to pack the wound, the ear, or the nose. Firm packing of the draining site will block the escape of cerebrospinal fluid and may increase the intracranial pressure, further damaging the brain. Cover a scalp wound and its draining cerebrospinal fluid with a sterile gauze to prevent further contamination, but do not bandage it tightly.

Change in Pupil Size

The nerves that control dilation and constriction of the pupils are very sensitive to pressure within the skull. An early sign of increased intracranial pressure is a change in the pupil's response to light. When a light is shined into the eye, the pupil should constrict promptly. Failure to constrict may indicate the development of increased intracranial pressure. Unequal pupil size may also indicate increased intracranial pressure on one side of the brain.

As soon as you have assessed the patient's level of consciousness, determine the reaction of each pupil to light. The pupils should constrict promptly when light is shined into the

eye. The size of the pupil and its ability to constrict in reaction to a bright light beamed into it are important clinical signs. You should make a sketch of the size of both pupils on the ambulance report form to indicate any difference in pupil size. Any change in the reaction of the pupil over time is an extremely important observation to record since it may be an indicator of progressive brain damage.

Convulsions

It is not uncommon for the patient who has a head injury to have a convulsion or seizure as a result of the injury. Immobilization of the cervical spine and maintaining an adequate airway are difficult to achieve during a convulsion. During the episode, protect the patient from further injury. If a convulsion occurs, administer 100 percent oxygen by a face mask to the patient to minimize the risk of hypoxia. After the convulsion, be prepared to clear and support the patient's airway to assure adequate ventilation.

Positioning the Patient

The ideal position for a patient with an isolated head injury is with the head of the stretcher elevated about 6 inches to promote the drainage of blood from the brain. Once the spine is adequately immobilized, the head of the spinal immobilization device should be elevated about 6 inches to minimize brain swelling.

Bleeding into the mouth or throat, vomiting, or the accumulation of excessive mucus may obstruct the upper airway. Use suction to clear any fluids that accumulate in the upper airway (Figure 20–7). The patient should be immobilized well enough to be turned on his or her side to facilitate clearing of the airway if necessary.

Many different patterns of head injury can occur. A thorough assessment of the patient will give you a good understanding of the extent and severity of most head injuries. You must remember to protect the cervical spine at all times. It is essential to establish an adequate

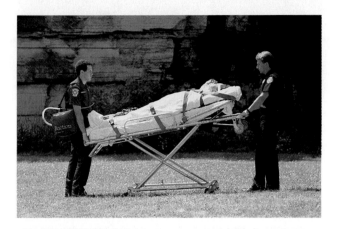

FIGURE 20-7

The patient with a head injury should be securely immobilized, with the head of the spinal immobilization device elevated about 6 inches. Suction must be available to clear any fluids that accumulate in the airway.

airway, ventilate the patient, and administer oxygen both to treat the patient and to minimize the risk of further loss of brain function. An initial assessment of the level of consciousness using either the AVPU or Glasgow Coma Scale with careful monitoring of the patient's level of consciousness will be of great assistance to the emergency department personnel in their eventual management of the patient.

YOU ARE THE EMT

1. Why is a brain contusion more serious than a brain concussion?
2. Why do you have to immobilize the patient with a head injury?
3. Why do you elevate the head of the stretcher during transport?
4. You have been called to treat a young man who is confused about where he is and is not making any sense when he talks. His mother tells you that he "walked away," apparently unhurt from an automobile accident five days ago. What kind of injury do you suspect? How serious could this problem be? How will you evaluate and treat this patient?
5. Why is it important to administer oxygen in all patients with head injuries?

INJURY TO THE SPINE

KEY TERMS

anesthesia (an"es-the'ze-ah) The loss of sensation from injury or from the administration of drugs.

intervertebral disc (in"ter-ver'tĕ-bral disk) A cushion between each two vertebral bodies.

neurogenic shock (nu"ro-jĕn'ik shok) Circulatory failure caused by paralysis of the nerves that control the size of the blood vessels, seen in spinal cord injuries.

spinal canal A tunnel formed by the back part of each vertebra that encloses and protects the spinal cord.

spinal cord An extension of the brain, composed of virtually all the nerves carrying messages between the brain and the rest of the body. It lies inside of and is protected by the spinal canal.

vertebra (ver'tĕ-brah) The 33 bones of the spinal column; there are 7 cervical, 12 thoracic, 5 lumbar, 5 sacral, and 4 coccygeal vertebrae.

Injury to the spine that damages the protection of the spinal cord can produce permanent paralysis. Over the past 15 to 20 years, since the advent of effective emergency medical services in the United States, there has been a gradual decrease in the incidence of paralysis from spinal injury. Most authorities agree that this decrease is a direct result of effective prehospital care of patients with spinal injury.

EMTs have learned how to recognize possible spinal injury even when the symptoms are not obvious. They have also learned how to clear and maintain the airway without endangering the spinal cord, how to remove helmets (and when *not* to remove them), and most important, how to splint spine injury patients. When these techniques are employed properly, they significantly minimize the risk of paralysis in the injured patient.

Chapter 21 first discusses fractures and dislocations of the spine. Next it describes the circumstances that are most likely to produce spinal injury and the symptoms and signs of spinal injury. Then the chapter explains how you decide whether spinal injury is present and how to treat spinal injuries. The last section of Chapter 21 discusses the complications of spinal cord injury.

GOALS

The goals of Chapter 21 are to
- describe fractures and dislocations of the spine.
- identify the symptoms and signs of spinal injury.
- become familiar with the circumstances that are most likely to result in a spinal injury.
- know how to diagnose spinal injury.
- learn the emergency treatment of spine injury patients.
- become familiar with the complications of spinal cord injury.

FRACTURES AND DISLOCATIONS OF THE SPINE

The spine is a segmented column of 33 **vertebrae,** which are stacked one on the next and extend from the base of the skull to the tip of the coccyx (Figure 21–1). Lying between each of the cervical, thoracic, and lumbar vertebrae are the **intervertebral discs.** The vertebrae are connected together by strong ligaments that allow a small amount of bending motion to occur between adjacent vertebrae. The ligaments, however, prevent excessive shifting of one vertebra onto the adjacent ones, creating a stable column that maintains the erect body posture. Posteriorly, each vertebra has a tunnel that extends from top to bottom (Figure 21–2). When stacked in the spinal column, the vertebrae create a bony **spinal canal** in which the **spinal cord** lies and is therefore protected.

Most injuries to the spine produce ligament sprains or nondisplaced fractures that heal well and have an excellent long-term prognosis. Sometimes, however, displaced fractures or dislocations of the spine damage the spinal cord or the nerve roots and cause permanent paralysis or even death. Distinguishing between those injuries that are not dangerous

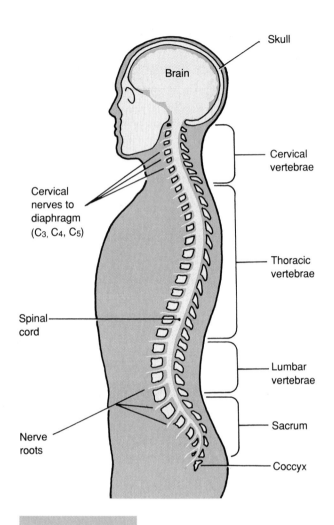

FIGURE 21–1

A lateral view of the spine shows the spinal cord lying inside the spinal canal.

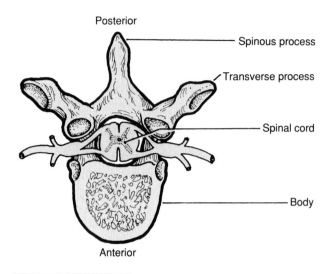

FIGURE 21–2

Top view of a typical thoracic vertebra showing how the spinal cord lies protected inside the bony spinal canal.

compress, pinch, or shear the spinal cord (Figure 21–3). This damage may make the difference between normal function and permanent paralysis. Therefore, it is imperative that no further motion occur in an unstable spine and that you provide rigid splinting of the injured spine at the scene.

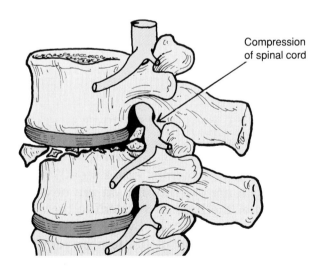

FIGURE 21–3

If the spine is unstable, even a small shift of one vertebra on the next may damage or even crush the spinal cord.

and those that may jeopardize the spinal cord is difficult and often requires special x-ray studies. At the scene of an accident you can never be certain whether the suspected spine injury is safe or dangerous, so it is best to consider *all* spine injuries as potentially dangerous and treat them as such.

If injury to the spinal column has made it unstable, it can no longer protect the spinal cord. The spinal cord fills most of the spinal canal. Even slight displacement of one vertebra on the next will narrow the spinal canal and pinch or shear the spinal cord. With an unstable fracture or dislocation, displacement of as little as one millimeter may be enough to

Recognizing a possible spinal injury is one of your major responsibilities. You should be suspicious of spinal injury when called to see any patient who has received a high-velocity injury. The types of trauma most likely to produce a spinal fracture in an adult are automobile and motorcycle accidents, gunshot wounds, shallow water diving injuries, falls from heights, and cave-ins. Children who fall from a height; fall from a bicycle, tricycle, or skateboard; or who have been struck by a moving vehicle are at high risk for a spine injury. In addition, any unconscious injured patient and any patient who has sustained a facial or scalp laceration or contusion must be assumed to have a spinal injury. Thus, when dispatched to an accident scene and when sizing up any of these injury situations, you must "think spinal injury."

The presence of a spine injury must be assumed with

- Violent impacts to the head, neck, torso, or pelvis.
- Sudden acceleration or deceleration accidents.
- Falls from a significant height with the patient landing on the head or feet.
- Gunshot wounds to the neck or trunk.
- All shallow water diving accidents.
- All unrestrained victims of a vehicular crash.

SIGNS AND SYMPTOMS OF SPINAL INJURY

You must be able to recognize those symptoms (complaints of the patient) and signs (those physical findings) that indicate the possibility of spinal injury. When combined with the circumstances surrounding the injury, the signs and symptoms enable you to manage the problem in a rational way.

Symptoms

Pain A conscious patient will be aware of pain in the spine and be able to direct your attention to the area of injury in the back or neck. However, with an unconscious patient, this most important and reliable symptom will *not* be present. Occasionally, a conscious patient with a spine injury will not complain of pain. This sometimes happens because the patient is lying very still ("splinting" the injury) or perhaps because other, more painful injuries are distracting the patient's attention from the spine injury.

Numbness, Tingling, or Weakness If the conscious patient complains of tingling, loss of feeling, or weakness in one or more of the extremities, spinal cord damage probably exists. Therefore, it is essential to evaluate and monitor the basic neurologic function of every injured patient at the scene.

Pain with Movement If the patient attempts to move the injured area of the spine, pain may occur or increase significantly. You should *never* try to test this increase in pain by moving the patient. Do not encourage anyone with neck or back pain to move. Proceed immediately with splinting.

Signs

Deformity Deformity of the spine is a certain indication that significant injury has occurred. However, most patients with spinal fractures and spinal cord injury do not have an obvious deformity. It occurs only in a severe injury with marked displacement of the bony fragments. Absence of a deformity in no way eliminates the possibility of a fracture or dislocation of the spine. When it is present, deformity is most often seen in the cervical spine with the head twisted or cocked to one side.

Tenderness Point tenderness over any portion of the spine is sufficient reason to suspect spinal injury. The spinous processes of all cervical, thoracic, and lumbar vertebrae can be palpated posteriorly in the midline. The spines of the seventh cervical (C_7) and the first thoracic (T_1) vertebrae are especially prominent at the base of the neck. Point tenderness anywhere along the spinous processes is a strong indication of a significant spinal injury.

Lacerations or Contusions Cuts and bruises are reliable signs that strong forces have been applied to the body. Almost all cervical spine fractures or dislocations result from a blow to the head. Therefore, any cut or bruise on the head or face is a very reliable indication that spinal injury may be present (Figure 21–4). Patients with serious injuries in other areas of the spine are likely to have bruises over the shoulders, the back, or the abdomen.

Paralysis or Anesthesia You should consider any weakness or **anesthesia** (loss of sensation) that can be demonstrated on physical examination to be a sign of spinal injury. You should touch the patient's fingers, toes, arms, and legs to assess feeling in these regions. Test muscle function through the strength of the grip by asking the patient to squeeze your fingers. You can test lower extremity strength by asking the patient to move his or her feet up and down. Assume that any injured patient who exhibits loss of sensation or weakness has a spinal cord injury.

Spinal cord injuries in the neck may cause paralysis of all four extremities as well as impairment of breathing. Spinal fractures at the level of the waist may cause numbness and/or paralysis below that level, but breathing as well

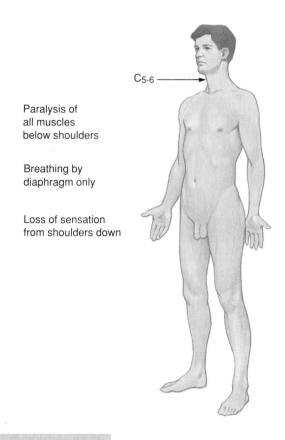

Paralysis of all muscles below shoulders

Breathing by diaphragm only

Loss of sensation from shoulders down

C5-6

FIGURE 21–5

The blue area indicates the region of numbness and paralysis from a spinal cord injury at the level of the fifth and sixth cervical vertebrae.

as strength and sensation in the upper extremities will not be affected (Figure 21–5).

DIAGNOSIS OF SPINAL INJURY

You should suspect a spinal injury whenever you arrive at an accident caused by any of the mechanisms described earlier. All patients so injured must be evaluated for the possibility of a spinal injury. In the conscious patient, you can take the following five steps to determine the presence of a possible spinal injury.

1. Ask the patient or witnesses about the nature of the accident.
2. Question the patient carefully about areas of pain, numbness, or weakness.
3. Look for contusions, lacerations, and abra-

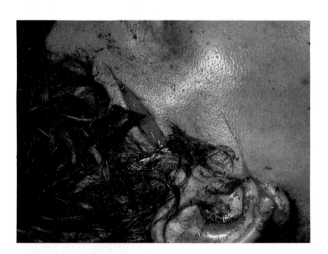

FIGURE 21–4

Lacerations of the head should make you suspect a spinal injury.

sions about the face, head, or trunk and look for any deformity of the spine.

4. Feel for any irregularity, deformity, or point tenderness along the spinous processes posteriorly. Check the arms and legs for decreased sensation.
5. Check for weakness or paralysis by asking the patient to wiggle his or her fingers and toes, unassisted.

If any one of these five signs or symptoms is present, you should assume that a spine injury has occurred and undertake appropriate splinting. No further manipulation of the spine by either the patient or you should be performed. The patient should not be allowed to move until spinal immobilization is complete.

Sometimes you will suspect a spinal injury in a patient who has been involved in a car wreck, shooting incident, fall from a great height, or some other high-velocity accident. Yet the patient does not complain of pain, numbness, or weakness, and no soft tissue injury or deformity is evident. No point tenderness can be elicited on palpation of the spine, and no numbness or weakness exists in the extremities. When this situation exists and you still suspect the presence of a spinal injury because of the mechanism of injury, the patient should be instructed to slowly and carefully move the spine to see whether motion produces pain at a specific location. Instruct the patient to bend his or her head forward, backward, and to each side gently and carefully. Then have the patient slowly bend forward from the waist. If any of these motions causes pain in this otherwise symptom-free patient, spinal injury must be considered a possibility. Of course, this step should never be performed if any of the other signs or symptoms described earlier are present or if the patient is unreliable or uncooperative.

The unconscious patient presents a more difficult problem. This person cannot cooperate with the full evaluation, and thus you cannot identify many of the signs and symptoms present in the conscious patient. Whenever unconsciousness has resulted from an accident that is known to be associated with spinal injury, you must assume that the patient has an associated spinal injury until proven otherwise.

EMERGENCY TREATMENT OF SPINAL INJURY

Proper emergency care of a spinal injury may prevent the need for extensive medical care and permanent disability. You have the opportunity to prevent paralysis and death. On the other hand, failure to diagnose a possible spinal injury or ineffective splinting of the unstable spine might cause significant, long-term problems for the patient.

The emergency care of spinal injury follows the same rules as emergency care for all other major injuries:

- Restore the patient's airway and ensure adequate ventilation.
- Control serious bleeding using local pressure dressings.
- Most importantly, splint the patient before you move him or her.

Restoring the Airway

You must always be aware of the danger of causing permanent paralysis through improper handling of the patient with a spine injury. However, this possibility should not prevent you from providing an open airway for the patient, because the patient will die if he or she remains unable to breathe. When a patient with a spine injury also has an obstructed airway, you should restore an adequate airway by using the trauma jaw-thrust or trauma chin-lift maneuver described in Chapter 20. The head-tilt/chin-lift maneuver should not be used, because it extends the neck and may cause further damage to the cervical spine. In the unconscious patient, you can lift or pull the tongue forward out of the pharynx to avoid any manipulation of the neck. If this maneuver is successful, maintain the airway with an oropharyngeal airway, but monitor it closely. Suctioning equipment must be available, because the airway will frequently need to be cleared of blood, saliva, or vomitus. Oxygen should be given to any patient with marginally effective respirations.

If these maneuvers do not relieve airway obstruction, you must improve the alignment of the neck to open the airway. Firmly grasp the patient's head with both hands and pull the head gently and firmly away from the trunk and turn it to the front, bringing the head to the "eyes forward" position (Figure 21–6). Then, maintain the head in the new in-line position while you repeat the jaw-thrust maneuver to open the airway. Alternatively, while one EMT maintains the in-line position, a second EMT can perform the trauma chin-lift maneuver to open the airway. Always avoid extreme extension and flexion of the head on the trunk, because these are the positions in which spinal cord damage is most likely to occur. Once the airway is open, hold the head in the new position with manual in-line support until it can be fully splinted.

Helmet Removal

Many patients with neck injuries are motorcyclists or football players who may be wearing protective helmets. In the majority of instances, the helmet does not need to be removed. Indeed, it is frequently fitted so snugly to the head that it can be secured directly to the spinal immobilization device. There are only four circumstances in which part or all of the helmet should be removed:

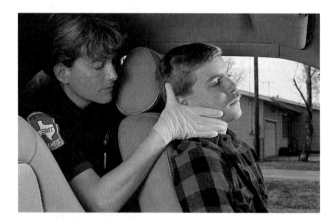

FIGURE 21–6

When alignment of the neck must be improved to establish an airway, grasp the head firmly with two hands and bring it back to the neutral in-line position.

- When the face mask or visor interferes with adequate ventilation or with your ability to restore an adequate airway.
- When the helmet is so loose that securing it to the spinal immobilization device will not provide adequate immobilization of the patient's head.
- When life-threatening hemorrhage under the helmet can only be controlled by its removal.
- When, because of the size of the helmet, using it as a part of the spinal immobilization will cause extreme flexion of the neck (this situation usually occurs in children).

When part of the helmet is interfering with ventilation, lift the visor of a motorcycle helmet away from the face or remove the face guard of a football helmet. Most football face guards are fastened to the helmet by four rubber clips. These clips can be cut easily with a sharp knife or scissors and the face guard removed (Figure 21–7). The chin strap should also be loosened to facilitate the chin-lift or jaw-thrust maneuvers. In most instances, exposing the face and jaw will allow access to the airway to secure adequate ventilation. Only when these steps do not allow adequate access to the airway should you remove the entire helmet.

The second indication for helmet removal is a loose helmet that cannot be adequately incorporated into the spinal immobilization device. Such a loose helmet can be removed quite easily. Severe uncontrolled hemorrhage from the face or scalp may occur on rare occasions beneath a helmet. In order to control the bleeding, helmet removal may be required.

Certain protective helmets are very large and, when secured to a spinal immobilization device, they will force the head to flex forward. Always avoid extreme flexion of the injured cervical spine. Such a helmet should be removed or a folded blanket or other sufficient padding should be placed between the patient's shoulders and the spine board to ensure that the spine is straight when immobilization is complete.

When, for one of these reasons, the helmet must be removed, the following specific proto-

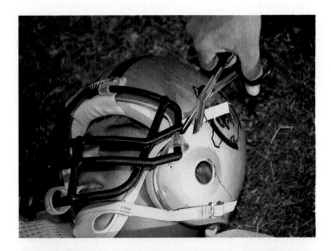

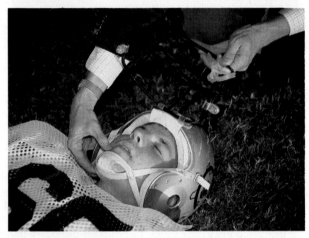

FIGURE 21–7

When airway access must be achieved in an injured football player, the face guard can be removed by (top) cutting the clips that attach it to the helmet and (bottom) lifting it out of the way.

col should be followed. Note that this procedure requires two EMTs.

1. First EMT: Stand or kneel above the patient's head and support the head in an in-line neutral position by placing a hand on each side of the helmet with your fingers on the patient's mandible or on the lower edge of a full face helmet (Figure 21–8a).
2. Second EMT: Cut or loosen the chin strap while the first EMT maintains head support (Figure 21–8b).

3. Second EMT: Place one of your hands on the patient's mandible with your thumb on one side and the long and index fingers on the opposite side. Place your other hand behind the patient's neck and apply firm pressure to the occipital region. This maneuver transfers the in-line support from the first to the second EMT (Figure 21–8c).
4. First EMT: Remove the helmet, remembering that it is usually egg-shaped and therefore must be expanded laterally to clear the ears. (Many football helmets have jaw pads that will be caught on the ears if they are not removed first.) If the helmet provides full facial coverage, it must be tilted backward first to avoid striking the nose. Once the nose is cleared, pull off the helmet from the head in a straight line (Figure 21–8d).
5. Second EMT: Throughout the removal process, maintain in-line support from below to prevent tilting of the head. As the helmet is removed, move your hand supporting the head superiorly so that it remains in contact with the edge of the helmet and fully supports the occiput as the head comes free (Figure 21–8e).
6. First EMT: After removing the helmet, place your hands on either side of the patient's head, firmly grasping the mandible and base of the skull, to provide stable in-line support until the patient is adequately splinted (Figure 21–8f, g).

During helmet removal, one EMT is always providing immobilization while the other EMT moves. Both EMTs never move at the same time. You should keep in mind that helmet removal is often not necessary. If adequate access to the airway can be obtained and maintained, and if the head is secure inside the helmet, the helmet can be left in place and secured to the spinal immobilization device to provide adequate splinting of the spinal injury. With large helmets or small patients, it may be necessary to place a support under the shoulders when the spinal immobilization device is applied to avoid flexion of the neck.

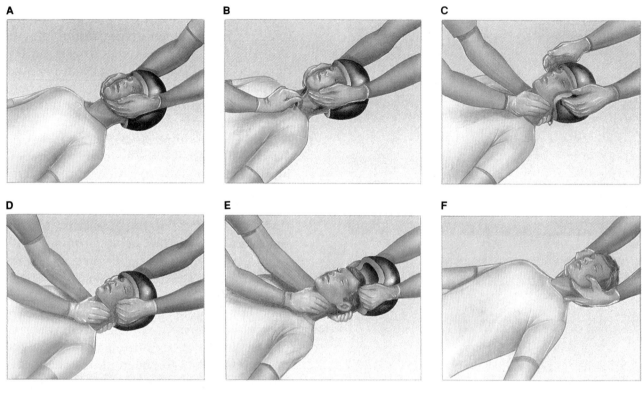

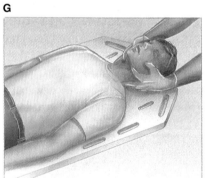

FIGURE 21–8

The proper steps of helmet removal are illustrated. (A) One EMT supports the head by placing a hand on each side of the patient's mandible. (B) The chin strap is loosened. (C) The second EMT places one hand on the mandible, the thumb on one angle, and the long and index fingers at the other angle. With the other hand, the second EMT supports the neck. (D) The first EMT removes the helmet with as little motion of the head as is possible. The helmet must be expanded to clear the ears and rotated to clear the nose. (E) The second EMT moves hand up to support occiput instead of neck. (F) After helmet removal, the first EMT resumes support of the head with hands on both sides of the patient's head, the palms over the ears, and the mandible supported by the fingers. (G) Head support is maintained until the patient is fully splinted.

Splinting of Spinal Injuries

Once you suspect a spinal injury, make all efforts to avoid damage to the spinal cord. Once the airway is secure, it is imperative for you to stabilize the head and trunk by manual in-line immobilization so that any displaced bone fragments will not impinge upon the spinal cord. Further abnormal motion—even as little as 1 millimeter—may cause significant spinal cord injury. Immediately, you must begin stabilization by holding the head firmly with two hands. Whenever possible, get behind the patient and place each hand around the base of the skull, supporting the mandible with the index and long fingers and the occiput with the thumbs and palms (Figure 21–9). Gently lift the head to the position where the patient's eyes are looking straight ahead and the head and torso are in line. *At no time* should the head or neck be twisted or excessively

A

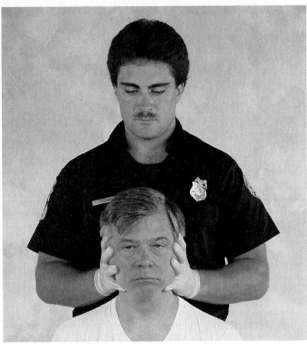

B

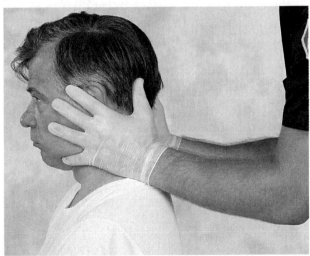

FIGURE 21–9

(A and B) Manual in-line immobilization is accomplished by placing both hands on the patient's ears with the thumbs and palms against the back of the skull. The little fingers are placed under the angle of the mandible.

flexed or extended. Moving the head to this neutral in-line position will facilitate splinting. Once accomplished, this neutral in-line position must be maintained until the patient is

examined in the hospital. Manual support must continue until the patient is completely secured to the spinal immobilization device.

In certain circumstances, movement of the head to the neutral in-line position should not be pursued. You should not force the head into this position if

- Neck muscle spasm occurs.
- Pain increases.
- Numbness, tingling, or weakness develops.
- The airway or ventilations become compromised.

In these circumstances, stop and immobilize the patient in the deformed position.

Cervical Collars Preliminary, partial cervical spine immobilization is provided by an appropriately sized, firm extrication collar. Although cervical collars are used routinely in spinal immobilization, they do not fully immobilize the cervical spine. They only provide partial support. Therefore, manual support must continue even after the collar is applied and until the patient is completely secured to a spinal immobilization device.

A cervical extrication collar should be rigid and be of the correct size for the patient. You must carry a variety of sizes to ensure proper fit for all patients. The collar should rest on the shoulder girdle and provide firm support under both mandibles. It must not prevent the patient or you from opening the mouth to clear the airway and it should never obstruct ventilation in any way (Figure 21–10). While one EMT provides continuous in-line support of the head manually, a second EMT selects and applies the appropriately sized collar.

Full Spinal Immobilization After the cervical extrication collar is in place, you should proceed to immobilize the entire spine as one unit using a spinal immobilization device. Many effective devices are available for use. You must be thoroughly familiar with the devices available in your EMS system. With all devices, the following general principles should be followed:

1. Maintain and support an adequate airway and ventilation at all times.

A

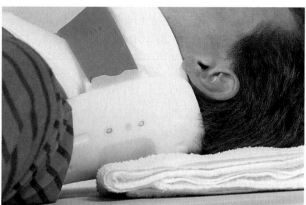

B

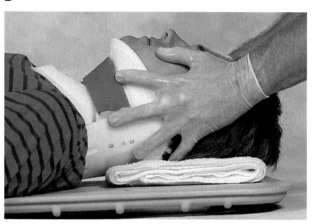

FIGURE 21–10

(A and B) An appropriately sized firm extrication collar provides partial support of the cervical spine.

2. Ensure and maintain in-line support of the entire spine throughout the entire splinting process.
3. Apply a properly sized cervical extrication collar as described previously.
4. Secure the patient's torso to the spinal extrication device before securing the head.
5. Avoid hyperextension or hyperflexion of the neck when you secure the head. In most adults, the neutral in-line position will create a space between the head and the spinal immobilization device. Adequate padding should be placed between the head and the device (Figure 21–11). In contrast, small children will need padding placed between the shoulders and the device to prevent

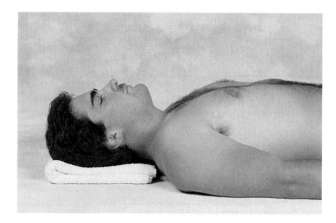

FIGURE 21–11

An adult usually requires some padding placed under the head to avoid excessive neck extension.

hyperflexion of the neck when secured to the device. This situation occurs because the child's head is relatively large, and securing the child to a flat surface naturally forces the head to flex on the trunk (Figure 21–12).
6. Secure all straps snugly to minimize motion; however, they should not restrict chest expansion or circulation to the limbs.
7. Be certain that the patient's mouth can be opened to clear the airway.
8. Secure the patient well to the spinal immobilization device with the head, torso, and

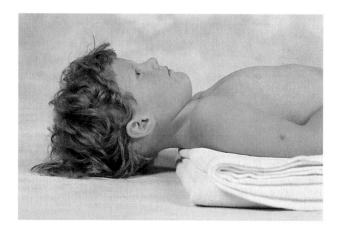

FIGURE 21–12

A child usually requires some padding placed under the shoulders to avoid excessive neck flexion.

pelvis aligned so that no motion will occur between any of these parts during movement and transport. The patient should be so well secured that the entire unit can be turned to one side to facilitate airway management or vertical extrication if necessary (Figure 21–13).

The specific details of complete spinal immobilization will depend on the particular devices used by your EMS system. Two commonly used methods, one with the patient lying down and the other with the patient seated, are described here.

The patient who is found lying down can be effectively immobilized using a long spine

A

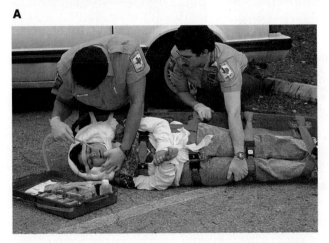

B

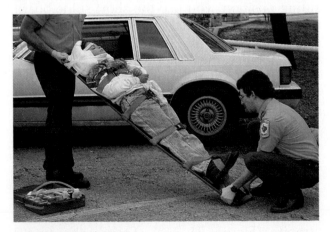

FIGURE 21–13

(A and B) When properly secured to the spinal immobilization device, the patient may be safely turned on one side or lifted vertically.

board. While one EMT continuously supports the head manually, a second EMT places a firm extrication collar around the neck to provide some stability (Figure 21–14a). Remember that the extrication collar provides some support, but it will not replace the support given by your hands. Maintain manual support of the head until the patient is fully secured to the spine board.

When found lying prone, the patient is turned as a unit, with one EMT supporting the head to be certain that the entire head-torso-pelvis complex moves in unison. Then, using the *four-person log roll* (or the *straddle slide* if necessary) as described in Chapter 46, the patient is transferred as a unit to the board, avoiding any rotation of the head, shoulders, or pelvis. Bystanders can be recruited to assist if necessary, but you must instruct them fully before the patient is moved.

Once the patient is centered on the long spine board, secure the upper torso to the board with long straps (Figure 21–14b).

Using a strap over the iliac crests or groin loops, secure the pelvis to the long board (Figure 21–14c).

Place padding under the head (adult) or under the shoulders (child) so that the body is entirely supported in the in-line position (Figure 21–14d).

Secure the head to the board with two straps: one over the forehead and the second over the pads and the cervical collar (Figure 21–14e).

Secure the legs to the board with straps above and below the knees (Figure 21–14f).

Place the arms securely under the pelvic straps so that they do not flop around during transport (Figure 21–14g). Alternatively, the patient's wrists can be tied loosely together with a cravat or soft rolled bandage (Figure 21–14h).

Remember that with small children padding may be needed under the shoulders to avoid flexion of the neck. In addition, because of their small size, blanket rolls should be placed between the child and the sides of the adult size board to prevent the child from slipping to the side (Figure 21–15). Appropriately sized pediatric spine boards are also available for children.

A

B

C

D

E

F

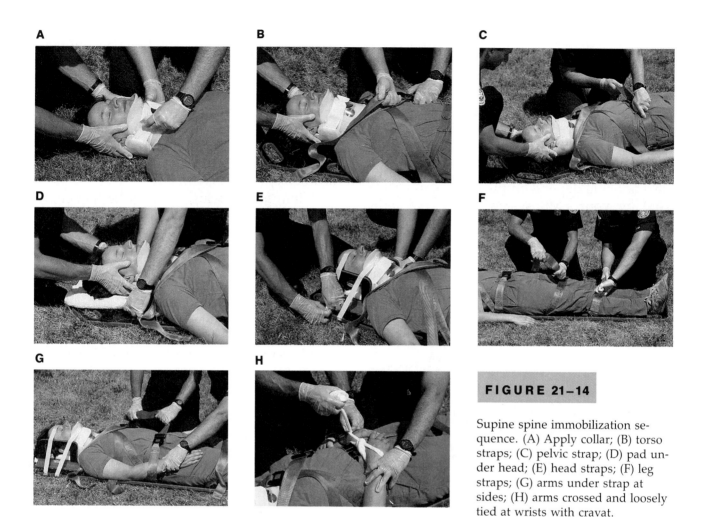

FIGURE 21-14

Supine spine immobilization sequence. (A) Apply collar; (B) torso straps; (C) pelvic strap; (D) pad under head; (E) head straps; (F) leg straps; (G) arms under strap at sides; (H) arms crossed and loosely tied at wrists with cravat.

G

H

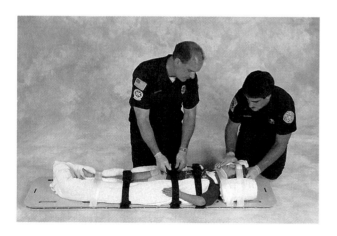

FIGURE 21-15

Place blanket rolls between a child and the sides of a spine board to prevent slipping.

When a spine injury patient is found in a sitting position, you use the short spine board or other short spinal extrication devices to splint the cervical and thoracic spine. First, you must stabilize the head with two hands and secure the airway. Gently bring the head to the "eyes-forward" position if pain or resistance is not encountered. Then apply the firm extrication collar while you continue in-line support of the head (Figure 21–16a). Then wedge the spinal extrication device between the patient's buttocks and the seat (Figure 21–16b). Open the side flaps and place them around the patient's torso, under the arms snugly in the armpits (Figure 21–16c). Secure the upper torso straps. Next, secure the midtorso straps (Figure 21–16d). Position and fasten both groin

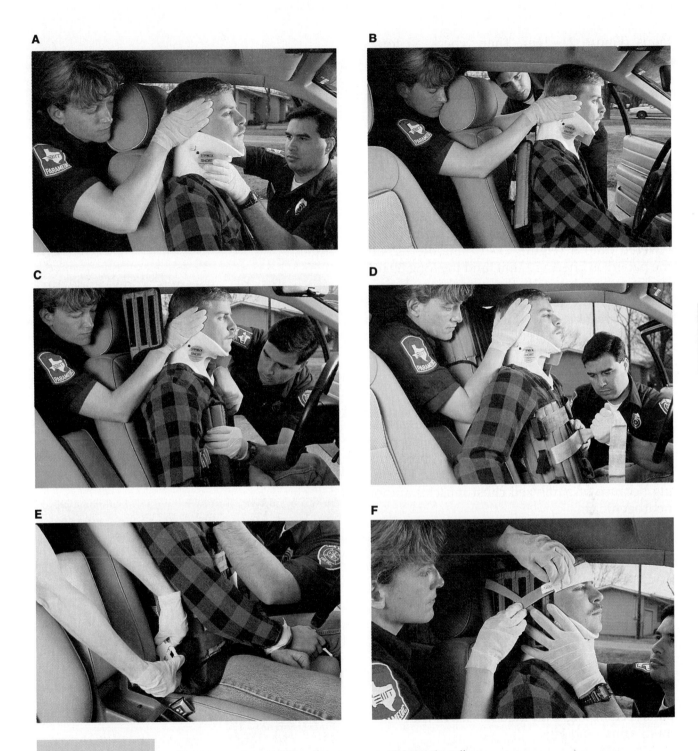

FIGURE 21—16 Seated spine immobilization sequence. (A) Apply collar.
(B) Wedge device behind patient. (C) Position side
straps. (D) Secure torso straps. (E) Secure groin loops.
(F) Secure head straps.

loops (Figure 21–16e). Then, check all torso straps to be certain they are secure. Next, pad any space between the occiput and the upper portion of the device. Secure the forehead strap and then the lower head strap around the cervical collar (Figure 21–16f).

The next step is to place the partially immobilized patient on the long spine board. The long board is placed next to the patient's buttocks, perpendicular to the trunk (Figure 21–17, top). The patient is turned to a parallel position with the long board and then slowly lowered onto it (Figure 21–17, middle). Then the patient is lifted as a unit, and the long board is slipped underneath the extrication device. The extrication device and the long board are then secured together (Figure 21–17, bottom).

COMPLICATIONS OF SPINAL CORD INJURY

In addition to paralysis and numbness, the patient with a spine fracture and spinal cord injury may develop two specific problems before reaching the hospital: impaired breathing because of paralyzed chest muscles and/or neurogenic shock.

Impaired Breathing

The motor nerves which supply the diaphragm branch off the spinal cord high in the neck (C_3, C_4, and C_5), and are rarely injured by fractures or dislocations of the cervical spine (see Figure 21–5). However, the nerves that control the chest wall muscles leave the spinal cord below the neck region. If the spinal cord is damaged at the midcervical level, these nerves will be paralyzed, along with the muscles of the abdomen, arms, and legs.

A patient with a spinal cord injury whose chest wall muscles and abdominal muscles have been paralyzed can breathe only with the diaphragm. As you observe the pattern of breathing in this patient, the chest wall will move only slightly. In contrast, because of the motion of the diaphragm, the abdomen will move in and out with each respiration. The respirations will be weak and rapid so that the

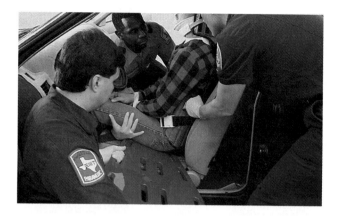

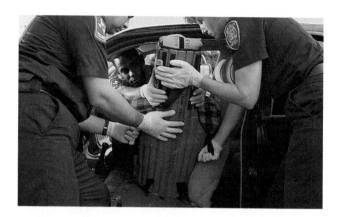

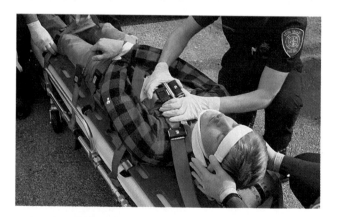

FIGURE 21–17

Once secured to the short board, the patient is placed on the long board for transport to the hospital. The long board is placed perpendicular to the patient's buttocks (top). The patient is turned and lowered onto the long board (middle). The two boards are then secured together (bottom).

patient may seem to be panting. These signs indicate the diaphragm is the only muscle supporting respiration. When the diaphragm is unable to substitute adequately for the paralyzed chest and abdominal muscles, the person with spinal cord damage will have respiratory insufficiency. You should monitor the patient's breathing, suction as necessary, and provide high-flow oxygen-enriched air. If the nerves to the diaphragm are injured as well, complete ventilatory support will be required for the patient to survive.

Neurogenic Shock

Neurogenic shock results from paralysis of the nerves that control the size of the blood vessels. The arteries and veins of a paralyzed person increase in size (dilate), particularly in the abdomen and lower extremities. This dilation of the blood vessels increases the volume of the circulatory system and consequently decreases the blood pressure. The circulatory system may fail, because not enough blood can be returned to the heart. This problem will be made even worse by hemorrhage at another site of injury.

The treatment for neurogenic shock is to splint the spine and put the patient in the *Trendelenburg* (shock) *position* by elevating the foot of the long spine board. This position will help blood to drain from the enlarged vessels in the abdomen and lower extremities and return to the heart for active circulation. The foot of the spine board should be elevated about 12 inches. Excessive elevation should be avoided, because it may cause the bowels and other abdominal organs to fall against the underside of the diaphragm and compromise the patient's principal remaining breathing mechanism. Twelve inches of elevation is sufficient to assist blood in its return to the heart and will not significantly impair the work of the diaphragm.

YOU ARE THE EMT

1. How can you determine whether a spinal injury is minor or serious? What are the major signs and symptoms of possible spinal injury?
2. What are the most common circumstances associated with a spinal injury?
3. You restored the airway and carefully splinted a spine injury patient. During transport she develops impaired breathing. What could be causing this problem, and how will you treat it?
4. You are "on duty" at the local football game. One of the players is down and you are evaluating him. He does not have any numbness, tingling, or weakness in his fingers or toes. He says he just had the wind knocked out of him and feels fine now. He wants to get up and walk back to the bench. What will you do?
5. What is neurogenic shock? How should you treat it?
6. What are the important differences between adults and children that must be considered when you are immobilizing the spine?

CHAPTER 22

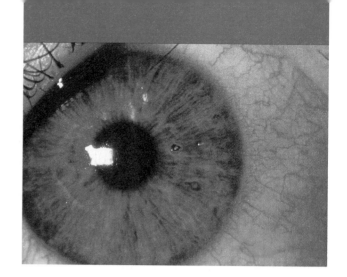

INJURIES OF THE EYE

KEY TERMS

blowout fracture Fracture of the orbit (eye socket) or of the bones that support the floor of the orbit.

conjunctiva (kon"junk-ti'vah) The delicate membrane that lines the eyelids and covers the exposed surface of the eye.

conjunctivitis (kon-junk"tĭ-vi' tis) Inflammation of the conjunctiva.

cornea (kor'ne-ah) The transparent tissue layer in front of the pupil and iris of the eye.

globe The eyeball.

hyphema (hi-fe'mah) Bleeding into the anterior chamber of the eye, obscuring the iris.

iris (i'ris) The muscle and surrounding tissue behind the cornea that dilate and constrict the pupil, regulating the amount of light that enters the eye.

lacrimal system (lak'rĭ-mal sis'tem) The tear glands and ducts of the eyes.

lens The transparent part of the eye, through which images are focused on the retina.

optic nerve (op' tik nerv) A cranial nerve that transmits visual sensations to the brain.

orbit The eye socket.

pupil The circular opening in the middle of the iris of the eye.

retina The light-sensitive area of the eye where images are projected; a layer of cells at the back of the eye that changes the light image into electrical impulses, which are carried by the optic nerve to the brain.

retinal detachment A condition in which the retina is separated from its attachments at the back of the eye.

sclera (skle'rah) The white portion of the eye; the tough outer coat of the eye that gives protection to the delicate, light-sensitive inner layer.

OVERVIEW

The eye is an organ of special sense, developed for vision. It is an optical system similar to that of a camera. The lens focuses an image on the retina, where special sensory cells change it into an electrical message carried by the optic nerves to the optic centers of the brain. The brain receives and interprets this sensory message. This entire process is what is called vision or sight. Accidents involving the eyes are frequent—sport, car, industrial, household, or environmental. Eye injury is serious, often painful, and potentially disabling. Correct initial emergency treatment by you will minimize pain and may very well help prevent permanent loss of vision. The first part of Chapter 22 presents the anatomy of the eye. The major part of the chapter is devoted to explaining the emergency treatment of injuries of the eye caused by foreign bodies, burns, lacerations, or blunt and penetrating trauma. Eye abnormalities that alert the EMT to suspect underlying head injury are discussed next. In the last section, contact lenses and eye prostheses are considered.

GOALS

The goals of Chapter 22 are to
- know the anatomy of the eye.
- know how to recognize and suspect various eye injuries.
- know the principles of correct emergency treatment for each type of injury: foreign bodies, burns, lacerations, blunt or penetrating wounds, and impaled objects.
- recognize abnormalities of the eyes that may indicate underlying head injury.
- know how to recognize the existence of an artificial eye or contact lens and what to do with it.

ANATOMY OF THE EYE

Like a fine camera, the eye has many intricate parts; all are important if the eye is to function properly (Figure 22–1). The eye is globe-shaped and approximately 1 inch in diameter. The shape of the **globe** (the eyeball) is maintained by the pressure of the fluid contained within it. The fluid toward the back of the eye, behind the lens, is clear and jellylike and is called the *vitreous humor*. The fluid in front of the lens is more watery and is called the *aqueous humor*. When the globe is lacerated, one or both of these fluids may leak out.

The **cornea** (surface covering the front part of the globe) is clear and transparent so that light may enter the eye. The rest of the surface of the globe, the white part of the eye, is made of a tough tissue called the **sclera**. In the visible portion of the eye, the sclera is covered by a smooth moist membrane called the **conjunctiva**. The conjunctiva also covers the undersurface of the eyelids. Thus, when the lids move, the two smooth, moist conjunctival surfaces slide over one another. Inflammation of the conjunctiva gives the eye a characteristic red color that is called **conjunctivitis** ("pink eye").

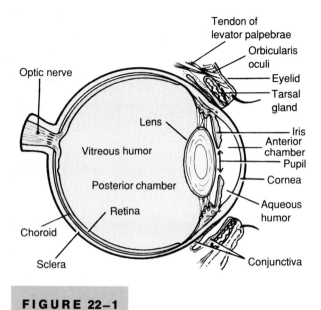

FIGURE 22–1

The major components of the eyeball (the globe).

A circular muscle lies just behind the cornea with an opening in its center. Just like a camera, this muscle adjusts the size of the opening to regulate the amount of light that enters the eye. The circular muscle and its surrounding tissue are called the **iris.** The amount of pigment in this tissue gives the eye its characteristic brown, green, or blue color. The circular opening in the middle of the muscle is called the **pupil.** The pupil becomes smaller in bright light and larger in dim light. The pupil also becomes smaller when an individual is viewing near objects and larger for those farther away. These automatic adjustments occur almost instantaneously when the individual is looking at any object.

Behind the iris is the **lens,** which focuses an image on the light-sensitive layer at the back of the globe, the **retina.** The retina is composed of several layers of cells at the back of the eye which change the light image into electrical impulses that can be carried by the **optic nerve** to the brain. Between the retina and the sclera at the back of the globe is a layer of blood vessels that nourishes the eye, especially the

retina. This layer is called the *choroid.* The retina and choroid are held against the sclera by the pressure of the vitreous humor.

The upper and lower eyelids protect the eyes. Recall that the inside of the eyelids is covered with the very smooth conjunctiva, which is continuously moistened by tears. The upper eyelid covers most of the surface of the eye and is shaped by a tough internal fibrous plate (the *tarsal plate*).

The **lacrimal system** consists of *lacrimal (tear) glands* and *tear ducts* (Figure 22–2). This system is important for protection of the eye. Lacrimal glands produce tears that act as a lubricating substance to prevent the conjunctiva covering the front of the eye from drying. Tears also flush foreign material from the surface of the eye. Small tear glands are located in the conjunctiva, and a large gland is located beneath the upper outer eyelid. Tear ducts are located on the inner side of the eye along the upper and lower lids. They drain the tears into the nose.

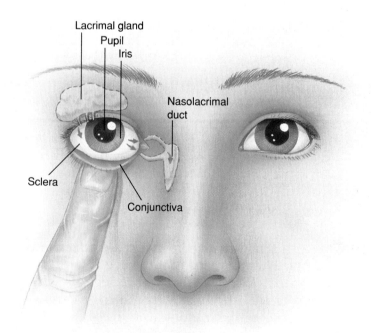

FIGURE 22–2

The lacrimal system (shown in beige) consists of tear glands and ducts. Tears act as lubricants and keep the front of the eye from drying out.

INJURIES OF THE EYE

Eye injuries are common, particularly in sports (Figure 22–3). Following an eye injury, a substantial proportion of patients may develop severe complications including blindness. Proper emergency care of the injured eye first requires a thorough examination to determine the extent and nature of any damage. The examination should be performed with great care to avoid aggravating the problem. Correct initial emergency treatment will minimize pain and may very well help prevent permanent loss of vision.

Following an injury to the eye, you must look for certain specific abnormalities or conditions. Swollen or lacerated eyelids can be produced by blunt or penetrating injury. The conjunctiva frequently becomes bright red from bleeding soon after irritation or injury. The damaged cornea readily loses its smooth, wet appearance.

In a normal, uninjured eye, the entire circle of the iris is visible; the pupils are round and equal in size; both eyes move together in the same direction when following your moving finger; and each pupil reacts equally with the other when exposed to light. After injury, pupil reaction or shape and eye movement are often disturbed. When any of these conditions is observed, you must suspect an injury of the globe or its associated tissues. Sometimes, abnormalities of pupillary reaction signify brain rather than eye injury; if there is no evidence of brain injury, an abnormal pupillary response is a good sign of eye damage.

Principal elements of the history are important. Always note and record:

- The patient's eye complaints (their severity and duration).
- The details of how the injury occurred.
- Any reported changes in vision.
- The use of any eye medications.
- The history of any previous eye operations.

Foreign Bodies in the Eye

Although large objects may be prevented from penetrating the eye by the bony **orbit** (eye

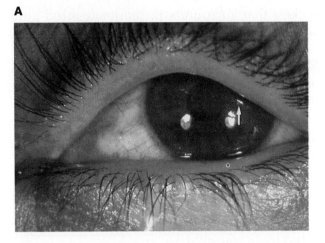
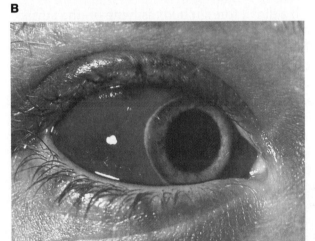
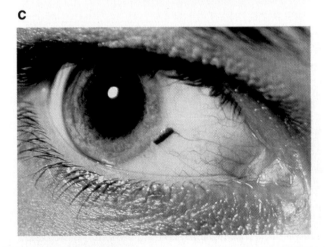

FIGURE 22–3

Common eye injuries include: (A) Corneal abrasion (white arrow), (B) subconjunctival hemorrhage, (C) foreign body on the conjunctiva.

socket) that surrounds it, moderate-sized and smaller foreign bodies of many different types can enter the eye and cause significant damage. Even a very small foreign body such as a grain of sand lying on the surface of the conjunctiva of the eye may cause severe irritation. The conjunctiva becomes inflamed and red almost immediately (Figure 22–4). The eye will begin to produce tears in an attempt to flush out the irritating object. Intense pain is produced by irritation of the cornea or conjunctiva. The patient may have difficulty keeping the eyelids open because the irritation is further aggravated by bright light.

If a small foreign body is lying on the surface of the patient's eye (Figure 22–3c), the eye should be irrigated gently with a normal saline solution. Irrigation with 500 to 1,000 ml of saline will frequently flush away loose, small particles. If a small bulb syringe is at hand, use it; a round nasal airway or cannula can be used to direct the saline into the affected eye. Always flush from the nose side of the eye toward the outside, to avoid flushing material into the other eye. After it is flushed away, a foreign body will often leave a small abrasion on the surface of the conjunctiva that will cause the patient to continue to complain of irritation

although the particle has been removed.

Foreign bodies stuck to the cornea or lying under the upper eyelid usually do not wash out with gentle irrigation. The undersurface of the upper eyelid may be examined for the presence of a foreign body. The upper lid should be everted (pulled forward) and upward away from the eyeball. If a foreign body is found on the undersurface of the lid, it can often be removed with a moist, sterile, cotton-tipped applicator (Figure 22–5). Never attempt to remove a foreign body that is stuck to the cornea.

Foreign bodies ranging in size from a pencil to a sliver of metal may be impaled in the eye (Figure 22–6). They must be removed by a physician. Bandage the object in place to support it. Cover the eye itself with a moist, sterile dressing and then surround the object by a collar fashioned from roller gauze or a small gauze pack. The object and the gauze collar can be stabilized by a roller bandage surrounding the head (Figure 22–7). If a significant length of foreign object is visible, it must be well stabilized to avoid any further leverage damage of the eye. Even though only one eye is injured, cover the other eye with a sterile eye pad and eye shield, too (Figure 22–7e). Because the eyes move together, covering both will keep each quiet and will prevent undue motion on the injured side.

A person with both eyes covered obviously cannot see and may become frightened. This situation is especially true in children. Covering both eyes without a warning may be unwise, because the patient may become uncooperative and struggle, causing more damage. Sometimes, the disorientation may cause more problems than the benefit attained from limiting eye movement. In these instances, leave the uninjured eye open. Calm reassurance and a quiet matter-of-fact explanation of why both eyes are being covered temporarily are both essential before you proceed. Once both eyes are covered, the patient will need assistance and continuous reassurance during transport. Tell the patient what is happening. A gesture as simple as holding the patient's hand will

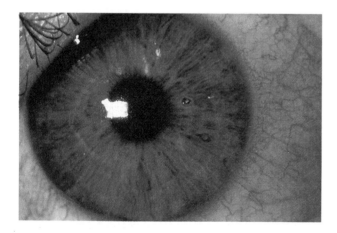

FIGURE 22–4

Conjunctivitis often is associated with a foreign body—in this case corneal—on the eye.

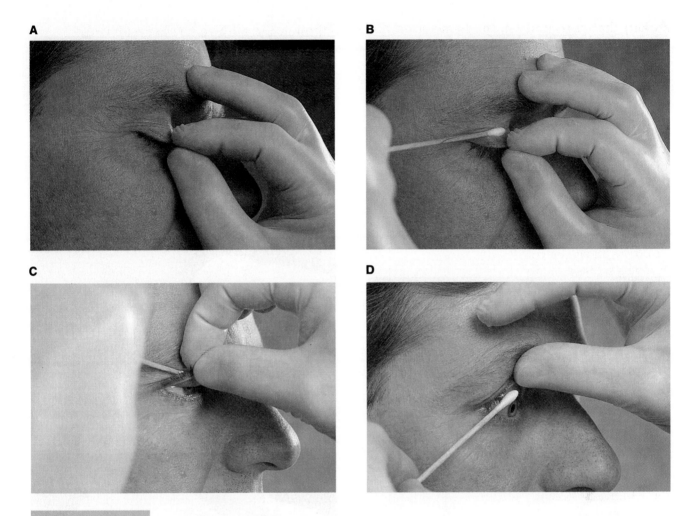

FIGURE 22-5   Removal of a foreign body from under the upper eyelid. (A) The patient is told to look downward while the eyelashes of the upper lid are grasped with the thumb and index finger and gently pulled away from the eyeball. (B) A cotton-tipped applicator is placed horizontally along the center of the outer surface of the upper lid. (C) The lid is pulled forward and upward, which causes it to roll or fold back over the applicator, exposing the undersurface of the lid. (D) If a foreign body is seen, it is gently removed with a moistened, sterile, cotton-tipped applicator.

often provide the needed support and reassurance.

On occasion, foreign bodies can come to lie entirely within the eye itself. Frequently, they are small metal fragments. Not infrequently, the patient may not be aware of the cause of the problem. Suspect such an injury when the history includes metal work (hammering, exposure to splinters, or vigorous filing) and when there are other signs of ocular injury. These situations must be handled by the ophthalmologist as urgent emergencies. X rays and special equipment may be needed to find the foreign body.

A

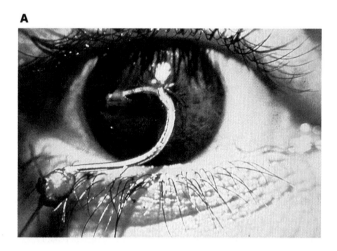

B

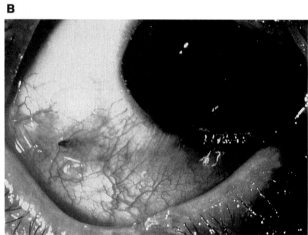

Impaled ocular foreign bodies include a wide variety of objects; (A) a fishhook, (B) a sharp metal sliver.

A

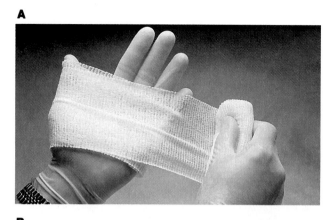

B

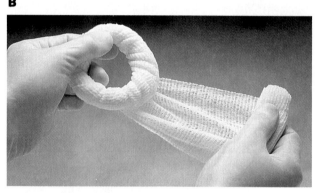

C

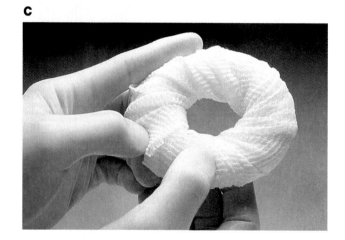

D

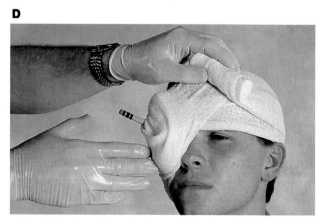

E

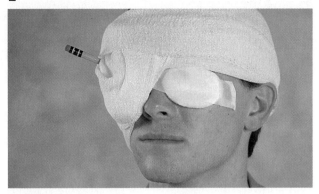

FIGURE 22–7

Bandage an impaled ocular foreign body with a surrounding dressing. (A) Preparing a doughnut ring. Wrap 2-inch roll around fingers and thumb seven or eight times. Adjust diameter by spreading your fingers. (B, C) Wrap the remainder of the roll, working around the ring. (D) Place doughnut dressing over the eye to hold impaled object in place, then secure it with gauze dressing. (E) Patch the uninjured eye.

Burns of the Eye

The eye can be burned by chemicals, heat, and light rays. The delicate tissues of the eye may be permanently damaged very easily. Prompt emergency care must be directed at stopping the burn and preventing further damage.

Chemical Burns Chemical burns require immediate emergency care to prevent permanent damage. Chemical burns are caused principally by acid or alkaline solutions. The only emergency treatment for chemical burns is flushing the eye with water or a sterile saline irrigation solution. Any clean water that is available can be used if sterile saline is not at hand.

The best techniques direct the greatest amount of irrigant as gently as possible into the eye. Use a bulb or irrigation syringe, a nasal cannula, or any item that will enable you to control the flow. Circumstances may necessitate pouring water into the eye, holding the patient's head under a gently running faucet, or even having the patient blink rapidly with the face immersed in a large pan or basin of water (Figure 22–8). A shower, if it is available, can be very effective. Irrigate for at least 5 minutes for any chemical spilled into the eye; if the burn has been caused by an alkaline solution or a strong acid, irrigation should last at least 20 minutes. Strong acids and all alkaline solutions can penetrate deeply; thus, a prolonged flush is necessary. You cannot use too much irrigant. Because opening the eye spontaneously may cause the patient pain, you often must force the lids open gently to irrigate the eye adequately. During irrigation it is especially important to protect the uninjured eye, and to prevent irrigation fluid from running into it.

After irrigation is completed, apply a clean dry dressing to cover the eye and transport the patient promptly to the hospital for further care. If the eye irrigation can be carried out satisfactorily in the ambulance, it should be done en route to save time.

Thermal Burns When a patient suffers burns of the face in a fire, the eyes usually close rapidly because of the heat. This reaction is a natural reflex to protect the eye from further injury. However, the eyelids remain exposed and are frequently burned (Figure 22–9). Burns of the eyelids require very specialized care. It is best to transport the patient who has burned eyelids promptly to the hospital without further examination. Both eyes should be covered with a sterile dressing moistened with sterile saline prior to transport. Eye shields may be applied over the dressings.

Light Burns Exposure to extremes of light can cause significant damage of the eye. The rays of light become focused on the retina, and the sensory cells can be damaged significantly. Infrared rays, eclipse light (if the patient has looked directly at the sun), and laser burns cause injuries of the retina that are generally not painful but may result in permanent visual damage.

Ultraviolet rays from an arc welding unit, light from prolonged exposure to a sun lamp, or a bright snow-covered area (snow blindness) can all cause a superficial burn of the eye. This kind of burn often is not painful initially, but

A

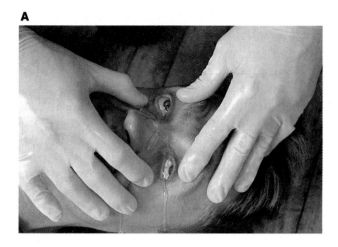

B

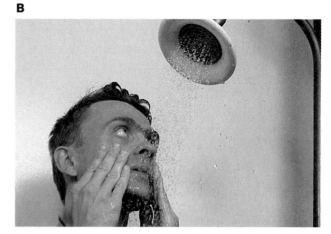

C

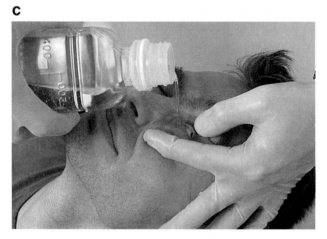

D

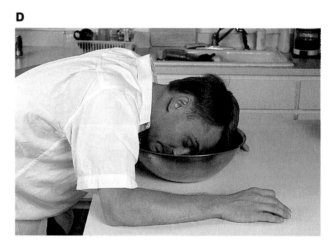

E

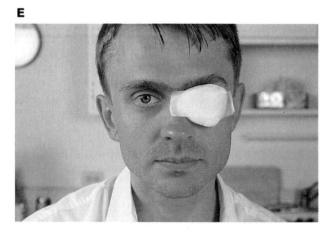

FIGURE 22–8

Four effective methods of eye irrigation: (A) Nasal cannula, (B) shower, (C) bottle, or (D) basin. Note in each that care is necessary to protect the uninjured globe from the irrigating solution. Irrigation should be carried out for at least 5 minutes with any chemical agent and for up to 20 minutes with alkali and strong acids. It may be necessary that you hold the eye open to irrigate it effectively. (E) Patch the damaged eye after irrigation is complete.

extreme discomfort may be experienced 3 to 5 hours later as the damaged cornea responds to the injury. The patient usually develops a severe conjunctivitis with redness, swelling, and excessive tear production. The pain from these corneal burns may be eased by covering each eye with a sterile, moist pad and an eye shield, and having the patient lie down during transport to the hospital. Protect the patient from further exposure to bright light and arrange that he or she be examined by a physician as soon as possible.

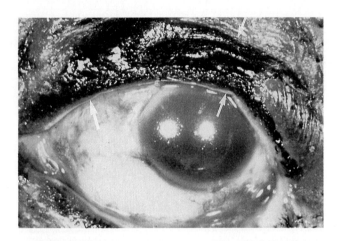

FIGURE 22–9

Occasionally, thermal injury will include significant damage of the eyelids. In this figure some 3rd-degree burns are evident (arrows). Protect the eye with a moist, sterile dressing and an eye shield and transport the patient promptly. It is wise to cover the other eye also.

Lacerations and Blunt Trauma of the Eye

Lacerations Lacerations of the eyelids require very careful repair to restore both appearance and function. Bleeding from a lacerated eyelid may be profuse, but it usually can be controlled by gentle manual pressure. If there is a laceration of the globe itself, apply no pressure to the eye; compression can interfere with the blood supply to the back of the eye and result in loss of vision from damage of the retina. Furthermore, pressure may squeeze the vitreous humor, the iris, lens, or even the retina out of the eye and cause irreparable damage or blindness.

Penetrating injuries of the eye should be treated following these four important guidelines:

1. Never exert pressure on or manipulate the injured eye (globe) in any way.
2. If part of the eyeball is exposed, gently apply a moist, sterile dressing to prevent drying.
3. Cover the injured eye with a protective metal eye shield.
4. Cover the opposite eye with a bandage to decrease movement on the injured side.

On rare occasions following a serious injury, the eyeball may be displaced out of its socket.

No attempt should be made to reposition it. It should be covered and stabilized with a moist, sterile dressing. The patient should be transported to the hospital lying in the supine position.

Blunt Trauma Of The Eye Blunt trauma can cause a number of serious injuries of the eye ranging from the common "black eye," a result of bleeding into the tissue around the orbit, to a severely damaged globe. One injury that is seen from time to time is **hyphema** (bleeding into the anterior chamber of the eye) that obscures part or all of the iris. This injury is common in blunt trauma (Figure 22–10) and may seriously impair vision in that eye. It may also indicate a more serious injury to the globe.

Blunt trauma can also cause a fracture of the orbit, particularly of the bones that form its floor and support the globe. This injury is called a **blowout fracture.** The fragments of fractured bone can entrap some of the muscles that control eye movement. Because of the altered eye motion, secondary to the muscle entrapment, the patient may experience double vision (Figure 22–11). Any patient who complains of pain, double vision, or decreased vision following a blunt injury about the eye should be placed on a stretcher and transported promptly to the emergency department. Protect the eye from further injury with a metal shield; cover the uninjured eye to minimize movement on the injured side.

Another result of blunt eye injury is **retinal detachment**—a condition in which the retina is separated from its attachments at the back of the eye. This injury is often seen in sports, especially boxing. It is painless but produces flashing lights, specks, or "floaters" in the visual field, and a cloud or shade over the patient's vision. This injury requires prompt medical attention to preserve vision in that eye, because the retina is separated from its nourishing layer, the choroid.

HEAD INJURY

Abnormalities in the appearance or function of the eyes often occur following a closed head

A

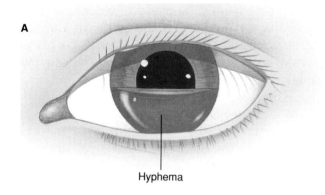

Hyphema

B   C

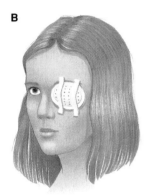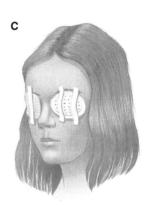

FIGURE 22-10

(A) Blunt trauma to the eye often produces a hyphema with blood accumulating in the anterior chamber overlying the iris. (B) Patients with blunt trauma to the eye should have an eye shield applied. (C) The opposite eye should be patched to minimize motion.

injury. Careful examination of the eyes may lead you to suspect a head injury. Any of the following eye findings should alert you to that possibility:

- One pupil larger than the other.
- The eyes not moving together or pointing in different directions.
- Failure of the eyes to follow the movement of your finger upon command.
- Bleeding under the conjunctiva which obscures the sclera (white portion) of the eye.
- Protrusion or bulging of one eye.

Record any of these observations along with the time that they are made.

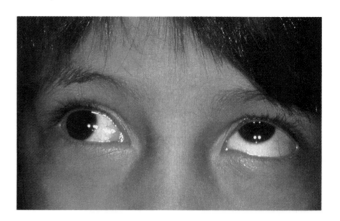

FIGURE 22-11

In the patient with a blowout fracture of the orbit, the eyes do not move together because of muscle entrapment. The patient, thus, sees two pictures of any object (double vision).

In an unconscious patient, remember to keep the eyelids closed. Drying of the ocular tissue can cause permanent injury and may result in blindness. The lids can be covered with a moist gauze or gently held closed with clear tape. Normal tears will then keep the tissues moist.

CONTACT LENSES AND ARTIFICIAL EYES

Contact lenses can be small, hard, plastic ones that are usually tinted or large, clear, soft ones that are very difficult to see. Never attempt to remove a contact lens if there is any question of an injury of the eye. Manipulation of the lens can aggravate the damage. The only time that contact lenses should be removed immediately in the field is in the case of a chemical burn of the eye. The lens can trap the chemical and make dilution with an irrigation solution difficult. If it is necessary to remove a hard contact lens, a small suction cup, the end moistened with saline, can be used (Figure 22-12a). Soft contact lenses are removed by placing a couple of drops of saline onto the lens and gently pinching it between the thumb and index fingers; it can then be lifted from the surface of the eye (Figures 22-12b and c).

In general—and particularly following injury of the eye—do not attempt to remove contact lenses. Emergency department personnel should always be advised of the presence of contact lenses so that proper care can be provided in the hospital.

The patient may be wearing an eye prosthesis (artificial eye). You should suspect the presence of an artificial eye when it does not respond to light, move synchronously with the opposite eye, or appear quite the same as its mate. Sometimes it is quite difficult to distinguish a prosthesis from a natural eye. If you suspect the patient has an artificial eye, ask the patient about this possibility so that there is no misleading or incorrect information about the patient's eye function. With regard to the emergency care, no harm will be done if an artificial eye is given the same care as a normal one.

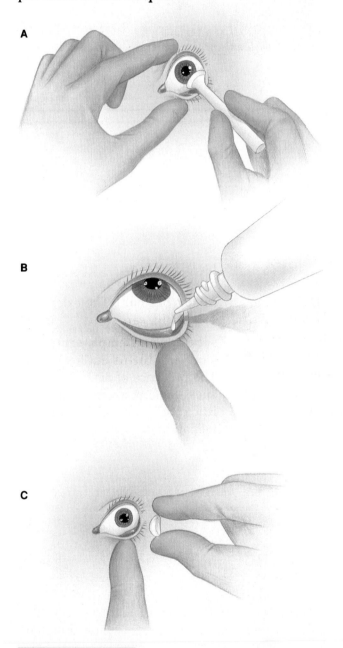

A

B

C

FIGURE 22–12

(A) A special suction cup, moistened with saline, is convenient for removing a small, hard contact lens. (B) To remove a soft contact lens, one or two drops of saline or irrigating solution are applied, and (C) the lens is pinched off with the thumb and index finger.

YOU ARE THE EMT

1. Describe the major anatomical elements of the eye.
2. Describe how an injured eye differs in appearance from a normal one.
3. From what part of the eye can foreign objects be flushed easily?
4. Describe the treatment for impaled objects.
5. How would you manage a patient with chemical eye injuries? Thermal injuries? Suspected light injuries?
6. What findings in the eyes would make you suspect an underlying head injury?
7. Why must you be careful not to exert any pressure on the eye when you treat penetrating eye injuries?
8. What are the treatment principles to follow when you treat lacerations and blunt injuries of the eye?
9. Describe the safe removal of contact lenses and the situation when you should attempt it.

CHAPTER 23

INJURIES OF THE FACE AND THROAT

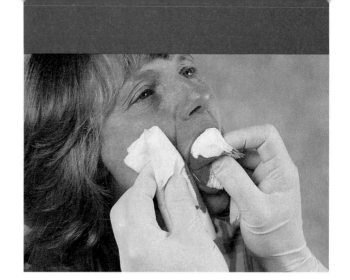

KEY TERMS

avulse (ah-vuls′) To pull or tear away.

deciduous teeth (de-sid′u-us tēth) Baby teeth.

external auditory canal (eks-ter′nal aw′dĭ-to″re kah-nal′) The ear canal.

mandible (man′dĭ-b′l) The bone of the lower jaw.

maxilla (mak-sil′ah) The bone that forms the upper jaw on either side of the face; it contains the upper teeth, the orbit of the eye, the nasal cavity, and the palate.

pedicle (ped′ĭ-k′l) An elongated, somewhat slender anatomical structure resembling the stalk of a plant.

pinna (pin′nah) The external part of the ear.

subcutaneous emphysema (sub″ku-ta′ne-us em″fĭ-se′mah) The presence of air in soft tissues, causing a very characteristic crackling sensation on palpation.

The face contains many specialized and important structures. Because of their prominence, these structures are vulnerable to injury that may cause permanent loss or damage of critical functions. The basic anatomy and categories of eye injuries are covered in Chapter 22. Injuries to other structures of the face present special problems. The most serious underlying problem with all injuries is partial or complete upper airway obstruction. Facial or neck injuries also are often associated with cervical spine damage. You must understand that the emergency treatment of injuries of the face and throat very often is associated with the management of the respiratory tract and spinal injuries. The first section of Chapter 23 focuses on injuries of the face, including soft tissue wounds, injuries of the nose and ear, and facial fractures. The second section discusses injuries of the throat and neck. General considerations for dental injuries conclude the chapter.

GOALS

. . . .

The goals of Chapter 23 are to

- understand how all facial or throat injuries can cause upper airway obstruction.
- know how to treat soft tissue wounds of the face, injuries of the nose and ear, and facial fractures.
- know how to manage foreign bodies in the nose and ear canal.
- understand how to treat patients with injuries of the neck and throat, including fractures of the larynx and trachea.
- know the proper handling of injured and loose teeth.

. . . .

INJURIES OF THE FACE
. . . .

The face and neck are particularly vulnerable to injury because of their relatively unprotected positions. Soft tissue injuries and fractures of the bones of the face occur commonly. These injuries will vary greatly in severity. Some may be potentially life-threatening and many will leave disfiguring scars if not treated properly. When you treat a person with a facial injury, it is most important to remember that a spinal injury may also have been sustained in the same accident. You must be careful to protect the spine and immobilize the potential injury adequately.

Injuries about the face frequently lead to partial or complete obstruction of the upper airway. Several factors may contribute to upper airway obstruction:

- Bleeding from facial injuries can be profuse, producing large blood clots in the upper airway.
- Loosened teeth or dentures may be dislodged into the throat. They may be swallowed or aspirated (Figure 23–1).
- Injuries of the mouth and nose may produce significant deformity of the upper airway.
- Soft tissue injury may produce severe swelling of the tissues that blocks the airway.

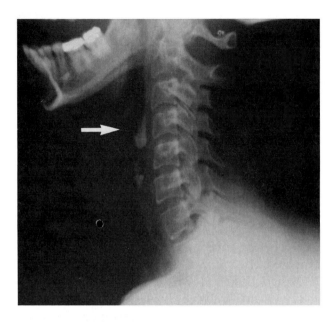

FIGURE 23–1

A tooth lying in the esophagus (arrow) is shown.

- In the semiconscious or unconscious patient, the head often is turned or twisted to one side, obstructing the airway passage.
- Direct injury of the larynx or trachea causes local bleeding and swelling and predictable airway obstruction.
- Associated brain injury may interfere with the control of breathing.

Soft Tissue Wounds

Soft tissue injuries of the face and scalp are common. Contusions usually cause local swelling. Some contusions of the scalp and forehead may produce a fairly large hematoma that forms a definite lump under the skin. Abrasions of the facial skin sometimes cause a significantly disfiguring scar. Lacerations and avulsion injuries are especially common. Frequently, a flap of skin is peeled back **(avulsed)** from the underlying muscle and fascia (Figure 23–2). Because these areas are well supplied with arteries and veins, even trivial soft tissue wounds of the face and scalp may bleed a lot.

The emergency care of soft tissue injuries of the face and scalp is identical to the treatment of soft tissue injuries elsewhere. Applying ice locally will help to control the swelling of contused soft tissues. Bleeding is controlled by applying direct manual pressure with a dry, sterile dressing. A circumferential wrap of roller gauze around the head will hold a pressure dressing in place. Do not apply excessive pressure to a scalp laceration if you suspect a skull fracture.

When penetrating injury exposes the brain, the eye, or other important structures, cover the exposed parts with a moist, sterile dressing to protect them from further damage. When a laceration extends through the cheek directly into the mouth, it may be necessary to apply pressure with a sterile dressing against both the inside and the outside of the cheek in order to control the bleeding (Figure 23–3). Objects penetrating the cheek usually must be removed before the bleeding can be controlled.

You should always check for bleeding inside the mouth in instances of facial injury. Broken teeth and lacerations of the tongue may cause profuse bleeding. If most of the blood is swallowed, hemorrhage may not be apparent at all outside the mouth. Inspect the inside of

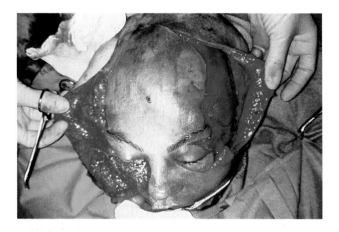

FIGURE 23–2

A major avulsion injury of the face is shown. Flaps include scalp and tissue of both cheeks.

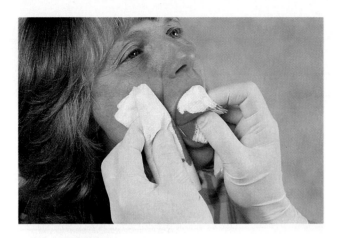

FIGURE 23–3

A penetrating laceration "through and through" the cheek may require a pressure dressing over both wounds to control bleeding.

the mouth of all persons who have sustained facial trauma for bleeding and hidden injuries.

Blood draining into the throat can produce both vomiting and airway difficulties. You must open and clear the airway (often with suction). Because this patient may have sustained a cervical spine injury, take care to avoid all airway maneuvers that may cause damage of the spinal cord. Use the trauma jaw-thrust or trauma chin-lift maneuver to open this patient's airway. Stabilize the spine initially; then turn the patient to one side so that any blood or vomitus can drain out of the mouth rather than pool in the pharynx and obstruct the airway.

With any facial injury, you must check whether any tissue is missing. Frequently, pieces of skin will be avulsed and can be found lying near the patient. Recover any free piece of tissue; wrap it in a moist, sterile dressing and place it in a plastic bag, kept cool. Take it to the emergency department with the patient. These pieces of skin often can be replaced surgically.

Flap-type avulsion injuries of the skin occur frequently on the face and scalp. As with flap injuries in other parts of the body, fold the flap of tissue back to its normal position before you apply a dry, sterile dressing to it. If the flap is left in a twisted or kinked position, a compression dressing applied to it may compress the

vessels entering through the **pedicle** (stalk) and cut off its blood supply. Fold the flap back into the bed from which it was avulsed. You can then apply a dry sterile compression dressing in a standard manner to hold it in place and control bleeding.

Injuries of the Nose

Soft tissue injuries of the nose usually result from blunt trauma and produce bleeding. An ice pack applied over the bridge of the nose or pinching the nostrils together, when the patient can tolerate it, may control the bleeding. A roll of gauze packed between the upper teeth and upper lip will sometimes help exert pressure on the blood vessels that supply the nose to help control the nosebleed (Figure 23–4).

Objects inhaled or stuffed into the nose may cause severe pain and occasionally bleeding. Generally, they do not cause complete airway obstruction. Such foreign bodies should be removed only by a physician in the emergency department. Attempting to remove them in the field will often result in their being pushed farther back into the nose, making later removal more difficult.

Injuries of the Ear

The ear is frequently injured. Bleeding usually is not excessive and can be easily controlled with local pressure. Bandaging the ear tight against the underlying scalp is extremely painful for the patient. You must always place a soft, padded dressing between the ear and scalp before you apply a roller dressing for pressure (Figure 23–5).

Occasionally, pieces of the ear or an entire **pinna** (exterior ear) are avulsed or cut off. If they can be found, you should wrap them in moist, sterile gauze and transport them with the patient to the emergency department. Use a plastic bag for the tissue packet and keep it cool.

The **external auditory canal** (ear canal) is a favorite place for children to place foreign bodies. They should be removed by a physician in the emergency department. Often such

A

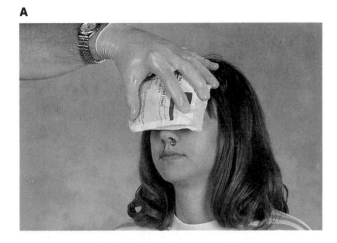

B

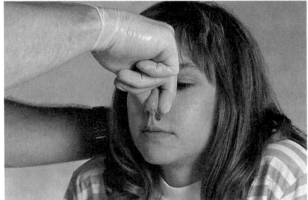

C

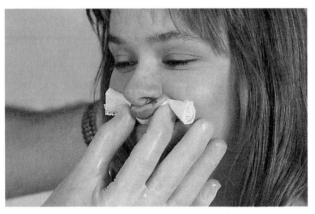

FIGURE 23–4

Bleeding from the nose following injury can be controlled in a number of ways. (A) Ice pack; (B) pinching the nostrils together; or (C) a gauze pack placed under the upper lip.

A

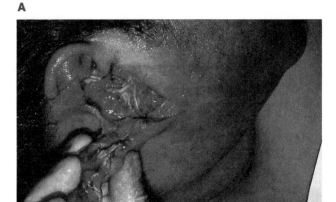

B

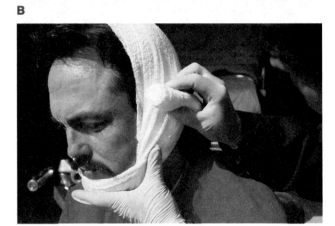

FIGURE 23–5

(A) A major lacerating injury of the ear is shown. (B) Proper dressing for this wound includes a soft, sterile pad behind the ear, between it and the scalp; a soft, moist dressing over the laceration itself; and a roller gauze wrap about the head to include the entire ear.

items are nuts, grains of corn, or seeds that may absorb water and swell. In such instances, prompt transport to the hospital is in order to allow treatment before much swelling has occurred. Do not manipulate this foreign body, because you may press it farther into the ear canal.

Facial Fractures

Fractures of the facial bones commonly result from a blunt impact— for example, collision of the patient's head with a steering wheel or windshield. The fracture may involve the nose, the orbit (eye socket), the **maxilla** (the upper jaw), or the **mandible** (the lower jaw). Fractures about the nose and mouth produce deformity, loose bone fragments, swelling, and bleeding that may combine to cause airway obstruction. Consider any patient who has sustained a direct blow on the mouth or nose as one with a facial fracture. Many times these fractures are not evident on the first examination, as the patient may only have some swelling and local pain. Other clues to the possibility of a fracture are

- Irregularity of the bite (the fit of the teeth).
- Absent or loose teeth.
- The inability to swallow or talk.
- Increased salivation.
- Bleeding in the mouth.
- Obviously, loose or mobile bone fragments.

In all of these injuries, use extreme care to avoid obstruction of the airway. The patient with a significant facial fracture is at continuous risk for developing airway obstruction as further bleeding and swelling occur. Clear the upper respiratory passages of any obstructing material; maintain the airway and assist ventilation during transport to the hospital.

INJURIES OF THE THROAT

Soft tissue wounds of the neck may also produce severe bleeding and swelling that may result in upper airway obstruction. The primary consideration in patients with injuries of the throat is the adequacy of the upper airway. You must establish and maintain it. Bleeding should be controlled with direct manual pressure with a dry, sterile dressing. Stabilize the cervical spine to protect it from further injury.

Occasionally, you will be required to treat a patient with a foreign object impaled in the neck. The object must be stabilized and bandaged in place with a soft gauze collar or doughnut dressing (Figure 23–6). Foreign objects in the neck are removed only on the operating table (Figure 23–7).

The larynx or trachea may be fractured in any crushing injury of the anterior aspect of the

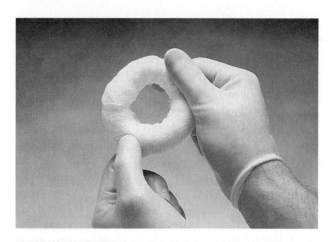

FIGURE 23–6

Doughnut dressings useful in stabilizing impaled objects should be available in all ambulances.

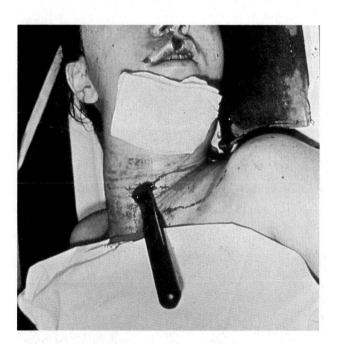

FIGURE 23–7

This patient was assaulted and raped at home by an intruder; a butcher knife was left in place. No major vessels or nerves were found injured. The knife was removed at operation.

neck. Impact against a steering wheel, attempt at suicide by hanging, or a clothesline injury sustained while riding a bicycle all are ways that the trachea can be fractured. When this injury occurs, loss of voice, severe—and sometimes fatal—airway obstruction, and leakage of air into the soft tissues of the neck result. The presence of air in the soft tissue produces a very characteristic crackling sensation on palpation called **subcutaneous emphysema** (Figure 23–8). Fracture of the cervical spine is often present with these injuries.

Some other signs of major injury in the neck, whether penetrating or blunt, include the following:

1. A hematoma that is visibly expanding or is pulsatile indicates major arterial bleeding.
2. Hoarseness may suggest direct damage of the larynx or of its nerve supply.
3. Inability to shrug the shoulders or loss of sensation or motor function in an arm may indicate spinal injury.

Each of these findings points to a major injury involving the vessels or nerves of the neck and signals a need for prompt transportation to the emergency department.

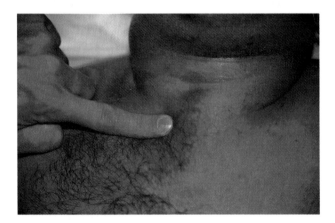

FIGURE 23–8

Fractures of the larynx or trachea can cause air to leak from the airway into the subcutaneous tissue. Although one cannot see it unless the tissues are extremely swollen, subcutaneous emphysema has a characteristic crackling sensation upon palpation.

Emergency care of injuries of the larynx and trachea consists of securing the upper airway, administering supplemental oxygen by face mask, and splinting the cervical spine. Keeping the patient calm and breathing slowly may be lifesaving, because rapid breathing usually makes the situation worse. Oxygen inhalation should be used whenever this injury is suspected; however, do not use positive pressure ventilation (with a bag-valve-mask) because air may be forced out of the injured trachea into the soft tissues and produce subcutaneous emphysema, compounding the problem. These are very serious, life-threatening injuries, and the patient must be transported rapidly to the hospital for treatment. Application of a pressure dressing for major bleeding from the neck is shown in Figure 23–9.

DENTAL INJURIES

Commonly, major injuries of the mouth, face or throat, are all associated with some dental damage. You, as an EMT, can do very little to treat major dental injuries. Often, they require rather complex reconstruction over fairly long periods of time. You must, however, address some of the common results of dental injuries in the field. The following are appropriate steps to take:

1. Remember that loose teeth are common and can cause airway obstruction at several points: the back of the throat, the larynx, or the trachea. They may be inhaled into the lung or swallowed. Clear the upper airway of all loose and freely movable teeth.
2. Save any removed teeth and transport them with the patient to the emergency department. The American Dental Association recommends that loose teeth be replaced in their sockets immediately or carried with the patient to the hospital in a dental preserving medium.
3. With the severely injured or unconscious patient who cannot cooperate, place the

A

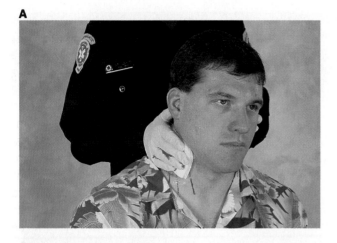

B

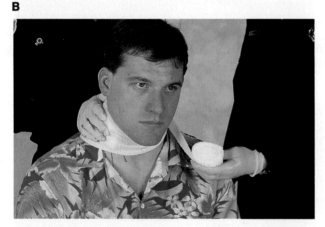

C

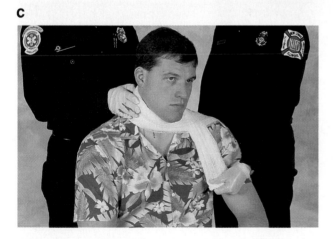

FIGURE 23–9

For a severe neck laceration, (A) control bleeding with manual pressure. (B) Secure the pressure dressing with a roller gauze wrapped loosely around the neck, then (C) firmly through the opposite axilla.

tooth (teeth) in a special packet (commercially available) which contains a tooth preserving medium and a net in which the tooth can be placed. This packet will hold the tooth and maintain its viability for up to 12 hours.

4. If the packet is not available, place the tooth (teeth) in whole fresh milk in a sealed plastic container. This medium will preserve tooth viability for a maximum of 2 hours.

5. *Do not* place teeth in tap water, dry gauze, or any other dry tissue.

6. If the patient is alert and cooperative, the tooth (teeth) may be placed under the tongue or in the *buccal vestibule* (the gum/cheek pouch).

In dental reconstruction, the use of the patient's own teeth is greatly superior, and much less expensive for the patient. Current surgical techniques may allow the reimplanting of some teeth, especially if it can be done within two hours after an injury (Figure 23–10). Certainly, the availability of native teeth will help dentists to assess color match and contour. Otherwise, the principles underlying the basic treatment of associated fractures and soft tissue injuries will be the guides for your treatment in this area. Broken teeth that remain firmly implanted in the socket must be left for the dentist to repair. They constitute no additional risk for the patient.

Deciduous (baby) **teeth** in children need not be recovered or replaced. However, if the child is 6 years or older, an injured or loose tooth may be a permanent one and should be preserved.

FIGURE 23–10

(A) Traumatic loss of a prominent tooth is shown. (B) The reimplanted tooth provides an excellent repair.

A

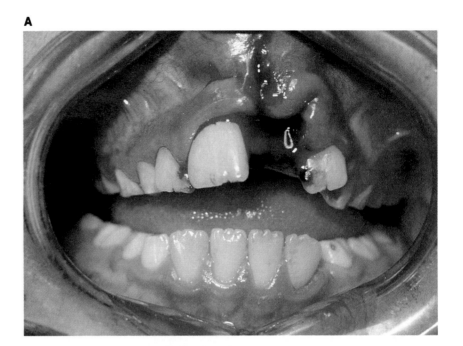

B

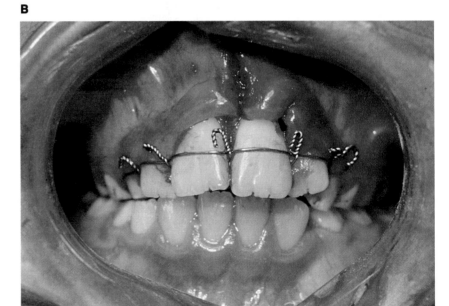

YOU ARE THE EMT

1. Why must you be concerned about possible spinal injuries when you see a patient with facial trauma?

2. The patient's head hit the windshield in an automobile accident. He is not obviously bleeding. What injuries should you expect? What symptoms will be evident?

3. How will you treat an avulsion injury that begins in the forehead and extends into the scalp?

4. Identify five causes of upper airway obstruction from injuries about the face.

5. What clues help you to suspect a facial fracture?

6. Children often push foreign bodies into the nose or ears; how do you handle this situation and why?

7. What methods can you use to bring loose teeth to the emergency department?

8. Review the methods of protecting yourself from contracting an illness from these patients.

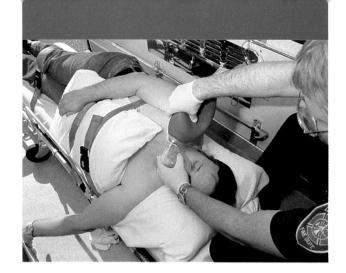

CHAPTER 24

INJURIES OF THE CHEST

KEY TERMS

dyspnea (disp'ne-ah) Difficult breathing.

flail chest A blunt chest injury in which three or more ribs are fractured in two or more places or in association with a sternal fracture so that a segment of chest wall is effectively detached from the rest of the thoracic cage.

hemoptysis (he-mop'tĭ-sis) The expectoration of blood or blood-tinged sputum; the coughing up of blood.

hemothorax (he″mo-tho'raks) A collection of blood in the pleural cavity.

myocardial contusion (mi″o-kar'de-al kon-tu'zshun) A bruise of the heart muscle.

paradoxical motion (par″ah-dok'se-kal mo'shun) The motion of the flail segment of a flail chest that is opposite to the normal chest wall movement.

pericardial tamponade (per″ĭ-kar'de-al tam″pon-ād') Acute compression of the heart due to a buildup of fluid or blood in the pericardial sac.

pericardium (per″ĭ-kar'de-um) The fibrous sac that surrounds the heart.

pleura (ploor'ah) The serous membrane covering the lungs and lining the thoracic cavity, completely enclosing a potential space known as the pleural space.

pleurisy (ploor'ĭ-se) Inflammation of the pleura.

pleuritic pain (ploo-rit'ik pān) Pain in the chest with respirations.

pneumothorax (nu″mo-tho'raks) An accumulation of air or gas in the pleural cavity.

pulmonary (pul'mo-ner″e) Of the lung.

pulmonary contusion (pul'mo-ner″e kon-tu'zhun) A bruise of the lung.

sucking chest wound An open or penetrating chest wall wound through which air passes during inspiration and expiration.

tension pneumothorax (ten' shun nu″mo-tho'raks) An accumulation of air or gas in the pleural cavity that progressively increases and causes a rise in intrathoracic pressure.

OVERVIEW

Injuries of the chest are serious because of the high likelihood of damage to the heart, lungs, or great vessels. Unless properly and promptly treated, a chest injury may be rapidly fatal.

Because the body has no capacity to store oxygen, any injury that interferes with normal breathing must be treated without delay to prevent permanent damage to those tissues that depend on a continuous supply of oxygen. Another major problem with chest injuries may be internal bleeding. Blood from lacerations of the thoracic organs or major blood vessels can collect in the chest cavity, compressing the lungs. Additionally, air can enter the chest cavity through the chest wall or the airways and collect within it to prevent expansion of the lungs—a function vital to the breathing process. All of these life-threatening injuries require you to act fast. A few minutes is often all that separates life and death in these emergencies.

Chapter 24 first describes the signs and symptoms of chest injury. It then covers the general principles of treatment for all chest injuries. Specific types of chest injury and their emergency care are considered as are common complications that can occur following any chest injury. You should carefully review Chapter 6 on the normal anatomy and function of the respiratory system before reading this chapter.

GOALS

The goals of Chapter 24 are to
- identify the signs and symptoms of chest injury.
- know the general principles of the care of all chest injuries.
- be able to recognize specific chest injuries and know their emergency care.
- know the complications that can accompany chest injuries.

SIGNS AND SYMPTOMS OF CHEST INJURY

Chest injuries are considered in two categories: open or closed. Open chest injuries are those in which the chest wall has been penetrated by some object such as a knife or bullet. An open chest injury may also be caused by a fractured rib in which the broken end of the bone lacerates the chest wall and the skin.

In closed chest injuries the skin is not broken. These injuries are generally caused by blunt trauma, as when the patient strikes a steering wheel, is tackled, or is struck by a falling object. Lacerations of the contents of the chest may occur in closed injuries, caused directly by broken ribs or when vital structures are torn from their attachments in the chest cavity, but the skin and chest wall are not penetrated.

The important signs of chest injury, either open or closed, are these:

- Pain at the site of the injury.
- Pain localized around the site of an injury that is aggravated by or occurs with breathing (**pleuritic pain** or **pleurisy**).

- **Dyspnea** (difficult breathing, shortness of breath).
- Failure of one or both sides of the chest to expand normally with inspiration.
- **Hemoptysis** (the coughing up of blood).
- A rapid, weak pulse and low blood pressure.
- Cyanosis (a bluish discoloration, most profound around the lips or fingernails).

Following an injury of the chest, any change in the normal pattern of breathing is a particularly important sign. A healthy, uninjured person usually breathes from 10 to 20 times per minute without difficulty and without pain. Respiratory rates of less than 10 breaths per minute or in excess of 24 breaths per minute usually indicate respiratory distress. The patient with an injury of the chest will have *tachypnea* (increased respiratory rate) and will breathe in shallow gasps because it hurts to take a deep breath.

As with any other injury, pain and tenderness are commonly noted at the point of impact as the result of a bruise or fracture. The pain is usually aggravated by the normal process of breathing. Irritation or damage of the pleural surfaces causes a characteristic sharp or sticking pain with each breath when these normally smooth surfaces must slide on one another. Review the mechanics of breathing in Chapter 6 to be certain of the function of the **pleura** in respiration. This sharp pain with each respiration is called pleuritic pain or pleurisy.

In the injured patient, dyspnea has many different causes. It may occur because

- The patient's chest is not expanding properly due to the loss of the normal nervous control of breathing.
- The airway is obstructed.
- The lung itself is being compressed from within the chest by accumulated blood or air.
- The chest wall is damaged.

Dyspnea in the injured patient indicates significant compromise of the function of the lung(s) that requires prompt, vigorous support and treatment.

Carefully observe the chest wall in patients who have sustained an injury. Failure of the chest wall on each side to expand when the patient inhales is an extremely important sign. It indicates that the muscles of the thorax have lost their ability to work appropriately. Loss of muscle function may be the result of a direct injury of the chest wall, or it may be related to an injury of the nerves that control those muscles.

Hemoptysis usually indicates that the lung itself or the air passages have been damaged. With a laceration of the lung, blood can enter the bronchial passages and is coughed up as the patient tries to clear the airway.

A rapid, weak pulse and a low blood pressure are major signs of hypovolemic shock. Shock following chest injury may result from insufficient oxygenation of the blood by the poorly functioning lung(s). This condition can also result from extensive bleeding from lacerated structures within the chest cavity.

Cyanosis, seen most readily around the lips and fingernails, indicates that blood is not being oxygenated sufficiently. Cyanosis in the patient with a chest injury indicates inadequate ventilation. This patient is unable to provide a sufficient supply of oxygen to the blood through the lungs and requires supplemental oxygen and respiratory support immediately.

Many of these signs and symptoms occur simultaneously. When any one of them follows chest injury, you must realize that the patient requires hospital care promptly. Also recall that the major reason for grave concern with chest injuries is that the body has no means of storing oxygen; it is supplied and used continously, even during sleep. Any interruption in this supply can be lethal and must be aggressively treated.

GENERAL PRINCIPLES OF THE CARE OF CHEST INJURIES
· ·

Despite the many types of chest injuries, almost uniformly, they require the same initial care. For this reason, this section reviews the general principles of the emergency treatment of chest injuries regardless of their cause.

The effectiveness of emergency medical care is directly related to the ability of the patient to breathe; therefore, your initial attention must be given to the airway and respiration. The upper airway must be cleared and maintained using the trauma jaw-thrust or chin-lift maneuver, which maintains the cervical spine in a neutral in-line position to protect it (Figure 24-1).

Ventilatory support and oxygen should be administered to the patient whenever respiratory distress exists. If the ventilatory rate is less than 12 or greater than 20 breaths per minute, supplemental oxygen should be given.

If the ventilatory rate is less than 10 or greater than 30 breaths per minute, assisted ventilation is needed. Your overriding first consideration is to provide adequate oxygen to those tissues, particularly the brain and heart, that need a continuous supply in order to function properly.

Cover open chest wounds with a dry, sterile dressing. Control bleeding from the chest wall with direct manual pressure. Bandage impaled or protruding objects—knives and the like—in place with a collar or support dressing to stabilize them and to minimize their movement. Impaled objects should not be removed in the field.

If you suspect a rib fracture, make the patient comfortable and quiet so that the possibility of further damage of the lungs, heart, or chest wall from the broken bone is minimized. Fractured ribs may be splinted using several types of external support. The most commonly used and simplest device is a sling and swathe (Figure 24-2). Applying adhesive tape or other nonyielding straps to the chest wall is harmful; tight strapping limits the capacity of the chest to expand and may interfere with the patient's respiratory effort.

A

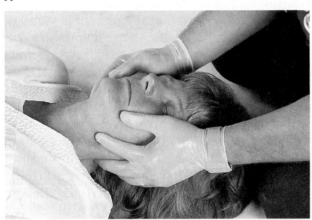

B

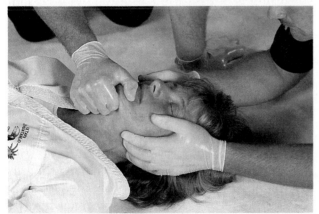

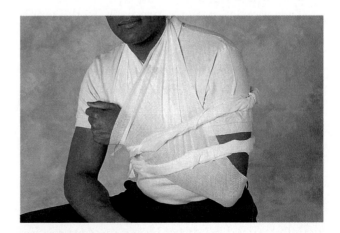

FIGURE 24–1

(A) The trauma jaw-thrust and (B) the trauma chin-lift techniques should be used to open and maintain the airway in an injured patient. Both techniques allow you to protect the cervical spine. The head is placed in a neutral in-line position and not hyperextended.

FIGURE 24–2

A sling and swathe will provide support for most fractured ribs. The humerus is used as a splint to support the injured ribs and decrease motion. Full immobilization of the ribs is difficult to achieve and may be harmful to the patient.

Observe and record the patient's vital signs frequently. They are the only means you have to diagnose and follow the course of internal bleeding and shock, and to monitor the patient's respiratory function.

Any critically injured patient with a significant chest injury should be transported rapidly to the hospital. Maintain the patient's airway, administer oxygen, assist ventilation, and attempt to control bleeding en route to the hospital.

Follow these steps in order to handle patients with chest injuries:

1. Be certain the airway is clear and maintain it using the trauma chin-lift or jaw-thrust maneuver to protect the cervical spine.
2. Use supplemental oxygen and be prepared to give respiratory support with mechanical aids, if necessary.
3. Control all sites of obvious external bleeding.
4. Cover penetrating wounds of the chest cavity promptly.
5. Observe, record, and monitor vital signs.
6. Carefully monitor the vital signs and the effect of treatment and be ready to transport the patient promptly, because his or her status may deteriorate quite rapidly at any time following a chest injury.
7. Transport all patients promptly to the emergency department and notify the hospital in advance of the type and severity of the injury sustained.

SPECIFIC CHEST INJURIES AND THEIR EMERGENCY CARE

Rib Fractures

Rib fractures are seen very frequently. They are usually caused by direct blows or compression injuries of the chest. Violent force is not always required to cause a rib fracture, particularly in the elderly. The upper four ribs are rarely fractured, because they are protected by the shoulder girdle. The fifth through tenth ribs are those most commonly broken. Only rarely are the eleventh and twelfth ribs (floating ribs) fractured, because they are small, have greater freedom of movement, are not attached to the sternum, and are deeply embedded in muscle.

A common finding in all patients with a single or multiple rib fractures is pain localized at the site of the fracture. By asking the patient to place one finger on the exact area of the pain, you can often determine the location of the injury. There may be a rib deformity, a chest wall contusion, or a laceration in the area. Deep breathing, coughing, or any movement is usually quite painful. The patient generally tries to remain still and will take rapid shallow breaths. Often the patient leans toward the injured side and places a hand over the area to "splint" the fracture and ease the local pain.

You must be sure that the patient is ventilating adequately by assessing the respiratory rate and other vital signs. Isolated simple rib fractures usually do not require any external support or splinting. Place the patient in a comfortable position on the litter and transport him or her promptly to the hospital. A patient with multiple rib fractures will be made more comfortable and find it easier to breathe if the chest wall is immobilized with a sling and swathe (see Figure 24–2). This maneuver uses the arm as a splint for the damaged chest wall. Do not wrap the swathe so tightly as to compress the chest and compromise the patient's ability to breathe.

Occasionally, the end of a fractured rib may puncture or lacerate the patient's lung or the chest wall (Figure 24–3), causing a **hemothorax** (a collection of blood in the pleural space), or a **pneumothorax** (a collection of air within the pleural space), compressing the lung. These two complications are discussed later in this chapter. Anterior fractures of the lower ribs (8–11) on the right or left are commonly associated with lacerations of the liver or spleen, respectively. These abdominal injuries must be suspected in all such instances of rib fracture.

Flail Chest

When three or more ribs are broken, each in two or more places, the segment of the chest wall lying between the fractures becomes free-

A Laceration of chest wall

B Perforation of lung

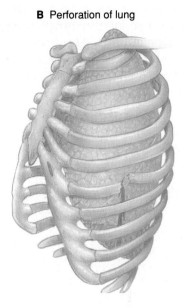

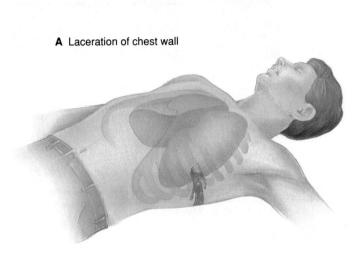

FIGURE 24–3   (A) A displaced rib fracture fragment may penetrate through the chest wall and create an open fracture. (B) More commonly, the fragment may penetrate (puncture) the lung and produce a hemothorax or a pneumothorax.

floating. This segment will collapse inward rather than follow the normal outward expansion of the chest wall each time the patient attempts to inhale. When the patient exhales, the segment will protrude slightly while the rest of the chest wall contracts. Thus, the motion of this floating segment is opposite to the normal movement of the rest of the chest wall. It is therefore called **paradoxical motion.** The portion of chest wall lying between the fractures is called the flail segment (Figure 24–4). Several terms are used to describe this injury. The proper one is **flail chest.** Other commonly used terms are crushed chest or stove-in chest. Ordinarily, considerable pain is associated with this injury and with the paradoxical motion of the flail segment.

Flail chest is a particularly serious injury. The lung immediately underneath the flail segment does not expand properly when the patient inhales, thus decreasing the efficiency of ventilation. Much more important, the amount of force that must be exerted on the chest wall to cause a series of ribs to fracture in several places and produce the flail segment almost

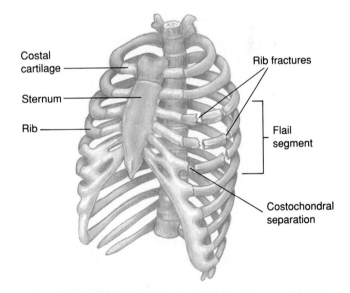

Costal cartilage

Sternum

Rib

Rib fractures

Flail segment

Costochondral separation

FIGURE 24–4

A flail chest results when several adjacent ribs are fractured in two or more places (third through fifth ribs on the left). With respiratory efforts, this segment will move paradoxically. Almost always this injury also results in severe contusion of the underlying lung.

always produces a severe **pulmonary contusion** (bruise of the lung) directly underneath the flail segment. The lung swells and experiences marked loss of respiratory function.

You can diagnose flail chest by closely observing the chest wall. You will notice that the chest does not rise properly, despite the patient's most desperate efforts to inhale deeply. In some patients with this injury, severe hypoxia and cyanosis rapidly result, requiring immediate, rapid transport of the patient to the emergency department.

The emergency treatment of a flail chest requires maintenance of the airway, vigorous respiratory support, and the administration of supplemental oxygen. Pain associated with the injury and the paradoxical motion of the flail segment will limit the patient's voluntary breathing. Stabilize the flail segment by applying firm support to it. The patient may breathe more comfortably if positioned with the flail segment against some external support such as the surface of the litter or a firm pillow. Frequently, the flail segment will involve the central portion of the anterior chest wall with a fracture of the sternum and fractures of ribs on both sides of the sternum. In this circumstance, the patient may breathe more readily when grasping a pillow and holding it up against the flail segment (Figure 24–5). Such support may lessen paradoxical motion and pain. Monitor the patient's vital signs closely; give respiratory support and oxygen to maintain adequate ventilation. Transport these patients as promptly as possible to the hospital.

Penetrating Injury

If driven with enough force, any sharp object can produce a penetrating chest injury. Common examples of these types of injury are stab wounds and gunshot wounds (Figure 24–6). Occasionally the force will cause a rib fracture. Penetrating injury usually produces varying degrees of hemothorax, pneumothorax, or both. Sucking chest wounds are frequently created by these injuries. All of these complications of chest injury are described separately later in this chapter.

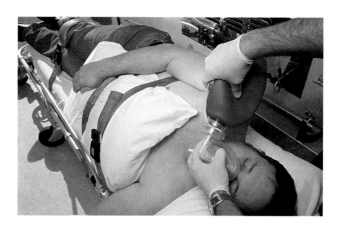

FIGURE 24–5

A flail anterior chest wall segment can be stabilized by having the patient hold a pillow firmly against the chest wall.

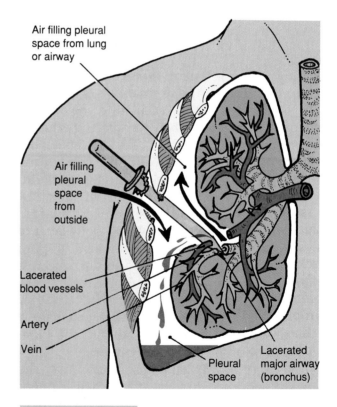

FIGURE 24–6

Damage to the lung, the heart, the great vessels, or the major airways may occur with a penetrating injury.

A penetrating object may injure any structure within the thoracic cavity. Gunshot wounds often have points of entrance and exit that give some clue about their route of transit and the structures injured. There is significant danger of laceration of the heart or the great vessels with each penetration. In such instances bleeding may be massive but rarely visible outside of the body, because it remains contained within the chest cavity. The patient, in addition to having respiratory distress from the injury, may be in shock from severe, rapid blood loss. Thus, a penetrating injury of the chest is a critical injury and may be fatal. Secure and maintain the patient's airway at once and administer ventilatory support and oxygen promptly. Treat the patient for hypovolemic shock by elevating the feet and controlling all obvious external bleeding. Rapid transportation to the hospital is necessary to save this critically injured patient's life.

Compression Injury

Sometimes a patient sustains sudden, severe circumferential compression of the chest, which produces a rapid increase in intrathoracic pressure. Such injuries occur commonly when the chest is crushed by a heavy object, such as a collapsed ceiling. Multiple fractures of the ribs can occur; a flail chest may result. This condition is called *traumatic asphyxia*. In addition, because of the sudden increased intrathoracic pressure that is transmitted to the heart and major veins in the chest, the upper part of the body may become cyanotic and swollen; the neck veins may be distended, and the eyes appear to bulge. Severe intrathoracic injury is common following this type of circumferential compression. It includes chest wall damage, pulmonary contusion, and cardiac injury; death is often immediate. Vigorous respiratory support and prompt transport to the hospital are both necessary.

Injuries of the Back of the Chest

Direct blows on the back of the chest can produce contusions or rib fractures. Other common injuries of the back are muscular strains and lacerations. Any patient who complains of pain in the back following injury should be examined very carefully for a spinal injury. In addition, it is imperative to monitor the patient's airway and ventilatory status closely.

An uncommon injury of the back of the chest is a fracture of the scapula. The scapula is covered by very large muscles. Consequently, if a fracture of this bone is suspected, you must assume that the patient has sustained a particularly severe blow. This degree of force will usually injure the underlying chest wall and lung. If you observe a significant contusion, abrasion, or laceration of the shoulder, some respiratory difficulty may also accompany this injury; be alert for it.

Direct blows to the lower posterior rib cage in the region of the tenth through twelfth ribs can cause an injury of the kidney on that side. This problem is described in Chapter 26.

COMPLICATIONS OF CHEST INJURIES

Many of the injuries just described have similar results, even though the causes of the injury may be different. You must be aware that any of these injuries may cause one or more of the complications considered in this section. The treatment of each of these complications is also described.

Pneumothorax

Pneumothorax (the presence of air within the chest cavity in the pleural space but outside the lung) is a condition in which the lung has been separated from the chest wall and is said to be "collapsed" (Figure 24–7). The volume of the lung is diminished, and the amount of air that can be inhaled into it is thus reduced. As a result, hypoxia will occur. As the degree of pneumothorax increases, respiratory distress becomes more severe. Pneumothorax can result from an open injury when air enters the pleural space through a wound in the chest wall. It can also be caused by air leaking from

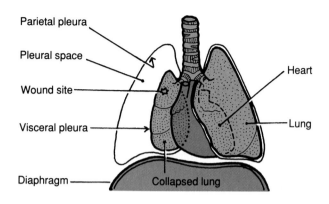

FIGURE 24–7

Pneumothorax occurs when air leaks into the pleural space from an opening in the chest wall or the surface of the lung itself. The lung collapses as air fills the pleural space and the two pleural surfaces are no longer in contact.

the lung or bronchus into the pleural space following a laceration of either one by a fractured rib or a penetrating instrument.

In a pneumothorax, the normal mechanism by which the lung expands (the fluid adhesion of the pleural surface of the lung to the pleural surface of the chest wall) is lost, and the affected lung cannot expand during inhalation (see the description of mechanics of breathing in Chapter 6). For patients with an open wound of the chest, the amount of pneumothorax that develops can be minimized by rapidly sealing the open wound prior to transport so that air will not be sucked into the chest through the wound.

In treating the patient suspected of having a pneumothorax, your sequence of treatment consists of clearing and maintaining the airway; administering oxygen; covering any open wound with a sterile, occlusive dressing; and transporting the patient to the hospital promptly.

Spontaneous Pneumothorax

In some people, congenitally weak areas exist on the surface of the lungs. Occasionally, such a weak area will rupture (blow out) spontaneously, allowing air to leak into the pleural space. Usually this event, called spontaneous pneumothorax, is not related to any major injury but simply happens with normal breathing. The patient experiences sudden sharp chest pain and increasing difficulty in breathing. The affected lung collapses, losing its ability to expand normally. The amount of pneumothorax that develops will vary, and the patient with this problem may be in no, mild, moderate, or severe respiratory distress.

You should suspect a spontaneous pneumothorax in a patient who develops the sudden onset of chest pain and shortness of breath without a specific known cause. The treatment of this patient is the same as for the patient with a traumatic pneumothorax.

Tension Pneumothorax

A patient with a pneumothorax that results from trauma or from a spontaneous rupture of the lung may develop a **tension pneumothorax.** In this condition, air continuously leaks out of the lung into the pleural space, expanding within the space with every breath the patient takes. The air, trapped in the pleural space, cannot escape. Hence, with each breath the affected lung collapses more until it is completely reduced in size to a very small ball 2 or 3 inches in diameter. At this point, pressure in the affected chest cavity begins to rise, and the collapsed lung is pressed against the heart and the lung on the opposite side; hence the term *tension pneumothorax.* The remaining uninjured lung in turn becomes compressed. As the pressure in the chest cavity rises further, it may exceed the normal pressure of blood in the veins returning to the heart (Figure 24–8). Blood can then no longer travel to the heart to be pumped to the lungs for oxygenation and then to the body. Death can follow rapidly.

Tension pneumothorax cannot exist without an intact or well-sealed chest wall. However, it is not limited to closed chest injuries. A patient with an open chest wound and a severe lung laceration may develop a tension pneumothorax after the external chest wound has been effectively bandaged and sealed (by you). In this situation, the lung may continue to leak air into the now closed pleural space, and a tension pneumothorax may develop.

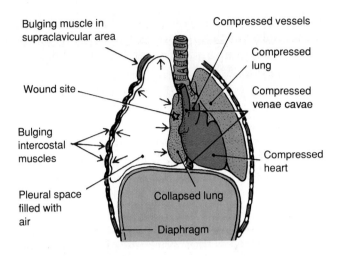

Bulging muscle in supraclavicular area

Compressed vessels

Compressed lung

Wound site

Compressed venae cavae

Bulging intercostal muscles

Compressed heart

Pleural space filled with air

Collapsed lung

Diaphragm

FIGURE 24–8

A tension pneumothorax develops when air, leaking from a lung or bronchus, or through the chest wall, becomes trapped in the pleural space and cannot escape to the outside. With each breath, more air accumulates in the pleural space. The trapped air compresses the injured lung and eventually the uninjured lung, the heart, and the great vessels. A tension pneumothorax can occur if a penetrating chest wound is bandaged tightly and air from a damaged lung cannot escape. It then accumulates within the pleural space.

The signs of a tension pneumothorax are severe, progressive respiratory distress, a weak pulse, rapidly falling blood pressure, bulging of the tissues of the chest wall between the ribs and above the clavicle, distension of the veins in the neck, and cyanosis. The condition may be rapidly progressive, causing death within a very few minutes.

Your treatment of a tension pneumothorax is directed at relieving the increasing pressure within the pleural space as soon as possible. In patients with closed chest injuries, decompression is accomplished by a physician or other appropriately trained person with advanced medical skills by placing a large bore needle into the pleural space to relieve the pressure.

If a tension pneumothorax develops following the bandaging of an open chest wound, simply releasing the dressing is often effective in relieving the problem. The air accumulated under pressure in the pleural space will rush from the wound once the dressing is released. Occlusive dressings for chest wounds can, according to local protocol, be applied with one edge not taped to allow air to escape from the injured chest, but not be drawn back in.

It must be emphasized that tension pneumothorax is one of the very few truly minute-by-minute emergencies. Prompt treatment of this patient will be lifesaving. Administer oxygen and transport the patient rapidly to the hospital.

Hemothorax

Hemothorax (the presence of blood in the chest cavity within the pleural space) may occur in open or closed chest injuries (Figure 24–9a). It is frequently accompanied by a pneumothorax

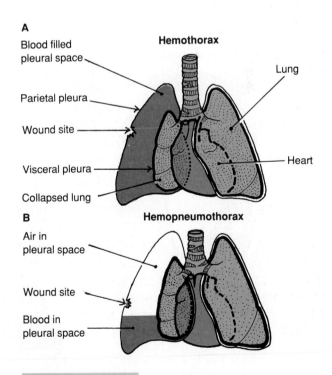

A

Hemothorax

Blood filled pleural space

Lung

Parietal pleura

Wound site

Visceral pleura

Heart

Collapsed lung

B

Hemopneumothorax

Air in pleural space

Wound site

Blood in pleural space

FIGURE 24–9

(A) A hemothorax is a collection of blood in the pleural space produced by lacerated blood vessels within the chest cavity. (B) Often hemothorax and pneumothorax coexist.

(Figure 24–9b). The bleeding may come from lacerated vessels in the chest wall, from lacerated major vessels within the chest cavity itself, or from a laceration of the lung. The air usually comes from a laceration of the lung or the chest wall. If the bleeding into the chest cavity is severe, the patient may develop hypovolemic shock.

In hemothorax, as in pneumothorax, the chest cavity becomes filled with something other than the lungs. Normal lung expansion cannot occur, and the lung itself is compressed. Less air can be inhaled. In addition, there may be significantly less blood available in the circulation to carry this reduced amount of oxygen to the patient's vital organs.

The patient with a hemothorax will have signs and symptoms very similar to the patient with a pneumothorax; in addition, the patient may be in hypovolemic shock as a result of the blood loss. You must remember that the blood loss will not be obvious, because it accumulates out of sight within the chest cavity.

The patient with a hemothorax requires immediate ventilatory support, the administration of oxygen, and prompt transportation to the hospital.

Sucking Chest Wound

An open chest wall injury may produce a sucking chest wound. In this condition, outside air is sucked through the open wound when the patient inhales (Figure 24–10a). Ordinarily, the pressure inside the chest cavity is slightly less than that of the atmosphere. Inhalation further reduces this pressure. If there is an open wound in the chest wall, air will move through the wound just as easily as it moves through the nose and mouth during normal respiration. The air that enters through the wound remains in the pleural space (a pneumothorax), and the lung does not expand. When the patient exhales, air passes back through the wound. Such open wounds are called **sucking chest wounds** because each time

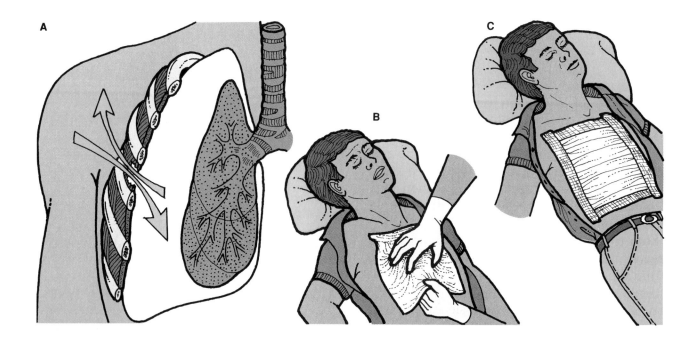

FIGURE 24–10   (A) With a sucking chest wound, air passes from the outside into the pleural space and back out with each breath—creating the sucking sound. (B) A sucking chest wound should be sealed with a large airtight dressing of aluminum foil or Vaseline gauze. (C) The dressing should be secured to the chest wall with tape.

the patient breathes there is a sucking sound at the wound caused by the passage of air.

As an initial emergency step, you must seal sucking chest wounds with an airtight dressing (Figure 24–10b and c). The purpose of the airtight dressing is to seal the wound and prevent air from passing through it. Several sterile materials, including aluminum foil, Vaseline gauze, or a folded universal dressing, may be used to seal the wound. A large enough cover must be used so that the dressing itself will not be sucked into the chest cavity. Secure the dressing to the chest wall with tape to prevent any air leakages around its edges. When a lung injury exists, remember that the patient with an occlusive bandage can develop a tension pneumothorax. Should the signs of a tension pneumothorax develop, release one edge of the occlusive dressing to allow the air under tension to escape from the pleural space.

Subcutaneous Emphysema

Laceration of the lung or disruption of any part of the tracheobronchial tree may allow air to escape into the soft tissue of the chest wall or neck. The air will spread into these tissues much as blood spreads into them following a contusion. Small bubbles of air come to lie in the subcutaneous tissue. This condition is called subcutaneous emphysema. When you palpate the area you will feel a crackling sensation under your fingertips as the bubbles of air are pushed about. In very severe instances, subcutaneous emphysema can involve the entire chest, neck, face, and head. Fractured ribs, with laceration of the lung, are the most common cause of this condition. The presence of subcutaneous emphysema may indicate a significant loss of respiratory function. After you begin ventilatory support and oxygen, transport the patient promptly to the hospital for evaluation and treatment.

Pulmonary Contusion

A pulmonary contusion is a bruise of the lung. It occurs in much the same way as bruises of any other tissue in the body. The lung is very fragile and quite susceptible to contusion.

When the blood vessels in the lung are injured, a considerable amount of blood oozes into the tissue around them; edema fluid also accumulates in the injured area. In the contused area of the lung, the exchange of oxygen and carbon dioxide between the alveolus and the capillaries of the blood vessels cannot take place normally because of the accumulation of blood and fluid.

Pulmonary contusion is almost uniformly associated with major blunt injuries of the chest, such as those that occur in automobile accidents and severe falls. It occurs commonly after a direct blow on the chest and may cause severe respiratory distress, depending on the extent of lung involved. The size of the contusion is the most important factor in determining its effect on the patient's ability to breathe. Pulmonary contusion of a significant degree will result in severe hypoxia. The patient may be in significant respiratory distress with rapid respirations and even cyanosis. You must then administer full ventilatory support and oxygen. Prompt transportation to the emergency department is mandatory.

Myocardial Contusion

Blunt injuries of the chest may produce **myocardial contusion,** or bruising of the heart muscle itself. This injury may not be detectable until fairly sophisticated laboratory and electrocardiographic studies have been done on the patient. Ordinarily, a severe myocardial contusion disturbs the electrical conduction system that controls the heart rate. In these circumstances, the heart becomes irritable. The sign of such irritability is extra heartbeats, which irregularly interrupt the normal cardiac rhythm. The patient with a myocardial contusion will have an irregular pulse with occasional pauses and occasional beats coming very close together.

There is no specific treatment in the field for myocardial contusion. However, in any patient who has sustained a chest injury, you must check the pulse carefully. Report any abnormality in the pulse rate or rhythm promptly to medical control, along with your suspicion of a possible myocardial contusion. Any sign of a myocardial contusion requires prompt transportation of the patient to the hospital because persistent irregularity of the heartbeat may result in a major abnormal rhythm that could lead to death.

Pericardial Tamponade

In **pericardial tamponade,** blood or other fluid collects in the pericardial sac **(pericardium)** that surrounds the heart, thereby squeezing on the heart. In patients with chest injuries, the condition almost always results from penetrating wounds of the heart that have opened one of its chambers so that, with each heartbeat, blood leaks out into the sac. The pericardial sac is a very tough, fibrous membrane that cannot stretch. When blood leaks out of the heart, it is caught within this unyielding sac. As blood accumulates within the pericardial cavity, it compresses the heart so that its chambers can no longer hold the blood normally returned to them through the veins.

The signs of pericardial tamponade are

- Very soft and faint heart tones (hard to hear even with a stethoscope).
- A weak pulse.
- Blood pressure readings in which the systolic and diastolic pressures come closer and closer together during successive readings (called a narrowing of the pulse pressure).
- Congested and distended veins in the upper part of the body, particularly the veins of the neck.

Pericardial tamponade is a rapidly progressive and life-threatening condition. The pressure of the blood accumulating within the pericardial sac must be relieved quickly or death will occur very rapidly. After you initiate vigorous respiratory support and oxygen, transport the patient rapidly to the hospital. Notify the hospital of the diagnosis of pericardial tamponade so that preparations can be made for its immediate treatment upon arrival.

Laceration of the Great Vessels

The chest contains several large blood vessels: the superior vena cava, the inferior vena cava, the main pulmonary artery, four main pulmonary veins, and the aorta with its major arteries distributing blood throughout the body. Injury of any of these vessels may be accompanied by massive, rapidly fatal hemorrhage. Any patient with a chest wound who is in hypovolemic shock may have an injury to one of these vessels. Frequently, the loss of blood is not obvious, because it remains within the chest cavity.

Emergency treatment of laceration of the great vessels includes pulmonary resuscitation with ventilatory support and the administration of oxygen. Here, particularly, rapid transport of the patient to the hospital may be lifesaving. A few minutes have meant the difference between life and death for some of these patients.

YOU ARE THE EMT

1. Describe the difference between a hemothorax and a pneumothorax. What is the treatment for each? How does each interfere with breathing?
2. One of the signs of chest injury is pleuritic pain. What is pleuritic pain? What are five other signs of chest injury?
3. Why is a flail chest injury such a serious problem? What is the emergency treatment of flail chest?
4. How is tension pneumothorax treated in a closed chest injury? In an open chest injury?
5. Define the term pulmonary contusion and state why it is important in chest injury.
6. What is a myocardial contusion? How would you identify its presence?
7. What is the mechanism by which pericardial tamponade produces death?

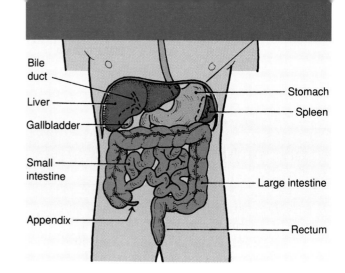

CHAPTER 25

THE ABDOMEN AND GENITALIA

KEY TERMS

abdomen (ab-do'men) The more inferior of the two major cavities, lying between the thorax and the pelvis and containing the major organs of digestion and excretion.

digestion (di-jest'yun) The chemical conversion of food into simple sugars, fats, and proteins that can be absorbed into the body and used by cells for energy.

hollow organs Tubes through which material passes, such as the stomach, intestines, ureters, and bladder.

hormone (hor'mōn) Chemical substance produced in the body by a gland that has special regulatory effects on the activities of another distant organ.

menstrual cycle The period of the regularly recurring changes in the endometrium that result in blood and mucus being shed intermittently, usually every 28 days.

mesentery (mes'en-ter"e) The delicate tissue formed by the peritoneum that suspends the organs within the abdomen and carries blood vessels and nerves to all these organs.

mucous membrane (mu'kus mem'brān) The lining of body cavities and passages that communicate directly or indirectly with the environment outside the body.

pelvic cavity The space within the walls of the pelvis.

peristalsis (per"ĭ-stal'sis) The wavelike movement by which the alimentary canal or other tubular organs propel their contents.

peritoneum (per"i-to-ne'um) The membrane lining the abdominal cavity (parietal peritoneum) and reflected inward over the abdominal organs (visceral peritoneum).

peritonitis (per"ĭ-to-ni'tis) Inflammation of the peritoneum.

referred pain Pain felt in an area of the body other than where the cause of pain is located.

solid organs Solid masses of tissue where much of the chemical work of the body takes place: in the liver, spleen, pancreas, and kidneys.

The abdomen is the lower of the two major body cavities. It extends from the diaphragm to the pelvis. It contains several organs that make up the digestive, the urinary, and the genital systems. Although all of these organs may be injured, some are better protected than others. You must know where these organs are located within the abdominal or pelvic cavities. You must also understand their functions so that, when an illness or injury occurs, you can assess its seriousness.

Chapter 25 begins with a description of the abdominal cavity—its boundaries and the organs that lie within it. Then the organs that make up the digestive system are more fully described. Peristalsis, the wavelike contraction that propels food through the digestive tract, is explained next. The component organs of the urinary system are presented. The chapter concludes with a description of the male and female reproductive systems. An explanation of the normal menstrual cycle in women is included.

The goals of Chapter 25 are to
- identify the boundaries, the bony landmarks, and the location of organs in the various quadrants of the abdominal cavity and in the pelvis.
- know the function of the various organs of the digestive system and how food is converted into nutrients for use by the body's cells.
- understand how food is propelled through the digestive tract by peristalsis; describe peristalsis.
- describe the location and functions of the organs of the urinary system.
- describe the organs of the male and female genital systems and understand their role in the reproductive process.
- identify the steps of the normal menstrual cycle.

THE ABDOMINAL CAVITY
. . . .

The abdominal cavity is the lower of the two major body cavities of the torso (trunk). It is divided into two parts: the **abdomen** and the pelvis.

The superior boundary of the abdomen is the diaphragm (the muscle separating the abdomen and the thorax); the inferior boundary is an imaginary plane between the pubis and the sacrum (pelvic bones). The anterior and posterior boundaries are the musculoskeletal body walls (Figure 25–1). The entire abdominal cavity is lined by the **peritoneum**, a glistening smooth layer of cells that covers the organs of the cavity and also lines the cavity wall.

The abdominal cavity contains the liver, gallbladder, bile ducts, spleen, stomach, and intestines (Figure 25–2). Immediately behind the peritoneum and between it and the major back muscles lie the kidneys with their drainage tubes (the ureters), the adrenal glands, the pancreas, and part of the duodenum, of the small intestine. In this same area between the peritoneum and the back muscles (the retroperitoneal space) lie two major blood vessels,

A

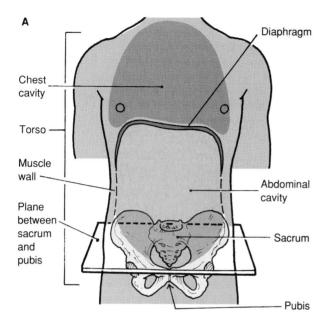

B

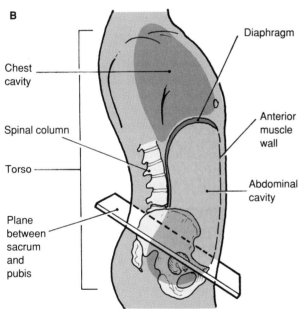

FIGURE   25-1

The boundaries of the abdomen are the anterior and posterior abdominal cavity walls, the diaphragm, and an imaginary plane between the pubis and the sacrum. (A) An anterior view; (B) a lateral view.

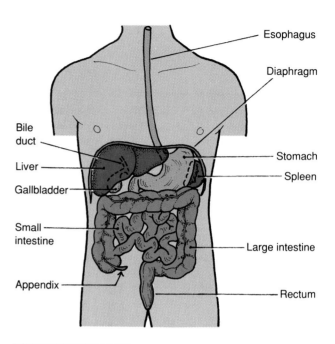

FIGURE   25-2

The major organs of the abdomen.

the aorta and the inferior vena cava. Many nerves and lymph glands lie near these large vessels (Figure 25–3).

The lower portion of the abdominal cavity, below the imaginary plane running from the pubis to the sacrum, is the pelvis (or **pelvic cavity**). In it lie the rectum, the urinary bladder, and in the female, the reproductive organs (Figure 25–4).

Nearly all of the organs within the abdomen are suspended from the body wall by sheets of tissue called **mesentery** (Figure 25–5). The mesentery is a very delicate tissue formed from the peritoneum. The mesentery carries blood vessels and nerves to all of the organs. The organs hang fairly freely from their mesenteric attachments, which allows them some movement within the abdominal cavity. This mobility is necessary for the normal continuous muscular activity of the bowel.

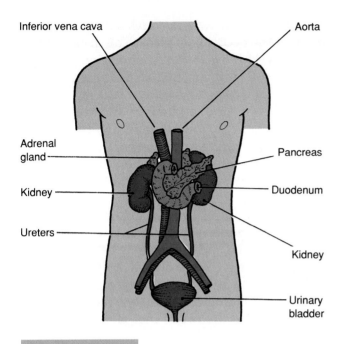

FIGURE 25-3

The major organs of the retroperitoneal space between the peritoneum and the back muscles; the aorta and inferior vena cava also lie in this plane.

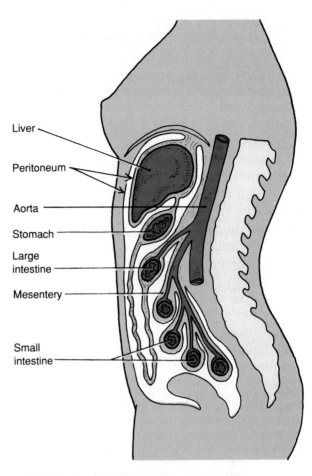

FIGURE 25-5

The abdominal organs are suspended from the body wall by tissue called mesentery. Within the mesentery are blood vessels that nourish the abdominal organs.

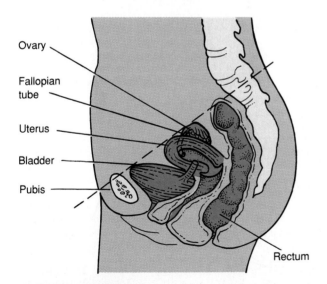

FIGURE 25-4

In the female, the major organs of the pelvic cavity include the reproductive organs.

The peritoneum lining the abdominal cavity, like all other tissues, has a nerve supply. The peritoneum lining the walls of the abdomen can perceive the same sensations as the skin can; however, the peritoneum forming the mesentery and covering the organs of the abdomen cannot localize a source of pain and can perceive only tension or stretching. The dual innervation of the two parts of the peritoneum gives rise to the phenomenon of **referred pain,** which is discussed in Chapter 33.

In general, the organs of the abdominal cavity and in the retroperitoneal space are either hollow or solid. **Hollow organs** are tubes through which material passes. For example, the stomach and intestines conduct food through the body; the ureters and bladder conduct and store urine until it is expelled. The stomach, duodenum, small intestine, large intestine (colon), rectum, appendix, gallbladder, bile ducts, urinary bladder, ureters, uterus, and Fallopian tubes are the hollow organs of the abdomen (Figure 25–6). **Solid organs** are solid

masses of tissue where much of the chemical work of the body takes place. The liver, spleen, pancreas, kidneys, ovaries, and adrenal glands are the solid organs of the abdomen (Figure 25–7).

Injuries to the abdomen and pelvis can damage either hollow or solid organs. In general, hollow organs discharge their contents into the abdominal cavity when they are lacerated, whereas solid organs tend to bleed copiously. Spilled content from the hollow organs usually sets up an intense inflammatory reaction, called **peritonitis,** which is very painful. Bleeding from solid organs may be rapidly fatal and frequently causes shock. Mesentery supporting hollow organs can be lacerated. In such instances bleeding from the torn mesentery can be severe, and the organ that is torn away will lose its blood supply.

The topographic anatomy of the abdomen was presented in Chapter 4. Bony landmarks, the major features of topography, in the abdomen include the symphysis pubis, the costal

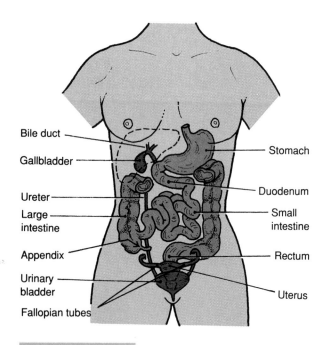

FIGURE 25–6

The hollow organs of the abdominal cavity, the retroperitoneal space, and the pelvic cavity.

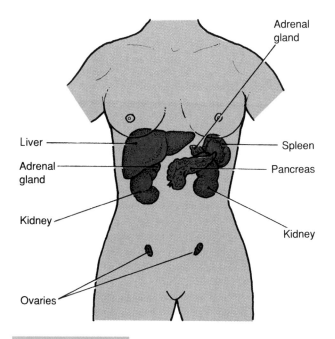

FIGURE 25–7

The solid organs of the abdominal cavity and the retroperitoneal space.

arch, the iliac crests, and the anterior superior iliac spines. The major soft tissue landmark is the umbilicus, which overlies the fourth lumbar vertebra. The abdomen is divided arbitrarily into quadrants by two perpendicular lines that intersect at the umbilicus (Figure 25–8).

THE DIGESTIVE SYSTEM

The digestive system is composed of the gastrointestinal tract (stomach and intestines), mouth, salivary glands, pharynx, esophagus, liver, gallbladder, pancreas, rectum, and anus (Figure 25–9). The function of this system is **digestion**—the processing of food that nourishes the individual cells of the body. Digestion of food, from the time it is taken into the mouth until essential compounds are extracted and delivered by the circulatory system to nourish all of the cells in the body, is a complicated chemical process. In succession, different secretions, primarily enzymes, are added to the food by the salivary glands, the stomach, the

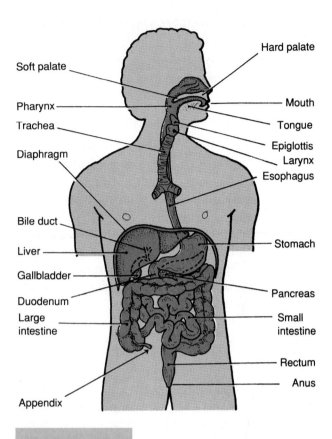

FIGURE 25–9

The digestive system lies within the head, thorax, abdomen, and pelvis. The many organs involved pass ingested food from mouth to anus and convert sugar, fat, and proteins to glucose and fatty and amino acids by a complex chemical process called digestion.

liver, the pancreas, and the small intestine to convert the food into basic sugars, fatty acids, and amino acids. These basic products of digestion are carried across the wall of the intestine and transported through the portal vein to the liver. In the liver, the products are processed further and then stored or transported to the heart through veins draining that organ. The heart then pumps the blood with these nutrients throughout the arteries and then to the capillaries where the nutrients pass through the capillary walls to nourish the body's individual cells.

Digestion also produces many chemical compounds that are poisonous. They cannot be passed safely into the general body circulation

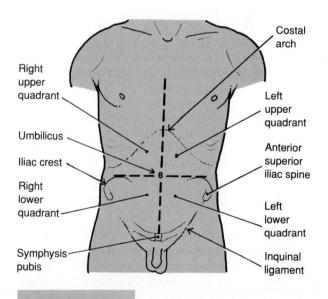

FIGURE 25–8

The bony landmarks and the major soft tissue landmark (the umbilicus) of the abdomen. The abdomen is divided into four quadrants.

until the liver has transformed them. All blood leaving the intestine must pass first through the portal vein to the liver to ensure protection for the body against such compounds.

Mouth and Salivary Glands

The mouth consists of the lips, cheeks, gums, teeth, and tongue. A **mucous membrane** lines the mouth. The roof of the mouth is formed by the hard and soft palates. The hard palate is a bony plate lying anteriorly; the soft palate is a fold of mucous membrane and muscle that extends posteriorly from the hard palate into the throat. The soft palate is designed to hold food that is being chewed within the mouth and to help initiate swallowing.

Paired salivary glands are located under the tongue, on each side of the lower jaw, and on each cheek. They produce nearly 1.5 liters of saliva daily. Saliva is approximately 98 percent water. The remaining 2 percent is composed of mucus, salts, and organic compounds. Mucus serves as a binder for the chewed food being swallowed and as a lubricant within the mouth.

Ptyalin, the only enzyme in saliva, initiates the digestion of starches. Otherwise, food is converted into a soft mush in the mouth and is mixed with mucus and saliva for easy swallowing.

Pharynx

The pharynx, or throat, is a tubular structure about 5 inches long that extends vertically from the back of the mouth to the esophagus and trachea. The trachea lies just in front of the esophagus. It is connected with the pharynx by the larynx, or voice box. The larynx is covered by a leaf-shaped valve called the epiglottis. An automatic movement of the pharynx during swallowing lifts the larynx to permit the epiglottis to close over it so that liquids and solids are moved into the esophagus and away from the trachea.

Esophagus

The esophagus is a collapsible tube about 10 inches long. It extends from the end of the pharynx to the stomach and lies just anterior to the spinal column in the chest. Contractions of the muscle in the wall of the esophagus propel food through it to the stomach. Liquids will pass with very little assistance.

Stomach

The stomach is located in the left upper quadrant of the abdominal cavity, largely protected by the lower left ribs. Muscular contraction in the wall of the stomach and gastric juice, which contains much mucus, convert ingested food to a thoroughly mixed semisolid mass. The stomach produces approximately 1.5 liters of gastric juice daily for this process. The major function of the stomach is to receive food in large quantities intermittently, store it, and provide for its movement into the small bowel in regular, small amounts. In 1 to 3 hours the semisolid food mass derived from one meal is propelled by muscular contraction into the duodenum, the first part of the small intestine. Poisoning or any reaction to trauma may paralyze gastric muscular action and cause retention of food in the stomach for prolonged periods. In these situations, vomiting is the only way the stomach can empty itself. Only one digestive enzyme, pepsin, is produced in the stomach and secreted into the gastric juice. This agent initiates the digestion of protein.

Pancreas

The pancreas, a flat, solid organ, lies below and behind the liver and stomach and behind the peritoneum on the spine and muscles of the back. It is firmly fixed in position, deep within the abdomen, and is not easily damaged. It contains two kinds of glands. One set of glands secretes nearly 2 liters of pancreatic juice daily. This juice contains many enzymes that aid in the digestion of fat, starch, and protein. Pancreatic juice flows directly into the duodenum through the pancreatic ducts.

The endocrine gland called the islets of Langerhans is the other kind of gland. It does not connect to any duct but secretes its products into the bloodstream across the walls of the capillary vessels. The islets produce a

hormone, insulin, that regulates the amount of sugar in the blood.

Liver

The liver is a large solid organ that takes up most of the area immediately beneath the diaphragm in the right upper quadrant. It is the largest solid organ in the abdomen and consequently one of the most often injured. The liver has several functions. Poisonous substances produced by digestion are brought to it by the blood and are rendered harmless. Factors necessary for blood clotting and for the production of normal plasma are formed here. Between 0.5 and 1 liter of bile is made by the liver daily to assist in the normal digestion of fat. The liver is the principal organ for the storage of sugar or starch for immediate use by the body for energy. It also produces many of the factors that aid in the proper regulation of immune responses.

Anatomically, the liver is a large mass of blood vessels and cells, packed tightly together. It is fragile and, because of its size, relatively easily injured. Blood flow in the liver is high, because all of the blood that is pumped to the gastrointestinal tract passes into the liver, through the portal vein, before it returns to the heart. In addition, the liver has a generous arterial blood supply of its own. Ordinarily, approximately one-quarter of the cardiac output of blood (1.5 liters) passes through the liver each minute.

Biliary System

The liver is connected to the intestine by the bile ducts. The gallbladder is an outpouching from the bile ducts that serves as a reservoir and concentrating organ for bile produced in the liver. Together, the bile ducts and gallbladder form the biliary system. The gallbladder discharges stored and concentrated bile into the duodenum through the common bile duct. The presence of food in the duodenum triggers a contraction of the gallbladder to empty it. The gallbladder usually contains 2 to 3 ounces of bile. Stones can form in the gallbladder and can pass into the common bile duct and obstruct it. This obstruction will produce jaundice.

Small Intestine

The small intestine, the major abdominal hollow organ, is so named because of its diameter in comparison with the large intestine. The small intestine is composed of the duodenum, the jejunum, and the ileum.

The duodenum, about 12 inches long, passes from the stomach to the jejunum. Most of this organ lies behind the peritoneum and closely curls around the pancreas. The duodenum is that part of the small intestine that receives food from the stomach. Here the food is mixed with secretions from the pancreas and liver for further digestion.

The jejunum and ileum together measure more than 20 feet on the average to make up the rest of the small intestine. The jejunum is the first or upper half, and the ileum is the second or lower half. The small intestine empties into the large intestine through the ileocecal valve between the ileum and cecum, the first part of the large bowel. This valve directs the passage of bowel contents in only one direction—into the colon. The junction of the small and large bowel is normally in the right lower quadrant of the abdominal cavity. The appendix is attached to the cecum at this point.

The small intestine hangs freely within the abdomen, dependent on its mesentery. Arteries from the aorta to the intestine and veins carrying blood to the liver lie in this mesentery. The cells lining the small intestine produce more enzymes and mucus to aid in digestion.

Bile, produced by the liver and stored in the gallbladder, is emptied as needed into the duodenum. It is greenish black but through changes during digestion, it gives feces their typical brown color. Its major function is in the digestion of fat. Enzymes from the pancreas and the small intestine carry out the final processes of digestion. More than 90 percent of the products of digestion (amino acids, fatty acids, and simple sugars), together with water, ingested vitamins, and minerals are absorbed across the wall of the lower end of the ileum into veins to be transported to the liver.

In normal routine activity, without any food or fluid ingestion at all, between 8 to 10 liters of fluid are secreted daily into the gastrointestinal tract. This fluid comes from the salivary glands, stomach, liver, pancreas, and small bowel. In a normal adult, about 7 percent of the body weight is delivered as fluid daily to the gastrointestinal tract. If significant vomiting or diarrhea occurs for more than 2 or 3 days, the patient will lose a very substantial portion of body composition and become severely ill.

Large Intestine

The large intestine, another major hollow organ, consists of the cecum, the colon, and the rectum. About 5 feet long, it encircles the outer border of the abdomen around the small bowel. The major function of the colon, the portion of the large intestine that extends from the cecum to the rectum, is to absorb the final 5 to 10 percent of digested food and water from the intestine to form solid stool, which is stored in the rectum and passed out of the body through the anus.

Appendix

The appendix is a small tube that opens into the cecum (the first part of the large intestine) in the right lower quadrant of the abdomen. It is 3 or 4 inches long. It may easily become obstructed and, as a result, inflamed and infected. Appendicitis, which is the term for this inflammation, is one of the major causes of severe abdominal distress. The appendix has no known function.

Rectum and Anus

The lowermost end of the colon is the rectum. It is a large hollow organ that is adapted to store quantities of feces until they are expelled. At its terminal end is the anus, a canal lined by normal skin and approximately 2 inches long. The rectum and anus are supplied with a complex series of circular muscles called sphincters that control, both voluntarily and automatically, the escape of liquids, gases, and solids from the digestive tract.

The Spleen

Smaller than the liver, the spleen is a major solid organ. It, too, is primarily composed of blood vessels and cells and is even more fragile than the liver. The spleen is found in the left upper quadrant of the abdomen, just beneath the diaphragm and immediately in front of the ninth to eleventh ribs. It is fixed in position by three strong ligaments. Although it is well protected by the ribs, the supporting ligaments can easily be torn from the spleen in a blunt injury. Bleeding from the lacerated spleen may be very severe, controllable only by its removal. Injuries that produce fractures of the eighth through twelfth ribs on the left side are likely to cause lacerations of the spleen.

The spleen is not required for life, nor is it associated with the functions of the digestive tract. The major function of this organ lies in the normal production and destruction of blood cells. After the spleen is removed, its function is assumed by the liver and the bone marrow.

PERISTALSIS

There are two layers of involuntary (smooth) muscle throughout the entire gastrointestinal tract from the esophagus to the rectum. The outer layer of smooth muscle is oriented longitudinally, and the inner layer is circular (Figure 25–10). Contraction of these muscles is stimulated when they are stretched by food that is swallowed. This muscular contraction is called **peristalsis.** Peristalsis starts at the esophagus and proceeds in a coordinated wavelike fashion to the anus, propelling food through the whole tract (Figure 25–9). Once started, a wave passes entirely through the system.

When peristaltic waves are especially strong or when they are interrupted by an obstruction so that the contents cannot be propelled along smoothly, the contraction causes a painful

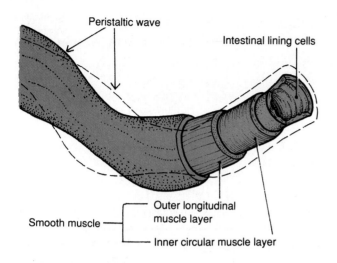

FIGURE 25-10

Peristalsis is a rhythmic, wavelike contraction of the smooth muscles in the wall of the intestine.

cramp that is called *colic*. Normal peristalsis is responsible for the bowel sounds that can be heard if one listens to the abdomen with a stethoscope. The sounds represent the passage of gas and fluid through the narrow, hollow digestive organs. Normally, peristalsis never ceases. It can, however, be abolished by peritonitis, abdominal injury, poisoning, or some diseases.

Discharge of gastrointestinal contents to some degree is controlled by two sets of sphincter muscles surrounding the anus. One of these muscles is involuntary and provides the major control of fecal passage; the other is voluntary and allows the individual to sense and control the passage of feces. Thus, the healthy person can control the time and rate of release of the products of digestion from the rectum.

THE URINARY SYSTEM

The urinary system controls the discharge of certain waste materials filtered from the blood by the kidneys. In the urinary system the kidneys are solid organs; the ureters, bladder, and urethra are hollow organs (Figure 25–11).

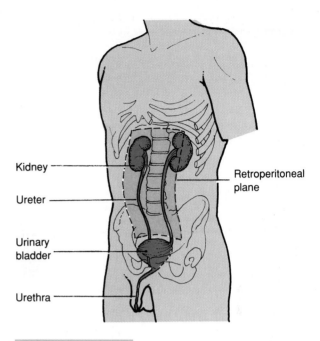

FIGURE 25-11

The urinary system lies in the retroperitoneal space behind the organs of the digestive system. The kidneys are solid organs, and the ureter, bladder, and urethra are hollow organs.

Ordinarily, we consider the urinary and genital systems together, because they share many organs in common. For clarity, the two systems are divided in this text. Figures 25–12 and 25–13 show the systems together.

Kidneys

The body has two *kidneys*. They lie on the posterior muscular wall of the abdomen behind the peritoneum in the retroperitoneal space. These organs rid the blood of toxic waste products and control its balance of water and salt. If the kidneys are destroyed or can no longer function adequately, a condition known as uremia occurs. Wastes accumulate within the bloodstream. The balance of salt and water is disturbed, and death will result.

Blood flow in the kidneys is high. Nearly 20 percent of the output of blood from the heart

FIGURE 25-12

The male genitourinary system.

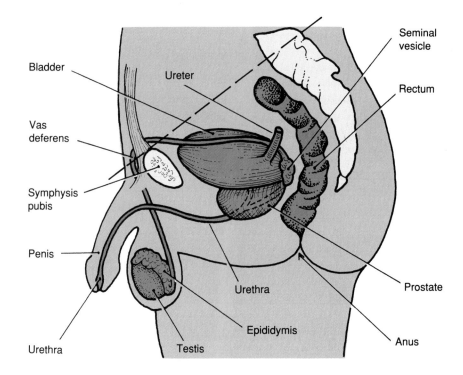

Seminal vesicle

Bladder

Ureter

Rectum

Vas deferens

Symphysis pubis

Penis

Urethra

Prostate

Urethra

Epididymis

Anus

Testis

FIGURE 25-13

The female genitourinary system.

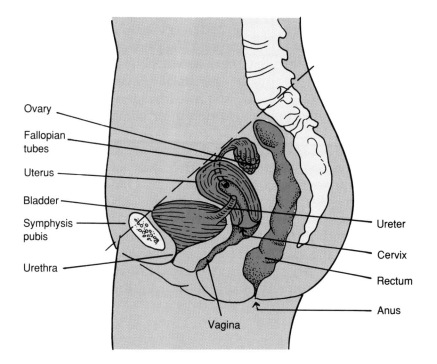

Ovary

Fallopian tubes

Uterus

Bladder

Symphysis pubis

Ureter

Cervix

Rectum

Urethra

Anus

Vagina

passes each minute through the kidneys. Large vessels attach the kidneys directly to the aorta and the inferior vena cava. Waste products and water are constantly filtered from the blood to form urine. The kidneys continuously concentrate this filtered urine by reabsorbing the water as it passes through a system of specialized tubes within them. The tubes finally unite to form the renal pelvis, a cone-shaped collecting area that connects the ureter and the kidney. Normally, each kidney drains its urine into one ureter through which the urine passes to the bladder.

Ureters

A *ureter* passes from the renal pelvis of each kidney along the surface of the posterior abdominal wall behind the peritoneum to drain into the urinary bladder. The ureters are small (diameter 0.5 centimeter), hollow, muscular tubes. Peristalsis occurs in these tubes to move the urine to the bladder.

Urinary Bladder and Urethra

The *urinary bladder* is situated immediately behind the pubic symphysis in the pelvic cavity. The two ureters enter posteriorly at its base on either side. The bladder empties to the outside of the body through the *urethra*. In the male, the urethra passes from the anterior base of the bladder through the *penis* (Figure 25–12). In the female, the urethra opens at the front of the *vagina* (Figure 25–13).

The bladder is formed of smooth muscle with a specialized lining membrane. Urination is largely an automatic function that can, however, be controlled voluntarily. Just as around the anus, there are muscular sphincters around the urethra over which we have some voluntary control. When the bladder reaches a critical point of fullness, sensory cells in its wall send messages to the brain signifying that the bladder must empty. The sensation is perceived as an urge or need to *void* (urinate). Under voluntary control, the sphincter muscles are relaxed, and the bladder involuntarily contracts to force urine through the urethra to the

outside of the body. The normal adult forms 1.5 to 2 liters of urine every day. This waste is extracted and concentrated from the 1,500 liters of blood that circulate through the kidneys daily.

THE GENITAL SYSTEM

The *genital system* controls the reproductive processes from which life is created. The male genitalia, except for the prostate gland and the seminal vesicles, lie outside the pelvic cavity (Figure 25–12). The female genitalia are contained entirely within the pelvis (Figure 25–13). The male and female reproductive organs have certain similarities and, of course, basic differences. They allow the production of *sperm* and *egg cells* and appropriate hormones, the act of *sexual intercourse* and reproduction.

Male Reproductive System and Organs

The male reproductive system includes the *testicles, vasa deferentia, seminal vesicles, prostate gland*, urethra, and penis (Figure 25–12). Each testicle contains specialized cells and ducts. Certain cells produce male hormones; others develop sperm. The hormones are absorbed directly into the bloodstream from the testicles. The vasa deferentia travel from the testicles up beneath the skin of the abdominal wall for a short distance. They then pass through an opening into the abdominal cavity and into the prostate gland to connect with the urethra. The vasa deferentia carry the sperm from the testicles to the urethra. The seminal vesicles are small storage sacs for sperm and seminal fluid. The vesicles also empty into the urethra.

Semen, also called *seminal fluid*, contains sperm cells carried up each vas from each testicle to be mixed with fluid from the seminal vesicles and prostate gland. The prostate gland surrounds the urethra where it emerges from the urinary bladder. Fluids from the prostate gland and from the seminal vesicles mix during sexual intercourse. During intercourse, special mechanisms in the nervous system prevent the passage of urine into the urethra. Only seminal fluid, prostatic fluid, and sperm pass from the penis into the vagina during ejaculation.

The penis contains a special type of tissue called *erectile tissue*. This specialized tissue is largely vascular; and, when filled with blood, causes the penis to distend into a state of erection. As the vessels fill under pressure from the circulatory system, the penis becomes a large rigid organ that can enter the vagina. Certain spinal injuries, and some diseases, can cause a painful continuous erection called *priapism*.

Female Reproductive System and Organs

The female reproductive organs include the *ovaries, Fallopian tubes, uterus, cervix,* and vagina (Figure 25–13). The ovaries, like the testicles, produce sex hormones and specialized cells for reproduction. The female sex hormones are absorbed directly into the bloodstream. A specialized *ovum* or egg cell is produced regularly during the adult female's reproductive years. The ovaries release a mature egg approximately every 28 days. This egg travels through the Fallopian tubes to the uterus.

The Fallopian tubes connect with the uterus and carry the ovum into the cavity of this organ. The uterus is pear-shaped and hollow, with muscular walls. The narrow opening from the uterus to the vagina is the cervix. The vagina is a muscular distensible tube that connects the uterus with the *vulva* (the external female genitalia). The vagina receives the male penis during sexual intercourse, when semen and sperm are deposited in it. The sperm may pass into the uterus and fertilize an egg, causing pregnancy. Should the pregnancy come to completion at the end of nine months, the baby will pass through the vagina and be born. The vagina also channels the menstrual flow from the uterus out of the body.

Menstrual Cycle

The menstrual period is the end of the monthly female reproductive cycle. From the start of her first menstrual period at about age 12, until she passes through *menopause* at about age 50, a woman has monthly periods of *menstruation*. Each month the *endometrium* (lining of the uterus) is stimulated by the female sex hormones to form a special bed. This bed is prepared so that, if a sperm and ovum unite to make a fertilized egg, the uterus will be ready to receive it and provide a place for it to grow. Approximately 15 days after the menstrual period has ceased, an egg is produced by one of the ovaries. This egg travels into the uterus through the Fallopian tubes.

If a sperm is able to travel from the vagina through the cervix to fertilize the egg, either in the uterus or in the Fallopian tubes, the fertilized egg will settle in the uterus and begin to grow in the lining where a bed has been formed since the end of the previous menstrual period.

If a fertilized egg does not embed in the lining of the uterus, a menstrual period will occur. During this period, the uterus sheds its recently formed special lining, a thin layer of cells and blood. The lining, in the form of the menstrual flow, passes out of the uterus through the cervix, into the vagina, and out of the body. The flow will last about 5 days. At the end of this time, the menstruation will cease; the uterus begins to prepare a new lining as a bed to receive a new egg; the cycle is repeated.

YOU ARE THE EMT

1. Distinguish between hollow and solid organs and give several examples of each.
2. Most people think of the pancreas as the organ that supplies insulin. What is insulin and what does it do?
3. What other products does the pancreas secrete and what are their roles?
4. Name at least three major functions of the liver.
5. Name the hollow organs of the digestive tract.
6. What are the solid organs of the urinary tract?
7. Can one live without a spleen or appendix?
8. Normally, how much fluid is secreted into the digestive tract each day by its components? Is this a significant figure in terms of body weight?
9. Describe the normal menstrual cycle.
10. What does the term menopause signify?

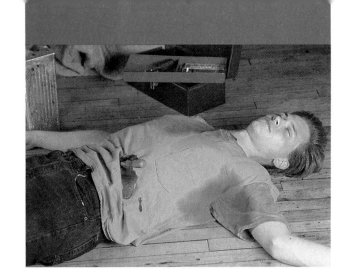

CHAPTER 26

INJURIES OF THE ABDOMEN AND GENITALIA

KEY TERMS

closed (blunt) abdominal injury Any injury of the abdomen caused by a nonpenetrating instrument or force in which the skin remains intact.

evisceration (e-vis"er-a'shun) Disembowelment; the displacement of organs outside of the body.

hematuria (hem"ah-tu're-ah) The discharge of blood in the urine.

hollow organs Tubes through which materials pass, such as the stomach and intestines, ureters and bladder.

open (penetrating) abdominal injury Any injury of the abdomen caused by a penetrating or piercing instrument or force in which the skin is lacerated or perforated and the cavity itself opened to air.

peristalsis (per"i-stal'sis) The wavelike movement by which the alimentary canal or other tubular organs propel their contents.

peritoneal cavity (per"ĭ-to-ne'al kav'ĭ-te) The abdominal cavity.

peritonitis (per"ĭ-to-ni'tis) Inflammation of the peritoneum.

rape Sexual intercourse without consent and chiefly by force or deception.

solid organs Solid masses of tissue where much of the chemical work of the body takes place: in the liver, spleen, pancreas, and kidneys.

Injuries to the abdomen may result from blunt or penetrating trauma. The blow from a steering wheel or dashboard in a motor vehicle accident or the force of a football tackle may be severe enough to injure the organs that lie in the abdominal cavity. Penetrating injuries, especially from a knife or gunshot wound, can result in damage to any abdominal organ.

Male and female external genitalia can also be injured. Although not life-threatening, injuries of the external genitalia are painful and frightening to the patient. You must reassure, as well as treat the patient. In instances of rape, treatment of injuries and reassurance must be combined with the need to procure information and protect the patient. You must show great understanding and attempt to provide some privacy for rape victims. You must learn to honor the patient's desires in these instances.

The first part of Chapter 26 describes blunt and penetrating abdominal injuries—how they are classified, how they are evaluated, and how you treat them. Next, the chapter contains a description of the handling of genitourinary injuries. The chapter concludes with a discussion of steps in assisting victims of sexual assault and rape.

GOALS

The goals of Chapter 26 are to
- know how to classify, evaluate, and treat abdominal and genitourinary injuries.
- know how to manage impaled or retained foreign bodies in the abdomen or urethra.
- know how to handle an eviscerated wound.
- understand the special problems in dealing with victims of sexual assault and rape.

INJURIES OF THE ABDOMEN

Classification of Abdominal Injuries

Abdominal injuries may be closed or open, and they may involve hollow or solid organs. **Closed (blunt) abdominal injuries** are those in which the abdomen is damaged by a severe blow, such as striking a steering wheel or being tackled in football; the skin, however, remains intact (Figure 26–1). **Open (penetrating) abdominal injuries** are those in which a foreign body has entered the abdomen and opened the peritoneum-lined cavity to the outside. Stab wounds or gunshot wounds are examples of open injuries (Figure 26–2).

Some penetrating injuries may only lacerate the abdominal wall. It may be hard for you to tell whether penetration extends through the peritoneum and into the abdominal cavity. Thus, when the injury is a gunshot or stab wound, you must always assume that the bullet or knife has penetrated the peritoneum and entered the abdominal cavity. Always provide emergency care as if that were the case. In treating penetrating abdominal wounds, the only certain way to determine whether organs have been injured is for a surgeon to explore the abdomen and look at each one.

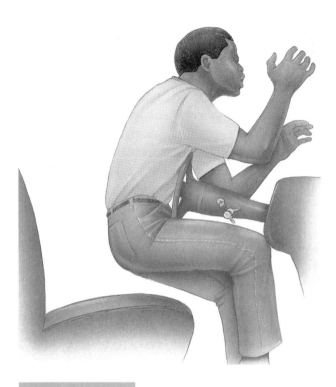

FIGURE 26-1

Striking the steering wheel is a common mechanism of blunt abdominal injury. Even though this contact causes a closed injury, it may result in a ruptured hollow organ, a lacerated spleen or liver, or a torn mesentery.

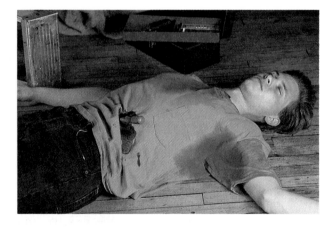

FIGURE 26-2

A means of producing a penetrating abdominal injury is shown. Having no knowledge of the length of the penetrating instrument or the patient's position at the time of injury, you must assume that penetration and visceral injury have been sustained.

Emergency medical care for penetrating abdominal wounds is based on the assumption that penetration has occurred and that one or several organs may have been injured.

The abdomen contains both hollow and solid organs, any of which may be damaged. The **hollow organs** usually contain the stream of food in the process of being digested, urine that is being passed to the bladder for release, or bile. Rupture or laceration of these organs will allow their contents to spill into the **peritoneal cavity,** where an intense inflammatory reaction (peritonitis) will be caused by the bowel contents (food, gastric juice, and digestive enzymes), urine, or bile. **Peritonitis** produces prompt and severe abdominal pain, tenderness, and muscular spasm. Paralysis of bowel muscular activity follows and the abdomen will become distended and firm to touch.

The **solid organs** are those where much of the chemical work of digestion, excretion, and energy supply for the body takes place. They have a rich blood supply; injuries of these organs usually cause severe hemorrhage. Laceration of the aorta or inferior vena cava with either closed or open abdominal injuries may also cause severe or fatal hemorrhage. Blood within the peritoneal cavity is not very irritating. Thus, pain and tenderness may not be prominent with major intraabdominal bleeding. Signs of these injuries may first be changes in pulse and blood pressure, together with the other signs that indicate shock: an ashen, pale color and cool, moist skin.

Evaluation of the Injured Abdomen

Abdominal injuries may be very simple to perceive or quite subtle. In general, the overriding complaint of a patient with abdominal injury is pain. For people who have sustained a blunt injury, bruises or other visible injuries may give clues as to the nature of the wounding agent (Figure 26-3). Patients with penetrating injuries generally have abdominal wounds that are evident when you visually inspect the abdomen. Some external bleeding may be present; and a large wound may have bowel or fat protruding from it. In addition to the complaint of pain, patients are often nauseated and may have to vomit following any type of abdominal injury. Generally, patients who are developing peritonitis prefer to lie perfectly still with their legs drawn up because it hurts them to move.

The signs of abdominal injury are usually more definite than the patient's symptoms. Abdominal tenderness, particularly localized, is a very important clinical sign. Difficulty in moving because of abdominal pain and firmness to palpation are other important clinical signs. Obvious entry and exit wounds are excellent clues for injuries; so are bruises. Altered vital signs such as low blood pressure; a rapid pulse; and rapid, shallow respirations are also important signs.

The method of evaluating an abdominal injury is the same for blunt and penetrating problems. Make the patient lie supine as comfortably as possible, with the knees slightly flexed and supported. Remove or loosen clothes. Assess and record the patient's vital signs first. Many abdominal emergencies, aside from those that cause severe bleeding, can cause a rapid pulse and low blood pressure. It is absolutely essential that a record of vital signs be made as early as possible and that they be recorded periodically thereafter to help the physicians evaluate the progress and severity of the problem when the patient arrives in the emergency department.

A rapid assessment of the patient's condition can be made by simple inspection. You should first note how the patient is lying. The patient with severe abdominal disease or injury prefers to lie still, usually with the knees drawn up. Rapid, shallow breaths prevent excessive movement of the abdominal contents. Motion of the body or the abdominal organs irritates the inflamed peritoneum and causes additional pain, which the patient instinctively tries to avoid.

Next, inspect the abdomen for skin wounds through which bullets, knives, or other missiles may have entered. When an entry wound is found, you should always check for corresponding exit holes in the patient's back or sides. Occasionally, if a very high-velocity

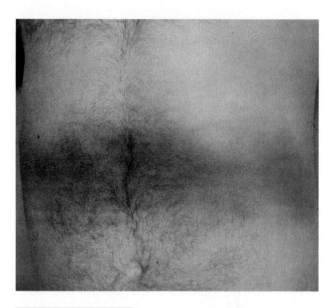

FIGURE 26–3

The seat belt has caused a bruise above the umbilicus.

missile has been the wounding agent, you will see a small, often harmless looking entrance wound with a huge, gaping exit wound on the patient's back or side. Impaled objects such as knives should be left in place and stabilized with supportive bandaging. Bruises or other visible injuries, as mentioned earlier, are important clues to the cause and severity of any blunt injury. Steering wheels, seat belts, and arm rests can cause characteristic patterns of bruising on the abdomen or chest. The location of bruises or wounds provides a clue to the underlying organs that may be injured. With severe lacerations of the abdominal wall, internal organs may be protruding through the wound. This condition is called **evisceration** (Figure 26–4).

The patient may tell you how and where the abdomen hurts, may feel nauseated, or may vomit. A patient with abdominal injuries may have a stomach full of food or drink. If vomiting occurs, especially in a patient who is unconscious or nearly so, it is imperative for you to keep the throat clear of vomitus so that it is not aspirated into the lungs. Turn the patient's head to one side and try to keep it

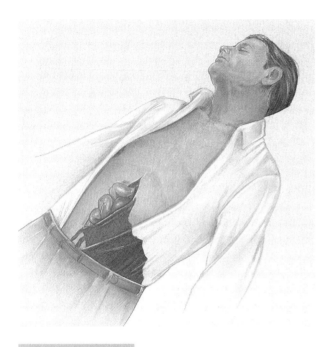

TABLE 26–1	Abdominal Injuries (Blunt or Penetrating)
Signs	**Symptoms**
Bruises	Pain (abdominal)
Tire or seat belt marks	Pain (referred)
Entry and exit wounds (bullets)	Nausea
Lacerations or stab wounds	Anxiety
Decreased blood pressure	Desire not to be moved
Increased pulse	
Rapid, shallow respirations	
Ashen color	
Local or diffuse abdominal tenderness	
Distension	
Shock	
Vomiting	

FIGURE 26–4

A large laceration of the abdominal wall allows some abdominal contents to protrude through the defect (evisceration).

lower than the chest. It is important that you note what has been vomited—undigested food, blood, mucus, or bile.

The purpose of the initial evaluation is to determine the type of injury—open (penetrating) or closed (blunt), its possible extent, and the presence of shock. Table 26–1 lists the signs and symptoms that occur with abdominal injuries.

Treatment of Abdominal Injuries

Blunt Abdominal Wounds Blunt abdominal wounds may cause severe bruises of the abdominal wall. Within the abdomen, the liver and spleen may be lacerated. The intestine may be ruptured. Supporting mesenteries may be torn, with injury of the vessels within them. The kidneys may be ruptured or torn from their arteries and veins. The bladder may be ruptured, especially in a patient who has been drinking heavily and thus has a full and

distended bladder. These patients may have severe intraabdominal hemorrhage as well as peritoneal irritation and inflammation from the ruptured hollow organs.

Place the patient who has sustained a blunt abdominal injury supine in a comfortable position with the head turned to one side. Clear the mouth and throat of vomitus. Monitor the vital signs for any indication of shock: pallor, cold sweat, rapid thready pulse, or low blood pressure. Institute all the appropriate measures to combat shock. You may have to assist respiration by clearing the airway and using oxygen when needed. You must provide prompt transportation to the emergency department.

Injuries from Seat Belts and Shoulder Belts Many thousands of injuries have been prevented and many lives have been saved by the use of seat belts. Patients who otherwise would have been thrown out of a smashed car owe their survival to the use of seat belts. However, the improper application of a belt occasionally causes a blunt injury of the abdominal organs.

Lap seat belts must be worn so that they lie below the iliac crests, snugly up against the hip joints and below the anterior superior iliac spines of the pelvis. If the seat belt lies too high, sudden deceleration or an abrupt stop of the vehicle may cause an injury of the abdominal organs or of the great vessels as the belt squeezes them against the spine (Figure 26–3 and Figure 26–5). Occasionally, fractures of the lumbar spine have been reported as a result of improper use of seat belts. Although these injuries do occur, remember that the use of the belt in many cases converts what could have been a fatal injury into a manageable one.

In all current model automobiles, the lap and diagonal (shoulder) seat belts are combined into one so that they may not be used independently. In some older cars still in use, only lap belts or two separate belts are provided. Used alone, diagonal shoulder safety belts can cause injuries of the upper part of the trunk, such as a bruised chest, fractured ribs, a lacerated liver, or even decapitation. Far fewer head and neck injuries are seen, however, when this belt is used in conjunction with the lap belt and a head rest.

Obviously, the inflatable air bag is a great advance in automotive safety. Its use is standard on only some vehicles today, but it has the potential of being a genuine lifesaver for individuals involved in head-on automobile collisions. The principles of its use are substantially the same as those governing seat belts: to restrain the driver or passenger in a cushioned seat during an accident. Continued use and experience will probably result in adoption of this safety feature on all vehicles.

Penetrating Abdominal Injury The penetrating abdominal wound presents a special problem. It is usually impossible to determine for certain without an operation whether an instrument or a missile has penetrated the abdomen; and, if it has, what organs are injured. You must assume that major damage has occurred even if no obvious signs are present immediately. Signs of intraabdominal injuries may develop slowly. In penetrating wounds, hollow organs are usually lacerated,

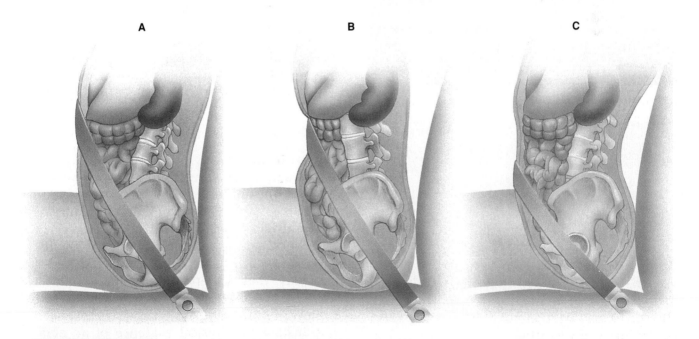

A   B   C

FIGURE 26–5 (A) Injury may occur if the seatbelt is placed too far above the iliac crest. (B) A sudden stop could cause compression of organs between the belt and the spine. (C) The proper location of the seat belt is at the hip joints.

and their contents discharge into the abdominal cavity and produce peritonitis.

If major blood vessels are cut or if major solid organs are lacerated, hemorrhage may be rapid and severe. All of the steps taken for the care of a blunt abdominal wound should also be carried out when abdominal penetration has occurred. Inspect the patient's back and sides for exit wounds. Apply a dry, sterile dressing to all open wounds. If the penetrating object is still in place, leave it and apply a stabilizing bandage of soft roller gauze around it to control external bleeding and to prevent movement of the object (Figure 26–6).

A

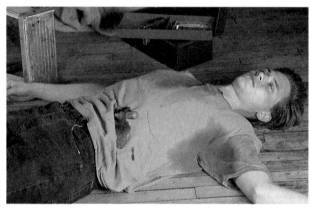

B

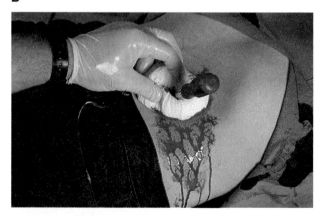

FIGURE   26–6

Stabilization of an abdominal penetrating foreign body is shown.

Evisceration Extensive lacerations of the abdominal wall may allow some organs to protrude through the wound (eviscerate). Do not try to replace them within the abdomen. Cover them with sterile gauze compresses moistened with sterile irrigating solution and secured with a sterile dressing. Because the open abdomen radiates body heat very effectively, and since exposed organs lose fluid rapidly, you must also address these issues in treating eviscerations. Covering the organs and keeping them moist and warm are thus of utmost importance. Never cover extruding organs with any material that clings or loses its substance when wet, such as toilet paper, facial tissue, paper towels, or absorbent cotton. If there are no gauze compresses, the organs may be covered with a sterile dressing that can itself be covered with sterile aluminum foil secured in place with a bandage and tape. The edge of aluminum foil can cut organs, but it is a good insulator, retaining both moisture and heat (Figure 26–7). Give other necessary emergency medical care as already described and transport the patient promptly to the emergency department. Eviscerations are first priority emergencies.

INJURIES OF THE GENITOURINARY SYSTEM

Injuries of the Kidney

Injuries of the kidney are not common. They may result from either blunt or penetrating trauma. The intensity of a blow required to damage a kidney is such that the injury is almost always associated with a fractured rib or other severely injured intraabdominal organs. The kidneys lie in such a well-protected area of the body that a penetrating wound almost always involves other organs as well as the kidney.

A history or physical evidence of an abrasion, laceration, ecchymosis, or a penetrating wound in the region of the lower rib cage (the flank) or the upper abdomen should make you suspect kidney damage. The patient found to

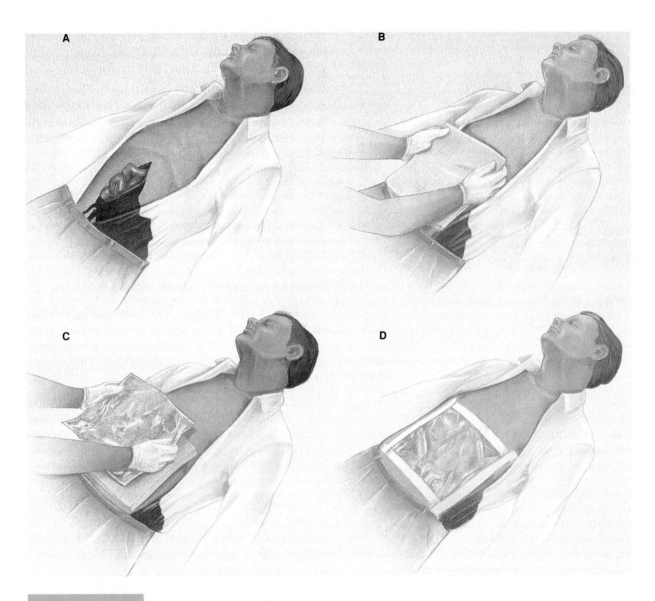

FIGURE 26–7   A moist, sterile dressing should be applied to all exposed tissues following abdominal evisceration. Aluminum foil can be secured over the dressing to keep the tissues moist.

have fractures on either side of the lower rib cage or of the lower thoracic or upper lumbar vertebrae may also be considered a likely candidate for a kidney injury (Figure 26–8).

Except for the signs of severe injury on the skin, such as bruises or lacerations, evidence of damage to the kidney will not be obvious on the external examination of the patient. Shock may be seen when the injury is associated with significant blood loss. Because the function of

the kidney is the formation of urine, an injury will usually be associated with blood in the urine, **hematuria.** Thus, any urine passed by the patient while under your observation must be measured and saved for a detailed microscopic examination at the hospital.

When the nature of the injury makes you suspect kidney damage, or blood has been passed in the urine, place the patient at total rest. Monitor vital signs carefully until arrival at

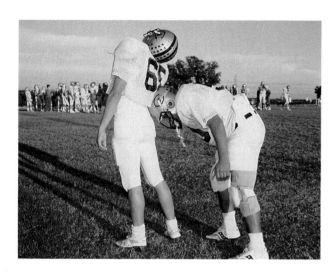

FIGURE 26-8

Blunt trauma to the lower rib cage or the flank can result in kidney injury.

the emergency department. Shock or other associated abdominal injuries may be present. The patient should be transported promptly to the hospital.

Injury of the Urinary Bladder

Injury of the urinary bladder, either blunt or penetrating, usually results in its rupture. Urine is spilled into the surrounding tissues. Any urine that passes through the urethra is likely to be bloody. Blunt injuries of the lower abdomen or pelvis frequently cause an explosive rupture of the urinary bladder, particularly when it is full and distended. Fractures of the pelvis are commonly associated with rupture or perforation of the urinary bladder, which is torn by sharp, bony fragments (Figure 26–9).

In the male, sudden deceleration can literally shear the bladder from the urethra. Penetrating wounds of the lower midabdomen or the *perineum* (the pelvic floor and associated structures that occupy the pelvic outlet) can directly involve the bladder. A history of any of these types of injury; evidence on physical examination of trauma in the lower abdomen, pelvis, or perineum; or blood at the urethral opening

each points to a possible injury of the urinary bladder. Save any urine passed by a patient with suspected bladder injury for a detailed analysis in the emergency department. A small amount of blood in the urine will not cause it to turn red. Only microscopic examination will show the abnormal presence of red blood cells.

When the possibility of an injury of the urinary bladder exists, keep the patient at rest and monitor the vital signs. The presence of associated injuries or of shock will dictate the urgency of transporting the patient to the emergency department.

Injuries of the External Male Genitalia

Injuries of the external male genitalia include all types of soft tissue wounds. Rarely are they life-threatening. They are uniformly extremely painful and generally a source of great concern to the patient. Avulsion (tearing away) of the skin of the penis, particularly in the uncircumcised male, can occur, especially in industrial accidents. When such an injury is encountered, wrap the denuded penis in a soft, sterile dressing moistened with sterile saline solution before prompt transport of the patient to the emergency department. Make a concentrated effort to salvage the avulsed skin and preserve it; but do not delay treatment or transport for more than a couple of minutes to salvage a remnant of damaged tissue.

Amputation, partial or complete, of the penile shaft demands immediate attention to blood loss, which can be effectively managed with use of local pressure with a sterile dressing on the remaining stump. If a complete amputation has occurred, it is important that you make an effort to locate the amputated part so that it can be used for surgical reconstruction. Wrap the recovered part in a moist, sterile dressing, place it in a plastic bag, and transport it in a cooled container. On very rare occasions, you may see a patient who has amputated his own penis. This violent gesture is usually associated with severe mental disease. Treatment for this situation is as just noted. You must also provide appropriate care for this very disturbed patient.

FIGURE 26–9

Fracture of the pelvis frequently results in laceration of the full bladder by the sharp fracture fragments. Urine then leaks into the pelvic cavity.

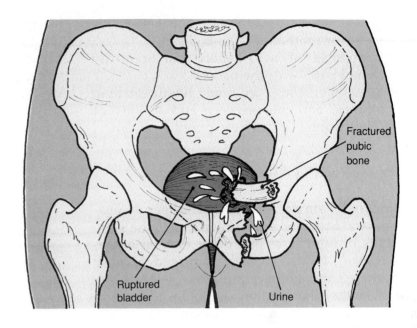

Fractured pubic bone

Ruptured bladder

Urine

The acute angulation of the erect penis with respect to the anterior abdominal wall can result in a "fracture" of the penis—disruption of the supporting erectile tissues of this organ. The injury may occur during particularly active sexual intercourse. It is always associated with intense pain, bleeding into the tissues, and fear. Prompt transport to the emergency department is indicated, because operative repair may be required.

Laceration of the skin about the head of the penis is an accident that usually occurs when the penis is in an erect state. These lacerations can be associated with profuse bleeding. Local pressure with a sterile dressing is usually sufficient to stop the hemorrhage.

The foreskin sometimes is caught in the zipper of trousers, a situation usually seen in children. If only one or two teeth of the zipper are involved, attempt to unzip the trousers. If the child is agitated or a long segment of skin is trapped, you should cut the zipper out of the trousers and make the patient more comfortable for prompt transport to the emergency department.

Urethral injuries in the male are uncommon. Lacerations of the urethra can result from straddle injuries, pelvic trauma, or penetrating wounds of the perineum. They can be associated with brisk bleeding. Direct pressure with a

dry, sterile dressing usually controls hemorrhage. Because the urethra is the channel for urine, whether the patient can void and the presence or absence of hematuria are facts of utmost importance. Save any voided urine for a later examination at the hospital. Foreign bodies protruding from the urethra should be left for removal in a surgical setting.

Avulsion of the skin of the *scrotum*, with or without associated damage of the scrotal contents, can occur. When possible, you should recover and preserve the skin in a moist, sterile dressing for possible use in reconstruction. Wrap the denuded scrotal contents or the perineal area with a sterile, moist compress. Control bleeding with a local pressure dressing. Transport this patient promptly to the emergency department.

Direct blows on the scrotum and its contents can result in rupture of a testicle or significant accumulation of blood about the testes. You should apply an ice pack to the scrotal area while the patient is being transported.

A few general rules apply to the treatment of injuries involving the external male genitalia:

- These injuries are extremely painful. Make the patient as comfortable as possible.
- Use sterile, moist compresses to cover denuded areas; sterile, dry dressings will help control bleeding.

- Never move or manipulate impaled instruments or urethral foreign bodies.
- If possible, always identify and bring detached parts with the patient.
- Remember, these are rarely life-threatening injuries, and the presence and severity of other wounds dictate the priorities of care.

Injuries of the Female Genitalia

Internal Female Genitalia The uterus, ovaries, and Fallopian tubes are subject to the same kinds of injuries as any other internal organ; however, they are rarely damaged because they are small and well protected by the pelvis. Unlike the bladder, they do not lie adjacent to the bony pelvis and are usually not injured when it is fractured.

An exception is the pregnant uterus. As pregnancy progresses, the uterus becomes substantially enlarged and rises out of the pelvis. Both penetrating and blunt injuries may involve this organ. Each is particularly severe because the uterus has a substantial blood supply during pregnancy. Additionally, you must realize that another life—that of the unborn child—is at risk. Expect to see the signs and symptoms of shock with these patients; be prepared to provide all necessary support. Notify the emergency department of the nature of the injury and the existence of the pregnancy. Transport this patient promptly. If it is possible, determine the progress of the pregnancy (such as the expected date of delivery) and report it to the emergency department personnel.

External Female Genitalia

The external female genitalia include the vulva, the clitoris, and the major and minor labia (lips) at the entrance of the vagina. The female urethra enters the anterior vagina.

Injuries of the external female genitalia can include all types of soft tissue injuries. These genital parts have a rich nerve supply; injuries are, thus, very painful. Lacerations, abrasions, and avulsions should be treated with moist, sterile compresses, local pressure to control bleeding, and a diaper-type bandage to hold the dressings in place. You must, under no circumstances, pack or place dressings into the vagina. Leave foreign bodies in place after you stabilize them with bandages. Transport these patients promptly to the emergency department. Contusions and other blunt injuries all require careful in-hospital evaluation.

In general, although these injuries are painful, they are usually not life-threatening. Bleeding may be copious, but it can usually be controlled by local compression. Priorities of need for transport to the emergency department are dictated by associated injuries, the amount of hemorrhage, and the presence of shock.

SEXUAL ASSAULT AND RAPE

Instances of sexual assault and **rape** are all too common. Often you can do little beyond soothing and calming the patient and providing transportation to the emergency department. Do not examine the genitalia unless obvious bleeding requires the application of a dressing. Advise the patient not to wash, douche, urinate, or defecate until after a physician has had the opportunity to make an examination in the emergency department. Treat all other injuries according to appropriate procedures and note that they dictate the urgency of transport to the emergency department. You must obtain and record as clear a history of the incident as possible. Questioning and all necessary treatment must be handled quietly, as rapidly as possible, and away from onlookers. A calm, professional manner is appropriate, with no display of personal curiosity.

You must be aware that the patient has the right to refuse assistance and to refuse to be taken to the emergency department. Such refusal sometimes occurs in cases of rape or sexual assault because the patient wishes to avoid publicity. It is not unusual for assistance to be refused after you arrive at the scene, even though help may originally have been requested. This choice, too, is the patient's prerogative. Referral to a rape counseling center can often be helpful in these circumstances.

YOU ARE THE EMT

1. What special problem does a penetrating abdominal wound present? How should you treat such a wound?
2. What two signs are suggestive of kidney injury?
3. What abdominal organ is commonly ruptured or perforated in conjunction with a fracture of the pelvis? How should you treat this injury?
4. What is peritonitis? What kinds of abdominal injuries would cause peritonitis? What characteristic symptoms does a patient with peritonitis exhibit?
5. Distinguish between the effects of injury on hollow and solid organs.
6. What structures would you expect to find injured on a patient with a perineal wound?

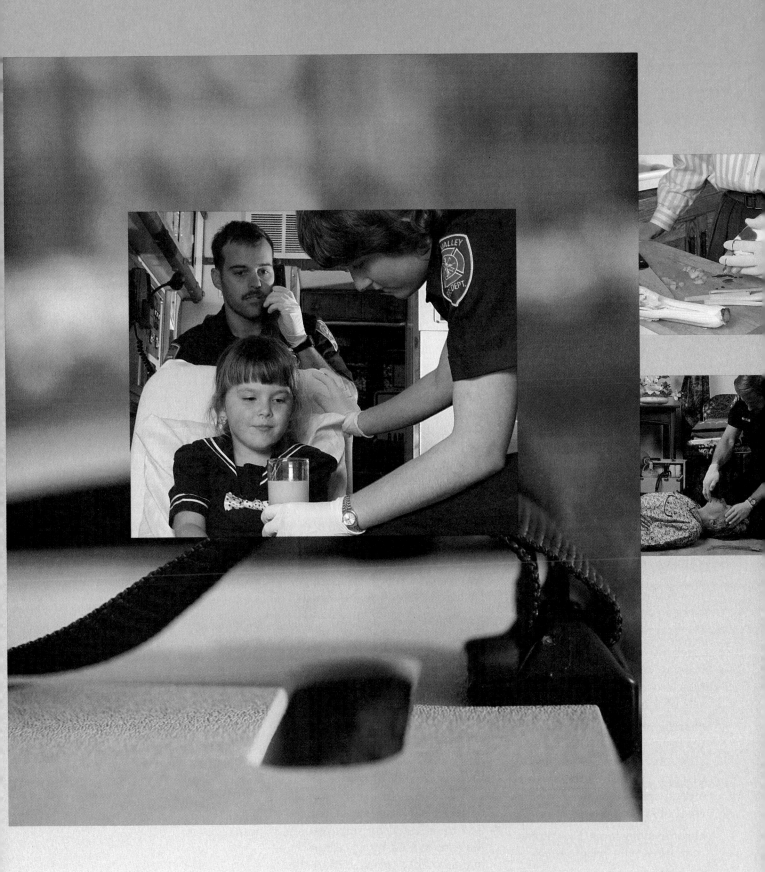

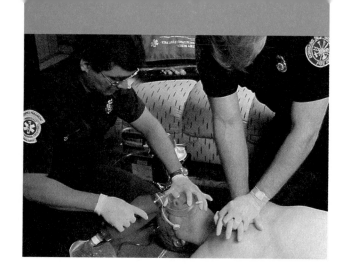

CHAPTER 27

MEDICAL EMERGENCIES

KEY TERMS

acute myocardial infarction (AMI) Heart attack; specifically, death of the heart muscle from obstruction of its blood flow.

acute symptoms Symptoms of sudden onset.

cerebrovascular accident (CVA) Stroke; a sudden lessening or loss of consciousness, sensation, and voluntary movement caused by rupture or obstruction of an artery in the brain.

cerebrovascular disease (ser"ĕ-bro-vas'ku-lar dĭ-zēz') Arteriosclerosis involving the vessels of the brain.

chronic obstructive pulmonary (or lung) disease (COPD) A slow process of dilation and disruption of the airways and alveoli caused by chronic bronchial obstruction.

chronic symptoms Symptoms that are slowly progressive.

congenital defect (kon-jen'ĭ-tal de'fekt) An imperfection, failure, or absence existing at and usually before birth.

diabetes mellitus (di"ah-be'tēz mel'i-tus) A metabolic disorder in which the ability to metabolize carbohydrates is impaired, usually due to a lack of insulin.

emphysema (em"fĭ-se'mah) Disease of the lungs in which there is extreme dilation and eventual destruction of pulmonary alveoli with poor exchange of oxygen and carbon dioxide. Also called chronic obstructive pulmonary disease (COPD).

endocrine gland (en'do-krĭn gland) Gland that produces hormones that regulate specific bodily functions.

epilepsy (ep'ĭ-lep"se) A condition manifested by seizures that are caused by an abnormal focus of activity within the brain, producing severe motor responses or changes in consciousness.

hormone (hor'mōn) Chemical substance produced in the body by a gland that has special regulatory effects on the activity of another distant organ.

hypertension (hi"per-ten'shun) Abnormally and persistently high blood pressure.

idiopathic disease (id"e-o-path'ik dĭ-zēz') A disease of unknown cause.

insulin (in'su-lin) A hormone produced by the pancreas that enables sugar in the blood to enter the cells of the body; insulin is used in the treatment and control of diabetes mellitus.

neoplasm (ne'o-plazm) Any new and abnormal growth such as a tumor.

periodic symptoms Symptoms that recur at intervals.

OVERVIEW

In the United States, the leading cause of death of people between the ages of 1 and 45 years is trauma. For this reason, much of the training for an EMT focuses on the management of injuries and extrication. Many calls to any emergency medical service, however, have nothing to do with injury, accident, or violence. These calls are about medical emergencies—about people who have become suddenly and unexpectedly ill or who are experiencing symptoms brought about by the progress of a given disease.

You are generally called to deal with medical emergencies at least as often as you have to respond to various instances of injury or accident. Frequently, knowing the exact cause of a given complaint is difficult. The diagnosis of a specific condition is not your job. Rather, your responsibility lies in recognizing the existence of a significant medical complaint and instituting appropriate support and transportation procedures.

Chapter 27 describes some of the more common causes of medical emergencies. Initially, it focuses on the major causes of medical illness and disease: degenerative processes, infections, neoplasms, endocrine diseases, obstructions, congenital defects, the environment, and obscure causes. The symptoms and clinical signs of illness and disease are defined next. Finally, a description of the chronology of medical illness and disease is presented. It will help you to decide whether a medical emergency is acute or has resulted from a chronic or a periodic disease and to assess the patient's needs accordingly.

GOALS

The goals of Chapter 27 are to
- state and describe eight major classes of problems that can result in a patient developing a medical emergency.
- be able to relate each of the causes of disease in the major classes to a specific condition that you might see.
- distinguish between symptoms and clinical signs and state the value of each in diagnosis.
- know examples of acute, chronic, and periodic medical problems that may cause medical emergencies.

CAUSES OF MEDICAL ILLNESS AND DISEASE

Medical emergencies usually result when a given disease progresses to cause specific symptoms. Medical diseases result from one of the following eight causes, discussed in turn in this chapter:

- *Degeneration* (deterioration) of healthy, normal tissue.
- *Infection* (invasion) of tissue by some type of organism (*virus, bacterium, fungus,* or *parasite*).
- *Neoplasm* (new growth or *cancer*) that both invades and destroys tissue.
- *Endocrine* disturbances that alter tissue function by the specific effects of an agent (a hormone) secreted in the body.
- Obstruction of hollow organs.

- *Congenital defects,* which are the absence of a part of the body or imperfect formation of part of the body at birth.
- The environment.
- Unknown or obscure causes.

Degenerative Processes

As the population of the United States ages, we become increasingly aware of degenerative diseases that destroy tissue. No part of the body is immune to degeneration of normal, healthy tissue. Joints, for example, wear out in a process called *degenerative arthritis* (inflammation and destruction of the joint) and often require surgical replacement. As the joint gradually deteriorates, the patient develops pain and loss of function. Years of smoking, or simply inhaling city or industrial fumes, can destroy both lung and airway tissue, resulting in **chronic obstructive pulmonary (or lung) disease (COPD),** or **emphysema** (air entrapment and small airway obstruction in the lung). Poor diet, smoking, high blood pressure, and a relatively sedentary existence, combined with genetic and other factors can result in one of the most common degenerative processes of all, *arteriosclerosis* (hardening of the arteries). This disease destroys small and large arteries in all tissues of the body and commonly causes heart disease or *stroke* (a sudden loss of cerebral function). Because arteriosclerosis damages blood vessels in the legs, arms, and the internal organs, it can cause a wide range of problems in many areas of the body. The symptoms become more severe as the blood vessel degeneration progresses.

Heart disease is common today and ranges from the person who suffers mild chest pain after exertion to the person who suddenly dies from a heart attack. The major cause of this problem is progressive degeneration and obstruction of the arteries that supply blood to the heart. The usual symptoms are chest pain, an irregular pulse, anxiety, and shortness of breath. This problem is considered in detail in Chapter 29.

Degeneration of the blood vessels in the brain is referred to as **cerebrovascular disease.** If one of the arteries feeding the brain is blocked or a damaged vessel within the brain ruptures, the blood supply to that part of the brain may be suddenly interrupted. This interruption of blood flow to an area of the brain causes a stroke. Strokes may result in a temporary or permanent loss of certain functions such as swallowing or speech, *hemiplegia* (paralysis of one-half of the body), coma, or even death.

Vascular disease in the legs makes it increasingly difficult for patients to run, walk long distances, or climb stairs. Similarly, if vascular disease involves internal organs such as the stomach, bowel, or kidney, symptoms and clinical signs can be related to those organs as well.

Quite often, you must take care of a person experiencing a heart attack or a stroke (Figure 27–1). Treatment must be directed at the function most damaged and causing the most symptoms. Often, basic life support must be instituted to restore or maintain breathing and circulation during transport.

Other areas of the body involved with severe vascular disease rarely cause the sudden and devastating problems seen with the heart and brain. Ordinarily, in these situations, symptoms are relentlessly progressive until they require the patient to seek medical help.

Infectious Processes

Communicable (infectious) diseases (a disease transmitted from person to person) are all around us. They range in severity from the common cold or viral "flu" to life-threatening infections such as *meningitis* (inflammation of the membranes covering the brain) or *hepatitis* (inflammation of the liver). Much progress has been made in this century to control infectious diseases. Smallpox, for example, has been virtually eliminated in civilized countries, and tuberculosis is under strict control. New diseases take their places, however. *AIDS (acquired immunodeficiency syndrome),* a life-threatening

FIGURE 27–1

Many patients are victims of heart disease or stroke.

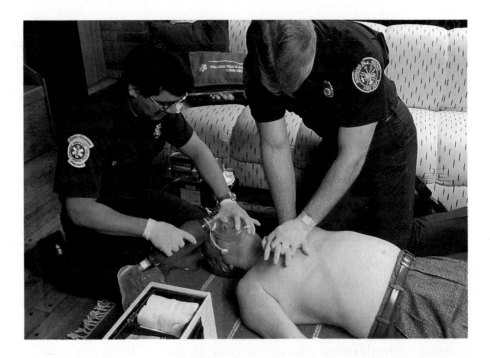

viral infection, was unknown in 1975. It has become a major medical threat in the 1990s.

The human body provides an excellent environment for the growth of bacteria, viruses, fungi, and parasites. The rapid growth of infectious organisms saps the body's energy as they invade and destroy normal tissue (Figure 27–2). The body responds to infection in many different ways. Fever and chills are general responses of the body as a whole. Nausea, vomiting, diarrhea, the coughing up of sputum, shortness of breath, abdominal pain, and local soft tissue swelling and redness are only a few of the many signs and symptoms that may accompany infection of specific body areas. The presenting complaints depend on the specific organ infected and the severity of the infection.

Most patients with infections require prompt medical treatment. Thus, you must be aware of the signs and symptoms indicating infection to facilitate proper transportation. Additionally, you must be careful to protect yourself, your other patients, and your vehicle from becoming contaminated while transporting an infected individual.

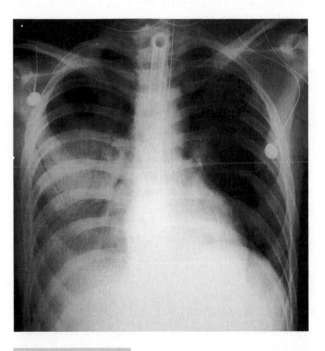

FIGURE 27–2

Chest X ray of a patient with pneumonia, a bacterial infection of the lung. Note the destruction (whitened areas) of the right lung compared with the clear left lung.

Chapter 35 reviews the common communicable diseases. Some are easily transmitted; some are not. Chicken pox is easily transmitted to the susceptible individual by airborne vectors. Tuberculosis is similarly airborne, but much more difficult to contract. AIDS is not easily transmitted casually; transmission requires direct contact of your blood with some fluid or secretion of the patient. The needed defense is provided by keen attention to simple and well-known protective measures: handwashing, masks, gloves, cleansing of all surfaces, and (occasionally) protective clothing.

A host of infective diseases exist, and the chances are great that you will encounter them from time to time.

Neoplastic Processes

The word **neoplasm** means new growth. In the body, new growths may be *benign* or *malignant.* Neoplasms always produce tumors or masses in tissue. Benign (nonmalignant) neoplasms tend to grow and expand locally, in the area of their origin. As they grow, they crowd and press onto adjacent organs. The symptoms of a benign neoplasm are those of a developing, usually painless, mass or of altered function of the involved organ or adjacent structures. Usually they grow slowly; rarely are they the cause of an emergency problem.

Malignant, or cancerous, neoplasms also develop as masses at their sites of origin; they, too, compress adjacent organs. Unlike benign neoplasms, however, they invade these adjacent organs and travel to distant parts of the body through veins and lymphatic vessels. In these distant areas, they can take root, grow, and eventually invade other tissues. Malignant tumors destroy organs and tissues by invasion and replacement of healthy tissue as well as by pressure.

From time to time, you will treat a patient with *cancer.* The symptoms depend on the location of the tumor and the extent of its growth. Although any tissue may develop a malignant neoplasm, the common cancer sites are the lung, the colon, the breast, and the internal female genitalia. When cancer spreads, the most frequently involved organs are lymph nodes, bone, liver, and lungs. Cancer is not a contagious disease. It does appear with some predictability in certain families. There is also some indication that a few cancers are caused by viruses. Cancer is not, however, passed from one person to another like a common infection. In general, your responsibility toward a cancer patient is to provide appropriate support for the most severely compromised functions, such as breathing or circulation, during transport to the hospital.

Complex Endocrine Processes

Some medical problems have a wide range of symptoms because they are the result of too much or too little hormone production by the **endocrine glands.** Each specific endocrine gland produces one or more hormones. Each **hormone** has a specific effect on some organ, tissue, or process. Disease states are caused from over- or underproduction of each of these substances. With endocrine diseases, specific bodily functions are increased, decreased, or absent. Several endocrine glands exist in the body, and each produces one or more hormones related to the control of a specific function. Table 27–1 contains a summary of those glands, their locations and the body functions each regulates.

Diabetes mellitus is a common problem. Because production of the hormone **insulin** is deficient, the body is unable to use sugar normally. This disease also damages the small blood vessels in the body. The tissue damage that results from the blood vessel destruction is as much a part of diabetes as is the difficulty in regulating the amount of sugar in the blood.

Among all the endocrine diseases, you will most frequently deal with diabetes (Chapter 32), because it is a fairly common problem and can cause diabetic coma or insulin shock. Other complex endocrine problems are rarely the cause of acute emergencies.

Obstructive Processes

The body contains many different hollow organs and tubes that carry blood, lymph, nutrients, air, and waste products. Stones, blood

Table 27-1   Endocrine Glands

Endocrine Gland	Location	Function	Hormones Produced
Pituitary	Base of skull	Regulation of all other endocrine glands	Multiple
Thyroid	Neck (over the larynx)	Regulation of metabolism	Multiple
Parathyroid	Neck (behind the thyroid) (3-5 glands)	Regulation of serum calcium	Single
Adrenal Cortex (rim)	Atop kidney (2 glands)	Regulate salt, sugar, and sexual function	Multiple
Adrenal Medulla (central core)	Atop kidney (2 glands)	Regulate blood pressure and response to stress	Multiple
Ovary	Female pelvis (2 glands)	Regulate sexual function, characteristics, and reproduction	Multiple
Testes	Male scrotum (2 glands)	Regulate sexual function, characteristics, and reproduction	Multiple
Islets of Langerhans	Pancreas	Regulate sugar metabolism and other functions	Multiple-insulin and other hormones

clots, tumors, foreign bodies, or scar tissue can obstruct these hollow structures. Substances that flow through the organ or vessel slow or stop, causing it to bulge (distend) behind the point of obstruction (Figure 27-3). A characteristic cramping pain *(colic)* almost always occurs as a result of such an obstruction, because the muscle in the wall of the distended organ tries to overcome the obstruction by contracting violently. Infection of a structure often develops behind the block and may persist or become very severe.

When the ureter is obstructed by a kidney stone, a prompt and specific colicky pain usually occurs in the affected flank and is often accompanied by fever and other signs of infection. In the lungs, the bronchi sometimes become obstructed by mucus, a foreign body, or a tumor; if the obstructive process is not treated promptly, pneumonia may result. Obstruction in the gastrointestinal tract usually produces visible distension of the abdomen and colicky abdominal pain. When a blood vessel is obstructed, as with arteriosclerosis, the tissue it supplies may die.

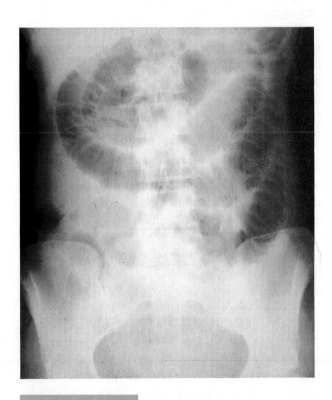

FIGURE 27-3

X ray of patient with an acute bowel obstruction. Note the small intestine distended with gas.

Often, you must transport patients with pneumonia, bowel obstruction, kidney stones, or some other obstructive process. Treatment for these patients depends on the organ involved and the specific functions that have been lost.

Congenital Processes

Each year, thousands of children are born with **congenital defects.** A congenital defect is a physical abnormality or deficiency that is present at birth. Some congenital defects are inherited; others develop as the fetus matures in the uterus. There is general agreement that the use of alcohol, tobacco, or drugs by the pregnant mother, especially in the first weeks of pregnancy markedly increases the chance of a defect in the child. The use of specific drugs in the first *trimester* (the first three months of pregnancy) as well as some diseases, such as German measles, in this time period are associated with the development of certain congenital defects.

Congenital defects can involve any organ or system of the body. They range from the most common problem, *inguinal hernia,* to the rare absence of a given organ or part of the body. Most such defects are surgically corrected immediately after birth and before an infant leaves the hospital. Some, however, are not. Among the late symptoms they can produce are vomiting, *jaundice* (yellow discoloration of the skin), a "blue baby" (from certain heart defects), or difficulties with swallowing.

Rarely do these defects create an extreme emergency. Such patients must, however, be transported promptly to the hospital for proper diagnosis and treatment.

Environmental Causes

Apart from the weather, water-related injuries, and electrical hazards, a great many medical emergencies have environmental causes. They are grouped in Chapter 28 as "Poisons, Stings, and Bites." In all likelihood, you will see many such problems. For example, many common household items are poisonous when inhaled or ingested. Stings and bites from snakes, bees, wasps, dogs, and other animals occur almost daily. The variety of allergies to pollens, food, injected toxins, and other agents is endless.

Symptoms and the extent of injury are directly related to the toxicity of the agent, the sensitivity of the patient to the substance, and the degree of exposure to the agent. Emergency treatment ranges from protecting individuals from environmental hazards to providing cardiopulmonary resuscitation (CPR) to severely ill patients. Because of the frequency of medical emergencies due to environmental hazards, you must become familiar with the symptoms and treatment of injuries and illnesses that result from poisons, stings, bites, exposure to *allergens* (agents causing allergic reactions), and the use or abuse of common agents.

Unknown or Obscure Causes

The cause of some medical emergencies is unknown or uncertain. Some diseases do not have clear-cut causes. **Epilepsy** (seizures), for example, is one such disease. Often it follows a specific brain injury, but it may be caused by a stroke, a brain tumor, or a high fever. More often, there is no cause that can be specifically identified. It is considered in Chapter 37. The causes of peptic ulcer disease, on the other hand, are well known. The particular factor causing an ulcer in a given patient may, however, remain obscure. Not all medical emergencies can be categorized by specific cause.

SYMPTOMS AND CLINICAL SIGNS OF MEDICAL ILLNESS AND DISEASE
· ·

A symptom is a complaint voiced by the patient. It is subject to the patient's interpretation and is often heightened by his anxiety. The same symptom can be presented very differently by different individuals. It also is subject to interpretation by the person to whom it is related: doctor, nurse, EMT, or paramedic. Examples of common symptoms include pain, difficulty with such functions as swallowing, breathing, and urinating, and strange sensations (such as a hollow or empty feeling, numbness, or tingling), or almost anything the patient can relate. Sometimes fear itself becomes a symptom.

A clinical sign is a physical finding that can be elicited or detected by one or more of the examiner's five senses. It is a sure, tangible finding that can be seen, heard, felt, smelled, or tasted. Examples of common clinical signs are swelling and redness, respiratory wheezes, broken bone ends felt just under the skin, and an acetone or fruity odor on a patient's breath. In most cases, signs are more reliable than symptoms because they can be seen and evaluated by more than one person and they can be obtained even when the patient is unconscious or unresponsive. Table 27–2 summarizes common symptoms and signs of typical medical emergencies.

CHRONOLOGY OF MEDICAL ILLNESS AND DISEASE

Many diseases progress slowly over several years and produce few, if any, symptoms during their early years. As the disease progresses, symptoms may become more frequent and more severe, usually forcing the person to seek medical treatment. Some diseases are periodic and a few, acute. For the

Table 27–2   Medical Emergencies: Common Symptoms and Signs

Organ or System	Symptoms	Clinical Signs
General Body (Systemic)	Malaise (feeling unwell) Dizziness Nausea Chills	Fever Change in pulse rate Change in skin color Change in skin texture Hypotension
Cardiovascular	Chest pain Dyspnea (shortness of breath)	Pulse abnormality Hypotension Frothy or bloody sputum Cyanosis (bluish color of skin)
Neurological	Headache Dizziness Weakness	Alteration of consciousness Paralysis Loss of specific function Numbness Changes in pupil size
Gastrointestinal	Abdominal pain Nausea	Diarrhea Vomiting Blood in stool or vomitus Distension Abdominal tenderness Abdominal masses
Respiratory	Dyspnea (shortness of breath) Chest pain	Change in respiratory rate Labored breathing Mucus production Frothy, bloody sputum Wheezing Rales
Genitourinary	Burning on urination Frequency	Blood in urine Changes in urinary flow Abdominal masses

EMT, these patients will either have **acute symptoms** (sudden onset), **chronic symptoms** (constantly present and slowly progressive), or **periodic symptoms** (recurring at intervals). A medical history of the patient and the disease process may aid you in discovering the cause of the symptoms. The history can be obtained from the patient, family, or friends at the scene.

Acute Medical Emergencies

Probably the best example of an acute medical emergency with acute symptoms is the **acute myocardial infarction (AMI),** or heart attack. It occurs suddenly, often without any identifying or preceding history, and produces severe symptoms and signs that require prompt, aggressive treatment. The disease causing the heart attack (coronary arteriosclerosis) may have been present for years but not evident until the heart attack occurs.

Chronic Disease

A chronic disease presents you with a different situation. The patient with chronic obstructive pulmonary disease or emphysema, for example, always has some difficulty in breathing and may have adapted well (compensated). Although never free from the basic disease, the person usually is able to manage if no complicating factor is added to the condition. However, a minor infection, a cold, too much fluid, or a mild allergic response, such as in hay fever, may trigger an acute decompensation in breathing. The decompensation and its symptoms may be sudden in onset, but they are associated with the chronic underlying disease.

Often, the patient can tell you that the symptoms and the decompensation were not a surprise, because such experiences occurred in the past. A person with chronic disease almost always has a medical history on record, which is invaluable to the doctors handling the case. An alert EMT can often obtain much of this history.

Periodic Illness

Some problems are periodic—that is, they recur at intervals with no manifestation of the disease during the intervening period. In contrast to the patient who is chronically ill, the person with periodic illness is well most of the time with only temporary episodes of disease. The person with epilepsy, for example, is normal save for the occasional seizure. An individual with a specific, severe allergy is similarly normal unless exposed to the substance that produces the allergic reaction. This patient may very well be able to tell you what caused the attack or symptoms and may even know the most effective treatment. Information from the patients in these instances may be very valuable.

Identification of a process as acute, chronic, or periodic may help you in assessing the need for care. Many patients with acute processes require immediate support or they will die. Some patients with chronic diseases may be at risk to die during an acute problem, but usually they will survive with good support. Those patients with periodic problems may be well when you see them. Your priorities of care and support are largely based on your assessment of the patient's problem.

YOU ARE THE EMT

1. You suspect the patient has cerebrovascular disease. Her symptoms are headache, dizziness, and weakness. Identify four or five clinical signs that might confirm your impressions.

2. Your patient says he has diabetes. Is this disease related to a neoplastic or an endocrine process? What is the specific function that is lost?

3. What are you noting when you examine a patient and record some systemic signs and symptoms? Give three examples of systemic signs or symptoms.

4. Why is it important to identify a patient's symptoms as being either acute, chronic, or periodic?

5. Give some specific examples of acute, chronic, and periodic diseases.

6. What are the eight general causes of medical diseases? Give a specific example from each category.

CHAPTER 28

POISONS, STINGS, AND BITES

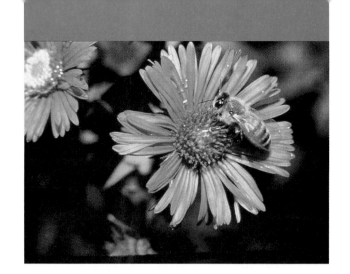

KEY TERMS

allergen (al'er-jen) A substance causing an allergic reaction.

antidote (an'tĭ-dōt) A specific substance to neutralize or counteract a poison.

antivenin (an"tĭ-ven'in) A substance produced to counteract the effect of an animal or insect venom.

cellulitis (sel"u-li'tis) A spreading redness and inflammation under the skin, the result of infection.

dyspnea (disp'ne-ah) Difficult breathing.

emesis (em'ĕ-sis) Vomiting.

envenomation (en-ven"o-ma'shun) The actual injecting of venom into a bite.

ignite Catch on fire.

ingestion Swallowing; taking a substance by mouth.

rabid (rab'id) An animal infected with rabies.

toxin A poison or harmful substance, produced by bacteria or animals or plants.

urticaria (ur"tĭ-kar'e-ah) Generalized itching, burning, and the development of multiple raised, reddened areas on the skin; hives.

vomitus (vom'ĭ-tus) Vomited material.

wheal (hwēl) A raised, whitish area on the skin resulting from an insect bite or allergic reaction.

OVERVIEW

Approximately 5 million children and adults swallow, inhale, inject, or come into surface contact with poisonous substances every year. These are usually accidental poisonings, although intentional poisonings and suicides also occur. EMTs have many responsibilities in dealing with poisoning cases. Chapter 28 examines these responsibilities, which range from identifying a toxic substance to treating various types of poisonings.

Chapter 28 also discusses insect and animal stings and bites and their associated complications. Although many stings and bites are painful, they are not usually serious. Some, however, are potentially dangerous, even life-threatening. For example, some people are highly allergic to the stings of bees, wasps, and hornets. Dog and other animal bites may cause rabies. Bites can occur from poisonous snakes, ticks, or spiders. Thus, much of this chapter is devoted to identifying symptoms of serious reactions to bites and stings and distinguishing poisonous snakes and spiders from nonpoisonous varieties. The last part of the chapter discusses human bites and marine animal injuries.

GOALS

The goals of Chapter 28 are to

- become knowledgeable about the problem of accidental and intentional poisoning and the location of area poison control centers.
- recognize the symptoms of a poisoning and identify the toxic substance involved.
- learn the emergency treatment for swallowed, inhaled, injected, and surface poisons.
- learn the emergency treatment for food poisoning and plant poisoning.
- identify the symptoms of stings from bees, wasps, hornets, and ants.
- become aware of the seriousness of an anaphylactic reaction to a bee, wasp, yellow jacket, or hornet sting.
- learn how to identify and treat scorpion stings and spider bites.
- distinguish poisonous snakes from nonpoisonous snakes and learn the emergency treatment for snake bites.
- know the diseases caused by tick bites and their emergency management.
- understand the seriousness of rabies and its link to certain animal bites.
- learn the emergency treatment for human bites and marine animal injuries.

POISONS

A *poison* is any substance that, when swallowed, inhaled, or absorbed, or when applied to, injected into, or otherwise introduced into the body, in relatively small amounts, by its chemical actions, may cause damage to structures or disturbances of function. The key elements of this definition are the statements "in relatively small amounts," and "by its chemical action." Very small amounts of a poison can cause much damage or death. The injury within the body is chemical and biolog-ical rather than physical as occurs with trauma. Poisons act by changing the normal metabolism of cells or by actually destroying them. Poisoning can result from several routes of contact: ingestion (swallowing), inhalation, injection, surface application, or absorption through the skin or mucous membranes.

Each year, some 5 million children and adults come into contact with a poison. Deaths from poisoning are fairly rare—the exact number is not well known, because conflicting data is published in the literature. Poisoning death rates for children have decreased progressively since the 1960s, probably due to the use of the safety cap on drug bottles and containers. However, there has been an increase in poisoning deaths in adults. Approximately two-thirds of poisoning fatalities are from drugs. Barbiturates (Nembutal® and seconal®) and opiates (heroin, morphine, demerol,® dilaudid,® and codeine) account for many of these deaths, but the introduction and widespread use of cocaine, crack, and newer "designer" drugs have created a whole new class of poisoning deaths. (Substance abuse is discussed in Chapter 36.) About one-third of all poisoning fatalities result from solid, liquid, or inhaled substances other than drugs.

Poison Control Centers

Several hundred poison control centers exist across the United States. Most of them are in the emergency departments of large hospitals, but some are independent, freestanding centers. The telephone numbers of these poison control centers are readily available. The personnel who staff the poison control centers have access to information concerning virtually all of the commonly used drugs, chemicals, and substances that could possibly be poisonous. Information for each of these agents includes a specific **antidote** (substance that will counteract the poison), if one is available, and the appropriate emergency treatment for that particular poison. Most of the centers are staffed 24 hours a day; contact them whenever your patient has a poisoning problem. In general, the poison control center can provide information for specific agents under both trade and generic names. You should know the location and telephone number of the nearest poison control center. Ordinarily, in an emergency situation, you should notify medical control about the nature of the specific case, including the fact that a poisoning has occurred; the size, weight, and age of the patient; and a description of the suspected agent. Dispatch will contact the poison control center and relay specific instructions.

Occasionally, the poison control center will recommend that you induce **emesis** (vomiting) by the use of syrup of ipecac. Give this drug according to the dose recommended by the poison control center, and proceed with arrangements to transport the patient. Generally, if one dose of syrup of ipecac does not produce results in 20 minutes, you will be requested to repeat the dose. However, you should *not* delay transport to wait to give a second dose.

Aggressive treatment of poisons, especially those that have been ingested, may be lifesaving. Your role is to provide immediate care and prompt transportation to the hospital emergency department.

Identifying Poisoning Victims and the Toxic Substances

Your primary responsibility is to recognize the likelihood that a poisoning has occurred. With even the slightest suspicion that someone has taken a poisonous substance, you should contact dispatch to relay information for the poison control center and begin emergency treatment. Some of the more common symptoms and signs of poisonings are nausea, vomiting, abdominal pain, diarrhea, dilation or constriction of the pupils, excessive salivation, sweating, **dyspnea** (difficulty breathing), depressed respirations, unconsciousness, and convulsions. If respiration is depressed or difficult, cyanosis may occur. Some chemical compounds will cause irritation or burns of the skin or mucous membranes. Redness, blistering, or even severe burns may result. The presence of such injuries about the mouth strongly suggests the ingestion of a poison.

You should next attempt to determine the nature of the poison. Objects at the scene such as overturned bottles, scattered pills, chemicals, or even an overturned or damaged plant may provide clues. The remains of any food or drink may also be important. Place any suspicious material in a plastic bag and take it to the hospital. If the patient vomits, collect the **vomitus** (vomited material) in a plastic bag and bring it to the hospital for analysis. Although it may be very unpleasant, collecting and bringing any suspicious materials, along with collected vomitus, may be the most important thing you can do after resuscitating and instituting emergency care for the patient.

Bring any containers for the poisonous materials that you collect. Specific ingredients are often listed on the labels. Also, for medications the number of pills originally in a bottle is usually specified, together with the name of the drug and its concentration. Information concerning the content of the substances can be of great help to the emergency department physicians. Knowing how much material is left in any container may give the physician some idea of how much has been ingested. Brand names are known at most poison control centers, and specific chemical contents can frequently be identified. Sometimes the manufacturer can be contacted for a specific description of the material in the container. By bringing the container with the patient, you may be able to speed up the proper treatment and thus help save a life.

Ingested, Surface, Inhaled, and Injected Poisons

Most poisons, regardless of what kind, do *not* have a specific antidote. Support for the patient may range all the way from reassuring an anxious parent to instituting cardiopulmonary resuscitation. However, in general, the most important treatment for poisons involves dilution and physical removal of the agent. This can be accomplished by surface flooding and washing for the skin, drinking water or milk and inducing vomiting for ingested poisons, or administering oxygen for inhaled poisons. Certain injected poisons may require a specific antidote. Injected poisons pose urgent problems, because they are difficult to remove or dilute.

Ingested Poisons Approximately 80 percent of all poisoning is by mouth (**ingestion**). The types of poison include drugs, drinks, household products, contaminated food, and plants. Poisoning in children and the elderly is usually accidental (Figure 28–1), whereas with the exception of contaminated food, ingested poisoning in adults is usually deliberate, employed as a method of committing suicide or murder. Drugs represent the majority of ingested poisons, but approximately one-third of poisonings are caused by other liquid or solid agents: cleaners, soaps, insecticides, acids, or alkalis. Plant poisonings are also common

among children who like to explore and often bite the leaves of various bushes or shrubs. Food poisoning, even though technically an ingested poison, and plant poisoning are covered in separate sections later in this chapter.

The emergency management of ingested poisons includes the rapid removal of as much of the poison as possible from the gastrointestinal tract and diluting or neutralizing the remainder. For the majority of poisoning victims, this emergency treatment is sufficient. Water or a glass or two of milk may be given to drink if the poison is acting as a stomach irritant. However, the use of large volumes of fluid to dilute or neutralize ingested poisons is controversial. Consult medical control before you proceed with the treatment of all poisoning victims.

Having the patient drink a suspension of activated charcoal in water will absorb many poisons. Powdered activated charcoal is mixed with fluid to make a slurry. The usual dosage is 25 to 50 grams (about 1 to 2 oz) of charcoal in a glass of water. Premixed, ready to use, containers of activated charcoal are also commercially available. A child may be afraid to swallow this inky, messy fluid, and you may have to do some coaxing to get the child to do so. However, you should never force the liquid into someone's mouth.

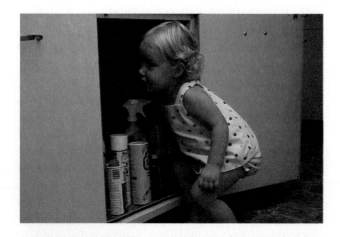

FIGURE 28–1

A curious child will try to taste or swallow almost any substance. A common victim of accidental ingestion of dangerous compounds is the unwatched toddler.

Physical removal of the poison can be done by inducing vomiting with syrup of ipecac. You should only induce vomiting in a patient who is completely alert. If not fully alert, the patient may aspirate the vomitus into the lungs. The poison control center will instruct you when to use syrup of ipecac. Two formulations of ipecac are commercially available—syrup of ipecac and ipecac extract. The extract is much more concentrated and should not be used in prehospital care. The usual dose of syrup of ipecac is 1 tablespoon (15 ml) in a glass of water for children between the ages of 1 and 5 years and 1 to 2 tablespoonsful (15 to 30 ml) in a glass or two of water for older children and adults. Advise medical control if your poisoning patient has one of these conditions before inducing vomiting. Vomiting will occur within 20 minutes of administration of syrup of ipecac in 90 percent of patients. If it does not occur, you will probably be instructed to repeat the dose once. Have the patient sit up; collect the vomitus. Be alert for any possible airway compromise or aspiration. If the patient cannot sit up, turn his or her head to the side.

There are certain situations in which vomiting may be dangerous. You should not attempt to induce vomiting under the following circumstances:

- If the patient is not fully alert or is unconscious, semiconscious, or having a convulsion.
- If the poison is corrosive, such as a strong acid or alkali (lye or drain cleaner), or has caused obvious burns on the lips or mouth. These agents may cause more injury when they are vomited back up.
- If the poison contains any petroleum product such as kerosene, gasoline, lighter fluid, or clear furniture polish. These agents will cause a serious chemical pneumonia if they are aspirated into the lungs or if their vapors are inhaled.
- Some authorities recommend not to induce vomiting in pregnant patients, infants under 1 year of age, or patients with severe cardiac disease.

Most ingested poisonings are from drugs. Many of them are opiates, sedatives, or barbiturates. In these circumstances you should expect central nervous system (CNS) depression and especially respiratory depression. These patients may require aggressive ventilatory support and even cardiopulmonary resuscitation, because absorption of some agents from the gastrointestinal tract is rapid. You must transport these patients to the emergency department promptly. Do not delay at the scene waiting for the patient to vomit. Gastric lavage, intravenous support, and other measures may be necessary to treat this patient in the hospital.

Surface Contact Poisons Many corrosive substances cause damage of the skin, mucous membranes, or eyes by direct contact. Acids, alkalis, and some petroleum or benzene products are very destructive. Contact with these agents will cause inflammation, chemical burns, or specific rashes or lesions in affected areas.

The emergency treatment for contact poisoning is to remove the irritating or corrosive substance as rapidly as possible. Dust off any dry chemical thoroughly, then wash the affected area with soap and water or flood the part under a shower. When a large amount of material has been spilled on a patient, flooding may be the most rapidly effective treatment. You should remove all clothing that has been contaminated with poisons or irritating substances as rapidly as possible so the skin may be cleaned with running water. Treat chemical agents in the eyes by rapid and copious irrigation for several minutes. You should irrigate the eyes for at least 5 minutes for acid substances and 15 to 20 minutes for alkalis. This problem is discussed further in Chapter 40. Many chemical burns occur in industrial settings, where showers and specific protocols for handling surface burns are available. If you are called to such a scene, there will usually be trained people there to assist you.

Do not spend time trying to neutralize substances on the skin. Rather, wash them off immediately with water. This procedure is faster and more effective than attempting to neutralize a substance chemically.

An exception to flooding the contact area with water is when the substance is one that chemically reacts violently with water. For example, phosphorus and elemental sodium are dry, solid chemicals that **ignite** (catch on fire) when they contact water. Fortunately, the incidence of exposure to these elements is rare. The emergency treatment is the same as for other dry chemicals. Dust the chemical off the patient. Remove the patient's clothing and apply a dry dressing to any burn area. Wear gloves and be especially careful to avoid contaminating yourself. Transport the patient promptly to the hospital for further care.

Inhaled Poisons For inhaled poisons—natural gas; certain pesticides; carbon monoxide, chlorine, or other gases—the emergency treatment is to move the patient into fresh air. Patients exposed to prolonged inhalation may require supplementary oxygen and basic life support. Because it is easy to inhale poisonous fumes in an emergency situation, you must be careful to protect yourself as well as your patients. Always use a self-contained breathing apparatus (SCBA) to protect yourself from inhalation poisoning.

Some inhaled poisons, such as carbon monoxide, are odorless and produce profound hypoxia without much irritation or damage to the lungs. Others, such as chlorine, are very irritating and produce airway obstruction and pulmonary edema. Administer oxygen whenever hypoxia, pulmonary edema, or airway obstruction results from inhaled poisons. Be ready to use supplemental suctioning and ventilatory support. Transport these patients to an emergency department as rapidly as possible, because some inhaled agents cause progressive lung damage, even after the patient is removed from direct exposure. Many times, these patients require two or three days of intensive care to reestablish normal lung function.

Injected Poisons Poisoning by injection is almost always the result of deliberate drug overdose—a problem that is discussed in Chapter 36. Other sources of injected poisons are the bites and stings of insects or animals. If the area around the site of an injection starts to swell, all rings, watches, or bracelets should be removed. Apply a constricting band above and

below the site of the injection. Adjust it just tightly enough to occlude (block) the flow of blood in the veins, creating a venous tourniquet. Do not cut off arterial flow, however, and ensure that the patient's pulse is still palpable distal to the constricting band. An ice pack or cold pack may decrease local pain and swelling about the injection.

In general, injected poisons are impossible to dilute or remove. Usually they are absorbed quickly into the body or cause intense local tissue destruction. In the case of rapid absorption, be prepared to offer basic life support. With severe local tissue damage, complex surgical procedures may be needed. Thus, prompt transport to the emergency department is mandatory.

Food Poisoning

The term "ptomaine poisoning" was coined in 1870 to indicate poisoning by a class of chemicals found in rotting food. This term is still used today in news accounts of episodes of food poisoning. Unfortunately, it is an incorrect term and indicates little about the problem. Food poisoning is almost always caused by the ingestion of food contaminated by bacteria. The food itself appears perfectly good and has no obvious decay or odor to indicate that it may be contaminated. There are two types: one type occurs when the bacteria themselves cause disease, and the other type occurs when the bacteria have produced **toxins** (poisons) that cause disease.

Food poisoning that results from the direct effect of the bacteria themselves is usually caused by a *Salmonella* bacterium. This condition is called *Salmonellosis,* and is characterized by severe gastrointestinal symptoms—nausea, vomiting, abdominal pain, and diarrhea—for up to 72 hours after ingestion. In addition to the gastrointestinal symptoms, patients suffering from *Salmonellosis* may be systemically ill with fever and generalized weakness from the bacteria. A variety of organisms in addition to can also produce milder intestinal *Salmonella* complaints. Only ingesting living bacteria can produce this disease. Usually, proper cooking kills bacteria, and proper cleanliness in the kitchen prevents the contamination of non-cooked foods. Some people are carriers of certain bacteria, and although they may not become ill themselves, they may transmit these diseases, particularly if they work in the food services industry.

The ingestion of preformed bacterial toxins is probably the commonest cause of food poisoning. The symptoms are not caused by the bacteria themselves, but rather by powerful toxins produced by the bacteria. The most frequent offender is food contaminated with *Staphylococcus*. This bacterium is responsible for the occasional episodes of food poisoning reported at church suppers or other large gatherings. It results from the advance preparation of food that has been kept warm for many hours so that the contaminating bacteria have a chance to grow and produce the toxins. Mayonnaise is a common vehicle for the development of staphylococcal toxins. Usually, staphylococcal food poisoning results in the onset of violent gastrointestinal symptoms (nausea, vomiting, and diarrhea) within 1 to 3 hours after ingestion. In general, the episode is over in 6 to 8 hours.

The most severe form of toxin ingestion is botulism. Frequently fatal, this disease usually results from eating improperly canned food in which the spores of *Clostridium* bacteria have grown and produced a toxin. The symptoms of botulism are neurologic: blurring of vision, weakness, and difficulty in speaking and breathing. Symptoms develop as long as 24 hours after ingestion. Untreated botulism poisoning may be fatal.

In general, you should not try to separate specific causes of acute gastrointestinal problems from one another; rather, you should transport the patient promptly to the hospital. In suspected botulism, you may have to assist respirations and give basic life support. In obvious instances of food poisoning where two or more individuals in one group have the same illness, you should bring along some of the suspected food.

Plant Poisoning

Several thousand cases of poisoning from plants occur each year; some are severe. Many household plants are poisonous if they are accidentally ingested, especially by children who like to nibble leaves. Some poisonous plants cause local irritation of the skin; others can affect the circulatory system, the gastrointestinal tract, or the central nervous system.

Circulatory Disturbances Thirty to 50 minutes after ingesting a poisonous plant that affects circulation, the patient may show the classic signs of circulatory collapse: tachycardia (a rapid heart rate); falling blood pressure; sweating; weakness; and cold, moist, clammy skin. There are no effective antidotes for plant poisonings that cause circulatory collapse. Treat the patient for shock. Lie the patient down with the legs elevated, administer oxygen, and transport him or her promptly to the hospital. Induce vomiting with syrup of ipecac in the alert and conscious patient. Save the vomitus and bring it to the hospital. Bring along the plant, or at least several leaves, for positive identification.

Mistletoe is one plant that has been thought to be a circulatory system poison if ingested. However, severe symptoms rarely occur from ingesting just a few mistletoe berries. The treatment is to induce vomiting, monitor and treat the patient for circulatory problems and transport him or her to the hospital.

Gastrointestinal (GI) Disturbances Small amounts of some plants can produce severe gastrointestinal disturbances. The usual symptoms of GI disturbance from plant ingestion are the same as those caused by any other toxic substance: vomiting, diarrhea, and cramps. Symptoms can occur within 20 to 30 minutes after ingestion. If the patient does vomit, you should collect the vomitus. Allow the patient to vomit as needed and transport him or her to the emergency department. The poison control center may direct you to induce vomiting if the plant has been positively identified.

Some agents in plants are locally irritating to the mucous membranes of the mouth and throat. In these instances, inducing vomiting may actually increase that irritation. If gastrointestinal symptoms occur soon after the ingestion, vomiting may help rid the patient of the substance; if symptoms are late, it is unlikely to do much good. Again, taking leaves or the whole plant to the emergency department may help identify the toxin.

A specific problem of skin or mucous membrane irritation occurs with dieffenbachia, a common houseplant (Figure 28–2). If a leaf of this plant is chewed, a severe irritation of the oral mucous membrane and the lining of the upper airway can occur. This irritation is enough to cause difficulty in swallowing, breathing, and speaking. Partial airway obstruction can occur; in rare instances the blockage becomes complete. For this reason the plant has been given the conversational name: "dumb cane." The emergency medical treatment involves maintaining an open airway, giving oxygen, and transporting the patient as promptly as possible to the hospital for respiratory support.

Central Nervous System Disturbances

Poisonous plants sometimes affect the central nervous system. Signs of such problems include depression, hyperactivity, excitement, stupor, mental confusion, or coma. Treat this type of poisoning with basic life support pro-

cedures. The poisoned patient may need complete ventilatory support during transportation. Do not induce vomiting in any patient who shows any signs of stupor or coma. Bring the patient promptly to the hospital, along with a sample of the plant or its leaves if possible.

Skin Irritants Skin irritation is the most common form of plant poisoning. Symptoms include itching, burning, and local blister formation. One of the most common plants to produce such reactions is poison ivy (Figure 28–3). In general, skin irritation occurs after direct contact with the plant and from a spreading onto the skin of the plant's sap or juice. Contact with these plants rarely produces systemic symptoms such as tachycardia, hypotension, or respiratory distress. The emergency treatment of skin irritants is thorough cleansing

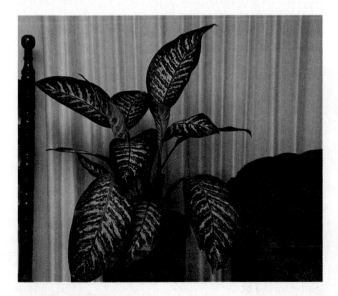

FIGURE 28–2

Dieffenbachia, also called "dumb cane," is a common houseplant that can cause severe irritation and swelling of the mouth and throat if ingested.

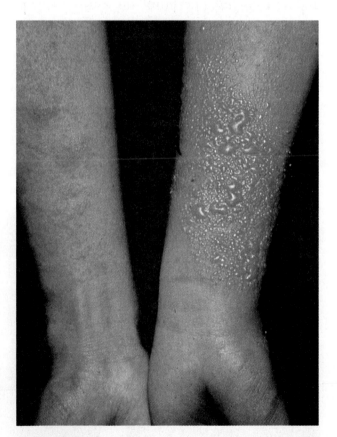

FIGURE 28–3

The sap or juice from poison ivy can cause itching, burning, and blister formation. Severe cases can become infected and require medical treatment.

with soap and water. This treatment is most effective if done within 30 to 60 minutes of exposure to the poison. Some patients occasionally need medical attention for prolonged symptoms.

STINGS

Many different kinds of insects can inflict pain from stings or bites. Some of these injuries are potentially dangerous. They are associated with stings or bites from bees, wasps, yellow jackets, hornets, certain ants, scorpions, and some spiders.

Bee, Wasp, Hornet, Yellow Jacket, and Ant Stings

There are over 100,000 species of bees, wasps, and hornets. Fatalities from this wide variety of stinging insects far outnumber those from snake bites; 65 percent are related to bee, wasp, and hornet stings. The stinging organ of most bees, wasps, or hornets is a small hollow spine that projects from the abdomen. Venom can be injected through this spine directly into the skin. The stinger of the honeybee is barbed so that the bee cannot withdraw it and must leave a part of its abdomen imbedded with the

stinger when it flies away, and then it dies. The honeybee, therefore, can only sting once. Wasps or hornets, with unbarbed stingers, can sting repeatedly (Figure 28–4). Identification of the stinging insect is often impossible, because it tends to fly away immediately after the injury.

Some species of ant, especially the fire ant, can bite repeatedly and often inject a particularly irritating toxin at the bite site. These bites usually occur on the feet and legs. It is not uncommon for the patient to sustain multiple bites within a very short period of time (Figure 28–5).

Symptoms associated with insect stings or bites usually occur at the site of injury. Local symptoms of stings and bites are sudden pain, swelling, heat, and redness about the affected area. Sometimes a **wheal** (whitish firm elevation of the skin) may occur, with itching (Figure 28–6). There is no specific treatment for these injuries; sometimes the application of ice may make them less irritating. The swelling that accompanies insect stings and bites may be considerable and sometimes frightens patients. However, the local manifestations of these stings are not serious.

The stinging organ of a honeybee with its attached muscle can continue to inject venom for up to 20 minutes after the bee has flown away, because the stinger remains in the wound.

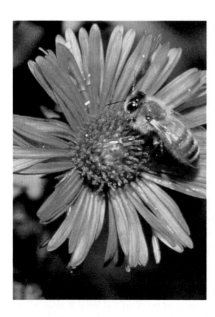

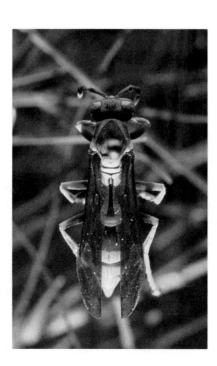

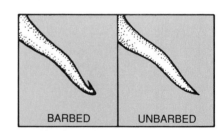

BARBED   UNBARBED

FIGURE 28–4

Most stinging insects inject venom through a small, hollow spine that projects from the abdomen. The stinger of the honeybee is barbed and cannot be withdrawn once the insect has stung someone with it. Wasps have unbarbed stingers and can withdraw the stinger and sting again and again.

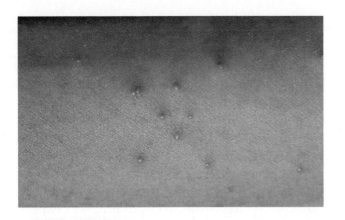

FIGURE 28–5

Fire ants, which come originally from Brazil, are becoming a serious health problem in the United States. They inject an irritating toxin. They can bite repeatedly, and some patients sustain multiple bites in a short time.

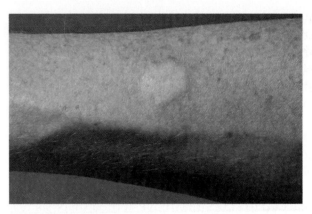

FIGURE 28–6

A wheal is a whitish, firm elevation of the skin that occurs after an insect sting or bite.

If you are assisting a person who has been stung by a honeybee, you should gently attempt to remove the stinger and that portion of the bee's abdomen by scraping it off the patient's skin. Do not use tweezers or forceps, as squeezing the stinger may only inject more venom into the patient.

Some insect bites are not noticed by the individual for some hours until **cellulitis** (a spreading redness and swelling of the skin) has developed. These patients require transport to the emergency department with immobilization of the injured area. Warm, moist packs may produce some comfort. Typically, fire ant bites produce an acute inflammation and ulcerations that are slow to heal.

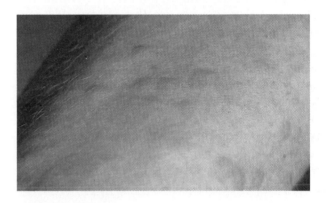

FIGURE 28–7

Urticaria (hives) that appears following a bee, hornet, or wasp sting is one of the warning signs of impending anaphylactic reaction.

Anaphylactic Reaction to Stings

Approximately 5 percent of all people are allergic to the venom of the bee, hornet, yellow jacket, or wasp. This allergy accounts for approximately 200 deaths per year. Honeybee venom is a common **allergen** (substance producing an allergic reaction) and can cause very severe reactions. In a person with such an allergy the sting of such an insect may result in a violent hypersensitivity reaction called *anaphylaxis* or *anaphylactic shock*. Generalized itching and burning, **urticaria** (hives) (Figure 28–7), swelling about the lips and tongue,

bronchospasm and wheezing, chest tightness and cough, dyspnea (difficult breathing), anxiety, abdominal cramps, and occasionally respiratory failure can all occur. If untreated, such a reaction can even proceed to death.

The rapid development of skin wheals and hives and wheezing respirations should alert you that a hypersensitivity reaction is taking place. Administer basic life support at once and transport this patient rapidly to the hospital. Administer oxygen and prepare to maintain an airway or give full cardiopulmonary resuscitation. If possible, place venous tourniquets (pulses palpable distal to the bands) above and below the site of the sting to localize the spread of toxin. Attempt to remove the stinger from the wound by gently scraping the site with the edge of a knife blade. An ice bag placed over the injury site may help to slow the rate of absorption of the toxin. However, speed is important in a patient with anaphylaxis. More than two-thirds of those who die from these reactions do so within the first hour after the sting.

Patients who have a history of severe allergic reaction to stings may have at their disposal bee sting kits (Figure 28–8). Commercially manufactured, they are usually prescribed specifically for the hypersensitive person by a physician. The kits usually contain the medication *epinephrine* prepared in a syringe and ready for injection. Epinephrine is a rapidly acting agent that produces bronchodilation to reverse the effects of the allergen on the airway. It has a short period of action and acts rapidly to produce acute relief. Most kits also contain some oral or intravenous *antihistamine*. These various agents are specific to counter the production of histamine, which is believed to be the specific substance produced by the body responsible for the attack. Usually, antihistamines are slower in onset of action and effective over a longer period than epinephrine.

If the patient is able to self-administer the agent, assist him or her in administering these lifesaving medications. Specific instructions for the use of epinephrine should be in the kit. In the absence of instructions, 1/2 ml of 1/1,000 epinephrine solution should be injected intramuscularly (into a muscle) or subcutaneously (just below the skin). Frequently, more than one injection over a period of time will be required as an anaphylactic reaction develops and progresses. Injections may be needed at intervals of 5 to 15 minutes. Having been injected with epinephrine, the patient will experience tachycardia and, on occasion, increased anxiety or nervousness. Complete the emergency care outlined earlier for support for this patient and transport him or her rapidly to the hospital.

Scorpion Stings

Scorpions and spiders are related, in that both are eight-legged arachnids from the same biological group (Arachnida). Scorpions are rare; they are found primarily in the Southwest and in deserts. Scorpions have a venom gland and a stinger at the end of their tail (Figure 28–9). Except for the sting of a specific scorpion in the Southwest, the Arizona scorpion, these injuries

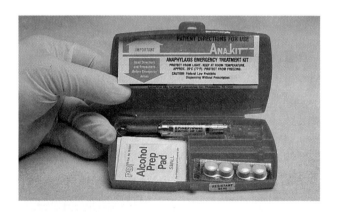

FIGURE 28–8

A typical prescription bee sting kit for a person known to be allergic to bee stings. The syringe is loaded with two premeasured doses of epinephrine. Instructions for proper administration, including self-administration, are included in the kit.

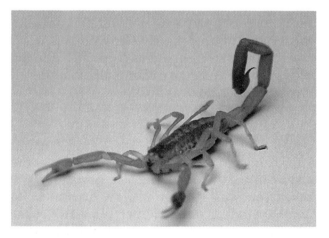

FIGURE 28–9

The sting of a scorpion is more painful than it is dangerous. The stinger and venom gland are located at the end of the scorpion's tail. Only the Arizona scorpion, which lives in the Southwest, is dangerous. Its venom can cause a severe reaction.

are ordinarily very painful but not dangerous. Only 4 percent of fatalities related to insect stings are associated with scorpions. Localized swelling, pain, and discoloration result from a scorpion sting. Arizona scorpion venom may produce a severe systemic reaction that brings about circulatory collapse, severe muscle contractions, excessive salivation, hypertension, convulsions, and cardiac failure. The emergency treatment for this sting is basic life support. **Antivenin** (a serum that contains antibodies that counteract the venom) is available but must be administered by a physician.

If you have a patient with a suspected sting from an Arizona scorpion, you should notify medical control as soon as possible. Administer all of the elements of basic life support and transport the patient to the emergency department as rapidly as possible. Remember, however, that only the Arizona scorpion can cause this serious reaction. This particular scorpion species does not reside anywhere else in the country.

BITES

Spider Bites

Spiders are numerous and widespread in the United States. Two species—the black widow spider and the brown recluse spider—are able to deliver serious, sometimes even life-threatening bites. Many other spiders bite, but these injuries do not produce serious complications.

Black Widow Spider The black widow spider is not large, measuring approximately 1 inch long with its legs extended. It is glossy black and has a distinctive, bright red-orange marking in the shape of an hourglass on its abdomen (Figure 28–10). Black widow spiders are found in every state except Alaska. They prefer dry, dim places around buildings, in woodpiles, and among debris.

A black widow spider bite is sometimes overlooked. The victim may not recall the bite itself, because the area may become numb after the bite. However, most patients bitten by a black widow spider will experience pain at the site of the bite. The danger of a black widow

spider bite is that the venom is neurotoxic (poisonous to nerve tissue), directly attacks spinal nerve centers, and causes systemic symptoms. Severe cramps, with boardlike rigidity of the abdominal muscles, tightness in the chest, and difficulty breathing occur over 24 hours. Other complaints include dizziness, sweating, vomiting, nausea, and skin rashes. Generally, the signs and symptoms subside over 48 hours, but the muscle cramps and ensuing pain can be agonizing.

Although painful symptoms following the bites are severe, death is not common (63 recorded in 10 years, from 1950 to 1960). A specific antivenin is available, but its use is accompanied by a high incidence of side effects. Its use is reserved for very severe bites, and for the aged or very feeble, and children under the age of 5. It will be administered, if necessary, by a physician.

In general, emergency treatment for a black widow spider bite is basic life support for the patient in respiratory distress. Much more commonly, the patient will require relief from pain. If the site of the bite can be identified, putting ice against it may slow the absorption of toxin. Transport the patient to the emergency department as soon as possible for

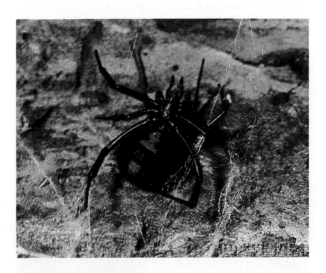

FIGURE 28–10

The black widow spider, shown here on its back, is distinguished by its glossy black color and bright red-orange hourglass markings on its abdomen. Its bite can cause severe, even life-threatening, injuries.

treatment of the symptoms of pain and muscle rigidity. It is also important for you, if possible, to identify the spider and bring it with the patient to the hospital.

Brown Recluse Spider Dull brown in color, the brown recluse spider is somewhat smaller than the black widow (Figure 28–11). It has a dark violin-shaped mark on its back, which can be easily seen from above. Although found mostly in the southern and central United States, it is currently moving to other areas. The spider takes its name from the fact that it tends to live in dark areas, corners, old unused buildings, under rocks, and in woodpiles. It has moved indoors in cooler areas and inhabits closets, drawers, cellars, and old piles of clothing.

The bite from the brown recluse, in contrast to the black widow, produces local rather than systemic symptoms. The venom of the brown recluse spider causes severe local tissue damage, which may produce a large, nonhealing ulcer if not treated promptly. Typically, the bite is not painful initially but becomes so within hours. The area becomes red, swollen, and tender, and it develops a pale, mottled cyanotic center. A small blister may form (Figure 28–12). Over the next several days, a large scab of dead skin, fat, and debris will develop and deepen to produce the large ulcer.

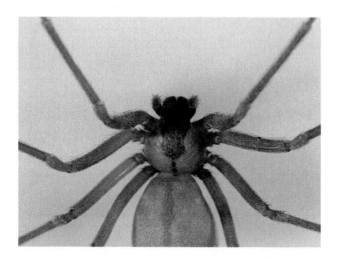

FIGURE 28–11

The brown recluse spider is dull brown in color and has a dark, violin-shaped mark on its back.

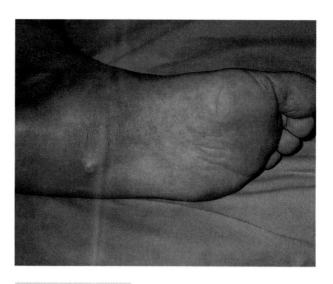

FIGURE 28–12

The venom from the sting of the brown recluse spider causes severe local tissue injury, which if not treated promptly can result in a large, nonhealing ulcer.

Systemic symptoms and signs from brown recluse spider bites rarely occur. When they do, the emergency treatment is basic life support and transportation to the emergency department. No specific antivenin exists for this toxin, and the only effective treatment to avoid the long-term painful ulceration is prompt surgical excision of the area. Thus, emergency treatment for a suspected brown recluse spider bite without systemic symptoms is also prompt transportation to the emergency department. Again, it is helpful if the spider can be identified and brought to the hospital along with the patient.

Snake Bites

Snake bites are a worldwide problem of some significance. More than 300,000 injuries from snake bites occur annually; 30,000 to 40,000 deaths result. The greatest number of the fatalities occur in Southeast Asia and in India (25,000 to 30,000) and in South America (3,000 to 4,000). Snake bites are fairly common in the United States: 40,000 to 50,000 are reported annually. Approximately 7,000 of them are caused by poisonous snakes. However, fatalities in the United States from snake bites are extremely rare—about 15 a year for the entire country.

Of the approximately 150 different species of snakes in the United States, only 4 are poisonous: the rattlesnake, the copperhead, the cottonmouth (water) moccasin, and the coral snake. Only Alaska, Hawaii, and Maine do not have at least one species of poisonous snake. As a general rule, these creatures are retiring and timid. They usually do not bite unless provoked, angered, or accidentally injured (as when one steps on them). There are a few exceptions to these rules. Moccasins are often rather aggressive snakes, and certainly very little provocation is needed to annoy a rattlesnake. Coral snakes, on the other hand, are very shy and retiring and usually bite only when they are being handled.

Most snake bites occur between April and October, when the animals are active. Most involve young males, and most occur within a very few states. Texas reports the largest number of bites. Other states with a major concentration of snake bites are Louisiana, Georgia, Oklahoma, North Carolina, Arkansas, West Virginia, and Mississippi. If you work in these areas, you should be thoroughly familiar with the emergency handling of snake bites. Remember that more than one snake may be in an area and that while you are working on a victim, you may accidentally encounter another snake and yourself become a victim.

When you respond to a snake bite, it is extremely important to identify whether **envenomation** (deposit of venom into the wound) has occurred. In one report of all snake bites throughout the United States, 27 percent were found to have had no envenomation at all, and an additional 37 percent had only minimal envenomation. Thus, only one-third of snake bites in general result in significant local or systemic injuries. There are several reasons why envenomation does not occur. Most commonly, the snake recently has struck another animal and has exhausted its supply of venom.

With the exception of the coral snake, poisonous vipers (snakes) in the United States all have hollow fangs in the roof of the mouth, which literally inject the poison from two sacs at the back of the head. The characteristic appearance of the poisonous snake bite, there-

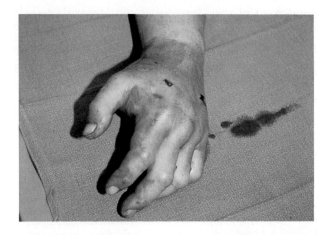

FIGURE 28–13

The presence of fang marks indicates a poisonous, pit viper snake bite. Swelling and discoloration of the hand indicate envenomation.

fore, is two small puncture wounds, usually about a half-inch apart, with surrounding discoloration, swelling, and pain (Figure 28–13). Some poisonous snakes have teeth as well as fangs. Nonpoisonous snakes can also cause bites, which usually leave a horseshoe shape of tooth marks. The mere presence of tooth marks does not necessarily mean that a poisonous snake attack could not have occurred. Fang marks, on the other hand, are a clear indication of a bite by a poisonous snake. In this situation you must look for signs of envenomation.

Pit Vipers Rattlesnakes, copperheads, and cottonmouth (water) moccasins are all pit vipers (Figure 28–14). The head of the pit viper is triangular and flat; there is a small pit located just behind the nostril and in front of each eye. The pupil of the eye is vertical and slitlike. The pit is a heat-sensing organ that allows the snake to strike accurately at any warm target, especially in the dark when it cannot see. Localization by the pits is much more accurate than that provided by the eye.

The fangs of the pit viper normally lie flat against the roof of the mouth. When the snake is striking, the mouth opens wide and the fangs extend, so that if the mouth strikes an object, the fangs will penetrate. The fangs are hollow, adapted teeth that act much like hypodermic needles. They are hinged to swing back and

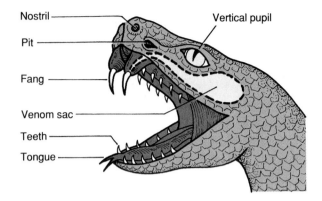

Nostril
Pit
Fang
Venom sac
Teeth
Tongue
Vertical pupil

FIGURE 28–14

Rattlesnakes, copperheads, and cottonmouth (water) moccasins all have hollow fangs in the roof of the mouth that inject poison from two sacs in the back of the head. These snakes are called pit vipers because they have small, heat-sensing organs (pits) located in front of their eyes that allow them to strike at warm targets, even in the dark.

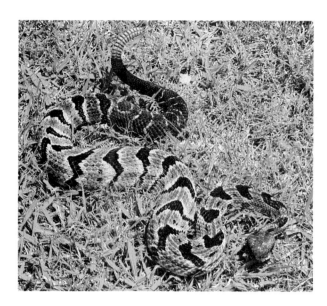

FIGURE 28–15

The rattlesnake is the commonest of the pit vipers. The "rattle" is actually layers of shed skin that lie against a small nubbin on the end of the tail.

forth as the mouth opens. They are connected to a sac containing a reservoir of venom, which in turn is attached to a poison gland. The gland itself is an adapted salivary gland, producing powerful enzymes that digest and destroy tissue. A purpose of the venom is to kill the small animal the snake attacks and also to start the digestive process prior to the animal's being eaten by the snake.

Among the pit vipers, the commonest is the rattlesnake (Figure 28–15). Several different species of rattlesnake exist. Apart from the features of the pit vipers in general, rattlesnakes can usually be identified by the rattle on the tail. The rattle is actually numerous layers of shed skin that come to lie against a small nubbin on the end of the tail. As the snake sheds its skin annually, the dried skin remnants that do not come off completely form the characteristic rattle. Rattlesnakes have many patterns of color, often with a diamond pattern. They can develop to 6 feet or more in length.

Copperheads are smaller than rattlesnakes. They are usually 2 to 3 feet long and have a characteristic reddish coppery color with brown or red cross-bands (Figure 28–16). Shyer than rattlesnakes, they inhabit woodpiles and abandoned dwellings, often close to areas of habitation. Although they account for most of

the venomous snake bites in the eastern United States, fatalities from copperhead bites are almost never seen.

Cottonmouth moccasins grow to about 4 feet. Also called water moccasins, these snakes are olive or brown, with black cross-bands and a yellow undersurface (Figure 28–17). They are

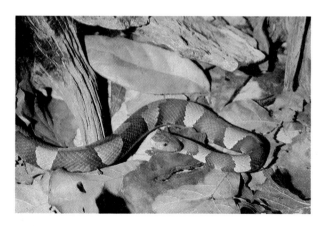

FIGURE 28–16

The copperhead is a reddish, copper-colored pit viper that accounts for most of the poisonous snake bites in the Eastern United States. Its bite is almost never fatal.

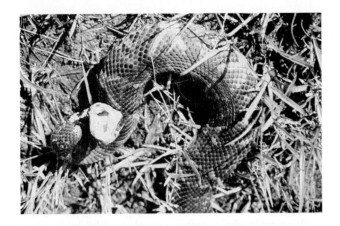

FIGURE 28–17

Cottonmouth (water) moccasins are pit vipers that live in the water. They get their name from their white mouth, as shown here. They are aggressive snakes whose bites can cause serious tissue injury.

water snakes with a particularly aggressive pattern of behavior. Although fatalities from these snake bites are rare, tissue destruction from the venom may be severe.

The signs of envenomation by a pit viper are severe burning pain at the site of the injury, followed by swelling and discoloration. These signs are evident within 5 to 10 minutes after the bite has occurred and spread slowly over the next 36 hours. Bleeding under the skin causes ecchymosis (bluish discoloration). An envenomated bite is painful and ecchymotic. Systemic signs, which may or may not occur, include weakness, sweating, fainting, and shock.

Occasionally, the patient bitten by a snake will faint from fright. Usually this situation is corrected promptly by lying the patient supine (flat on the back). Consciousness returns, and the episode is temporary. Do not confuse a fainting spell with shock, which, if it does occur, happens much later after the bite has occurred.

The venom of the pit viper causes localized destruction of all tissues. It can also interfere significantly with the body's clotting mechanism and cause bleeding at various distant sites. Tissue destruction locally starts from the moment of envenomation. If an hour has elapsed from the time the patient was bitten without local signs of envenomation (no swell-

ing, no discoloration, no severe local pain), it is safe to assume that envenomation has not occurred.

The emergency treatment of snake bites from pit vipers is directed primarily at local containment of venom and then at the systemic effects. Carry out the following steps to treat a bite from a pit viper:

1. Calm and reassure the patient. Place the patient supine and explain that staying quiet will decrease the spread of any venom through the system. Assure the patient that poisonous snake bites rarely cause death.
2. Locate the bite area; clean it gently with soap and water or a mild antiseptic.
3. Place venous tourniquets above and below the fang marks. Wrap soft rubber tubes about the extremity and tighten them just enough to occlude the venous circulation. The distal pulse in the extremity should not disappear. This maneuver will help limit the spread of the venom through the veins of the extremity.
4. Be alert for vomiting. Patients may often do so from anxiety rather than from the effects of the toxin itself.
5. Do not give anything by mouth, especially alcohol.
6. Immobilize the extremity with a splint.
7. In the relatively rare instance of the bite occurring on the trunk rather than on the extremity, it will be impossible to use tourniquets and splinting. Keep the patient supine and as quiet as possible and transport as quickly as possible.
8. Monitor the vital signs: blood pressure, pulse, and respiration.
9. If there are any signs of shock, place the patient in the shock position and give oxygen.
10. If the snake has been killed, as is often the case, bring it with you. Identification of the offending snake is extremely important in administering the correct antivenin.
11. Notify the hospital that you are bringing in a snake bite patient; and, if possible, describe the snake. Transport the patient promptly to the hospital.

If the patient shows no sign of envenomation, provide basic life support as needed, place a sterile dressing over the suspected bite area, apply venous constricting bands above and below the bite, and immobilize the injury site. The same procedure applies for the patient who shows early signs of envenomation but who can be delivered to the hospital in less than 30 minutes.

The patient who shows early signs of envenomation but cannot be delivered to a hospital in less than 30 minutes may require local removal of the venom by suction. This treatment should be carried out only on the specific instructions of a physician. After a bite, the venom remains locally in the tissue for about 30 minutes. Some of it can be mechanically removed by making a small, one-half-inch incision through the skin in the long axis of the extremity over the fang mark. The incision should be just deep enough to go through the skin so that subcutaneous fat is visible (one-quarter of an inch deep). To cut any deeper would risk injury of important tendons, nerves, or blood vessels. The suction cup from a snake-bite kit should be applied to suck out the poison mechanically.

This technique—incision and suction—should only be used on a bite of the extremity. It should never be used on the head or trunk, nor should it be done without the direction of medical control. It is applicable only for the patient showing definite signs of envenomation less than 30 minutes after the bite. This process has been criticized for two reasons: Many snake bites deposit venom much deeper than the skin and subcutaneous fat, and there is some evidence that the technique of incision and suction is not effective, and may only cause further injury and infection.

All patients with suspected snake bite patients should be brought to the emergency department whether they show signs of envenomation or not. Regardless of whether envenomation has occurred, treat these wounds like all other deep puncture wounds to prevent infection. If you work in an area where poisonous snakes are known to live, you should always keep a snake bite kit in the ambulance, you should know the local medical protocol for handling snake bites, and you should also know the address of the nearest facility where antivenin is available. It may be a nearby zoo,

the local or public state health department, or a local community hospital.

Coral Snake The coral snake is a small, very colorful reptile with a series of bright red, yellow, and black bands that completely encircle its body (Figure 28–18). Many harmless snakes have coloring similar to the coral snake. The difference is that the red and yellow bands of the coral snake are next to one another, completely encircling the body. There is a rhyme for remembering this fact: "Red on yellow will kill a fellow; red on black, venom will lack."

The coral snake is a rare creature. It lives primarily in Florida and in the desert Southwest. It is not found in the northern regions of the United States. The coral snake is not a pit viper; the head is not triangular, there are no pits, and there are no projecting fangs. A relative of the cobra, the coral snake has tiny fangs and injects the venom with its teeth by a chewing motion, not an injection. Because of its small mouth and teeth and limited jaw expansion, the coral snake usually bites its victims on a small part of the body, especially a finger or toe. Following the bite of a coral snake, one or more punctures or scratchlike wounds can be found in the area.

The danger of this particular snake is that its venom is a powerful toxin that causes paralysis

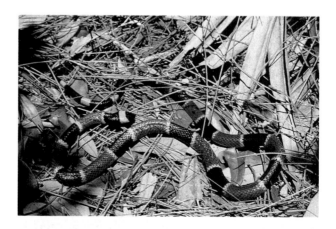

FIGURE 28–18

The coral snake is not a pit viper. It injects venom with its teeth. It is characterized by red and yellow bands next to each other circling its body completely.

of the nervous system. Usually, there are minimal or no local symptoms of a coral snake bite. However, within a few hours bizarre behavior will occur, followed by progressive paralysis of eye movements and respiration as a result of the toxic effects on the nervous system.

Treatment, either emergency or long term, depends on positive identification of the snake. Antivenin is available, but most hospitals or doctors must order it from a central supply area, often in another city. Therefore, you should notify the hospital of the need for it as soon as possible. The steps for emergency care of a coral snake bite are as follows:

1. Immediately quiet and reassure the patient.
2. Flush the area of the bite with one to two quarts of warm, soapy water to wash away any poison left on the surface of the skin.
3. Lightly apply venous tourniquets around the extremity above and below the bite.
4. Splint the extremity to minimize movement and the spread of venom at the site.
5. Check the patient's vital signs and continue to monitor them.
6. Keep the patient warm and elevate the lower extremities to help prevent shock.
7. Give artificial ventilation with oxygen if needed.
8. Transport the patient promptly to the emergency department, giving advance notice that the patient has been bitten by a coral snake.
9. Give the patient nothing by mouth.

The incision and suction technique is not done in the case of a coral snake bite, as there is little local effect from this injury. The danger is to the central nervous system from an absorbed neurotoxin. Antivenin is the most effective means of control.

Tick Bites

Tick bites are a special problem. Ticks can spread infectious diseases, so the problem with a tick bite is not from the bite itself, but from the infecting organisms that the tick carries. Two diseases—Rocky Mountain spotted fever, and Lyme disease—are commonly spread by ticks.

Rocky Mountain spotted fever occurs within 7 to 10 days after a bite by an infected tick. Its symptoms include nausea, vomiting, headache, weakness, paralysis and even cardiorespiratory collapse. Rocky Mountain spotted fever occurs all over the United States, not just in the Rocky Mountain area.

Lyme disease has received much publicity recently. It is, after AIDS, the second most rapidly growing infectious (contagious) disease in the United States. Originally seen only in Connecticut, Lyme disease has now been reported in 35 states. It occurs most commonly in the Northeast, the Great Lake States, and the Pacific Northwest. New York State reports the largest number of cases. Lyme disease is caused by a bacterium that is carried by a tick. Symptoms begin about 3 days after being bitten by an infected tick. A progressive red rash develops and may spread to several parts of the body. After a few more days or weeks, painful swelling of the joints, particularly the knees occurs. Lyme disease may be confused with rheumatoid arthritis and may result in permanent disability. However, if it is recognized and treated promptly with antibiotics, the patient may recover completely.

People who are bitten by ticks are not aware they have been bitten—the bite is painless. The tick attaches itself to the skin, where it sucks blood and becomes swollen with blood. Infections are spread through the saliva of the tick, which is injected into the skin at the time the tick attaches itself. Ticks are tiny insects, only a fraction of an inch long, and they can be mistaken for a freckle on the skin. When a tick swells with blood, it may reach a quarter inch in diameter. Ticks are found on brush, shrubs, trees, sand dunes, or on other animals. Ticks usually attach themselves directly to the skin. Tick bites occur most commonly during the summer months, when people are out in the woods wearing little protective clothing.

A person who goes into a high-risk area should wear light colored clothing (so that a tick can be easily spotted), tuck the pants cuff into the socks, and periodically examine himself or herself for ticks. Ticks like to attach themselves to the warm, moist parts of the body, particularly in skin folds. Clothing, as well as any pets that may have been in the area, should also be examined carefully. Remember these rules when you are engaged in rescue efforts in areas infested with ticks.

It takes at least 18 hours for the infection to be transmitted from the tick to the person it has bitten, so if you are called on to remove a tick, you should proceed carefully and slowly. Do not attempt to suffocate the tick with gasoline, vaseline, or burn it with a lighted match (you will only burn the patient!). These remedies were once thought to be effective by making the tick back out of the skin on its own. However, they do not work, and there is some evidence that by irritating the tick, as these techniques do, you only cause it to put more infecting bacteria into the skin.

Physically remove the tick. Using a fine tweezers, grasp the tick by the body and pull it straight out of the skin. This method will usually remove the whole tick. Even if part of the tick is left embedded in the skin, the part containing the infecting organisms has been removed. Once the tick is removed, paint the area with disinfectant and save the tick in a glass jar or similar container so that it can be identified. Do not handle the tick with your fingers.

All patients with tick bites should be seen by a physician. You should tell the patient that there are diseases that may be spread by ticks, and that he or she should see a physician within the next day or so. Remember that the symptoms of Rocky Mountain spotted fever or Lyme disease do not occur until a few days after the person has been bitten by an infected tick. If you are called to transport someone who has the symptoms of either of these diseases, you do not need to look for ticks. Provide any necessary supportive emergency care and transport the patient to the hospital.

Dog Bites and Rabies

The exact incidence of dog bites is unknown. Most people who are bitten by dogs do not report the bite to a physician and do not require the services of an EMT. Dog bites, however, are potentially serious problems. The animal's mouth is heavily contaminated with virulent bacteria, and serious infection may result from a bite. Consider all dog bites as contaminated and potentially infected wounds.

Often the patient is extremely upset and frightened. Most dog bites are not serious; therefore, calm reassurance on your part is extremely important. All dog bites should be treated by a physician. Tetanus prophylaxis may be necessary. The wound may or may not require sutures (stitches), and antibiotics are frequently given. Occasionally, dog bites result in mangled, complex wounds that require much surgical expertise for repair.

The prehospital treatment for dog bites of any severity is to place a dry, sterile dressing over the wound and promptly transport the patient to the emergency department.

A major concern with dog bites is the spread of *rabies*, an acute, virtually always fatal viral infection of the central nervous system. The virus is present in saliva of the infected animal and is transmitted by biting or by licking an open wound. All warm-blooded animals can be affected. Rabies can be prevented in a patient who has been bitten by a **rabid** animal (one infected by rabies) by administering a specific vaccine. Although rabies is extremely rare today, particularly with widespread inoculation of pets, it still exists. Stray dogs may not have been inoculated and could be carriers of the disease. Certain other animals—squirrels, bats, foxes, skunks, and raccoons—may also carry rabies. Each of these animals has been implicated as a cause of rabies after biting a human.

A rabid animal may act perfectly normally or may appear vicious, salivate excessively, appear wild ("mad dog") or show some other form of unusual behavior. You cannot tell whether an animal is rabid by its behavior. The vaccine that is used to prevent rabies in pets is very effective. If an animal has been inoculated against rabies, it ordinarily will have a tag so stating on its collar. It is, therefore, very important to identify this fact if the animal can be located. Usually, a dog is a pet and can be identified. If it does not have a rabies tag, it should be captured (not killed) by an animal control officer and turned over to the health department for observation. Unless you are specially trained in handling animals, you should not attempt to handle a strange dog or wild animal but instead call the local animal control officer. If the animal is then suspected of having rabies, it is killed and the brain studied. Results of this study will determine whether the animal was rabid.

When the animal cannot be found or identified, the patient usually is treated with rabies inoculations. If started early enough, these inoculations will prevent rabies from developing. Beginning in 1980, a rabies vaccine was developed from material grown in human tissue, and this substance is now in common use. You should know where the local rabies control center is located and also where the closest institution that has human rabies vaccine is located.

On occasion, you will be called to treat a child who has been attacked by a dog. Children, particularly young ones, may be seriously injured or even killed by dogs. The dog may be a stray, or it may even be the family pet. These dogs are not always vicious or rabid; sometimes the child unknowingly provokes the dog. Even though the dog may not appear rabid or even vicious, you must assume that it may turn on you and attack you as well. Therefore, do not enter the scene until the animal has been secured by either the police or the animal control officer of the community. Then, carry out the necessary emergency care and transport the child to the emergency department promptly.

Human Bites

A somewhat neglected area of emergency medical treatment is the human bite. It is relatively uncommon but potentially one of the most severe injuries seen today. The human mouth contains an exceptionally wide range of virulent bacteria, more so than the mouth of a dog. For this reason, any deliberate human bite that has penetrated the skin must be regarded as a very serious injury. Similarly, any laceration caused by a human tooth, such as may result on a hand from punching someone in the mouth, may result in a serious, spreading infection (Figure 28–19). The emergency treatment for human bites is prompt immobilization of the area with a splint or bandage, application of a dry, sterile dressing; and transport to the emergency department for surgical cleansing of the wound and antibiotic therapy. Remember

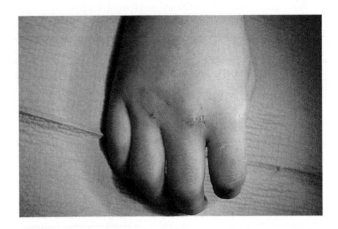

F I G U R E 28–19

The human bite is a very serious injury, because if left untreated it will become the source of a significant, dangerous, spreading infection.

when you are treating someone who has been punched in the mouth that the person who delivered the punch may also need treatment.

Injuries from Marine Animals

In recent years there has been a good deal of publicity concerning shark bites. They remain extremely rare. The emergency treatment of a large marine animal bite is the same as for any other major open wound. Get the patient out of the water, control hemorrhage, apply dressings and splints, treat for shock, and transport the patient to the emergency department promptly. If there are sharks in the area, be careful not to let any part of your body dangle over the boat or into the water.

Many other injuries may result from marine animals, but none of them are as dramatic or as potentially life-threatening as the large marine animal bite. With the exception of the shark and barracuda, most marine creatures are not aggressive and will not deliberately attack a human. Injuries from these animals occur when they are accidentally stepped on or otherwise provoked.

The most frequent injuries from marine animals occur from swimming into the tentacles of a jellyfish, stepping on the back of a stingray, or falling or stepping on a sea urchin. If you work near water, you should be familiar with the marine life in your locality.

Stings from the tentacles of a jellyfish, a Portuguese man-of-war, various anemones, corals, or hydras can be treated by removing the patient from the water and pouring rubbing alcohol on the affected area. Then sprinkle the area with meat tenderizer. Finally, dust the area with talcum powder. This treatment will inactivate the poison that has been deposited on the skin and usually is the only treatment necessary. Alcohol will fix or denature the toxins, and meat tenderizer will destroy them. On very rare occasions, a patient may have a systemic allergic reaction from the sting of one of these animals. Treat the patient for anaphylactic shock; give basic life support and transport the patient rapidly to the hospital.

Injuries from the spines of urchins, stingrays, or certain spiny fish such as a catfish can best be treated by immobilizing the affected area and soaking it in hot water for 30 minutes.

TABLE 28–1   Guide to Diagnosis and Emergency Treatment of Marine Animal Injuries

Type of Injury	Marine Animal Involved	Emergency Treatment	Possible Complications

Trauma (bites and lacerations)	Major wounds by
	  Shark
	  Barracuda
	  Alligator gar
		Control bleeding
		Prevent shock
		Give basic life support
		Splint the injury
		Secure prompt medical care
			Shock
			Infections

	Minor wounds by
	  Moray eel
	  Turtle
	  Corals
		Cleanse wound
		Splint the injury	

Sting (by tentacles)	Jellyfish Portuguese man-of-war Anemones Corals Hydras	Inactivate the toxin with alcohol, meat tenderizer, and talcum powder[1]	Allergic reactions Respiratory arrest
Puncture (by spines)	Urchins Cone shells Stingrays Spiny fish (catfish, toad, or oyster fish)	Inactivate with hot water[2]	Allergic reactions Collapse Infections Tetanus Granuloma formation
Poisoning (by ingestion)[3]	Puffer fish Scromboids (tuna species) Ciguatera (large colored fish) Paralytic shellfish	Give basic life support; prevent self-injury from convulsions	Allergic reactions Asthmatic reactions Paresthesia, numbness Temperature reversal phenomena Respiratory arrest and circulatory collapse

Miscellaneous:
  Shocks
  Skin rashes
	Electric fish
	Marine parasites
		No treatment required; injuries usually self-limiting	Electric fish or electric eel may precipitate a panic reaction

[1] The intense burning pain resulting from the sting of the jellyfish is produced by nematocysts (stinging cells) on the tentacles. Even when the sea creature is washed up on shore, the stinging cells can remain potent for as long as several days. In treating the sting, 95-percent alcohol "fixes" the nematocysts on the skin and prevents further stinging, and the meat tenderizer neutralizes the protein toxin of the nematocyst. Powder dries the area and causes the cells to stick together so they can be more readily removed by scraping.

[2] A toxin is introduced with some of the puncture wounds from this group.

In any case, the wounds are excruciatingly painful. It appears that the foreign material or poison introduced into the wound is heat-sensitive. Dramatic treatment results occur with soaking in quite hot water for thirty to sixty minutes. Be careful, however, not to scald the patient with water that is too hot, as the pain of the wound will mask the normal reaction to heat.

[3] Should ingestion of a poisonous fish be suspected, reference to Halstead's *Poisoning and Venomous Marine Animals of the World* or seeking immediate assistance from poison control centers is suggested.

The water should be as hot as the patient can stand without actually burning. Toxins from these animals are heat sensitive, and dramatic relief from local pain often occurs just from the application of hot water. Allergic reactions may occur following injections from these animals. As with any puncture wound, tetanus and other infections could develop. These patients should be transported to the emergency department.

Some sea animals, such as nonpoisonous water snakes, may cause injuries by minor bites. Treat these bites as any other bites with sterile dressings and transport for evaluation and tetanus prophylaxis.

Many fish are poisonous if eaten. The emergency treatment of such poisoning is the same as for any other poisoning: basic life support, prevention of injury from convulsions, and prompt transport of the patient to the emergency department.

Other rare conditions include shocks from electric eels or skin rashes from marine parasites. In general, these injuries are mild. Panic from contact with electric eels can be the most impressive part of this particular injury. Table 28–1 provides a quick reference for the management of common marine organism injuries.

YOU ARE THE EMT

1. What circumstances would lead you to suspect that a poisoning has occurred? What should you do?
2. Describe when you would induce vomiting, how you would induce vomiting, and when you would not induce vomiting.
3. Your patient has been stung by a wasp and she tells you she is allergic to "bees." List the symptoms of an anaphylactic reaction and the emergency treatment you should be prepared to give.
4. A camper has been bitten by a water moccasin. Is this snake poisonous? If so, how do you determine if envenomation has occurred? Describe the steps needed to treat this patient.
5. You are called to see a camper who says he was bitten by a tick and who shows you a tiny, brown insect on his leg. Should you remove it, and if so, how? What should you tell him about any diseases that he could get from the tick?

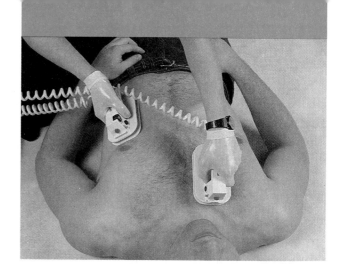

CHAPTER 29

HEART DISEASE

KEY TERMS

acute myocardial infarction (AMI) (ah-kūt mi″o-kar′de-al in-fark′shun) Heart attack; specifically, death of the heart muscle from obstruction of its blood flow.

angina pectoris (an-ji′nah pec′toris) Chest pain from heart disease that is brought on by excitement or exertion and relieved by rest and nitroglycerine tablets.

arrhythmia (ah-rith′me-ah) An irregular or abnormal heart rhythm.

asystole (ah-sis′to-le) Complete absence of heart activity.

bradycardia (brad″e-kar′de-ah) Slow but regular heart rhythm.

congestive heart failure (CHF) (kon-jes′tiv hart fāl′yer) A disease in which the heart loses its ability to pump blood, usually as a result of damage to the heart muscle.

dilation (di-la′shun) Widening of a tubular structure such as a coronary artery.

dyspnea (disp′ne-ah) Difficult breathing.

fibrillation (fi-brĭ-la′shun) A form of arrhythmia characterized by completely disorganized, ineffective quivering of the heart muscle.

infarction (in-fark′shun) Death of tissue, usually caused by interruption of its blood supply.

lumen (loo′men) The inside diameter of an artery or other hollow structure.

pedal edema (ped′al ĕ-de′mah) Edema of the feet, usually seen in congestive heart failure.

pulmonary edema (pul′mo-ner″e ĕ-de′mah) Fluid building up in the lungs, a result of congestive heart failure.

sputum (spu′tum) Fluid that is coughed or spit up from the lungs.

syncope (sin′ko-pe) Fainting.

tachycardia (tak″e-kar′de-ah) Rapid but regular heart rhythm.

OVERVIEW

Heart attacks and other forms of heart disease strike over 4 million people a year in the United States. Currently, heart disease causes more than 700,000 deaths annually. Although death rates in recent years have tended to level off rather than increase, heart disease remains a leading cause of death. In fact, about one-third of the population will die as a result of heart disease. For EMTs, these statistics mean that on many occasions you will be called to manage patients with some form of heart disease.

Chapter 29 begins with a basic definition of heart function and then explains how improper function results in heart disease. The chapter next describes angina (severe chest pain) and acute myocardial infarction (death of the heart muscle). You must become familiar with the symptoms of these two major types of heart disease and with the emergency treatments each type calls for. Chapter 29 also deals with the symptoms and treatment of chronic congestive heart failure. The final section of the chapter discusses the emergency treatment of patients who have had prior heart surgery or who have a cardiac pacemaker.

GOALS

The goals of Chapter 29 are to
- describe angina pectoris and learn how nitroglycerin is used to relieve the pain of angina.
- describe acute myocardial infarction (AMI) and its consequences.
- learn how to identify the signs and physical findings of AMI and how to approach the patient with suspected AMI.
- understand the causes and treatment of chronic congestive heart failure.
- learn how to treat AMI in the patient who has had previous coronary artery surgery.
- learn how to treat the patient with pacemaker failure.

CARDIAC FUNCTION AND ANATOMY

To carry out its pumping function, the *myocardium* (heart muscle) must have a continuous supply of oxygen and nutrients. When the heart must increase its work, as during periods of physical exertion and stress, the myocardium requires more oxygen and therefore more blood flow. In the normal heart, the increased need for blood is easily supplied by **dilation** (widening) of the coronary arteries, which increases blood flow. *Arteriosclerosis*, which is a thickening and destruction of the arterial walls caused by fatty deposits within them, interferes with the ability of the coronary arteries to dilate and to carry additional blood. Indeed, arteriosclerosis can cause complete *occlusion*, or blockage, of a coronary artery and thus cut off the supply of oxygen and nutrients to that part of the myocardium. Acute myocardial infarction (AMI), the death of the heart muscle, and **angina pectoris,** which is chest pain caused by an inadequate flow of blood to the heart muscle, are each conditions that occur from too little oxygen. Each represents a degree of coronary arteriosclerosis.

The coronary arteries are the arteries that supply the heart muscle. They originate at the first part of the aorta, just above the aortic valve. The right coronary artery supplies the right ventricle and, in most people, part of the left ventricle. The left coronary artery divides into two major branches, both of which supply the left ventricle (Figure 29–1).

Arteriosclerosis, the disease process that damages the coronary arteries, usually involves other arteries of the body as well. The disease begins when a deposit of fatty material, *cholesterol*, is laid down on the inside of an artery. Deposits may start accumulating as early as age 18. As a person ages, more of this fatty material is deposited, and the **lumen,** or the inside diameter of the artery, narrows. As these deposits grow, calcium deposits form, and the inner wall of the artery, which is normally smooth and elastic, becomes narrowed, rough, and stiff. Blood clots can form easily on this damaged blood vessel lining (Figure 29–2).

Damage of the coronary arteries may become so extensive as to limit their ability to increase blood flow at times of maximum need. Therefore, during physical activity or emotional stress, the oxygen supply to the heart can no longer meet the heart's requirement.

Arteriosclerosis is not just found in people over 40, even though in the United States, the peak incidence of heart disease occurs in the decades between 40 and 70. You must be aware, however, that heart attack and angina can occur any time from the teens to the 90s. A 28-year-old person with chest pain is not too young to have a heart attack.

Many factors have been identified that place a person at higher risk of a myocardial infarction. These are called risk factors. They are divided into two groups:

1. Factors that can be controlled or modified.
2. Factors that cannot be controlled or modified.

FIGURE 29–1

The coronary arteries carry the blood supply to the heart. The right coronary artery supplies the right ventricle and the larger left coronary artery supplies the correspondingly larger left ventricle.

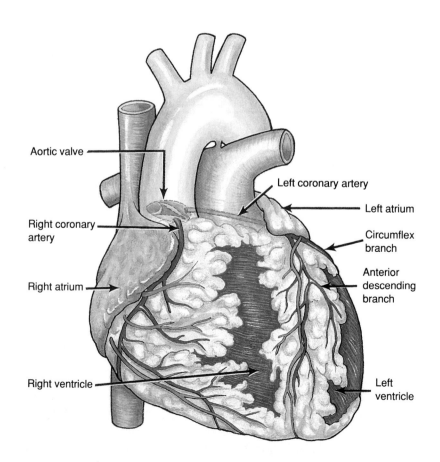

Aortic valve

Right coronary artery

Right atrium

Right ventricle

Left coronary artery

Left atrium

Circumflex branch

Anterior descending branch

Left ventricle

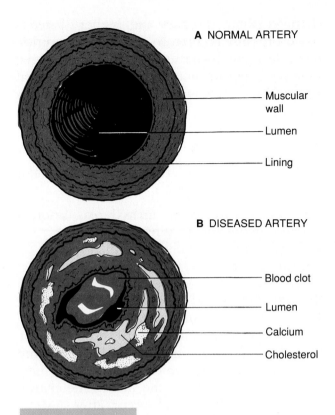

A NORMAL ARTERY

- Muscular wall
- Lumen
- Lining

B DISEASED ARTERY

- Blood clot
- Lumen
- Calcium
- Cholesterol

FIGURE 29–2

Cross section of a coronary artery: (A) the lumen of a normal artery is unobstructed, the walls are smooth and elastic; (B) the lumen of an artery with arteriosclerosis is narrow, the walls are thickened with cholesterol and calcium deposits, and are irregular and stiff. A blood clot can form in this artery.

The major controllable factors are cigarette smoking, high blood pressure, elevated cholesterol levels, elevated triglyceride levels, lack of exercise, obesity, stress, and blood sugar levels associated with diabetes. The major risk factors that cannot be controlled are age, sex, race, heredity, and the presence of diseases such as diabetes.

ANGINA PECTORIS

If the heart is deprived of adequate oxygen for its needs for more than several seconds, severe chest pain will occur. The pain is characteristically crushing—it takes the patient's breath away. Some people describe it as "squeezing" or "like somebody standing on my chest." This pain is called angina pectoris, or simply *angina*. Because the occurrence of angina pectoris indicates coronary artery disease, it is important to understand the pain and to recognize it.

Angina pectoris occurs when the need for oxygen by the heart exceeds the supply. It generally occurs at times when the heart is working hard—during periods of physical or emotional stress. The principal characteristic of angina pectoris is pain that comes on with exertion and is relieved by rest. The pain is usually felt under the sternum. It can radiate to the mandible, to the arms (especially the left arm), or to the epigastrium (the upper-middle region of the abdomen). The pain usually lasts from 3 to 8 minutes, and rarely longer than 10 minutes. It may be associated with shortness of breath, nausea, or sweating. It disappears promptly when the oxygen supply to the heart equals or exceeds the demand—that is, when stress lessens or ceases as the patient relaxes or when oxygen is given. Although angina pectoris is painful, it does not mean death of the myocardium, nor does it usually lead to the death of the patient or to permanent heart damage. It does, however, indicate that the person has some degree of coronary artery disease.

Patients with angina may show symptoms that are different than those just mentioned, and you must be familiar with them. Occasionally, a patient will not have pain as such but will admit discomfort—the "squeezing" sensation or tightness in the chest mentioned earlier, or perhaps difficulty in breathing. Sometimes the patient complains of discomfort or pain not in the chest, but at a point of referral, such as the mandible, left arm, or epigastrium. The patient may interpret these symptoms as gastrointestinal ("It's probably indigestion," or "My ulcer is kicking up"). Physical exertion is not the only cause of angina. Emotional stress, a large meal, or common anxiety may also trigger an attack. You must keep this in mind if you suspect angina pectoris.

Angina is treated with a medication called *nitroglycerin*. It comes in the form of a small white pill, about one-half the size of an aspirin tablet, as a spray, or as a skin patch applied to the chest (Figure 29–3). The pill is not swallowed but rather is placed sublingually (under the tongue). Nitroglycerin works in seconds, relaxing the muscle of blood vessel walls, dilating coronary arteries, and increasing blood flow and the supply of oxygen to the heart muscle. Nitroglycerin relieves the pain of angina pectoris. Nitroglycerin also relaxes and dilates blood vessels in the brain, sometimes causing a severe headache.

ACUTE MYOCARDIAL INFARCTION (AMI)

If the narrowing of the coronary artery by arteriosclerosis is very severe or a blood clot forms inside the coronary artery, the oxygen supply in the area of the heart served by that artery can be completely cut off or become so inadequate that the myocardium dies (Figure 29–2b). This condition is called **acute myocardial infarction (AMI).** AMI usually occurs in the left ventricle, the larger, thickwalled heart

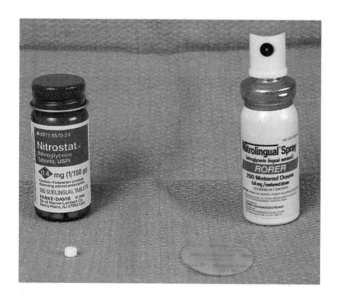

FIGURE 29–3

Nitroglycerin tablets are small, white pills, about half the size of a standard aspirin tablet. They are placed sublingually to relieve the pain of angina pectoris. Nitroglycerin can also be delivered by sublingual spray or chest skin patch.

chamber that produces the higher systemic blood pressure (Figure 29–4). The left ventricle requires more blood and much more oxygen than the lower-pressure right ventricle. The left ventricle therefore suffers the most from a lack of oxygen.

Consequences of AMI

Acute myocardial infarction has three major and serious consequences to the patient:

- Sudden death from arrhythmia (unorganized, ineffective beating of the heart).
- Congestive heart failure (CHF).
- Cardiogenic shock.

Sudden Death Approximately 40 percent of all patients who suffer AMI die before they reach the hospital. These deaths occur because of sudden abnormalities in the heart rhythm called **arrhythmias,** which prevent any effective pumping action of the heart. The chance that an arrhythmia will occur after AMI is greatest within the first hour after the event; it diminishes to a very small risk after three to five days. Arrhythmias may result in **fibrillation,** (ineffective, completely disorganized quivering) or **asystole** (no cardiac action at all) (Figure 29–5). In either case, the clinical appearance of the heart is *cardiac arrest.* These situations require cardiopulmonary resuscitation (CPR).

A wide variety of arrhythmias may be the result of AMI. These include:

Tachycardia: Rapid but regular beating of the heart.

Bradycardia: Unusually slow but regular beating of the heart.

Atrial flutter: Beating of the atria up to rates of 300/minute not associated with equal beating of the ventricles.

Atrial fibrillation: Disorganized, ineffective quivering of the atria.

Ventricular extrasystoles: Additional beats of the ventricle interspersed with the regular rhythm.

Ventricular fibrillation: Disorganized, ineffective quivering of the ventricles.

FIGURE 29–4

Acute myocardial infarction (AMI) usually occurs in the left ventricle after a blood clot obstructs the left coronary artery and prevents blood from reaching the left ventricle.

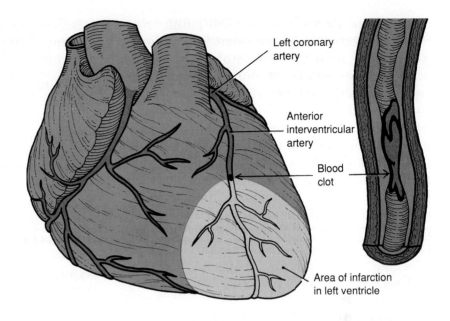

Left coronary artery

Anterior interventricular artery

Blood clot

Area of infarction in left ventricle

FIGURE 29–5

ECG (electrocardiogram) tracings show (A) normal cardiac rhythm, (B) arrhythmia from ventricular fibrillation, and (C) asystole.

A

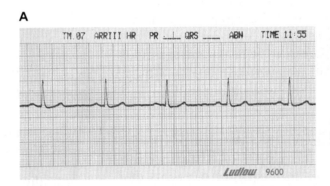

B

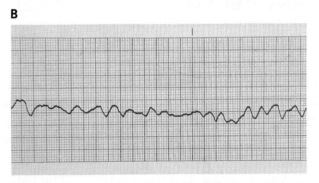

C

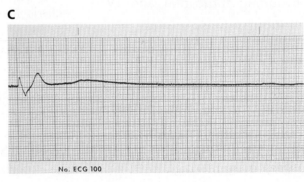

Congestive Heart Failure (CHF) Failure of the heart occurs when the heart muscle is so damaged by **infarction** (death of the tissue) or other diseases that it can no longer pump enough blood for the needs of the body. Congestive heart failure (CHF) can occur any time after a myocardial infarction, but it usually happens between the first few hours and the first few days after a heart attack. These patients may develop **pulmonary edema,** which means their lungs fill up with fluid. Frothy, pink **sputum** (fluid spit or coughed up from the lungs) is a sign of pulmonary edema. **Dyspnea** (shortness of breath) and generalized edema (swelling, particularly of the legs and feet) are also seen in patients with CHF.

Cardiogenic Shock Cardiogenic shock is an early complication of AMI that occurs within 24 hours of the event. It means that the heart has been so damaged that it is unable to sustain a normal systemic blood pressure, and shock results. Shock with AMI is an extremely serious complication and may result in death.

The Chain of Survival

The chain of survival is a descriptive concept that interrelates the aspects of emergency cardiac care to show the sequence of events that must occur to provide the best chance of survival from out-of-hospital sudden cardiac arrest. The links in the chain of survival are as follows:

- Recognition of early warning signs and early access and activation of EMS.
- Early BLS (within 4 minutes of cardiac arrest).
- Early defibrillation as soon as possible (within 10 minutes).
- Early ACLS, including intubation and IV medications.

Clinical Presentation of AMI

A patient with an acute myocardial infarction may show the following signs and symptoms:

- Sudden onset of weakness, nausea, and sweating without an obvious cause.
- Chest pain (crushing or squeezing).

- Sudden arrhythmia with fainting.
- Pulmonary edema.
- Sudden death.

Unfortunately, the first sign of heart disease may be sudden death; 40 percent of all patients with AMI never reach the hospital. Sudden death from AMI usually is the result of cardiac arrest from ventricular fibrillation. The chance to save such a patient exists only if someone defibrillates the heart (see Chapter 9) or begins cardiopulmonary resuscitation (CPR) within 4 minutes of the event. Ventricular asystole, or the lack of any heartbeat, may also be a cause of sudden death. This is a hard problem to detect because the outward appearance of a patient in asystole is the same as one in ventricular fibrillation, and many ventricular arrhythmias can rapidly produce asystole if no treatment is given.

In general, patients with fibrillation respond better to CPR than patients in asystole. Although risk of death is greatest at the instant of myocardial infarction, and this moment is the most dangerous time for the patient, rapid administration of basic life-support has successfully resuscitated many a patient with cardiac arrest from AMI.

The great majority of patients with AMI who do not die suddenly will develop chest pain. Classically, this pain exhibits the following characteristics:

- It is substernal.
- It is squeezing in character or felt as a heaviness or pressure.
- It lasts longer than 30 minutes.
- It is not related to exertion, nor is it relieved by rest or nitroglycerin.
- It is felt as radiating to the mandible, to the left arm, to both arms, or to the epigastrium.

The pain of AMI differs from that of angina pectoris in two ways. First, the pain of AMI lasts longer than that of angina pectoris. Anginal pain usually lasts no longer than from 3 to 10 minutes, and the pain of AMI may last from 30 minutes to several hours. Second, the pain of AMI, unlike that of angina pectoris, may not be related to exertion or mental or emotional stress. It is also not relieved by rest or nitroglycerin. The pain of AMI may come on at any time—perhaps waking the person from sleep or occurring when the individual is sitting quietly, reading.

About 90 percent of patients with AMI develop some sort of cardiac arrhythmia, usually extra beats in the damaged ventricle. These extra beats, called extrasystoles or premature ventricular contractions, may group together and produce a series of disturbed, rapid, continuous beats, called ventricular tachycardia. If ventricular tachycardia persists, it can develop into ventricular fibrillation—the totally ineffective quivering of the cardiac muscle. Some patients with AMI do not feel pain but may notice the irregularity of their heartbeat. The episodes of ventricular arrhythmia may cause **syncope** (fainting). Therefore, any patient who faints suddenly must be treated as suspect for AMI, especially if there was any chest pain or discomfort prior to or after the episode of syncope.

The sudden onset of left ventricular failure may cause pulmonary edema and dyspnea. Pulmonary edema may be the first sign of AMI. If the amount of damage caused by the infarction is great enough, the heart can no longer pump blood effectively. Because acute myocardial infarction occurs usually in the left ventricle, that ventricle will have a reduced pumping capability and cannot effectively handle the blood coming from the lungs. The undamaged right ventricle, however, will continue to pump blood into the lungs, pressure within the lung capillaries will rise, and fluid will then leak out from the pulmonary blood vessels into the pulmonary alveoli. The lungs literally fill with fluid, and the patient feels like he or she is drowning. Sometimes the fluid in the alveoli actually comes out of the mouth as a pink, frothy sputum (Figure 29–6). The patient cannot get enough oxygen from the air and experiences dyspnea.

If the patient has no past history of dyspnea or heart failure and if the pulmonary edema has come on suddenly, you should assume that the patient has had an AMI and provide the appropriate emergency care. Such care includes positioning the patient with the head up, clearing the airway, and administering supplemental oxygen.

When the left ventricular muscle is damaged by AMI, the amount of blood pumped per

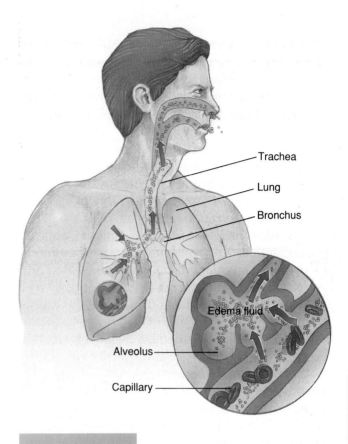

Trachea

Lung

Bronchus

Edema fluid

Alveolus

Capillary

FIGURE 29–6

The lungs of a patient with pulmonary edema fill with fluid, and the person exhibits dyspnea. Some of the fluid may exit the mouth and nose in the form of pink, frothy sputum.

minute falls. Occasionally, a patient who has not complained of pain and who is not experiencing an arrhythmia might suddenly experience extreme weakness and feel unable to stand or walk. This extreme weakness is probably the result of falling cardiac output. You should assume that this patient is having an acute myocardial infarction and treat him or her accordingly.

The Physical Findings of AMI

The physical findings of AMI are variable and depend on the extent and severity of heart muscle damage. The following are the most frequent physical findings in acute myocardial infarction:

■ *Pulse:* Generally, the pulse rate increases as a normal response to stress, fear, or the actual injury of the myocardium. Because arrhythmias are common in AMI, you may feel an irregularity of the pulse. In some cases of acute infarction, bradycardia (an abnormal slowing of the pulse) develops rather than tachycardia (an abnormally rapid pulse).

- *Blood Pressure:* Blood pressure falls as a result of diminished cardiac output and diminished capability of the left ventricle to pump.
- *Respiration:* Respirations are normal unless pulmonary edema occurs. In this case, rapid shallow respirations are seen.
- *General Appearance:* The patient appears frightened. A cold sweat is frequently present. The patient may feel nauseated and may vomit. The skin is often ashen gray as a result of poor cardiac output and the loss of skin perfusion. Occasionally, cyanosis (a bluish tint to the skin) may be observed as a result of poor oxygenation of the circulating blood. In acute congestive heart failure, you may observe distended neck veins that do not collapse when the patient sits up.
- *Mental State:* One of the unexplained aspects of acute myocardial infarction is that most patients have an almost overwhelming feeling of impending doom. They are convinced—almost resigned—that they are about to die.

Approach to the Patient with Suspected AMI

Take the following steps when you are treating a conscious patient in whom heart disease or acute myocardial infarction is suspected:

1. *Reassure the patient.* Act professionally. Be calm. Speak to the patient in a voice that is not too loud or too soft. Let the patient know that trained people—including yourself—are present to provide care and that he or she will soon be taken to the hospital. Remember, all patients are frightened. Some may act carefree, and some may be demanding; but all are frightened. Your professional attitude may be the single most important factor in securing the patient's cooperation. Patient agitation and anxiety may be directly related to the increased number and frequency of irregular or extra heartbeats. An arrhythmia may rapidly produce ventricular

fibrillation, asystole, and death. Apart from providing assurance and comfort, the calmness and poise with which you approach a patient may help prevent a fatal worsening of the condition.

2. *Take the patient's history.* Take a brief history from the patient. Friends or family members who are with the patient might have helpful information.

3. *Obtain and record vital signs.* As one EMT takes the history, the other should obtain and record vital signs—pulse, blood pressure, and respiratory rate. Note the exact time when the vital signs are taken. It is essential to monitor the vital signs closely, because the patient with an acute myocardial infarction is always at risk for sudden cardiac arrest. Should cardiac arrest occur, you must consider automatic defibrillation and institute CPR promptly.

4. *Position the patient.* If AMI is suspected, place the patient in a comfortable position, usually sitting and well supported. Make sure the patient has no difficulty breathing and has no airway obstruction.

5. *Administer oxygen.* Administer oxygen by face mask. Explain to the patient that you are giving oxygen before you position the face mask.

6. *Report to medical control.* Report to the hospital by radio. Give the patient's history, vital signs, medications being taken, and the treatment you are giving. Take care not to frighten the patient. Follow the instructions of your medical control.

7. *Transport the patient to the hospital.* Transport the patient promptly to the emergency department. Proper emergency handling and prompt transport to the hospital are critical. Some newer treatments for AMI use drugs to dissolve the blood clot. To be effective, this treatment must be started within 3 or 4 hours of the onset of the AMI. Alert the hospital emergency department as to the status of the patient and your estimated time of arrival. Describe the patient's condition to the emergency department staff on arrival and leave a copy of the ambulance report form for the patient's hospital records.

CHRONIC CONGESTIVE HEART FAILURE

Just as the pumping function of the left ventricle can be impaired by coronary artery disease; it can also be impaired by diseased heart valves or chronic hypertension. When the muscle can no longer contract well enough, the heart attempts in other ways to maintain adequate cardiac output. Two specific changes in heart function occur: the heart rate increases, and the left ventricle enlarges in an attempt to increase the amount of blood pumped each minute.

When these adaptations can no longer make up for the decreased heart function, **congestive heart failure** eventually develops. It is called ''congestive'' heart failure (CHF) because the lungs become congested with fluid once the heart fails to pump the blood effectively. Blood tends to ''back up'' in the pulmonary veins, which increases the pressure in the capillaries of the lungs. When the pressure in the capillaries exceeds a certain level, fluid (mostly water) passes through the walls of the capillary vessels and into the alveoli. This condition, you will recall, is called pulmonary edema. It may occur suddenly, as in AMI, or slowly over months, as in chronic congestive heart failure.

When damage of the muscle of the right side of the heart has occurred or the right ventricle can no longer pump against the back pressure of a failed left ventricle, swelling takes place elsewhere in the body. Usually this fluid collects in the feet and legs and is called **pedal edema.** It may occur suddenly over a few hours in acute problems or slowly over a long time. Beyond the sensation of uncomfortable swollen limbs, this swelling produces relatively few symptoms. Chronic pedal edema, however, even in the absence of pain or other symptoms, may indicate underlying heart disease.

Symptoms and Signs of CHF

Once fluid passes from the capillaries to the alveoli, the patient has a marked sensation of shortness of breath, or dyspnea. The fluid tends to make the lungs stiffer. Therefore, the patient breathes rapidly but with shallow respirations. The patient finds it harder to breathe lying down than standing or sitting. When the

patient is lying down, the return of blood to the right ventricle and to the lungs increases and causes further pulmonary congestion.

The patient with chronic congestive heart failure generally has marked dyspnea, shows mild or pronounced agitation, and insists on sitting upright. Chest pain may or may not be present. The patient often has greatly distended neck veins that do not collapse even when the patient is sitting erect, and swollen limbs from pedal edema (Figure 29–7). Checking the vital signs will reveal a normal or somewhat high blood pressure, a rapid heart rate, and rapid, shallow respirations. While listening to the patient's chest with a stethoscope, you may hear the sound of air bubbling

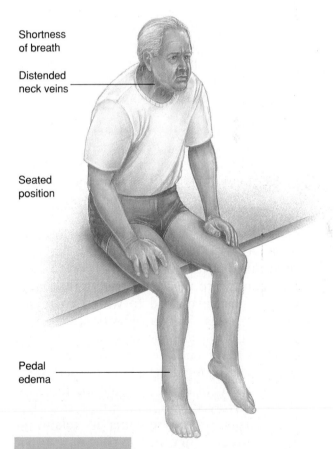

Shortness of breath

Distended neck veins

Seated position

Pedal edema

FIGURE 29–7

The patient with chronic congestive heart failure (CHF) will be dyspneic and prefer to sit to decrease the effort of breathing. Pedal edema and distended neck veins are common.

through the fluid in the alveoli and bronchi. This sound is called *rales,* a sound like rattles, and is an abnormal sound indicating disease within the respiratory system. It is a sound much like sand falling on an empty tin can. You might also hear wheezing. In severe congestive heart failure, these sounds can be heard from the apex to the base of the lung. They are best heard by listening at the back of the patient's chest.

Treatment of CHF

Treat the patient with chronic congestive heart failure the same way as the patient with AMI. Take the vital signs, monitor heart action, and give oxygen. Allow the patient to remain in an upright position with the legs down. It is important to reassure and calm the patient. Many patients for whom this situation is chronic have specific medications for its treatment. Gather these medications and take them along. Prompt transportation to the emergency department is, of course, essential.

PATIENTS WITH PRIOR HEART OPERATIONS AND PACEMAKERS

In 1987, over 300,000 operations were performed to bypass damaged coronary arteries in the heart. In the *coronary artery bypass graft (CABG)* operation, a vein from the leg or an artificial vessel is sewn directly from the aorta to a coronary artery beyond the point of the obstruction. More recently, a different kind of operation has been used to widen narrowed coronary arteries. In this operation, called an *angioplasty* or *balloon angioplasty,* a tiny balloon is attached to the end of a long thin catheter. It is introduced through the skin into a peripheral vein and then, under x-ray control, threaded into the narrowed coronary artery and then inflated. This procedure aims to dilate the coronary artery rather than bypass it. You will almost certainly have a patient with AMI or angina who has had such an operation.

Patients who have had a bypass graft will have a long surgical scar on their chests from the operation (Figure 29–8). Patients who have

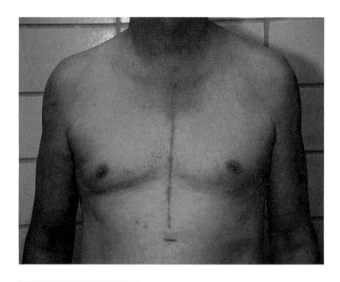

FIGURE 29–8

The surgical scar on this patient's chest implies a previous coronary artery bypass graft operation (CABG).

had an angioplasty will not. These operations produce quite good results in the treatment of angina: 80 percent of patients achieve full relief, and 15 percent improve. However, there is still some controversy as to whether either operation reduces the risk of subsequent myocardial infarction. Some studies indicate that if an infarction does not occur at the time of the operation or during the time the patient is hospitalized, there is much less likelihood that AMI will occur within the next two or three years. The debate over whether coronary artery surgery prolongs life significantly has not been settled.

In any event, AMI in a patient who has undergone a bypass procedure or angioplasty is treated exactly the same as one who has not. Carry out all of the previously described procedures and transport the patient promptly to the emergency department of the hospital. If CPR is required, carry it out in the usual way, regardless of the scar on the patient's chest.

Many people with heart disease in the United States have cardiac pacemakers. These battery powered devices maintain a regular cardiac rhythm and rate by delivering an electrical impulse through wires that are in direct contact with the myocardium. The generating

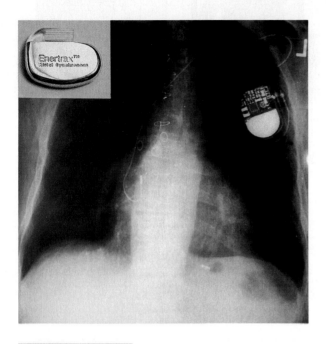

FIGURE 29-9

A pacemaker (inset) is a device implanted under the skin that delivers an electrical impulse to regulate the heartbeat. The wire electrode can be seen on the X ray running from the pacemaker to the heart.

unit is generally placed under a heavy muscle or a fold of skin (Figure 29-9). Pacemakers are inserted when the electrical control system of the heart is so damaged that it cannot function properly.

You will normally not be concerned with pacemaker problems. Modern technology is such that an implanted unit will not require change or battery charge for some years. Wires are well protected and rarely broken. In past years, pacemakers sometimes malfunctioned when a patient got too close to an electrical radiation source such as a microwave oven, but this is no longer the case. Every patient wearing a pacemaker should be aware of the precautions that must be observed for it to function properly. A properly functioning pacemaker will cause a cardiac rhythm that is absolutely regular and does not change with the patient's activity.

If a pacemaker does not function properly, the patient may experience syncope (fainting),

dizziness, or weakness. The pulse ordinarily will be slow (35 to 45) and irregular. In this situation, the heart is beating without the stimulus of the pacemaker and without the regulation of its own electrical system, which is damaged. The heart tends to assume a fixed slow rate that is not fast enough to allow the patient to function normally. A patient with a malfunctioning pacemaker should be promptly transported to the emergency department because repair of the problem may require an operation.

YOU ARE THE EMT

1. What role does arteriosclerosis play in the development of AMI or angina pectoris?
2. You have a patient with chest pain. How can you decide whether this person is suffering from angina or from an acute myocardial infarction (AMI)?
3. The patient is unconscious. You suspect AMI. What should you do? List the steps of emergency treatment.
4. You have a patient with congestive heart failure (CHF). What causes this condition and what are its symptoms?
5. A patient is having chest pain. You notice a long surgical scar on his chest. How will this change your management of AMI or angina?

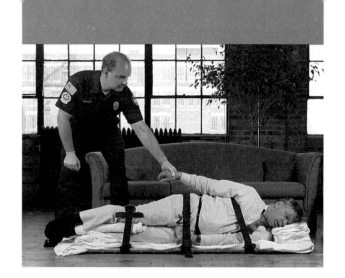

STROKE

aneurysm (an'u-rizm) A swelling or enlargement of a part of an artery, resulting from weakening of the arterial wall.

aphasia (ah-fa'ze-ah) Loss of speech.

arterial rupture Rupture of a cerebral artery.

cerebrovascular accident (CVA) (ser"ĕ-bro-vas'ku-lar ak'sident) Stroke; a sudden lessening or loss of consciousness, sensation, and voluntary movement caused by rupture or obstruction of an artery in the brain.

dysphasia (dis-fa'ze-ah) Difficulty in speaking.

embolus (em'bo-lus) A blood clot or other substance that has formed in one blood vessel or the heart that breaks off and travels to another blood vessel, where it causes blockage.

flaccid paralysis (flak'sid pah-ral'ĭ-sis) Paralysis in which the involved extremity or body part is limp.

hemiplegia (hem"e-ple'je-ah) Paralysis of one side (left or right) of the body.

lumen (loo'men) The inner diameter of an artery or other hollow structure.

monoplegia (mon"o-ple'je-ah) Paralysis of one extremity.

stroke The loss of brain function, usually the result of a cerebrovascular accident.

thrombosis (throm-bo'sis) The formation of a blood clot in a blood vessel.

thrombus (throm'bus) The blood clot that forms in a vessel.

OVERVIEW

Stroke, the common term for cerebrovascular accident (CVA), occurs when blood flow to the brain is interrupted long enough to damage the brain. The brain requires a continuous flow of oxygenated blood. If that flow is interrupted, for any reason, for more than four minutes, irreversible damage can occur to the part of the brain that has lost its blood supply. Because specific areas of the brain are responsible for specific functions of the body, the area of the brain destroyed will determine what function is lost. For example, interruption of blood flow to the motor control area on the right side of the brain will cause paralysis of the left side of the body, and interruption of blood flow to the speech center will result in aphasia (the inability to speak).

Although brain damage following a stroke may be extensive, stroke patients usually do not die. Most will gradually improve and experience partial or complete return of function.

Chapter 30 begins with a brief explanation of how blood circulates in the brain.

Then the three major causes of stroke (thrombosis, arterial rupture, or cerebral embolism) are described. The symptoms and signs of stroke are discussed next. The final section describes the emergency treatment of stroke patients. This treatment includes care and compassion on your part to help relieve the fear and anxiety that can accompany a stroke and may even worsen its effects.

GOALS

The goals of Chapter 30 are to
- understand how blood circulates in the brain.
- identify the three causes of stroke.
- recognize the symptoms and signs of stroke.
- learn the procedures for the emergency care of stroke patients.

CAUSES OF STROKE

The cerebral arteries that circulate blood to the brain originate close to the heart, directly from the subclavian artery. Two carotid arteries anteriorly and two vertebral arteries posteriorly supply the brain. The two vertebral arteries unite at the base of the brain to form one large vessel called the *basilar artery*. The basilar artery is linked to the two carotid arteries at the base of the brain to form a circle of vessels around the brain stem. This allows a constant blood supply for the vital functions of the brain (Figure 30–1).

A **cerebrovascular accident (CVA)** is the interruption of blood flow to the brain which results in the loss of brain function. **Stroke** is the set of symptoms and signs caused by any interruption of blood flow to the brain that lasts long enough to damage it. Men and women are equally affected by cerebrovascular accidents; most occur in elderly patients who have arteriosclerosis, heart disease, or hypertension (abnormally high blood pressure). It is sometimes

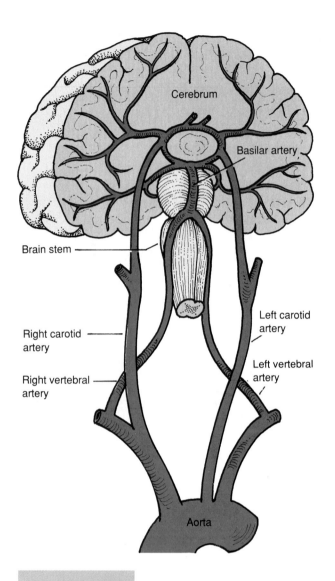

FIGURE 30–1

The brain receives a continuous supply of blood from the large carotid and vertebral arteries.

very difficult to identify the specific cause of a stroke in an elderly patient.

Interruption of cerebral blood flow may result from one of three events:

1. Thrombosis (clotting of the cerebral arteries).
2. Arterial rupture (rupture of a cerebral artery).
3. Cerebral embolism (obstruction of a cerebral artery by a clot that formed elsewhere in the body and traveled to the brain).

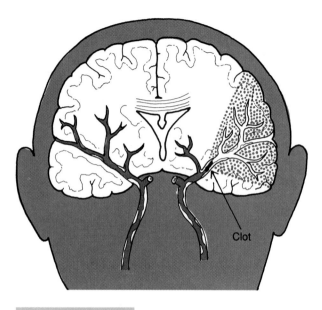

FIGURE 30–2

Arteriosclerosis can damage the wall of a cerebral artery, producing narrowing and thrombus (clot) formation. When the vessel is narrowed or completely blocked, blood flow to that part of the brain may be stopped, and a stroke results.

Thrombosis

Arteriosclerosis, with progressive narrowing and obstruction of the **lumen** (inner diameter) of the arterial wall, may occur in the cerebral arteries as well as arteries elsewhere in the body. This narrowing may cause the formation of a **thrombus** (clot inside the vessel), which can suddenly and completely cut off the flow of blood (Figure 30–2). **Thrombosis,** the formation of a thrombus, is the most common cause of stroke.

Arterial Rupture

Arterial rupture can cause hemorrhage into the brain itself or into the space around the brain. This hemorrhage may precipitate brain injury by means of several mechanisms. The leaking artery may go into spasm, further shutting off the circulation to that part of the brain. Hemorrhage directly into the brain tissue may cause damage by direct contact. Hemorrhage into the *subarachnoid space* (space surrounding the brain) may cause severe irritation to the meninges (membranes lining the brain), causing a form of meningitis. Lastly, bleeding may increase the intracranial pressure (pressure inside the skull), causing injury by literally squeezing the brain.

Generally, bleeding occurs at a weakened, dilated area of the wall of the blood vessel. This area of weakness, called an **aneurysm,** is usually a congenital lesion of an artery at the base of the brain, a weakened portion of the arterial wall that has been present since birth. Congenital arterial lesions are relatively common causes of stroke in young but otherwise healthy adults (Figure 30–3).

Arterial bleeding producing a stroke may also be caused by *hypertension* (high blood pressure). The bleeding may come from a weakened artery which is damaged by arteriosclerosis or may even come from a normal artery that has ruptured because of excessive internal pressure.

Cerebral Embolism

A blood clot that forms elsewhere, usually in the left side of the heart, may travel to a cerebral artery and obstruct it. A blood clot that passes from its point of formation to another point in the body through the vascular system is called an **embolus.** Blood clots often form on damaged or diseased heart valves. Irregular cardiac rhythms, particularly atrial fibrillation, also allow clots to form within the heart. These clots can break loose and travel as emboli to the brain (Figure 30–4).

An embolus is not always clotted blood. Anything that enters the bloodstream can travel from that point to another site through the blood vessels. Small particles from a degenerated arteriosclerotic blood vessel wall may break loose and travel as emboli to block a cerebral artery and cause a stroke.

SIGNS AND SYMPTOMS OF STROKE

The three different causes of interrupted blood flow to the brain can cause three distinct clinical

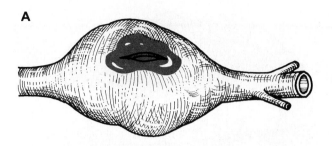

A

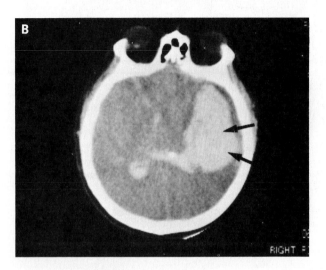

B

RIGHT

FIGURE 30–3

(A) An aneurysm is a weakened, dilated portion of an artery. It usually occurs at the base of the brain. An aneurysm can rupture, causing bleeding into the brain. (B) A CT scan of a ruptured cerebral aneurysm. The light area represents hemorrhage into the brain tissue (arrows).

pictures. Thrombosis of a cerebral artery causes specific losses of body functions, generally without pain or seizures. The functional loss represents the area of the brain to which blood flow is interrupted. Arterial rupture may also result in loss of a body function but is usually accompanied by a sudden, violently severe headache. The patient may rapidly lose consciousness. Cerebral embolism may cause a sudden seizure, paralysis, or loss of consciousness without headache or pain.

Regardless of its cause, a stroke may produce any of the following clinical signs or symptoms:

■ Paralysis of one **(monoplegia)** or both **(hemiplegia)** extremities on one side of the body. It

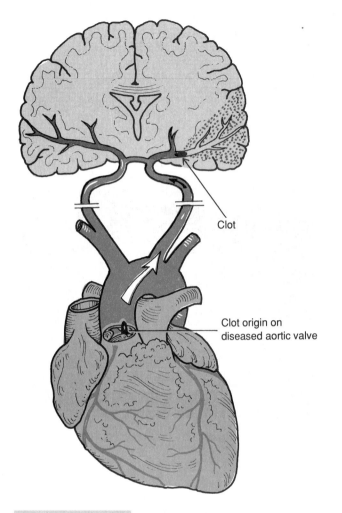

FIGURE 30-4

An embolus, a blood clot usually formed on a diseased heart valve, can travel through the body's vascular system, lodge in a cerebral artery, and cause a stroke.

is very rare for a stroke to cause paralysis of both sides of the body. You can determine the presence of paralysis by asking the conscious patient to move the feet simultaneously and to firmly squeeze your hands. Diminished or absent movement on one side of the body is usually indicative of a stroke. In the unconscious patient, detect hemiplegia by pinching the hands and feet to determine a lack of response on one side or the other. Note in your written report which part of the body became paralyzed first, in case it spreads later.

- Diminished level of consciousness, which may vary from confusion or dizziness to coma.
- Difficulty with speech or vision, which may vary from slight slurring to complete **aphasia,** and from temporary blurring to complete blindness.
- Seizures (although many individuals with epilepsy experience seizures from other causes without any damage of the brain).
- **Dysphagia** (difficulty with swallowing) or dyspnea (difficulty with breathing).
- Loss of facial expression or paralysis of facial motion, usually on one side of the face.
- Headache.

Although a stroke patient usually experiences more than one of the above effects, any one of these signs or symptoms is sufficient evidence to suspect a cerebrovascular accident and to begin appropriate treatment.

EMERGENCY CARE OF A STROKE PATIENT

When you respond to a stroke patient, you should carefully observe vital signs, respirations, and blood pressure. Are respirations regular or irregular? Certain characteristic hesitancies in the breathing rhythm occur in some stroke patients, whereas others may have very rapid, but not labored, respirations. Is the respiratory rate sufficient or will respiratory support be required?

Always make certain that the airway is clear. Paralysis of the throat muscles may occur following a stroke, and the patient may have difficulty maintaining an adequate airway. If there is any hint of airway obstruction, or if there is an irregular or slow respiratory rate, use supplemental oxygen, suction as needed, and prepare to establish an artificial airway. An artificial airway should not be necessary if your assessment shows that the patient is breathing well and the airway is clear. An artificial airway adds to the discomfort of a patient who does not need it.

Check the pulse both at the wrist and the neck. Observing early in the course of a stroke whether both carotid pulses (one on each side of the neck) are present can be helpful to the emergency department physician. The absence of a carotid pulse only on one side may indicate thrombosis of that vessel. When you palpate the pulse, note its rhythm. An irregular pulse may indicate underlying heart disease and therefore suggest embolism as a cause of the stroke.

Take the blood pressure. A very high blood pressure in combination with a slow pulse is often a sign of increased intracranial pressure. Because the brain is confined within the rigid bony skull, this pressure on the brain tissue may cause permanent damage. Such damage can occur in a matter of minutes, and cause death. The patient with increased intracranial pressure requires immediate transport to the hospital so that blood pressure and cerebral swelling can be controlled promptly. These patients should be given oxygen by face mask because the oxygen may help to control swelling of the brain.

Even though a stroke patient may be unable to speak and appear to be unconscious, he or she may still be able to hear and to understand what is taking place. Be very careful of what you say, avoiding all unnecessary or inappropriate remarks. Try to communicate with the patient by looking for signs indicating that he or she can understand you. Such indications may be very subtle—a glance, a gaze, motion or pressure with the finger or hand, efforts to speak, or nodding of the head. If you can establish effective communication, you will have a wonderful opportunity to help calm the patient. The loss of the ability to communicate is a frightening experience that can add to a patient's problems. Anything that you can do to relieve this fear will help in treatment.

Do not give a stroke patient *anything* by mouth. The muscles of the throat may be partly or completely paralyzed. Even a conscious patient may be unable to swallow. Frequently, these patients will be choking on saliva or mucus, especially if they cannot swallow. Clear the airway by suction and give oxygen. Occasionally you may need to use an oropharyngeal or nasal airway if the tongue is **flaccid** (soft and limp) and has fallen back into the throat and is obstructing the airway. When you insert the airway, be careful not to cause vomiting, which might cause greater airway obstruction.

TRANSPORTATION

Transport the stroke patient who has evidence of increased intracranial pressure as rapidly as possible. With this exception, you can transport other stroke patients promptly and gently. In general, you should transport the patient who is conscious on one side, with the paralyzed side down and the head elevated about six inches (Figure 30–5). This position has the added benefit of freeing the conscious patient's useful extremities. Take care, however, to adequately cushion and protect the paralyzed side from injury. In semiconscious or unconscious patients, ambulance transport on the right side may make adequate monitoring of the patient impossible, because the patient will be facing the wall of the ambulance. It may be necessary to reverse the position of the stretcher in the ambulance to ensure adequate

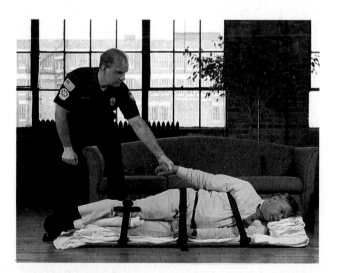

FIGURE 30–5

The semiconscious or unconscious stroke patient should be transported with the paralyzed side down and well protected with padding. The head should be elevated about 6 inches.

visual monitoring of the patient during transport. If this is not possible, it may be necessary to place the patient on the stretcher with the head at the foot of the stretcher.

The way you handle a patient with stroke as well as the patient's family is extremely important in the overall care. Avoid anything that will increase the anxiety of the patient. Too energetic or aggressive handling by you or the family may aggravate the effects of a stroke. The single most important aspect of the treatment for this patient is thoughtful, compassionate care. A stroke is a true crisis, and both the patient and the family need calm reassurance. This point cannot be emphasized too much. A calm, professional attitude will reassure both the patient and the family and do much to prevent further damage.

YOU ARE THE EMT

1. The patient is an elderly man, and his daughter tells you she thinks he has just suffered a stroke. How can you distinguish whether his condition was caused by a thrombosis or by a cerebral hemorrhage?
2. You suspect stroke because the patient is paralyzed on *one* side. What are the other signs and symptoms of stroke?
3. Once you are sure you are dealing with a stroke patient, how do you proceed with emergency treatment? List the steps.
4. What are the criteria for deciding how rapidly you must transport a stroke patient to the hospital?
5. Why shouldn't you give a stroke patient anything to eat or drink?

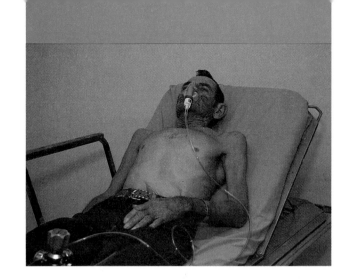

CHAPTER 31

DYSPNEA

asthma (az'mah) A disease of the lungs in which muscle spasm in the small air passageways and the production of large amounts of mucus result in airway obstruction.

bronchitis (brong-ki'tis) Irritation of the major lung passageways, either from infectious disease or irritants such as smoke.

carbon dioxide narcosis (kar'bon di-ok'sīd nar-ko'sis) A condition characterized by a chronically high blood level of carbon dioxide in which the respiratory center no longer responds to high blood levels of carbon dioxide.

chronic obstructive pulmonary disease (COPD) A slow process of dilation and disruption of the airways and alveoli, caused by chronic bronchial obstruction.

croup (kroop) An infectious disease of the upper respiratory system that may cause partial airway obstruction and is characterized by a barking cough.

embolus (em'bo-lus) A blood clot or other substance that has formed in one blood vessel or the heart that breaks off and travels to another blood vessel, where it causes blockage.

emphysema (em"fĭ-se'mah) Disease of the lungs in which there is extreme dilation and eventual destruction of pulmonary alveoli with poor exchange of oxygen and carbon dioxide. Also called chronic obstructive pulmonary disease (COPD).

epiglottitis (ep"ĭ-glot-ti'tis) An infectious disease in which the epiglottis becomes inflamed and enlarged and may cause upper respiratory obstruction.

hyperventilation (hi"per-ven"tĭ-la'shun) Rapid, deep breathing.

pleuritic chest pain Pain in the chest with respirations.

pneumonia (nu-mo'ne-ah) An infectious disease of the lung.

pulmonary edema (pul'mo-ner"e ĕ-de'mah) Fluid building up in the lungs, a result of congestive heart failure.

pulmonary embolism (pul'mo-ner"e em'bo-lizm) The condition whereby a blood clot breaks off from a large vein and travels to the lung.

rales (rahlz) Cracking, rattling breath sounds, in patients with fluid in the lungs.

rhonchi (rong'ki) Coarse breath sounds, in patients with chronic pulmonary disease.

stridor (stri'dor) A harsh, high-pitched respiratory sound, such as the inspiratory sound often heard in acute laryngeal obstruction.

Venturi mask A breathing unit that provides a specific concentration of oxygen through a delivery tube connected to a standard face mask.

wheezes (hwēz-ez) High-pitched, whistling breath sounds, characteristically heard on expiration in patients with asthma.

Dyspnea (difficult or labored breathing) is more commonly described as shortness of breath. It is a symptom; it is something that the patient feels. It may be accompanied by distinct signs of respiratory distress. Dyspnea may result from a variety of medical or traumatic causes. The traumatic causes of dyspnea are discussed in Chapter 24. This chapter deals with the medical, nontraumatic causes of dyspnea.

Chapter 31 begins by describing the physiology of the pulmonary system. The role of the lungs in exchanging oxygen and carbon dioxide is explained, along with the disorders that prevent or obstruct that exchange. Then the medical problems that produce dyspnea are described. These include infections of the upper or lower airway, acute pulmonary edema, chronic obstructive pulmonary disease, asthma or allergic reactions, airway obstruction, pulmonary embolism, hyperventilation, and spontaneous pneumothorax. The last part of the chapter discusses the treatment of dyspnea in relation to whatever medical problems are involved.

GOALS

The goals of Chapter 31 are to
- understand the physiology of the body's pulmonary system.
- identify the nontraumatic, or medical, causes of dyspnea.
- learn the proper emergency care for someone suffering from dyspnea.

PULMONARY PHYSIOLOGY

The major function of the lungs is respiration—the process of providing oxygen to the blood and removing carbon dioxide from the blood to be expelled in the air that is breathed out. To carry out this exchange of oxygen and carbon dioxide properly, there must be no obstruction of inspiration (the flow of air breathed in) and expiration (air breathed out) to and from the alveoli (microscopic pulmonary air sacs). There must also be no interference with the passage of those gases between the alveoli and the pulmonary capillaries.

The alveoli are microscopic, thin-walled air sacs. They lie against the pulmonary capillary vessels that connect the pulmonary arterioles and the pulmonary venules. The exchange of oxygen and carbon dioxide between air in the alveoli and blood in the pulmonary capillaries occurs rapidly and easily (Figure 31–1).

In most disorders of the lung, one or more of the following situations exists:

- The pulmonary vessels are actually separated from the alveoli by fluid or infection.
- The alveoli are damaged and cannot transport gases properly across their own walls.
- The air passages are obstructed by spasm or mucus.
- The pleural space is filled with air and the lung cannot expand.

All these conditions prevent the proper exchange of oxygen and carbon dioxide. In addition, abnormalities of the pulmonary blood vessels themselves may interfere with blood

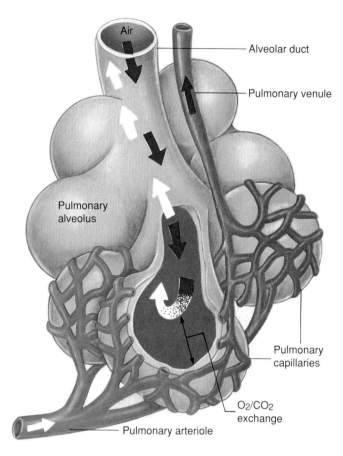

Air

Alveolar duct

Pulmonary venule

Pulmonary alveolus

Pulmonary capillaries

O_2/CO_2 exchange

Pulmonary arteriole

FIGURE 31–1

An enlarged view of a single alveolus (air sac) showing where the exchange of oxygen and carbon dioxide between air in the sac and blood in the pulmonary capillaries takes place.

flow and thus with the proper transfer of oxygen and carbon dioxide.

Any type of lung disease that causes too little oxygen to enter the blood or prevents carbon dioxide from being removed from the blood is harmful to the body. The major stimulus that causes a normal individual to breathe is the level of carbon dioxide in the arterial blood. If the level of carbon dioxide in the blood drops too low, the person automatically breathes at a slower rate and less deeply. This response, which causes less carbon dioxide to be expired, allows carbon dioxide to rise to a normal level in the blood. On the other hand, should the level of carbon dioxide rise above normal in the arterial blood, the patient breathes at a more rapid rate and more deeply, "blowing off" the

gas and thereby lowering its amount in the arterial blood. The arterial level of carbon dioxide is controlled breath by breath and is regulated so automatically that very little variation occurs in the normal, healthy person. Carbon dioxide is measured according to its presumed pressure: the normal value ranges from 40 to 46 millimeters of mercury (mm Hg).

The level of carbon dioxide in the arterial blood can rise for a number of reasons. The blowing off process itself may be impaired by various types of lung disease. Also, the normal body production of carbon dioxide may increase, either acutely in some diseases, or chronically over a long time.

If the arterial carbon dioxide slowly rises to a high level and remains there, the respiratory center (the area in the brain stem that senses the level of carbon dioxide and controls breathing) may become depressed, so that it no longer responds normally to a rise in arterial levels of carbon dioxide. This condition, called **carbon dioxide narcosis,** may be so severe and the respiratory center become so depressed that the patient has no stimulus to breathe at all from the increased arterial carbon dioxide concentration. Respiration will then stop unless a secondary drive to stimulate it exists. Fortunately, there is a second stimulus that develops in patients with chronically high blood carbon dioxide levels. That stimulus is a low level of oxygen in the blood, which will then cause the respiratory center to respond and stimulate respiration. This stimulus of low oxygen (the hypoxic drive) is not as strong as that of rising carbon dioxide *(hypercapnia).*

A certain physiologic danger exists when a patient has a chronically high carbon dioxide blood level. The respiratory center becomes used to this high level and will not respond to it. The respiratory center has, in fact, been "drugged" by the high carbon dioxide levels. With carbon dioxide narcosis, the only stimulus to breathe is the arterial hypoxia. If the arterial level of oxygen is then raised, such as happens when the patient is given additional oxygen, there is no longer any stimulus to breathe: both the high carbon dioxide and low oxygen drives are lost. Patients with chronic lung diseases frequently have a chronically high level of blood carbon dioxide, a condition that has developed slowly, over years. Giving too much oxygen to such a patient may actually depress, or completely stop, the respirations.

CAUSES OF DYSPNEA

Medical problems in which dyspnea is present include the following:

- Infections of the upper or lower airway.
- Acute pulmonary edema.
- Chronic obstructive pulmonary disease.
- Spontaneous pneumothorax.
- Asthma or allergic reactions.
- Mechanical obstruction of the airway.
- Pulmonary embolism.
- Hyperventilation.

Infection of the Upper or Lower Airway

Infectious diseases causing dyspnea may affect all parts of the airway. These diseases range from those causing mild discomfort to those showing signs of acute airway obstruction that require a full range of respiratory support. In general, in all of these situations the problem is obstruction, either to the flow of air in the major passages (colds, diphtheria, epiglottitis, and croup), or to the exchange of gases between the alveoli and the capillaries (pneumonia). The common cold is usually associated with swollen nasal mucous membranes and the production of fluid from the sinuses and from the nose. Dyspnea is not severe, and the common complaint is "stuffiness" or difficulty in breathing. Despite years of research, no sure treatment exists for colds; fortunately, they rarely cause a severe emergency.

Diphtheria, although well controlled in the past decade, is still highly contagious and severe when it occurs. A product of the disease is the formation of a membrane lining the pharynx that is composed of debris, inflammatory cells, and mucus. This diphtheritic membrane can rapidly and severely obstruct the passage of air into the larynx.

Acute **epiglottitis,** a bacterial infection of the epiglottis, can produce severe (two to three times normal) swelling of this flap over the larynx, especially in children (Figure 31–2).

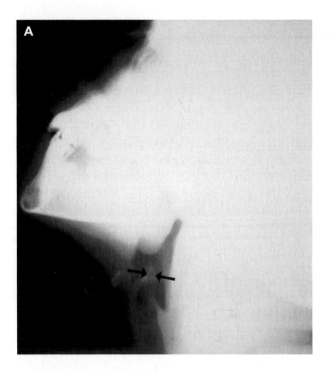

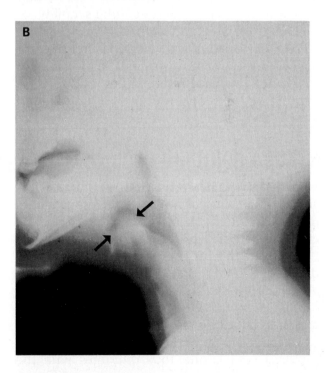

FIGURE 31–2

Acute epiglottitis. The epiglottis in (A) is normal; air is seen outlining the upper airway passages, and the size of the epiglottis (arrows) is normal. In (B), the epiglottis is massively swollen and almost fully obstructs the airway.

Acute and complete airway obstruction can occur from this swelling. Acute epiglottitis can occur in adults. It is frequently missed because it is thought of mainly as a disease of children. Acute epiglottitis in the adult is characterized by a severe sore throat. Respiratory obstruction may come on suddenly. Acute epiglottitis in children is further discussed in Chapter 38.

Croup is an inflammation and swelling of the lining of the larynx, where the airway is normally at its narrowest. The common sign of croup is **stridor,** a high-pitched, barking, rough sound heard on inspiration. Stridor signifies further narrowing of the air passage of the larynx, which occasionally may progress to significant obstruction.

Pneumonia is an acute bacterial or viral infection of the lung itself. The infection damages and destroys lung tissue. In addition, fluid accumulates in the surrounding normal lung tissue and separates the alveoli from their capillaries. As a result, the lung's ability to exchange oxygen and carbon dioxide is impaired. The breathing pattern does not indicate major airway obstruction but may show a tachypnea (increase in breathing rate) to compensate for the reduced amount of unimpaired lung tissue.

Acute Pulmonary Edema

Sometimes, the heart muscle is so injured after an acute myocardial infarction or other illness that it cannot circulate blood properly. In this case, the left side of the heart cannot remove blood from the lung as fast as the right side delivers it. Fluid then builds up within the alveoli and between them and the pulmonary capillaries in the lung tissue itself. This accumulation of fluid is called **pulmonary edema.** It physically separates alveoli from pulmonary capillary vessels and thus interferes with the exchange of carbon dioxide and oxygen (Figure 31–3). The patient usually experiences dyspnea with rapid, shallow respirations. There is not enough room left in the lung after fluid has been added to allow slow deep breaths. In very severe instances, a frothy pink sputum is apparent at the nose and mouth.

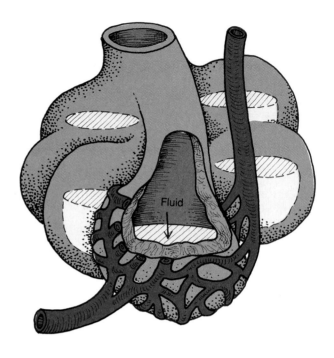

FIGURE 31–3

Pulmonary edema. Fluid fills the alveoli and separates the capillaries from the alveolar wall.

In some instances, you will see patients who have pulmonary edema without heart disease. Acute smoke inhalation, the inhalation of irritating toxic chemical fumes, or sudden compression injuries of the chest can all produce pulmonary edema. In these cases, pulmonary edema occurs from direct lung or bronchial damage or irritation. The result, however, is the same: fluid collects in alveoli and lung tissue.

Chronic Obstructive Pulmonary Disease

Chronic obstructive pulmonary disease (COPD) is a common problem of the lungs, affecting some 10 to 20 percent of the entire adult population in the United States. It is a slow process, which over several years results in disruption of the normal airways, the alveoli, and the pulmonary blood vessels. The process itself may be a result of direct lung damage from repeated infections, from the inhalation of toxic agents such as industrial gases, or, most commonly, from cigarette smoking. Although it is well known that cigarettes are a direct cause of lung cancer, their role in the development of chronic obstructive pulmonary disease is far more significant, and less well publicized. Tobacco smoke is itself a bronchial irritant and can create chronic **bronchitis** (irritation of the trachea and bronchi). Excess mucus is constantly produced and obstructs small airways and alveoli. Pneumonia easily occurs when these passages are persistently obstructed. Ultimately, repeated episodes of irritation and pneumonia cause scarring in the lung and dilation of the obstructed alveoli. This condition is called chronic obstructive pulmonary disease (COPD) or **emphysema** (Figure 31–4). Gradually, the patient's arterial oxygen level falls, and the carbon dioxide level rises.

If an acute infection of the lung is added to an already chronic lung condition, the arterial oxygen level may fall rapidly. In many patients, the arterial carbon dioxide level is high enough to produce carbon dioxide narcosis. Patients with COPD cannot handle pulmonary infections well because the existing airway damage makes them unable to cough up the mucus or sputum produced by the infection. The chronic airway obstruction makes it difficult to breathe deeply enough to clear the lungs. These patients require respiratory support and careful administration of oxygen.

Patients with COPD usually are older. They may or may not be cyanotic. However, they will have a history of recurring lung problems and are almost always long-term cigarette smokers. Cigarette habits for patients are measured in pack-years. 1 package of cigarettes per day per year is one pack-year, and 2 packs per day per year *or* 1 pack per day for 2 years is 2 pack-years. It is not uncommon to find a 60-year-old patient with a 100 pack-year history of cigarette use. There is a direct relationship between numbers of pack-years and incidence of chronic obstructive pulmonary disease. Chronic obstructive pulmonary disease patients may complain of chest tightness and constant fatigue.

Spontaneous Pneumothorax

When the surface of the lung is disrupted, air escapes into the pleural cavity. Normally, the negative pressure in the pleural space keeps the lung inflated. If air gets into the pleural space, the negative pressure is lost, and the natural elasticity of the lung tissue causes the lung to collapse. The accumulation of air in the

FIGURE 31–4

Chronic obstructive pulmonary disease. (A) A normal alveolus and bronchiole. (B) The bronchiole wall has become infected and thickened, narrowing its lumen. The alveolus is dilated. (C) A mucus plug completely obstructs the bronchiole and further dilates the alveolus.

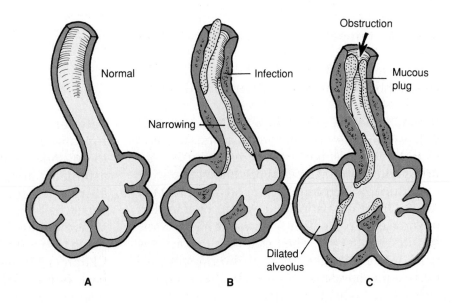

pleural space, which may be partial or complete, is called a pneumothorax. Most cases of pneumothorax are caused by trauma, but some medical conditions may cause it without any injury. In that case, the condition is called a spontaneous pneumothorax.

Patients with emphysema are at high risk for spontaneous pneumothorax, when a weakened portion of lung ruptures, often during coughing. Spontaneous pneumothorax may occur in certain chronic lung infections, or in young people born with weak areas of the lung. A patient with a spontaneous pneumothorax becomes dyspneic, and complains of pleuritic chest pain—pain that is worse during breathing—on one side. These patients are rarely cyanotic. By listening to the chest with the stethoscope, sometimes you can notice that the breath sounds are absent or decreased on the affected side. However, the altered breath sounds are very difficult to hear in a patient with severe emphysema. Spontaneous pneumothorax may be the cause of sudden dyspnea in a patient with underlying emphysema.

Asthma or Allergic Reactions

Asthma is an acute spasm of the bronchioles (smaller air passages) associated with excessive mucus production (Figure 31–5). Asthma is a serious, common disease. About 6 million Americans suffer from asthma, and some 4,000 to 5,000 die from it each year. It produces a characteristic wheezing as the patient attempts to exhale through the partially obstructed air passages. These same bronchioles open easily during inspiration. In other words, when the patient breathes in, the breathing is normal; the characteristic wheezing is heard only on expiration. Sometimes this wheezing is so loud that you can hear it without a stethoscope. In some instances, the actual work of exhaling is very tiring and the patient may become cyanotic.

Asthma, which can occur at any age, usually results from inhalation, ingestion, or injection of some agent to which the patient has become sensitized (allergic). The reaction in the airways is an intense exaggeration of the normal protective mechanisms set off by the allergens (agents to which the patient is sensitive).

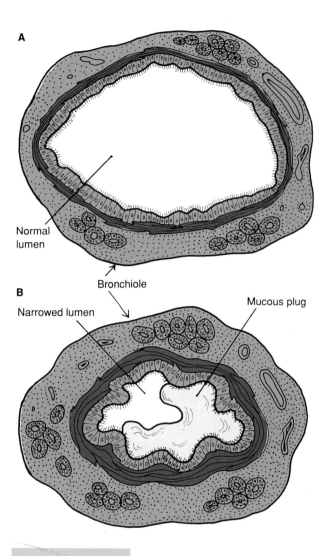

A
Normal lumen
Bronchiole

B
Narrowed lumen
Mucous plug

FIGURE 31–5

Asthma. (A) A cross section of a normal bronchiole. (B) The bronchiole in spasm; a mucus plug has formed and partially obstructs the bronchiole.

Between attacks, patients have normal lung function. An allergic response to a bee sting or to any other substance may produce an acute asthmatic attack. In its severest form, this allergic reaction can produce anaphylactic shock, which may cause respiratory distress severe enough to result in coma and possibly death. (Anaphylactic shock is also discussed in Chapters 12 and 28.) Asthma attacks may also be brought on by severe emotional stress or respiratory infections.

A much milder and much more common allergy problem is "hay fever." This is caused by an allergic reaction to pollen. In some areas of the country where pollen is present in the air throughout the year, it is almost a universal illness. Generally, it does not produce major emergency problems but does produce a number of difficulties in the upper respiratory tract, such as a stuffy or runny nose, and sneezing.

Mechanical Obstruction of the Airway

Mechanical obstruction of the airway may occur in semiconscious and unconscious individuals as a result of the position of the head, obstruction by the tongue, or aspiration of vomitus. Opening the airway with the head-tilt or chin-lift maneuver may solve the problem. You should perform the maneuver only after you have ruled out a head or neck injury. If simple opening of the airway does not correct the breathing problem, a search for upper airway obstruction must be made. Upper airway obstruction from a foreign body must be considered as a first diagnosis in any dyspneic patient who has been eating just before the onset of the problem or in young children, especially crawling babies, who might have swallowed and choked on a small object.

Strictly speaking, acute upper airway obstruction is much more often a traumatic cause of dyspnea than other causes, because it is rarely associated with disease. The techniques for handling the acutely obstructed airway, both in adults and children, are reviewed in Chapter 7. The most important consideration is for you to suspect the cause and move quickly to treat it.

Pulmonary Embolism

An **embolus** is anything in the circulatory system that passes from its point of origin to lodge at a distant site, remaining within the system. Circulation beyond the point of obstruction is cut off or markedly decreased. Emboli can be blood clots in the arteries or the veins. They can also be foreign bodies which enter the circulation, such as a bullet or a bubble of air. Embolism is the condition that results from obstruction of circulation by an embolus. Embolisms are very serious and can cause sudden death.

Pulmonary embolism is the passage of a blood clot formed in a vein that breaks off and circulates through the venous system, through the right side of the heart, and into the pulmonary artery, where it becomes lodged. Pulmonary emboli may occur as a result of slow blood flow, damage of the lining of vessels, or a tendency for blood to clot unusually fast. Usually they are seen in patients confined to bed when blood flow decreases and veins are often collapsed. They are a particularly important problem in patients for days or weeks after having had a hip fracture or hip reconstructive surgery. Almost always, emboli arise in the large veins of the legs or pelvis, thus affording the opportunity for a large, long clot to develop. Pulmonary embolism occurs when the clot is dislodged, so that it passes to the pulmonary artery. The large, long clot can significantly interrupt pulmonary artery blood flow.

The degree of patient awareness of this problem is directly related to the amount of lung tissue damaged. Complete, sudden obstruction of the right heart output results in sudden death. Damage of the lung, with inflammation of the pleural surface, frequently causes **pleuritic chest pain** (sharp, stabbing pain) with each breath. Significant obstruction of the pulmonary artery or its main branches means that, even though a lung is actively involved in inhalation and exhalation of air, no exchange of oxygen or carbon dioxide takes place in the areas of blocked blood flow because there is no effective circulation. In this circumstance, the level of arterial carbon dioxide usually rises, and oxygen may drop sufficiently to cause cyanosis.

Pulmonary emboli are fairly common and difficult to diagnose. In the United States, approximately 650,000 instances occur yearly; 10 percent are immediately fatal and 90 percent are not. Most often, pulmonary emboli are never noticed by the patient. Symptoms and signs, when they do occur, include dyspnea, acute pleuritic chest pain, hemoptysis (coughing up blood), cyanosis, and tachypnea. Almost anything that imposes undue inactivity or low blood flow on a lower extremity may predispose to a pulmonary embolus—bed rest, dehydration, a cast, traction, or a direct injury. However, most pulmonary emboli arise with hospitalization. Only rarely do they occur in active, healthy individuals.

Hyperventilation

Dyspnea occurring in a patient without lung abnormalities is called **hyperventilation.** Hyperventilation is described as overbreathing to the extent that the level of arterial carbon dioxide falls below normal. When excessive breathing "blows off" too much carbon dioxide, the blood pH (a measure of blood acidity) rises above normal. *Alkalosis* develops; it is the cause of many of the symptoms associated with hyperventilation. Hyperventilation is common in psychological stress—affecting some 10 percent of the total population at some time. Some of the symptoms can be self-induced by breathing as deeply and as rapidly as possible for 3 to 5 minutes; most people undergoing this exercise would not be aware that they had been hyperventilating. In general, the symptoms are numbness, tingling of the hands and feet; and, despite the rapid breathing, a sense of shortness of breath. Respiratory rates generally rise above 40 per minute. Recent studies indicate that this type of "panic attack" can be associated with significant differences in blood flow in specific areas of the right and left sides of the brain. A specific organic defect may exist to explain this reaction.

TREATMENT OF DYSPNEA

Infection of the Upper or Lower Airway

Dyspnea associated with acute infectious processes is quite common and, except for the patient with pneumonia, rarely serious. The acute congestion and stuffiness of a common cold rarely require emergency care. In fact, people with colds usually treat themselves with over-the-counter medications.

For patients with upper airway infections and dyspnea, administer supplemental, humidified oxygen that is warm and thoroughly saturated with moisture. Do not attempt to suction the airway or place an oropharyngeal airway in a patient with epiglottitis, because these maneuvers may cause complete airway obstruction. Transport the patient promptly to the hospital.

The dyspnea of pneumonia is not caused by upper airway obstruction but by the loss of effective lung volume and a need for more rapid air exchange. It will not be helped by the use of artificial airways but will improve with the administration of oxygen.

Acute Pulmonary Edema

Dyspnea caused by acute pulmonary edema usually is associated with a heart attack. The treatment is outlined in Chapter 29. When the problem is not associated with cardiac disease but with direct lung damage, the patient will require supplemental oxygen, clearing of the usually copious secretions from the airway, and prompt transport to the emergency department.

The best position for the conscious patient who has sustained a myocardial infarction or direct lung irritation is the one in which it is easiest to breathe. Usually that is a sitting-up position. Administer 100 percent oxygen, and carefully suction the airway of heavy secretions. You will rarely need to use an artificial airway, because no upper airway obstruction problem exists. The unconscious patient with acute pulmonary edema may require full ventilatory support, an airway, oxygen, and suctioning.

Chronic Obstructive Pulmonary Disease (COPD)

Patients with chronic obstructive pulmonary disease (emphysema or chronic bronchitis) are generally older. Their chests often have a barrel-like appearance, because air has been gradually and continuously trapped within the lung in increasing amounts; these patients usually are thin. They may be only semiconscious or unconscious from hypoxia or carbon dioxide narcosis, may appear in respiratory distress, and may be cyanotic. The patient with COPD may be using accessory muscles to breathe, including those in the neck and shoulders. The lips will be pursed in an attempt to puff air out (Figure 31–6).

The medical history of the person with lung disease usually reveals a sudden increase in shortness of breath with a long history of dyspnea; rarely, however, is there any history of chest pain. The patient often has had a recent "chest cold" and may remember having a recent fever as well as the inability to cough up mucus. The patient who can produce sputum will cough up thick, green or yellow sputum. The patient is almost always a smoker.

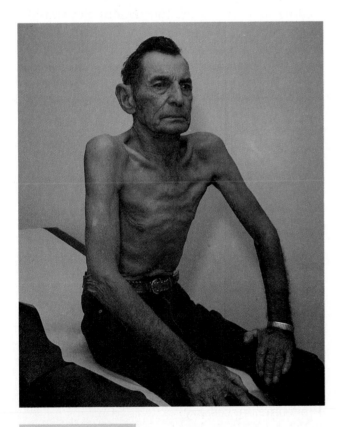

FIGURE 31–6

The typical appearance of a patient with chronic obstructive pulmonary disease. Notice the barrel-shaped chest, pursed lips, and the use of the accessory muscles of respiration.

The blood pressure of patients with COPD is normal. The pulse, however, is rapid and occasionally irregular. Pay particular attention to the respiratory rate. It may be rapid or very slow, as in carbon dioxide narcosis. When listening to the chest, you will hear abnormal breath sounds. **Rales** (crackling breath sounds), **wheezes** (whistling sounds), and **rhonchi** (rough, gravelly sounds) are some of the abnormal sounds you will hear. Sounds of breathing are frequently hard to hear and often are detected only high up on the posterior chest.

Note and record the patient's initial vital signs, paying particular attention to the respiratory rate. Speak with assurance and assume a concerned, professional approach. You will usually administer oxygen, although you must take great care to monitor the respiratory rate after you begin oxygen treatment. Reevaluate the respiratory rate and the patient's response to oxygen repeatedly—at least every 5 minutes—until the patient reaches the emergency department. This monitoring is important, because the supplemental oxygen may cause a rapid rise in the arterial oxygen level. This, in turn, can abolish the secondary respiratory oxygen drive while the carbon dioxide level remains high. If the patient is depending on a low oxygen level to sustain breathing, the rapid rise might abolish this stimulus and cause respiratory arrest. However, the patient will still need the oxygen, and you should not withhold oxygen for fear it will depress or even stop the patient's breathing. You should assist breathing if the respiratory rate slows. Slowing of the respiratory rate in a patient with chronic obstructive pulmonary disease who is receiving oxygen does not mean that the patient no longer needs it; he or she may need it even more.

For this reason, the best system to use when providing supplemental oxygen to a patient with COPD is a **Venturi mask** (Figure 31–7). With this system, 100 percent oxygen is delivered to a mask, usually at a low (2 to 5 liters per minute) flow. Inside the mask, the diameter of the tube widens. This widened tube diameter causes a low pressure within the mask. Room air is sucked through openings (ports) on the

A

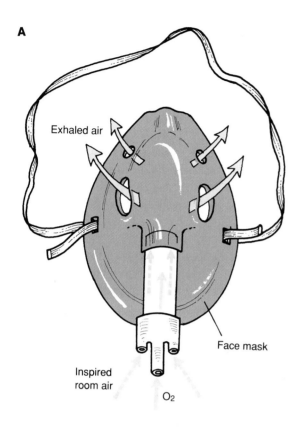

Exhaled air

Face mask

Inspired
room air

O₂

B

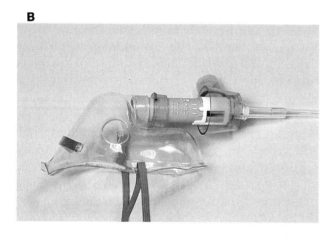

FIGURE 31–7

(A) A diagrammatic representation of a Venturi mask.
Room air is inhaled along with 100 percent oxygen. The
room air dilutes the pure oxygen, minimizing the risk of
exposure to high oxygen concentrations. (B) A Venturi
mask.

side of the mask to dilute the 100 percent
oxygen. Depending on the initial oxygen flow
and the size of the ports, a given concentration
of inspired oxygen can be administered (24
percent, 28 percent, 35 percent, and up to 50
percent). When you are in doubt as to what
concentration to use, start with a low concentration (24 percent) and gradually increase it
until the patient improves.

The advantage of the Venturi mask is the
production of a high volume and high flow of
inspired air at a controlled, fairly low concentration of inspired oxygen. It is impossible to
determine beforehand what concentration of
inspired oxygen may raise arterial levels
enough to interfere with the breathing drive, so
you must watch the patient's response very
carefully when you use this mask system. Be
prepared to give assistance when the respiratory rate declines, urge the patient to breathe
deeply, and transport the patient as promptly
as possible to the emergency department. Patients with chronic obstructive pulmonary disease find breathing difficult when lying down.
They should be allowed to assume a position of
comfort, usually sitting upright, during transport (Figure 31–8).

Spontaneous Pneumothorax

Patients with spontaneous pneumothorax may
have severe respiratory distress, or they may
have none at all and complain only of pleuritic
chest pain. Give supplemental oxygen, by
Venturi mask if the patient has underlying
COPD, and provide prompt transport to the
hospital. Like most dyspneic patients, those
with spontaneous pneumothorax are usually
more comfortable sitting up. Monitor the patient carefully. Be alert to any sudden deterioration of the patient's respiratory status and be
ready to establish an airway, assist respirations, and give full cardiopulmonary support if
it becomes necessary.

Asthma or Allergic Reactions

The asthma patient may be young or old.
Respiratory distress is obvious; you can often

hear the wheezing on expiration without your stethoscope. While the individual can breathe in without much difficulty, expiration is greatly impeded because of bronchospasm and mucus production. The obstruction causes the person literally to labor to push each breath out. The effort to breathe out is tiring and frightening. The history of the asthmatic is one of episodic attacks of shortness of breath, with the patient usually completely normal between them.

Because the public generally tends to call all lung trouble "asthma," it is important for you to confirm whether the patient has recurrent attacks of this nature but can breathe normally at other times. The patient or family should always be asked to describe what "asthma" means. Not all wheezing is asthma: some forms of heart failure, foreign body aspiration, or toxic fume inhalation may cause wheezing. The history of repeated episodes is critical to identifying the patient with true asthma.

Assess the vital signs. Chest pain is rarely present in asthma patients. The pulse rate will be normal or elevated. The blood pressure may be slightly elevated as a consequence of tension and anxiety experienced or from a medication

that the patient may have taken in an attempt to relieve the attack. The respiratory rate will be increased. Asthmatic reactions of the type that occur following a bee or wasp sting may progress rapidly to full anaphylactic shock. Thus, finding out what brought on the attack is very important. Many individuals wear or carry medical identification tags that may provide a clue in the most extreme cases.

Administer oxygen and allow the person to sit up, because breathing will be much easier in this position. As in other emergencies, reassurance from you will help to relieve the tension and anxiety that make these attacks worse.

Many persons with asthma or known sensitivities to bees or certain food products carry medications to take when an attack occurs. These medications should be obtained and administered with your help. Kits are now available for the subcutaneous or intramuscular injection of 1/2 ml of 1:1,000 epinephrine. The use of this agent may rapidly reverse or reduce an anaphylactic reaction. Many patients who know their sensitivities keep such kits readily available. You should know how to help the patient with a kit to administer the agent promptly; it may be lifesaving.

Epinephrine is a very potent agent that has a number of significant side effects, so the user must be certain of the diagnosis and clear as to the history of the episode. The person with full-blown anaphylactic shock may rapidly become unconscious and require assisted respiration as well as supplemental oxygen. All such patients require prompt transport to the emergency department.

You must be prepared to handle the production of large amounts of mucus with appropriate suctioning and then administer oxygen. If the patient is unconscious, airway maintenance may be needed. Occasionally, full CPR is required for an episode of anaphylaxis.

Occasionally, a patient has a prolonged asthmatic attack, unrelieved by epinephrine, and develops a condition known as *status asthmaticus*. This is a true emergency; the patient is frightened, frantically trying to breathe, using all the accessory muscles. This patient must be given oxygen and brought rapidly to the emergency department.

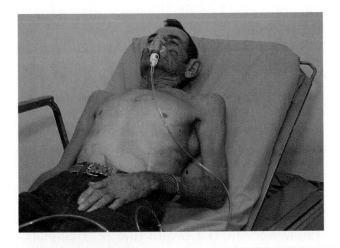

FIGURE 31–8

The patient with chronic obstructive pulmonary disease and dyspnea should be transported in the sitting position. A Venturi mask can provide supplemental oxygen at a controlled concentration, but you must check the respiratory rate every 5 minutes during transport.

The effort to breathe during an asthmatic attack is very tiring, and the patient may literally be exhausted by the time you arrive. He or she may no longer be anxious or even struggling to breathe because of exhaustion. Do not make the mistake of thinking that this patient is recovering and no longer needs your help. He or she is actually at a very critical stage and is likely to stop breathing. Aggressive airway management, oxygen administration, and prompt transport to the hospital are essential in this situation.

Obstruction of the Airway

In crawling children or patients known to have been eating just before dyspnea developed, you may assume that the acute breathing difficulty arose from an inhaled or aspirated foreign body. The first thing to do is clear the upper airway. Then administer supplemental oxygen and transport the patient promptly to the emergency department, especially if you are unsuccessful in clearing the air passage. Airway management from this cause is discussed in Chapters 7 and 38.

Pulmonary Embolism

Usually, pulmonary embolus is not a problem that you will be called on to manage, because it is most likely to occur in hospitalized patients. The common signs and symptoms are acute pleuritic chest pain, which may limit breathing; tachypnea; and occasionally, hemoptysis (coughing up blood). Varying degrees of hypoxia and carbon dioxide retention are also seen.

You will usually not need to clear the airway, because no obstruction exists. Since a considerable amount of lung tissue may not be functioning, supplemental oxygen is mandatory. Place the patient in a position of comfort, usually sitting, and assist the breathing. Hemoptysis, if present, is usually not severe, but it must be cleared. You should also expect an unusually rapid heartbeat, which may also be

irregular. Acute reflex responses to pulmonary emboli may produce cardiac arrest that will require full cardiopulmonary resuscitation. When this diagnosis is suspected, prompt transport to the emergency department is indicated, along with respiratory support as outlined.

Hyperventilation

The hyperventilating patient is often hysterical, terrified of dying, and has the feeling that it is impossible to get enough air into the chest, despite the fact that a larger quantity than usual is being exchanged. However, not all patients who hyperventilate fall into the hysterical category; the patient may be quite calm, although obviously hyperventilating. Dizziness is common. Often the person experiences a sensation of numbness or tingling in the hands and feet, which may also be described as "being cold." Sticking, stabbing chest pains that increase with respiration may occur. Vital signs reveal tachypnea and tachycardia, with normal blood pressure. Cyanosis is not seen, which may be the key indication to you that hyperventilation is the cause of the dyspnea.

Other illnesses may cause a reaction that looks like simple overbreathing. Alterations in the body's acid or alkali balance may produce hyperventilation. This may be seen in the untreated diabetic patient, in severe shock, or after ingestion of certain poisons. Pulmonary embolism may also produce hyperventilation.

It is important when you respond to a suspected case of hyperventilation to assess the patient's status and obtain a history. The presence or absence of chest pain, the coughing of blood, and a history of cardiac problems or diabetes may easily be noted.

In the absence of any other cause for hyperventilation, the best treatment begins with calm reassurance from a health care professional— you. Many of the symptoms seen in hyperventilation, such as tingling of the fingers and dizziness, are caused by the alkalosis secondary to low carbon dioxide in the blood. However, the blood carbon dioxide level will not reach a dangerously low level.

The traditional management of hyperventilation has been to have the patient breathe into a paper bag. This will force the patient to rebreathe the exhaled carbon dioxide, theoretically allowing the blood level to rise back to normal. However, a patient with underlying pulmonary disease may become severely hypoxic during this maneuver. Furthermore, there is some evidence that, even with rebreathing into a paper bag, the blood carbon dioxide level does not rise significantly. Therefore, there is some possible danger in rebreathing into a paper bag, and this "time-honored" technique may not even be effective. It is better to reassure the patient in a calm, professional manner, and provide prompt transport to the hospital. Although hyperventilation by itself is not a serious condition, patients who hyperventilate should be evaluated by a physician in the hospital. It is easy for even an experienced observer to make an incorrect diagnosis. All of these patients should be carefully examined to allow appropriate treatment.

YOU ARE THE EMT

1. Which of the causes of dyspnea can be quickly ruled out and why? Which of the causes must you focus on and why?
2. Why should you be particularly careful when you administer oxygen to an elderly patient with chronic obstructive pulmonary disease? What specific steps and equipment should you use?
3. You have been called to treat a patient who reportedly is hyperventilating. On arrival, you notice that someone is already holding a paper bag and telling the patient to breathe into it. Should you continue this treatment? Why or why not?
4. You are called to a patient who is having an asthma attack. What does that mean? What will you do if the attack progresses to anaphylactic shock?
5. You are called to a patient with the sudden onset of dyspnea. You conclude that he is in pulmonary edema. What information led you to this conclusion?

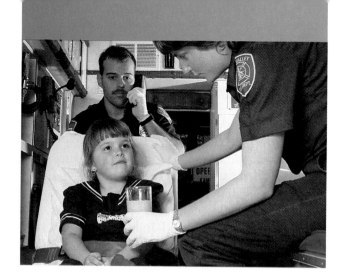

CHAPTER 32

DIABETES

KEY TERMS

acidosis (as"i-do'sis) A pathological condition resulting from the accumulation of acids in the body.

diabetes mellitus (di"ah-be'tēz mel'i-tus) A metabolic disorder in which the ability to metabolize carbohydrates is impaired, usually due to a lack of insulin.

diabetic coma Unconsciousness in uncontrolled diabetes caused by dehydration and acidosis.

diaphoresis (di"ah-fo-re'sis) Perspiration; especially profuse sweating.

glucose (gloo'kōs) D-glucose or dextrose; one of the basic sugars.

hormone (hor'mōn) Chemical substance produced in the body by a gland that has special regulatory effects on the activity of another, distant organ.

hyperglycemia (hi"per-gli-se'me-ah) Abnormally increased glucose level in the blood.

hypoglycemia (hi"po-gli-se'me-ah) Abnormally decreased glucose level in the blood.

insulin (in'su-lin) A hormone produced by the pancreas that enables sugar in the blood to enter the cells of the body; insulin is used in the treatment and control of diabetes mellitus.

insulin shock Unconsciousness in a diabetic patient caused by hypoglycemia; often the result of extensive exercise or failure to eat after a routine dose of insulin.

polydipsia (pol"e-dip'se-ah) Excessive thirst persisting for long periods of time.

polyuria (pol"e-u're-ah) The passage of an unusually large volume of urine in a given period.

type I diabetes The type of diabetic disease that usually starts in childhood and requires insulin for proper treatment and control.

type II diabetes The type of diabetic disease that usually starts in later life and is often treatable without the use of insulin.

Diabetes mellitus is a serious disease that affects approximately 6 percent of the population of the United States (13 to 15 million people). It is a progressive and permanent disease with many severe complications, including kidney failure, blindness, and blood vessel and peripheral nerve damage. Most diabetics try to balance their food intake with their insulin therapy and do so quite well. Sometimes the balance shifts—either too much or too little food is ingested, or insulin levels change. Then, problems develop. The patient may become disoriented, incoherent, convulsive, or unconscious.

Most people don't know what to do when they encounter a diabetic with these symptoms. Does the patient need sugar or insulin? Many think the patient may be intoxicated. Similarly, it is not easy for an EMT to treat these symptoms. They could indicate diabetic coma or insulin shock. Although both conditions are serious, insulin shock is life-threatening if not treated within minutes. Therefore, you must have a thorough understanding of the basic problem in diabetes in order to make an accurate assessment of a diabetic emergency and administer the proper lifesaving treatment.

Chapter 32 begins with some definitions of terms related to diabetes and an explanation of how glucose and insulin work in the body. After describing the different types of diabetes, the chapter focuses on the two emergency situations that can occur with diabetes—diabetic coma or insulin shock—and how to treat each condition. The chapter also explains what you should do when you are unable to make a distinction between diabetic coma and insulin shock, as is often the case. The use of devices for the rapid assessment of blood glucose is discussed, as is the similarity of diabetes and alcoholic intoxication. The chapter concludes with a consideration of all the tissues damaged by diabetes and a brief word concerning EMT safety in treating these patients.

GOALS

The goals of Chapter 32 are to

- understand the unique roles of glucose and insulin in the general metabolism of the body.
- know how diabetes mellitus is caused.
- distinguish between diabetic coma and insulin shock.
- know how to diagnose and treat diabetic emergencies.
- be able to relate diabetes to its effect on other tissues of the body.
- understand the differences between type I and type II diabetes.

HISTORY AND PREVALENCE OF DIABETES

Literally, the word *diabetes* means: "a passer through, a siphon." Medically, the term characterizes a disease that is associated with the passage of large quantities of urine containing glucose and accompanied by significant thirst and deterioration of the body. Diabetics come to the attention of the physician because of certain symptoms and signs: thirst, the consumption of much liquid, and the production of much urine. Left untreated, the disease produces a relentless wasting of body tissues, and death.

It is a common disease in the United States, affecting approximately 6 percent of the population, although effective treatment exists. Most patients can live an entire life span with diabetes; some may succumb to particularly aggressive forms of the disease. In general, however, it is a problem that can be fairly well understood and effectively treated by the patient who must cooperate in regulating his or her life, especially eating habits and activities.

Diabetes is a disease with two distinct patterns. It may become evident when the patient is a child or it may develop in later life—usually when the patient is middle aged. These two patterns of onset have given rise to a great number of definitions concerning diabetes. All are descriptive of some aspect of the disease. It is quite likely that you will hear or come to know some of these terms yourself even though current medical practice discourages using many of them.

Definitions

Diabetes mellitus: This term literally means sweet diabetes. It refers to the presence of sugar in the urine and serves to distinguish this problem from *diabetes insipidus,* a lack of the hormone regulating urinary fluid reabsorption.

Juvenile diabetes: The form of the disease which becomes evident in childhood. It is characterized by an absolute lack of insulin, which must be replaced daily for effective treatment. The term, as such, is no longer used.

Adult onset diabetes: The form of the disease that becomes evident as the patient ages. Ordinarily, it represents a partial deficiency in insulin supply and does not usually require insulin for its treatment. A synonym is *maturity onset diabetes.* Sometimes this disease may be called *mild diabetes.* These terms, as such, are no longer used.

Noninsulin-dependent diabetes: The form of the disease that can be managed without using insulin for control of blood sugar. Measures such as weight loss, the use of oral insulin stimulants, and diet are generally effective in its control.

Insulin-dependent diabetes: The state of the disease in which insulin must be used to control blood sugar.

Borderline diabetes: Jargon used to characterize the patient whose random blood sugar may be elevated or in whose urine sugar may be detected. It has little meaning and does not indicate the presence of the disease.

In 1981 the American Diabetes Association approved two new terms to describe diabetes: type I and type II diabetes. These terms are commonly used to describe the disease today.

Type I diabetes comprises diabetics who do not produce any insulin. Former terms referring to this type included juvenile diabetes or insulin-dependent diabetes. These patients more readily develop some of the metabolic problems of diabetes, such as ketoacidosis.

Type II diabetics have a different, equally serious, but more readily treatable form of the disease. They produce inadequate amounts of insulin or they produce insulin in fairly normal amounts, but its capacity to function is impaired. Although some of these patients may require some supplemental insulin, most can be treated with oral medication (hypoglycemic agents) or diet. This term in general replaces the previous terms adult (maturity) onset, and noninsulin-dependent diabetes.

Today, the terms *type I* and *type II* diabetes are preferred for routine medical use. Neither form of the disease is more or less serious. Each can affect many tissues and functions in the body aside from the glucose-regulating mechanism. Type II diabetes, because the patient remains able to produce some insulin, is easier to regulate. Each form is a lifelong disease requiring constant management.

Today, much more is understood about the cause of the disease. It is probably one of the group of *autoimmune* problems in which the body literally destroys its own tissues because it becomes allergic to them. The severity of diabetes relates to the amount of insulin-producing tissue damaged or destroyed and to the time of life at which the process started.

THE ROLE OF GLUCOSE AND INSULIN

All cells require **glucose,** or sugar, to function properly; some cells will not function at all without it. It is the major source of energy for the body. In the absence of glucose, or with very low levels, brain cells rapidly sustain permanent damage. A constant supply of sugar is as important to the brain as oxygen is.

Glucose is carried to all body cells in the arterial blood. However, glucose cannot enter a cell to provide the needed fuel or energy to live, without **insulin.** Insulin is a **hormone** produced by beta cells of the islets of Langerhans in the pancreas. The specific function of insulin is to allow glucose to enter the individual cells of the body (Figure 32–1). Thus, a constant

supply of insulin is absolutely necessary for the normal function of all body cells.

Diabetes mellitus is a disease in which the body is unable to use glucose normally as an energy source because of either a lack of insulin or poor function of the insulin that is present. When there is not enough effective insulin, glucose in the blood cannot be used by cells of the body normally because it cannot enter them. Ingested glucose remains in the blood and gradually rises to extremely high levels. At a sufficiently high concentration (usually two times normal—200 mg/deciliter or more), glucose is excreted by the kidney. The excretion of excess glucose by the kidney causes a constant and high loss of fluid in the urine, because a large amount of water is required to allow the sugar to be excreted. The loss of water in such large amounts, in turn, causes the classic symptoms of uncontrolled diabetes: **polyuria** (frequent and copious urination) and **polydipsia** (frequent drinking of liquid to satisfy continuous thirst).

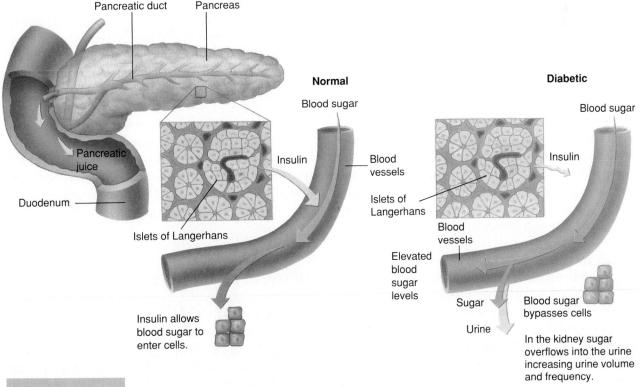

FIGURE 32–1   Insulin is required for cells to absorb sugar.

Without insulin, glucose cannot supply energy for cells; thus, other fuel sources must be found. Fat is the readily available resource in the body. Unfortunately, when fat is used as an immediate energy source, *acetone* and other chemicals, called *ketones* and *fatty acids*, are formed as waste products. (When glucose is used, the waste products are carbon dioxide and water, each of which is easily excreted.) Acetone, fatty acids, and ketones are not easily excreted and can be detected in the urine and the blood. As they accumulate in blood and tissue, they produce a dangerous situation, **acidosis,** seen in uncontrolled diabetes. Severe, uncontrolled diabetes causes diabetic ketoacidosis, the clinical signs and symptoms of which are vomiting, abdominal pain, and deep and rapid breathing. When the acid levels of the body become too high, individual cells cannot live and will cease to function. If the patient is not given proper fluid and insulin, ketoacidosis will progress to unconsciousness, diabetic coma, and eventually death.

Diabetes mellitus is treatable. When there is a total lack of insulin production by the pancreas, it can be replaced by a daily injection of the hormone that has been extracted from animals or, more recently, by synthetic insulin. "Insulin-dependent" diabetics take one or more injections of insulin every day. Children who have to take insulin every day have been called "juvenile diabetics." Now, we would refer to these patients as having type I diabetes.

All children with diabetes are insulin-dependent. However, not all adults who develop diabetes require insulin. Many adults have a more easily controlled form of the disease, but one that is equally serious. Insulin, in the diabetic whose disease becomes evident in later life, is usually still produced, but at a lower, and usually insufficient, level for the patient's regular diet and routine. Additionally, the action of the insulin that is produced may be less effective. Many of these patients can control their blood sugar by diet alone. For some, weight loss alone cures their diabetes. Others use pills that stimulate the pancreatic islet cells to produce more insulin. Some of these patients also require small doses of supplemental insulin. This form of diabetes was formerly called adult onset diabetes; now we refer to it as type II diabetes.

It should be apparent now that diabetes is a disease of balance. The patient requires glucose as an energy source and insulin to use it properly. The diabetic must balance the need for glucose against his or her available insulin supply. A variety of methods of treatment exist and one must be tailored for each patient depending on the severity of the disease.

Ordinarily, most diabetic patients check their urine daily for the presence of sugar and acetone. The balance of insulin and ingested food should be such that no sugar or only a trace of it and no acetone at all are detectable in the urine. Many patients now use *blood-glucose self-monitoring units* to measure the level of sugar in the blood. A drop of blood from the fingertip or ear lobe is placed on a thin strip of chemically treated paper. The color the paper turns can be compared with a standard color chart provided with the test strips. The patient thus has a measure of the amount of glucose currently present in the blood. This reading is a much more direct assessment than detecting sugar in the urine. The readings are in milligrams per deciliter of blood; the normal blood glucose level lies between 100 and 150 mg/deciliter. Devices for pricking the fingertip with a fine needle are now available, as well as standard tables for reading the strips (Figure 32–2a, b).

A more elaborate unit that provides a digital readout of the blood sugar level is also available. In this unit, the test strip of paper exposed to the patient's blood is placed in the unit and analyzed automatically (Figure 32–2c).

DIABETIC COMA AND INSULIN SHOCK

The patient with diabetes may develop an acute emergency situation because of either of two conditions: diabetic coma or insulin shock. The problem for you is that the symptoms of both conditions are quite similar. Therefore, you

A

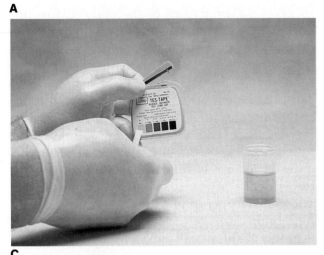

C

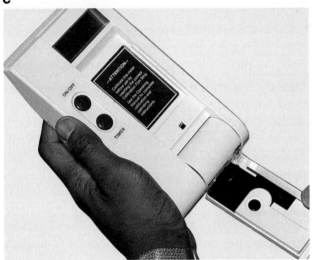

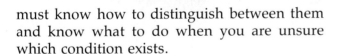

B

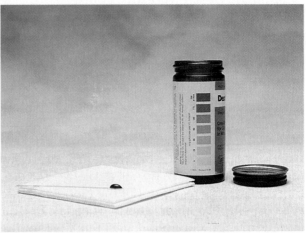

FIGURE 32–2

(A) Test strips for assessing the presence of glucose in urine are commercially available. (B) Test strips for assessing the level of glucose in blood are commercially available. (C) Blood-glucose self-monitoring unit. The patient obtains a drop of blood from the fingertip using a small, hand-held device. The chemically treated strip with the blood on it is inserted into the meter, which measures the amount of glucose currently present in the blood.

must know how to distinguish between them and know what to do when you are unsure which condition exists.

Diabetic Coma

The waste products from fat used by the body for normal energy needs markedly increase the acidity of blood and tissue. When this circumstance continues, individual cellular function in the body is impaired and eventually will stop. Additionally, if the loss of fluid from frequent urination is severe enough, marked dehydration will occur. Although the sugar level in the blood is very high (a condition called **hyperglycemia),** too much blood sugar does not directly cause diabetic coma. Ketoacidosis—the presence of acid waste products in the

blood—and the loss of body fluid together cause this condition.

Diabetic coma occurs in the patient with diabetes who is not under medical treatment, who takes insufficient insulin, who markedly overeats, or who, although well controlled, undergoes some sort of stress, such as an infection or illness. Usually, ketoacidosis develops over a long period of time—hours or days. The patient may ultimately be found comatose with the following physical signs:

- Air hunger, manifested by rapid and deep sighing respirations (*Kussmaul respirations*).
- Dehydration (excessive loss of body water) manifested by a dry, warm skin and sunken eyes.
- A sweet or fruity (acetone) odor on the breath caused by the waste products in the blood.

- A rapid, weak ("thready") pulse.
- A normal or slightly low blood pressure.
- Varying degrees of unresponsiveness.

Insulin Shock

Insulin shock occurs in the diabetic patient who has taken too much insulin, who has taken a regular dose of insulin but has not eaten enough food, or who has exercised vigorously and used up all available glucose. Sugar is rapidly taken out of the blood and into cells to supply their energy needs. In this situation, not enough sugar remains in the blood to provide the continuous supply needed for the brain. Because the brain requires as constant a supply of glucose as it does oxygen, unconsciousness and permanent brain damage can quickly occur if the blood sugar remains low.

Children who have diabetes may pose a particular management problem. Children have high activity levels and they may rapidly exhaust circulating glucose, after a normal insulin injection, with excessive play or activity. Additionally, children are likely to be less responsive to the demands of eating correctly and on time. Most learn such routines quickly, but insulin shock occurs in children more often and more severely.

Insulin shock develops much more quickly than diabetic coma—in some instances, in a matter of minutes. Insufficient sugar in the blood **(hypoglycemia),** is associated with the following signs and symptoms:

- Normal or rapid respirations.
- Pale, moist skin (clammy).
- **Diaphoresis** (sweating).
- Dizziness, headache.
- Full, rapid pulse.
- Normal blood pressure.
- Aggressive or unusual behavior.
- Hunger.
- Fainting, seizure, or coma.

Both diabetic coma and insulin shock produce unconsciousness and, in some instances, death. Diabetic coma is a complex metabolic disease that requires some time to develop and involves all the tissues of the body. Correction of diabetic ketoacidosis and diabetic coma may take many hours in a well-controlled hospital setting. Insulin shock is an acute condition. As blood sugar drops, the signs of insulin shock can become evident rapidly. Ordinarily, a diabetic patient who has taken his or her standard insulin dose and missed a meal, may be in insulin shock before the next meal. The very critical concern, in this situation, is the absolute dependence of the brain on an unending and adequate supply of glucose. Without it, permanent brain damage will occur. Giving glucose in a timely fashion will rapidly (within minutes) reverse insulin shock.

Diabetes and the Alcoholic

Occasionally, a patient who is diabetic is mistakenly identified by the police after an accident or incident as intoxicated and confined without treatment in a "drunk tank" for over 24 hours. Usually this patient dies. Certainly, diabetes and alcoholism can coexist in any patient. You must be alert to the fact that the signs and symptoms of acute alcoholic intoxication may be quite similar to those of diabetic coma or insulin shock. Sometimes, in situations such as this, an emergency medical identification bracelet, necklace, or card may help save the patient's life (Figure 32–3). Often, only a blood sugar test in the emergency department will allow final determination of the problem.

DIAGNOSIS AND TREATMENT OF DIABETIC EMERGENCIES

Most individuals with diabetes understand their disease well and keep their own treatment well controlled. The emergency situations arise with the complications of diabetes: diabetic coma, insulin shock, or other manifestations of the disease. Not infrequently, an unconscious patient may be an undiagnosed diabetic. In this instance, you will have no knowledge of the disease in this patient and you must treat him or her like any other unconscious individual.

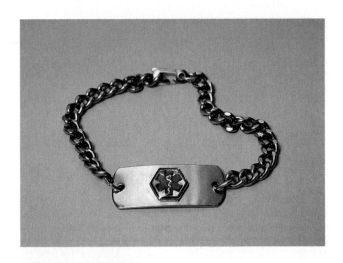

FIGURE 32–3

An emergency medical identification tag may be lifesaving for the patient.

Full life support and transport to the emergency department are appropriate for diagnosis as well as treatment.

It may be difficult for an inexperienced person, even one who knows the patient has diabetes, to tell the difference between diabetic coma and insulin shock. In either case, the patient who has not yet reached coma may feel sick or be semiconscious. Such a patient may be able to inform you about the exact cause of his or her condition.

If you know that the patient has diabetes and is ill, you must ask the patient or the family these two questions:

■ Have you taken your insulin today?
■ Have you eaten today?

If the patient has eaten but has not taken insulin, the problem is probably developing diabetic ketoacidosis. If the patient has taken insulin but has not eaten, the problem is probably insulin shock. The diabetic patient will often know what the trouble is. Listen carefully.

If the patient is unconscious and is a known diabetic, you must decide on the basis of the signs and symptoms just described whether the problem is diabetic coma or insulin shock.

This decision will determine, to a degree, the urgency of transport. The primary visible difference will be the patient's breathing: deep, sighing respirations in diabetic coma and normal or rapid respirations in insulin shock. The diabetic patient who is unconscious and having convulsions is more likely to be in insulin shock. All noticeable differences are compared in Table 32–1.

TABLE 32–1	Findings in Diabetic Emergencies	
	Diabetic Coma	**Insulin Shock**
History		
Food intake	Excessive	Insufficient
Insulin dosage	Insufficient	Excessive
Onset	Gradual	Rapid, within minutes
Skin	Warm and dry	Pale and moist
Infection	Common	Uncommon
Gastrointestinal Tract		
Thirst	Intense	Absent
Hunger	Absent	Intense
Vomiting	Common	Uncommon
Respiratory System		
Breathing	Air hunger	Normal or rapid
Odor of breath	Sweet, fruity	Normal
Cardiovascular System		
Blood pressure	Low	Normal
Pulse	Rapid, weak	Normal or rapid and full
Nervous System		
Headache	Absent	Present
Consciousness	Restless merging to coma	Irritability, seizure, or coma
Urine		
Sugar	Present	Absent
Acetone	Present	Absent
Treatment		
Response	Gradual, within 6 to 12 hours following medication and fluid	Immediate after glucose

When testing a patient with suspected signs of diabetes, you must first check whether the patient has an emergency medical identification symbol: a wallet card, necklace, or bracelet. It will advise whether the patient has a known problem and can probably aid your quick assessment and diagnosis. Remember, however, that just because a person is a known diabetic does not mean that diabetes is always causing the present condition. Diabetics can sustain other illnesses, such as a heart attack or stroke, just as well. Thus, a full, careful assessment is always required, paying attention to the ABCs.

The patient in diabetic coma (acidosis, dehydration, hyperglycemia) needs insulin, complex intravenous fluid treatment, and probably other medications. You must transport this individual to the hospital promptly for appropriate medical care.

The patient in insulin shock (rapid onset of coma, hypoglycemia) needs sugar immediately.

For the conscious patient, sugar cubes, granulated sugar, maple syrup, honey, candy, fruit juice (sweetened with granulated sugar if available), or sweetened soft drinks will reverse the reaction within several minutes (Figure 32–4). Do not be afraid to give too much sugar. The problem will not be treated with only a sip of juice or a pinch of sugar. An entire candy bar or a full glass of sweetened juice is needed. Remember, do not give sugar-free drinks sweetened with saccharin or synthetic sweetening compounds. They will have little or no effect. Even if the patient responds after receiving sugar, you must transport him or her to the hospital as soon as possible. Whether additional treatment is required is a decision for the physician to make.

When there is any doubt about whether a conscious diabetic patient is developing insulin shock or diabetic coma, *give sugar*, even though the final diagnosis may be diabetic ketoacidosis. The reason for giving sugar is that untreated insulin shock will certainly cause unconsciousness and can quickly cause significant brain damage or death. As a matter of priority, the patient in insulin shock is in a far more

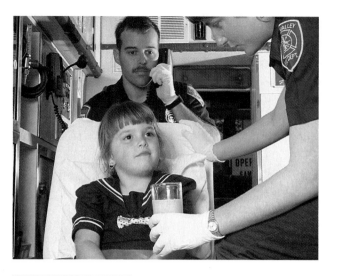

FIGURE 32–4

The child with diabetes may experience insulin shock more frequently than an adult, because activity level can vary greatly very quickly and inadequate attention may be paid to eating correctly or on time. This person needs lots of sugar administered quickly to offset the effects of too much insulin in the body. Pure sugar, candy, or fruit juice will reverse the reaction promptly.

critical condition and far more likely to develop permanent problems than the patient in diabetic ketoacidosis. Giving sugar to a conscious patient in insulin shock could save a life or prevent brain damage. If you give sugar in an emergency situation to a patient in diabetic ketoacidosis, there is very little risk of seriously worsening the condition. Permanent damage or death will occur, if at all, only after a long period. Diabetic coma requires hours of careful insulin and fluid therapy, which must be carried out only under a physician's care and in the hospital.

The patient suspected of being in insulin shock who is unconscious or who becomes unconscious during treatment cannot swallow. No attempt should be made to give this patient juice, sugar, or any such material by mouth, as it may be aspirated into the lungs. Intravenous glucose is needed and will be given in the emergency department. The basic EMT is not responsible for starting an intravenous solution; rather, your responsibility is to provide the most prompt transportation of the patient possible so that care may be given in this very urgent situation.

In the past it has been recommended that "instant glucose" (a prepared jelly) or glucose tablets be placed under the tongue or in the mouth of the unconscious patient. In general, this practice is not wise. Recent studies have indicated that very little sugar, given in this manner, is absorbed. The risk of choking or aspirating liquid into the lungs probably outweighs the benefits of providing such small amounts of glucose. The only way of giving sugar to these patients is intravenously. Prompt transportation to the emergency department is the appropriate step.

COMPLICATIONS OF DIABETES

Diabetes is a systemic disease affecting all tissues of the body. Thus, you are likely to be called to treat these complications of diabetes as well. The principal organs and structures damaged are kidneys, eyes, small arteries, and peripheral nerves. As a result of these problems, you may see a variety of problems, usually not acute emergencies, that arise from and are associated with diabetes. They will include patients with visual disturbances, renal failure, and ulcers or infections on the feet or toes. You must not forget that, although this disease is primarily one relating to metabolism and the capacity of the body to use sugar for energy, no tissue escapes its effect. Diabetes is a risk factor for cardiovascular disease. Individuals with diabetes should control their blood sugar levels and diet to modify the magnitude of the risk.

EMT SAFETY

In the management of problems related to diabetes, there is relatively little exposure of the EMT to potential risk. Obviously, obtaining and checking a blood or urine sample requires that you use gloves and wash your hands carefully. However, exposure to body fluids is generally very limited. Routine precautions, applicable to your contacts with any other patient, are appropriate and safe.

YOU ARE THE EMT

1. Distinguish between type I and type II diabetes. Which type is more easily managed than the other? Why?
2. You know that glucose is as important to the brain as oxygen. Explain why the combination of too much insulin and too little food deprives the brain of glucose.
3. Children with diabetes are much more likely to go into insulin shock than adults, even though their parents carefully control their diet and injections. Why?
4. Your patient is semiconscious, and you believe he is hyperglycemic. Describe some signs and symptoms that would lead you to conclude he is hyperglycemic. How will you treat this patient?
5. You have been called to a college party. One of the girls seems to have had too much to drink and is talking incoherently. Her friends are worried because they know she is a diabetic. What should you do?
6. Besides glucose metabolism, what are some of the other organ systems and functions that can be affected by diabetes?

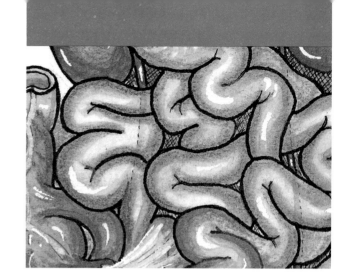

CHAPTER 33

THE ACUTE ABDOMEN

acute abdomen A condition of sudden onset within the abdomen demanding immediate medical treatment.

aneurysm (an'u-rizm) A swelling or enlargement of a part of an artery, resulting from weakening of the arterial wall.

anorexia (an"o-rek'se-ah) Lack or loss of appetite for food.

colic (kol'ik) Acute cramping abdominal pain.

emesis (em'ĕ-sis) Vomiting.

guarding The involuntary protecting of the inflamed abdomen by abdominal wall muscular contraction.

hernia The protrusion of a loop or knuckle of an organ or tissue through an abnormal body opening.

ileus (il'e-us) Paralysis of bowel motility arising from any of a number of causes.

peritoneum (per"i-to-ne'um) The membrane lining the abdominal cavity (parietal peritoneum) and reflected inward over the abdominal organs (visceral peritoneum).

peritonitis (per"i-to-ni'tis) Inflammation of the peritoneum.

referred pain Pain felt in an area of the body other than where the cause of pain is located.

strangulation (strang"gu-la'shun) Arrest of the circulation in a part due to compression or entrapment; a situation causing death of tissue.

OVERVIEW

Injuries or illnesses that affect the abdomen have one thing in common: They are very painful. They can also be very serious—often serious enough to require an emergency operation. Abdominal pain has many causes, the most obvious of which is injury. The less obvious causes are related to illness and disease. So difficult are these types of problems to diagnose that even skilled surgeons may have trouble pinpointing an exact cause. You are not expected to make such a diagnosis in a patient who has an acute abdomen. Instead, you must realize how serious an acute abdomen can be and recognize its existence.

The symptoms are usually sudden in onset and rapidly progressive. They may quickly result in death. The overriding principle in giving emergency care in these situations is to correct life-threatening problems and transport the patient to the hospital without delay.

Chapter 33 focuses on the acute abdomen caused by illness or disease. The chapter begins with a definition of the term "acute abdomen," and another less frequently used term, "abdominal catastrophe." The chapter then describes the signs and symptoms of the acute abdomen and its major causes. The last part of the chapter discusses the emergency care of the acute abdomen. Throughout, the emphasis is on recognizing the seriousness of the problem and the need for prompt transport.

GOALS

The goals of Chapter 33 are to
- define the terms "acute abdomen" and "abdominal catastrophe."
- describe the signs and symptoms of an acute abdomen.
- understand the causes of an acute abdomen.
- know the causes of referred pain and how to recognize it.
- know how to treat a patient with an acute abdomen.

DEFINITION OF ACUTE ABDOMEN

Acute abdomen is a medical term that indicates the presence of some process that causes a sudden irritation of the **peritoneum,** the thin membrane that lines the entire abdominal cavity. This condition, called **peritonitis,** causes a major symptom—severe pain. The major clinical signs are abdominal tenderness and distension. All penetrating abdominal wounds and all blunt injuries severe enough to damage abdominal organs produce the signs and symptoms of an acute abdomen. Many diseases can also cause an acute abdomen.

The term *abdominal catastrophe* is used less frequently to denote the most sudden and severe form of an acute abdomen. Neither term is exact, because neither refers to any specific disease or organ. Both mean the presence of a severe intraabdominal problem that causes peritonitis. Both mean that a combination of certain signs and symptoms exists in a patient, regardless of its cause.

Because many diseases in many different organs result in the same clinical signs and the subjective complaint of pain in the abdomen, it is possible to consider them all under the term *acute abdomen*. Frequently, even a skilled surgeon has difficulty determining exactly what is causing an acute abdomen. You need not know the exact cause of an acute abdomen, and you must not waste time attempting to make an exact diagnosis in this patient. Rather, your responsibility lies in being able to recognize the existence of this condition and to provide proper support and prompt transportation to the appropriate medical facility.

THE SIGNS AND SYMPTOMS OF AN ACUTE ABDOMEN

The following common signs and symptoms of an acute abdomen arise from irritation or inflammation of the peritoneum:

- Local or diffuse abdominal pain and/or tenderness.
- A rigid, quiet patient.
- A patient breathing rapidly with shallow breaths.
- Referred (distant) pain.
- Anorexia, nausea, vomiting.
- Tense, often distended, abdomen.
- Constipation.
- Tachycardia (rapid pulse).
- Hypotension (low blood pressure).
- Fever.

The patient with peritonitis always complains of abdominal pain, even when lying quietly. There is usually tenderness when the abdomen is palpated or when the patient moves. Thus, this patient is quiet and breathes with difficulty and rapidly, with shallow breaths, because it hurts. The degree of pain and tenderness usually is related directly to the severity of peritoneal inflammation.

The peritoneum can be separated anatomically into two divisions. *Parietal peritoneum* lines the walls of the abdominal cavity, and *visceral peritoneum* covers the surface of all the abdominal organs. The nerve supply to these two areas of peritoneum is different. Parietal peri-

toneum is supplied by the same nerves that innervate the skin of the abdomen. Sensations perceived by the parietal peritoneum are similar to those felt by the skin: pain, touch, pressure, heat, and cold. Thus, the sensory nerves of the parietal peritoneum can identify and localize a point of irritation well.

In contrast, visceral peritoneum is supplied by the autonomic nervous system. These nerves are far less able to localize any sensation. Furthermore, sensations that are felt are only those that arise from the activation of stretch receptors caused by distension or forceful contraction of the hollow abdominal organs. This type of sensation is usually interpreted as **colic,** a severe, intermittent cramping pain.

The autonomic innervation of the visceral peritoneum gives rise to the phenomenon of **referred pain.** This term means that an irritated peritoneal surface on a distended or inflamed organ may cause pain at a distant point on the surface of the body. Referred pain occurs because the body has two separate but connected nervous systems. The spinal cord supplies sensory nerves to the skin and muscles. The autonomic nervous system controls the abdominal organs and the blood vessels. Connecting nerves between the two systems allow the stimulation of the autonomic nerves to be perceived as stimulation of the spinal nerves. As an example of referred pain, *acute cholecystitis* (inflammation of the gallbladder) may cause pain in the right shoulder. The autonomic nerves serving the gallbladder lie at the same anatomic level near the spinal cord as the spinal sensory nerves that supply the skin of the shoulder (Figure 33–1).

Peritonitis always causes **ileus** or paralysis of the muscular contractions that normally propel material through the intestine. The retained swallowed gas and feces will cause abdominal distension. In the presence of such paralysis, nothing that is eaten will be passed normally out of the stomach or through the bowel. **Emesis** (vomiting) is the only way in which the stomach can empty itself. Peritonitis almost always is associated with nausea and vomiting. These complaints are not specific and are seen with almost every type of gastrointestinal disease or peritonitis. Nausea is nearly universal

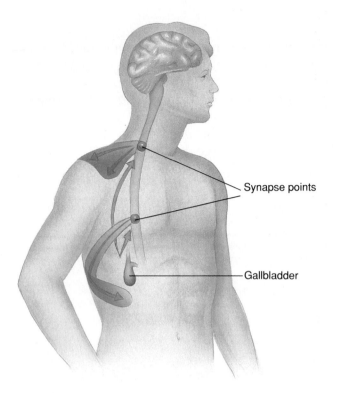

FIGURE 33–1

Acute cholecystitis causes referred pain in the shoulder as well as abdominal pain.

with bowel disease or injury; and it usually precedes emesis.

Similarly, **anorexia** (loss of hunger or appetite) is a nonspecific symptom. It, too, is an almost universal complaint in gastrointestinal and abdominal disease or injury. It is not specific for any one problem. Its absence usually indicates that the situation may not be as serious as one might think. Diarrhea is rarely seen in patients with an acute abdomen, because of the bowel paralysis. Varying degrees of constipation are much more frequent.

Peritonitis is always associated with a loss of body fluid into the abdominal cavity. The loss results in a decrease in the volume of the circulating blood and may eventually cause hypovolemic shock. Depending on the stage of the development of peritonitis, the patient may have normal vital signs or may have tachycardia and hypotension. If peritonitis is associated with hemorrhage, the signs of shock are much more apparent.

Depending on the cause of the acute abdomen, fever may be present. Patients with *diverticulitis* (an inflammation of small pockets in the colon) or cholecystitis may have substantial temperature elevations. On the other hand, patients with acute appendicitis may not have fever until the appendix has ruptured and an abscess starts to form.

An acute abdomen is characterized by abdominal pain and tenderness. Pain may be sharply localized or diffuse and may vary in its severity. Localized pain gives a clue to the organ or area causing it. Tenderness may be minimal or so great that the patient will not allow the abdomen to be touched.

Tenseness of abdominal muscles is also part of an acute abdomen. In some instances, the muscles of the abdominal wall become rigid. This boardlike muscle spasm, called **guarding,** can be seen with major problems such as a *perforated peptic ulcer* or *pancreatitis*. Usually, some degree of muscular guarding always overlies the irritated areas. Muscular spasm may be involuntary as the abdomen attempts to protect itself from further irritation. In some situations, patients can obtain comfort only by lying in one position. Thus, the position of the patient may provide an important clue. The patient with appendicitis may draw up the right knee. The patient with pancreatitis may lie curled up on one side. Each position tends to relax muscles adjacent to the inflamed organ and to lessen the pain.

Distension can easily be gauged by looking at the patient's abdomen, because it begins shortly after muscular contractions of the bowel have ceased. Pulse and blood pressure may undergo significant change or none at all. These findings usually reflect the severity of the process, its duration, and the amount of fluid lost into the abdomen.

EXAMINATION OF THE ABDOMEN

You can examine the abdomen quickly using the following steps:

1. Place the patient supine with the legs drawn up and flexed at the knees for relaxation.

2. Determine whether the patient is restless or quiet, whether motion causes pain, or whether any characteristic position, distension, or obvious abnormality is present.
3. Palpate the abdomen gently to see whether it is tense (guarded) or soft.
4. Determine whether the patient can relax the abdominal wall on command.
5. Determine whether the abdomen is tender when palpated.

Such an examination will yield much information, but it should not be prolonged. The physician will do a much more detailed examination in the hospital. Abdominal palpation should be done very gently. Occasionally, an organ within the abdomen will be enlarged and very fragile, and rough palpation could cause further damage.

CAUSES OF ABDOMINAL DISEASE

Gastrointestinal and Urinary Tracts

The abdominal cavity contains the solid and hollow organs that make up the gastrointestinal, genital, and urinary systems. You will recall that these organs are completely covered by peritoneum; parietal on the inside of the abdominal cavity, and visceral over the surface of the organs. The entire abdominal cavity normally contains a very small amount of peritoneal fluid bathing the organs. Any condition that allows pus, blood, feces, urine, gastric juice, intestinal contents, bile, pancreatic juice, amniotic fluid, or other material to lie within or adjacent to this cavity can give rise to the signs of an acute abdomen (Figure 33–2).

Among the common diseases that produce signs of an acute abdomen are acute appendicitis, perforated peptic ulcer, cholecystitis, and diverticulitis. The list of diseases that can produce an acute abdomen includes nearly every abdominal problem. The more common emergency problems and the location of the direct and referred pain produced are listed in Table 33–1.

Because the parietal peritoneum is richly supplied with very sensitive nerves, disease or

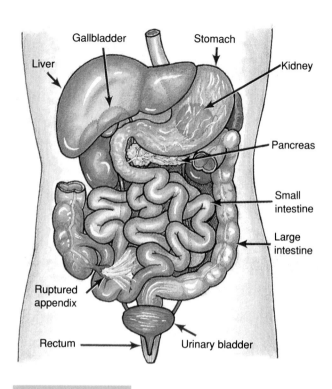

FIGURE 33–2

Pus from a ruptured appendix has entered the abdominal cavity and caused peritonitis.

inflammation of organs that lie behind or beneath the abdominal cavity can also cause the signs of peritonitis. These signs and symptoms are similar to those produced by actual inflammation within the abdominal cavity itself. Pancreatitis, for example, can produce a severe reaction that is hard to distinguish from a perforated ulcer. Kidney stones that cause ureteral colic are frequently associated with ileus (paralysis of bowel action). Infections of the urinary tract may also cause peritoneal irritation.

Internal Female Genitalia

Gynecologic problems are a common cause of acute abdominal pain and were described in Chapter 27. You must be aware that the woman with lower abdominal pain and tenderness may very well have a problem related to her ovaries, Fallopian tubes, or uterus.

Table 33–1	Common Diseases That Cause Acute Abdomen and Localization of Pain

Disease	Localization of Pain
Appendicitis	Around navel (referred); right lower quadrant (direct)
Cholecystitis	Right shoulder (referred); right upper quadrant (direct)
Duodenal ulcer	Upper mid-abdomen or upper back
Diverticulitis	Left lower quadrant
Aortic aneurysm (ruptured)	Low back and right lower quadrant
Cystitis (bladder inflammation)	Lower mid-abdomen (retropubic)
Kidney infection	Costovertebral angle
Kidney stone	Either right or left flanks, radiating to genitalia (referred)
Pelvic inflammation (female)	Both lower quadrants
Pancreatitis	Upper abdomen (both quadrants); back

The normal menstrual cycle was described in Chapter 25. Many abdominal problems in women are related to this cycle. A common lower abdominal pain, often confused with appendicitis but fairly short lived, is called *mittelschmerz*. It is associated with the release of an egg from the ovary. Characteristically, it occurs in the middle of the menstrual cycle, between periods. It signifies to the patient that an egg that can be fertilized has been discharged. Some women also experience painful cramps at the time of their menstrual periods. In some, the discomfort may be crippling and the menstrual flow may be severe. Each of these conditions causes abdominal pain, and mittelschmerz may be associated with some lower abdominal tenderness.

A common cause of an acute abdomen in the female is *pelvic inflammatory disease (PID)*, an infection of the Fallopian tubes and the surrounding tissues of the pelvis. With pelvic inflammatory disease, the lower abdominal

signs of acute pain and tenderness may be intense with an associated high fever. This condition warrants prompt transport to the emergency department for treatment.

Between one and two percent of all pregnancies are ectopic. The term *ectopic pregnancy* means that an ovum, after being fertilized by a sperm cell, has come to lie in an area outside of the uterus. Usually, the egg comes to lie in the Fallopian tube and grows and develops there. The Fallopian tube is simply not large enough to support the growth of the fetus and placenta for more than about six to eight weeks. Then it commonly ruptures, often producing massive internal hemorrhage and the rapid development of abdominal pain. In this situation, the acute abdomen may be associated with the rapid onset of hypovolemic shock. This combination mandates immediate transport to the hospital as a priority one emergency.

Other Systems and Areas

The aorta lies immediately behind the peritoneum on the spinal column. In older people the wall of the aorta sometimes develops weak areas that swell to form an **aneurysm.** The development of an aneurysm is rarely associated with symptoms, because it occurs slowly; but, if the aneurysm ruptures, massive hemorrhage may occur. The signs of acute peritoneal irritation may then be evident, along with severe back pain, because the peritoneum is rapidly stripped away from the body wall by the hemorrhage. In such instances, peritoneal signs are usually associated with profound shock because of the associated bleeding. Again, the association of acute abdominal signs and symptoms with shock requires prompt transportation.

Pneumonia, especially in the lower parts of the lung, may cause both ileus and abdominal pain. In this instance, the problem lies in an adjacent body cavity; but the intense inflammatory response can affect the abdomen. Treat and transport this patient like any other with abdominal pain.

A **hernia** is a protrusion of an organ or tissue that normally should lie within a body cavity through a hole in the body wall containing that cavity. Virtually every organ or tissue in the body has been described as herniating through its covering membranes. Hernias can occur in association with congenital defects (as around the umbilicus), after operations where a wound has failed to heal well, or in areas where some natural weakness exists such as in the groin. Hernias always produce a mass or lump that the patient can describe. At times, the mass will disappear back into the body cavity where it belongs. In this case, the hernia is said to be *reducible*. If the mass cannot be pushed back within the body, it is said to be *incarcerated*.

As long as a hernia is reducible, it constitutes little risk to the patient, and some individuals live with them for years. When a hernia is incarcerated, its contents may become seriously compressed by the surrounding tissue to the extent that the blood supply is compromised. This situation, called **strangulation,** is a serious medical emergency and warrants immediate surgical intervention for removal of the dead tissue and repair of the hernia.

The signs and symptoms that would indicate a serious hernia problem are these:

- The existence of the hernia itself.
- A clear statement that a mass that was reducible is no longer able to be pushed back inside the body.
- Pain at the hernia site.
- Tenderness when the hernia is palpated.
- Skin discoloration (red or blue) over the hernia.

The presence of these signs and symptoms warrant the prompt transport of the patient to the emergency department.

EMERGENCY CARE OF THE PATIENT WITH AN ACUTE ABDOMEN

The signs and symptoms of an acute abdomen justify a working diagnosis of some serious abdominal surgical emergency. Do not delay in transporting the patient to the emergency department. Carry out the following steps as quickly as possible prior to transport:

1. Do not attempt to make a specific diagnosis of the cause of the acute abdomen.
2. Clear and maintain the airway.
3. Anticipate vomiting.
4. Give oxygen.
5. Do not give the patient anything by mouth (NPO = Nil Per Os, Latin meaning "Nothing by mouth").
6. Do not administer any sedative or analgesic agent.
7. Record all pertinent information: onset, type, severity, and duration of symptoms.
8. Anticipate the development of hypovolemic shock.
9. Position the patient comfortably for transport.

Vomiting is common in these patients, because the emergency frequently develops just after the patient has eaten a large meal or had much to drink. Clear the patient's throat and airway of vomited material and keep them clear. Pain often makes breathing physically difficult. Thus, you should administer supplemental oxygen to compensate for a small respiratory volume.

Under no circumstances should you give a patient with acute abdominal signs anything to eat or drink. Food or fluid will only aggravate many of the symptoms. In the presence of peritoneal irritation and intestinal paralysis, food does not pass out of the stomach. If an emergency operation is required, the presence of food in the stomach will make the operation much more dangerous.

No matter how much pain the patient is experiencing, do not give any medication to relieve pain or sedate the patient. The examining physician must know exactly where and how severe the pain is. Medication frequently masks these findings and may delay an ultimate diagnosis until it is too late to correct the problem easily or safely.

In cases of acute abdomen, you must not attempt to diagnose the patient's disease. Rather, you should listen to the description of the location of pain and tenderness and the severity of the patient's symptoms. Note the presence of abdominal tenderness, distension, or guarding. Record the patient's description of how the process started, along with the vital signs, so that the physician may know what these were when the patient was first seen. Close monitoring of vital signs is important, because they may change quickly. The development of shock is common in these cases and must be recognized early. Its presence makes prompt transport to the hospital even more imperative. Make the patient as comfortable as possible; conserve body heat using blankets; treat for shock in instances where it is evident; and transport the patient gently and promptly to the emergency department.

YOU ARE THE EMT

1. You believe the patient's severe abdominal pain may be from acute cholecystitis. The patient also has right shoulder pain. Does this pain confirm your suspicions? Explain why the patient is experiencing referred shoulder pain.
2. You were complimented for recognizing acute appendicitis and getting the patient to the hospital before his appendix ruptured. Why is a ruptured appendix considered such a serious medical emergency?
3. Identify eight body substances that could, by their presence within the abdominal cavity, cause an acute abdomen.
4. Your patient has all the signs and symptoms of an acute abdomen. Describe the emergency treatment you will administer.
5. Describe some gynecologic disorders that can cause an acute abdomen.
6. Name four causes other than those arising within the abdominal cavity itself that can cause an acute abdomen.

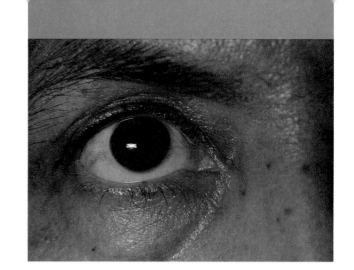

CHAPTER 34

COMMON MEDICAL COMPLAINTS

KEY TERMS

cirrhosis (sir-ro′sis) A disease of the liver marked by progressive destruction of liver cells often causing jaundice.

colic (kol′ik) Acute cramping abdominal pain.

diarrhea (di″ah-re′ah) Abnormal frequency and liquidity of bowel movements.

dysphagia (dis-fa′je-ah) Difficulty in swallowing.

dysuria (dis-u′re-ah) Painful or difficult urination.

emesis (em′ĕ-sis) Vomiting.

geriatric (jer″e-at′rik) Pertaining to the aged or elderly.

hematemesis (hem″ah-tem′ĕ-sis) The vomiting of blood.

hematuria (hem″ah-tu′re-ah) The discharge of blood in the urine.

hiccup A sudden inspiration of air that is rapidly checked by closure of the glottis causing a characteristic sound.

incontinence (in-kon′tĭ-nens) Involuntary emptying of bowels or bladder.

jaundice (jawn′dis) The deposition of bile pigment in the skin and mucous membranes resulting in a yellow appearance of the patient.

nocturia (nok-tu′re-ah) Excessive urination at night.

purulent (pu′roo-lent) Consisting of or containing pus.

tinnitus (tĭ-ni′tus) Ringing in the ear.

vertigo (ver′tĭ-go) Dizziness.

OVERVIEW

An EMT attends many patients who have not been injured in an accident or become severely ill with one of the diseases described in this text. These patients may have any one of a number of less severe complaints that are serious enough, however, to interfere with their normal daily activities.

Complaints involving the gastrointestinal tract include difficulty in swallowing, vomiting, vomiting blood, diarrhea, passage of blood in the stool, jaundice, colic, heartburn, constipation, and the eating disorders bulimia and anorexia nervosa. Complaints involving the urinary tract include pain or burning during urination, passage of blood in the urine, frequency of urination, lack of bladder control, urinary retention, renal stones, and renal colic.

In the female genital tract, common complaints include vaginal spotting, bleeding or discharge, pregnancy outside the uterus, mittelschmerz, pelvic inflammation, and prolapse of various structures. In the male, urethral discharge, hernias, hydroceles, and testicular tumors may be encountered.

Vertigo, headaches, and hiccups are separate problems that are also encoun-tered occasionally. While generally not life-threatening, many of these problems are perceived as serious by the patient and thus require attention.

Elderly patients are especially upset by many of the symptoms of these and other problems. The chapter therefore includes a discussion of the special concerns of geriatric patients and concludes with a note on EMT safety.

GOALS

The goals of Chapter 34 are to
- know and be able to describe common gastrointestinal complaints not associated with injury or an acute abdomen.
- know and be able to describe common urinary and genital complaints not associated with injuries.
- define vertigo and hiccup and describe their causes.
- understand the special concerns of geriatric patients.
- know the common principles underlying EMT safety measures for all these complaints.

THE GASTROINTESTINAL TRACT

As an EMT, you will often be called to attend many patients with a wide variety of medical complaints who have not been injured nor have a life-threatening medical emergency. Only rarely will these complaints be accompanied by a life-threatening situation such as hemorrhage. A good grasp of the spectrum of these conditions is essential for your success as an EMT. The complaints can be grouped according to anatomical systems.

Dysphagia

Dysphagia is the sensation of sticking or discomfort when swallowing. It is caused by obstructing lesions in the esophagus, which can range from swallowed foreign bodies to tumors. The condition may be severe and acute, as with a foreign body, or slowly progressive, as with cancer. In general, the patient complains of a sensation of food sticking under the sternum or at the back of the throat.

Dysphagia is a complaint ignored by many people until the problem becomes serious. For example, at first only chunks of meat may have given problems. Most individuals can treat such swallowing difficulties with a drink of water at meals. They then tend to forget about the problem until the next meal, because dysphagia usually does not cause pain. Eventually, however, only liquids or very soft foods can be tolerated. When the person finally consults a physician, the problem is often severe and has interfered with the patient's nutrition.

You must recognize that when a patient complains of dysphagia, it has either come about because of a long-standing disease that has recently become intolerable or has come on quickly and is thus an acute problem. In either instance, professional help must be obtained promptly. Although not usually an emergency condition in itself, dysphagia is often associated with serious illness that has been neglected or ignored. It becomes an emergency once the patient can no longer swallow. Then, there is a danger that food or saliva will be aspirated into the lungs. Prompt transportation to the emergency department for diagnosis and treatment is indicated.

Vomiting and the Aspiration of Vomitus

One of the commonest gastrointestinal complaints is vomiting, or **emesis.** It is the response of the stomach to a noxious stimulus—irritation, infection, or obstruction. It is to be distinguished from *regurgitation,* which is a "burp" of air or fluid that comes up as the result of the stomach being too full.

Vomiting has many causes. One is any situation that produces peritonitis or an acute abdomen that can stop peristaltic contraction in the gastrointestinal tract. When the muscles that propel the contents of the intestine through the tract stop working, vomiting becomes the only way the stomach can empty.

Any disease that causes inflammation of the inside lining of the gastrointestinal tract, especially the stomach, may cause extreme muscle contractions with vomiting. *Gastroenteritis,* a viral or bacterial infection of the stomach and intestine, is a common cause of vomiting. The ingestion of irritating agents, especially alcohol, can also cause emesis. Alcohol is a stimulator of gastric juice production as well as an irritant of the stomach lining. Food poisoning often causes vomiting as the stomach attempts to rid itself of the noxious agent. Alcohol and contaminated food are not the only irritants. The excessive use of certain drugs such as aspirin may also cause inflammation of the stomach lining and result in vomiting. Mechanical obstruction to the passage of material through the gastrointestinal tract will also cause vomiting. Mechanical obstruction can be produced by tumors or by swallowed foreign bodies.

Vomiting is common among children. Often, a baby's contented "burp" after a full bottle will produce a "swallowful" of regurgitated milk and much air. This response is normal. Other infants, however, may experience severe, unremitting and forceful vomiting from a condition called *pyloric stenosis,* an obstruction of the outlet of the stomach. Most of the time, vomiting in children is from a bacterial or viral gastroenteritis.

Vomiting is always serious, because you have no real knowledge of its cause. It may be a much more complex problem than gastroenteritis or "too much to drink." In adults, vomiting that continues for several days may result in a dangerous loss of water, nutrients, and body salts. Serious metabolic problems can then occur, particularly dehydration. In infants and small children, vomiting may produce these changes within 24 hours. In such situations, the patient may actually be in shock because of the significant fluid and salt loss. This type of shock is considered in Chapter 12.

The alert patient who is vomiting because of illness is rarely, if ever, in danger of aspirating the vomitus. All the protective reflexes of the airway are active. However, a very small drop of irritating saliva or gastric juice aspirated into the larynx may cause laryngospasm and usually triggers violent coughing. The patient who is vomiting must be assisted to vomit as is necessary to avoid aspiration and then placed in a position of comfort. You must be alert for more vomiting during transport. An emesis basin or other receptacle and clean towels should be immediately available to the patient.

The sleepy, unconscious, or drunken patient may aspirate vomited material into the airway very quickly. Normal reflex protection in these patients is often depressed or absent. Once aspirated, material is rarely coughed out by the patient because the cough reflex is also depressed. Acidic gastric juice can destroy lung tissue rapidly. Alveoli and small bronchi can literally be digested. The remaining damaged lung tissue is easily infected, and a lung abscess usually follows.

In treating a vomiting patient who is not fully alert, you must pay special attention to maintaining a clear airway. Aspiration of vomitus can occur in a matter of seconds. Be prepared to clear and maintain the airway. This patient should be placed on one side, with the head lower than the feet. Nothing must be allowed to accumulate in the pharynx. Large-bore suction catheters should be at hand to clear vomitus as it occurs. Manually maintain the airway using the jaw-thrust or chin-lift technique (Figure 34–1).

At times, you may arrive after the patient has aspirated vomitus into the lungs. Sometimes this event produces few symptoms and signs. More often, however, the patient is breathing rapidly with some difficulty and produces a large volume of tracheal secretions. This patient may also be cyanotic. In this instance, prompt transport to the emergency department is absolutely essential. En route, administer supplemental oxygen. Full ventilatory support, including assisted breathing, may be required. Removal of the aspirated vomitus at the hospital within 30 to 60 minutes may save the patient's life or prevent abscess formation in the lungs.

The vomiting patient who is in shock (dehydrated; lethargic; hypotensive; with a rapid, thready pulse) as a result of emesis alone is seriously ill and demands prompt hospital care. This patient has lost as much fluid, electrolytes,

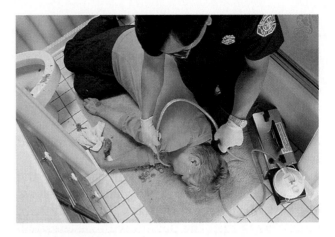

FIGURE 34–1

The airway must be kept clear, particularly in the semi-conscious patient. Here, the EMT is using a large-bore suction catheter to keep the airway clear.

and plasma as the patient with a severe burn or with extensive hemorrhage. After all the necessary measures for airway protection and initial support have been completed, the patient should be given oxygen and transported as promptly as possible to the emergency department. In each of these instances, you must note the contents and appearance of the vomited material, its frequency, its volume, and the character of the vomiting process (forceful, projectile, or regurgitant).

Hematemesis

The vomiting of blood, called **hematemesis,** is a particularly disturbing event for the patient. In general, it is associated with disease in the esophagus or stomach. The three most common disorders causing hematemesis are ulcers of the stomach or duodenum, ruptured *esophageal varices,* or *gastritis.*

Ulcers have a variety of causes. Most patients will have a history of upper abdominal pain and may be taking antacids or other medication to relieve these symptoms. Some ulcers also are associated with stomach cancer. Many patients have had a previous history of vomiting blood.

Esophageal varices are dilated veins in the wall of the esophagus that develop in patients with liver disease. Scarring in the liver blocks its normal venous blood flow, which is then shunted to the veins in the esophagus. The veins become quite enlarged, and their very thin walls rupture easily. Bleeding from esophageal varices is sudden, heavy, painless, and frequently fatal.

Gastritis (inflammation or irritation of the stomach lining) is produced by emotional stress or by chemical irritants such as alcohol, aspirin, and other drugs. The patient with gastritis will usually have vague, moderately severe, upper abdominal pain and mild left upper quadrant tenderness.

Hematemesis can be manifested as "coffee-ground" vomitus in relatively small quantities or as large quantities of very bright red blood. Coffee-ground vomitus is so called because the material produced looks like coffee grounds suspended in the clear mucus and liquid of normal gastric juice. It indicates a very slow rate of bleeding into the stomach. The small quantities of blood are digested and turn dark brown in the stomach. Large quantities of bright red blood, on the other hand, mean that very brisk bleeding is taking place.

With either form of hematemesis—bright red bleeding or coffee-ground vomitus—the patient should be transported promptly to the emergency department. The amount of blood vomited should be estimated and recorded. If possible, a sample of the vomitus should be collected and taken with the patient to the hospital. Monitor vital signs closely; protect and maintain the airway; and expect further vomiting while en route to the hospital.

Diarrhea

Just as there are a number of causes of vomiting, so are there a number of causes of **diarrhea,** which is a term describing an abnormally large number of bowel movements of abnormally liquid character. Anxiety, gastroenteritis, the common viral "flu," severe bacterial infections such as typhoid fever, or parasitic infestation can all cause diarrhea. A number of inflammatory diseases in the bowel for which causes are unknown, such as *ulcerative colitis,* can also cause diarrhea. In the elderly person, one of the most common causes is a partial obstruction of the bowel by a fecal impaction. In this apparently contradictory situation, the fecal impaction allows only watery material to pass, producing the complaint of diarrhea.

Rarely is diarrhea the cause of an acute emergency problem. If it has been present for several days and if the patient has been unable to take sufficient food or fluid to balance the amount lost, dehydration and lethargy may be present. This patient, just like the patient who has been vomiting excessively, may have unstable vital signs and may be developing hypovolemic shock. You must recognize that uncontrolled diarrhea or vomiting, if it has lasted over a period of several days or more, may result in serious metabolic changes. The patient with diarrhea serious enough to necessitate an emergency call should be transported to the emergency department for an assessment of the cause of the problem.

Melena and Hematochezia

The term *melena* is derived from a Greek word meaning black. It describes a dark, black stool that is very tarry or sticky in consistency. It has a characteristic, particularly foul odor. The black color is caused by the presence of blood that has been digested within the gastrointestinal tract. In general, melena is caused by slow, continuous bleeding in the upper part of the gastrointestinal tract from ulcers, polyps, or tumors. Some medications (bismuth and iron-containing compounds) may give the same dark color to the stool, but neither the tarry consistency nor the foul smell is present after such medication. Melena is not an emergency situation unless it has persisted and been ignored for a long time. Under those circumstances the patient may exhibit signs of hypovolemic shock. Melena is, however, a cause for grave concern, because the bleeding source must be identified as soon as possible.

The passage of bright red blood in the stool is called *hematochezia.* Hematochezia has a number of causes that range from the very serious problem of colon or rectal cancer to the common problem of hemorrhoids. Keep in mind that sometimes patients mistake vaginal bleeding for rectal bleeding. Bright red blood in the stool is not ordinarily an emergency medical problem, although it may be very alarming to the patient. Except in very few instances, the bleeding customarily is not massive. It is, however, a distinctly abnormal situation that requires prompt medical evaluation to diagnose the cause.

In the treatment of a complaint of melena or hematochezia, monitor the patient's vital signs and then transport the patient to the emergency department for appropriate examination and diagnosis. An accurate description of the characteristics and the volume of the bloody stool passed will be helpful to the evaluating physician.

Jaundice

Occasionally, you will be called to see a patient with **jaundice.** The term is derived from a French word meaning "yellow." It is not a disease; rather, it describes a yellow color of the skin. Many problems may cause jaundice, almost all of them related to some malfunction of the liver or the biliary tract. The liver produces bile, a brownish yellow compound that plays an essential role in the digestion of fat in the gastrointestinal tract. Bile is excreted from the liver into the duodenum through the biliary tract. A considerable portion of the excreted bile is reabsorbed in the intestines and returned to the liver. The rest is excreted. It is responsible for the normal brown color of feces.

Any disease that interferes with the normal function of the liver so that bile cannot be made or excreted will cause jaundice. Common causes of abnormal liver function are infection (hepatitis) and poisoning of liver cells from alcohol and other toxic substances. Chronic alcohol abuse causes permanent liver damage, which is called **cirrhosis.** Any situation in which the outflow of bile from the liver to the gastrointestinal tract is blocked will cause jaundice. For example, a gallstone that forms in the gallbladder can block the biliary tract; cancers of the bile duct, pancreas, or duodenum can also block the biliary tract.

Although severe jaundice is evident by simply looking at the patient, the early and mild stages may not be visible or can be seen only by using good lighting to look at areas of the body that are normally white. The best place to look for jaundice is the sclera of the eye, particularly in darkly pigmented individuals (Figure 34–2). When examining any patient, you should routinely check the sclera for *scleral icterus* (yellow color).

Jaundice always indicates a serious medical condition. All patients with jaundice must receive a thorough medical evaluation by a physician. Because the jaundice may be caused by hepatitis, which can be highly contagious, you must be particularly careful when handling the patient.

Colic

Colic is a characteristic, abdominal pain that is caused by obstruction of one of the hollow organs. The pain is intermittent; it rises sharply to an excruciating peak and then goes away fairly suddenly as the muscle in the wall of the organ relaxes. Colic occurs in individuals with obstruction of the gastrointestinal tract by tumors, polyps, foreign bodies, or adhesions.

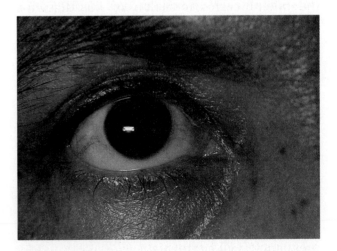

FIGURE 34–2

Careful inspection of the sclera, or normally white portion, of the eye in good lighting may reveal even mild degrees of jaundice.

Obstruction in the small bowel is generally noted as colic located around the umbilicus. In the right or left colon, obstruction produces a pain that is felt in the same flank. Individuals who have a kidney stone obstructing a ureter experience a characteristic radiation of pain from the flank into the genitalia. The pain from a kidney stone is severe.

Colic is a common complaint among children, where it represents very active peristalsis in the gastrointestinal tract. It is also a relatively frequent complaint in the adult in association with "flu" syndrome and vigorous diarrhea. Again, in this situation, it is associated with extreme activity of the gastrointestinal tract. Frequently, the patient will describe colic as a cramp or a "gas pain."

You must be familiar with colic and be able to recognize the characteristic pain when it is described. It is a very distressing complaint for the patient. Generally, although colic is not an acute emergency, you must transport these patients to the emergency department because the cause must be assessed by a physician.

Heartburn (Esophageal Reflux)

The esophagus is lined with tissue that is similar to the skin. Because it does not produce mucus, it has no capacity to protect itself from the potent corrosive action of the digestive enzymes in gastric juice. Occasionally, gastric juice will reflux into the lower esophagus and attack its lining. The damage to the lining can range from mild irritation to deep ulcers and even perforation of the esophagus in extreme cases. Esophageal reflux causes a typical burning pain referred to as heartburn, under the sternum. Usually, the pain occurs after heavy meals, drinking to excess, or at night when a person is lying in bed. It occurs most frequently in the obese, short patient and is aggravated by straining, squatting, or lifting. Anything that increases the intraabdominal pressure (such as pregnancy) will aggravate it.

Esophageal reflux and heartburn are commonly associated with a specific anatomic abnormality, *sliding hiatal hernia*. In this situation the junction of the esophagus and stomach herniates, or slides, into the chest through the hiatus or opening in the diaphragm. In this position, gastric juice can easily irritate the esophagus, causing heartburn. This problem is complex and must be addressed by a physician.

Esophageal reflux is a common problem but not an emergency. However, the symptom of substernal chest pain can be caused by other, more serious, disorders. You must be alert to the patient complaining of "indigestion" or "heartburn" whose symptoms may be due to an acute myocardial infarction, a peptic ulcer, or acute gallbladder disease.

Transport patients with any substernal pain to the emergency department promptly to allow a physician to diagnose the exact cause.

Bulimia and Anorexia Nervosa

Bulimia is defined as an abnormal increase in the sensation of hunger. Bulimia results in significant overeating followed by self-induced vomiting. In this way, the bulimic individual maintains a relatively normal weight.

Anorexia nervosa, in contrast, is defined as lack or loss of appetite. Characteristically, the patient takes less and less food and may become seriously emaciated and malnourished.

Bulimia may occur at any age, but it is rare in older individuals. Anorexia nervosa is much more common in younger women. Neither is a strict emergency situation, although you may be called if anorexia nervosa has caused severe problems in nutrition. Each situation is a manifestation of a rather severe underlying psychological disorder. Each requires skilled treatment for a prolonged period of time. You must recognize the need for this type of care in these patients. Emergency transport ordinarily will be needed only by the neglected, severely dehydrated, and starved anorexic patient or by the bulimic individual who is experiencing a specific problem related to vomiting.

A warning for the EMT is that significant instances of drug abuse with syrup of ipecac, a drug traditionally used to induce vomiting in patients who have swallowed a poisonous substance, are now being reported in bulimic patients. Drug abuse of this type is rarely suspected. Ambulance supplies of this medication should therefore be carefully supervised.

Constipation

Constipation in the older individual is a frequent and generally progressive phenomenon. As patients become less and less physically active, bowel activity similarly tends to decrease. Much more important is that the older person's diet tends to become softer and include fewer fresh fruits, vegetables, and foods with high levels of bulk. If such a person loses teeth, he or she may have some difficulty in chewing and swallowing. Automatically, the patient with fewer teeth prefers softer and mushier foods. This type of diet produces a very small, hard stool that takes considerable effort to pass. Many individuals, especially those bedridden or in nursing homes, cease to make the effort to have regular bowel movements.

After some time, the colon (large bowel) becomes greatly distended with accumulated feces. Ironically, constipated patients may develop a watery diarrhea, which is caused by a substantial fecal impaction. In this situation, the only material that can pass down the gastrointestinal tract and around the impaction is liquid; the liquid literally flows around the obstruction. Fecal impaction is one of the more common problems of the older patient. It is often a cause of partial bowel obstruction.

Unfortunately, in the older patient the rather common complaint of chronic constipation frequently masks a very serious cause of progressive constipation and obstruction—cancer of the colon. A common presenting complaint of colon cancer is difficulty passing stools, up to and including complete obstruction. For this reason alone, the elderly patient who complains of increasing and severe constipation should be taken to the hospital emergency department for diagnosis.

THE URINARY TRACT

Dysuria

Dysuria is a sensation of pain, burning, or itching that occurs during urination. It generally indicates an inflammatory process or infection within the lower urinary tract, which includes the external urethral opening, the urethra, and the bladder. Dysuria is a relatively common symptom in females because of their higher frequency of urinary tract infections. Although dysuria is symptomatic of a problem that should be evaluated and treated, it is not a significant emergency situation. Patients should be advised to consult with their physicians.

Hematuria

The passage of blood in the urine is called **hematuria.** Occasionally there is enough of it to be visible to the naked eye. More frequently, however, it is identified only by microscopic examination of a urine specimen. Hematuria has a number of causes: tumors of the urinary tract, stones causing abrasions and bleeding from the kidney or the ureters, and trauma are some of the more common causes. If called for this problem, you should transport the patient to the emergency department for an appropriate diagnostic workup. Except following an injury, hematuria is not an emergency situation. However, if it is easily evident to the unaided eye, it may point to a very serious problem within the urinary tract. Expeditious diagnosis is demanded, especially if the patient has no pain. Hematuria associated with pain, burning, or itching usually means infection. Hematuria caused by trauma is discussed in Chapter 26.

Any urine passed by the patient with significant urinary complaints should be brought to the emergency department for analysis. Frequently, it can provide the necessary clue for diagnosis.

Frequency

The term *frequency* describes an abnormally high number of voiding (urinating) episodes during any 24-hour period. Frequency associated with dysuria usually indicates a bladder infection. Infection usually causes the passage of very small quantities of urine at very frequent intervals. Generally, the urine associated with a bladder infection has a foul odor.

In the aging male, the prostate gland, which surrounds the upper portion of the urethra as it joins the bladder, commonly enlarges. As this gland grows, it squeezes on the urethral passage and partially obstructs it. A sign of this obstruction is urinary frequency, which persists not only during the day but throughout the night as well. The passage of urine at night is called **nocturia.** Congestive heart failure is another problem which can often cause frequency and nocturia in the older patient.

Urinary frequency is not an emergency situation, but you should recognize that its presence signifies an underlying disorder that requires treatment.

Incontinence

The uncontrolled passage of urine or feces resulting in soiling of one's clothing is called **incontinence.** It may occur in several emergency conditions. For example, the patient undergoing an epileptic seizure frequently experiences incontinence during the seizure. In this situation incontinence does not indicate significant urinary or bowel disease. The patient with a spinal cord injury resulting in paraplegia has lost control of the muscular sphincters that control both urinary and fecal discharge.

Episodic incontinence is frequently associated with unconsciousness or semiconsciousness, as in an alcoholic binge. The elderly patient may be incontinent as a result of generalized senile degeneration of the brain cells that provide control.

Incontinence that is sudden, unexpected, and not associated with any obvious cause may signal the presence of a significant disorder in the lower urinary tract or rectum. Such incontinence is a reason to transport the patient to the hospital for diagnosis.

Renal Colic

A fairly common clinical problem is the formation of kidney stones. Once formed, the stones usually cannot be dissolved in the body. As long as the stones are in the kidney they do not cause pain. At the most, they may produce

hematuria, which may not be apparent unless the urine is examined microscopically for red blood cells.

A stone that passes from the kidney into the ureter can obstruct this very small caliber tube. Urine is formed continuously in the kidney. Approximately 1 liter of it is passed out of each kidney through the ureters into the bladder every day. There is no reservoir for urine above the bladder and the capacity of the ureters and the collecting system of the kidney is very small. Therefore, this liter of urine must pass quickly through the ureter into the bladder without impediment. When a ureter becomes obstructed by a stone, a characteristic severe pain (renal colic) occurs as the muscular ureter tries to overcome the obstruction by very vigorous peristalsis close to the stone (Figure 34–3). The colic is perceived as an excruciatingly sharp cramping pain in the flank on the right or left side of the back. As the stone progresses down the ureter, the pain may radiate to the groin and the external genitalia. Once the stone enters the bladder, the renal colic ceases. Renal colic is one of the severest forms of pain known. Relief requires very vigorous treatment.

The patient suffering from renal colic can describe the type of pain, its location, and its radiation. This patient is generally restless and forever seeking a position of some comfort—getting up or lying down. An attack of renal colic is not a life-threatening situation for the patient. It is, however, an urgent one in which the patient demands and requires relief from pain. If your patient suffers from renal colic, transport him or her promptly to the emergency department. Ordinarily, no significant measures for support of other body systems are necessary. Any urine passed should be collected, saved, and presented for analysis at the hospital.

Acute Urinary Retention

Occasionally, and most often in the older male patient, you will encounter acute urinary retention. Ordinarily, this situation occurs as an event in a long history of urinary difficulty characterized by gradual loss of force of the

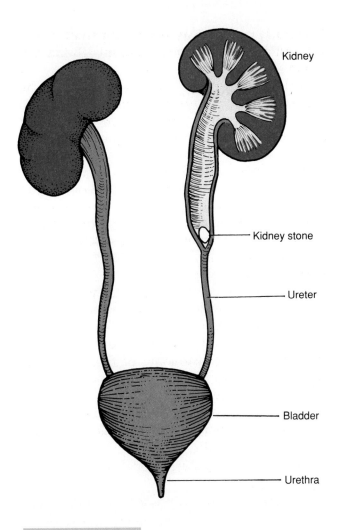

A kidney stone produces excruciating pain called renal colic when it passes from the kidney where it is formed and into the ureter. The stone obstructs the ureter and causes distension.

Kidney

Kidney stone

Ureter

Bladder

Urethra

urinary stream, increasing urinary frequency, and nocturia. Usually it results from a slowly progressive enlargement of the prostate gland so that the urethral outlet of the bladder becomes obstructed. This enlargement can be benign (prostatic hypertrophy) or malignant (prostatic cancer).

The discomfort of acute bladder distension is intense, and the urge to void is overwhelming. As more urine is produced by the kidneys, the bladder may enlarge up to the level of the umbilicus. This situation can develop over a matter of a very few hours and requires prompt

transport to the emergency department. Relief will be obtained only by *catheterization* (inserting a tube directly into the bladder). Catheterizing the patient will be done by personnel in the emergency department; in this situation, it can be a difficult procedure. Ordinarily, the catheter will be left in until the obstruction can be corrected.

THE FEMALE GENITAL TRACT

A number of gynecologic problems that cause acute pain have been described in Chapter 33. Some are reviewed here and additional ones, not causing severe discomfort, are presented.

Vaginal Spotting, Bleeding, and Discharge

A normal menstrual cycle produces a monthly, bloody vaginal discharge in all healthy, nonpregnant women after puberty and before menopause. The characteristics of the bleeding vary from individual to individual and are usually well known to the woman (length of flow, amount of material discharged, presence or absence of cramps, and onset and termination). Any other vaginal discharge is abnormal.

The most common causes of abnormal vaginal discharge are fungal or bacterial infections in the vagina. The complaint of vaginal discharge does not signify an emergency condition, and immediate transport to the hospital is not necessary. Medical care and advice should be recommended and sought.

Any bleeding from the vagina, other than menstrual, is abnormal. The most common and least serious cause relates to abnormalities of the menstrual cycle. However, vaginal bleeding may be the only sign of malignant disease within the female reproductive system, especially of the cervix or uterus. Bleeding after sexual contact may be an early sign of these tumors.

In general, vaginal bleeding is not an acute medical emergency because the volume of blood lost is usually quite small. Bleeding, however, indicates the likelihood of a serious problem requiring prompt diagnosis. Unfortunately, as with many other clinical signs, the patient tends to ignore bleeding if there is no pain. For this reason, you must encourage the patient to seek medical evaluation and even offer transport to the emergency department for diagnosis. You should not examine the female genitalia or vagina, or pack or put anything into the vagina.

Ectopic Pregnancy

Ectopic pregnancy, described in Chapter 33, is the development of a fetus in an abnormal location, usually in the Fallopian tube. It occurs on rare occasions when an ovum, after being discharged from the ovary, becomes fertilized early in its passage to the uterus through the Fallopian tube. The ovum sometimes comes to rest within the tube rather than in the cavity of the uterus. The Fallopian tube is a relatively thin-walled structure with little muscular content. It does not have the capacity to expand to encompass the developing fetus. If the fertilized ovum lodges there, the Fallopian tube can support the growth of the fetus and its placenta for approximately six to eight weeks. Then the tube, stretched beyond its capacity to expand, ruptures.

Rupture of the Fallopian tube with a contained pregnancy can cause severe bleeding into the abdominal cavity. The patient may have sudden, severe lower abdominal pain and tenderness and may rapidly develop hypovolemic shock.

Any woman who can give a history of appropriate sexual exposure, with one or two missed menstrual periods, who is in shock, and who may have a tender lower abdomen must be suspected of having an ectopic pregnancy.

The emergency medical treatment for this patient is based on anticipating and treating shock. All the measures needed for the correction of hypovolemic shock must be instituted. Prompt transportation to the hospital is mandatory, because the bleeding usually continues and may become life-threatening. This patient will require an emergency surgical procedure to control the problem.

THE MALE GENITAL TRACT

Urethral Discharge

Any material that passes out of the male urethra other than urine or semen is called a *urethral discharge*. It is an abnormal condition that requires medical attention. Urethral discharge is the most common indication, in the male, of sexually transmitted disease—an extremely widespread problem in the United States today. The penile urethral discharge may be thin and watery or it may be grossly **purulent** (containing pus).

If you are called for the patient whose only complaint is a urethral discharge, the situation is not an emergency. However, treatment for the cause of the discharge should be sought immediately, because some of these diseases can become chronic and produce devastating effects for the individual years later. Additionally, the individual is a carrier of and a potential transmitter of sexually related diseases.

External Genitalia

Hernias were described in Chapter 33. However, some conditions involving the scrotum and testes, although mimicking a hernia, are quite different.

The testis can develop a number of masses. A *hydrocele* is a sac of water that is trapped about the testis or the spermatic cord. Hydroceles are usually soft and painless. Although an operation may be required to repair the problem, it is not an acute emergency. Other masses of the testis may be tumors. They are not emergency situations but do require prompt, usually surgical, diagnosis and treatment.

Painful masses may represent *orchitis* (inflammation or infection of the testis) or *epididymitis* (inflammation or infection of a part of the spermatic cord). These situations are acute emergencies. Apart from the painful swollen mass that requires treatment, the patient may have fever and other signs of sepsis. Transport this patient, supine, to the emergency department for treatment as soon as possible.

In some younger males, the testis may twist on the spermatic cord and become swollen and very painful. This condition is called *testicular torsion*. It requires immediate treatment and mandates prompt transport to the emergency department.

VERTIGO, HICCUPS, AND HEADACHE

Vertigo

The problem of **vertigo** (dizziness) is relatively common, especially among the aging population. It usually is caused by arteriosclerosis of the cerebral blood vessels, which produces impaired circulation in the brain. Injuries or infections of the inner ear can also cause vertigo. In these cases, the vertigo is usually accompanied by **tinnitus** (ringing in the ear). Certain medications are available to counteract vertigo even when the exact cause is unknown.

In general, vertigo is not an acute emergency problem. It can be so severe, however, that the patient is literally confined to bed, unable to walk or sit safely. When vertigo is this severe, the cause must be identified. Transport this patient to the emergency department for diagnosis and care. It is not uncommon for these patients to be nauseated, so you must be alert for vomiting. Ordinarily, no care other than keeping the patient lying flat and comfortable is needed. Vertigo in which there is an actual sensation of rotating in space should be distinguished from lightheadedness or giddiness, which is a much more common complaint.

Hiccups

Hiccups, a common complaint that arises from a variety of causes, is a sudden inspiration of air that is rapidly checked by closure of the epiglottis of the larynx. In the healthy individual, it results from acute distension of the stomach, from anxiety, or, occasionally, from a central nervous system problem. Irritation of the diaphragm, particularly the presence of an abscess in a postoperative patient, will cause persistent hiccups. Rarely is this condition an emergency medical problem. It becomes so only if it has lasted for several hours or days and interferes with eating and sleeping. A number of hospital treatments exist, ranging from rebreathing inspired air to the use of intravenous sedative medication. In general, if the symptoms are severe and persistent enough to warrant calling an emergency medical service, transportation to the emergency department is indicated.

Headaches

One of the most common causes for emergency calls, visits to doctor's offices, or general patient concern is the headache. Some 90 percent of the population experience them; statistics concerning headaches are revealing. They are among the 10 top reasons for emergency department visits. In a recent survey, they accounted for 18 million visits to doctors in one year. Nearly 14 percent of men in the United States and twice as many women report headaches as a frequent experience.

In the practical management of this problem, you should divide headache into two categories: chronic and acute. Patients with chronic, recurrent long-standing headache problems will usually already have sought medical help. If you can ascertain that this is a long-standing problem (months or years) and the patient has not received nor sought help, he should be directed to his physician. A variety of well recognized causes of headache exist and effective treatment is often available.

An acute severe headache may be caused by many different problems. Stroke, brain tumor, tension, drug use, postconcussion states, sinusitis, arthritis of the temporomandibular joint, viral or bacterial infections, fever, facial or cervical spine lesions, and hunger are some of the more common causes. Your role will not be to diagnose the cause of this problem but to recognize its existence and gauge its severity.

The acutely affected patient should be transported to the emergency department for evaluation and treatment.

In the instance of headache associated with stroke or brain tumor, other neurological signs will also be present. In these instances, transportation of this patient is an urgent matter.

SPECIAL CONCERNS FOR GERIATRIC PATIENTS

Most of the problems discussed in this chapter occur in adults. A few of them are much more complicated in the **geriatric** (older) patient. Sudden changes or rapid moves from familiar surroundings may easily disorient or terrify elderly patients. They may respond with a combative attitude. Not infrequently, they stubbornly refuse to accept the most obviously needed methods of treatment. In these situations, the cooperation of friends and family, along with patience and a calm approach on your part, are all absolutely necessary. Generally, the wishes of the patient and the patient's family must be respected unless the emergency is obviously life-threatening.

The older patient's physiological response to disease is as important as the psychological reactions just described. In general, the older (over 70 years of age) individual's response to almost any disease is slower and less intense. Complaints of pain or tenderness are frequently denied by the patient until they become very serious. Consequently, symptoms are often ignored by those taking care of the geriatric person. Thus, it is not uncommon that any disease will have proceeded much further along its course in this group than in younger patients. You are likely to encounter more seriously ill patients with more systemic results of their problems, such as

- Signs and symptoms of developing shock.
- Dehydration.
- Generalized sepsis.

The result of this rather poor response to disease is that you must consider the older patient with a specific complaint as seriously ill,

requiring aggressive support and prompt transportation.

Two diseases that are much more common in the older patient are osteoporosis and vascular disease. You should be aware of how these two conditions can cause serious problems for the elderly patient.

Osteoporosis is a condition most commonly seen in the aging woman, but it affects older men as well. It is a gradual and progressive loss of calcium from all bones of the body. Bone so affected becomes weaker and is much more likely to fracture. Osteoporosis is a complex problem. Its cause and treatment are not fully understood at the present time. In some older patients, trivial injuries may result in complex fractures. Occasionally, the fracture may be spontaneous, caused simply by contraction of the patient's own muscles. Emergency treatment is the same for these patients as for those with any other similar fracture. You, as an EMT, cannot treat osteoporosis. You must, however, recognize the existence of the condition and suspect a fracture in the elderly patient even after insignificant trauma.

Vascular problems occur frequently in the elderly. Eventually arteriosclerosis will develop in all the blood vessels. The older population will be more at risk for a heart attack or stroke. The peripheral blood vessels in the extremities are particularly likely to develop arteriosclerotic disease. Cold extremities, ulcers or infections of the toes or feet, or an abscess following a trivial injury such as a torn toenail are not uncommon. Most of these situations do not pose significant emergency problems. You will, however, find some instances of severe foot infections that obviously have been neglected by the patient. In these instances, the patient will require hospital treatment to resolve the problem completely.

Older patients, especially those living alone, tend to neglect themselves. There are a number of reasons why this occurs.

- It is difficult to prepare three meals a day for only one person and many elderly people neglect to do so.
- The fear of spending money that may be "needed later" is sometimes very great for

people living on fixed incomes and leads to economies that may be detrimental to the patient.

- The effort required to circulate, socialize, and meet other people is often too strenuous for an older person.
- Long established habits are difficult to change.
- Many elderly patients are afraid or cannot afford to seek timely medical help.

As a result, it is not uncommon to receive an older patient in a hospital with a medical problem who is significantly malnourished, who has no family contact, and who may have several significant medical problems. You must be aware of these considerations in assessing and transporting the older, especially single, patient. They can significantly complicate matters for the patient.

EMT SAFETY

For most of the problems described in this chapter, you will not be exposed to any major extra risk. Hematemesis, hematochezia, and melena all involve your potential contact with the patient's blood. Gloves, masks, thorough handwashing and cleansing when the patient has been delivered will protect you best from the transmission of diseases such as AIDS. In all instances when you are exposed to the patient's excrement, be careful to wear gloves and masks and use good handwashing. The presence of jaundice should alert you to take special care with that patient because the jaundice may be caused by hepatitis.

YOU ARE THE EMT

1. The patient is in shock as a result of long hours of vomiting. Why is this condition as serious as that resulting from a severe burn or uncontrolled internal bleeding?
2. You have been called to a medical emergency in which a female patient is vomiting blood. Identify and describe three possible causes of hematemesis.
3. How does anorexia nervosa differ from bulimia? Why do you think it occurs most often among young females?
4. What are kidney stones, and why do they cause such terrific pain?
5. A male patient complains of a swollen painful testicular mass. What are some of the conditions that can cause this situation?
6. Define four terms descriptive of bleeding from the gastrointestinal tract and state the meaning of each.
7. An 80-year old woman and her 50-year old daughter have slipped and fallen on an icy sidewalk in winter. Would you expect the older woman to have sustained a fracture more readily than her daughter? Why?
8. The elderly person living alone is more likely to have medical problems in addition to a given emergency complaint than a younger person; give four reasons why.

CHAPTER 35

COMMUNICABLE DISEASES

KEY TERMS

body substance isolation (BSI) The procedure of using barriers for self-protection when handling blood and body fluids.

carrier An animal or person who may transmit an infectious disease but does not display any symptoms of it.

communicable (kŏ-mu'nĭ-kah-b'l) (contagious) Capable of transmitting disease.

contamination The presence of infective organisms on or in objects such as dressings, water, food, or on the patient's body.

hepatitis (hep"ah-ti'tis) An infection of the liver caused by a virus that causes fever, loss of appetite, jaundice, and fatigue.

HIV infection Acquired immunodeficiency syndrome (AIDS).

host The organism or individual attacked by the infecting agent (the host is infected).

incubation period (in"ku-ba'shun pe're-od) The time between exposure of the host to the infectious agent and the appearance of symptoms of that infection.

infection (in-fek'shun) The invasion of a host or host tissue by organisms such as bacteria, viruses, or parasites.

infectious disease Clinical disease resulting from an infection.

meningitis (men"in-ji'tis) An inflammation of the meningeal coverings of the brain; it can be caused by a virus or a bacterium.

transmission The manner by which an infectious agent is spread: contact, airborne, by vehicles, or by vectors.

tuberculosis (TB) (too-ber"ku-lo'sis) A chronic bacterial disease that usually affects the lungs. Signs and symptoms are cough, fatigue, weight loss, chest pain, and coughing up of blood.

universal precautions Protective measures developed by the Centers for Disease Control (CDC) for use when dealing with objects that might accidentally puncture the skin of a health care worker.

window phase of testing The time from exposure to a disease to the time lab tests note the presence of an antibody.

512

Communicable diseases go back to the origins of man. In epidemic proportions they have killed more people than wars or natural disasters. Smallpox, typhoid, and influenza have been catastrophic enough to change the course of history. Medical research, vaccines, and improvements in sanitation have eradicated many communicable diseases, but germs still exist and are transmitted to humans by other humans or by insects and animals. Old diseases have been replaced by new ones: Acquired immunodeficiency syndrome (AIDS), for example, is the communicable disease perhaps most feared today.

EMTs, doctors, nurses, and other medical personnel are sometimes exposed to communicable diseases. It is very important for these personnel to become knowledgeable in lessening the risk of exposure and taking preventive actions after exposure. Chapter 35 explains how communicable diseases are transmitted and how to prevent their transmission. Part of prevention is identifying patients with contagious diseases—often a difficult task. The chapter next describes five communicable diseases that are apt to cause problems for EMTs and other care providers: hepatitis, herpetic whitlow, meningitis, tuberculosis, and HIV infection. The last section of Chapter 35 reviews risk and prevention procedures that should be followed by all EMTs.

GOALS
. . . .

The goals of Chapter 35 are to

- understand communicable diseases and the infectious process.
- understand the role of the EMT in treating a patient with a communicable disease.
- become familiar with the characteristics and basic epidemiology of common communicable diseases.

ROUTES OF TRANSMISSION
. . . .

The term **communicable** disease refers to an illness that can be transmitted from one person to another. The *mode of transmission* (method of transfer) can take place in one of four ways (Figure 35–1):

- *Contact transmission.* There are two methods of contact: direct and indirect. Direct physical contact takes place between an individual and the infected person. Indirect physical contact takes place between an individual and inanimate objects that may have infectious organisms on them—for example, vehicle surfaces, dressings, equipment, or linens. Such objects are said to be **contaminated.**
- *Airborne transmission.* The infective organism is introduced into the air by a patient who is coughing or sneezing. Droplets of mucus that carry bacteria or other organisms can then be inhaled by another individual.
- *Vehicle transmission.* The infective organism is introduced directly into the body through the

A

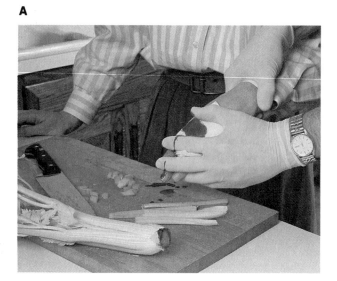

B

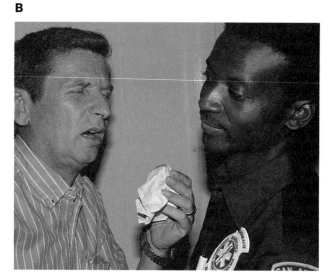

C

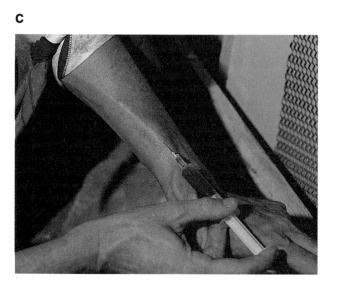

D

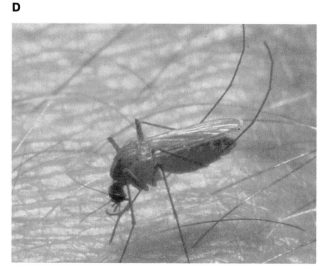

FIGURE 35–1   There are four major methods of transmission of infectious disease: (A) Contact—touching materials contaminated by infectious organisms; (B) airborne—inhaling droplets containing infectious organisms; (C) vehicle—using contaminated needles or other instruments; and (D) vector—being bitten by an animal or insect that is carrying disease.

ingestion of contaminated food, or water, or by the infusion of contaminated drugs, fluid, or blood.

■ *Vector transmission.* The infective organism is transmitted to an individual by animals; for example, mosquitoes transmit malarial parasites, and ticks transmit Rocky Mountain spotted fever. Vector-borne diseases rarely

present a great risk to prehospital care providers.

Vehicle and vector transmission present little additional risk for an EMT. The greatest opportunity for acquiring a communicable disease is through direct or indirect contact. When rendering care, care providers often do not take the time to wash their hands thoroughly after contact with a patient or contaminated materials. When this simple procedure is omitted, the opportunity for infection increases, especially if the care provider engages in hand-to-nose or hand-to-mouth treatment.

Airborne transmission can present a risk of infection; but it is less likely than with direct or indirect contact. The method of organism transfer and the duration of exposure to the patient play major roles. In general, there must be contact with a coughing or sneezing patient, direct contact with sputum produced, or prolonged exposure to the patient. In most areas, transport times and conditions do not fulfill these requirements. For instance, if you transport a patient and later find out that the patient had tuberculosis, the risk to you is minimal.

Whether an **infection** develops depends on four factors:

- The amount of the organism present.
- The degree to which the organism survives when exposed to light and air, or its *virulence*.
- The individual's resistance to infection.
- The portal of entry into the body.

These factors can best be related by the following formula:

$$\text{infection} = \frac{\text{dose} \times \text{virulence} \times \text{portal of entry}}{\text{resistance of the host}}$$

Each part of this formula should be considered when you evaluate exposure in a particular situation. In most instances, transporting a patient with a communicable disease does not place you at risk. The actual risk, in any situation, arises when you have direct contact with the infective organism for a given disease. In general, actual risk is much less than perceived risk in any infectious situation. Knowledge of how each disease is spread and how to block the spread is your major protective measure.

PREVENTION

All persons involved in the care of patients are at risk for acquiring an infectious or communicable disease. The risk can be minimized, however, by using basic protective measures. EMTs are responsible for protecting themselves, other personnel, and other patients.

Prevention begins with maintenance of your personal health. Regular annual health examinations should be required for all personnel. A history of all of your childhood **infectious diseases** (for example, measles, mumps, whooping cough, or chicken pox) should be recorded and kept on file. If you have not had one of these diseases, obtain the appropriate immunizations. Immunizations should be kept up to date and recorded in your health file. Recommended immunizations include:

- Measles vaccine.
- Rubella (German measles) vaccine.
- Tetanus-diphtheria boosters.
- Mumps vaccine.
- Influenza vaccine (yearly).
- Hepatitis B vaccine.

All EMTs should be skin tested for tuberculosis (PPD testing) prior to employment to identify those who have been exposed to the disease in the past. PPD testing should be repeated every year.

Knowing beforehand that a patient to be transported has a communicable disease is a definite advantage. This is when your health record will be valuable. If you have already had the disease or been vaccinated against it, of course, you are not at risk. Otherwise, you must take appropriate protective measures. Not all patients with a communicable disease will be identified initially, however. Therefore, preventive measures must be practiced whenever possible.

Many times patients can be **carriers** of diseases and not exhibit symptoms. For example, you may treat a patient who is bleeding and not realize that the patient has hepatitis. If you have an open cut anywhere, the virus can enter and cause infection. Handwashing is the single most important measure for self-protection. It should be carried out before and as soon after contact as possible. Some handwashing agents, such as those that have an alcohol base, do not require running water. They are a good first line of defense until you can perform a proper handwashing (Figure 35–2).

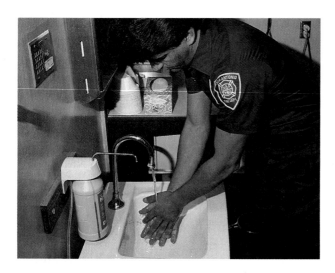

FIGURE 35–2

The single most important measure for self-protection against contagious disease is thorough handwashing.

TABLE 35–1	Protective Measures Against Possible Signs and Symptoms of Communicable Disease
Signs and Symptoms	**Protective Measures**
Presence of fever and rash	Mask
Diarrhea	Handwashing, use disposable gloves when in contact with stool; wash hands after gloves are removed.
Draining wounds (pus or blood oozing)	Handwashing; use disposable gloves when touching drainage; wash hands after gloves are removed; apply dressing to wound.
Jaundice (yellow tinge to the skin or sclera of eyes)	Handwashing; use disposable gloves when touching blood or secretions; wash hands after gloves are removed

IDENTIFICATION OF COMMUNICABLE DISEASE PATIENTS

Identifying a patient as having a possible communicable disease is often difficult. Ordinarily, you do not have an established diagnosis when you answer a call and must respond based on presenting symptoms. Table 35–1 details general protective measures that are appropriate when communicable disease could be a threat. **Universal precautions** using **body substance isolation (BSI)** should be instituted as a routine procedure.

In any instance in which exposure is documented or suspected, there should be an established protocol for you to follow. The protocol should list the steps to be followed to ensure proper follow-up. Care should begin with the completion of an incident report to document the specific events. Specific information regarding the patient will be available from the hospital. The infection control practitioner at each hospital is a valuable resource person who can review the events of the exposure, evaluate your contact with the patient, and provide initial information regarding the need for additional follow-up. Follow-up and docu-

mentation of work-related illnesses or exposure are each very important.

You should not take field exposures lightly. An example of a field exposure that is often ignored by the care provider or the hospital is a needle stick injury. A puncture wound from a needle stick should never be ignored. The needle may itself be contaminated, and the risk of contracting hepatitis is high. Every hospital has a needle stick protocol. You must be familiar with the procedures followed in your area and make sure they are followed whenever a needle stick injury occurs.

DISEASES THAT CAUSE CONCERN

Several communicable diseases raise concern among prehospital care providers. They include, among others, hepatitis, herpetic whitlow, meningitis, tuberculosis (TB), and AIDS.

In most cases, the risk to the prehospital care provider is minimal.

Hepatitis

Hepatitis can be caused by chemicals, alcohol, or drugs as well as by viruses. The first three forms of the disease are not communicable and are relatively common. Several viral types of hepatitis also exist and are communicable.

- Type A (viral or infectious).
- Type B (serum).
- Type non-A, non-B (Type C or transfusion).

Hepatitis A is a disease usually seen in children. Most children who have it do not show any symptoms. They do pass it to their parents (during close contact, especially diaper changes). Hepatitis A does not have serious complications, and the patient usually recovers without difficulty. Hepatitis A can also be acquired by the ingestion of the virus through contaminated shellfish or water.

Hepatitis B, also known as serum hepatitis, is caused by a virus that is spread through blood-to-blood contact (transfusion, needle stick), mucous membrane (saliva or sputum contact), or sexual contact. The virus is hardy; it can survive for long periods of time in the environment. It has been found alive on surfaces for six weeks and longer.

The primary symptoms and signs are nausea, vomiting, fatigue, abdominal pain, and jaundice. The patient with hepatitis B can be very hard to identify, because many individuals who have the disease do not demonstrate the primary symptoms or signs. Many individuals will have only "flu" symptoms, which are often overlooked. The **incubation period** for hepatitis B is very long—from 42 to 200 days after exposure.

Serum hepatitis is a disease that has been shown to have long-term serious effects for many of the individuals who acquire it. Many patients become carriers or develop chronic hepatitis. A relationship has been established between the incidence of hepatitis B and liver cancer. Thus, you can appreciate the efforts to eradicate this disease through vaccination in high-risk groups. There is no specific treatment for hepatitis B nor is there a cure for the disease once it has been acquired.

Because prehospital care personnel have a high degree of contact with blood from patients, vaccination for them is recommended. To protect against exposure to hepatitis B, you should carry out the following steps:

1. Practice good handwashing techniques.
2. Wear disposable gloves whenever you have contact with blood or oral secretions.
3. Clean blood-contaminated areas in the vehicle with a bleach solution.
4. Use proper technique for needle disposal. Do not recap needles and do not cut them; dispose of them in a puncture-resistant container.
5. Participate in a hepatitis B vaccination program.

Non-A, non-B hepatitis (NANB) presents itself in a similar manner as the other forms of hepatitis. It is currently believed that there are two different viruses in the NANB group, because there appears to be two different incubation periods—one long and one short. It is felt that the majority of cases of this disease are related to blood transfusions. This form has now been named hepatitis type C. Thus, contact with blood and/or needlestick injury poses a risk for NANB hepatitis. In December 1990, a test became commercially available to screen blood for hepatitis type C (NANB) prior to transfusion. However, due to the **window phase of testing,** even with this screening test, all blood given in transfusions will not be 100 percent free of NANB.

Herpetic Whitlow

Another recognized occupational health risk is *herpetic whitlow*. Herpetic whitlow is a herpes viral infection of the finger. It is acquired when a care provider has breaks in the skin of the hands and has direct contact with the oral secretions of a patient actively infected with herpes virus. Like other herpes viral infections, there is no cure for this disease. It will recur from time to time. The incubation period is 2 to

12 days following exposure, but it may vary among individuals. The symptoms are redness, swelling, pain, and nerve impairment of the finger or hand. Treatment is supportive, to relieve the pain. There is no cure, so prevention is especially important. Measures for protection include good handwashing, especially if there are breaks in the skin, and the use of disposable gloves for any contact with a patient's oral secretions.

Meningitis

Meningitis, an inflammation of the meningeal coverings of the brain, may be caused by either a virus or a bacterium. The patient who has viral meningitis does not present a significant risk to you. The viral form of the disease is usually transmitted via food or water. Bacterial meningitis does carry a risk for **transmission,** especially if there is direct contact with nasopharyngeal secretions from suctioning the patient, from giving mouth-to-mouth ventilation, or from the patient's coughing into your face. Even under these circumstances, only a few forms of meningitis from very specific bacteria are transmitted—and these only rarely. In each of these instances, there would be a recommendation for follow-up care. You should also follow the local guidelines for exposure to communicable diseases.

Tuberculosis

Tuberculosis (TB) is another disease that creates concern for those involved in the care of the patient. However, TB is not a highly communicable disease. The organism that causes tuberculosis is known to reside in the lungs. If the patient is not coughing and creating droplets, the disease is not communicable. Risk occurs only through direct contact with a coughing patient, or the patient's sputum. Simply transporting a patient does not create a high risk. Care providers who work in an area where the incidence of tuberculosis is high should undergo skin testing and follow-up.

HIV Infection/AIDS (Acquired Immunodeficiency Syndrome)

HIV infection is caused by the human immunodeficiency virus (HIV), which was discovered in 1983. HIV attacks and destroys certain white blood cells of the immune system, the T4 lymphocytes. The loss of these cells makes the HIV-infected individual prone to *opportunistic infections* (infection by organisms that do not commonly cause disease in humans). The virus does not survive outside of the body in sufficient numbers to cause infection and is easily killed by drying and most commonly used disinfectants.

Epidemiologic studies since 1981 have shown that HIV is transmitted by direct contact with HIV-infected blood, semen, or vaginal secretions; it can also be transmitted across the placenta to offspring of HIV-infected mothers. In addition, it is likely that cerebrospinal, pericardial, joint, and amniotic fluids may be capable of transmitting the HIV infection. There is no scientific documentation that HIV infection is caused by contact with tears, sweat, saliva, sputum, urine, feces, vomitus, or nasal secretions, *unless* those fluids contain grossly visible blood. HIV infection is *not* transmitted by handshaking, kissing, toilet seats, telephones, hot tubs, swimming pools, or mosquitoes. It is possible, but unlikely, that a human bite could transmit the HIV infection. However, the Centers for Disease Control (CDC) advises EMTs who come in contact with body fluids in situations where distinguishing fluid types is difficult, "to treat all body fluids as potentially hazardous" and use body substance isolation procedures.

The natural history of HIV infection/AIDS is described as occurring in stages, depending on how the immune system is impaired by the disease. Once HIV infection has occurred, the body begins to produce antibodies to the virus. These antibodies can be detected by the ELISA blood test 6 to 12 weeks after infection. In some cases, the ELISA test is incorrectly positive for HIV infection: a false-positive. Therefore, a positive ELISA test should be confirmed by another test, the Western Blot test. Another test, an antigen test, is designed to directly detect the virus. Combined with the ELISA and Western Blot tests, this antigen test should yield more conclusive information.

The CDC has divided HIV infection into four clinical classes:

- *Group 1: Acute Infection:* Individuals experience a flu-like illness and the ELISA and Western Blot tests subsequently become positive ("seropositive");
- *Group 2: Asymptomatic Infection:* Individuals are "seropositive" and have changes in T4 cell counts;
- *Group 3: Persistent Generalized Lymphadenopathy:* Patients have swollen lymph glands at two or more sites which persist for more than three months; and,
- *Group 4: Other Illnesses:* Patients experience one or more of the following: mental disorientation (dementia), muscle wasting and weakness (myelopathy), peripheral nerve numbness and weakness (neuropathy), fever, and/or diarrhea for more than one month, and/or more than 10 percent weight loss.

Over 95 percent of all HIV infections are found among intravenous (IV) drug users who share needles, homosexual and bisexual men, and sexual partners of HIV-infected persons. Other high-risk groups are hemophiliacs, people who have received transfusions of HIV-contaminated blood, and infants born to HIV-infected mothers. According to the CDC's statistics on health care workers exposed to HIV, the maximum chance of contracting HIV infection from a known AIDS patient by occupational exposure (needle stick) to blood is less than 0.5 percent. As of May 1989, only one paramedic has become HIV infected as a result of occupational exposure; that case is listed in the "undetermined" risk category by the CDC.

To minimize the risk of HIV (and other) infection, you should be familiar with the concept of universal precautions. This modern concept accepts the premise that certain body fluids may cause the spread of certain infectious agents. The concept implies that EMTs should take certain precautions universally when treating all patients. The concept of universal precautions can be best addressed by following these body substance isolation (BSI) procedures:

1. Wear gloves when you handle any patients. When you clean contaminated equipment, general-purpose utility gloves (e.g., rubber household gloves) are recommended. Heavy leather or "bunker gloves" are recommended for use where you are likely to encounter broken glass and sharp edges, such as when you extricate automobile accident victims.
2. Wear protective eyewear and a face mask when body fluid splatter is anticipated.
3. Do not recap, cut, or bend used needles; place them directly into a puncture-resistant container designed for "sharps."
4. Follow cleaning and infection control protocols closely.
5. Wear gowns if possible when uniforms may become extensively soiled with body fluids.
6. Change contaminated clothes and wash exposed skin thoroughly.
7. Use face shields, pocket masks, or other airway adjuncts.
8. Wash hands after you remove gloves as a means of self-protection. Change gloves between patients.

If contact with a patient's high-risk body fluids occurs on an unprotected area of the body, inform the responsible medical authority and follow appropriate local protocols. These protocols should include:

1. Submitting an incident report.
2. Notifying the appropriate medical adviser.
3. Obtaining counseling for the pre-HIV test and informed consent for baseline testing.
4. Retesting at 6 weeks, 12 weeks, and 6 months.
5. Obtaining post-test counseling.

The most difficult aspect of this disease is that there are no outward markers. A patient with AIDS looks no different than any other patient suffering from a chronic debilitating illness. You cannot discriminate against any patient, because to delay or refuse care is not only unethical but is gross negligence, abandonment, and malpractice. With universal precautions, there should be little fear of increased risk in caring for HIV-infected patients.

Actual Risk and Prevention Procedures

Consideration of the hepatitis viruses and HIV clearly demonstrates the importance of handwashing and careful handling of blood-related problems. Clean blood-contaminated equipment and work areas as a first step in infection control. Clean blood-covered areas with a fresh solution of 1 part bleach to 10 parts water (1:10). Always wear gloves during these cleaning procedures.

Routine rescue vehicle cleaning is an essential part of the prevention and control of communicable diseases. Cleaning will remove surface organisms and should be accomplished after each run and on a daily basis. "High contact areas" are those that were in direct contact with the patient's blood/body fluids or those that you touch after contact with the patient. These areas must be cleaned after each run.

Cleaning solutions recommended by the CDC are either an Environmental Protection Agency (EPA)-approved germicide that is effective against tuberculosis (TB) bacterium or a 1:10 solution of household bleach. Avoid the use of aerosol spray products. A solution in a bucket or a pistol-grip spray bottle is recommended. Alcohol is not a recommended cleaning solution. Personal protective equipment and gear should be employed as recommended on the solution's material safety data sheet (MSDS).

Contaminated disposables (paper sheets, needles, dressings, and other medical waste) should be handled in strict accordance with local health department procedures. Hospital infection control personnel or the local medical director should be consulted, and written protocols should be followed. EMTs should be aware of the local infection control regulations and procedures.

Handwashing is extremely important. It should be completed as soon as practical after treatment. It is recommended that a waterless antiseptic hand cleanser should be kept on responding units to use when handwashing facilities are not available, but handwashing with soap and water should be accomplished as well as soon as practical after every patient contact.

The probability that a rescuer will become infected with HBV or HIV as a result of performing CPR is minimal. Transmission has only been documented as a result of blood exchange or penetration of the skin by blood-contaminated instruments. Transmission of

TABLE 35–2   Common Childhood Diseases

Disease	Signs and Symptoms	Mode of Transmission
Bacterial meningitis	Fever, severe headache, stiff neck, sore throat	Direct contact with oral, nasal secretions
Chickenpox (varicella)	Fever, rash, cutaneous vesicles	Airborne, direct contact with vesicle drainage
German measles (rubella)	Fever, rash	Airborne, direct contact with oral secretions
Hepatitis A	Fever, loss of appetite; jaundice, fatigue	Direct contact with urine, stool, or oral ingestion of virus
Measles (rubeola)	Fever, rash, bronchitis	Airborne, direct contact with secretions
Mumps	Fever, swelling of salivary glands (parotid)	Airborne, direct contact with saliva
Whooping cough (pertussis)	Violent cough at night, whooping sound when cough subsides	Airborne, direct contact with oral secretions
Scarlet fever	Fever, headache, nausea, vomiting	Airborne, direct contact with oral secretions

Knowledge of disease processes and the consistent following of infection control protocols remain your best defenses against communicable disease. Tables 35–2 and 35–3 summarize this information for common childhood and adult diseases.

TABLE 35–3 Common Adult Diseases

Disease	Signs and Symptoms	Mode of Transmission
HIV infection	Fever, night sweats, weight loss, cough	Sexual contact, blood, needles
Gonorrhea	Discharge from urethra or vagina, lower abdominal pain, fever	Sexual contact
Hepatitis B	Fever, fatigue, loss of appetite, nausea, headache, jaundice	Blood, sexual contact
Hepatitis Non A–Non B	Fever, headache, fatigue, jaundice	Blood
Malaria	Cyclic fever, chills, fever	Blood-mosquito vector
Mononucleosis	Fever, sore throat, fatigue	Mouth-to-mouth kiss
Pneumonia	Fever, cough	Airborne
Syphilis	Genital and cutaneous lesions, nerve degeneration (late)	Sexual contact, blood
Tuberculosis	Fever, night sweats, weight loss, cough	Airborne

YOU ARE THE EMT

1. Malaria is a vector-borne disease that is transmitted to humans by mosquitoes. Identify three other modes of transmission of communicable diseases. Give an example of a disease spread by each mode.
2. You have just suffered a needle stick injury in the field. What should you do?
3. You just found out that one of the patients you transported yesterday has serum hepatitis. You're not worried, because you have followed all the steps to protect against exposure. What are they?
4. AIDS is not only a serious disease; it is also a controversial social issue that is at the forefront of media attention. What are the facts concerning the mode of transmission of this disease? How can you protect yourself against infection from an AIDS patient?

HBV and HIV infection during mouth-to-mouth resuscitation has not been documented. Transmission of herpes while performing CPR is very rare. However, transmission of bacterial meningitis and tuberculosis is theoretically possible, and the emergence of multidrug-resistant tuberculosis is cause for concern. EMTs with impaired immune systems are also at increased risk.

CHAPTER 36

SUBSTANCE ABUSE

KEY TERMS

addiction (ah-dik′shun) A state characterized by an overwhelming desire or need (compulsion) to continue the use of a drug or agent and to obtain it by any means, with a tendency to increase the dosage.

delirium tremens (DTs) (de-lēr′e-um tre′mens) A clinical withdrawal syndrome characterized by restlessness, fever, sweating, disorientation, agitation and convulsions seen in alcoholics who are acutely deprived of their source of supply.

dependency (de-pen′den-se) The total psychophysical state of an addict in which increasing doses of the drug are required to prevent the onset of abstinence symptoms.

depressant (de-pres′ant) An agent that reduces functional activity.

drug Any chemical or biological substance given to patients to aid in the diagnosis, treatment, or prevention of disease.

fetal alcohol syndrome A condition of the children of alcoholic mothers characterized by growth retardation (low birth weight), failure to thrive, mental retardation, and a variety of specific congenital abnormalities.

hallucinogen (hah-lu′sĭ-no-jen″) An agent that produces false perceptions in any one of the five senses.

hypnotic (hip-not′ik) Sleep inducing.

narcotic (nar-kot′ik) An agent producing insensitivity or stupor.

sedative (sed′ah-tiv) A substance that allays activity and excitement.

sensitivity An overreaction or allergy to a substance.

stimulant (stim′u-lant) Any agent producing excitation.

substance abuse The knowing misuse of any substance to produce some desired effect.

tolerance (tol′er-ans) The ability to endure large doses without ill effect, such as the ability to endure the continued or increasing use of a drug.

OVERVIEW

The term substance abuse has been introduced in recent years because the rate of abuse of medical and nonmedical preparations today far exceeds that of past years. Formerly, substances that were abused usually were limited to alcohol, nicotine, and some narcotic drugs. The abuse of readily or illegally obtained materials involves millions of persons and billions of dollars and has spread into every level of American life. The indirect cost of substance abuse to society cannot be calculated. You will treat many patients whose problems can be traced to some type of substance abuse. A major problem in the United States today is the use of a central nervous system stimulant, cocaine, in various forms. Additionally, "designer drugs," illegally made from standard chemical precursors with actions similar to those of legitimate medications, have become widely popular.

Chapter 36 begins by defining the terms an EMT must know in order to understand the range of problems of substance abuse. The chapter then describes the two major forms of substance abuse: alcohol and various drugs. The symptoms of alcoholism, the effects on the body of too much alcohol, and the treatment of alcohol intoxicated patients are all discussed.

"Drug abuse" is a broader subject that begins with a description of the various types of drugs that are abused and progresses to the specific problems of drug abuse and the emergency treatment of the drug abuser. The chapter concludes with a brief discussion of other forms of substance abuse: specifically, aspirin, anabolic steroids, laxatives, vitamins, and food.

GOALS

The goals of Chapter 36 are to
- know the scope of alcohol abuse as a problem in society today.
- know the general effects of alcohol on a patient and those that require specific emergency treatment.
- be familiar with the emergency treatment for injuries and illnesses that occur as a result of alcohol abuse.
- know the scope of and the general problems related to drug abuse in the United States.
- become familiar with the nature of the several types of drugs used, their routes of administration, and the tolerance and sensitivity that can develop in a drug user.
- know the specific acute treatment for the major problems associated with the several types of drug use described.
- know the problems that arise with drug withdrawal.
- become familiar with other forms of substance abuse.

THE MEANING OF SUBSTANCE ABUSE

The term **substance abuse** calls to mind a specific **drug** addiction. Although drug use and addiction are major social and public health problems in the United States today, they are by no means the only form of substance abuse. Alcohol, food, laxatives, emetics, and routine medications such as aspirin and vitamins are all significantly abused (Figure 36–1). A common

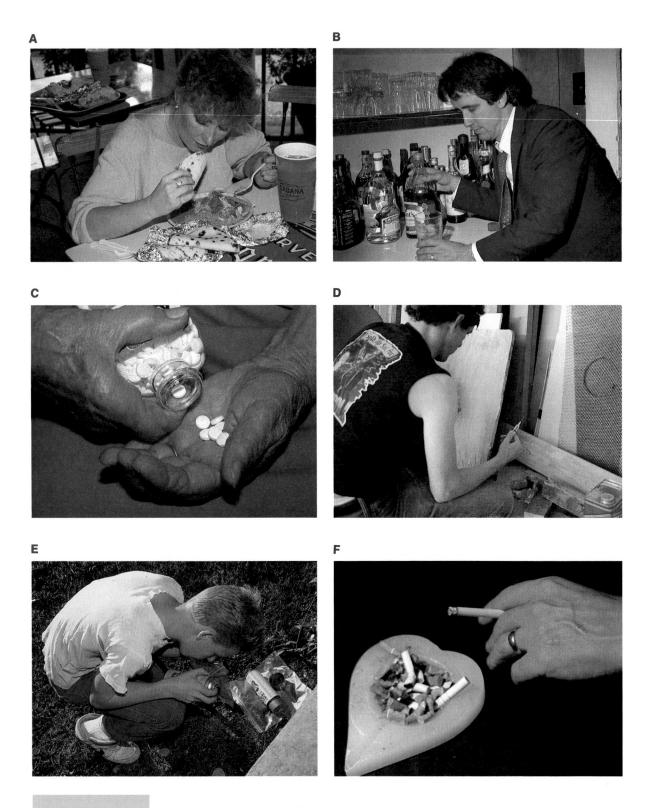

A

FIGURE 36–1   Substance abuse is not limited to narcotics addiction. It can also include abuse of (A) food, (B) alcohol, (C) aspirin, (D) drugs, (E) solvents, and (F) nicotine.

thread uniting all the agents used is that they are self-administered without medical control or consideration for proper or sterile preparation or dosage. The agents are self-prescribed by the user for certain desired effects. Usually, the user loses control over the amount of substance consumed as time passes. Generally, no medical indication for the use of the agent exists. In time, continued compulsive use produces an absolute need for increasing the amounts of an agent used to achieve the same result. This is called **addiction.**

An unfortunate result of the widespread use of drugs is that many crimes are committed by individuals who need money to purchase them. Many agents in widespread use are freely available and inexpensive. Others can only be obtained legally with a prescription. Still others cannot be obtained legally at all. Fulfilling the demand for this group has produced a flourishing black-market drug trade that provides traffickers with an annual profit of several billion dollars. Into this trade have come substances with little or no medical use, such as *marijuana*, as well as legitimate drugs like Seconal® or *morphine*.

The indiscriminate use of drugs has produced varying degrees of **dependency** and addiction to them. Addicts have a compulsion to use their drug and are willing to exhaust any means to obtain it. In general, the treatment of addiction and substance abuse is similar to the management of a patient with any chronic disease. The treating professional must have patience, persistence, and dedication.

Most agents that are knowingly misused are taken for their effects on the mind: they can be described as stimulatory, depressant, hallucinatory, hypnotic, sedative, or narcotic. In the United States the use of such agents proliferated widely in the late 1960s and 1970s; 40 percent of military personnel serving in Viet Nam are said to have experienced significant drug use in that country. In the 1980s, illegal drug purchases in the United States exceeded $80 billion annually—a figure that surpassed the combined expenditure for food, clothing, and education. In the early part of the final decade of the twentieth century, there is a constant flow of newer agents such as *crack*,

and *designer drugs.* Multiple drug use, where some are used to counteract the bad effects of others, is being seen more frequently.

Several patterns of initial drug contact are known. Sometimes the drugs are prescribed for a bonafide medical reason, such as the treatment of pain. Sometimes the drugs are used for recreational purposes or in response to group or peer pressure. The general pattern is for drug use to be tapered or stopped by an individual. Use itself is not equated with addiction. In fact, most initial users do not become addicts.

Overall, substance abuse presents many different patterns and a wide spectrum of effects. One common theme, however, is that it is detrimental to individuals and society. Direct costs related to alcohol abuse alone have been estimated at $60 billion annually. Indirect costs in other lives affected, opportunities lost, toxic effects on newborn children, and other hidden costs are incalculable.

ALCOHOL ABUSE

The most commonly abused drug in the United States is alcohol. It affects more than 12 million people directly annually (10 percent of all males and 3 percent of all females) and causes more than 200,000 deaths. It is the third greatest national health problem after heart disease and cancer. Alcoholism is not limited exclusively to destitute drunks. Executives, housewives, business-people, and laborers can all become victims of this agent and its addiction. Alcohol is a powerful central nervous system (CNS) depressant. It interferes with the capacity of the individual to think, to function well, and to face situations rationally. More than 50 percent of all traffic fatalities or injuries involve drivers who have abused alcohol; 67 percent of murders and 33 percent of suicides involve users of alcohol. Alcohol has been, and still is, a major danger in society.

Effects of Alcohol

Alcohol, like all other drugs, produces tolerance. Patients who are addicted to it require more and more alcohol over time to produce the same effect. In general, as a **depressant,** alcohol dulls the sense of awareness, slows reflexes, and increases reaction time. Patients under the acute influence of alcohol may exhibit the same signs as those with physical injuries or illnesses, such as head trauma, toxic reactions, or uncontrolled diabetes.

When you attend a patient who may be suffering from the acute effects of alcohol, always bear in mind that the patient could have a physical illness or injury as well. A patient should be brought to the emergency department if there is the slightest question that illness or injury is involved, in addition to the direct, observable effect of alcohol. Sometimes, the physician has difficulty sorting out the effect on a patient of injury or illness from that of alcohol. Often the family or an acquaintance can provide some information about the patient's drinking habits up to the time of the emergency situation.

The drunken patient may behave aggressively and inappropriately, fall easily, or be combative. Self-injury is common and often is not perceived by the inebriated patient. You may have to seek out injuries and fractures. Occasionally, a patient will have consumed so much alcohol that signs of serious central nervous system depression appear. In such cases complete respiratory support may be necessary. Death can and has resulted from this degree of excessive consumption of alcohol.

Alcohol ingested in large amounts irritates the stomach. Patients who have consumed too much alcohol may vomit, usually forcefully, as a result of this irritation and the production of excess gastric juice. Sometimes these patients will vomit blood (hematemesis). Hematemesis can occur when the lower part of the lining of the esophagus is lacerated by repeated forceful vomiting and bleeds at the point of the tear. It can also be caused by direct irritation and gastritis (ulceration of the lining of the stomach). Rupture of dilated veins in the lower esophagus (esophageal varices) that have developed because of cirrhosis (alcoholic liver disease) is also a common cause of hematemesis in the chronic alcoholic.

Long-term alcohol abuse produces *ataxia* (muscular incoordination), memory loss, apathy, and other signs of chronic brain deterioration. Alcohol can also cause fetal damage in pregnant women. **Fetal alcohol syndrome** characterizes children of alcoholic mothers. Low birth weight, certain congenital anomalies, failure to thrive, and mental retardation of the newborn child are all common parts of this syndrome. Although the developing fetus may be exposed on a long-term basis to alcohol, acute withdrawal in the newborn is not a major problem.

A very specific syndrome occurs when a patient who is used to a constant supply of alcohol withdraws from it. This condition may occur if a patient can no longer buy alcohol, becomes ill, is injured, or for some other reason is cut off from the routine daily source. Alcohol withdrawal may manifest itself as alcoholic hallucinations (hallucinosis) or as **delerium tremens (DTs).**

An alcoholic hallucination can be the visual perception of fantastic figures or the auditory perception of odd voices with an otherwise fairly clear mental state. Hallucinations may be frightening to the patient, but are usually transient. They may or may not be associated with withdrawal. They often precede delirium tremens, a much more severe complication.

Delirium tremens may occur from one to seven days after alcohol withdrawal. It is characterized by restlessness, fever, sweating, confusion, disorientation, agitation, delusions, hallucinations, and occasionally, convulsions. A history of chronic alcohol ingestion, followed by a period of one or more days of withdrawal, can generally be obtained from the patient's family or acquaintances. Patients with DTs are extremely ill; the mortality rate from this problem alone, in the absence of any associated illness or injury, has been estimated at 10 to 15 percent.

Treatment of Alcohol Abuse

Given the widespread use of alcohol, an acute episode of alcoholic intoxication is not usually reason for emergency medical care. Patients whom you are called to treat will usually be acutely intoxicated and have another major problem such as CNS depression, respiratory insufficiency, vomiting, pulmonary aspiration, hematemesis, or an injury. Transport these patients to the emergency department after you address the major associated medical problem. Occasionally, complete ventilatory support is needed. You must always be alert for vomiting and its consequences with these patients. Injuries or bleeding are treated as noted elsewhere in this text.

Individuals suffering from hallucinations or DTs are acutely ill patients. Hallucinations and restlessness may precede the development of convulsions and complete delirium. Should convulsions occur, they should be treated like any other seizure. The patient should not be restrained, although adequate protection must be provided to prevent self-injury. Oxygen should be given and the patient watched carefully for vomiting. In general, isolated seizures in the alcoholic are treated like any other episode of seizure activity.

These patients may be hypovolemic from sweating, fluid loss, insufficient fluid intake, or vomiting. Should signs of hypovolemic shock develop, transport the patient promptly. You must elevate the feet slightly, clear the airway, and turn the head to one side to minimize the chance of aspiration. Generally, these patients are irrational and may respond inappropriately to suggestions or conversation; however, they are frequently frightened. Each one should be approached in a calm and relaxed manner with reassurance and the necessary emotional support.

In the United States, most states have developed a legal definition of acute alcoholic intoxication. You must be familiar with the one that applies in your area. Usually it is a blood alcohol level of 0.10 percent. This percentage means that 0.1 gm (100 mg) of alcohol exists in each 100 ml of circulating blood. Each ounce of 86 proof whiskey adds approximately 25 mg of alcohol for each 100 ml of blood.

At 0.05 percent levels, motor skills start to deteriorate. At a level of 0.10 percent alcohol, there is a seven percent chance of any driver having an automobile accident as a result of the depressant effect of alcohol. At 0.16 percent, the accident probability exceeds thirty percent. An acute level of 0.3 percent is associated with the development of coma and respiratory depression; few survive levels of 0.4 percent. Because alcohol is an addictive agent to which individuals develop **tolerance,** you will often see reports of survival of patients with very high blood alcohol levels (0.5 percent to 1.5 percent). These figures are seen in the long-term chronic user of alcohol who has become habituated to the drug.

The chronic alcoholic patient rarely needs emergency support unless mental deterioration leads to an injury or to unusual exposure such as falling asleep in an unprotected, exposed area. This type of patient also frequently requires emergency care for the problems of chronic alcohol use, such as hematemesis. In these circumstances, treatment and transport are dictated by the associated illness or injury and not by the alcohol abuse which will be treated later.

DRUG ABUSE

Types of Drugs

Aside from alcohol, drugs that are abused for their subjective effects on a person's mental state include the following:

1. Opium compounds.
2. CNS depressants.
3. CNS stimulants.
4. Nicotine.
5. Marijuana.
6. Hallucinogens.
7. Inhalants.

Opium Compounds The *opium analgesics* (pain relievers) are natural or synthetic derivatives of opium from poppy seeds. They include *heroin, morphine,* Demerol®, Dilaudid®, and methadone. The very mild agent *codeine* is also in this group. In general, these drugs are all pain relievers and have a wide range of legitimate medical application. Individual use may have started with an appropriate medical prescription or as a recreational venture.

Of these **narcotic** agents, the use of heroin is absolutely illegal in the United States. The remainder can be obtained by medical prescription. In most, but not all of the United States, codeine and a few other agents, such as opium and morphine, are *exempt narcotics*. This term means that small quantities of the drugs, as prescribed by law, may be sold over the counter without a prescription and may be refilled. As such, codeine is the basic drug in many nonprescription preparations for cough and mild headache or pain relief. Morphine is a basic agent in several antidiarrheal remedies. Usually, these narcotics are contained in mixtures to treat specific problems. Some states have abolished the exempt status of codeine and other agents because of drug abuse problems. You should know which narcotic agents may be purchased locally without prescriptions in your area.

Intravenous administration of these drugs is associated with a characteristic "high" or "kick." These agents are, however, all CNS depressants and can cause severe respiratory depression. Tolerance develops rapidly with their use so that massive doses are being taken by some users. In general, emergency medical problems related to opium compounds are caused by respiratory depression and general CNS malfunction.

In the early 1980s, the use of heroin and analogous agents began to decline. It is rising again as individuals who use crack and cocaine will sometimes use heroin to help them control the intoxication and withdrawal from these agents. Thus, you may frequently be faced with patients in whom the stimulating effects of a drug such as cocaine are seen concurrently with the depressant effects of heroin. The clinical picture is justifiably often unclear. All elements of support may be required on a rapidly changing, minute-to-minute basis.

Within the past decade, a family of opium-like compounds, all derived from the same parent substance, *thebaine*, and all used to relieve pain, has been developed. The compounds are all chemically similar and are all

based on the oxycodone nucleus. A variety of combinations of these agents with less potent analgesics is legitimately available. Some of the more common trade names are Percocet®, Percodan®, and Vicodin®. Each of the codones is legitimately prescribed and used for the treatment of moderate to severe pain. Each codone is a CNS depressant, and each can be highly addictive.

CNS Depressants The *barbiturates* and other **hypnotic** (sleep-inducing) drugs are CNS depressants and generally have effects remarkably similar to those of alcohol. They depress the central nervous system. They do not relieve pain, nor do they produce a specific "high." Frequently, they are used in combination with alcohol or with the opium analgesics to increase the effects of another agent. There are over 30 street names for barbiturate products based largely on the color of the legitimately made preparation (Figure 36–2). Table 36–1 lists many of these common names.

In general, the barbiturates are categorized by two properties: the rapidity of their onset of action and the duration of their effect. Some agents such as thiopental® (sodium pentothal) have a very rapid onset (15 to 30 seconds after

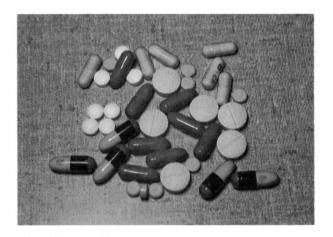

FIGURE 36–2

"Goof Balls" (barbiturates), "Yellow Jackets" (pentobarbital), "Red Devils" (secobarbital), and other CNS depressants alter the state of consciousness so that the individual appears drowsy or peaceful.

an intravenous dose) and are fully eliminated in 30 to 60 minutes. This agent is used to induce over 70 percent of the general anesthetics given in the United States. Some, like *phenobarbital*, at the other end of the spectrum, are slow in onset and prolonged (up to 24 hours) in effect. Table 36–2 lists the commonly used barbiturates and their lengths of action.

Barbiturates have been a part of legitimate medicine for over a century. They are easy to obtain and relatively cheap. It is not unknown for a given individual to solicit prescriptions from several physicians for the same or a variety of barbiturates. A typical user is middle-aged, in a highly productive and consequently stressful job or home situation; relaxation is the

TABLE 36–1   Most Commonly Abused Barbiturates and Their Street Names

Amobarbital (Amytal)	Pentobarbital (Nembutal)	Secobarbital (Seconal)	Equal parts: Secobarbital and Amobarbital (Tuinal)
Blue angel	Nebbies	F-40s	Double trouble
Blue birds	Nembies	Mexican reds	Gorilla pills
Blue bullets	Yellow bullets	M and Ms	Rainbows
Blue devils	Yellow dolls	RDs	Reds/blues
Blue dolls	Yellow jackets	Red birds	Tootsies
Blue heavens	Yellows	Red bullets	Trees
Blues		Red devils	Tuies
Blue tips		Red dolls	
		Red lilies	
		Reds	
		Seccies	
		Seggies	

TABLE 36–2   Classification of Barbiturates by Duration of Effects

Ultra-Short 1–4 Hours	Short-Acting 3–6 Hours	Intermediate-Acting 6–12 Hours	Long-Lasting 12–24 Hours
Pentothal (thiopental)	Amytal (amobarbital)	Butisol (sodium butabarbital)	Luminal (phenobarbital)
Brevital (methohexital)	Seconal (secobarbital)		
	Nembutal (pentobarbital)		

purpose of using the agent. Barbiturate use is high, but pure addiction to barbiturates is infrequent.

In general, the shorter-acting agents pentobarbital ("Yellow Jackets") and secobarbital ("Red Devils") are preferred over the long-acting, more stable phenobarbital. Addiction to the very short-acting agents is almost unknown and probably would only be seen in patients with access to anesthetic agents. Similarly, addiction to the long-acting agents is uncommon.

There are many other nonbarbiturate depressant drugs: *meprobamate, glutethimide,* the *benzodiazepines,* (*Halcion®, Ativan®, Valium®* and its analogs), *Librium®, Haldol®, methaqualone* and various other antianxiety, **sedative,** and hypnotic agents. These agents all depress CNS activity and alter the state of consciousness so that the individual may appear drowsy or peaceful. In general, the agents are taken by mouth or by injection. Intravenous use of these agents is not common, but it does exist. Contents of capsules can be suspended or dissolved in water and injected to produce a rather sudden state of ease and contentment. Unfortunately, this use of depressant drugs induces tolerance quickly; and successive doses with time must be larger and larger. Depressants are popular as drugs in combination with others. They help users of stimulants to sleep and to cope with their agitation. Used with alcohol, their effect is markedly increased.

In general, the treatment of those overdosed with barbiturates must be aimed at support for general depression: airway clearance, ventilatory assistance, and transport. Today, with a much more common practice being multidrug use, the given picture in a specific patient may not be clear. Treatment must be directed at obvious injuries or illnesses with the thought that drug use may complicate any picture and make the requirement for full life support mandatory.

Finally, like alcohol, barbiturates can pass across the placenta into a developing fetus. As such, the child of an addicted mother is likely to require much extra postnatal care and may have specific developmental problems.

CNS Stimulants The effect of CNS **stimulants** on the individual depends on the route of administration, the drug, its dose, and the circumstances. *Amphetamines* are commonly taken orally by truck drivers, students, and others to produce a general mood elevation, improve task performance, suppress appetite, or prevent sleepiness. They may just as well produce irritability, anxiety, and lack of effective concentration. A host of these agents exist. Amphetamine, methamphetamine, and Benzedrine or ("bennies") are the characteristic drugs. They are frequently known as speed or "uppers." Caffeine, found in coffee and cola drinks, is a mild stimulant, as are certain antiasthmatic drugs such as Adrenalin™ and *aminophylline.* Nasal decongestants, such as *ephedrine* and *isoproterenol,* are also mild stimulants. These drugs will cause tachycardia, increased blood pressure, rapid breathing, an excited state, agitation, headaches, sleeplessness, and a sense of euphoria or well-being. Disorganized behavior may also accompany the use of these agents. Taken as prescribed for specific medical problems, they can be beneficial. When they are used in an uncontrolled fashion, they all can become addictive.

Two variations of amphetamine compounds, "*Ecstasy*" and "*Eve*," have come to the fore in the recent years. Ecstasy was a legal drug for medical use until 1985, when its potential for abuse was determined to be higher than its medical benefit. Eve has a similar chemical structure and chemical effect. Recent reports link its use with possible deaths from cardiac arrhythmias.

When attending a patient who has taken large doses of stimulants over a rather brief period, you will usually find an agitated individual who exhibits irrational or paranoid behavior. Occasionally, the patient experiences chest pain after ingesting large doses of stimulants. The individual who has taken large doses of stimulants for three or four days in succession ("a run") and is forced to stop because of the effects may fall into a deep sleep to awaken hungry, lethargic, and depressed. Sudden withdrawal may also produce coma.

In general, addiction to stimulants is among

the hardest to treat medically. The emergency care of these patients depends on the stage of addiction at which the patient is found. If you are called to see an individual during the actual use of stimulants, you will probably find an agitated, suspicious, combative, frightened patient who is tachycardic, hypertensive, and tachypneic. Reassurance, protection of the patient from self-injury, and prompt transportation are needed. If you are dealing with the patient in acute withdrawal, you may face the "crash" stage after acute stimulation. This patient may be depressed, suicidal, incoherent, sleepy, or near coma. Full basic life support may be needed.

In the family of CNS stimulants, at the present time, it is proper to consider cocaine separately. Unquestionably, it is one of the most popular illegal drugs being used in the United States. Between 30 and 60 tons of cocaine are imported into the country annually.

The use of the drug has vastly increased in the past decade. Presently, at least 25 million Americans are estimated to have had some experience with the agent; 3,000 to 4,000 people each day are initiated into its use; 4 million use it regularly. Between the mid-1970s and 1980s, emergency department visits for cocaine-related problems rose 300 percent. There was an observed 400 percent increase in deaths related to cocaine and a 450 percent increase in referrals to treatment programs. More recent evidence indicates that cocaine use is spreading beyond urban areas and involving increasingly younger individuals. Unfortunately, cocaine is fairly cheap and thus is readily available to anyone. The use of cocaine transcends all boundaries in society in the United States, involving everyone from top executives to the unemployed. Typically, the addict is male, in his early 20s, with a history of drug abuse involving other agents, and a habit of multi-agent addiction.

Raw coca leaves are extracted with hydrochloric or sulfuric acid to produce either the sulfate or chloride salt of the active agent, cocaine. This resulting white powder is the standard street form of cocaine. If this powder is dissolved with an alkali (base) like sodium bicarbonate (weak) or sodium hydroxide (strong) and an organic solvent such as ether is added to the solution, the base will separate the sulfate or chloride from the cocaine which is then soluble in the ether. The ether, containing pure cocaine, is easily separated from the water/base solution. Evaporating the ether leaves relatively free crystalline cocaine whose purity depends on the initial product used and the care with which the extraction is carried out. The crystalline product, pure cocaine, is commonly called "crack" because of the popping or cracking sound the crystals make when they are smoked in a pipe. This process produces free cocaine by treating the raw cocaine salt with a base and extracting this solution with ether; hence the term *free base*. Free-basing is often taken to mean the smoking of the cocaine crystals produced by the chemical extractions just described.

The following street terms have been used to identify cocaine:

- Coke
- Crack
- Crystal
- Ice (also used to denominate a smokable form of amphetamine)
- Free Base
- Snow
- Tool
- Lady
- Blow
- Flake
- Nose Candy
- Happy Trails
- Green Gold
- Gold Dust
- Star Spangled Powder
- Rock

Cocaine in combination is sometimes called

- Liquid Lady (cocaine and alcohol), or
- Speed Ball (cocaine and heroin for IV use)

Cocaine may be taken in a number of different ways. Classically, it has been inhaled into the nose to be absorbed through the nasal mucosa. This route of use produces direct tissue damage, nosebleeds, and ultimately destruction of the nasal septum. Although it is now rarely seen, the clinical hallmark of the cocaine addict was a perforated nasal septum. The drug can be injected intravenously or "popped" subcutaneously. The major advantage to the user of the crack crystal is that it is pure cocaine, which melts at 93 degrees F. It vaporizes at a slightly higher temperature and thus can be mixed with tobacco and smoked. In this form, it reaches the vast capillary network of the lung and can be absorbed in seconds. The immediate outflow of blood from the heart spreads the drug to the brain promptly, and its effect is felt almost at once.

Cocaine can be absorbed through all mucous membranes and even across the skin. The duration of action for a given dose in the body is less than one hour. Obviously, smoked crack produces the most rapid means of absorption possible and hence the most potent effect.

Cocaine is a major stimulant of the central nervous system, causing a profound sympathetic discharge. The immediate results are excitement, euphoria, talkativeness, and agitation. Occasionally, hallucinations occur. Anxiety and worries fade away. The user truly feels good. Once the effect of the cocaine dose has worn off, profound lethargy and depression (a crash) occurs. Many people now use cocaine with other drugs to alleviate the effects of the crash or to relieve the agitation it induces.

You will likely encounter many patterns of cocaine use. An individual who has used one or two doses only may be seen in the giddy, euphoric stage or in the crash phase when he is depressed and irritable. No specific emergency treatment beyond careful observation is needed in these instances.

Cocaine overdose can occur with any form of the drug and any route. The adult fatal dose is thought to be 1200 mg. However, there are reported fatalities from major cocaine-induced cardiac arrhythmias with doses of as little as 25 to 30 mg (the usual amount taken in a run of snorting or inhaling).

The acute overdose patient presents a genuine emergency. Such a patient may be psychotic, hyperactive, or paranoid. Threatened, these patients may be hostile or combative.

Physically you will note tachycardia, tachypnea, an irregular pulse, hypertension, muscle tremors, and occasionally a seizure. Chest pain is not uncommon. In extreme cases, fatal cardiac arrhythmias and intracerebral bleeding have occurred.

In the crash phase, these patients may be disturbed and suicidal, particularly if they have experienced hallucinations which can be visual or auditory and frightening. Coma and paralysis may ensue and death can occur. Obviously, in this complex series of presentations, you must be prepared to offer full basic life support as well as management of the acute psychological reactions. Immediate transport is needed because of all of the inherent risks for this patient.

Nicotine Cigarette smoking is so widespread and such a common phenomenon in the United States today that no one takes it other than as a routine activity. In fact, it does fit all the criteria for drug dependence and should be regarded as an addictive practice. There is general agreement that nicotine is the agent that contributes to the continuing use of cigarettes by many. Nicotine is a mild CNS stimulant. Compulsive smokers report a range of withdrawal effects from no particular problems to irritability, hostility, and depression.

Your role in dealing with this problem is in handling the effects of long-term smoking on the tracheobronchial system. Smoking is by far the most common cause of chronic obstructive pulmonary disease (COPD) because cigarette smoke is a bronchial irritant. The long-term chronic smoker is continuously exposing the lining of the airways to material that keeps them filled with mucus and secretions which impede airflow. The "smoker's cough" is a direct result of this chronic inflammation.

Side effects of smoking are linked to lung, airway, bladder, and oral cancer, and the aggravation of peripheral vascular disease. Approximately 1,000 persons in the United States die of smoking-related diseases daily. Although none of these effects is directly related to nicotine, it is the major effective agent that keeps people smoking—even those who wish they could stop.

Marijuana A variety of names are associated with the active agent from the flowering hemp plant called *Cannabis sativa.* In the United States, the extract from the flowers of the plant top is called marijuana or "pot" (Figure 36–3). In Africa, the Far East, and India, the term *hashish* refers to extracts of the stalks of a related plant, *Cannabis indica.* "Bhang and charas" refer to less powerful extracts from the stems and leaves of Cannabis sativa or Cannabis indica.

Inhaling marijuana as smoke from a cigarette produces euphoria, relaxation, and drowsiness. The drug does impair short-term memory and the capacity to do complex work. In some people, euphoria can give way to depression and confusion. An altered perception of time is common, and anxiety approaching panic can occur. With very high doses, patients experience hallucinations. Marijuana use is common; estimates are that, in the United States, one-quarter of the population has used this drug, and 20 million people continue to use it daily. Marijuana remains the most popular and most used illegal drug in the United States today.

No known beneficial medical effect is associated with marijuana use; although, recently, extracts of the active agent in marijuana have been found to control nausea in patients undergoing long-term chemotherapy treatment for cancer.

In view of the widespread popularity of marijuana, you will undoubtedly encounter problems associated with its use—probably acute anxiety and the hallucinations the drug can produce. Both conditions should be treated in the same way that problems arising from the use of hallucinogens or stimulants are treated. Users may, unknowingly, purchase marijuana that has been mixed with crack, cocaine, or phencyclidine. In these cases, the clinical presentation may be confused by the use of two agents.

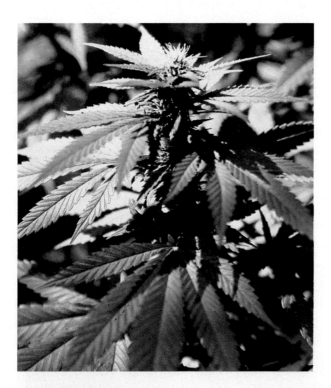

FIGURE 36–3

Marijuana is known as "pot" in the United States and "hashish" in other parts of the world. Extracts obtained from the plant tops are inhaled as cigarette smoke and produce euphoria, relaxation, and drowsiness. Despite its popularity, marijuana is known to produce acute anxiety, impaired memory, and hallucinations.

Hallucinogens Hallucinogens (psychedelic agents) cause an alteration of the patient's sense of perception. Their use is common; nearly 10 million Americans report some experience with them; and 1 million claim regular use.

The use of these drugs induces hallucinations, intensifies visual or auditory perceptions, and separates the user from reality. In the southwestern United States and in Mexico, these agents have been used for centuries in Indian religious rituals, although the active factors were not isolated from native cactus plants and mushrooms until the 1950s.

The list of such agents is relatively short and includes

- Lysergic acid derivatives ("LSD," "Acid," "Big D," "Sugar," "Brown Dol").
- Phenylethylamine derivatives such as mescaline, peyote ("Big Chief" and "Cactus").
- Indole analogs.
- Psilocybin or psilocin ("Magic Mushrooms").
- Phencyclidine ("PCP" and "Angel Dust").

The major historical hallucinogens are LSD, mescaline, and psilocybin. Users develop and lose tolerance fairly rapidly and thus true addiction is rare. The actual hallucinogenic effects experienced by individual users vary with their individual psychic makeup. Lethargy, drowsiness, vertigo, and nausea occur commonly. Most such agents are taken orally and produce effects lasting up to six hours.

Individuals requiring treatment for the ingestion alone may show fear or signs of euphoria. Abdominal pains, nausea, and vomiting are seen frequently. Beyond careful observation, protection of the patient, and prompt transport, there is little you have to offer this individual.

Many people ingest hallucinogens unknowingly and thus neither expect nor can cope with the results. Others have been driven to attempt physical feats such as flying or leaping great distances while under the influence of the agent. In these circumstances, treatment for the "bad trip" includes close observation, reassurance, and protection of the patient from self-injury. Do not leave such a patient alone. Obviously, priority treatment must be given to any injuries that a user may have sustained.

Phencyclidine is frequently used to "cut" or mix with other agents, thus producing a mixed reaction for the patient. It is not infrequently mixed with cocaine with unpredictable results.

Inhalants An additional problem, outside the realm of specific drug use, is associated with the inhalation of agents to produce an intoxicating effect. Inhalants include solvents, such as acetone or toleune that are found in glues, cleaning compounds and lacquers, gasoline, various halogenated hydrocarbons that are used as propellants in aerosol sprays, and Freon®. None of these agents is a pharmacologic item. They all produce CNS effects remarkably similar to those of alcohol. They are all CNS depressants.

Individual users have devised a variety of improvised containers to allow inhaling; some are as simple as breathing vapors within plastic bags (Figure 36–4); and some are quite elaborate. Most often, you will be handling a "sniffer" who appears to be drunk. If, however, the patient has become unconscious while sniffing, the apparatus that was used

may have caused significant or complete airway obstruction. In this case, you may have a patient with profound hypoxia and its associated problems, including cardiopulmonary arrest.

Long-term effects of the use of inhalants include destruction of liver cells—as seen in the various forms of hepatitis that are caused by exposure to toxic organic compounds—and destruction of cells in the central nervous system. At this time, it is unclear whether central nervous system damage is due to the inhaled agent itself, to the resultant hypoxia, or to both.

Emergency medical care should include basic life support, airway establishment and maintenance, ventilatory assistance, possibly cardiac resuscitation, and prompt transportation.

General Problems with Drug Abuse

Problems arising from drug abuse relate to the specific nature of the drug taken, its effect on the patient, the route of administration, and the combined effect of other agents used at the same time. Certainly, individual tolerance and sensitivity of the user to a given agent have a major bearing on the severity of the problem.

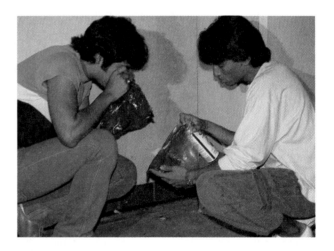

F I G U R E 36–4

Inhalants such as paint spray are "sniffed" using improvised, closed containers. The simplest device is a plastic bag. Inhalants are CNS depressants that can destroy liver cells as well as cells in the central nervous system.

Nature and Effect of the Drug Itself Almost every patient who abuses drugs does so because drugs alter the state of consciousness. Many of these agents cause CNS depression. You are likely to see all stages of depression, from mild drowsiness to coma. Other potential problems include the likelihood of vomiting and subsequent aspiration, respiratory depression or arrest, and self-injury. Sometimes, patients fall asleep in odd positions, with an arm or leg curled under their body or hanging over a chair or couch. Compression of blood vessels can reduce circulation in these extremities, sometimes for hours. The decreased blood flow can result in permanent damage and even loss of the limb. Nerves can be compressed, causing paralysis. Sometimes severely depressed patients fall and sustain injuries of which they are unaware. These injuries may be neglected for long periods of time.

Stimulants induce restlessness in the user and sometimes severe anxiety. When this state is unmanageable, it becomes similar to an acute psychosis with paranoia. You may encounter a patient with an acute fright reaction who exhibits paranoid or totally wrong thinking. Acute depression may be evident in the patient who has suddenly stopped using stimulants. Convulsions also may occur with abuse of some stimulants.

Hallucinogens induce very specific perceptual alterations that are related to sound, sight, or the other senses. The user, of course, anticipates that the altered sensory state will be pleasurable. Frequently, this situation does not happen; instead, the induced hallucination may be terrifying. You are almost certain to encounter someone who is having this type of a "bad trip."

Route of Administration Many agents are taken by mouth. Ordinarily, the oral route of administration poses no particular problem for the patient. Other agents are injected by needle, intravenously, subcutaneously (just under the skin), or into muscles. Illegally obtained drugs are usually not prepared with regard for sterility or proper composition for injection. They are frequently "cut" or diluted by agents such as sugar or other drugs that are not sterile.

Addicts are endless experimenters who are willing to take any drug by any route to experience a new "high." Thus, many agents not designed for injection are being given by needle. Frequently, a group of addicts will share the same needle. Usually, one individual will reuse a single needle for several injections.

The results of such practices can be devastating. Tissue can be destroyed by the direct action of the injected material on it. Bacteria with resulting infection can be introduced into a vein, subcutaneous tissue, or muscle at each injection. Phlebitis (an inflammation of the vein with or without direct bacterial infection) or both superficial and deep subcutaneous abscesses commonly occur. Even more lethal to the patient are the severe systemic infections, hepatitis, brain abscess, or endocarditis (infection of the valves and the lining membrane of the heart) that can develop. An additional risk is acquired immunodeficiency syndrome (AIDS), a life-threatening viral infection that can be transmitted through direct blood contact. When many individuals use one needle with no sterile precautions, they are at a high risk for contracting any of these diseases if only one among them has or is carrying it.

Other Agent Use Using more than one agent at one time is an increasingly common practice among all addicts. Generally, these drugs will have a complementary effect, such as alcohol and tranquilizers together. Occasionally, stimulants and depressants are mixed, or hallucinogens are used with each. Much more frequently now, a second agent is used to treat the anticipated bad effects of the primary drug used. The results for many patients are completely unpredictable. When you encounter such a situation, gather as much evidence and information about the agents used as possible. Often, it is very difficult for the physicians at the emergency department to assess the major problem because of the confused clinical picture.

Tolerance and Sensitivity Tolerance to some agents rapidly develops in users. Additionally, cross-tolerance to other agents may occur. The result of tolerance is that the chronic abuser comes to use extremely large doses of a given drug to achieve the desired effect. During a period when the drug is not used, tolerance is often lost as rapidly as it developed (usually within weeks). Thus, a user returning to an accustomed habit after a period of abstinence or withdrawal may dangerously overdose on what was previously a "routine" amount of drug. You will certainly see instances of this effect and note greatly exaggerated (for the patient) results of a single "routine" dose.

Any individual may have or may develop **sensitivity** to any drug or to any of the materials mixed with it. In the most acute form, an allergic or sensitivity reaction to an agent may result in *anaphylaxis*. Anaphylaxis is characterized by the rapid development of itching and burning on the skin, urticaria (hives), chest tightness, a nasal itch and sneezing, cough, respiratory wheezing, and dyspnea. It can occur following the administration of a substance by any route (orally, intravenously, subcutaneously, or otherwise). The major response in anaphylaxis is bronchospasm and a copious outpouring of mucus into the airway. Respiration is difficult and may become impossible. Anaphylaxis is a relatively rare occurrence in the addicted population; however, it is a constant risk with the use of any substance.

Treatment of the Drug Abuser

Assessment A few general rules apply when you are faced with a situation of drug abuse. Information is absolutely necessary for the emergency department physician. Bottles, needles, and whatever appliances or drug paraphernalia are about the patient should be collected and brought with the patient to the hospital. Unprescribed use of controlled substances is illegal in the United States. Each state has regulations about turning the equipment over to police. In some states, the sale of equipment for the preparation of cocaine and other agents is legal, although the use of the drug is not. You must be thoroughly knowledgeable about your own state laws as well as federal regulations.

When you suspect drug use, look for signs that will identify the substance. The presence of spoons, lamps, or pipes may give a clue that an agent is indeed being used (Figure 36–5). Examination of the patient may reveal further clues. The chronic user of the opium analgesics, for example, usually has small constricted pupils that do not constrict any further with light. Barbiturate users have dilated pupils, again relatively insensitive to light. The presence of intravenous puncture sites or multiple, small, cutaneous abscesses on the arms or legs is also a sign of a chronic drug abuser (Figure 36–6).

Depressants The moderately depressed patient who has ingested a depressant should be stimulated by talking, gentle pinching, or light shaking. You cannot know whether the patient is on the way to further depression or is awakening from a deeper coma. The danger in further depression is that it may produce respiratory arrest. Thus, the patient should be kept awake during transport to the emergency department. Be ready to assist respiration and be alert for vomiting. The use of oxygen is beneficial. Even if you are certain that the agent was taken orally, you should never induce vomiting in a semiconscious or drowsy patient. Transport this patient promptly and make any information that you can gather available to the appropriate personnel in the emergency department. The patient with respiratory depression needs ventilatory support and must be transported as quickly as possible while receiving it.

Stimulants The anxious, excited, or paranoid patient on stimulants should be handled in a calm, professional manner. Often a quiet attitude and gentle approach will help "talk down" such a patient. Gaining the patient's confidence with a pleasant manner often works. Restraints should not be used unless the patient is likely to injure others or self. Applying restraints is usually difficult and may require more than two EMTs. At the very least, restraints will increase a patient's anxiety, fear, and hyperactivity. The patient on stimulants

FIGURE 36–5

Drug paraphernalia may provide a clue to identifying the substance when you suspect drug use. Any bottles, needles, and appliances should be brought to the hospital with the patient.

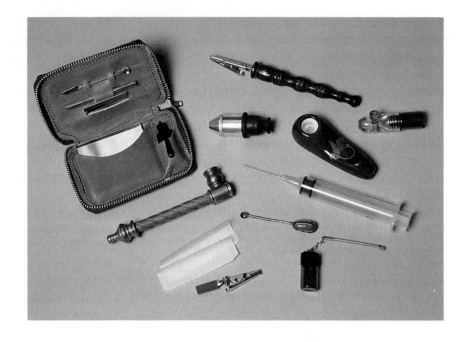

FIGURE 36–6

Signs of a chronic drug abuser: (A) Small constricted pupils (an opium user); (B) large dilated pupils (a barbiturate user); (C) intravenous needle marks or small cutaneous abscesses on the arms or legs.

A

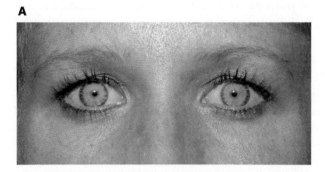

B

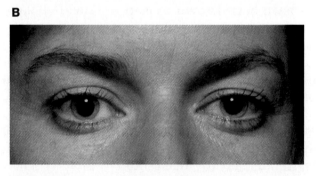

C

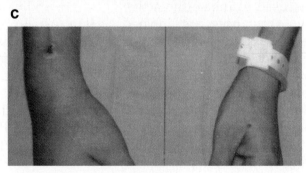

must never be left alone during transport or even placed alone in the ambulance where difficult behavior cannot be controlled.

The patient on stimulants who is convulsing must be protected from self-injury. Oxygen should be given and the airway kept clear with gentle suction. This patient will require complex, intravenous drug treatment at the hospital and must be taken there as quickly as possible. Occasionally, the patient taking stimulants will undergo severe reactive depression if withdrawn suddenly from any drug. Usually, the withdrawal symptoms include listlessness, apathy, and hunger. They may progress to coma and profound respiratory depression requiring full life support. You must be prepared to treat this eventuality, especially with the multidrug user.

Hallucinogens The patient who is experiencing a bad trip from a hallucinogenic agent is treated just like the one on stimulants. Individuals rarely take a dose sufficient to induce coma or significant depression. The usual direct effect of the agent is past in a few hours. These patients require a calm, mature manner and much emotional support. Unless absolutely needed, restraints should not be used. These patients must never be left unattended. Hallucinations or odd perceptions can occur suddenly, and patients have been known to leap from vehicles or windows under the influence of various agents. They must be carefully watched until your arrival at the emergency department. General support measures and observation are usually all that is needed.

Inhalants The patient in severe distress from inhalants is usually hypoxic. Hypoxia is often caused by the device, usually of makeshift construction, that is used to inhale the active vapors. Frequently, substances are inhaled from within a closed plastic bag that collapses and obstructs the airway. With the resulting hypoxia, you must be prepared to render all possible support: oxygen, artificial ventilation, and even cardiopulmonary resuscitation. In the absence of severe hypoxia, the patient should be treated as one with an overdose of a CNS depressant. Vomiting should be expected and

treated. Oxygen may be needed. The patient should be transported to the emergency department along with the agent inhaled, if possible. The agent may be housed in an aerosol can, a bottle of glue, or a tin of gasoline. Some agents, such as glycols, have very specific tissue toxicity (kidney or liver). Their rapid identification by emergency department personnel may aid in the start of treatment to protect these organs.

Injuries A rapid assessment of the physical status of the drug user is absolutely essential. Injuries not sought are often overlooked. Fractures must be splinted. The swollen cyanotic limb that has been compressed must be splinted and positioned as naturally and comfortably as possible. Head injuries must be recognized promptly because their effects frequently mimic drug use and vice versa. Prompt transportation with all appropriate support is indicated for the drug user who has sustained any injury.

Infections In addition to the effects of the drugs, the drug user may develop major systemic or local infectious problems. The local problems are almost always abscesses or cellulitis. Cellulitis is characterized by redness, swelling, warmth, and tenderness of soft tissue. It usually occurs in an extremity at the site of a drug injection. An infected limb should be splinted and the patient transported promptly because hospitalization and intravenous antibiotic treatment will probably be required. Abscesses, especially if they have ruptured spontaneously and are draining, should be dressed with sterile bandages and treated with all the precautions for open draining wounds (see Chapter 35).

The individual with a major systemic infection usually shows signs of that problem. Seizures, coma, or other neurological manifestations, and fever occur with a brain abscess; acute cardiac failure and fever occur with endocarditis; jaundice is a hallmark of hepatitis. These patients require prompt transport to the hospital. Procedures for handling the jaundiced patient with suspected hepatitis or AIDS are described in Chapter 35.

Multiple Drug Use You must be alert to the fact that a drug user may have used as many as three or four different agents. The use of drugs in conjunction with alcohol also occurs frequently. In situations in which the drugs complement one another, the effects on the patient are generally much greater than when each drug is used alone. Sometimes drugs with opposite effects are taken. In general, unless a given agent is a specific antagonist of one drug, opposing effects do not cancel each other. They usually result in panic reactions from acute stimulation that has been imposed on an altered mental state. Sometimes, they can produce profound depression.

Unfortunately, multiple drug use is becoming the norm today and the clinical picture produced is often confusing indeed.

Anaphylaxis A drug user undergoing an acute anaphylactic reaction is a priority-one emergency patient who requires major respiratory, ventilatory, and cardiac support. The most expeditious transport to the emergency department is indicated together with all available life-support measures. Treatment for anaphylactic shock is considered in Chapter 12.

Drug Withdrawal

Patients who are addicted to drugs—that is, who are psychologically and physically dependent on a constant supply of a drug—usually experience a severe reaction when the drug is withdrawn. These reactions are characterized by anxiety, nausea and vomiting, convulsions, delirium, profuse sweating, tachycardia, hallucinations, and severe abdominal cramps. Ordinarily, you are not required to treat acute withdrawal. However, if a patient has suddenly become unable to procure a regular supply, acute withdrawal may occur and may become an emergency problem. Often the patient can tell you the exact situation.

Individuals experiencing acute withdrawal are as urgently ill as those suffering from a drug overdose. They should be transported promptly to the emergency department, where controlled withdrawal can be instituted with constant medical and psychological support.

Except for nicotine, planned withdrawal is rarely attempted on an ambulatory or outpatient basis.

OTHER FORMS OF SUBSTANCE ABUSE

Virtually anything that can be taken as an agent, eaten or drunk, has been used to excess. There are compulsive water drinkers, steroid abusers, over-the-counter "pill poppers," and abusers of a variety of agents and foods. You will undoubtedly meet people who exhibit this type of behavior. In every instance, the characteristic is the obsessional, compulsive need of the patient to do whatever it is that is being done, even if it is to the patient's obvious detriment. Some specific problems are described here.

Aspirin

One of the most widely used and useful medications available today is aspirin (acetylsalicylic acid). Found in a variety of compounds, it is an effective pain reliever. Because of its availability, many people take aspirin for a wide variety of reasons. Despite its usefulness, aspirin can produce two specific toxic effects on the body. It can irritate the lining of the stomach and the small intestine, which can cause inflammation and ulcers that bleed. It can also interfere with platelet function and impair the blood-clotting mechanism. You may be called to see a patient with hematemesis (vomiting blood) caused by too much aspirin. The emergency treatment is the same as that described for all upper gastrointestinal bleeding (Chapter 34).

Anabolic Steroids

The term *anabolism* means the building of body tissue from simpler substances. A steroid is one of a variety of hormones produced by the adrenal cortex. Commonly, today, anabolic steroids are taken by would-be and even professional athletes to build muscle mass or improve athletic performance. Unfortunately, although users believe that greater athletic prowess is the result, there is no clear evidence that it comes about by virtue of better body tissue, more muscles, or better health. The improved athletic response may be from more aggressive behavior by the individual or from a sensation of less fatigue with exertion.

What is not realized by most users of anabolic steroids is their harmful side effects, which include aggression, violent outbursts, rage, and depression. No less disturbing are the physical effects. In men, they include breast enlargement, testicular atrophy, diminished sperm production, and impotence. In women, clitoral enlargement, baldness, beard growth, voice changes, and breast atrophy can occur. In both sexes a distinct pattern of antisocial behavior known as "roid rage" is seen in addition to an increased risk of developing coronary artery disease, stroke, liver tumors, jaundice, accelerated bone growth and maturation (leading to a short stature), acne, hypertension, and diabetes. Long-term use of these agents has become associated with withdrawal syndromes similar to those seen when CNS stimulant use is stopped.

Ordinarily, this form of abuse does not concern the EMT. It may, however, be a complicating factor in many situations.

Laxatives

A variety of laxatives and stool softeners, both potent and mild, are available without prescription. Some individuals use them to the extent that significant diarrhea occurs and is sustained. In these instances, you must focus on the result of the laxative use. For example, a patient may be in profound dehydration as a result of the diarrhea. Emergency transportation then is indicated, with treatment directed at metabolic shock (Chapter 12). Usually, these situations do not pose significant emergency problems.

Vitamins

Nearly every pharmacy and supermarket has a huge stock of every available vitamin. Well-described disease states are associated with excessive use of as well as lack of vitamins. Sometimes the clinical picture of vitamin abuse

is indeed bizarre. Ordinarily, vitamin abuse is not a concern of the EMT; however, it is a widespread problem in the United States.

Food Abuse

In the United States, morbid obesity as a result of food abuse involves millions of individuals. Many of these patients routinely consume in excess of 5,000 calories per day. Many seek and require surgical or medical control of their obesity. Emergency problems for this group of people occur when individual weight reaches a level that interferes with normal breathing or other activities. The compulsion to eat may not be controllable by the individual and has been likened to an uncontrollable alcohol addiction.

Some individuals with a compulsion to eat control their weight with vomiting, a disorder called *bulimia*. For them, a second addiction to syrup of ipecac or other emetics in addition to that for food is becoming recognized. Other individuals, concerned with figure and weight, literally starve themselves, a condition called *anorexia nervosa*. They often become addicted to a variety of appetite suppressants. Chapter 34 describes eating disorders in detail.

SUMMARY

One of your responsibilities as an EMT is to recognize the widespread nature of substance abuse in the United States and the great variety of presentations it can have. It is likely that, in a few months of routine work, you will encounter more than one instance of substance abuse. Each situation has a specific treatment pattern and each must be met logically for support to be effective. In general, the problems of substance abuse represent for the patient severe, deep psychological needs. The EMT who is aware of the spectrum of disability associated with substance abuse can more easily cope with its manifestations.

EMT SAFETY

Nowhere in emergency work is your protection as necessary as in dealing with the population of substance abusers. Although individuals whose problems involve food, vitamin, aspirin, steroid, or proprietary laxatives, pose little health threat, the drug and alcohol abusers form a different group.

The group of drug-abusing patients is one in which the likelihood of serious and unrecognized infections (AIDS or hepatitis) is fairly high. The patients may be combative to the extent of biting, hitting, or otherwise injuring you. Open and draining abscesses are commonly seen. Especially with the alcoholic, one of the major emergency problems may be copious bleeding. As a result, virtually every

avenue is open for contact with the body fluids of an infected patient.

Any barrier that can be placed between you and the patient, about whom you know little, is appropriate: gloves, goggles, a jump suit, and mask. Your actual handling of the patient, to allay fear and panic and to defuse frightening situations, may enable him or her to be less aggressive and combative. You must learn to expect the unexpected with these patients continuously and to keep your own protection always in mind. The drugs used, in general, pose no great threat to you. The drug user does.

YOU ARE THE EMT

1. You have been called to treat a patient who "passed out" at a beer bash. His friends were going to let him "sleep it off," but they don't think he looks normal. What are some of the problems you should be looking for?
2. You are called to see a patient who has overdosed on "Goof Balls." Are these a central nervous system depressant or stimulant? What kinds of problems is this patient likely to experience? This patient is a known diabetic. Does this disease have any bearing on the present problem?
3. Your patient is on a "bad trip." He thinks he is Superman. What type of drugs is he probably taking? How should you treat him?
4. Your patient is a 15-year-old girl who is screaming that her family is trying to kill her. Her parents tell you she has never been on drugs, but her younger sister pulls out some pills she says she

found in her sister's room. What will you say to the parents? What kind of drugs does her behavior indicate she might be using? How will you treat this patient?
5. You are called to help with a young man found in a rooming house, alone and unconscious. Drug paraphernalia is apparent in the room. Both arms have multiple needle puncture sites. The right arm appears swollen and discolored (red). It is tender, causing him to moan when it is touched or moved. A small amount of pus is seen at one of the injection sites. Describe your overall care for this patient and state some of the problems he may have.
6. You are involved with a known drug-abusing patient who, at this time, in addition to his acute drug problem, is febrile (102 degree F) and jaundiced. What are appropriate precautions for you to take?

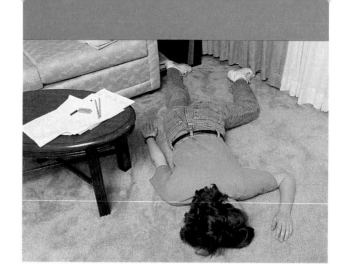

CHAPTER 37

UNCONSCIOUSNESS
AND EPILEPSY

. . . .

KEY TERMS

. . . .

anaphylaxis (an"ah-fĭ-lak'sis) An unusual or exaggerated allergic reaction of the organism to foreign protein or other substance.

arrhythmia (ah-rith'me-ah) An irregular or abnormal heart rhythm.

aura (aw"rah) A subjective sensation or phenomenon that precedes and marks the onset of a seizure.

convulsion (kon-vul'shun) A seizure.

epilepsy (ep'i-lep"se) A condition manifested by seizures that are caused by an abnormal focus of activity within the brain, producing severe motor responses or changes in consciousness.

heat stroke A life-threatening condition caused by exposure to excessive heat, natural or artificial, and marked by dry skin, dizziness, headache, nausea, and muscle cramps.

hypothermia (hi"po-ther'me-ah) A condition in which the internal body temperature falls below 95 degrees F after prolonged exposure to freezing or near-freezing temperatures.

postictal state (post-ik'tal stāt) After an epileptic attack.

seizure (se'zhur) Generalized, uncoordinated muscular activity associated with loss of consciousness; a convulsion.

status epilepticus (sta'tus ep" ĭ-lep'ti-kus) A series of rapidly repeated epileptic convulsions in one individual without any periods of consciousness between them.

stroke The loss of brain function, usually the result of cerebrovascular accident.

triage (tre'ahzh) Sorting. A technique of establishing treatment and transportation priorities in any event where the number of casualties is greater than the emergency facility can handle.

OVERVIEW

The unconscious patient is at a decided disadvantage. Unable to talk and often showing no obvious signs of illness or injury, the unconscious patient cannot tell you whether the problem is a heart attack, insulin shock, or just a simple fainting spell. Therefore, you must know how to proceed when faced with unconsciousness.

The first step in the care of an unconscious patient is to provide basic life support when it is needed. Then, you must attempt to determine the cause of the unconscious state. Finally, treat the unconsciousness, basing your approach on its presumed cause. For some patients unconsciousness is the result of cardiopulmonary arrest; for others it may be brought on by injury, emotions, environmental causes, drugs, or neurological disease.

The first half of Chapter 37 briefly describes the problems that can cause unconsciousness and then refers to the chapter in this text that deals with the specific problem in more detail. The second half of Chapter 37 focuses on one of the neurological diseases that commonly causes unconsciousness—epilepsy. A condition characterized by episodic sei-zures, the rate of epilepsy is on the increase because more people are surviving the events that cause it, such as head injury, meningitis, or brain abscess. Chapter 37 describes the various types of seizures—most of them now controlled by medication—and explains how you should manage the various manifestations of seizure activity. A final paragraph outlines some considerations for EMT safety.

GOALS

The goals of Chapter 37 are to
- know how to assess the basic pressing needs of the unconscious patient.
- know how to determine the various causes of unconsciousness.
- become familiar with the treatment for each of the various causes of unconsciousness.
- recognize the various types of epileptic seizures and know how to manage them.

INITIAL EMERGENCY CARE OF UNCONSCIOUSNESS

All unconscious patients require similar emergency medical treatment, regardless of the specific cause of the unconsciousness. In general, you must follow these six steps when you are treating an unconscious individual:

1. Secure and maintain an airway.
2. Institute cardiopulmonary resuscitation (CPR) when necessary.
3. Observe the incident; record the history when it is available; note any items that might serve as evidence regarding the cause of the unconscious state.
4. Attempt to define the specific cause of unconsciousness in this patient.

5. Periodically observe and record the patient's vital signs and level of consciousness.
6. Transport the patient promptly to the emergency department.

For every unconscious patient, the first and foremost treatment is to ensure an open airway and to provide respiratory support when necessary. A supine (lying flat) unconscious patient is in danger of aspirating vomitus or other oral contents, or of suffocating from an obstructed airway. Open the airway and place the unconscious patient on one side with the head about six inches lower than the feet; maintain an open airway (Figure 37–1). Transport the patient in this position with continued monitoring of respiration and vital signs. If you suspect a neck injury after an accident in a patient who is not conscious, the first step in emergency care is to stabilize the spine (Chapter 7 and Chapter 21). Then, you may direct your attention to the airway.

The head downward position is not beneficial to the unconscious patient with a head injury. In this situation, you must balance the need for controlling and maintaining the airway against the possibility of aggravating the head injury. In general, the first priority is management of the airway. When the patient sustaining a head injury has a clear airway and is breathing well, do not transport him or her with the head lower than the feet.

When the unconscious patient has sustained a full cardiopulmonary arrest and when it is known that this state has lasted fewer than 10 minutes at normal body temperature, you must begin cardiopulmonary resuscitation (CPR) (Figure 37–2). Many patients with an acute myocardial infarction (AMI or heart attack) have been saved by the timely and vigorous application of CPR immediately after the attack.

Once cardiopulmonary function has been restored and stabilized, a medical history should be obtained (Figure 37–3). You are in an excellent position to obtain information about the cause of a patient's problem. You should question relatives and bystanders about the onset of the unconsciousness. When did it start? Did it come on suddenly or gradually? Did the patient complain of headache, weakness or numbness? Did a seizure occur? Has the patient had previous episodes of unconsciousness, epilepsy, or any other medical illness? Is there a possibility of drug use or drug overdose, or any type of poisoning? If the

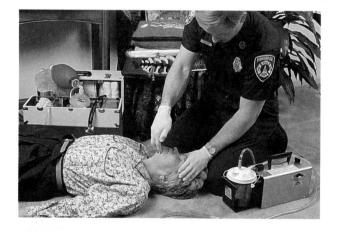

FIGURE 37–1

Securing and maintaining the airway and adequate respiration is the first and most important treatment for the unconscious patient.

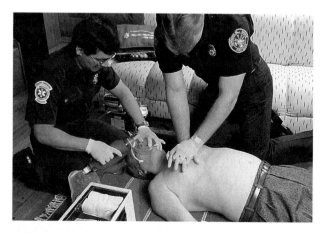

FIGURE 37–2

Start CPR on an unconscious patient who has sustained a full cardiopulmonary arrest for less than 10 minutes at normal body temperatures.

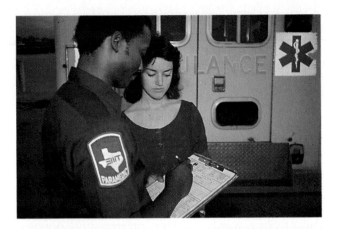

FIGURE 37-3

Any information concerning the patient's medical history that you can provide will help emergency department personnel.

patient rouses during transportation, question him or her. You must also look for medical identification symbols (emergency medical bracelet, necklace, or card) that might suggest the cause of the unconscious state. Environ-

mental causes of unconsciousness, such as an *electrical shock* or exposure to excessive heat or cold, should be noted. Evidence of head injury should be sought. Note and gather any bottles, evidence of drugs, plant material, or any other items that might be linked to the patient's unconsciousness and take them along with the patient to the emergency department (Figure 37-4). These items might help emergency department personnel to complete the patient's medical history.

Record vital signs; note and describe any injuries. Note the time of the onset of unconsciousness and whether it developed suddenly or slowly, as well as all subsequent changes. Assess the patient's level of consciousness and record it using the AVPU scale described in Chapter 20. The Glasgow Coma Scale (Figure 37-5) is another simple and easy to use scale which measures the level of consciousness. Many EMS systems employ it routinely. Note whether the pupils of the eyes are constricted or dilated and record the pupillary response to light. Transport the patient promptly to the emergency department.

A rather lengthy list of duties attends the initial treatment of the unconscious patient.

FIGURE 37-4

Unconsciousness can be caused by injuries, epilepsy, injected or ingested agents, environmental causes, diseases, and emotions.

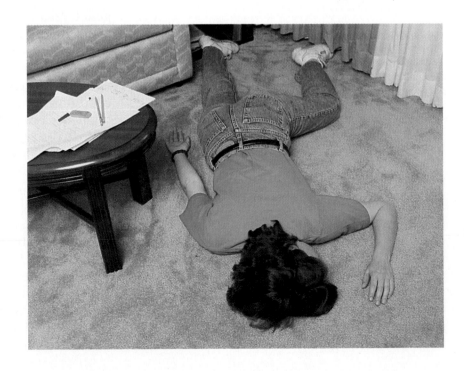

GLASGOW COMA SCALE

Eye Opening	Spontaneous	4
	To Voice	3
	To Pain	2
	None	1
Verbal Response *	Oriented	5
	Confused	4
	Inappropriate Words	3
	Incomprehensible Words	2
	None	1
Motor Response **	Obeys Command	6
	Localizes Pain	5
	Withdraws (pain)	4
	Flexion (pain)	3
	Extension (pain)	2
	None	1
Glasgow Coma Score Total		

TOTAL GLASGOW COMA SCALE POINTS	
14 - 15 = 5	CONVERSION = APPROXIMATELY ONE-THIRD TOTAL VALUE
11 - 13 = 4	
8 - 10 = 3	
5 - 7 = 2	
3 - 4 = 1	

FIGURE 37–5

The Glasgow Coma Scale, based on eye opening, verbal, and motor responses, is a practical means of monitoring changes in level of consciousness. If response on the scale is given a number, the responsiveness of the patient can be expressed by summation of the figures. *Lowest* score is 3; *highest* is 15.

* Arouse patient with painful stimulus if necessary.

** Apply knuckles to sternum; observe arms.

Some priorities do exist. This patient belongs in an emergency department. If you have difficulty supporting the airway, breathing, and circulation, your first and most pressing duty is to get him or her to the emergency department rapidly. If the vital functions are stable, taking a few moments to gather the foregoing information will probably help emergency department personnel greatly.

CAUSES OF UNCONSCIOUSNESS AND ITS TREATMENT

After resuscitation of an unconscious patient, you should try to determine the cause of the unconsciousness. Unconscious patients take highest priority in **triage** and transportation. It is important to determine the cause of unconsciousness because, once it has been determined, medical treatment designed to reverse the condition can be started. Unconsciousness can be caused by diseases, injuries, emotions, the environment, injected or ingested poisonous agents, and epilepsy (see Figure 37–4). Table 37–1 lists some of the more common problems causing unconsciousness, and their treatment.

Diseases

The common diseases that may produce unconsciousness are diabetes mellitus and arteriosclerosis.

In diabetes, unconsciousness may quickly occur if too much insulin is taken without enough food, causing the blood sugar level to drop (insulin shock). In this situation, not enough glucose is available for normal brain function. A headache, followed by unconsciousness, develops rather quickly. Emergency treatment must be given promptly to avoid permanent brain injury. In the opposite state—that is, when the blood sugar is too high because of insufficient insulin—unconsciousness results after a long period of time. This condition is known as diabetic ketoacidosis (diabetic coma). Unconsciousness in this situation occurs because of excessive fluid and sugar loss from the kidneys, which produces dehydration and a gradual accumulation in the blood and body tissue of acidic metabolic waste products. Insulin shock and diabetic coma are more fully discussed in Chapter 32. You must be thoroughly familiar with the emergency medical care for each situation and remember that both can cause unconsciousness.

Arteriosclerotic vascular disease can attack every artery in the body. When the disease damages and subsequently blocks the arteries that supply the heart, a heart attack may

Table 37-1   Causes of Unconsciousness and Emergency Medical Management

Problem	Cause	Mechanism	Management	Chapter
Diseases:				
Diabetic coma	Hyperglycemia and acidosis	Inadequate use of sugar, acidosis	Transport, complex treatment for acidosis	32
Insulin shock	Hypoglycemia	Excess insulin	Sugar, transport	32
Myocardial infarction	Damaged myocardium	Insufficient cardiac output	Oxygen, CPR, transport	29
Stroke	Damaged brain	Loss of arterial supply to brain or hemorrhage within brain	Support, gentle transport	30
Injury:				
Hemorrhagic shock	Bleeding	Hypovolemia	Control external bleeding, recognize internal bleeding, CPR, transport	12
Respiratory insufficiency	Insufficient inspired O_2	Paralysis, chest wall damage, airway obstruction	Clear airway, supplemental O_2, CPR, transport	7
Cerebral contusion, concussion, or hematoma	Blunt head injury	Bleeding into or around brain, concussive effect of blow	Airway, supplemental O_2, CPR, careful monitoring, transport	20, 37
Emotions:				
Psychogenic shock	Emotional reaction	Sudden drop in cerebral blood flow caused by vasodilation	Place supine, make comfortable, observe for injuries	37
Neurological problems:				
Epilepsy	Brain injury, scar, genetic predisposition, disease	Excitable focus of motor activity in brain	Support, protect patient, transport in status epilepticus	37
Injected or ingested agents:				
Alcohol	Excess intake	Cerebral depression	Support, CPR, transport	36
Drugs	Excess intake	Cerebral depression	Support, CPR, transport (bring drug)	36
Plant poisons	Contact, ingestion	Direct cerebral or other toxic effect, local irritant effect	Support, recognition, CPR, identify plant, local wound care, transport	28
Animal poisons	Contact, ingestion, injection	Direct cerebral or other toxic effect, local irritant effects	Recognition, support, CPR, identify agent, local wound care, transport	28
Environment:				
Heatstroke	Excessive heat, inability to sweat	Brain damage from heat	Immediate cooling, support, CPR, transport	42
Anaphylaxis	Acute contact with agent to which patient is sensitive	Allergic reaction, bronchospasm, excess bronchial secretions	Intramuscular epinephrine, support, CPR, transport	28
Electrical shock	Contact with electrical current	Cardiac abnormalities (fibrillation, standstill)	CPR, transport, do not treat until current controlled	40

(continued)

Table 37-1	Causes of Unconsciousness and Emergency Medical Management			
Problem	**Cause**	**Mechanism**	**Management**	**Chapter**
Systemic hypothermia	Prolonged exposure to cold	Diminished cerebral function, cardiac arrhythmias	CPR, rapid transport, warming on the way	42
Drowning	$O_2 \downarrow$, $CO_2 \uparrow$, breath holding, H_2O inhalation	Cerebral damage	CPR, rapid transport	43
Air embolism	Intravascular air	Obstruction to arterial blood flow by air bubbles	CPR, transport, recompression	43
Decompression sickness	Intravascular nitrogen	Obstruction to arterial blood flow by nitrogen bubbles	CPR transport, recompression	43

follow. Loss of consciousness may be sudden because of an acute **arrhythmia,** a sudden disordered beating of the damaged heart. In this situation, CPR may be lifesaving. Heart attack is more fully discussed in Chapter 29.

Similarly, when arteriosclerotic vascular disease damages the arteries that supply blood to the brain, thrombosis (clotting in the vessel) or actual rupture of a damaged or diseased vessel may cause a **stroke.** Unconsciousness in these patients may be preceded by a seizure or sudden headache. Although a stroke rarely causes sudden death, it may result in partial or complete loss of consciousness. The methods of handling the patient with a stroke, partially conscious or unconscious, are unique to this condition and are presented in Chapter 30.

Injuries

Many types of injury result in a loss of consciousness. All injuries that cause excessive blood loss may bring about hypovolemic shock. In this situation, not enough blood is left in the vascular system to supply the brain and heart. Loss of consciousness from hypovolemic shock occurs only after much of the circulating blood volume has been lost, because the body tries to maintain blood pressure in order to preserve blood flow in the heart and brain as long as possible. Thus, the injured patient who has a low blood pressure will require the most rapid possible transport to a source of medical care.

Chest injuries often produce unconsciousness as a result of insufficient oxygen intake. Injuries of the chest wall, for example, cause severe pain restricting breathing and limiting the body's supply of oxygen. As described in Chapter 24, a hemothorax or pneumothorax reduces the capacity of the lung to accept and transport oxygen. Cervical spinal cord injuries result in a paralysis of some or all of the muscles of respiration. With all of these injuries, your primary responsibility is to ensure an open airway and to give supplemental oxygen and provide respiratory support as needed.

Injury of the head is probably the most common traumatic cause of loss of consciousness. After you resuscitate the patient with a head injury, it is essential to assess the level of consciousness and monitor it carefully until the patient reaches the hospital. Often, changes in the level of consciousness occur quickly in these patients. For this reason alone, a person with a head injury should be transported to the emergency department rapidly. Frequently, an immediate operation to correct the cause of the unconsciousness is necessary. During transport, maintain the airway, protect the cervical spine, give oxygen, and support respirations.

Emotions

The common faint is an emotional reaction that results in a temporary but sudden general dilation of blood vessels without any increase in cardiac output. Momentarily, an adequate blood supply for the brain is lost and its function impaired. In general, consciousness returns promptly once the patient becomes supine. You must be alert for injuries that might have occurred when the patient fell during a fainting episode. In general, these associated injuries are the pressing reasons for emergency care after a common fainting episode.

Environmental Causes

Environmental causes of loss of consciousness include excessive heat or cold, electrical shock, water, the exposure to gases under extreme pressure, certain work-related injuries, and extreme allergic reactions. Generally, unconsciousness due to extremes of heat (**heat stroke**) or cold (systemic **hypothermia**) are easily diagnosed by virtue of the circumstances and the patient's body temperature. Vigorous, general support of the patient is mandatory, in addition to appropriate cooling or warming. Specific details of these problems are contained in Chapter 42.

With patients who have sustained electrical shock, you must think first of self-protection. The patient, if still in contact with the source of the current may, if touched, transmit the full volume of current to you. Control of the electric current must be achieved before any treatment can be given. The patient may have sustained a cardiopulmonary arrest as a result of the electrical shock and require CPR as an initial step. A detailed review of handling the patient injured by electricity is contained in Chapter 40.

In general, drowned patients require basic life-support measures and rapid transport to the nearest emergency department. CPR may be required and, for hypothermic patients, warming may be necessary. A detailed description of the treatment for drowning and other water-related problems is presented in Chapter 43.

The very special situation of **anaphylaxis** is a manifestation of an allergic reaction in its most extreme form. It results from acute contact either by injection, ingestion, or inhalation of a foreign substance. Anaphylactic shock can produce death from respiratory failure in a matter of minutes. Severe spasm of the bronchi combined with a flood of mucus into these airways make breathing (especially exhalation) difficult. A great number of patients who are sensitized to specific agents know it and carry kits for the intramuscular or subcutaneous injection of epinephrine as an antidote. Anaphylaxis is discussed in detail in Chapters 12 and 28.

Injected or Ingested Toxic Substances

Many different substances, including alcohol, drugs, and plant and animal poisons, may be injected or ingested. Some are very toxic in very small amounts. Some, such as alcohol, are used in moderation as routine substances by a large portion of the population but are used to great excess by others. Many of these agents have a direct toxic effect on the brain. Usually, emergency medical care for injection or ingestion of toxic agents includes cardiorespiratory support and prompt transport to the emergency department. Note the size of the pupils of the eyes in these patients. Widely dilated pupils are characteristic of an overdose with drugs such as barbiturates; constricted pupils, on the other hand, occur with the use of narcotics such as heroin, morphine, and Demerol. If it is possible to do so quickly and without jeopardizing the care of the patient, you should try to identify the agent causing the unconsciousness. Bring it with the patient or report its existence to the emergency department personnel.

The medical treatment for all toxic overdoses—alcohol, drugs, or other agents—is support of the patient's basic life functions until the drug has been cleared (metabolized) by the body. In some cases, medical treatment may include the use of a specific antagonist to the toxic substance. In some other situations, the patient may require the use of an artificial kidney to rid the body of the substance.

Usually, the drug overdose patient will spend some time in the hospital (in an intensive care unit) until physicians are certain he or she is free from the agent. Detailed discussions of substance abuse are contained in Chapter 36.

EPILEPSY

Epilepsy is a relatively common condition that is characterized by recurrent episodes of **seizures.** One out of every 200 people has some form of epilepsy. Its frequency is increasing as more individuals survive episodes of head injury, meningitis, or brain abscess. The seizures are usually easily controlled by medication. Uncontrolled, epilepsy causes periodic seizures. In general, most people take the term *seizure* to mean generalized, uncoordinated muscular activity associated with a loss of consciousness. However, seizures occur in a variety of forms from a severe convulsion to simply ''blacking out'' for a few seconds.

Seizures may occur as a result of a recent or old head injury, a brain tumor, an embolus that is causing an acute block of blood flow within the brain, brain hemorrhage, infection, fever, or simply a genetic predisposition. They are usually caused by an abnormal focus of electrical activity in the brain that produces the severe motor activity and changes in the level of consciousness.

Most seizures involve altered states of consciousness that last for variable periods of time. Many seizures are followed by a **postictal state** of sleepiness or unconsciousness that lasts for a varying length of time. During the postictal state, transitory weakness or paralysis on one side of the body or in one limb may provide a clue to the location in the brain of the lesion causing the seizure. If observed and recorded, this information can be valuable for the physician. Patients with epilepsy who have recurrent seizures frequently carry some medical identification tag or card. Close questioning of family members or friends will also usually confirm this diagnosis.

Not all seizures are due to epilepsy; many other serious illnesses can cause them. It is especially important to determine the cause in the patient who has had no history of previous seizure activity. Identification of the cause may require an extensive medical work-up in the hospital.

Classification of Seizures

Seizures are generally classified according to the degree and location of abnormal electrical activity in the brain. Seizure episodes are placed in one of two categories: generalized seizures and partial seizures. In a *generalized seizure* (also called convulsive or tonic-clonic seizure), most of the brain is involved in the abnormal electrical discharge. Usually all extremities are involved in the muscular activity and the patient becomes unconscious. There are usually three phases of a generalized seizure: the aura, the convulsion itself, and the postictal state.

The **aura** is a sensation perceived by the patient that something is about to happen; it precedes the convulsion in many patients with epilepsy. It can take many forms (a sound, a twitch, a feeling of dizziness or anxiety, or the perception of an unusual odor). For an epileptic patient, it is often the same for each attack and serves as a warning that a seizure is about to begin. The aura lasts only a short while and is immediately followed by the convulsion. Sustained, tonic (rigid) muscular contractions, which can cause odd posturing of the body, may last several minutes. Clonic (repetitive) muscular activity, or spasms, may be superimposed on the rigid muscular contractions.

During the **convulsion,** the jaw muscles contract, occasionally causing the patient to bite the tongue or lips. Loss of bowel or bladder control is common during a generalized seizure, and involuntary urination or defecation often takes place.

After one to several minutes, the convulsive phase ends and is followed by the postictal state. This phase is a period of exhaustion and recovery following the convulsion. During this phase, which may last for 10 to 30 minutes, the patient's level of consciousness is depressed, the airway may become obstructed by mucus, vomitus, or the relaxed pharyngeal muscles, and respirations may be slowed. Localized transitory weakness or paralysis may be present.

Partial seizures involve less extensive and very specific areas of the brain. Therefore, the seizure activity is limited to one extremity or one side of the body. Usually, the patient remains conscious and aware of the event. This type of seizure is called a simple partial seizure. Simple partial seizures can progress to generalized seizures in which the abnormal motor activity extends from one side of the body to the other. In this situation, consciousness is usually lost. In another type of seizure, the complex partial seizure, the patient is unresponsive or displays automatic behavior, such as chewing, fumbling with clothing, walking aimlessly, or muttering. A summary of these types of seizures is contained in Table 37–2.

TABLE 37–2   Classification of Seizures

Name (Synonyms)	Manifestation	Emergency Care	Other Conditions Taken for it	Complications
Generalized Seizure (Tonic-clonic Convulsive Grand mal Major motor seizure)	Aura; muscular contraction with spasms; postictal state; or depressed consciousness; patient is unaware of seizure and depressed after it	Observe, protect, and do *not* restrain patient; do *not* force mouth open; do *not* put hand in mouth; O_2 and airway clearing after convulsion; transport for seizure >10 min, for status epilepticus, or for new seizures	Stroke; heart attack; any other sudden emergency	Aspiration during postictal phase; self-injury
Nonconvulsive Seizure (Petit mal)	Sudden stare; lack of attention; common in children; short (seconds); prompt return of full awareness	None; if not diagnosed may need medical evaluation	Inattention; day dreaming	Poor learning if not diagnosed and recognized
Simple Partial Seizure	Patient awake and alert; experiences an involuntary jerking which progresses to involve one entire side or one limb	None; unless it progresses to a generalized seizure	Odd mental behavior	None
Complex Partial Seizure (Psychomotor seizure)	Patient is confused; shows random repetitive actions; may start or stare; generally unresponsive with altered consciousness; usually short (2–5 minutes); no memory of seizure; long post-seizure period	None; reassure; remain with and protect patient; do not restrain, startle or command; suggest and guide	Drug or alcohol induced behavior; mental disease	None

Management of Seizures

The important first step in the management of a generalized seizure is to prevent self-injury during the attack. When an epileptic patient says that a seizure is about to occur (the aura), take immediate action. Help the patient lie down on the ground away from danger to minimize the chances of injury during the seizure. Protect the patient's head, arms, and legs, but do not rigidly restrain them. Tight clothes should be loosened. Nothing should be forced into the patient's mouth, especially if the teeth are clenched or if the patient is convulsing. Padded ''bite sticks'' made by taping tongue depressors together have been popular to prevent biting of the lips, cheeks, or tongue. Sometimes, however, they have been bitten in two by the patient or have lodged in the pharynx and actually obstructed the airway. If an object is used to prevent biting, it should be placed between the molars, not the front teeth. It is, however, rarely needed. Never put your fingers into the patient's mouth.

Contraction of the chest muscles may cause the patient to appear to have an airway obstruction and to become cyanotic. The return of normal respiration almost always follows a seizure. Lack of respiration during the attack rarely presents a problem unless several convulsions follow one another in quick succession. The airway can best be kept open by putting the patient on one side, head down, so that gravity will aid in keeping the tongue out of the pharynx and any vomited material will not be easily aspirated.

Following the phase of excessive muscular activity, the patient will be drowsy, perhaps disoriented, and only partially conscious (the postictal phase). At this point you should assess the airway; any mucus or vomitus should be cleared and the airway adequately maintained until the patient is fully awake. Once vital signs are assessed and recorded, a secondary survey of the patient should be performed. Look for any injuries that may have occurred during the seizure and assess the level of consciousness.

The patient who has a history of epilepsy and who has frequently recurring seizures usually achieves complete recovery of function soon after the seizure. Transportation of such a patient to the hospital is not necessary. Following the seizure, this patient requires a period of rest to allow full recovery. Patients without a history of previous seizures, however, must have a thorough medical evaluation in the hospital. If your evaluation during the postictal state reveals any abnormality (airway difficulty or injury as a result of the seizure), even the patient with a history of seizures should be transported to the hospital for continued evaluation and treatment. Because most seizure patients take some type of medication, all drugs being taken by the patient should be brought to the hospital.

A few patients with epilepsy experience **status epilepticus,** in which one seizure closely follows another, with no return of full consciousness between them. Potentially, this situation is very serious, because the patient does not have time to breathe well or to recover from the stress of the initial seizure. The same problem can occur if a single seizure lasts longer than 10 minutes.

When you are faced with a prolonged convulsive spell (lasting longer than 10 minutes) or repeated seizures closely following one another (status epilepticus), you must give supplemental oxygen and transport the patient promptly to the hospital. Under these circumstances, the seizure may not be controlled without specialized hospital treatment. This patient should be placed in the highest priority category for triage and transport; status epilepticus can be life-threatening.

In the management of partial seizures, the same general rules apply as for convulsive seizures. A problem may arise in diagnosing a complex partial seizure, because it may be mistaken for intoxication, drug abuse, or another medical condition causing abnormal behavior. A cardinal rule concerning the handling of a patient with abnormal behavior is that the patient should not be physically restrained unless it is essential for his or her own safety or the care of others. A patient may react violently to restraint. During a complex partial seizure, which may last 15 minutes or longer, the patient is in a confused state but usually responds to suggestions and comments given in a friendly manner. Stay with the patient, provide reassurance, and observe the vital functions carefully until the abnormal behavior ceases. A thorough medical evaluation in the hospital may be needed to diagnose the cause of this type of seizure.

EMT SAFETY

In general, the unconscious patient poses little immediate risk to you as an EMT by virtue of the unconsciousness. The injured or bleeding patient poses the risk of blood and body fluid contact. Relatively few causes of unconsciousness are related to easily transmitted diseases such as hepatitis, the various "flu" syndromes, or the acute infectious problems of childhood. Routine attention to handwashing, the use of masks and gloves and standard ambulance cleansing will protect you and your vehicle from infection and contamination.

YOU ARE THE EMT

1. You have responded to a construction accident. A worker has fallen off a ladder and is unconscious. What are the first three steps you should take in administering emergency care?
2. As you know, stroke can cause unconsciousness because the supply of blood to the brain is interrupted. Explain how the following problems can cause unconsciousness: insulin shock, hemorrhagic shock, and epilepsy.
3. With epilepsy, how can you tell whether the patient is having a tonic-clonic seizure or a partial seizure? How would you manage each type?
4. The patient has just suffered an epileptic seizure and is in a postictal state. What does that mean? What should you do during this time?
5. What is the major difference between simple and complex partial seizures?
6. Give three examples of other disorders that can be easily confused with simple or complex partial seizures.

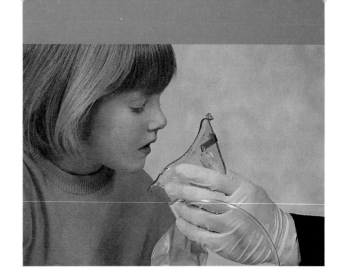

CHAPTER 38

PEDIATRIC EMERGENCIES

KEY TERMS

croup (krōōp) An infectious disease of the upper respiratory system that may cause partial airway obstruction and is characterized by a barking cough.

dehydration (de″hi-dra′shun) Loss of water from the tissues of the body.

epiglottitis (ep″ĭ-glot-ti′tis) An infectious disease in which the epiglottis becomes inflamed and enlarged and may cause upper respiratory obstruction.

febrile convulsion (feb′ril konvul′shun) A seizure, usually of short duration and not dangerous, that sometimes accompanies high fevers in children.

gastroenteritis (gas″tro-en-ter-i′tis) A viral or bacterial infection of the lining of the stomach and/or the intestines.

meningitis (men″in-ji′tis) An inflammation of the meningeal coverings of the brain; it can be caused by a virus or a bacterium.

neonate (ne′o-nāt) A newborn infant.

pediatrics (pe″de-at′riks) Medical practice devoted to the care of children up to age 15.

sudden infant death syndrome (SIDS) Death from unknown cause occurring during sleep in an otherwise healthy infant; also called crib death.

OVERVIEW

One of the most difficult emergencies for the EMT is having to respond to an injured, ill, or physically or sexually abused child. At the same time, perhaps no part of the EMT's job is as rewarding, because saving a child's life or rescuing a child from permanent, disabling injury means giving back to that child the promise of years of productive activity.

Children differ from adults in more than just body size and build. Several diseases, particularly certain infections, occur more frequently in children. Trauma is the leading cause of death in children over the age of 1 year. Although the basic principles of management of injuries and illnesses in children are similar to the treatment principles used with adults, certain differences do exist.

Chapter 38 begins with a description of the pediatric patient and the common diseases and illnesses of childhood. The chapter next discusses the techniques of basic life support, the procedures for relieving airway obstruction, and the management of trauma resulting from injuries. The chapter then presents a number of specific pediatric emergencies. These include fever, abdominal pain, poisoning, contagious childhood diseases, and sudden infant death syndrome (SIDS). Also discussed are two special pediatric emergencies—the problems of child abuse and sexual abuse. Chapter 38 concludes with a section on transporting the pediatric patient—not an easy task when dealing with a young and frightened child.

GOALS

The goals of Chapter 38 are to
- describe the pediatric patient.
- know how to administer basic life support to a child.
- know how to clear an obstructed airway in a child.
- know the principles of management of trauma in children.
- become familiar with specific pediatric emergencies, including fever, abdominal pains, poisoning, contagious diseases, and sudden infant death syndrome (SIDS).
- recognize the special pediatric problems of child abuse and sexual abuse.
- learn how to transport infants and children.

THE PEDIATRIC PATIENT

An entire segment of professional medical practice, called **pediatrics,** is devoted to the care of the young. Many health problems in children are unique, and similarly, many common health problems of adults simply do not exist in children. Thus, medicine has come to consider the unique areas peculiar to pediatrics as a separate discipline.

Handling a sick or injured child can be extremely difficult. It is almost always a trying emotional experience to confront a seriously ill or injured child, and not everyone is comfortable doing so. You must approach a child with a calm, professional manner; hard as it is, personal feelings must be kept firmly in check. Parent and crowd anxiety are amplified in the behavior and response of pediatric patients to the stress of injury or disease. Although helping ill or injured children may not be easy, it has rewards that few other activities can match. In most situations, the management of a pediatric patient involves managing both the child and the parent.

Traditionally, pediatrics pertains to children up to age 15. Recently, however, interest has been expressed in extending the upper age limit to the time of entrance into college. This is the age at which many children sever family ties. Further, it seems reasonable to provide an individual with continuous care from infancy to adulthood. Within this long time span, some specific divisions exist. The neonatal period covers the first 30 days after birth. In the **neonate,** the commonest causes of death are problems related to the birth (prematurity, for example) or congenital defects. Until the age of 1 year, a child is regarded as an infant; among these pediatric patients, congenital defects are the major cause of death. From age 1 to age 8, the individual is considered a young child; and from 8 to 15, an older child. Among these latter groups, the most common cause of death is trauma from motor vehicle accidents, falls, household accidents, and poisonings.

Pediatric diseases are by no means limited to the common infectious problems such as measles, mumps, or chicken pox. Cancer, while uncommon in children, is a real and very serious problem. Some viral and bacterial infections can also be severe. Injury, accidental or not, is another common and potentially serious childhood problem.

BASIC LIFE SUPPORT

Like adults, children cannot tolerate cerebral hypoxia (lack of oxygen) for more than a few minutes before permanent brain damage occurs. Therefore, the rules of basic life support are no different for children than for adults. The techniques of basic life support must be adapted because of the child's size and meta-

bolic requirements. Review Chapters 7 and 9 to refresh your understanding of the principles of basic life support. Figures 38–1 and 38–2 are American Heart Association CPR and ECC Performance Sheets for pediatric patients that can help you refresh your understanding of these important principles and skills.

Cardiopulmonary arrest in an adult is usually caused by heart attack. In contrast, primary heart disease is rare in children unless there is a major congenital defect. Such defects are usually identified at birth. In the majority of instances, infants and children first sustain a respiratory arrest. Then they may undergo cardiac arrest as a result of the lack of oxygen produced by the respiratory problem. It is, therefore, very important for you to secure and maintain an adequate airway and to ventilate the child who has respiratory problems. Some causes of cardiopulmonary arrest in children include

- Suffocation caused by the aspiration of a foreign body.
- Drowning.
- Infections of the airway such as croup (acute bacterial or viral laryngitis) or acute epiglottitis (viral or bacterial infection resulting in acute swelling of the epiglottis).
- Injuries about the head and neck.
- Accidental poisonings.
- Sudden infant death syndrome (SIDS).

The basic difference in the management of a child with cardiopulmonary arrest as contrasted to an adult is the size of the patient. This factor dictates the specific techniques of resuscitation. For children above 8 years of age, techniques used in an adult are effective. In patients under the age of 8 (infants and younger children), you must use modified techniques of resuscitation. These divisions are not rigid; for example, a small 9- or 10-year-old usually should be managed as a child. The specific techniques for cardiopulmonary resuscitation (CPR) in infants, children, and adults are described in Chapters 7 and 9.

Skill Performance Sheet
Child One-Rescuer CPR

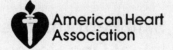

American Heart Association

Student Name _____ Date _____

Performance Guidelines	Performed
1. Establish unresponsiveness. If second rescuer is available, have him or her activate the EMS system.	
2. Open airway (head tilt–chin lift or jaw thrust). Check breathing (look, listen, feel).*	
3. Give 2 slow breaths (1 to 1½ seconds per breath), watch chest rise, allow for exhalation between breaths.	
4. Check carotid pulse. If breathing is absent but pulse is present, provide rescue breathing (1 breath every 3 seconds, about 20 breaths per minute).	
5. If no pulse, give 5 chest compressions (100 compressions per minute), open airway with chin lift, and provide 1 slow breath. Repeat this cycle.	
6. After about 1 minute of rescue support, check pulse.* If rescuer is alone, activate the EMS system. If no pulse, continue 5:1 cycles.	

*If victim is breathing or resumes effective breathing, place in recovery position.

Comments _____

_____

_____

Instructor _____

Circle one: Complete   Needs more practice

FIGURE 38–1   Child one-rescuer CPR performance sheet.
*Reproduced with permission. Basic Life Support Heartsaver Guide, 1993. Copyright ©
American Heart Association.*

Skill Performance Sheet
Infant One-Rescuer CPR

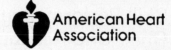 American Heart Association

Student Name _____ Date _____

Performance Guidelines	Performed
1. Establish unresponsiveness. If second rescuer is available, have him or her activate the EMS system.	
2. Open airway (head tilt–chin lift or jaw thrust). Check breathing (look, listen, feel).*	
3. Give 2 slow breaths (1 to 1½ seconds per breath), watch chest rise, allow for exhalation between breaths.	
4. Check brachial pulse. If breathing is absent but pulse is present, provide rescue breathing (1 breath every 3 seconds, about 20 breaths per minute).	
5. If no pulse, give cycles of 5 chest compressions (rate, at least 100 compressions per minute) followed by 1 slow breath.	
6. After about 1 minute of rescue support, check pulse.* If rescuer is alone, activate the EMS system. If no pulse, continue 5:1 cycles.	

*If victim is breathing or resumes effective breathing, place in recovery position.

Comments _____

_____

_____

Instructor _____

Circle one: Complete   Needs more practice

FIGURE 38–2   Infant one-rescuer CPR performance sheet.
*Reproduced with permission. Basic Life Support Heartsaver Guide, 1993. Copyright ©
American Heart Association.*

AIRWAY OBSTRUCTION

Airway obstructions can usually be relieved by placing the child supine, tilting the head, and lifting the chin in the usual fashion (the head-tilt/chin-lift maneuver). In infants and some small children forced hyperextension of the neck will actually obstruct the airway because of the suppleness of the neck and the shape of the infant airway. These children may breathe better if the neck is held straight (in the "sniffing position") rather than hyperextended (Figure 38–3). If the child has vomited, you should clear the pharynx with finger or suction and turn the head to one side. The airway must be clear before assisted ventilation can be given. Because neonates and infants are nose breathers rather than mouth breathers, you must pay particular attention to keeping their nasal passages clear and open.

Obstruction of the airway by a foreign body is an especially common problem in young children, particularly among those who are crawling and exploring their environment. Sometimes the foreign body is aspirated into the lung and must be removed under anesthesia at the hospital. If a foreign body is only partially obstructing the airway, the child usu-ally will still be able to breathe in and out, although with some difficulty. If the foreign body is clearly visible in the mouth and can be easily removed, you should do so. However, if it is lodged in the upper airway, cannot be easily seen, or cannot be easily dislodged with a finger, it should not be removed if the child can still breathe air past the obstruction. Improper manipulation of a foreign body can turn a partial obstruction into a complete one.

Transport children with partial airway obstruction promptly to the hospital. Administer oxygen by gently placing the oxygen mask over the child's mouth and nose. Children are often afraid of anything placed over their mouths or faces. You should explain what the mask is and how it will help the youngster to breathe. It should not be held close to the face to achieve an airtight seal. Rather, it should be held a bit away, with a high flow of oxygen, so that the inspired air is substantially enriched (Figure 38–4).

You should only attempt to dislodge a foreign body when there is a complete airway obstruction or when there is a partial obstruction with poor air exchange that does not improve with the use of 100 percent oxygen (when cyanosis persists). In children, as in

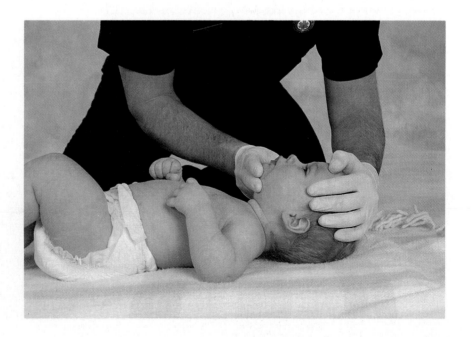

FIGURE 38–3

Relieve airway obstruction in a young child or infant by keeping the neck straight rather than hyperextended.

adults, a foreign body can only be dislodged by applying energy to it. An abdominal-thrust maneuver reliably imparts the most energy, in the right direction, to dislodge the obstructing object. The abdominal-thrust maneuver, modified for size, is the best method of dislodging a foreign body in the airway of a child.

To remove a foreign body from the airway of a conscious child or infant which results in complete obstruction or persisting cyanosis, follow these steps or refer to the 1993 American Heart Association standard skill sheets for foreign body airway obstruction (Figures 38–5 and 38–6):

1. First attempt to pull the foreign body out of the airway with your fingers only if it can be directly visualized and doing so will not risk pushing the object further down the airway.
2. If direct manual extrication does not work, use the abdominal thrust maneuver in children.
3. If the foreign body is obstructing the airway of an infant, place the infant face down supporting the head and neck with one hand and placing the trunk over your forearm or thigh. The infant's head should be lower than the chest. Deliver 4 back blows, forcefully, between the shoulder blades with the heel of the hand. While supporting the head, sandwich the infant between your hands and turn it to a supine position. Deliver 4 chest thrusts in the midsternal region in the same manner as external chest compressions, but at a slower rate. (Figure 38–7).
4. Once the obstructing foreign body has been dislodged using one of these methods, open the airway again using the tongue-jaw-lift maneuver and remove the dislodged foreign body with your fingers.
5. Maintain the open airway and assist ventilation as necessary. If the infant or child begins to breathe spontaneously, give oxygen and transport the patient promptly to the hospital, even if the foreign body appears to have been completely removed.
6. If these maneuvers fail to dislodge the foreign body or to open an adequate airway, repeat a full series once and arrange to transport the child or infant as quickly as possible to the emergency department. Continue maneuvers while en route to the hospital.
7. For management of an unconscious child or infant or one that becomes unconscious refer to Chapter 7.

FIGURE 38–4

Hold an oxygen mask slightly away from a child's face instead of tightly over the mouth or face. A high flow of oxygen will enrich the air the youngster breathes.

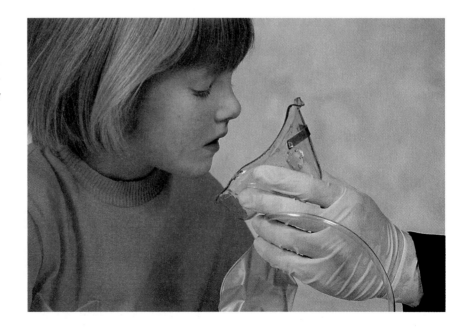

Skill Performance Sheet
Child Foreign-Body
Airway Obstruction —
Conscious

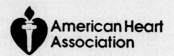

Student Name _____ Date _____

Performance Guidelines	Performed
1. Ask "Are you choking?"	
2. Give abdominal thrusts.	
3. Repeat thrusts until effective or victim becomes unconscious.	
Child Foreign-Body Airway Obstruction — Victim Becomes Unconscious	
4. If second rescuer is available, have him or her activate the EMS system.	
5. Perform a tongue-jaw lift, and if you see the object, perform a finger sweep to remove it.	
6. Open airway and try to ventilate; if still obstructed, reposition head and try to ventilate again.	
7. Give up to 5 abdominal thrusts.	
8. Repeat steps 5 through 7 until effective.*	
9. If airway obstruction is not relieved after about 1 minute, activate the EMS system.	

*If victim is breathing or resumes effective breathing, place in recovery position.

Comments _____

_____

_____

Instructor _____

Circle one: Complete   Needs more practice

FIGURE 38–5   Management of a foreign body obstructed airway in a conscious child. *Reproduced with permission.* Basic Life Support Heartsaver Guide, *1993. Copyright © American Heart Association.*

Skill Performance Sheet Infant Foreign-Body Airway Obstruction — Conscious

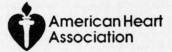

American Heart Association

Student Name _____ Date _____

Performance Guidelines	Performed
1. Confirm complete airway obstruction. Check for serious breathing difficulty, ineffective cough, *no* strong cry.	
2. Give up to 5 back blows and 5 chest thrusts.	
3. Repeat step 2 until effective or victim becomes unconscious.	
Infant Foreign-Body Airway Obstruction — Victim Becomes Unconscious	
4. If second rescuer is available, have him or her activate the EMS system.	
5. Perform a tongue-jaw lift, and if you see the object, perform a finger sweep to remove it.	
6. Open airway and try to ventilate; if still obstructed, reposition head and try to ventilate again.	
7. Give up to 5 back blows and 5 chest thrusts.	
8. Repeat steps 5 through 7 until effective.*	
9. If airway obstruction is not relieved after about 1 minute, activate the EMS system.	

*If victim is breathing or resumes effective breathing, place in recovery position.

Comments _____

_____

_____

Instructor _____

Circle one: Complete   Needs more practice

FIGURE 38–6   Management of a foreign body obstructed airway in a conscious infant.
Reproduced with permission. Basic Life Support Heartsaver Guide, *1993. Copyright ©*
American Heart Association.

Croup and Epiglottitis

Two illnesses may cause airway obstruction in children because of swelling of the tissues of the airway itself. **Croup** is a viral illness that causes acute swelling of the lining of the larynx below its opening. Acute **epiglottitis** is a bacterial infection that produces severe swelling of the epiglottis, the flap of tissue that protects the opening to the larynx (Figure 38–8). Children with these illnesses have fever, show progressive respiratory difficulty, and generally have a barking, brassy cough and hoarseness. There is a progressive and excessive muscular effort with breathing.

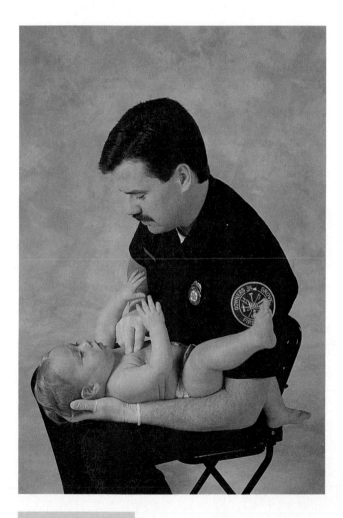

FIGURE 38–7

In the infant with complete airway obstruction, the foreign body can be expelled by applying five chest thrusts with the infant held in the position shown.

You should never put a tongue blade, a finger, or an artificial airway into the mouth of such a child. This type of intervention may cause spasm of the larynx and complete airway obstruction. Airways (oral or nasal) are designed to support a flaccid tongue—not to bypass a swollen epiglottis—and they do not help in croup, because the obstruction in this condition is far below the reach of the device. Back blows and chest thrusts—the techniques for dislodging a foreign object—obviously will be of no benefit in these children and should be avoided. Instead, the infant or child should be placed in a "sniffing" position with the head and neck forward on the chest (Figure 38–9). Under medical protocol, warm, moist oxygen should be administered for epiglottitis, but a cool mist is most appropriate for croup. Gently remove any secretions from the mouth with suction. The child should be transported as promptly as possible to the hospital for treatment. Either of these conditions is very frightening to both the child and parents. Both should be reassured and kept calm because excessive agitation of the child will only aggravate the breathing problem.

Airway Maintenance

An unconscious infant or child should have an appropriately sized oropharyngeal airway inserted between the tongue and the palate. The proper length of the oropharyngeal airway for these patients is roughly equal to the distance from the corner of the patient's mouth to the earlobe (Figure 38–10). A semiconscious child may accept an airway or may expel it. The child who expels it can probably breathe adequately without it. This child has retained adequate reflex responses to protect the airway. Skill must be developed in the use of infant and child sizes of bag-valve-mask and other adjuncts to assist ventilation.

TRAUMA

The automobile is the major killer of American children today. Children are injured as pedestrians, on bicycles, on motorcycles, or as pas-

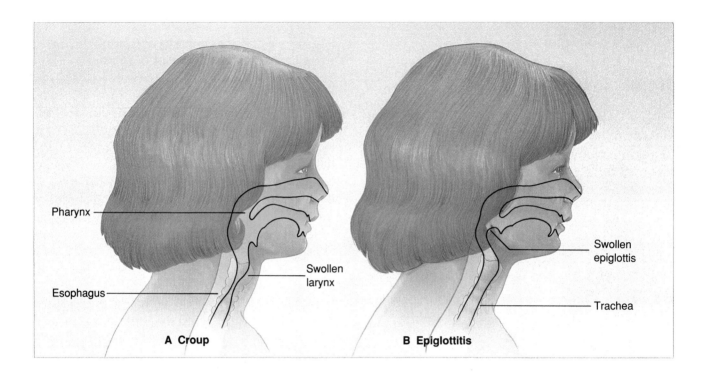

FIGURE 38–8   (A) Airway obstruction caused by croup, a viral illness that causes extensive swelling of the lining of the larynx. (B) Epiglottitis, a bacterial infection that produces severe swelling of the epiglottis.

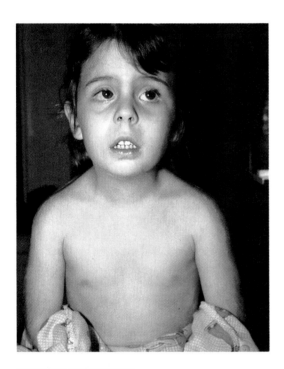
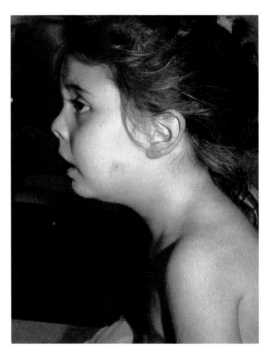

FIGURE 38–9   The "sniffing position" usually provides the most comfortable position for breathing in the child with croup or epiglottitis.

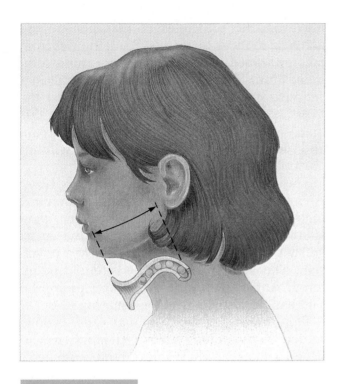

Technique of approximating the proper size of oropharyngeal airway to insert in a child. The length of the airway should be equal to the distance from the corner of the mouth to the earlobe.

sengers in cars. Occasionally, a serious injury results from athletics or recreational activity. The basic principles that apply to the management of trauma in adults also apply to trauma in children: establish an airway, protect the cervical spine, control bleeding, and splint musculoskeletal injuries.

Shock

Shock in an injured child almost always results from blood loss. Because a child has a smaller blood volume, a pediatric patient can tolerate far less actual blood loss than can an adult. The total circulating blood volume in an infant is only 300 to 500 ml. Delayed capillary refill in a peripheral extremity is a good indicator of early shock. A late indicator of shock is a low systolic blood pressure. If the systolic blood pressure is below 50 in a child under 5 years of age, under 60 in a child between 5 and 12, or under 70 in a teenager or young adult, the patient is defi-

nitely in shock. Remember, many other physiologic changes precede the actual fall in blood pressure. When the blood pressure finally becomes low, the condition is extremely serious. To measure the blood pressure properly, three different sizes of pediatric blood pressure cuffs should be available at all times. Use a cuff that will cover about three quarters of the distance between the elbow and the axilla on the back of the arm.

Treatment for the child in shock consists of controlling the airway, protecting the cervical spine, dressing any obvious wounds to stop bleeding, splinting fractures, elevating the feet, and handling the patient gently. Do not give the child who has been in an accident anything by mouth. If the child needs an emergency operation, the stomach should be completely empty. Often the children will ask for water, particularly if they are in shock. You must say "no" in a kindly way.

Head, Neck, and Spinal Injuries

Injuries of the head, neck, and spine usually are caused by vehicular accidents, falls, or diving mishaps. You should assume that any unconscious child who has been involved in an accident has sustained a neck injury. The child should be treated and transported in the same manner as any other patient with suspected spinal fractures:

1. Do not flex the neck or back. Remember to pad under the shoulders of an infant or small child to compensate for the disproportionately larger head size.
2. Secure an adequate airway and immobilize the head, neck, and trunk on a spine board before moving the child.
3. Offer assisted ventilation as the need arises and be alert to control vomiting.
4. Avoid the urge to pick up and cradle an injured child unless there is an overriding need to move quickly, such as a fire or other threatening environmental problems.
5. Transfer children with head injuries with the head slightly elevated and supported on the spine board. All the basic rules for managing the patient with a head injury (Chapter 20) apply equally in children.

6. Monitor the patient's level of consciousness. This is one of the most important duties after resuscitation and control of injuries. From the time you first see the patient until you deliver the patient to the emergency department, make periodic notations regarding the patient's level of consciousness. Use the AVPU or Glasgow Coma Scale to record your observations every 5 minutes. Report and record any change in the level of consciousness. A patient with a head injury may pass from an alert state to a comatose state in a few minutes and require an urgent, lifesaving operative procedure. Assessing the level of consciousness and its change is the single most important measure you can take in the management of patients with pediatric or adult head injury.

Extremity Injuries

In general, extremity injuries are not life-threatening. Treat open soft tissue wounds with a dry, sterile compression dressing. Open fractures tend to bleed considerably in children as well as in adults. Prompt control of bleeding is especially important in children. Bleeding can almost always be controlled by local compression. In those rare circumstances when a tourniquet must be used to control bleeding, the same rules apply as for an adult (see Chapter 11). If a blood pressure cuff is used as a tourniquet on a child, inflation of the cuff to 100 mm Hg will usually secure complete control of the bleeding.

Splint a child's extremities in the same manner as for an adult. Of course, the small extremity of a child requires appropriately sized splints. A supply of pediatric splints must be maintained in the ambulance (see Chapter 16). Before you place a splint or align an injured extremity, assess the distal neurovascular function (pulse, capillary refill, sensation, and motor function). Continue to monitor the neurovascular status after you apply the splint until the patient reaches the hospital.

Injuries of the Trunk

Penetrating abdominal or chest injuries are uncommon in children. When they occur, however, the principles of management are identical to those for adults. Blunt injuries from falls or vehicular accidents are far more common. Blunt abdominal trauma may result in a serious internal injury such as rupture of the liver, spleen, or kidney. The child with this kind of injury may complain of abdominal pain and develop signs of shock, even without obvious external blood loss.

These injuries are often difficult to diagnose. A child who has sustained a blunt abdominal injury and is complaining of abdominal pain should be transported promptly to the emergency department to be examined by a physician. The vital signs must be carefully monitored. Anticipate shock and treat it promptly. You should also be alert for vomiting.

Blunt injuries of the chest may cause serious cardiac or pulmonary injury. All children who have sustained a chest injury require immediate transport to the emergency department. Prehospital care is identical to that for adults.

SPECIFIC PEDIATRIC EMERGENCIES

A few emergency situations occur in children that do not exist or are seen only rarely in adults. They include high fevers with convulsions, certain conditions that cause abdominal pain, poisoning by various household substances, specific contagious diseases, and SIDS. Any of these conditions may be quite serious, and all will be frightening to the parents.

Fever

A child responds to many illnesses by very rapidly developing a high fever. Temperatures of 103 degrees F (39.4 degrees C) and higher are common in children. In general, you should not attempt to measure rectal temperature in small children or infants. The rectum is small and can be damaged easily by the thermometer. In these patients, high fever is usually obvious. The child is flushed, crying, and feels warm to the touch. In older children, oral or rectal temperatures should be taken using the appropriate type of thermometer.

Fever is not a disease itself, but rather the sign of an underlying problem, usually infectious. Most fevers in children are not serious and do not cause permanent brain injury. About 5 percent of children with fever develop **febrile convulsions.** These seizures are of short duration, usually are not dangerous, and require no special treatment beyond airway maintenance. The underlying cause of the fever must be determined by a physician so that proper treatment of the principal disease can be instituted.

The most dangerous fevers in children are those caused by *heat stroke.* In the treatment of heat stroke, the same principles apply for the care of children as for adults (see Chapter 42). The temperature of the body must be reduced as quickly as possible. A child who has been in the sun, in an extremely warm, poorly ventilated room, or in a closed, parked car, and who has hot, dry skin may be suffering from heat stroke. These children should be undressed, cooled in a tub of cold water, and transported promptly to the emergency department. Covering the child with cool, wet sheets and using fans will also help lower temperature quickly. Children with heat stroke must be monitored carefully. The surface area of a child is large with respect to child's volume, and the body temperature may change rapidly.

Occasionally, a child who has *epilepsy,* a seizure disorder, may have a fever and develop a prolonged seizure. The child with epilepsy whose attack is triggered by fever needs a prompt diagnosis of the cause of the fever. In contrast to the usual febrile seizures, which are brief, lasting one to two minutes, epileptic seizure will last longer. When a child who is having a seizure becomes cyanotic, you must attempt to restore the airway. You should never place your fingers in the mouth, because the convulsing child may bite. You should not attempt to pry the jaws open; it will usually do more harm than good. Gentle extension of the neck will open the airway partially. Ventilation through the nose in the patient with clenched teeth should be facilitated by keeping the nasal passages clear with suction. Administer oxygen by face mask. Following the seizure, the child will be in a postictal state, with an altered level of consciousness and slow respirations. The child may be difficult to awaken. You should maintain the airway, continue to administer oxygen, and transport this child promptly to the hospital. The general treatment for patients with epilepsy is outlined in Chapter 37.

Another cause of febrile convulsions in children is **meningitis,** a viral or bacterial infection of the covering membranes of the brain and spinal cord. This is an extremely serious disease but not usually a very contagious one. These children will be hot and obviously sick. A sore throat or upper respiratory problem may have preceded the current illness. Headache and a stiff neck are common. Children with these symptoms should be transported to the emergency department as quickly as possible.

Abdominal Pain

The most serious cause of abdominal pain in childhood is *appendicitis.* Although it can occur at any age, appendicitis is usually seen between the ages of 10 and 25. The older child may give a history of progressive abdominal pain. It starts over the umbilicus and is crampy in nature. It moves to the right lower quadrant of the abdomen in a matter of hours and becomes steady and severe. Usually the child is nauseated and has no appetite. Occasionally, vomiting occurs. The child tends to be irritable or fussy, and fever is common.

The major difficulty in identifying appendicitis in pediatric patients occurs with the younger child or infant who can give no clear history. In this situation, the clinical picture is almost identical with viral or bacterial **gastroenteritis** ("flu"). Diagnosis is difficult for the doctors and may be delayed. A good rule for you to follow is to transport every child with a sore or tender abdomen to the emergency department, if only for appropriate diagnosis. You should never attempt to make a distinction between appendicitis and gastroenteritis.

Dehydration (loss of body fluids) is a common problem in infants and children. It is frequently seen in association with situations that cause abdominal pain. Diarrhea or vomiting can each bring about dehydration in small patients much more quickly than in adults. Sometimes gastroenteritis produces diarrhea that persists for days before medical aid is sought. Dehydration may be a cause of shock in infants and children. The dehydrated child may be lethargic with dry skin and mucous membranes. Because of the potential for shock, the dehydrated child must be transported to the emergency department promptly.

Poisoning

Little children are curious and like to sample the contents of brightly colored bottles or cans, thinking that they contain something good to eat or drink. Sometimes a considerable amount of a substance is swallowed before the child or parent realizes that a dangerous substance has been ingested. Many common household items are poisonous. When responding to a poisoning, you should take these steps:

1. If caustic (irritating) material has been spilled on the child, wash it off with lots of water. If it has spilled on the child's clothes, remove them. If any of the material is in the child's eyes, flush the eyes thoroughly with water for several minutes.
2. If the child has swallowed tablets from a medicine bottle, gather any spilled tablets and replace them in the bottle so that the number can be counted. The emergency department physician will then have an idea of how many tablets the child may actually have taken.
3. If the child has swallowed any substance, identify it, attempt to estimate the amount taken, and gather the remainder. Bring any bottle or any other container of the substance to the emergency department.
4. As soon as you are certain that a poisoning has occurred, notify dispatch and medical control. Identify the patient, the child's age and size, the ingested agent, and the suspected amount taken. The dispatch center will contact the local poison control center and relay specific treatment instructions to you. Your job is to care for and transport the patient safely and promptly and to gather critical information about the ingested substance for emergency department personnel.

5. If the poison control center recommends that vomiting should be induced, give 1 tablespoon of syrup of ipecac in a glass of water and transport the child promptly to the hospital. If the child does not vomit in 20 minutes, the dose may be repeated once. If the level of consciousness deteriorates, do not give any more ipecac. Do not delay transport to await the onset of vomiting.
6. Do not attempt to induce vomiting in a child who has swallowed strong acid or strong alkali (such as lye or Drano®), or any petroleum product.
7. Do not attempt to induce vomiting in a child who is unconscious or partially conscious. The danger of vomitus being aspirated into the lungs is too great. If the poisoned child does vomit, suction the material out of the mouth and pharynx and collect it for analysis at the hospital.
8. Transport the patient to the emergency department promptly. Be prepared to give all needed support up to and including full CPR. Many ingested items, especially medications, promptly produce respiratory depression. In all children who have ingested poisonous substances, close monitoring of respiration is critical and support of impaired breathing is essential. Anticipate vomiting in these patients also. Many substances that are ingested are very irritating to the stomach and induce vomiting by themselves.

A description of the proper emergency treatment for various poisonous agents is contained in Chapter 28.

Contagious Diseases

Occasionally, you must transport a child who is suffering from one of the common infectious childhood diseases for some other medical reason. A contagious disease is usually easy to spot. Measles (rubeola), German measles (rubella), and chicken pox produce specific types of rash; mumps causes swelling and tenderness of the parotid glands directly in front of the ears.

You should notify the hospital that a child is arriving who appears to have a contagious disease. Masks can serve a useful purpose if the child has fever and a rash. As a general rule, however, children with these diseases are not a particular threat of infection, because you probably have had the disease or have been immunized against it. Careful handwashing, cleaning of exposed surfaces and equipment in the vehicle, and appropriate use of masks will usually protect you. Specific information regarding a variety of contagious diseases is contained in Chapter 35.

Sudden Infant Death Syndrome (SIDS)

Approximately 10,000 infants die each year in the United States from SIDS. The exact cause is unknown, but it is suspected to be a viral infection. It usually occurs during sleep in an otherwise healthy infant between the ages of 2 and 6 months and thus has been called "crib death." In such a situation, you are going to encounter anguished, severely disturbed parents. Some time and effort must be spent on comforting the parents. At the same time, however, every effort must be made to revive the baby, even if the infant's death preceded your arrival by some prolonged period of time. Basic life-support measures should be instituted before and during transportation to the hospital, even if the baby seems to be dead. Resuscitation efforts should be continued until the baby is pronounced dead by a physician. The emergency department should be notified in advance of the nature of the problem.

SPECIAL PEDIATRIC PROBLEMS

Child Abuse

The exact incidence of child abuse is unknown. What is known, however, is that child abuse is a far greater problem than was once suspected. The deliberate, intentional injury of a child physically and emotionally is, unfortunately, not rare in our society today. Child abuse is progressive—that is, the child may be continually abused with increasing severity, until death ultimately results. Child abuse can occur in any family and is found at all socioeconomic levels.

An abused child is often brought to the hospital for medical attention, or EMS is called because of a supposed accidental injury. Child abuse should be suspected if the history given by the person who called does not appear to fit the child's injury. Characteristically, the abused or battered child will have many injuries, all at different stages of healing. The child may appear withdrawn, fearful, or hostile, and may be undernourished. Occasionally, the child's parent or caretaker reveals a history of several "accidents" in the past. The abuser may be a parent, relative, or babysitter. Sometimes, particularly if the child is living with a single parent, the abuser is an acquaintance of that single parent.

When you suspect child abuse, you should not attempt to make a diagnosis. Instead, what history is given should be carefully recorded and the child transported promptly to the hospital, even if the injuries appear relatively trivial. Most states have laws requiring health care personnel to report cases of suspected child abuse to various social service or police agencies. Ordinarily, this responsibility lies with the physician. Thus, when you have special information or suspect child abuse, you should report it to the physician at the hospital. Often a child who is a suspected victim of abuse will be admitted to the hospital for protection, even though the injuries alone are not severe enough to warrant hospitalization.

However, you cannot bring the child to the hospital without the parent's consent. Sometimes the parents can be persuaded if you tell them that the child may need special X rays or tests. You should not accuse anyone of child abuse, even if it appears obvious. Maintaining a professional approach is not easy, as an obvious case of child abuse arouses strong emotions and challenges one's ability to think and act clearly. If the parent refuses transport, and you are concerned, the police should be consulted.

The ultimate determination of child abuse is made in the courts, often after a long and complicated legal process. The responsibility of all health care professionals is to identify suspicious instances of child abuse so that necessary steps can be taken. You should be knowledgeable about the specific laws in your state regarding the reporting of child abuse.

Sexual Abuse of Children

Sexual abuse is another problem that can occur in children as well as adults. It may occur in infants, young children, adolescents, and to both boys and girls. Most victims of rape are over 10 years of age, although, unfortunately, younger children are sometimes victims as well. You should not examine the young child's genitalia unless there is obvious bleeding or other injury that must be treated. An examination that allows you to place the proper dressing for the injury is sufficient. Sometimes a child will have been beaten and will also have bruises or even fractures. These injuries should be treated appropriately.

When sexual abuse is suspected, the child should not wash, urinate, or defecate before an examination is carried out by the physician at the emergency department. If the molested child is a girl, a male EMT should enlist the aid of a female EMT or police officer to assist him. Professional composure should be retained throughout. A concerned, caring approach to these children is extremely important. They should be shielded from onlookers and curious passersby. As much history as is possible

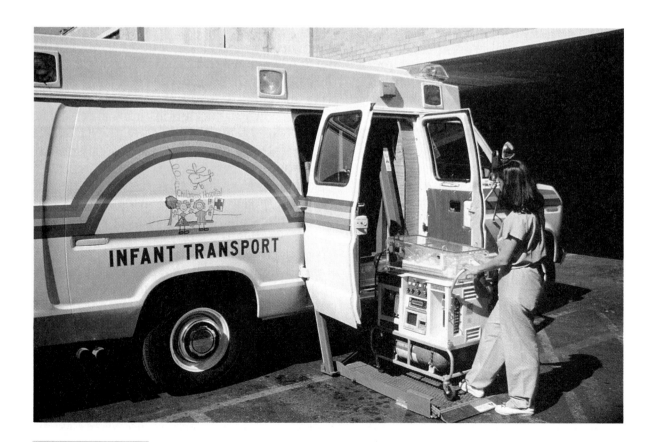

FIGURE 38–11   A specialized vehicle for the emergency transportation of premature, ill, or high-risk infants.

should be obtained from the child and any witnesses. The child may be hysterical or unwilling to give any story at all, especially if the abuser is a sibling, relative, or family friend. You are in the best position to retrieve the most accurate first-hand information concerning the incident, so you must record any information carefully and completely. All information should be written in clear and accurate detail on the ambulance report form. All child victims of sexual assault should be transported to the emergency department. You should carry the local phone numbers of agencies in your area that specialize in addressing these problems. Sexual molestation of children is a crime, and you should cooperate with law enforcement officials in their investigations.

Transportation of Children

Infants and small children are very susceptible to temperature changes. Their body surface area is very large in relation to their total body volume. Thus, they lose body heat more rapidly than adults and must always be transported well wrapped in blankets. Very young and sick children are also extremely susceptible to infection. You should thus avoid breathing or coughing directly on a small, sick child. The child should be as isolated as possible from bacterial contamination, particularly from your own nose, mouth, and hands. An infant carrier should provide access to the child so that the airway may be kept clear and artificial ventilation maintained if necessary. If oxygen is given, it should be warm. Carriers and their accessories are described in Chapter 39.

Newborns should be transported in special incubators that will allow oxygen enrichment and control of humidity and temperature. If an incubator is not available, the newborn should be wrapped in blankets except for the face and carried in a warm ambulance. Many large medical centers maintain specially equipped vehicles for the transportation of infants and small children. You should know the location and availability of these vehicles (Figure 38–11).

An older child may comprehend, to some degree, that an emergency is taking place but not the exact nature or severity of the problem.

Children are easily frightened, and, as such, often behave in a belligerent or hysterical fashion. Whenever possible, the child should have a familiar person or familiar object close by. Parents, relatives, or close friends are invaluable in dealing with frightened children. Treasured objects such as dolls, teddy bears, or a blanket may be necessary to help secure the cooperation of these young patients. The child should be allowed to take such objects to the hospital. The parents should remain close to the child whenever possible. The child's siblings should be assigned to the care of a responsible neighbor or relative who can keep them informed and safe, yet away from the patient during transport and treatment.

YOU ARE THE EMT

1. Your patient is a young child with croup who is gasping for breath. Should you insert an artificial airway, give oxygen, or both? Why?
2. What are the common causes of shock in a child? How do you treat a child in shock?
3. You have been called to treat a child with a very high temperature. The mother is perplexed because the youngster did not seem to be sick. You notice the child has a sunburn and you suspect heat stroke. What are the other symptoms of heat stroke? What emergency care will you give this patient?
4. Your patient is 2-year-old child who has fallen out of his crib. After a thorough examination, you are confident that he has no broken bones or head injuries, but you have noticed lots of "old" bruises. You begin to suspect child abuse, but there is no real evidence. What will you do?

CHILDBIRTH

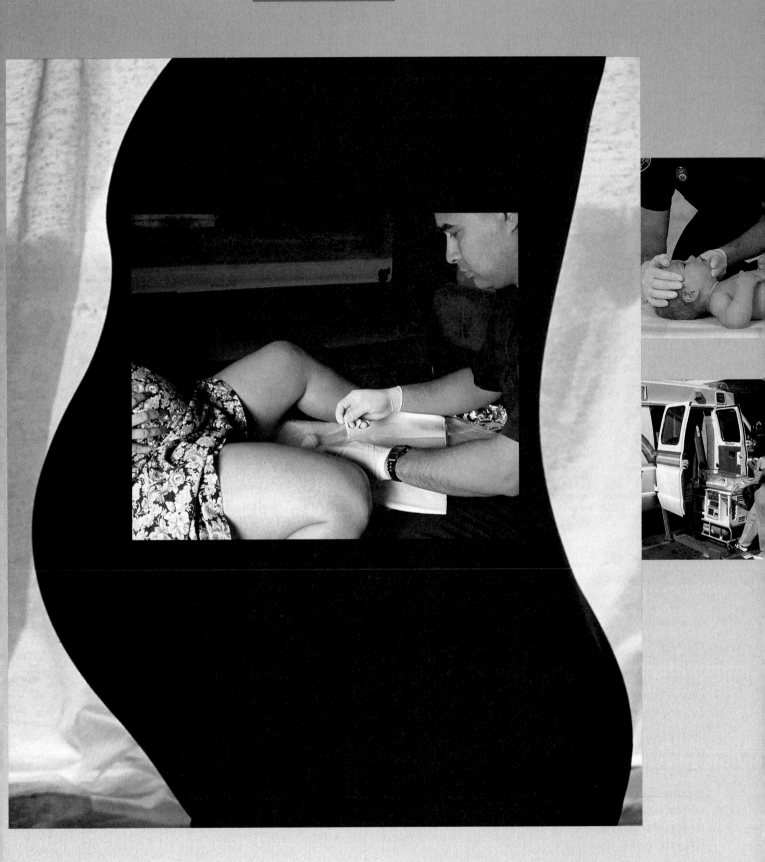

CHAPTER 39

CHILDBIRTH

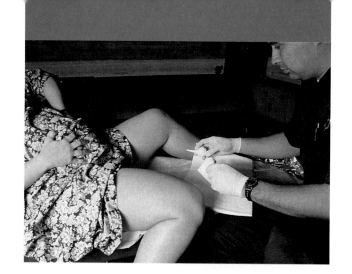

KEY TERMS

abortion (ah-bor'shun) Miscarriage.

amniotic sac (am-ne-ot'ik sak) The fluid-filled cavity that grows around the developing fetus, inside the uterus.

Apgar score A measure of a baby's condition at birth.

bloody show The appearance of a small blood and mucus plug from the vagina, often signaling the beginning of labor.

cervix (ser'viks) The opening or mouth of the uterus.

crowning The appearance of the baby's head at the cervix during labor.

eclampsia (ĕ-klamp'se-ah) A convulsive disorder of pregnancy associated with severe hypertension.

ectopic pregnancy (ek-top'ik preg'nan-se) A pregnancy where the fetus develops outside of the uterus, usually in a Fallopian tube.

fetal alcohol syndrome A condition of the children of alcoholic mothers characterized by growth retardation (low birth weight), failure to thrive, mental retardation, and a variety of specific congenital abnormalities.

fetus (fe'tus) The developing baby in the uterus.

miscarriage (mis-kar'ij) Delivery of fetus and placenta before 20 weeks gestation, for any reason.

multigravida (mul″tĭ-grav'ĭ-dah) A woman who has been pregnant more than one time.

placenta (plah-sen'tah) The afterbirth that grows during pregnancy, through which all the nutrients for the fetus pass during development.

presentation (pre″zen-ta'shun) The manner in which a baby is born; the part of the baby that appears first.

primigravida (pri″mĭ-grav'ĭ-dah) A woman who is pregnant for the first time.

umbilical cord (um-bil'ĭ-kal kord) The tissue connecting the placenta with the fetus.

uterus (u'ter-us) The womb.

vagina (vah-ji'nah) The birth canal.

OVERVIEW

Childbirth, especially the not-making-the-hospital-in-time version, has for years been the subject of TV drama. The woman is in agony, the relatives and friends are frantic, there is always a storm, and then someone comes to the rescue and starts calling for boiling water. Finally, with great fuss and fanfare, a healthy baby is born. Everyone is delighted, and the stand-in doctor—the father or the star of the show—is particularly proud at what he has accomplished.

In real life, this situation occurs infrequently. Most babies in the United States are born in hospitals. Rarely is the EMT called to see a pregnant woman when the birth process is well along and there is not time to get her to a hospital. However, it does happen, and you must be prepared to move quickly and efficiently. You will need a sterile emergency delivery pack rather than boiling water, and you must be aware of a number of potential problems. The umbilical cord could be wrapped around the baby's neck. The baby could have difficulty breathing. The mother might have excessive bleeding. Fortunately, most emergency births are trouble free, but even so, you must be very knowledgeable about the whole process of childbirth. Childbirth is an exciting, drama-filled event.

Chapter 39 begins with a description of the developing fetus and an explanation of what can go wrong during pregnancy. The chapter next describes the onset of labor and how you can decide whether an emergency delivery is needed. The three stages of labor are then presented in detail. The last part of the chapter discusses abnormal deliveries and complications, including failure of the amniotic membrane to rupture, breech deliveries, prolapsed umbilical cord, excessive bleeding, abortion or miscarriage, twins, delivery without sterile supplies, and premature infants. In addition, there is a discussion of babies born to mothers who are victims of substance abuse, and the measures necessary for your own safety during emergency childbirth are presented.

GOALS

The goals of Chapter 39 are to
- understand the basic anatomy of the developing fetus.
- recognize the complications of pregnancy.
- identify the onset of labor.
- know how to assess the need for an emergency delivery of a baby.
- describe the three stages of labor and the role of the EMT in assisting the mother during the childbirth process.
- know the steps to take with the newborn baby.
- know the procedures for handling both abnormal deliveries and complications of childbirth.

THE DEVELOPING FETUS

The **fetus** (developing baby) grows inside the mother's **uterus** (womb) for nine months. During this time, the mother's abdomen grows larger as the uterus enlarges with the growing fetus. As the fetus grows, it requires more and more nourishment. The **placenta** (afterbirth) develops on the wall of the uterus and is connected to the fetus by the **umbilical cord.** The close attachment of the placenta to the wall of the uterus allows oxygen and other nutrients to cross from the mother's circulation into the placenta and then along the umbilical cord to support the fetus as it grows. The fetus develops inside a fluid-filled, bag-like membrane called the **amniotic sac** (Figure 39–1).

COMPLICATIONS OF PREGNANCY

Most pregnant women are healthy, but some may have medical diseases along with being pregnant. You may safely treat any heart or lung disease in the mother with oxygen without harm to the fetus.

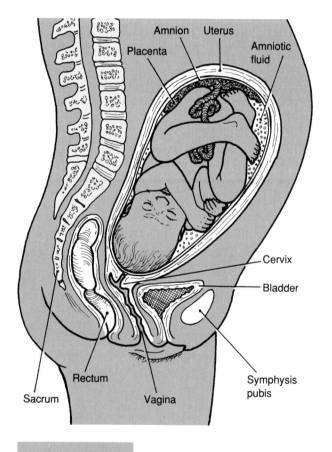

FIGURE 39–1

Anatomic structures of the pregnant woman.

As the time for delivery nears, certain complications can occur. **Eclampsia** (convulsions that result from severe hypertension) is treated by laying the mother on her side, maintaining an airway, and providing supplemental oxygen. If vomiting occurs, you must suction the airway. Transport the pregnant patient with convulsions promptly to the hospital.

Hemorrhage from the **vagina** (birth canal) that occurs before labor begins may be very serious. In early pregnancy, bleeding may be a sign of an abortion **(miscarriage)** or of an **ectopic pregnancy** (a pregnancy developing outside of the uterus). Ectopic pregnancy is covered in detail in Chapter 34. In the later stages of pregnancy, hemorrhage may indicate problems with the placenta, among them placenta abruptio and placenta previa. In *placenta abruptio*, the placenta separates prematurely from the wall of the uterus. In *placenta previa*, the placenta develops over and covers the mouth of the uterus (the **cervix).** In both instances, sudden, often painless, bleeding will result. Any bleeding from the vagina in a pregnant woman is a serious sign and should be treated in the hospital promptly. If the patient shows signs of shock, she should lie on her side during transportation. A pregnant woman is usually more comfortable lying on her side than on her back. Place a sterile pad or sanitary napkin over the vagina and replace it as often as necessary. Save the pads so that the hospital personnel can estimate how much blood has been lost. Do not put anything into the vagina. Save any tissue that may be passed from the vagina.

When a pregnant woman is involved in an automobile accident, the situation can be very serious, because severe hemorrhage may occur from injuries to the pregnant uterus. The result can be severe injury to the fetus from oxygen deprivation. A pregnant woman who has been in an accident should be evaluated and transported to the hospital promptly. Support the airway, and if there is any sign of bleeding, administer oxygen. Transport her on her left side, rather than on her back, because this will relieve pressure of the uterus on intraabdominal organs.

THE ONSET OF LABOR

The onset of labor is the beginning of the delivery process. It begins with the characteristic labor pains, which are contractions of the uterus. The total time of labor varies greatly, but it is usually longer in a **primigravida** (a woman who is having her first baby) and becomes progressively shorter with each successive baby. (A pregnant woman who has previously given birth is called a **multigravida.**) Other signs indicating the beginning of labor are the appearance of the **bloody show** and rupture of the amniotic sac (breaking of the *bag of waters*). These events may occur before the onset of labor pains. The bloody show is a small plug of blood-stained mucus that forms in the cervix and is expelled when labor begins. Rupture of the amniotic sac allows the amniotic fluid to gush out of the uterus through the vagina. At term, there is normally about one liter of amniotic fluid.

Labor pains become stronger and more regular as the baby begins to move down the birth canal. The mother will feel increasing pressure in her lower abdomen and may feel she has to move her bowels. This sensation is normal and means that the baby's head is pressing on the rectum. As delivery nears, the cervix of the uterus dilates (opens), so that the baby's head can pass through into the vagina.

There are three stages of labor. The first stage begins with the onset of labor pains and ends when the cervix is fully dilated. The second stage begins when the cervix is fully dilated and ends when the baby is born. The third stage begins with the birth of the baby and ends with the delivery of the placenta. During the first stage there is usually time to transport the mother to the hospital. During the second stage you will have to make a decision to deliver the mother at home or transport her to the hospital. If the third stage is occurring and the baby has been born, the placenta will usually deliver within 30 minutes, and you will usually not transport the mother during that time.

ASSESSING THE NEED FOR AN EMERGENCY DELIVERY

Once you have determined that the patient is indeed in labor, the next major decision is whether to have her deliver at the scene or to transport her to the hospital. Consider delivering the mother at the scene under the following circumstances:

- When delivery can be expected within a few minutes.
- When the hospital cannot be reached because of a natural disaster or traffic accident.
- When there is no transportation available.

You can make a determination of whether the delivery is going to occur within a few minutes by asking the mother certain questions and looking for **crowning** (the phase of labor when the baby's head is visible). Ask if the patient is a multigravida. If so, she may be able to tell you if she is about to deliver. If she says yes, make immediate preparations for delivery. If she has to move her bowels, the baby's head is pressing on the rectum and delivery is about to occur. You should also inspect the vagina to determine whether crowning has occurred. Spread the mother's legs apart gently, reassuring her that this is being done in order to help decide whether she should be delivered immediately or transported to the hospital. Crowning means that delivery is about to occur (Figure 39–2).

Once labor has begun, there is no way it can be slowed down or stopped. Never attempt to hold the mother's legs together. To do so would only complicate the delivery. Do not let the mother go to the bathroom. Instead, reassure her that the sensation of needing to move her bowels is normal and that it means she is about to deliver.

THE FIRST STAGE OF LABOR

Once you have made the decision to deliver the baby at the scene, move quickly but calmly. Delivery will usually require the assistance of

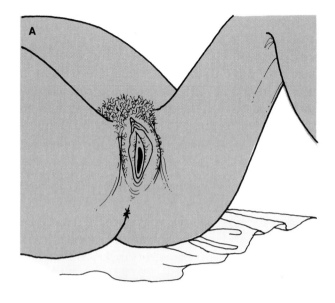

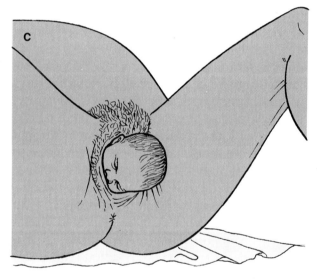

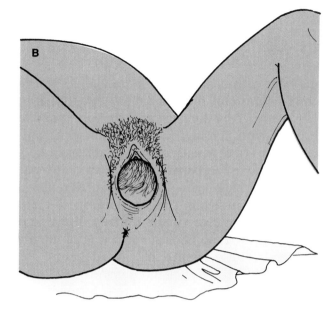

FIGURE 39–2

The vagina during the progress of labor. (A) The normal vagina is closed before labor begins. (B) During crowning, the head of the baby is visible at the opening of the vagina. The vaginal tissue is thin and must stretch enough during contractions for the baby's head to come through. Sometimes this tissue tears. (C) The head is delivered, usually with the baby's head pointing to the right or left, and posterior.

two people. If you are the only EMT available, you must seek assistance from a nurse, police officer, or even a family member or neighbor who may have had experience in childbirth. Never leave your patient once the decision has been made to deliver her at the scene. Someone else should seek outside help if it is needed. Remember, the mother, *not you*, delivers the baby. Your part is to help, guide, and support the baby as it is born.

Your emergency vehicle should always be equipped with a sterile emergency delivery pack containing the following items:

- 1 pair of surgical scissors.
- 3 hemostats or special cord clamps.

- Umbilical tape.
- Small rubber bulb syringe.
- 5 towels.
- 1 dozen 4 × 4 gauze sponges.
- 3 or 4 pairs of rubber gloves.
- 1 baby blanket.
- Sanitary napkins.
- An infant size breathing bag and face mask.
- Goggles.

Place the mother on a spine board that is padded with blankets, folded sheets, or towels. Put a pillow under her hips. Sometimes it is better to put the pillow under one hip to allow the mother to turn to one side; this may make suctioning the baby easier when it is born. If delivery is occurring in an automobile, the mother should lie on the seat, with one foot on the floor and the other on the seat, with the knee and hip bent (Figure 39–3).

If the emergency delivery is occurring at home, you should move the mother to a sturdy table if possible. You will find it easier to work there than if the mother is in bed. Flex both her hips and knees, and support her head with one or two pillows. Spread her legs apart. Place newspapers or sheets on the floor around the delivery area to help soak up the amniotic fluid that will be released when the amniotic sac ruptures (Figure 39–4).

Your assistant should be at the mother's head to comfort and soothe her and to reassure

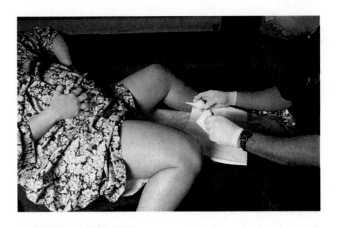

FIGURE 39–3

The set-up for an emergency delivery in an automobile.

FIGURE 39–4

The initial set-up for an emergency delivery at the scene. The set-up shown is for a right-handed EMT. Note the projection of the surface just beyond the mother's vagina so that the baby can be placed there after delivery.

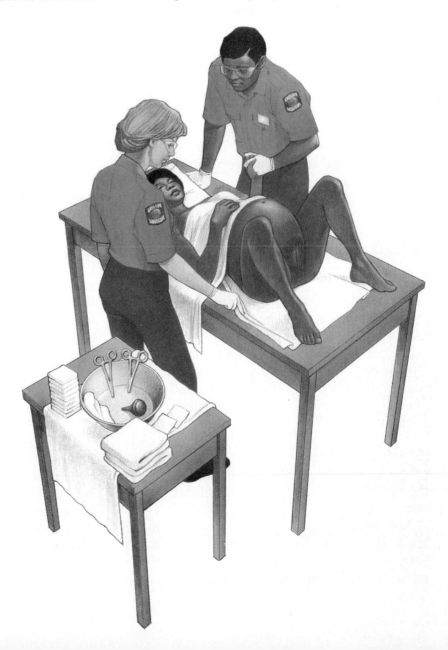

her during the delivery. The patient may want to grip someone's hand. She may have to vomit. In that case, have your helper turn her head to the side so that her mouth and airway can be cleared. Position yourself at the mother's right side if you are right-handed or at her left side if you are left-handed. About 2 feet of the table should extend beyond the mother's buttocks. This will be a convenient surface on which to place the newborn baby.

Place the emergency delivery pack on a chair or table close to the patient so that you can reach it easily. Open the delivery pack carefully so that its contents remain sterile; thoroughly wash your hands, put on the goggles, and then put on the sterile gloves. Then, using a gloved hand, place one sterile, folded towel under the patient's buttocks; place another sterile towel between her legs, just below the vagina; and spread a third towel across her abdomen.

Stand so that you can see the vagina at all times. Time the mother's contractions from the beginning of one to the beginning of the next. In between contractions, encourage the mother to rest. Remind her not to strain with the contractions and to breathe deeply through her mouth.

THE SECOND STAGE OF LABOR

Delivery

Watch the head as it exits the vagina. Once it is obvious that the head is coming out farther with each contraction, you should place your right hand (or your left hand if you are left-handed) over the emerging head and exert very gentle pressure on it. This will allow the head to come out smoothly and prevent the head and baby from suddenly popping out of the vagina during a strong contraction, possibly causing injury. You may move to the end of the table so that you are standing between the mother's legs while the actual delivery is occurring.

The head is usually tilted to one side or the other rather than straight up and down. A baby's head has two soft areas—one near the brow (front of the head) and one near the occiput (back of the head). They are called the *fontanelles*. The brain is covered only by skin and membranes at these places. You must be particularly careful not to push your finger or thumb into one of the fontanelles. Hold the head carefully in your palm, maintaining gentle pressure during contractions and decreasing the pressure slightly between contractions. It may take two, three, or more contractions for the delivery of the head to occur from the time it presents (Figure 39–5).

The head has to be supported as it is born. As soon as the head is delivered, you can use the index finger of your other hand to feel whether the umbilical cord is wrapped around the neck. A cord that is wound tightly around the neck could cause the baby to strangle and must therefore be released from the neck immediately (Figure 39–6). Usually, you can slip it over the baby's shoulder. If not, and if it feels tightly wound around the neck, it must be cut. Clamp the cord with two clamps placed about 2 inches apart. Cut the cord between the clamps. Then you can unwrap it from around the neck. The cord is fragile and easily torn. Handle it very carefully. Do not let the clamps come off until the ends of the cord have been tied (tying the cord will be discussed later in this chapter). Usually, the cord is not around the baby's neck and does not have to be cut until after the birth.

Support the baby's head with one hand as the mother continues to deliver the baby. As soon as the chin, and, therefore, the whole head, is born, the baby's face will turn sideways. At this point, once the whole face is visible, suction the infant's mouth and nose. Squeeze a bulb syringe and gently insert it into the baby's mouth about 1½ inches; any accumulated mucus, blood, water, or amniotic fluid is sucked out and squirted onto the towel across the mother's abdomen. Repeat the suctioning two or three times in the mouth and two or three times in each nostril. The newborn baby is a nose breather, so you must pay particular attention to clearing the nose (Figure 39–7).

By the time suctioning is finished, the upper shoulder will be visible in the vagina. The baby's head is the largest part of the body.

FIGURE 39–5

A side view as the baby's head is born. The face is pointed posteriorly and to one side. Note the position of the hands for a right-handed EMT. A left-handed EMT would have the hands reversed. The hands support and exert gentle pressure to prevent rapid delivery of the baby.

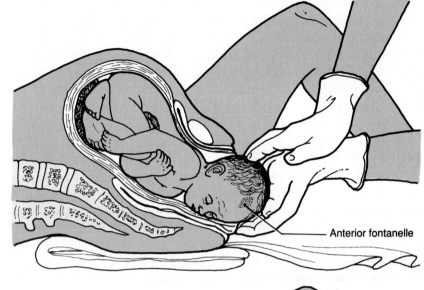

Anterior fontanelle

FIGURE 39–6

If the umbilical cord is wrapped tightly around the baby's neck, you must free, clamp, and cut it.

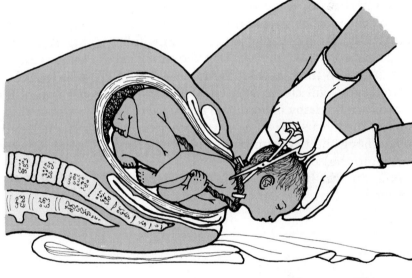

FIGURE 39–7

Once delivery of the head is complete, you should suction the baby's mouth and nostrils for the first time, using the bulb syringe.

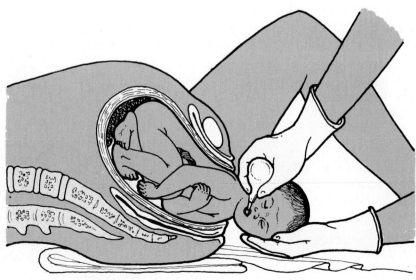

Once it is born, the rest of the baby usually delivers easily. Support the head and upper body as the shoulders deliver. Then the abdomen and hips will appear and be delivered. Once the abdomen and hips deliver, support them with your other hand so that now the baby is being well supported with both hands. Handle the baby firmly but carefully. It will be slippery. Take particular care not to squeeze the neck or chest (Figure 39–8).

As soon as the entire baby is born, place it immediately on a towel, on its back, on the space on the table or bed that was set aside for this purpose. Keep the baby's head slightly lower than the rest of its body and turn it slightly to one side. Use a sterile gauze pad to wipe the baby's mouth and again suction its mouth and nose. Keep the baby at the same level as the mother's vagina. If the baby is held higher than the mother's vagina, blood will be siphoned from the baby through the umbilical cord back into the placenta (Figure 39–9).

Next, you will clamp and cut the umbilical cord. Once the baby is born, the umbilical cord is of no further use to either the mother or the baby. Using the two clamps in the emergency kit, clamp the cord about halfway between the mother and the baby. Place the clamps about 2 to 6 inches apart. Once they are firmly in place,

you should cut the cord between them using the sterile scissors. There is no rush to cut the cord once it is clamped. Do this part of the procedure with great care, because the cord is fragile and easily torn. If it is handled too roughly, it could be torn from the baby's abdomen, resulting in a fatal hemorrhage. Once you have cut the cord between the two clamps, you should tie the end coming from the baby. If the cord was cut earlier to remove it from around the baby's neck while the head was being delivered, now is the time to tie it. The emergency childbirth kit contains special umbilical tape for tying the cord. Do not use ordinary string or twine, because it will cut through the soft, fragile tissues of the cord. Place a loop of the tape around the cord about 1 inch nearer to the baby than the clamp. Tighten the tape slowly so that it doesn't cut the cord and then tie it firmly with a square knot. Cut the ends of the tape but do not remove the clamp. Do not remove the clamp on the end of the cord coming out of the mother's vagina. This part of the cord is attached to the placenta and will be delivered when the placenta delivers (Figure 39–10).

Wrap the baby in a blanket or towel so that only the face is exposed. The baby can be cradled in your arm while its mouth and nose

FIGURE 39–8

Support the baby's head with one hand, and its trunk with your other hand. Remember that the baby is slippery, and you must hold it firmly but gently.

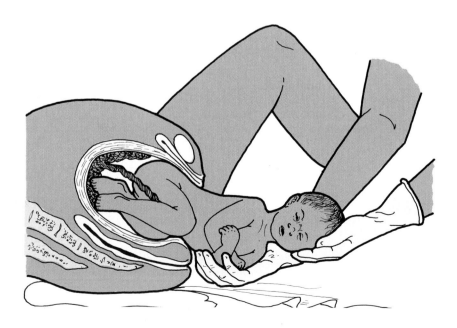

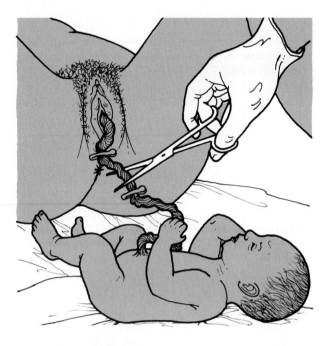

FIGURE 39–10

Clamp the umbilical cord with two sterile clamps, about 3 inches apart, placed halfway between the baby and the mother's vagina. Cut the cord between the 2 clamps. As an extra safeguard, tie the cord near the baby's navel with the special umbilical tape. Leave the clamps on the cord.

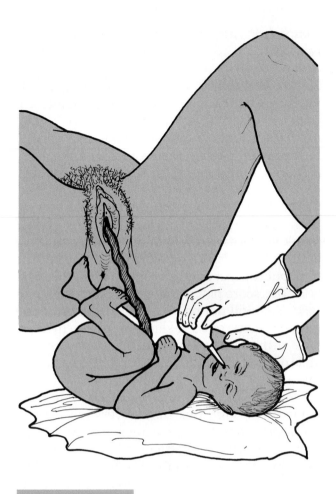

FIGURE 39–9

After delivery, place the baby at the level of the vagina, with its head lowered slightly. Clear the airway with the bulb syringe a second time.

are being suctioned, rather than leaving it on the flat surface. Newborn babies are very sensitive to cold, so if it is at all possible, you should keep the blanket warm (to about 90 degrees F) before you use it. By now the baby should be pink and breathing on its own.

Evaluating the Newborn

A rough guide to the status of the newborn baby can be obtained using the **Apgar score.** This system assigns a number value to each of five areas of activity of the newborn baby: cardiac rate (pulse), respirations, muscle tone,

reflex irritability, and color. The numbers are then totaled. A perfectly healthy baby will have a total score of 10, but most babies will have a score of 7 or 8 at 1 minute after birth. The Apgar score should be calculated at 1 and 5 minutes after birth. By 5 minutes, most babies have a score of 8 to 10 (Figure 39–11).

Cardiac Rate The pulse rate of the newborn should be over 100 beats per minute. If a stethoscope is unavailable, you can measure the pulsations in the umbilical cord using your fingers. The score for a pulse over 100 is 2. If the pulse is below 100, the score is 1. If the pulse is absent, the score is 0. Absence of pulse, of course, indicates absence of cardiac activity and the need for immediate cardiopulmonary resuscitation (CPR).

APGAR SCALE	1 min.	5 min.
Cardiac Rate (>100 = 2, < 100 = 1, 0 = 0)	2	2
Respiratory Rate (Rapid = 2, Slow = 1, Absent = 0)	2	2
Muscle Tone (Good = 2, Fair = 1, Absent = 0)	1	2
Reflex Irritability (Strong = 2, Weak = 1, Absent = 0)	2	2
Color (All pink = 2, Some pink = 1, No pink = 0)	1	2
TOTAL	8	10

FIGURE 39–11

The Apgar score is calculated for each birth at 1 and at 5 minutes. In this example, the baby had only fair muscle tone, and some cyanosis of the feet at 1 minute, giving an Apgar score of 8. However, by 5 minutes, muscle tone and color had improved, giving an Apgar score of 10, which is perfect.

Respiratory Effort Normally, the newborn's respirations are regular and rapid, with a good strong cry. If the respirations are slow, shallow, or labored, or if the cry is weak, respiratory insufficiency may exist. Complete absence of respirations or crying is obviously a very serious sign. The score for rapid respirations is 2, and for slow respirations, 1. If respirations are completely absent, the score is 0.

Muscle Tone The degree of muscle tone indicates the oxygenation of the baby's tissues. Normally, the hips and knees are flexed, and, to some degree, the baby will resist attempts to straighten them out. If this is the case, the score is 2. If the baby has some muscle tone but only weakly resists attempts to straighten out the knees or hips, the score is 1. If the baby is completely limp, with no muscle tone, the score is 0.

Reflex Irritability This part of the Apgar scale measures the baby's response to a stimulus. It calls for snapping a finger against the sole of the baby's foot. If the baby cries and tries to move the foot away, the score is 2. A weak cry is scored 1, and no cry or reaction is scored 0.

Color Most babies are blue at birth but become pink very rapidly. The feet and lips should "pink up" within a few minutes of birth. If the entire baby is pink, the score is 2. If the body is pink but the feet and lips remain blue, the score is 1. The score is 0 if the entire baby is blue or pale. You will not be able to use skin color as a guide in black or dark-skinned babies. Instead, look at the lips and tongue. They may be blue at birth but should "pink up" within a few minutes.

On occasion, you may be called to assist a delivery and find that the delivery has already taken place and that the baby is in trouble. The first thing you should do is to quickly calculate the Apgar score to establish a baseline evaluation of the baby's vital functions. One way to help remember the five components is to use the name Apgar as follows:

A   Appearance (color)
P   Pulse
G   Grimace (reflex irritability)
A   Activity (muscle tone)
R   Respirations

THE THIRD STAGE OF LABOR

The third stage of labor begins after the baby is delivered. Give the baby, wrapped in a warm blanket, to your assistant, and turn your attention back to the mother. You will now assist the mother with delivery of the placenta. The placenta will be attached to the end of the umbilical cord that is coming out of the mother's vagina. The placenta, like the baby, delivers itself; you only assist. The placenta usually delivers itself within a few minutes of the baby's birth, but it may take as long as 30 minutes. Delivery of the placenta may be speeded up by gently massaging the mother's abdomen with a firm, circular motion. The abdominal skin will be wrinkled and very soft. You should be able to feel a firm, grapefruit-sized mass in the lower abdomen. This is the uterus, with the placenta inside. As the uterus is massaged, it will contract and become firmer. If the baby is breathing well and is in good condition, place it at the mother's breast and allow it to nurse. This will also stimulate the uterus to contract and help to deliver the placenta. Never pull on the end of the umbilical cord in an attempt to speed delivery of the placenta. You may tear the cord, or the placenta, or both, and cause serious, perhaps life-threatening, hemorrhage.

Some bleeding, usually less than 250 cc, occurs before the placenta delivers. Once the placenta delivers, bleeding, except for a few drops, should stop. If any of the following three emergency situations occurs during the third stage of labor, the mother should be transported promptly to the hospital:

- If more than 30 minutes elapse and the placenta has not delivered.
- If there is more than 250 cc of bleeding before delivery of the placenta.
- If there is significant bleeding after the delivery of the placenta.

Transport the baby with the mother. Place a sterile pad or sanitary napkin over the vagina, place the mother in the shock position, administer oxygen, and monitor her vital signs closely. Never put anything into the vagina.

Once the placenta delivers, inspect it carefully. The normal placenta is round, measures about 7 inches in diameter, and is about 1 inch thick. One surface is smooth and covered with a shiny membrane; the other surface is rough and lobulated (Figure 39–12). Place the entire placenta and cord into a plastic bag and bring them to the hospital. Hospital personnel will examine the placenta to make certain that the entire placenta has been delivered and that no part has been retained. If a piece of the placenta has been retained, it could cause persistent bleeding or infection.

Before proceeding to the hospital, place a sterile pad or sanitary napkin over the vagina

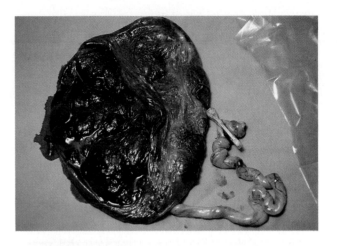

FIGURE 39–12

The normal placenta is round, and measures about 7 inches in diameter and 1 inch in thickness. One side is smooth, the other is rough. Place the entire placenta in a bag and bring it to the hospital.

and lower the mother's legs. Before taking her, the baby, and the placenta to the hospital, you should take a minute to thank anyone who assisted, congratulate the mother, and record the time of birth for the record-of-live-birth form. Remember to also record the Apgar scores at one and five minutes.

ABNORMAL DELIVERIES AND COMPLICATIONS

Failure of the Amniotic Membrane to Rupture

Usually, rupture of the amniotic membranes is one of the first signs that labor is beginning. The membranes may also rupture during contractions, signaled by the resulting gush of fluid. On rare occasions, the membranes will not rupture at all, and the baby will be born still covered by the membranes. As the head presents, a saclike membrane will cover the head and face. This situation is serious, for the membranes will suffocate the baby if they are not removed. You should therefore break the membranes immediately, using your fingers, a sterile clamp, or scissors. If you do use an instrument, be very careful not to cut the baby.

The amniotic fluid will gush out when the membranes are ruptured. Clear the baby's nose and mouth immediately, using the bulb syringe and gauze sponge, and proceed with the rest of the delivery.

Resuscitation of the Newborn

A newborn baby will usually begin breathing spontaneously within 30 seconds after birth. If it does not breathe spontaneously or it is limp and its Apgar score is low, you should institute resuscitation, following these steps:

1. Suction the airway again, as you did previously.
2. Place the baby on its side with the head lower than the rest of the body.
3. Stimulate the baby. Gently slapping or flicking the soles of the baby's feet or rubbing its back provides adequate stimulation and should yield results within 10 to 15 seconds. If unsuccessful, and the baby still does not breathe spontaneously, begin mouth-to-mouth-and-nose resuscitation.
4. Using the infant breathing bag and mask in your delivery kit, cover the baby's nose and mouth and begin respirations. Use enough gentle pressure to make the infant's chest rise with each breath. It may be necessary to bypass the pop-off valve in order to ventilate initially. After the initial resistance, the pressures required to inflate the chest should be no more than 30 to 40 cm H_2O. The volumes required are 6 to 8 mL/Kg. The assisted respiratory rate is 40 to 60 breaths/min. Watch for bilateral chest wall expansion and the presence of breath sounds. Prolonged use of a bag-valve-mask resuscitator can result in gastric distension. If you do not have an infant bag and mask available, you can perform mouth-to-nose-and-mouth breathing. Cover the baby's mouth and nose with your mouth and breathe with the same force you would use to exhale a breath of fresh air. This should be just enough force to make the baby's chest rise. Do not use a lot of pressure and make sure that air is getting into the baby's nose. Babies are nose breathers rather than mouth breathers. Start the resuscitation with two breaths delivered slowly (1 to 1½ seconds each) and watch for inflation of the lungs and motion of the chest wall. If the baby starts to breathe spontaneously, attach an oxygen tubing to the infant mask and let the baby breathe the oxygen until it becomes pink. After 15 to 30 seconds of assisted respirations, assess the heart rate. It should be at least 100 beats per minute if assisted respirations are to be discontinued. If 2 minutes go by, and the baby is still not breathing spontaneously, begin full CPR.

5. Cardiac compression is performed with the baby lying on a firm surface or cradled in one arm while you apply cardiac compressions with the other hand. In the infant, the heart lies just below an imaginary line drawn between the nipples on the middle third of the sternum. Cardiac compression is done with the index and middle fingers. Select a point in the midline of the sternum one finger breadth below the line between the nipples. Place the more superior finger (the one closer to the baby's head) at this point. The other finger will then lie on the lower part of the sternum. Press the two fingers gently against the lower half of the sternum. The sternum and rib cage of the newborn are flexible and easily compressed. Use only enough force to compress the sternum ½ to 1 inch.

   Chest compressions should be done if the heart rate is less than 60 beats per minute, or between 60 and 80 beats per minute and not rising despite adequate ventilation with 100 percent oxygen for 30 seconds. These should be continued at a rate of 100/min. Chest compressions may be discontinued when the baby's heart rate becomes 80 beats per minute or more. Ventilation is done during a pause every third compression. The goal is to achieve 120 actions (combined ventilations and compressions) per minute. The ratio is 3:1—90 compressions to 30 ventilations per minute. Recall that ventilation is as absolutely vital in performing CPR in the newborn as it is in the adult, and cardiac compression alone, without ventilation, is worthless (Figure 39–13).

6. Continue CPR while transporting the baby

A

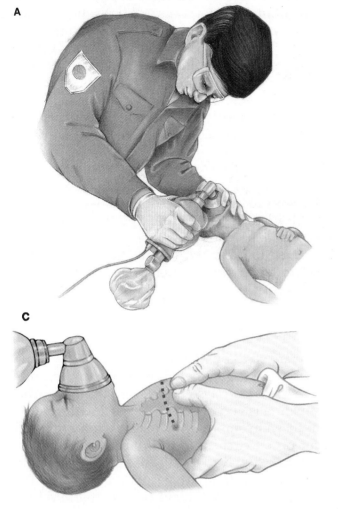

C

B

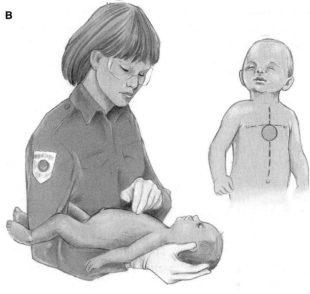

FIGURE 39-13

Cardiopulmonary resuscitation is different for a baby than for an adult. (A) Use an infant mask and bag; cradle the baby as shown and use just enough force to make the chest rise with each breath. (B) Cardiac compression in the infant is done with the index and middle fingers; the inset shows the location on the infant's chest. (C) Side-by-side placement for chest compressions in newborns. Overlap the thumbs for very small newborns.

to the hospital. You will have to get help to transport the mother and baby, because you must maintain continuous cardiopulmonary resuscitation. Continue your efforts at resuscitation until the baby breathes spontaneously or is pronounced dead by a physician. Do not give up! Many babies have survived and developed without brain damage even after long periods without spontaneous breathing if they have been given effective CPR.

7. Keep the baby warm, but not hot, at all times. The baby is not yet able to regulate its body temperature well and must be kept in a warm environment.

8. If the baby is obviously dead when born and is covered with blisters, has a foul smell, and the head is soft, then, and only then, should

you not attempt CPR. If there is any doubt in your mind that the baby has a chance for survival, you should start resuscitation.

Breech Delivery

Most babies are born with a vertex **presentation** (the head coming out first). Occasionally, the buttocks come out first. This delivery is called a *breech presentation*. You will not be able to determine whether a breech presentation is occurring ahead of time, and will only be able to identify it when you see the buttocks, rather than the head, appear at the vaginal opening. Breech deliveries are usually slow, so that there is time to get the mother to the hospital. However, if the buttocks have already passed through the vagina, delivery is underway and the emergency procedures just outlined should be followed.

The preparations for a breech delivery are the same as for a vertex delivery. Position the mother, unwrap the emergency delivery kit, and place yourself and your partner as you would for a normal delivery. Allow the buttocks and legs to deliver spontaneously. You can support them with your hand to prevent rapid expulsion. The buttocks will usually come out easily. Let the legs dangle on either side of your arm as you support the trunk and chest as they are born. The head is almost always face down and should be allowed to deliver spontaneously. As the head is delivering, you should keep the baby's airway open by putting a gloved finger into the vagina and keeping the walls of the vagina from compressing the baby's airway. Note that this is one of only two circumstances when you should put your fingers into the vagina.

During a breech delivery, you should never try to pull the head out. If the head is stuck in the vagina and fails to deliver, you should apply firm pressure to the uterus with the hand that is not supporting the infant. This is done by applying pressure to the lower abdomen, just above the pubic symphysis. You may be able to feel the head through the mother's abdominal wall. This maneuver will frequently enable the head to be delivered spontaneously.

If the head delivers spontaneously, the delivery can continue as for a normal birth. If the head does not deliver spontaneously within three minutes, another EMT or an assistant will have to transport the mother and baby rapidly to the hospital while you hold the baby's airway open (Figure 39–14).

On very rare occasions, the presenting part of the baby is neither the head nor buttocks, but a single arm or leg or foot. This is called a *limb presentation*. You *cannot* successfully deliver such a presentation in the field; these babies must be delivered in a hospital. If you are faced with a limb presentation, you must transport the mother to the hospital immediately. If a limb is protruding, cover it with a sterile towel. Never try to push it back in. Place the mother on her back and transport promptly.

Prolapsed Umbilical Cord

On rare occasions, the umbilical cord may come out of the vagina before the baby, a presentation called *prolapse of the umbilical cord*. This situation is very dangerous, because the baby's head will compress the cord during birth and cut off all circulation to the baby. Prolapse of the umbilical cord usually occurs early in labor, so there is time to get the mother to the hospital. Do not attempt to push the cord back into the vagina. This complication must be

FIGURE 39–14

In breech delivery, the buttocks come out first, then the legs. Usually the baby is easily delivered. The head, which is the largest part of the baby, delivers last, and may be difficult. Provide an adequate airway for the baby with your fingers while it is still in the vagina as shown and support the trunk as it delivers with your other hand.

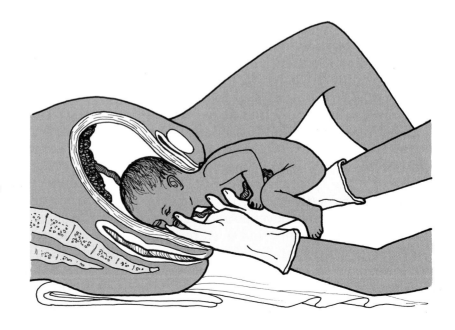

treated in the hospital. Your job is to try to keep the baby's head from compressing the cord. Place the mother on a spine board in the Trendelenburg (shock) position, with her hips elevated on a pillow or folded sheet. Carefully insert your sterile gloved hand into the vagina and gently push the baby's head away from the umbilical cord. Note that this is the only other occasion that you should actually place a hand into the vagina. Wrap a sterile towel moistened with saline around the exposed cord. Give the mother oxygen and transport her rapidly to the hospital.

Excessive Bleeding

Some bleeding always occurs with delivery. However, bleeding that exceeds approximately 250 cc (soaking more than 5 pads) is considered excessive. There are several possible causes for excessive bleeding, all of which may be serious and require emergency care. Treat excessive bleeding by covering the vagina with a sterile pad, and changing the pad as often as necessary. Do not discard these blood-soaked pads because the hospital personnel will use them to estimate the amount of blood that has been lost. Save any tissue that may have passed from the vagina as well. Place the mother in the shock position, administer oxygen, monitor vital signs frequently, and transport her immediately to the hospital. Never hold the mother's legs together in an effort to stop the bleeding, and never "pack" the vagina with gauze pads in an attempt to control bleeding.

Bleeding may occur at any time during pregnancy. Early in the pregnancy, it is usually slight, and, while it may indicate that a serious problem is occurring, does not usually mean an immediate, life-threatening complication. However, bleeding that occurs during the third trimester (the last 3 months before delivery) near the end of pregnancy is much more dangerous. At term (the time when the baby is ready to deliver), the blood vessels supplying the uterus and placenta have grown very large, and any disruption of these vessels may cause massive hemorrhage. Third-trimester bleeding may be caused by either placenta previa or placenta abruptio. Any bleeding that occurs during the third trimester is potentially life-threatening to both the mother and the baby. Therefore, you should transport any patient who exhibits third-trimester bleeding to the hospital rapidly, positioning the patient in the shock position, collecting any blood soaked pads, and alerting medical control that you are bringing in a pregnant woman with third-trimester bleeding.

Abortion (Miscarriage)

Delivery of the fetus and placenta before 20 weeks is called miscarriage or **abortion.** Abortions may be spontaneous (without any obvious known cause) or deliberate. Deliberate abortions may be self-induced (by the mother herself) or by someone else. Deliberate abortions may be planned and performed in a hospital or clinic setting. Regardless of the reasons for the abortion, complications can occur that you may be called on to treat.

The most serious complications of abortion are bleeding and infection. Bleeding may result from portions of the fetus or placenta being left in the uterus (incomplete abortion) or from injury to the wall of the uterus (perforation of the uterus and possibly the adjacent bowel or bladder). Infection can result from such perforation, as well as from the use of unsterile instruments to cause the abortion. If the patient is in shock, treat her for shock and transport her promptly to the hospital. Collect any tissue that passes through the vagina and bring it to the hospital. Never try to pull any tissue out of the vagina; rather, cover it with a sterile pad. In rare instances, massive bleeding may occur from an abortion and cause severe hypovolemic shock. Consider the use of the pneumatic antishock garment (PASG) in such a situation. However, remember that the use of the PASG is controversial, and you should consult medical control before applying it.

Twins

Twins occur about once in every 80 births. Sometimes there is a family history of twins. The mother may suspect she is having twins because she has an unusually large abdomen.

Twins are usually, but not always, diagnosed early in pregnancy using modern ultrasound techniques.

Twins are smaller than single babies, and the delivery is usually not difficult. Twins should be suspected if the baby is small or if the mother's abdomen remains fairly large after the birth. If twins are present, the second one will usually be born within 45 minutes of the first. About 10 minutes after the first birth, labor pains will begin again, and the birth process will repeat itself.

The procedure for delivering twins is the same as for single babies. Clamp and cut the cord of the first baby as soon as it has been born and before the second baby is delivered. The second baby may deliver before or after the first placenta. There may be only one placenta or there may be two. When the placenta has been delivered, check whether there is one or two umbilical cords. If two cords are coming out of the placenta, the twins are *monozygotic* (identical) and there will only be one placenta. If only one cord is coming out of the placenta, then the twins are *dizygotic* (fraternal), and there will be two placentas. Occasionally, the two placentas of fraternal twins are fused together, so that you may think you are dealing with identical twins.

It is important to remember that if you only see one umbilical cord coming out of the first placenta, there is still another placenta to be delivered. On the other hand, if both cords are attached to one placenta, there will not be a second placenta, and the delivery is over. Remember, monozygotic twins must both be the same sex; twins of different sexes are always dizygotic. Dizygotic twins may be of the same sex or of different sexes. Record the time of birth and the Apgar score of each twin separately. Twins may be so small as to be premature; handle them very carefully and keep them warm. Use the Apgar score as a guide in the same way as you would use it for a single birth.

Delivery of a Baby of an Addicted Mother

Unfortunately, more and more babies are being born to mothers who are addicted to drugs or alcohol. These mothers often have had little or no prenatal care. Their babies will show the effects of the addiction; they may be premature, have low birth weights, irritability, low Apgar scores, and severe respiratory depression. Some will die. **Fetal alcohol syndrome** is a term used to describe the babies of alcoholic mothers.

You may be called to handle a delivery of a drug- or alcohol-addicted mother. In addition to the usual measures you take for delivery, pay particular attention to your own safety. Be particularly careful not to cut or stick yourself with any sharp object, and wear goggles and sterile gloves at all times. Some clues that you are dealing with an addicted mother will be the presence of drug paraphernalia, empty wine or liquor bottles, and statements made by neighbors or by the mother herself. The newborn baby of an addicted mother will likely need immediate hospital care. Carry out the delivery as outlined earlier, but be prepared to support the baby's respirations and administer oxygen while transporting it and the mother to the hospital. Do not judge or lecture the mother; your job is to help deliver the baby as best you

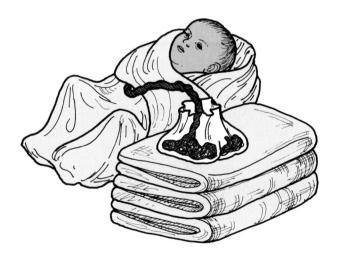

FIGURE 39–15

When sterile supplies are not available and you cannot cut the umbilical cord, keep the placenta, still attached to the cord, at the same level as the baby during transport to the hospital.

can, and get both the infant and the mother to the hospital.

Delivery Without Sterile Supplies

On rare occasions, you may have to deliver a baby without a sterile emergency delivery pack. If you can, use clean sheets and towels that have not been used since they were laundered. Even if you do not have a sterile pack, you should always have goggles and sterile gloves with you. Put these on; they are for your own protection as well as that of the mother and baby. Carry out the delivery as if sterile supplies were on hand. As soon as the baby is born, you should wipe out the inside of its mouth with your finger to clear the mouth of blood and mucus. Without the delivery pack, you should not cut or tie the cord. Instead, as soon as the placenta is born, wrap it in a clean towel or put it in a plastic bag and transport it with the baby. Always keep the placenta and the baby at the same level so blood does not drain from the baby into the placenta (Figure 39–15). Keep the baby warm, and transport the mother, baby, and placenta to the hospital promptly.

Premature Infant

The usual *gestation period* (period for the development of a baby) is 9 calendar months or 40 weeks. A normal, single baby will weigh approximately 7 pounds at birth. Any baby that delivers before 8 months gestation or weighs less than 5½ pounds at birth is considered premature. This determination isn't always easy to make. Often, the exact gestation time cannot be determined; and you probably have no scale to weigh the baby. A premature baby is smaller and thinner, and its head is proportionately larger compared with the rest of its body than a full-term baby (Figure 39–16).

Premature babies need special care to survive. With such care, even babies as small as one pound have survived and developed into

FIGURE 39–16

A premature infant (right) is smaller and thinner, than a full-term baby (left). In addition, the premature baby's head is larger compared with the rest of its body than is the full-term infant's.

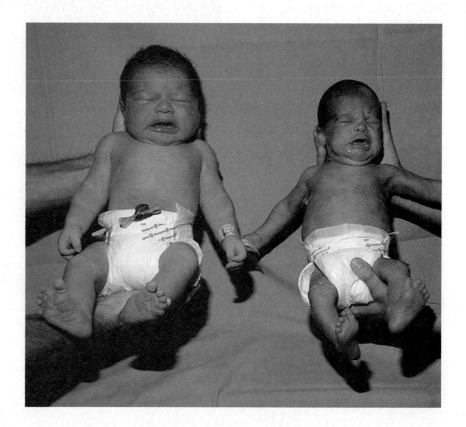

normal children. You should follow certain, specific procedures when you are handling a premature infant:

1. *Keep the baby warm.* Wrap it in a warm blanket as soon as it is born. Keep the face exposed, but keep the head covered. Keep the baby in a place where the temperature is between 90 and 95 degrees F.
2. *Keep the mouth and nose clear of mucus.* Like all newborn babies, premature ones are nose breathers, and the small nasal passages can be obstructed easily. Use the bulb syringe to suction the mouth and nostrils frequently. Handle the baby and all its parts very gently.
3. *Carefully observe the cut end of the cord attached to the baby and be sure that it is not bleeding.* The loss of even a few drops of blood can be very serious.

4. *Give oxygen.* Open the valve on your oxygen cylinder slowly to give a steady stream of oxygen (about 70 to 100 bubbles per minute through the water bottle that is attached to the oxygen tank). Do not direct the stream of oxygen directly into the baby's mouth, but make a small tent over the baby's head using a blanket or a piece of aluminum foil, and direct the oxygen into the tent. Although there may be some danger to a premature baby from receiving very high concentrations of oxygen, there is no danger if it is given over a short period of time in this manner.
5. *Do not infect the baby.* Premature babies are very susceptible to infection. Protect them from contamination. Do not breathe directly into the baby's face. Keep everyone else as far away from the baby as possible.

FIGURE 39–17

A mobile infant carrier is used by large hospitals for transporting premature infants and other high-risk babies.

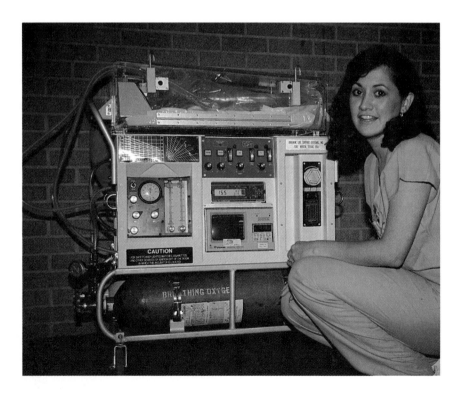

6. *Notify the hospital.* Do this before transporting the baby and mother. Bring a family member with you to the hospital.

Some large medical centers have mobile infant carriers for the transportation of high-risk infants (Figure 39–17). If such a vehicle is available, the hospital personnel may want to send it rather than have you transport the baby in the ambulance. If such a vehicle is not available, you should transport the baby in a special carrier. The premature infant carrier has supplies that can be used for the immediate care of the premature infant as well as for its transport. These items include a quilted pad, baby blanket, diaper, thermometer, suction tube and suction bulb, sterile Kelly clamp, and, most important, hot water bottles and an oxygen cylinder with the necessary attachments.

Fill the hot water bottles and pad them well so they don't come in direct contact with the infant's skin. Place them in the carrier so that one is on the bottom and on each side of where the baby will lie. Once you have wrapped the baby in a blanket and placed it inside the carrier, secure the carrier inside the vehicle. Keep the temperature of the vehicle at 90 to 95 degrees F while the baby and mother are being transported to the hospital.

YOU ARE THE EMT

1. The patient tells you she is in labor and too far along to get to the hospital in time. How will you decide whether to take her in the ambulance or help her to deliver at the scene?

2. Should you cut the umbilical cord before or after the placenta delivers? Why?

3. You have just evaluated the baby you helped deliver. Its Apgar score is a perfect 10. Describe the areas of activity that are measured, and how you scored each one to get a 10.

4. You arrived just in time to help a woman deliver an eight-week premature baby girl. Although tiny, her color is good and she is crying. What steps will you take in the care of this newborn that you wouldn't normally have to take with a healthy full-term baby?

5. You have just helped deliver a healthy baby boy. While you are waiting for the placenta to deliver, the mother tells you that labor pains are starting up again. You notice that her abdomen is still quite protuberant. What should you be prepared for next?

6. You are called to assist a woman who is obviously in labor. Your assessment shows that she is crowning. A neighbor tells you that the woman uses crack regularly. How will you handle this delivery differently than you would a normal one? What particular risks are there to this baby?

SECTION 8

ENVIRONMENTAL EMERGENCIES

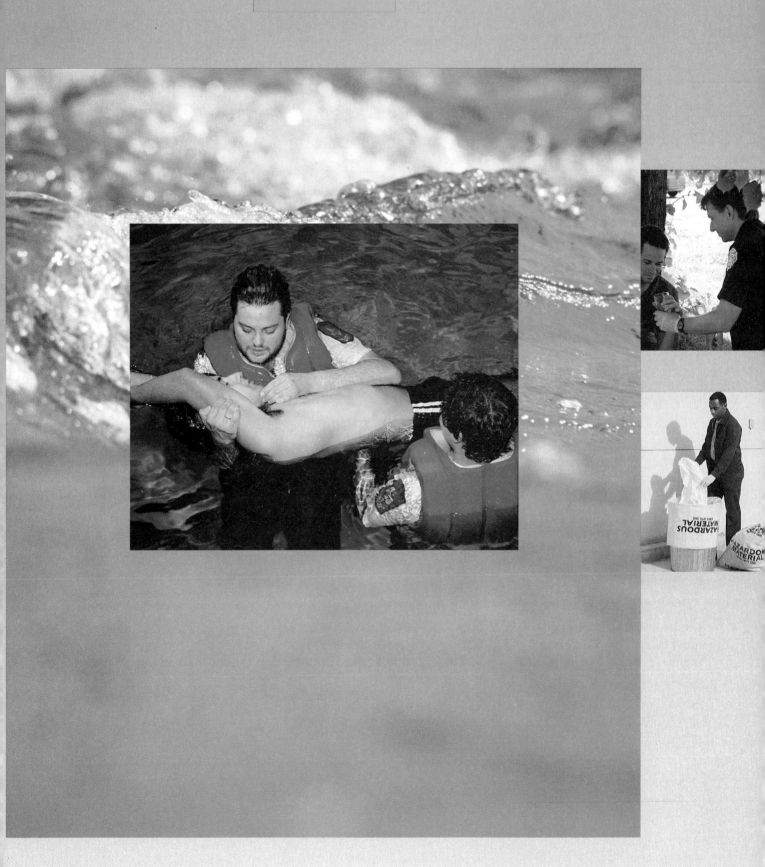

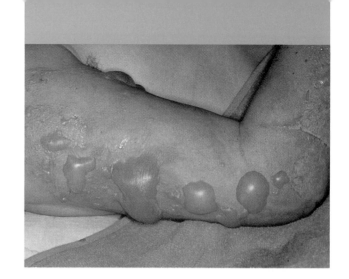

BURNS

chemical burn A burn that results from any toxic substance that contacts the body.

conductor Any substance that allows an electrical current to flow through it.

decontamination (de"kon-tam-ĭ-na'shun) The orderly process by which radiation or chemical hazards can be removed from clothing, equipment, vehicles, and personnel.

insulator (in'su-la"tor) Any substance that prevents an electrical current from flowing.

ionizing radiation (i'on-īz-ing ra-de-a'shun) Nuclear radiation that has the capacity to alter body cells.

Radiation Emergency Assistance Center/Training Site REAC/TS A facility in Oak Ridge, Tennessee that serves as a worldwide hotline for advice about and assistance following radiation accidents.

radioactivity The spontaneous release of energy by particles that make up atoms.

roentgens/rads (R) (rent'gens) The units of measurement for gamma and X ray radiation.

thermal burn (ther'mal bern) A burn that is caused by heat.

OVERVIEW

Burns are among the most serious and most painful of all injuries. Burns occur when the body, or a part of it, receives more energy than it can absorb without injury. The sources of this energy include heat, toxic chemicals, electricity, and nuclear radiation. The severity of a burn is usually rated by the amount of injury to the body tissues. The actual depth of the burn and the amount of the body surface involved are calculated together to determine the seriousness of the burn.

When treating a burn, you may be faced with other problems in addition to the burned patient. The fire that caused the burn may have to be extinguished. The toxic substance may have to be removed. The patient may be experiencing shock or respiratory arrest caused by the burn, especially in the case of an inhalation injury or a lightning strike. The patient may have sustained fractures from falling, especially after an electric shock. And, you yourself may be at risk from the heat, the live wire, the toxic fumes, or the radioactivity that caused the burn.

Chapter 40 begins with a review of skin anatomy. It then describes how the most common type of burn—the thermal burn—is evaluated for degree of seriousness and how thermal burns should be treated. The chapter next addresses chemical and electrical burns. The last section discusses radiation injuries. These include burns from solar radiation and injuries resulting from exposure to radioactivity.

GOALS

The goals of Chapter 40 are to
- review the anatomy of the skin.
- identify the features of first-, second-, and third-degree burns and learn how to estimate the depth and extent of the burn.
- determine the severity of a thermal burn.
- learn the emergency management of a thermal burn.
- identify the various types of chemical burns and learn how to treat them.
- understand how electrical energy, including lightning, enters and exits the body and how to treat electrical burns and injuries.
- describe the effects of exposure to solar radiation and nuclear radiation.
- learn the emergency medical care for exposure to radioactive materials.

ANATOMY OF THE SKIN: A REVIEW

The anatomy of the skin is presented fully in Chapter 14. There are two layers of the skin: the epidermis and the dermis. The epidermis is the tough, outer layer. Its cells are constantly being worn away and replaced as new cells are produced. The dermis, the layer just below the epidermis, contains the structures that give the skin its characteristic appearance. These are the hair follicles, sweat glands, sebaceous glands that secrete the oil that lubricates the skin, blood vessels, and nerve endings.

Deep to the skin are the subcutaneous tissue and the muscle fascia. The subcutaneous tissue is the fatty layer that varies in thickness in different parts of the body and from person to person. The final and deepest layer, below the

Layers of the skin. A burn may extend through some or all of these layers.

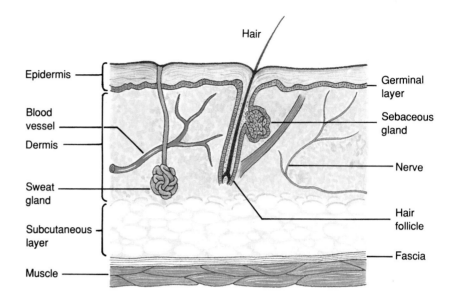

subcutaneous layer, is the fascia, which covers the muscles (Figure 40–1). A burn may extend through some or all of these layers.

The skin is an organ, not merely a tissue. It serves many functions. It keeps bacteria out of the body. It maintains the water content of the body. It serves as insulation and helps control the body's temperature. Through the nerve endings, the skin is the organ that reports to the brain on the body's environment and on the many sensations with which the body comes in contact. Any break in the skin destroys this protective envelope and allows bacterial invasion and infection, fluid loss, and loss of temperature control, any of which may cause serious illness and death.

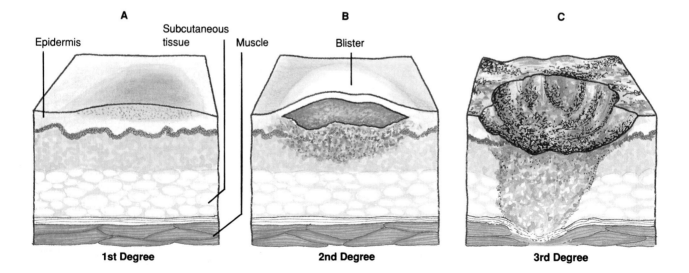

Three common degrees of thermal burn injury. (A) A first-degree burn causes epidermal injury with redness of the skin. (B) A second-degree burn causes partial destruction of the dermis and is characterized by blisters. (C) A third-degree burn causes complete epidermal and dermal destruction, and may extend even deeper.

THERMAL BURNS

You will be frequently called to evaluate or treat burn injuries. Burns are the second most common cause of accidental death in the United States, accounting for over 10,000 deaths a year, most of them in children under the age of 6 years. Proper emergency care following a burn may make the difference in survival and decrease long-term disability. The most common type of burns, **thermal burns,** are caused by heat. The seriousness of the burn may be estimated by observing the damage to the skin and calculating the extent of the body surface area that has been burned. The terms first-, second-, and third-degree burns are used as a measure of the depth of the burn to the skin (Figure 40–2).

First-degree burns occur when only the superficial part of the epidermis has been injured. The skin turns red (erythematous) but does not blister or actually burn through (Figure 40–3). A sunburn is a good example of a first-degree burn.

Second-degree burns occur when the epidermis and a varying extent of the dermis are burned, but the entire thickness of the dermis is not destroyed and the subcutaneous tissue is not injured. The second-degree burn is characterized by blister formation (Figure 40–4).

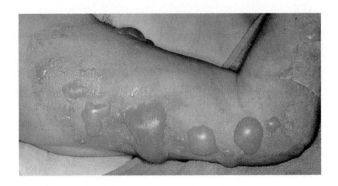

FIGURE 40–4

In a second-degree burn the epidermis and part of the dermis are injured. Blister formation characterizes the second-degree burn.

Third-degree burns extend through the dermis and into, or beyond, the subcutaneous fat. The burned area is dry, leathery, and discolored (charred or chalk white). Thrombosed (clotted) blood vessels may be visible under the burned skin, or the subcutaneous fat may be visible. The severely burned area may be without feeling, because the nerve endings have been destroyed, although the surrounding less severely burned areas may remain extremely painful (Figure 40–5).

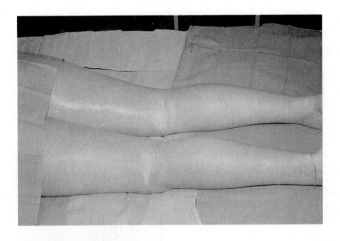

FIGURE 40–3

In a first-degree burn only the superficial part of the epidermis is injured. The skin will be red and very painful, as is often the case after a day at the beach.

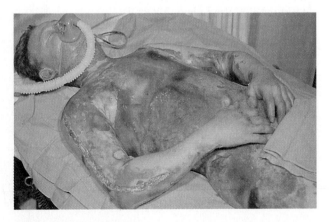

FIGURE 40–5

In a third-degree burn, the epidermis and the dermis are injured. Because superficial nerve endings are destroyed, the burned area may not have feeling. The surrounding areas, however, are extremely painful.

It may be impossible to accurately estimate the depth of a particular burn in the field. Even experienced burn surgeons may underestimate or, more commonly, overestimate the extent of a particular burn. Some burn centers no longer use the terms first-, second-, and third-degree burns. Centers now use a simpler classification: full thickness or partial thickness. A partial-thickness burn does not go down into the subcutaneous tissue, a full-thickness burn does. The outlook for a partial-thickness burn to heal without scarring is better. For calculating the severity of a burn, assume that first- and second-degree burns are partial thickness, and a third-degree burn is full thickness. You should be familiar with the terminology used in your area for describing the depth of a burn.

The extent of the burn, or the amount of surface area involved, may be calculated using the Rule of Nines. This system divides the surface of the body into sections, each of which is approximately 9 percent of the total body surface area. Remember that in infants and small children, the head is relatively larger than it is in adults, and the legs are relatively smaller. As a result, the Rule of Nines is calculated differently in small children than in adults. Using the Rule of Nines, you can make a rough estimate of the surface area that has been burned (Figure 40–6).

Seriousness of Thermal Burns

It is important to try to estimate the seriousness of a burn injury, because doing so will assist medical control in directing you to the proper treatment facility, such as a specialized burn center.

Five factors determine the seriousness of a thermal burn:

- The depth (first-, second-, or third-degree).
- The amount of surface area (Rule of Nines).
- Involvement of critical areas (hands, feet, face, or genitalia).
- The patient's age (very young or very old).

FIGURE 40–6

The Rule of Nines. In the adult, most areas of the body can be divided roughly into portions of 9 percent, or multiples of nine. This division, called the Rule of Nines, is used to estimate the percentage of body surface damage sustained in a burn. In a small child, relatively more area is taken up by the head and less by the lower extremities. Accordingly, the Rule of Nines is modified.

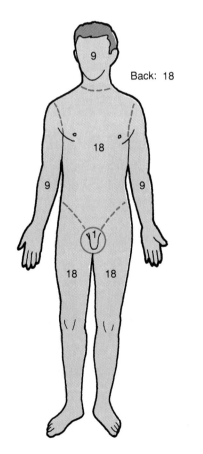
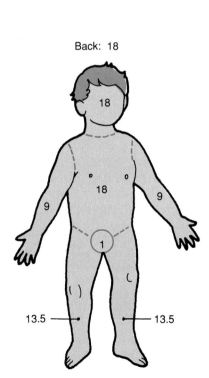

- The patient's general health (are other injuries or illnesses present?).

These five factors will enable you to determine whether the burn is critical, moderate, or minor.

Critical burns are the most serious. They include

- All burns complicated by fractures.
- Any degree of respiratory injury.
- Third-degree burns that involve the hands, feet, genitalia, or face.
- Third-degree burns that involve more than 10 percent of the body surface.
- Second-degree burns that involve more than 25 percent of the body surface.
- Any otherwise moderate burn in an elderly or critically ill patient.

Moderate burns are less serious than critical burns but are still serious injuries. They include

- Third-degree burns that involve 2 to 10 percent of the body area (excluding the hands, feet, face, or genitalia).
- Second-degree burns that involve 15 to 25 percent of the body surface area.
- First-degree burns that involve 50 percent or more of the body surface area.

Minor burns include third-degree burns that involve less than 2 percent of the body surface area or second-degree burns that involve less than 15 percent of the body surface area.

A different system is used to determine critical burns in children. Any third-degree burn in a child is considered a critical burn. Any second-degree burn of more than 20 percent of the body surface is also a critical burn in a child. A second-degree burn of 10 to 20 percent of the body surface area would be a moderate burn, and a second-degree burn of less than 10 percent of the body area would be considered a minor burn.

Emergency Care of a Thermal Burn

There are four goals in the emergency care of a thermal burn:

1. Stop the burning process and prevent further injury.

2. Cover the burned area with a dry, sterile dressing to decrease heat loss and decrease the risk of infection.
3. Support the patient's vital functions.
4. Transport the patient promptly to a hospital that has the necessary capabilities to treat a burn.

Your first responsibility when responding to a burned patient is to stop any further burning from occurring—in other words, put out the fire. Move the patient away from a burning area to prevent further injury from the heat or from smoke inhalation. If the patient's clothing is still on fire, wrap him or her in a blanket, or use a dry chemical fire extinguisher to put out the flames. Remove any smoldering clothing. If the skin and clothing are still hot, immerse them in cool water or cover them with a wet, cool dressing. This will relieve pain and stop any further burning. Do not immerse the burned area for more than 10 minutes, however. If the burning has stopped before you get to the patient, then immersing the part in water is not necessary. Immerse the part only if it is still burning. The greatest danger with a burn is infection, and immersing it in water may increase the risk of infection. Clean dressings and clean or sterile water should always be used to minimize the risk of infection.

An extensive burn can result in hypothermia (the loss of body heat). Do not allow any extra heat loss to occur except to put out the fire.

Rapidly estimate the extent and severity of the burn. Cover the burned area with a dry dressing. Sterile gauze is best if the burned area is not too extensive, or you may use a clean sheet if there is not enough sterile dressing material. Most importantly, do not put anything else on the burned area. Use a dry, sterile dressing only. Never use ointments, lotions, or antiseptics of any kind. If the patient has sustained a critical burn, administer oxygen as well. The patient may also need to be treated for shock before being promptly transported.

More people die in fires as a result of smoke inhalation than from burns of the skin. The patient who has sustained burns about the face or has inhaled smoke or fumes may develop respiratory distress. Any patient in respiratory distress needs oxygen and prompt transport

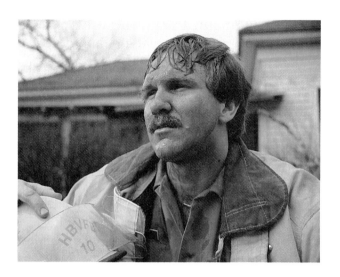

FIGURE 40–7

Suspect a burn injury to the respiratory system in any-one who has burns about the face or who has inhaled smoke or fumes.

(Figure 40–7). Sometimes respiratory problems do not develop immediately. Be aware that a burn patient who at first appears to be breathing well may suddenly develop severe respiratory distress.

Equally dangerous as a respiratory burn is poisonous gas inhalation during a fire. There are two particularly dangerous poisonous gases that are produced in fires: carbon monoxide and cyanide. If a person has been trapped in a burning building or room, there is a good chance that he or she has inhaled carbon monoxide. Carbon monoxide has no odor or taste and does not irritate the respiratory tract; a patient who has inhaled carbon monoxide does not always cough or bring up sputum, and may not be aware of the inhaled toxin. Cyanide gas is produced by the burning of a variety of plastics. It has a characteristic odor of burnt almonds. However, a person may not recognize the odor and be unaware of the inhaled cyanide.

Both carbon monoxide and cyanide gases act as poisons by interfering with the ability of red blood cells to transport oxygen. Move the patient whom you suspect has inhaled poison gas out of the burning area as rapidly as possible. Remember that you are at risk from

inhaling poison gas if you do not use the proper mask system. Never enter an area where you suspect toxic fumes or poisonous gases without wearing a properly functioning mask system. Once the patient has been moved to an open area, treat any burns, and immediately administer 100 percent oxygen through a nonrebreathing mask. Transport the suspected carbon monoxide or cyanide poisoning patient rapidly to the hospital.

Patients who have sustained critical burns should be treated in a burn center. Alert medical control that a patient with a critical burn is being brought in so that medical personnel can organize prompt and appropriate triage. Know the location of the nearest burn center(s) in your area.

CHEMICAL BURNS

A **chemical burn** may occur from any toxic substance that comes in contact with the body. Most chemical burns are caused by strong acids or strong alkalis that get on the skin or clothing. Sometimes the fumes of strong chemicals can cause burns, especially to the respiratory tract. The eyes are particularly vulnerable to chemical burns.

Most chemical burns occur in industrial settings—factories or laboratories. Places where such chemicals are used usually have some facilities for treatment of accidental chemical burns. Employees often have some training in emergency measures to be used in accidental chemical burns; however, this is not always the case. You may be called to a scene of a chemical burn and find that no emergency measures have been carried out.

The emergency care of a chemical burn is basically the same as that of a thermal burn. To stop the burning process, the chemical itself must be removed from contact with the patient. With very few exceptions, this means the area must be flooded with gallons of water. ("The solution to pollution is dilution" is the best rule to follow in most instances of chemical burns.) Except in very rare instances, do not try to find something to neutralize the chemical, but flood the area with water immediately. Most industrial plants have special showers or hoses for this purpose. Flood the area of burn with water. Do not direct a forceful stream of water from a hose on the patient because the extreme water pressure may add mechanical injury to the burned skin. Remove the clothing from the affected area while the skin is being flushed (Figure 40–8). Often the patient will tell you that the burning pain has stopped once the flooding begins. Nonetheless, you should continue flooding the area with gallons of water for 10 minutes after the burning pain has stopped. Many chemicals, particularly strong alkalis, have a delayed reaction and will continue to cause injury even though the patient feels no further pain. Once you have completed the flooding, cover the burned area with a dry, sterile dressing just as you would do with a thermal burn. Then, transport the patient to the hospital.

Chemical Injuries of the Skin

Chemical (acid and alkali) burns may cause severe skin injury. Strong alkalis, such as concentrated sodium hydroxide or potassium hydroxide, may cause more severe burns than strong acids because they penetrate more deeply into the tissues. The treatment for liquid acid or alkali burns is to flood the area with copious amounts of water. If a solid substance such as lime has been spilled on the patient, you should brush it off before flushing the area. A dry chemical (Figure 40–9) may be activated by contact with water and will cause more damage to the skin than when it is dry. Remove the patient's clothing, including shoes, stockings, and gloves, because residual amounts of chemicals are retained in the creases of the clothes. Be particularly careful not to get any chemical, dry or liquid, on you or your uniform

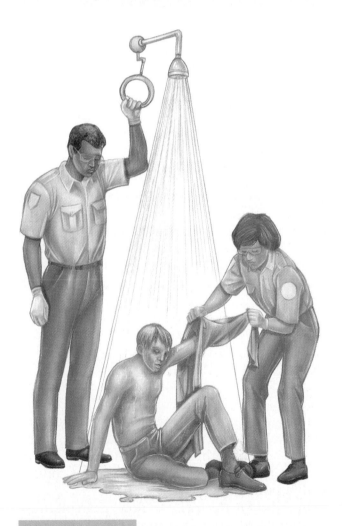

FIGURE 40–8

Chemical burns are treated by flooding the area with water. Remove the clothing as the flooding is taking place. Continue the flooding, with gallons of water, for 10 minutes after the burning pain has stopped.

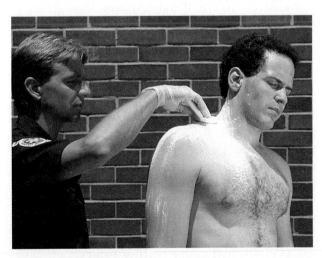

FIGURE 40–9

Always brush dry chemicals off of the skin and clothing before the area is flooded. Dry chemicals are activated when they mix with water and cause a more severe burn than when they are dry.

when you are treating someone who has chemical burns.

Burns that are caused by phenol (carbolic acid), may require special handling. You should first flood the burned area with water, as you would do for any other chemical burn. However, phenol is not very soluble in water; therefore, medical control may direct you to then wash the skin with a phenol solvent, such as polyethylene glycol, propylene glycol, or glycerol. This allows the phenol to dissolve better in water. You may then be asked to continue flooding the area with large amounts of water. Controversy exists about the emergency treatment of a phenol burn. If you work in an area where this chemical is widely used, you should consult your local medical authorities for their protocol on how to manage a patient with a phenol burn.

Chemical Injuries of the Eyes

Chemical burns of the eye are particularly serious. Permanent blindness can result from these injuries, even after a very brief exposure to the chemical. The basic principle in the emergency management of these injuries is the same as for a chemical burn to the skin: flood the area with water. The normal reaction of the eye to any injury is to close tightly, so you must hold the eyelids open while flooding the eye. Use a gentle stream of water, taking care not to wash the chemicals into the uninjured eye (Figure 40–10). Continue flooding for at least 5 minutes for an acid burn and 10 to 20 minutes for an alkali burn. You may have to support the patient's head under the faucet during the flushing process. When you have completed flushing, cover both eyes with soft pads and transport the patient promptly to the hospital. Do not put any substances other than water into the eyes, regardless of the chemical that has caused the burn. Any chemical added to the eye will just cause further injury.

Chemical Inhalation Injuries

Inhalation injuries from chemical fumes are particularly serious. If the patient complains of *dyspnea* (difficult breathing), if there are obvious fumes that you can smell in the air, or if the

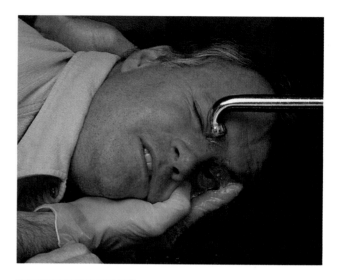

FIGURE 40–10

Chemical burns to the eye are serious. Flood the affected eye with a gentle stream of water. Hold the eyelids open, which is hard to do because the patient's natural reflex is to keep the eye shut. Take care to prevent any of the chemical from getting into the other eye during flushing.

patient says he or she has inhaled fumes, you should assume that an inhalation injury has occurred. Give oxygen and transport the patient promptly to the hospital. Even if a patient who has inhaled fumes has no obvious signs of respiratory distress, he or she still could have had a significant respiratory injury and may at any moment develop respiratory difficulty.

ELECTRICAL BURNS

Electrical burns may occur as a result of contact with high- or low-voltage electricity. Ordinary household current is powerful enough to cause severe burns. High-voltage burns may occur in electrical utility workers or from direct contact with a power line.

In order for electricity to flow, a circuit must be completed from the source of the electricity to the ground. Any substance that prevents an electrical circuit from being completed is called an **insulator**. Rubber, for example, is an insulator. Any substance that allows a current to flow through it is called a **conductor**. Water and most metals are conductors. The human body, which is largely composed of water, is also a good conductor. Electrical burns occur when the body, or a part of it, completes a circuit connecting a power source with the ground (Figure 40–11).

Two dangers are specifically associated with electrical burns. First, the amount of deep tissue injury may be very great. Despite the small size of the skin burn wounds, severe damage may occur to deeper tissues. Second, the burn may be accompanied by cardiopulmonary arrest from the electrical shock, which further complicates the patient's injury.

Electrical energy is capable of producing severe tissue injury. In order to cause injury, the electricity must flow through the body. It must enter the body at one point and exit at another point. There is always a wound (a burn) where the electricity went into the body, and another at the point of exit. The entrance wound may be quite small, but the exit wound may be extensive and deep (Figure 40–12).

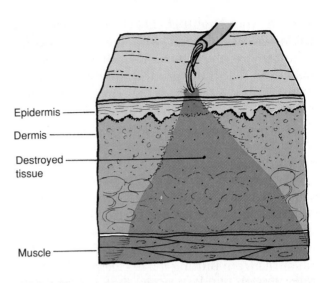

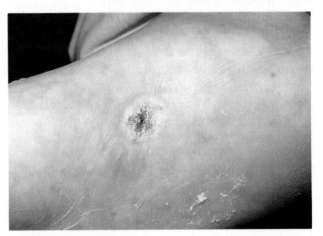

FIGURE 40–12

(A) Electrical burns can cause severe tissue damage. Although the surface burn at the point of entry may be very small, the exit wound may be extensive and deep. (B) A typical small entrance burn wound on the foot.

High-voltage electrical energy can destroy muscles and skin to such an extent that amputation may become necessary.

Electric Shock Injuries

The energy from a high-voltage electrical current passing through the body may disrupt the normal electrical rhythm of the heart and cause cardiac arrest. Also, the electrical current may cause violent muscle contractions that could result in fractures or dislocations. Compression fractures of the vertebrae and posterior disloca-

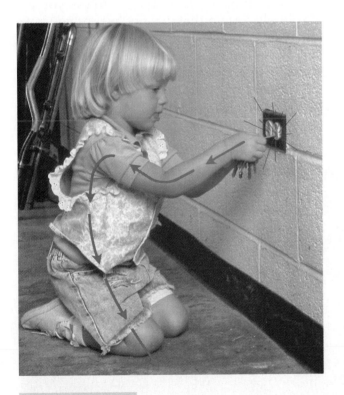

FIGURE 40–11

The human body is a good conductor of electricity. An electrical burn usually occurs when the body, acting as a conductor, completes a circuit.

tion of the shoulder are injuries that are characteristically seen with electrical shocks. Furthermore, the electrical shock will cause the patient to fall to the ground, often resulting in further injury. Therefore, when you are called to the scene of an electrical accident, you must be prepared to assess and treat a patient who is in cardiac arrest, has multiple injuries, and has severe burns.

Most electrical burns in the home occur from faulty electrical equipment or the careless use of appliances. Remember that ordinary house current (115 volts) is enough to cause death by electrocution. Small children can suffer electrical burns from putting a live electrical cord into their mouth. Make certain that the power is turned off before approaching anyone who may still be in contact with an electrical wire or appliance. Touching someone who is still in contact with a live electrical wire will result in your completing the circuit and receiving an electrical injury as well (see Figure 40–11).

Electrical burns outside the home often occur from accidental contact with a downed power line or from accidental contact with a power line by a construction worker doing excavation work. You may respond to a call involving a downed power line. Assume that any downed power line is live unless the power company has shut it off. Power lines may have anywhere

from 115 to 50,000 volts running through them. Telephone lines and television cable lines have a much lower voltage but still enough to cause a shock. Unless you are absolutely certain that a downed line is a low-voltage line, assume that it is a live, high-voltage line and do not touch it.

If an electrical line has fallen across a car and there are people inside, they are safe as long as they stay inside the car. The rubber tires of the car will insulate them. They should be told to stay in the car until the power company can shut the power off (Figure 40–13). In very rare instances this situation is compounded by a danger from fire or oncoming traffic. If passengers' lives are in danger, they should be instructed to jump clear of the car, making certain that they do not touch the car and the ground at the same time. Small children should be tossed out of the car to you first. As always, you must take particular precautions for your own safety when you are responding to such an accident scene.

Never move a downed wire unless you are absolutely certain that it is not live, or you have had special training and have the necessary special equipment to handle live electrical wires. EMTs responding to emergency calls have been fatally injured from accidental contact with electrical wires.

FIGURE 40–13

Do not touch a downed power line until the utility company has shut off the power. If a live wire has fallen across a car, warn the passengers to stay inside. If they have to escape because of a fire, they must jump clear of the car without touching the ground and the car at the same time.

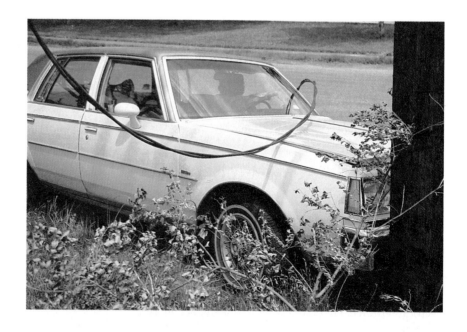

Treatment of an electrical injury calls for instituting cardiorespiratory resuscitation if needed, placing dry, sterile dressings on all burn wounds, and splinting suspected fractures. All electrical burns are potentially severe injuries that require further treatment in the hospital. CPR may have to be prolonged in these cases, but success rates are higher when CPR is begun promptly and then sustained.

Lightning Injuries

Lightning causes over 1,000 injuries and 200 deaths each year in the United States—more than any other weather phenomenon. Lightning strikes contain massive amounts of energy (up to 50 million volts), and may cause temperatures in excess of 50,000 degrees F.

Lightning may cause injury in four different ways:

- *Direct strike.* The lightning hits the person directly, usually conducted through a metal object such as a golf club, or umbrella, or a work tool. This is the most serious form of lightning injury.
- *Flashover.* The lightning current travels over the surface of the person on its way to the ground. Flashover usually occurs when the person is wet, and it causes less severe injury.
- *Side flash.* The lightning strikes near someone and "splashes" through the air to the person.
- *Stride potential.* Lightning strikes the ground near someone then travels up one leg and down the other into the ground.

Side flash and stride potential may involve more than one person, and can be the cause of multiple patients being injured in a lightning strike.

A lightning injury is different from a high-voltage electrical injury caused by a power line. Although there is much greater energy from a lightning injury, its duration is usually only a fraction of a second. As a result, lightning strikes rarely cause deep tissue injury. The major types of injuries that result from lightning are cardiac arrest, neurologic injuries, blunt trauma, and superficial burns.

The most serious injury, cardiopulmonary arrest, results from electrical injury to the heart's conducting mechanism. Frequently, cardiac activity may reestablish itself spontaneously, but often respiratory activity does not resume.

Neurologic injuries usually include unconsciousness and may include temporary paralysis, confusion, and amnesia.

Blunt trauma to any area of the body may occur if the force of the strike literally hurls the person across the ground.

Characteristics of Lightning Burns Burns from lightning are very characteristic. They are superficial and have a spidery, feathery, branching appearance. There is almost never an entrance or exit wound as seen in high-voltage electrical line burns. Thermal burns, however, may occur if the person's clothes catch on fire.

Emergency Care of Lightning Injuries There are two major points to keep in mind when you treat patients struck by lightning: prolonged resuscitation may be needed, and, if many people are injured, you should use a special system of triage. First, if at all possible, move the patient(s), and yourself, out of danger from further lightning strikes. Lightning can strike twice in the same place, and you cannot help anyone if you are hit by lightning yourself. It is safe to touch someone who has been struck by lightning, because no electrical charge will remain by the time you arrive.

A person struck by lightning may be in complete asystole (cardiac standstill) or ventricular fibrillation. If there is no detectable heartbeat or spontaneous respirations, begin basic life support immediately, taking care to protect the cervical spine when you insert an airway support. Lightning victims are often young with healthy cardiovascular systems. Therefore, start CPR even if the patient has fixed and dilated pupils, because there are reports of lightning victims recovering completely when emergency cardiopulmonary resuscitation has been prompt and persistent. Once heartbeat is restored, or if it is present at the start, continue to assist ventilation until the patient breathes spontaneously. Continue to monitor the cardiopulmonary system while you complete the remainder of the assessment. Splint any obvious or suspected fractures, dress any thermal burns, and transport the patient promptly to the hospital.

If you are called to a scene where several people have been struck by lightning, you must modify the usual triage protocols. In other mass casualty situations, patients who have no spontaneous cardiac or respiratory activity are given a low priority for treatment. In a lightning strike, however, you should direct your highest priority to those very patients—those in cardiac or respiratory arrest—because they can virtually all be saved by prompt and effective cardiopulmonary resuscitation. Other victims who are breathing spontaneously and have a palpable pulse can generally wait for treatment and transportation because they rarely have other life-threatening injuries.

NUCLEAR RADIATION INJURIES

The energy produced from nuclear reactions can cause injury in several ways. Burns similar to thermal burns can occur from exposure to solar radiation (the sun) or from the heat of an atomic explosion. In addition, exposure to **radioactivity** (the spontaneous release of energy by particles that make up atoms) can cause many different injuries ranging from acute burns to chronic illness and even death.

Radiation Burns

The energy from the sun is produced by a continuous nuclear reaction (fusion). This energy is in the form of heat, light, and radiation. The ozone layer of our atmosphere protects the earth from most of this radiation energy. However, prolonged exposure to the sun can cause a radiation injury: a *solar burn*. Solar burns are usually not serious. They are similar to thermal burns and are only rarely more severe than first-degree burns. The pigment in the skin (*melanin*) protects it from some of the solar radiation. Therefore, darker-skinned people have less risk for solar burns than do fair-skinned people. However, if a large percentage of the skin is involved, such a burn may cause significant discomfort and occasional systemic symptoms due to mild hypotension. When

these symptoms are present, you should transport the patient to the hospital.

Nuclear radiation burns can also occur from the heat of an atomic detonation. Such injuries would be commonplace in a nuclear mass casualty situation, one in which you hope never to be involved. The most common concern in regard to nuclear radiation injury occurs from exposure to radioactive chemicals and radioactive leaks from nuclear energy plants.

Nuclear Radiation Exposure

Humans have always been exposed to small amounts of nuclear radiation through cosmic rays and naturally occurring radioactive materials, but the risk of accidental exposure has increased greatly in recent years. With the development of nuclear power, many people now work with highly radioactive materials. Radioactive chemicals are being used increasingly in biomedical research and industry. The manufacture and transportation of nuclear fuels and radioactive chemicals, and the disposal of used radioactive material provide increasing sources of accidental exposure or contamination.

Although many safety systems are in place for managing nuclear emergencies and preventing nuclear exposure, these systems can become disabled or misused. There is a chance that you may be called to the scene of a nuclear accident. For that reason, some knowledge of nuclear radiation and its effects on the body is necessary.

Nuclear radiation is the result of energy produced by radioactivity. Nuclear radiation that has the ability to alter body cells is called **ionizing radiation**. Nuclear radiation and ionizing radiation are both forms of energy transmission.

There are three types of ionizing radiation: *alpha radiation*, *beta radiation*, and *gamma radiation*. Alpha rays possess very low energy. They are easily stopped by paper, a few inches of air, or light clothing. Thus, they pose little danger. Beta rays are commonly emitted from laboratory chemicals and are widely used in biomedical research and in industry. Beta rays can penetrate to a greater depth than alpha rays but are effectively stopped by clothing, glass, or a thin metal shielding. The great danger from beta rays is from accidental spilling or ingestion of beta-radioactive chemicals that can be absorbed into the bloodstream and then emit radioactivity into the body for a prolonged time. Gamma rays are much more powerful and thus more dangerous than alpha or beta rays. Gamma rays can penetrate through the human body. Heavy shielding such as lead or concrete is necessary to protect against these rays. X rays are similar to gamma rays (Figure 40–14).

The amount of radioactive energy that a person receives depends on several factors:

- The distance that the person is from the source of the radiation.
- The strength of the radiation source.
- The duration of the exposure.
- The extent of the body area exposed.
- The amount of shielding between the source and the person.

The amount of radioactivity that someone receives decreases rapidly as the distance from

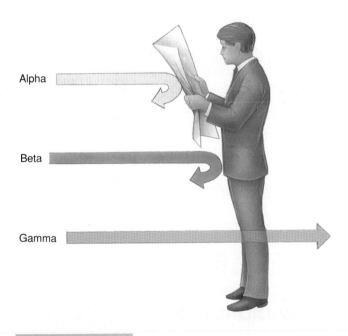

FIGURE 40–14

The three basic types of ionizing radiation are alpha, beta, and gamma. Alpha rays are easily stopped by paper. Beta rays are stopped by clothing. Gamma rays are very powerful and can penetrate through the body. They can be stopped only by heavy shielding such as lead or concrete.

the source increases. A person who is standing 6 feet away from a radioactive source will receive only one-quarter the radiation the person would receive from 3 feet away, and if the person were 12 feet away, he or she would receive one-sixteenth as much.

Measurement of Nuclear Radiation

Gamma and X ray radiation is measured in **roentgens (R)** or in **rads**. Although these two terms differ slightly, the differences are so small that they may be used interchangeably. You may encounter situations in which the radiation has been measured in either roentgens or rads. Radiation from beta particles is measured in *Curies* or, because the amounts of radiation are usually very small, in *millicuries* or *microcuries*. You may encounter these terms if you are called to a laboratory where a radiation accident has taken place.

A Geiger counter or similar instrument is used to measure the level of radioactivity, usually gamma rays or X rays in the environment. Beta radiation is usually so low that it can only be measured by very sensitive instruments. Alpha radiation is rarely measured.

The Effect of Nuclear Radiation on the Body

Nuclear radiation, which disrupts the structure of individual atoms within body cells, will alter and even destroy the ability of cells to function normally. Exposure to exceedingly large doses of radiation over a short time span will produce radiation burns as described earlier in this chapter. More commonly, exposure to low doses of radiation occurs over a long period of time. The biological effects of this type of radiation are delayed for periods of from a few days to many years, depending on the dose, the type of radiation received, and whether part or all of the body has been exposed. The most striking long-term results of radiation overexposure include *leukopenia* (decrease in the white blood cells), *alopecia* (loss of hair), malignant diseases (cancers and leukemia), cataracts, sterility, or congenital defects of offspring of exposed persons.

With short-duration overexposure, the acute effects may be seen in a matter of hours, days, or weeks. When a low grade of exposure occurs over a prolonged period of time, the accumulated effects may not be seen for years.

Accidents Involving Radiation Hazards

The vast majority of accidents involving radioactive materials occur in facilities that use these materials daily. You should seek and follow the professional advice that is readily available in these centers. Accidents occasionally happen where professional guidance is not available, and in these cases, you should be able to do the following:

- Recognize indications of radioactivity.
- Obtain the necessary assistance.
- Initiate appropriate emergency medical care while you exercise caution.
- Minimize your exposure to the radiation.
- Avoid spread of radioactive contamination.

Radioactive substances are supposed to be kept in labeled and shielded containers. Any radioactive materials shipped by interstate commerce must be labeled. Vehicles used to transport radioactive materials must be marked with a placard indicating a radioactive shipment (Figure 40–15).

In order to distribute advice about handling a radioactive accident, a national plan has been developed. Called the *Interagency Radiological Assistance Plan (IRAP)*, it may be activated by a telephone call to the appropriate regional coordinating office. Assistance can range from expert technical advice on the telephone to the dispatch of an emergency team or expert to the scene. Your dispatch center should become familiar with the location and telephone number of your regional coordinating offices of IRAP.

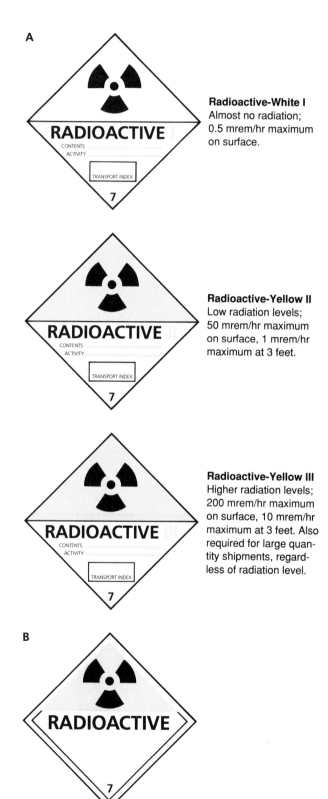

Radioactive-White I
Almost no radiation; 0.5 mrem/hr maximum on surface.

Radioactive-Yellow II
Low radiation levels; 50 mrem/hr maximum on surface, 1 mrem/hr maximum at 3 feet.

Radioactive-Yellow III
Higher radiation levels; 200 mrem/hr maximum on surface, 10 mrem/hr maximum at 3 feet. Also required for large quantity shipments, regardless of radiation level.

FIGURE 40–15

(A) Required labels for packages containing radioactive materials. (B) Typical warning placard on any vehicle that transports radioactive materials.

In addition, a nationwide center, the **Radiation Emergency Assistance Center/Training Site (REAC/TS),** located in Oak Ridge, Tennessee, is available. REAC/TS is supported by the US Department of Energy (DOE) and the Federal Emergency Management Agency (FEMA), and serves as a worldwide hotline for advice about and assistance after radiation accidents. REAC/TS will not send a team to the scene, but will give up-to-the-minute advice on how to handle the situation. The REAC/TS telephone, answered 24 hours a day, is 615–482–2441.

Emergency Medical Care for Radiation Accidents

Only rarely is radioactivity a continuing problem when you arrive on the scene of a radiation accident. Exposure to gamma rays or X rays does not make the patient radioactive. There is a risk of further radiation exposure when

- the source of radiation is still present and active or
- radioactive material has spilled on the patient.

Before you enter an area where radiation is still being produced, you must put on the necessary protective clothing. Then rapidly move the patient out of the area of danger just as if he or she had been in a traffic accident and was in the path of oncoming cars. Then begin patient assessment and emergency care. If radioactive material has spilled onto the patient, it must be removed. In this case, you are at risk from radiation injury if you get any of the spilled material on you. You must wear the necessary protective clothing and rubber gloves. Remove the victim's clothes and place them in a container specially designated for radioactive waste. Doing so will contain up to 70 percent of the radioactivity. Then carry out the necessary assessment and emergency care procedures. After you have stabilized the patient, remove any protective clothing that you have put on and place it in a separate radioactive waste container. Facilities that handle radioactive materials are required to have special disposal containers for this purpose. Dur-

ing transport try to protect the other ambulance personnel and the vehicle itself from contamination. Notify the hospital that you have a patient who has been in a radiation accident and transport the patient to the hospital.

After you have transported a patient who has been contaminated by contact with radioactive materials, you must decontaminate the vehicle as well as yourself. Most hospitals have a radiation safety officer who will be able to provide guidance as to the specific techniques for proper **decontamination.**

YOU ARE THE EMT

1. Which is more severe—a first- or a third-degree burn? How would you determine whether a patient was suffering from a first-, second-, or third-degree burn?
2. Your patient is a 2-year-old youngster who spilled his mother's hot tea over himself. Wearing only a diaper, he received second-degree burns on his chest, stomach, and thighs. Is this a critical, moderate, or minor burn? What factors can you use to determine the degree of seriousness?
3. What two dangers are associated with electrical burns? How should you treat an electrical burn?
4. How would you carry out triage on several victims of a lightning strike? How would it differ from the triage of victims of other injuries?
5. Explain the difference between nuclear radiation and ionizing radiation. What are gamma rays?

CHAPTER 41

HAZARDOUS MATERIALS

KEY TERMS

absorption A process of decontamination whereby the material is removed, usually from equipment, by special filters or materials designed to absorb the contaminants.

CHEMTREC Chemical Transportation Emergency Center: a service organized by the chemical industry to assist emergency personnel in identifying and handling hazardous material spills.

decontamination (de-kon-tam-ĭ-na'shun) The orderly process by which radiation or chemical hazards can be removed from clothing, equipment, vehicles, and personnel.

dilution (di-lu'shun) A process of decontamination whereby the contamination is washed off with floods of water.

Hazmat Rule of Thumb A guide to how close you can come to a hazardous material spill before you know what the hazardous material is.

protection level A measure of the amount of protective equipment that someone must have to avoid injury during contact with a hazardous material.

self-contained breathing apparatus (SCBA) A respiratory aid that does not require outside air.

toxicity level (tok-sis'ĭ-te lev'el) A measure of the risk that anyone is subjected to by contact with a certain hazardous material.

triage (tre-ahzh') Sorting. A technique of establishing treatment and transportation priorities in any event where the number of casualties is greater than the emergency facilities can handle.

OVERVIEW

A great number and variety of hazardous materials pass through the streets, over the railways, and through the air of every city in the country every day. The exact extent of this traffic is not known, but accidents do occur that involve vehicles carrying hazardous materials. Hazardous materials may be of many different types, including chemicals, radioactive materials, and poisons, in the form of solids, liquids, or gas. They are appropriately named because they represent a hazard to everyone exposed—rescue personnel and the public, as well as to an injured person or persons.

When you are responding to a hazardous materials incident, you cannot follow those "move-fast-take-action-save-lives" instincts that are an EMT's trademark. Instead, you must take time to accurately assess the scene. That means identifying the size of the hazard area, finding a safe location to which patients can be removed, and taking self-protective measures against contamination. Safety is your prime consideration in this situation. If a hazardous materials accident is not carefully handled, a lot of people, including rescue personnel themselves, can become casualties.

Chapter 41 stresses the safety precautions you must take when responding to a hazardous materials incident. The chapter begins with a description of the assessment process that you must carry out. This assessment includes identifying the hazardous material and establishing a hazard zone. Then, specific ways of obtaining information and assistance in managing the hazardous accident are presented. The chapter next addresses decontamination—for the patient and rescue personnel. The last portion of Chapter 41 deals with triage in a hazardous materials accident—that is, sorting and assigning treatment priorities when the number of casualties is greater than emergency facilities can handle.

GOALS

The goals of Chapter 41 are to

- stress the importance of assessing the scene of a hazardous materials incident, which includes identifying the hazardous material and establishing a hazard zone before you institute emergency treatment.
- describe CHEMTREC—how you will contact it and methods you will use to identify the specific hazardous material and how to obtain assistance in managing it.
- understand the various toxicity and protection levels you must be familiar with in order to handle a hazardous materials incident.
- describe the process of decontamination—for you as well as for your patient or patients.
- explain what triage is and how it works in a major hazardous materials accident.

PRELIMINARY ASSESSMENT OF A HAZARDOUS MATERIALS INCIDENT

Sometimes when you deal with hazardous materials, the hazard is obvious; other times, it is not. Sometimes the dangerous nature of the situation is not recognized until many people have been needlessly exposed or injured. This is particularly true in cases where odorless poisonous gases or vapors have been released. Rescuers have lost their lives or become permanently disabled because of a lack of understanding and appreciation of the potential dangers of hazardous materials. Failure to set up the necessary hazardous materials zone has often resulted in serious and sometimes fatal situations.

EMTs and rescue personnel are taught that rapid response at the scene of an accident can be lifesaving and is of great importance. You and your co-workers pride yourselves on the ability to make quick decisions and to act on them. Even so, you are sometimes criticized for taking too much time at the scene of an accident. However, when you arrive at the scene of an accident where hazardous materials may be present, you must first step back and assess the situation. Safety—for you, for the

patient, and for the public—is of primary concern. You will be able to carry out the necessary emergency care only after you have assessed the situation, discovered critical information about the hazardous material, put on any necessary protective equipment, and established a safety zone. As in other situations where you may be at risk, you must not allow yourself to become a casualty!

Only those people trained in the management of hazardous materials should come near the hazard zone. Some hazardous materials accidents involve small quantities of toxic materials; others, however, involve barrels, boxes, tanks, or even carloads of harmful substances. An important first step in controlling the scene is to identify the danger zone, where exposure to the toxic substances may occur. The **Hazmat Rule of Thumb** is one way to determine the size of the danger zone. To use this method, hold your arm straight out, with your thumb pointing up. Center your thumb over the hazardous area. Your thumb should completely cover the hazardous area from your view (Figure 41–1). If it doesn't, move back, try the rule of thumb again, and keep doing so until your thumb completely blocks the hazardous area from view. Take special care when

According to the Hazmat Rule of Thumb, at arm's length your thumb should entirely cover the hazard zone.

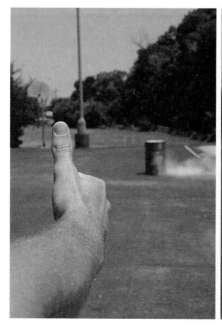
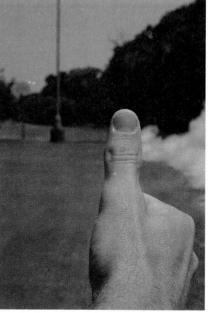

toxic fumes are present. The safe area will be upwind from the site of the spill. But remember, wind direction can change quickly.

Identifying Hazardous Materials

The single most important step in any hazardous materials incident or accident is to identify the substance(s) involved. Accurate identification of the materials is critical. Such information should be prominently displayed on all boxes or cartons that contain a hazardous material, on all vehicles that transport it, and in all factories that produce it. Manufacturers and transporters are required by law to display a four-digit identification number on the ends of a tank, vehicle, or rail car used to carry hazardous substances (Figure 41–2). This same four-digit identification number (some are preceded by the letters UN or NA) can also be found on the shipping paper or packaging of the material (Figure 41–3). Frequently, the name of the substance will also be displayed,

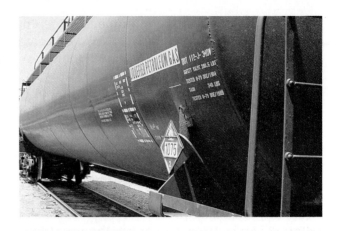

FIGURE 41–2

Any tank, vehicle, or rail car that carries hazardous materials is required by law to display a four-digit identification number on the end of the vehicle. In case of an accident, these numbers can be matched up against a list of toxic substances so that the hazardous material can be quickly identified.

FIGURE 41–3

A typical shipping bill for a hazardous substance. The material is listed by name, classification, and identification number. This number can be matched against a list of toxic substances so that the hazard can be identified, the toxicity and protection levels determined, and appropriate treatment and decontamination can be accomplished.

CONTAINS HAZARDOUS MATERIALS
FOR HELP IN CHEMICAL EMERGENCIES INVOLVING SPILL, LEAK, FIRE OR EXPOSURE CALL TOLL-FREE 1-800-424-9300 DAY OR NIGHT

STRAIGHT BILL OF LADING
ORIGINAL—NOT NEGOTIABLE

Shipper's No. _____

Carrier's No. _____

SCAC _____ Date _____

(NAME OF CARRIER)

	TO:		FROM:	
Consignee		Shipper		
Street		Street		
Destination	Zip	Origin		Zip
Route			Vehicle Number	

No. Shipping Units	HM	Kinds of Packages, Description of Articles (IF HAZARDOUS MATERIALS—PROPER SHIPPING NAME)	HAZARD CLASS	I.D. NUMBER	WEIGHT (subject to correction)	RATE	LABELS REQUIRED (or exemption)
1 TC	X	ACETONE	Flammable Liquid	UN1090	85,000		Flammable
		SHIPPING NAME	CLASSIFICATION	ID NUMBER			

along with the identification number. Different kinds of hazardous materials have different colored and shaped labels to help in identification (Figure 41–4).

When you first arrive at the scene of a hazardous materials incident, you should first try to read labels and identification numbers from a distance, using binoculars if necessary. Do not go into the area and risk exposure to yourself at this time unless you are absolutely certain that no hazardous spill has occurred. Relay any information to your dispatch center where it can be used to identify the hazardous material.

Identifying Hazardous Materials: CHEMTREC

The Chemical Manufacturers Association has established the Chemical Transportation Emergency Center **(CHEMTREC)** in Washington, D.C. This center operates 24 hours a day, 7 days a week. Its toll-free number is 1–800–424–9300 from anywhere within the continental United States except the District of Columbia. In the District of Columbia, the number is 483–7616, and in Alaska, call that number collect: 0–202–483–7616. CHEMTREC will provide hazardous information, warnings and guidance for proper emergency management and treatment if the DOT identification number (described later), the chemical name, or the product name of the hazardous material is given. The information must be accurate, however, if CHEMTREC is to help. CHEMTREC cannot identify an "unknown" substance. In addition, the U.S. Department of Transportation's guide entitled *Hazardous Materials: The Emergency Response Guidebook* (DOT P 5800.4, 1987), lists all hazardous materials and the proper emergency action to take with regard to control of the scene and emergency care of ill or injured patients. Several similar publications are also available. Some state and local government agencies may also have pertinent information regarding hazardous materials found frequently in their areas. A copy of the guidebook and other information relevant to your local area should be readily available in the dispatch center so that you may carry out the

proper emergency management as soon as the hazardous material is identified.

Once you have identified the hazardous substance by name, or by the number on either the package, vehicle, or papers, dispatch should then call CHEMTREC for positive identification and information about how to manage the spill. The DOT guidebook or a similar publication should then be consulted regarding the specific hazards, proper treatment protocols, and the necessary steps to take for your own protection.

Hazardous materials are classified according to **toxicity levels** and according to **protection levels.** These levels are used in many of the publications dealing with the handling of hazardous materials. The toxicity level—designated 0, 1, 2, 3, or 4—is a measure of the risk that the substance poses to anyone coming in contact with it. The higher the number, the greater the toxicity. Level 0 indicates those materials whose exposure would cause little if any health hazard. Levels 1 and 2 indicate those materials that are only slightly hazardous, but require that you wear a **self-contained breathing apparatus (SCBA).** Level 3 indicates those materials that are extremely hazardous to health, for which you must wear full protective clothing with none of your skin surface exposed. Level 4 indicates those substances that are so hazardous that minimal contact will cause death. For Level 4 substances, you need specialized gear designed for protection against that particular hazard.

The protection level—lettered A, B, C, or D—is a measure of the amount and type of protective gear that you need to prevent injury from the particular hazardous substance. Level A is the most hazardous. It requires encapsulated protective clothing and offers full body protection as well as special equipment that is sealed.

FIGURE 41–4

Some hazardous materials warning labels.

Hazardous Materials Warning Labels

DOMESTIC LABELING

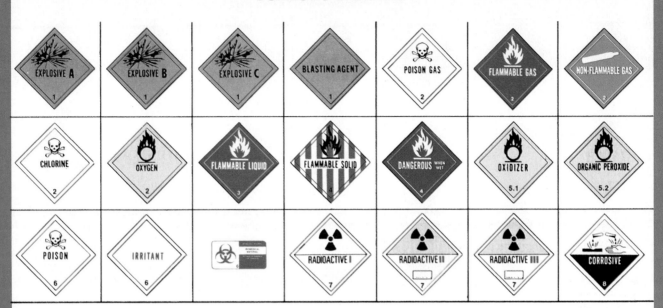

General Guidelines on Use of Labels
(CFR, Title 49, Transportation, Parts 100-177)

- Labels illustrated above are normally for *domestic shipments.* However, some air carriers *may* require the use of International Civil Aviation Organization (ICAO) labels.

- Domestic Warning Labels *may* display UN Class Number, Division Number (and Compatibility Group for Explosives only) [Sec. 172.407(g)].

- Any person who offers a hazardous material for transportation MUST label the package, if required [Sec. 172.400(a)].

- The Hazardous Materials Tables, Sec. 172.101 and 172.102, identify the proper label(s) for the hazardous materials listed.

- Label(s), when required, must be printed on or affixed to the surface of the package near the proper shipping name [Sec. 172.406(a)].

- When two or more different labels are required, display them next to each other [Sec. 172.406(c)].

- Labels may be affixed to packages (even when not required by regulations) provided each label represents a hazard of the material in the package [Sec. 172.401].

**Check the Appropriate Regulations
Domestic or International Shipment**

Additional Markings and Labels

HANDLING LABELS

Cargo Aircraft Only
172.402(b)

Bung Label
172.402(e)

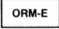

ORM-E
172.316

INNER PACKAGES
COMPLY WITH
PRESCRIBED
SPECIFICATIONS
173.25(a)(4)

Package
Orientation
Markings
172.312(a)(c)

Fumigation
173.9

EMPTY

173.427

Here are a few additional markings and labels pertaining to the transport of hazardous materials. The section number shown with each item refers to the appropriate section in the HMR. The Hazardous Materials Tables, Section 172.101 and 172.102, identify the proper shipping name, hazard class, identification number, required label(s) and packaging sections.

Poisonous Materials

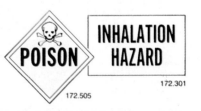

POISON
172.505

INHALATION
HAZARD
172.301

Materials which meet the inhalation toxicity criteria specified in Section 173.3a(b)(2), have additional "communication standards" prescribed by the HMR. First, the words "Poison-Inhalation Hazard" must be entered on the shipping paper, as required by Section 172.203(k)(4), for any primary capacity units with a capacity greater than one liter. Second, packages of 110 gallons or less capacity must be marked "Inhalation Hazard" in accordance with Section 172.301(a). Lastly, transport vehicles, freight containers and portable tanks subject to the shipping paper requirements contained in Section 172.203(k)(4) must be placarded with POISON placards in addition to the placards required by Section 172.504. For additional information and exceptions to these communication requirements, see the referenced sections in the HMR.

U.S. Department of Transportation
**Research and Special Programs
Administration**

Copies of this Chart can be obtained by writing
OHMT/DHM-51, Washington, D.C. 20590.

Hazardous Materials Warning Placards

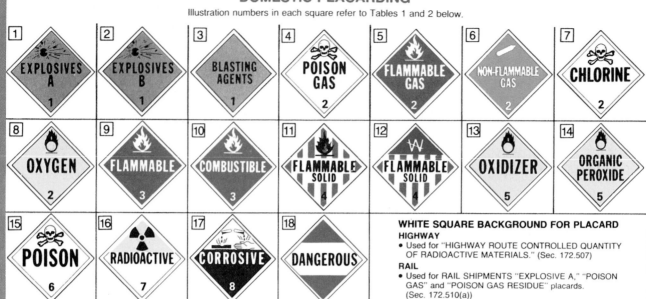

DOMESTIC PLACARDING

Illustration numbers in each square refer to Tables 1 and 2 below.

1 EXPLOSIVES A — 1	2 EXPLOSIVES B — 1	3 BLASTING AGENTS — 1	4 POISON GAS — 2	5 FLAMMABLE GAS — 2	6 NON-FLAMMABLE GAS — 2	7 CHLORINE — 2
8 OXYGEN — 2	9 FLAMMABLE — 3	10 COMBUSTIBLE — 3	11 FLAMMABLE SOLID — 4	12 FLAMMABLE SOLID — 4	13 OXIDIZER — 5	14 ORGANIC PEROXIDE — 5
15 POISON — 6	16 RADIOACTIVE — 7	17 CORROSIVE — 8	18 DANGEROUS			

WHITE SQUARE BACKGROUND FOR PLACARD

HIGHWAY
- Used for "HIGHWAY ROUTE CONTROLLED QUANTITY OF RADIOACTIVE MATERIALS." (Sec. 172.507)

RAIL
- Used for RAIL SHIPMENTS "EXPLOSIVE A," "POISON GAS" and "POISON GAS RESIDUE" placards. (Sec. 172.510(a))

Guidelines
(CFR, Title 49, Transportation, Parts 100-177)

- Placard any transport vehicle, freight container, or rail car containing any quantity of material listed in Table 1.
- Materials which are shipped in portable tanks, cargo tanks, or tank cars must be placarded when they contain any quantity of Table 1 and/or Table 2 material.
- Motor vehicles or freight containers containing packages which are subject to the "Poison-Inhalation Hazard" shipping paper description of Section 172.203(k)(4), must be placarded POISON in addition to the placards required by Section 172.504 (see Section 172.505).
- When the gross weight of all hazardous material covered in TABLE 2 is less than 1000 pounds, no placard is required on a transport vehicle or freight container.
- Placard freight containers 640 cubic feet or more containing any quantity of hazardous material classes listed in TABLES 1 and/or 2 when offered for transportation by air or water (see Section 172.512(a)). Under 640 cubic feet see Section 172.512(b).

TABLE 1

Hazard Classes	No.
Class A explosives	1
Class B explosives	2
Poison A	4
Flammable solid (DANGEROUS WHEN WET label only)	12
Radioactive material (YELLOW III label)	16
Radioactive material:	
Uranium hexafluoride fissile (Containing more than 1.0% U^{235})	16 & 17
Uranium hexafluoride, low-specific activity (Containing 1.0% or less U^{235})	16 & 17

Note: For details on the use of Tables 1 and 2, see Sec. 172.504 (see footnotes at bottom of tables.)

TABLE 2

Hazard Classes	No.
Class C explosives	18
Blasting agent	3
Nonflammable gas	6
Nonflammable gas (Chlorine)	7
Nonflammable gas (Fluorine)	15
Nonflammable gas (Oxygen, cryogenic liquid)	8
Flammable gas	5
Combustible liquid	10
Flammable liquid	9
Flammable solid	11
Oxidizer	13
Organic peroxide	14
Poison B	15
Corrosive material	17
Irritating material	18

UN or NA Identification Numbers

MUST BE DISPLAYED ON TANK CARS, CARGO TANKS, PORTABLE TANKS AND BULK PACKAGINGS

PLACARDS OR ORANGE PANELS

1090 and FLAMMABLE 3

Appropriate Placard must be used.

1090 3 | 1017 2 | 1993 3

- When hazardous materials are transported in Tank Cars (Section 172.330), Cargo Tanks (Section 172.328), Portable Tanks (Section 172.326) or Bulk Packagings (Section 172.331), UN or NA numbers must be displayed on placards, orange panels or, when authorized, plain white square-on-point configuration.
- UN (United Nations) or NA (North American) numbers are found in the Hazardous Materials Tables, Sections 172.101 and 172.102.
- Identification numbers may not be displayed on "POISON GAS," "RADIOACTIVE," or "EXPLOSIVE A," "EXPLOSIVE B," "BLASTING AGENTS," or "DANGEROUS" placards. (See Section 172.334.)
- In lieu of the orange panel, identification numbers may be placed on plain white square-on-point configuration when there is no placard specified for the hazard class (e.g., ORM-A, B, C, D, or E) or where the identification number may not be displayed on the placard. See Section 172.336(b) for additional provisions and specifications.
- When the identification number is displayed on a placard the UN hazard class number must be displayed in the lower corner of each placard (see Section 172.332 (c)(3)).
- Specifications of size and color of the Orange Panel can be found in Section 172.332(b).
- NA numbers are used only in the USA and Canada.

Additional Placarding Guidelines

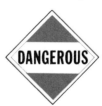

DANGEROUS

A transport vehicle or freight container containing two or more classes of material requiring different placards specified in Table 2 may be placarded DANGEROUS in place of the separate placards specified for each of those classes of material specified in Table 2. However, when 5000 pounds or more of one class of material is loaded therein at one loading facility, the placard specified for that class must be applied. This exception, provided in Section 172.504(b), does not apply to portable tanks, tank cars, or cargo tanks.

CAUTION: Check each shipment for compliance with the appropriate hazardous materials regulations — Proper Classification, Packaging, Marking, Labeling, Placarding, Documentation — prior to offering for shipment.

In an emergency, call Chemtrec, 1-800-424-9300

Level B requires nonencapsulated protective clothing, that is, clothing designed against a particular hazard, usually made of nonpermeable material (material that only limited amounts of moisture and vapor can pass through). In addition, Level B requires breathing devices that do not use outside air, but contain their own air supply, such as a SCBA, and eye protection.

Level C, like Level B, requires the use of nonpermeable clothing and eye protection. Face masks that filter all inhaled outside air must be used.

Level D requires structural firefighting clothing. *All* levels of protection require the use of gloves. You should wear two pairs of rubber gloves, so that you can remove one pair if it becomes heavily contaminated, and still be protected.

Establishing a Hazard Zone

While the process of identifying the hazardous material is going on, you should establish and secure a hazard zone. Using the Hazmat Rule of Thumb, identify and isolate the danger area. Remain upwind of the area and avoid low areas where toxic fumes may tend to settle. Keep bystanders away. Often, well-meaning people try to help, but unless people are specifically trained for such situations, you should keep them away. On the other hand, experienced, knowledgeable people such as company safety officers may be able to offer valuable assistance. If you are not specially trained in Hazmat, you should let one of these experts take charge of the scene. This individual can then coordinate information from the dispatch center, CHEMTREC, and other resources.

Management of the Injured in a Hazardous Materials Accident

If an accident has resulted in injury to one or more people, you must first remove the injured from the area to avoid further exposure. This is the most dangerous time in any hazardous materials accident—dangerous to the injured people and dangerous to the rescuers. Very little information about the nature of the haz-ardous materials or the extent of the danger may be available.

Never enter the area until you are adequately protected. The level of protection will depend on the toxicity level and protection level of the substance or substances involved. If the injury has taken place in a closed space, remember that you are particularly at risk from toxic smoke and fumes. When you are ready to enter the area, make certain that you have a way out through a safe escape route.

Emergency treatment of exposure to hazardous materials is primarily aimed at supportive care. There are very few specific antidotes or treatments for most injuries due to hazardous materials, and different people may respond differently to contact with the same hazardous material. Most fatalities and serious injuries from hazardous materials result from airway and breathing problems. You must first remove the patient from the hazardous area. Specific extrication techniques are described in Chapter 47. Once the patient is clear of the area, you should then monitor the respirations closely. Maintain the airway and give supplemental oxygen at the rate of 4 to 6 liters per minute. Monitor the vital signs closely.

Brush off any solid material that may remain on the patient's clothes. Remove the clothing, collecting it in a container specifically designed for this purpose. Try to avoid getting any of the substance on yourself. Treat the patient for a chemical burn by removing the clothing (and collecting it in a special container), then flooding the skin with water. By doing this, you are starting the process of decontamination. The management of chemical burns is described more fully in Chapter 40.

If the patient has swallowed a toxic material, and the material can be positively identified, medical control may direct you to induce vomiting with syrup of ipecac, or to give a suspension of activated charcoal. Never induce vomiting in a patient unless he or she is fully alert. Treat the patient as you would for poisoning. The management of poisoning is described in Chapter 28.

Dress any wounds. Splint all spine and limb injuries and package the patient for transport. Avoid getting any material on yourself. If further decontamination is not needed, transport the patient to the hospital. Notify the emergency department of the patient's condition, what the hazardous material is, and what measures you have already taken.

DECONTAMINATION

Many people involved in a hazardous materials incident will need to undergo **decontamination** (the process of removing and properly disposing of hazardous materials from the patient, rescue equipment, and rescue personnel). Failure to decontaminate adequately and promptly will result in prolonged exposure, perhaps causing more serious injury to your patient. It may expose other EMT, rescue, and hospital personnel to the hazardous materials as well. However, there will be times (such as blunt abdominal trauma or a crushed chest) when the patient's traumatic injuries may be more life-threatening than is the contamination. You will have to determine whether it is more important to decontaminate the patient or provide transport to the hospital quickly. Medical control can provide guidance in these situations. In some circumstances, decontamination and emergency care of injuries may proceed simultaneously. However, if you must make a choice, consider that a patient is "better blistered and living than decontaminated and dead." In such cases, notify the hospital not only that you are bringing in a critically injured patient but that the patient is contaminated as well. The hospital may have to set up a decontamination zone for this patient.

Decontamination begins as soon as you know you are going on a run that may involve hazardous materials. Before transporting a contaminated patient in your ambulance, you should tape the cabinet doors shut, and cover the floor and sidewalls with plastic sheeting. This will minimize the amount of decontamination you will have to perform later.

Once at the scene, begin by establishing a decontamination zone. All contaminated personnel, patients, clothing, and equipment should be kept within this zone until decontaminated. Trained crews should be available to help set up the decontamination zone and take charge of it. Cooperate with the crew, while remembering your primary mission of providing emergency care. The decontamination zone should be well marked with plastic, tape, or other warning devices to control traffic. Special containers to receive contaminated clothing should be available (Figure 41–5).

The decontamination zone should include Hot, Warm, and Clean zones. The Hot zone should have a primary decontamination zone, a secondary decontamination zone, and a minimum exposure zone. The Warm zone should have a disrobing area, and a personnel decontamination area. The Clean zone should be, as its name implies, free of contamination. It should lead away from the decontamination site. Personnel should not travel into the Hot zone from the Warm zone, but the other way around: from Hot to Warm to Clean.

There are four accepted methods of decontamination: dilution, absorption, chemical wash, and disposal and isolation.

- **Dilution** means flushing the contaminated person or equipment with water.
- **Absorption** is the use of special filters and chemicals to absorb the hazardous material.

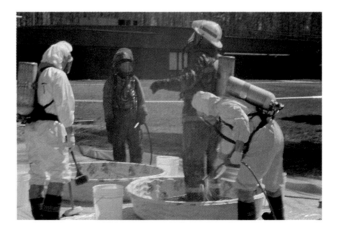

FIGURE 41–5

A decontamination zone. Note that the perimeter of the zone is clearly marked.

- Chemical washes are specific chemicals used to neutralize the hazardous material.
- Disposal and isolation is used when materials are more easily disposed of (thrown away) than decontaminated. Sometimes clothing and equipment cannot be decontaminated. Special containers are then used for disposal (Figure 41–6).

The following are the 10 basic steps in decontamination:

1. Set up the entry point to the decontamination zone. Remove outer gloves and place them in the proper disposal container.
2. Remove obvious surface contamination, with brushing and flooding with water.
3. Remove any contaminated breathing apparatus from anyone who must return to a contaminated area (they will get clean apparatus once they get there).
4. Remove all protective clothing and decontaminate, dispose of, or store it as necessary.
5. Remove the rest of the clothing. Remember that the clothing of someone who has been exposed to toxic gas may be heavily contaminated, even though you do not see any obvious chemicals—the clothing will have absorbed the gas.
6. Wash the body with floods of water from a hose or an overhead shower if available.
7. Dry the body and receive clean, dry clothing.
8. Perform a medical evaluation of everyone who has gone through the decontamination process.
9. All personnel going through decontamination should be seen in a hospital for further complete medical evaluation.
10. Clean up and dismantle the decontamination site.

TRIAGE IN A HAZARDOUS MATERIALS ACCIDENT

Triage is the sorting of casualties when the number of casualties is greater than the emergency facility can handle simultaneously. Tri-

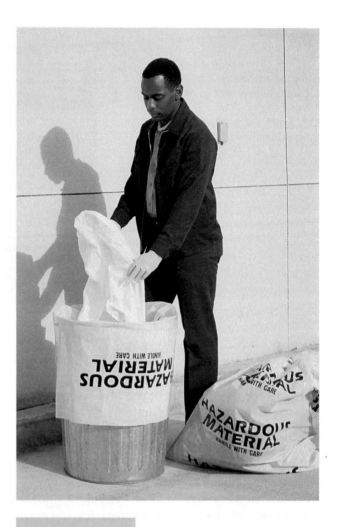

FIGURE 41–6

All clothing exposed to hazardous materials must be placed in special sealed containers to avoid further spread of the hazardous substance.

age is frequently discussed in mass casualty and disaster planning. Most disaster drills focus on such mass casualty situations as an airplane crash or a natural disaster, where large numbers of people are killed and seriously injured. Hazardous materials incidents occur commonly and can also create a mass casualty situation, exposing many people to possible injury or contamination (Figure 41–7). In addition, a hazardous materials accident will cause concern and even hysteria among the public. This means that you will have to carry out triage to separate the truly injured from those

FIGURE 41-7

A hazardous material spill can occur in any community, and may involve the need for triage. The EMS system must be prepared to respond to these situations.

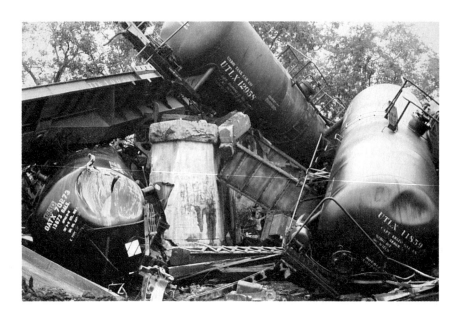

who may have been contaminated and from those who are simply anxious and worried. In that case, triage should have one major function: to identify victims who truly have an acute injury from the hazardous materials incident. Remove those patients from the area, decontaminate them as necessary, provide the proper emergency care, and transport them to the hospital. Send people who have had a "possible exposure" to a separate area for observation. If delayed symptoms of exposure do occur, you can then transport these patients to the hospital after the more seriously injured have been taken care of. In most cases, patients who do not develop symptoms do not require evaluation at a medical facility.

Transporting patients who have been injured in a hazardous materials incident may pose many problems. The number of injured may be far greater than the transportation system can handle. Although the initial triage decisions will usually determine the priority of transportation, you must constantly reevaluate patients awaiting transportation so that if a patient's condition deteriorates, he or she can be moved to a higher priority for transport. Make sure that any patient you transport is properly decontaminated unless the injuries

are so severe that any delay to decontaminate him or her would be life-threatening. It is very dangerous to the patient and the rescue personnel to place a poorly decontaminated patient inside an ambulance or helicopter and then close the doors. Any toxic fumes given off by the patient or by the clothing can contaminate the inside of the transport vehicle, perhaps causing injury to the EMT, other attendants, the driver, or the pilot. Be certain that any bags of contaminated clothing and other personal effects are properly sealed if they are going with the patient. Notify the receiving hospitals of the impending arrival of patients who have been involved in a hazardous materials accident. This will alert hospital triage teams so that appropriate precautions can be taken once the patients begin to arrive.

After the incident is over, all patients are cared for, and all personnel and equipment are decontaminated, you and your crew should evaluate the incident, critique it, and make plans for the next incident, so that you can improve your performance. Your EMS system should have a prearranged protocol for the handling of a hazardous materials incident. Based on your experience, you may want to suggest modifications in that protocol.

YOU ARE THE EMT

1. You have been warned on countless occasions not to rush into the area of a hazardous materials accident until you have assessed the situation. What exactly should this assessment consist of?

2. How will you identify a hazardous material that has spilled out of a truck that has been in an accident? List the steps you will take. What further information do you then need to protect yourself and your patient from further exposure to a hazardous material?

3. You have to enter an established hazard zone to treat and rescue injured persons. What kind of self-protective measures should you take before entering the area?

4. Describe three hazardous materials accidents that could require triage procedures. Briefly describe the steps you would take if you were the triage officer at one of these accidents.

5. Decontamination is an important part of any hazardous materials incident. How will you prevent contamination from spreading to you, the ambulance, and other rescue and hospital personnel? What decontamination procedures will you follow after you have transported the patient to the hospital?

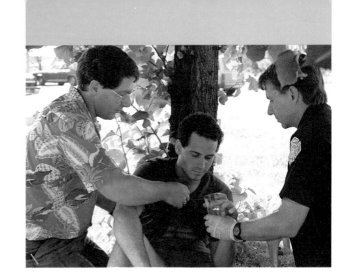

CHAPTER 42

HEAT AND COLD EXPOSURE

KEY TERMS

ambient temperature (am'be-ent tem'per-ah-tūr) The temperature of the environment that is surrounding the body.

conduction (kon-duk'shun) The loss of heat by direct contact of a body part with a colder object.

convection (kon-vek'shun) The loss of heat through moving air, from the body to a colder environment.

core temperature The temperature of the central part of the body, the heart, lungs, and vital organs.

electrolytes (e-lek'tro-līts) Salts dissolved in body fluids and cells.

evaporation (e-vap"o-ra'shun) Conversion of water from a liquid to a gas.

frostbite Damage to tissues as the result of exposure to low environmental temperatures.

heat cramps Painful muscle cramps associated with activity that occurs in a warm or hot environment.

heat exhaustion A form of heat injury in which the body loses fluid and electrolytes from heavy sweating. (Also called heat prostration or heat collapse.)

heat stroke A life-threatening condition caused by exposure to excessive heat, natural or artificial, and marked by dry skin, dizziness, headache, nausea, and muscle cramps.

hypothermia (hi"po-ther'me-ah) A condition in which the internal body temperature falls below 95 degrees F after prolonged exposure to freezing or near-freezing temperatures.

radiation The loss of heat from the body through still air to a colder environment.

OVERVIEW

Environmental emergencies due to heat or cold exposure may be encountered in any part of the country and at any time of year. These emergencies may occur in the inner city, suburbs, or farms. They can occur indoors, outdoors, in office buildings, homes, or farm buildings. Proper care of patients who are suffering from the effects of heat or cold exposure will help to minimize their injuries and speed their recovery. On the other hand, improper treatment of these emergencies can result in serious consequences, even death. Therefore, it is important to have a thorough understanding of the effects of heat and cold on the body, as well as the emergency management of these injuries.

The first half of Chapter 42 is about heat exposure. The chapter begins with an explanation of what happens when the body becomes overwhelmed by heat. Next, the three forms of heat exposure—heat cramps, heat exhaustion, and heat stroke—are discussed.

The second half of Chapter 42 is about cold exposure. This section begins with an explanation of how the body reacts to cold temperatures, and how systemic injuries (hypothermia) and local injuries (frostnip or frostbite) occur. The chapter describes the five stages of hypothermia and the treatment for hypothermia. The chapter concludes with a warning about how you can avoid exposure yourself.

GOALS

The goals of Chapter 42 are to
- describe the three forms of heat exposure: heat cramps, heat exhaustion, and heat stroke.
- identify the five ways the body can lose heat.
- describe the stages, symptoms, and treatment of hypothermia.
- learn how to treat local cold injuries, specifically frostnip and frostbite.
- understand the importance of self-protection against cold exposure.

HEAT EXPOSURE

Illness will result when the body is exposed to more heat energy than it can deal with. The normal body temperature of 98.6 degrees Fahrenheit (F) or 37.0 degrees centigrade, or Celsius (C), is maintained by complicated mechanisms. This internal temperature remains constant, regardless of the temperature of the environment (the **ambient temperature**). When the body is in a hot environment, or when excessive body heat is produced by vigorous physical activity, the body will attempt to rid itself of the excess heat. As described in Chapter 14, you can use several mechanisms to decrease body heat. The body's own most efficient mechanisms are sweating (and evaporation of the sweat) and dilation of skin blood vessels, which brings blood to the skin surface to increase the rate of radiation of heat from the body. In addition, the person who becomes overheated will remove clothing and attempt to move to a cooler environment.

Ordinarily, the heat-regulating mechanisms of the body work very well, and people are able to tolerate significant temperature changes quite well. Illness from heat exposure occurs when the normal regulatory mechanisms are overwhelmed and the body is no longer able to tolerate the excessive heat. Illness from heat exposure can take three forms: heat cramps, heat exhaustion, and heat stroke. However, the three forms of heat illness may be present in the same patient; untreated heat exhaustion may progress to heat stroke.

People who are at greatest risk for heat illnesses include children, the elderly, patients with cardiac disease or neurologic impairment, and those with limited mobility. Certain drugs, when taken for other conditions, may make a person susceptible to heat illnesses as well. Medications that decrease the ability of the body to sweat, (such as certain antidepressant drugs) and alcohol predispose the user to heat illness. When you are treating someone for a heat illness, always obtain a history of the use of drugs or medication.

Heat Cramps

Heat cramps are painful muscle spasms that occur after vigorous exercise. Heat cramps do not occur only in hot environments. They may be seen in factory workers or even well-conditioned athletes. The exact cause of heat cramps is not well understood. It is known that sweat produced during strenuous exercise, particularly in a warm environment, causes a change in the body's salt (electrolyte) balance and may result in the loss of essential **electrolytes** from the cells. If the muscles are working vigorously, their cells will be vulnerable to this electrolyte loss. As of yet, however, there is no proof that the muscles that develop cramps have actually lost electrolytes. Dehydration may also play a role in the development of muscle cramps. Large amounts of water can be lost from the body as a result of excessive sweating. This loss of water may affect muscles that are being stressed and cause them to go into spasm.

Heat cramps usually occur in the leg or abdominal muscles. When the abdominal muscles are involved, the pain and muscle spasm may be so severe that the patient appears to have an acute abdominal problem. A history of sudden onset of abdominal cramps as a patient has been exercising vigorously in a hot environment is the best clue to a diagnosis of heat cramps.

Treat heat cramps in the field using the following steps:

1. Remove the patient from the hot environment. Loosen any tight clothing.
2. Rest the cramping muscles. Have the patient sit or lie down until the cramps subside.
3. Replace fluids by mouth. Use water or a diluted (half-strength) balanced electrolyte solution (such as Gatorade®). Do not give salt tablets or solutions high in salt concentration. The patient will have an adequate amount of electrolytes circulating; they are just not distributed properly. With adequate rest and fluid replacement, the body will adjust the distribution of electrolytes and the cramps will disappear.

If, after these measures, the cramps do not go away, you should transport the patient to the hospital. Once the cramps have resolved, the patient may resume activity. For example, an athlete can return to play once the heat cramps have disappeared. However, if he or she resumes heavy sweating, the cramps may recur.

Heat Exhaustion

Heat exhaustion, also called *heat prostration* or *heat collapse,* is the most common serious illness caused by heat. It occurs when the body loses so much water and electrolytes through very heavy sweating that hypovolemia (fluid depletion) occurs. For sweating to be an effective cooling mechanism, the sweat must be able to evaporate from the body. If evaporation does not occur, cooling will not take place. The body will continue to produce sweat, with further loss of body water. Persons standing in the hot sun with several layers of clothing on (football fans or parade watchers, for example) may sweat profusely but experience little body cooling. High environmental humidity will also decrease the amount of evaporation that can occur. Thus, persons who exercise vigorously and those who wear heavy clothing in a warm, humid environment are particularly prone to heat exhaustion.

Patients who have developed heat exhaustion are in mild hypovolemic shock. The signs and symptoms of heat exhaustion are those of hypovolemia. The patient will often admit to working hard or exercising in a hot, humid environment and sweating heavily. The skin is usually cold and clammy and the face gray. This patient may also complain of feeling dizzy, weak, or faint, with accompanying nausea or headache. The vital signs may be normal, although the pulse is often rapid. The body temperature is usually normal or slightly elevated, but on rare occasions it may be as high as 104 degrees F (40 degrees C).

Treat the patient for mild hypovolemic shock. Remove him or her promptly from the hot environment. Loosen any tight clothing and remove any excessive layers of clothing (Figure 42–1). Encourage the patient to lie down. If the patient is fully alert, you should encourage him or her to drink up to a liter of water or a diluted, commercially available balanced salt solution. Never force fluids by mouth on a patient who is not fully alert, because the patient could aspirate the fluid into the lungs.

In most cases these measures will reverse the patient's symptoms, and he or she will feel better within 30 minutes. However, if the symptoms do not clear promptly, the level of consciousness decreases, or the temperature remains elevated, you should transport the patient to the hospital promptly for more vigorous treatment, such as intravenous fluid therapy and close monitoring.

Heat Stroke

Heat stroke is the least common but most serious illness caused by heat exposure. It occurs when the body is subjected to more heat than it can handle and the normal mechanisms for getting rid of the excess heat are overwhelmed. The body temperature then rises rapidly to the level where tissues are destroyed. Untreated heat stroke will result in death. Heat stroke may occur during vigorous physical activity. It may occur outdoors or in a closed, poorly ventilated, humid space. Heat stroke is likely to occur during heat waves among people (particularly the elderly) who live in buildings without air conditioning or good ventilation. It may occur in children left unattended in a locked car on a hot day.

The symptoms of heat exhaustion often precede heat stroke. If not treated, heat exhaustion can develop into heat stroke. A patient with heat exhaustion whose temperature is elevated may be developing heat stroke.

Many heat stroke patients have hot, dry, flushed skin because their sweating mechanism has been overwhelmed. However, early in the course of heat stroke, the patient may still be sweating and the skin may be moist or wet. Remember that a patient can have heat stroke even if he or she is still sweating. The body temperature rises rapidly in heat stroke patients. It may rise up to 106 degrees F (41 degrees C) or more. As the body **core temperature** (the temperature of the heart, lungs, and vital organs) rises, the patient's level of consciousness falls.

Often the first sign of heat stroke is a change in behavior. However, the patient then becomes unresponsive very quickly. The pulse is usually rapid and strong at first, but as the patient becomes increasingly unresponsive, the pulse becomes weaker and the blood pressure falls.

Heat stroke is a life-threatening emergency; untreated heat stroke will always result in

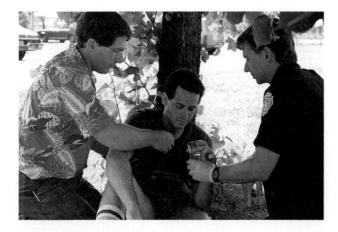

FIGURE 42–1

Remove the patient who is suffering from heat exhaustion to a cool environment. If the patient is fully alert, give him water or a diluted electrolyte solution to drink.

death. You must be able to identify the patient with heat stroke as early as possible. Recovery of a patient with heat stroke depends on the speed and vigor with which treatment is administered. The emergency treatment of heat stroke is to get the body temperature down by any means that are available. Get the patient out of the hot environment and into the ambulance with the air conditioning set to maximum cooling. Remove the patient's clothing, cover him or her with wet towels or sheets, and direct a fan toward the patient. Transport the patient rapidly to the hospital. Notify the hospital of the problem so that preparations can be made for the immediate treatment of the heat stroke patient on your arrival.

COLD EXPOSURE

Normal body temperature (98.6 degrees F or 37 degrees C) must be maintained within a very narrow range to allow chemical reactions in the body to work efficiently. The mechanisms that regulate body temperature can maintain it in hot or cold weather. However, if the body, or a part of it, is exposed to freezing or near-freezing temperatures, these mechanisms may be overwhelmed and cold exposure will result. Cold exposure may cause injury to individual parts of the body or to the body as a whole. When the entire body temperature falls, the condition is called **hypothermia.** Sometimes only parts of the body such as the feet, hands, ears, or nose may suffer cold injury. This condition is called frostbite.

Heat always travels from a warmer place to a cooler place. Because the body is usually warmer than its surroundings, the body will tend to lose heat. The body generates heat through the metabolism of food as it uses the food to do work. In this way, the body can usually replace heat that is lost to the surrounding environment. The body can lose heat in the following five ways:

- **Conduction.** Conduction is the direct transfer of heat from a part of the body to a colder object. Conduction occurs when a warm hand touches a cold piece of metal or comes into contact with ice or snow. Conduction

heat loss occurs when the body or a part of it is immersed in water with a temperature of less than 98 degrees F (37 degrees C). Heat passes directly from the body to the colder substance.
- **Convection.** Convection occurs when heat is transferred, through air moving across the body surface, to a cooler area. An individual wearing light clothing who is standing outside loses heat to the environment by convection.
- **Evaporation.** The conversion of any liquid to a gas is called evaporation. This conversion requires energy (heat). When sweat or water evaporates from the skin surface, the heat necessary for this process is taken from the body. Swimmers coming out of the water will feel a sensation of cold as the water evaporates from their skin. Evaporation is the natural mechanism by which sweating cools the body.
- **Radiation.** Heat always travels from a warm object to a cooler one, even if the objects are not in contact with each other. A warm object will give off (radiate) heat to a cooler environment. A person standing in a cold room will lose heat by radiation.
- **Respiration.** With normal breathing (respiration), the warm air in the lungs is exhaled into the atmosphere and body heat is lost.

The rate and amount of heat loss by the body can be modified in a variety of ways: increasing heat production, moving to an area where heat loss is decreased, or wearing insulated clothing. One way for the body to increase its heat production is by increasing the rate of metabolism of its cells. This increased activity occurs most obviously in muscles as shivering. Moving out of a cold environment and seeking shelter from winds is another way to decrease heat loss from radiation and convection.

Protective, insulated clothing serves in several ways to decrease heat loss. Insulators are materials which do not conduct heat. Dry, still air is an excellent insulator. Thus, layers of clothing that trap air and wool, down, or synthetic foams that have small pockets of entrapped air are good insulators. Protective clothing also traps perspiration and does not allow evaporation to occur.

Sweating without evaporation will not result in cooling. Covering the head is also important in decreasing radiation. A great deal of body heat can be lost by radiation from the uncovered head. Covering the head will minimize radiation heat loss by up to 70 percent.

Hypothermia

Hypothermia means, literally, low temperature, and is diagnosed when the inner (core) temperature of the body falls below 95 degrees F (35 degrees C). Generalized, progressive cooling of the body results in hypothermia. It can develop quickly, as when someone is immersed in cold water, or more gradually, as when a lost hunter is exposed to the cold environment for several hours or more. Hypothermia does not always occur in rural or remote areas; it is a problem in the cities as well. Nor does the temperature have to be below freezing for it to occur. In winter, homeless persons and those who lack heating for their homes may develop hypothermia. Hypothermia may occur in the summer, as when a swimmer remains in the water for a long period of time. As with all heat and cold injuries, hypothermia is more common among elderly and ill individuals, who are less able to accommodate to temperature extremes.

The body can usually tolerate a drop of a few degrees of internal body temperature. However, when the core temperature falls below 95 degrees F (35 degrees C), symptoms of hypothermia will occur. The body loses its ability to regulate its temperature and to generate body heat. Progressive loss of body heat then begins to occur.

Symptoms of Hypothermia The symptoms of hypothermia become progressively more severe as the core temperature falls. Hypothermia progresses through five general stages (Table 42–1). Although there is no clear distinction between the stages, you should be able to estimate the severity of the problem by knowing the signs and symptoms present in each stage. When you evaluate a hypothermic patient in the field, you should be able to distinguish between mild and severe hypothermia.

Mild hypothermia occurs when the core temperature is between 90 and 95 degrees F (32 and 35 degrees C). The patient is usually alert and shivering. Shivering is an attempt to generate more heat through muscular activity. In addition, jumping up and down and stamping the feet will occur as the patient tries to produce more heat. More severe hypothermia occurs below 90 degrees F (32 degrees C).

TABLE 42–1   Systemic Hypothermia

	Core Temperature				
	95°F	90°F	85°F	80°F	78°F and Below
Degree of Hypothermia	Mild	Mild	Moderate	Severe	Severe
Signs and Symptoms	Shivering; foot stamping	Loss of coordination	Lethargy	Coma	Apparent death
Cardiorespiratory Response			Slow pulse	Weak pulse; arrhythmias; slow respirations	Ventricular fibrillation; cardiac arrest
Level of Consciousness	Withdrawn	Confused	Sleepy	Irrational	Unconscious

Shivering stops, and muscular activity decreases. At first small, fine muscle activity—for example, coordinated finger motion—ceases. Eventually, as the temperature falls further, all muscle activity stops. As the core temperature drops to 85 degrees F (29 degrees C), the patient becomes lethargic. He or she may lose interest in combating the cold environment. If the temperature continues to fall to 80 degrees F (27 degrees C), decreased vital signs become apparent. The pulse slows and becomes weaker. Respiration slows and cardiac arrhythmias may occur. Below 80 degrees F all cardiorespiratory activity may cease, and the patient may appear dead.

Never assume that a cold, pulseless patient is dead. Patients may survive even after severe hypothermia, if proper emergency measures are carried out.

Treatment of Hypothermia Even mild degrees of hypothermia can have serious consequences and complications. It is therefore necessary to have all hypothermia patients evaluated and treated in the hospital. Management of hypothermia in the field, regardless of the severity of the exposure, consists of two steps: stabilizing the vital functions and preventing further heat loss. All hypothermic patients should be transported rapidly to the hospital. When there is an unavoidable delay in transport or the hospital is a long distance away, it is essential to minimize further loss of body heat.

Do not try to rewarm a hypothermic patient in the field. This may cause an irreversible and fatal cardiac arrhythmia. Rather, your goal of treatment is to prevent further heat loss. Definitive rewarming should only be done in the hospital where the patient can be monitored closely and maximum resuscitation can be provided when necessary. Remove the patient immediately from the cold environment. If your ambulance is nearby, place the patient in it, warmed to room temperature of about 70 degrees F. If there will be a delay in getting the patient out of the cold, try to prevent further heat loss by moving him or her out of the wind and away from contact with any object that will conduct heat from the body.

If the patient is alert and is shivering, you may assume that the hypothermia is mild. You may give the patient warm fluids by mouth. Remove all wet clothing and cover the patient with a blanket. Notify the hospital of the patient's condition so that preparations can be made for rewarming to begin as soon as the patient arrives.

When the patient is not shivering, moderate or severe hypothermia is present. A standard thermometer cannot be used to measure body temperature accurately in such patients, because it does not register low enough temperatures. A special low-temperature thermometer is required. The patient with a more severe form of hypothermia will have a core temperature below 90 degrees F.

There is controversy about whether to perform basic life support (BLS) on the hypothermic patient who appears to be pulseless. Although patients who are severely hypothermic may appear pulseless, they may actually have a pulse rate of only one or two beats per minute. If you cannot feel a radial pulse, gently palpate for a carotid pulse and wait for a full minute before you decide that a patient is truly pulseless. Even such a slow pulse is an indication of cardiac activity, and such a patient does not need BLS. Cardiac activity may spontaneously recover once the core is warmed. A hypothermic patient may be assumed to be in a "metabolic ice box," and attempting BLS may upset a balance that the body has achieved. On the other hand, there is evidence that, correctly done, BLS will increase blood flow to the critical parts of the body. Some authorities thus recommend starting BLS on a pulseless, hypothermic patient. If you are in an area where hypothermia is a common problem, you should have prearranged protocols for dealing with this situation. In all cases, consult medical control before proceeding with BLS in the severely hypothermic patient.

The American Heart Association recommends that CPR be started if the patient has no detectable pulse or breathing. Ventilation with warm, humidified oxygen should also be started. Wet clothing should be removed, and the patient protected from the cold and wind. Warm packs may be placed at the neck, groin, and in the armpits.

Management of Cold Exposure in a Sick or Injured Person

All patients who are severely injured will have some degree of hypothermia. When you are evaluating a multiply injured patient, remember that in addition to the injuries, this patient is hypothermic.

You may also encounter a sick or injured person who has been trapped in a cold environment. This patient may develop hypothermia or already have problems related to the cold exposure. Remember, an injured or sick person is more susceptible to cold injury than is a healthy one. Take the following steps promptly to prevent further cold injury:

1. Remove wet clothing and keep the patient dry.
2. Prevent conduction heat loss. Do not allow the patient to lie against any wet or cold surfaces (such as a car frame).
3. Insulate all exposed body parts (especially the head) by wrapping them with a blanket or any other dry, bulky material that is available.
4. Prevent convection loss by erecting a wind barrier around the patient.
5. Remove the patient from the cold environment as promptly as possible.

Regardless of the nature or severity of the cold injury, remember that a seemingly dead person may be very much alive, and although the patient may not be responding, he or she may be able to hear you. There have been reported cases of patients having heard themselves being pronounced dead by someone who had forgotten the old saying: "No one is dead unless he is warm and dead."

Local Cold Injuries

Most injuries from the cold are localized to exposed parts of the body. The extremities, particularly the feet, are especially vulnerable to cold injury. When exposed parts of the body become very cold but not frozen, the condition is called frostnip, chilblains, or immersion foot (trench foot). When the parts become frozen, the injury is called **frostbite.** There are three

important factors that determine the severity of a local cold injury:

- The duration of the exposure.
- The temperature to which the body part was exposed.
- The wind velocity during exposure.

The following six factors may make a person more susceptible to localized cold injury:

- Inadequate insulation from cold or wind.
- Restricted circulation from tight clothing or shoes, or circulatory disease.
- Fatigue.
- Poor nutrition.
- Alcohol or drug abuse.
- Hypothermia.

In hypothermia, blood is shunted away from the extremities in an attempt to maintain the temperature of the body core. This shunting of blood increases the risk of local cold injury to the extremities. Thus, the patient with hypothermia may also develop frostbite or other local cold injury. The reverse is also true. You must remember that both local and systemic cold exposure problems can occur in the same patient.

Frostnip and Immersion Foot

Frostnip occurs after prolonged exposure to the cold. Freezing of the skin may be present but freezing of the deeper tissues has not occurred. Because this condition is usually not painful, the patient often is not aware that a cold injury has occurred. The skin becomes pale (blanched). Exposed parts of the body, particularly the ears and nose, are commonly affected. *Immersion foot*, also called *trench foot*, occurs after prolonged exposure to cold water. It is particularly common in hikers or hunters who stand for a long time in cold water. The skin of the foot is wrinkled, pale, and cold to the touch.

The emergency treatment of these less severe local cold injuries includes removing the patient from the cold, wet environment and rewarming the part. With frostnip, contact with a warm object such as your hands or the patient's body, or blowing warm breath onto the part may be all that is needed. During rewarming, tingling and redness of the affected part will occur. With immersion foot, remove wet shoes, boots, and socks and rewarm the foot gradually, protecting it from further cold exposure.

Frostbite

Frostbite is the most serious local cold injury, because the tissues are actually frozen. Freezing permanently damages cells, although the exact mechanism by which the damage occurs is not known. The presence of ice crystals within the cells may cause physical damage to them. The change in the water content in the cells may also cause changes in the concentration of critical electrolytes, which produce permanent changes in the chemistry of the cell. When the ice thaws, further chemical changes occur in the cell. As a result, the damaged cells die and *gangrene* occurs or they become permanently damaged. If gangrene occurs, the dead tissue must be surgically removed, sometimes by amputation. If less severe damage occurs, there will still be permanent changes in the injured part. It becomes reddened, tender to touch, and cannot tolerate further exposure to cold.

Frostbite can be identified by the hard, frozen feel of the affected tissues. Much like a burn, the depth of damage to the skin will vary. Frostbite may be superficial or deep. With superficial frostbite only the skin is frozen, and with deep frostbite the deeper tissues are frozen as well. It may be impossible to differentiate superficial from deep frostbite in the field, and even an experienced surgeon in a hospital setting may not be able to tell until several days have gone by. Most frostbitten parts are white, yellow-white, or blue-white. They are hard and cold to the touch (Figure 42-2).

The emergency treatment of frostbite in the field should include the following steps:

1. Remove the patient from further exposure to the cold.
2. Handle the frostbitten part gently. Protect it from further injury. Never rub it with anything. Rubbing injured tissues just causes further damage to them. Do not allow the patient to stand or walk on a frostbitten foot.

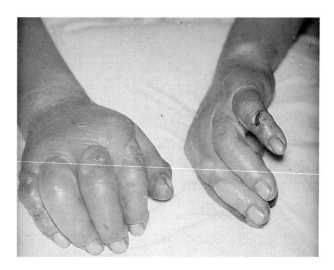

FIGURE 42-2

Frostbitten tissue may be white, yellow-white, or blue-white and is hard and cold to the touch, because the tissues are actually frozen. The exact depth of injury cannot be determined in the field and may take several days to become obvious.

3. Remove any wet or restricting clothing and cover the injured part loosely with a dry, sterile dressing.
4. Evaluate the patient's general condition for the signs or symptoms of systemic hypothermia.
5. Support the patient's vital functions as necessary and transport the patient promptly to the hospital.

Rewarming of the frostbitten extremity is rarely done in the field. You can cause a great deal of further injury to a frostbitten part by attempts to rewarm it. Never try to heat a frostbitten part with something warm such as the exhaust from the ambulance engine or, even worse, an open flame. This will only cause further damage to the fragile tissues. Rewarming is best accomplished under controlled circumstances in the emergency department. If prompt hospital care is not available and your medical control or prearranged protocol instructs you to institute rewarming in the field, it is best accomplished in a warm-water bath. Immerse the frostbitten part in water at a temperature of between 100 degrees and 112 degrees F (38 degrees and 44.5 degrees C). Check the water temperature with a thermometer before the limb is immersed and frequently during the rewarming process. The water temperature should never exceed 112 degrees F (44.5 degrees C). Keep the frostbitten part in the water bath until it feels warm and the color (redness) has returned.

Do not attempt rewarming if there is any chance that the part may freeze again before the patient reaches the hospital. Some of the most severe consequences of frostbite (gangrene and amputation) have occurred in parts that were thawed and then refrozen.

Cover the frostbitten part with soft, padded, sterile cotton dressings. If blisters have formed, do not break them. Remember, you cannot accurately predict the outcome of a case of frostbite early in its course. Even body parts that are blue and appear gangrenous may recover if given proper emergency and hospital treatment.

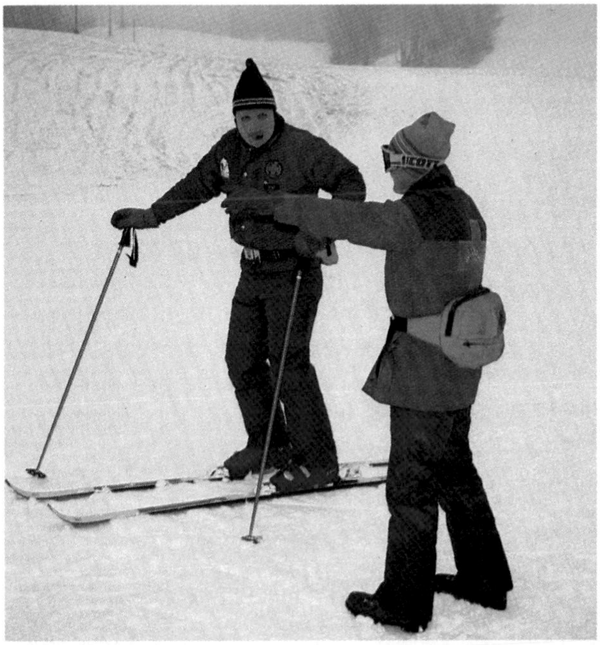

Cold Exposure and the EMT

When working in a cold environment, you are also at risk for becoming a hypothermia patient. Specific survival training and precautions should be given to EMTs who work in regions where cold-weather search-and-rescue operations may be needed. You must be thoroughly familiar with the specific conditions in your assigned areas, be aware of existing weather conditions, and stay tuned to forecasts of predicted weather changes. Proper clothing should be available and worn at all times (Figure 42–3). The vehicle must be properly equipped and maintained for a cold environment. As with many other hazards, you must be concerned with self-protection in order to remain capable of helping others. Never allow yourself to become a casualty!

FIGURE 42–3

An EMT who works in a cold environment must wear proper clothing to protect against hypothermia and frostbite, especially during search-and-rescue operations.

YOU ARE THE EMT

1. What causes heat cramps? Why shouldn't you give salt tablets to patients who are suffering from the muscle spasms of heat cramps?
2. It's the end of August and football practice has just started. You are called to treat a 16-year-old boy who has collapsed in the 80-degree heat. After ruling out medical problems and injuries, you realize he has collapsed from the heat. How will you decide whether he has heat exhaustion or heat stroke? How should each condition be treated?
3. Why shouldn't you attempt to rewarm a hypothermic patient in the field? What measures should you take in the field?
4. What is the difference between frostnip and frostbite?

CHAPTER 43

WATER HAZARDS

KEY TERMS

air embolism (ār em'bo-lizm) A condition caused by a bubble of air in the blood stream.

bradycardia (brad"e-kar'de-ah) Slow but regular heart rhythm.

breath-holding blackout Loss of consciousness due to a decreased stimulus for breathing.

decompression sickness (the bends) (de"kom-presh'un sik'nes) A situation seen in divers in which gas, especially nitrogen, forms bubbles in blood vessels, obstructing them.

diving reflex Slowing of heart rate caused by submersion in cold water.

drowning Death from suffocation by submersion in water.

hypothermia (hi"po-ther'me-ah) A condition in which the internal body temperature falls below 95 degrees F after prolonged exposure to freezing or near freezing temperature.

laryngospasm (lah-ring'go-spazm) A severe constriction of the vocal cords.

near drowning Survival, at least temporarily, after suffocation in water.

pulmonary edema (pul'mo-ner"e ĕ-de'mah) Fluid building up in the lungs, a result of congestive heart failure.

recompression chamber (re"kom-presh'un chām'ber) A single-person or multiperson capacity compressed air tank that is used by an experienced medical team to restore the body to a high pressure environment.

self-contained underwater breathing apparatus (SCUBA) A system that delivers air to the mouth and lungs at various atmospheric pressures, increasing with the depth of the dive.

Each year in the United States, water accidents claim approximately 9,000 lives. Drowning is the third leading cause of deaths from injury, surpassed only by motor vehicle and fall-related deaths. The U.S. Department of Health and Human Services has prepared a national objective to reduce crude death rate for drowning by over 50 percent.

Many persons in danger of drowning can be saved by prompt, appropriate emergency care. This care may be as simple as removing the patient from the water and clearing the airway, or resuscitation may require advanced life support (ALS) measures and high-technology equipment for deep water rescue.

In any water hazard emergency, the patient has a much better chance of survival if the EMT knows how to start artificial ventilation in the water, prevent further injury to the spine in diving accidents, and begin cardiopulmonary resuscitation once the patient is out of the water.

Chapter 43 begins with an explanation of how submersion in water affects the lungs. The chapter then discusses the emergency care of near-drowning victims, including those patients with suspected spinal injuries. The chapter next describes diving problems, especially those hazards associated with scuba divers, including ruptured eardrums, air embolism, and decompression sickness. The final section of Chapter 43 briefly discusses other water hazards.

GOALS
. . . .

The goals of Chapter 43 are to

- understand why drowning and near drowning occur after a patient is submerged in water.
- learn the emergency care for near-drowning victims.
- learn how to identify and treat suspected spinal injuries associated with near-drowning accidents.
- become familiar with diver associated problems, especially air embolism and decompression sickness (the "bends").
- recognize other water hazards, including hypothermia and breath-holding blackout.
- become familiar with strategies to prevent immersion accidents.

. . . .

DROWNING AND NEAR DROWNING
. . . .

Drowning is death from suffocation by submersion in water; **near drowning** is defined as survival, at least temporarily, after suffocation in water. Drowning usually results from a cycle of events that result in panic in the water (Figure 43–1). Panic can set up a cycle that will end in death, and it can affect someone who is submerged in water for even a short period of time. The victim struggles to the surface or the shore and becomes fatigued or exhausted. This panic-driven effort only causes the person to sink deeper into the water.

The mechanism of death by drowning differs in fresh water, such as a swimming pool, from that in salt water, such as the ocean. Statistics show that in most drowning cases (85 percent to 90 percent) significant amounts of water enter the lungs of the victim. Fresh water is

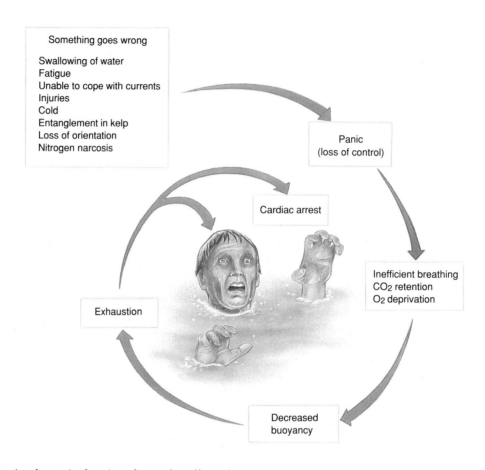

Something goes wrong

Swallowing of water
Fatigue
Unable to cope with currents
Injuries
Cold
Entanglement in kelp
Loss of orientation
Nitrogen narcosis

Panic
(loss of control)

Cardiac arrest

Inefficient breathing
CO_2 retention
O_2 deprivation

Exhaustion

Decreased
buoyancy

FIGURE 43–1   A schematic drawing shows the effect of panic in water accidents where it can contribute to the death of the person who loses self-control.

quickly absorbed across the walls of the alveoli of the lung into the bloodstream. This water then dilutes electrolytes in the body and causes red blood cells to rupture. Additionally, rupture of the alveoli may cause irreversible damage to lung tissue. Salt water, if it enters the lungs, causes injury through a different mechanism. Highly concentrated sea water literally pulls the body water from the lung capillaries into the alveoli, causing **pulmonary edema.** As a result, it is difficult to transport oxygen across the wall of the alveolus into the blood. Contaminants in the water such as bacteria or chemicals will cause additional lung injury and further complicate resuscitation efforts.

The inhalation of very small amounts of either fresh or salt water can severely irritate the larynx and send muscles of the larynx and the vocal cords into spasm. This phenomenon is called **laryngospasm.** Laryngospasm pre-

vents more water from entering the lungs. It is important to note that the patient's lungs cannot be ventilated when significant laryngospasm is present. Progressive hypoxia occurs until the victim becomes unconscious. At this point, the spasm relaxes and rescue breathing will become effective.

EMERGENCY CARE IN DROWNING ACCIDENTS—ACCEPTED TREATMENT PROTOCOLS

Treatment begins with rescue and removal from the water. You must take care to stabilize and protect the victim's spine because associated cervical spine injuries are possible, especially in diving accidents. Artificial ventilation should begin as soon as possible by the rescuer, even before the victim is removed from the water. In most cases, you should use mouth-to-mouth ventilation with the head in a neutral position opening the airway with the jaw-thrust or chin-lift maneuver. If there is evidence of upper airway obstruction by foreign matter, remove the obstruction manually, by suction (if available), or (if necessary) by application of a subdiaphragmatic abdominal thrust (the Heimlich maneuver) followed by continued rescue breathing.

Check for the victim's pulse immediately after the victim emerges from the water. The pulse may be difficult to find due to peripheral vasoconstriction and low cardiac output. If the pulse is absent, CPR should be started immediately. Remember: transport to the hospital is mandatory in all near-drowning victims, even if initial field resuscitation appears completely successful, because fluid aspiration may lead to delayed complications that may last for days or weeks.

If the patient is conscious and still in the water, a water rescue is necessary. Throw a rope, life preserver, or any available object that will float to the victim. A swimming rescue should not be attempted unless you have been trained and are experienced in the techniques. When attempting a swimming rescue, always wear a personal flotation device. Well-meaning, inexperienced people have themselves become victims while attempting a swimming rescue. Many items can be floated out to the victim. For example, an inflated spare tire, rim and all, will float well enough to support two people in the water. The basic rule of water rescue can be remembered by this old adage: "Throw, tow, row, and *only then* go!" (Figure 43–2).

The EMT who works in a recreation area near lakes, rivers, or the ocean front must have a prearranged plan for water rescue. This plan must include access to and cooperation with

FIGURE 43–2

Swimming rescues must not be attempted by untrained personnel who cannot handle panic-striken persons in the water. Always follow this sequence: throw a flotable object, or tow the swimmer in by pole or rope. If these approaches fail, try to use a boat. Only when these courses have been exhausted, and only if you wear a personal flotation device and are capable of a swimming rescue should you attempt it.

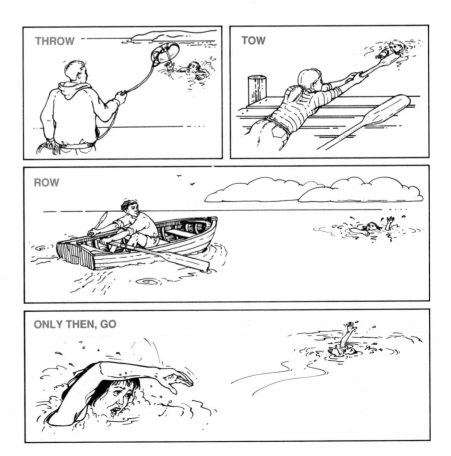

local personnel who are trained and skilled in water rescue and who can assist in developing a preplanned protocol for water rescue. Immediate access to life jackets and other rescue equipment is vitally important because the success of any water rescue depends on how rapidly the victim is removed from the water and proper ventilation procedures are initiated.

SPINAL INJURIES IN DROWNING ACCIDENTS

Spine fractures and spinal cord injuries may complicate drowning accidents. You must assume that spinal injury exists if the drowning has resulted from a diving accident; if the patient is unconscious; or if the patient is conscious but complains of weakness, paralysis, or numbness in the arms or legs. Most spinal injuries in diving accidents affect the cervical spine. When spinal injury is suspected, the neck must be protected from further injury. The suspected injury must be stabilized while the patient is still in the water.

When you suspect a spinal injury and the patient is face down in the water, perform the following accepted treatment steps:

1. *Turn the patient face up.* Two rescuers are required to turn the patient safely. The entire upper half of the patient's body must be rotated as a unit. Twisting only the head, for example, may aggravate any injury to the cervical spine.
2. *Restore the airway and begin ventilation,* as soon as the victim is face up in the water, using the mouth-to-mouth method or with available adjunctive equipment. The head and trunk should be supported as a unit by one rescuer while the other rescuer opens the airway and begins artificial ventilation. Immediate ventilation is the primary treatment of all drowning and near-drowning patients (Figure 43–3).
3. *Float a buoyant spine board under the patient.* The head and trunk should then be secured to the board to eliminate motion of the cervical spine. Remember, do not remove

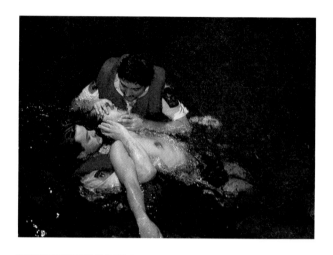

FIGURE 43–3

Artificial ventilation, the primary treatment of all drowning and near-drowning patients, should be started as soon as the patient is face up in the water.

the victim from the water until he or she is secured to the spine board.

4. *Remove the patient from the water on the board and begin CPR.* Effective cardiac compression or full CPR cannot be carried out in the water.

Remember: always prevent further heat loss by keeping the patient warm with blankets.

RECOVERY TECHNIQUES

On occasion, you may be called to the scene of a drowning and find that the victim is not floating or visible in the water. An organized rescue effort must then be carried out by personnel experienced with equipment (scuba gear, snorkels, and mask) and recovery techniques. As a last resort when standard procedures for recovery are unsuccessful, a grappling iron or large hook may be used to drag the bottom for the victim. Although the hook has the potential to seriously wound the patient, it may be the only effective method of bringing the patient to the surface for resuscitation efforts.

RESUSCITATION EFFORTS

You should *never* give up on resuscitating a drowning victim. When a person is submerged in water colder than body temperature, heat will be conducted from the body to the water, lowering the body temperature. Particularly in water colder than 70 degrees F (21 degrees C), **hypothermia** will occur and protect the vital organs from the lack of oxygen. Furthermore, in some circumstances exposure to cold water will induce certain reflexes, which may preserve basic body functions for prolonged periods. Recent literature reports survival, with good neurological recovery, in a 2½-year-old girl who was submerged in cold water for at least 66 minutes. Full resuscitation efforts should be maintained until the victim recovers or is pronounced dead by a physican at the scene or in the hospital.

DIVING PROBLEMS

Most serious water-related injuries are associated with dives, with or without scuba gear. Some of these problems are related to the nature of the dive; others result from panic. Panic is not restricted to the person who is unfamiliar or frightened by water; it happens to the experienced diver or swimmer as well. The **diving reflex** can occur in people who dive or jump into very cold water. A sudden reflex involving the vagus nerves may cause immediate **bradycardia** (reflex slowing of the heart rate); this person may lose consciousness and drown. However, because of hypothermia and a related lowered metabolic rate, the victim may be able to survive for an extended period of time under water. Full resuscitation efforts should be undertaken and continued, regardless of the length of submersion.

There are over three million **self-contained underwater breathing apparatus (SCUBA)** sport divers in the United States with approximately 200,000 new divers being trained annually. Medical problems relating to scuba diving techniques and equipment are becoming increasingly common. These problems are separated into three phases of the dive: descent, bottom, and ascent.

Descent Problems

Descent problems are usually due to the sudden increase in pressure on the body as the person dives deeper into the water. Some body cavities cannot adjust to the increased external pressure of the water, resulting in severe pain. The usual areas affected are the lungs, the sinus cavities, the middle ear, the teeth, and the area of the face surrounded by the diving mask. Usually, the pain caused by these "squeeze problems" forces the diver to return to the surface to equalize the pressures, and the problem alleviates itself. A diver who continues to complain of pain after returning to the surface, particularly in the ear, should be transported to the hospital.

A person with a ruptured eardrum may develop a problem while diving. If cold water enters the middle ear through a perforated tympanic membrane (ruptured eardrum), the diver may lose his or her balance and orientation. The diver may then shoot to the surface and sustain ascent problems.

Bottom Problems

Problems related to the bottom of the dive are rarely seen. Most of them are due to faulty connections in the diving gear and result either from inadequate mixing of oxygen and carbon dioxide in the air the diver breathes or from poisonous carbon monoxide accidentally fed into the breathing apparatus. All of these situations can cause drowning or rapid ascent, and all require emergency resuscitation and transport of the patient.

Ascent Problems

Most of the serious injuries associated with diving are related to ascending from the bottom and are referred to as ascent problems. These emergencies usually require vigorous resuscitation. Two particularly dangerous medical emergencies are **air embolism** and **decompression sickness** (also called **the bends**).

Air Embolism The most common and most dangerous emergency in scuba diving is air embolism. It may occur on a dive as shallow as 6 feet. Air embolism results when the diver holds his or her breath during a rapid ascent. The air pressure in the lungs remains at a high level while the external pressure on the chest decreases. As a result, the air inside the lungs expands rapidly. This rapid expansion causes the alveoli in the lungs to rupture. The air released from this rupture can cause injury in several areas. Air may enter the pleural space and create a pneumothorax (air in the pleural space that compresses the lungs). It can also enter the mediastinum (the space within the thorax that contains the heart and great vessels), causing a condition called *pneumomediastinum*. Or it may enter the bloodstream and create bubbles of air in the vessels called *air emboli*.

Pneumothorax and pneumomediastinum both result in pain and severe dyspnea. A bubble of air in the bloodstream (air embolus) will act as a "plug" and prevent the normal flow of blood and oxygen to a specific part of the body. The brain and spinal cord are the organs most severely affected by air embolism because they require a constant supply of oxygen (Figure 43–4).

The following are signs and symptoms of air embolism.

1. Blotching (mottling of the skin).
2. Froth (often pink or bloody) at the nose and mouth.
3. Severe pain in muscles, joints, or abdomen.
4. Dyspnea and/or chest pain.
5. Dizziness, nausea, and vomiting.
6. Dysphasia (difficulty in speaking).
7. Difficulty with vision.
8. Paralysis and/or coma.

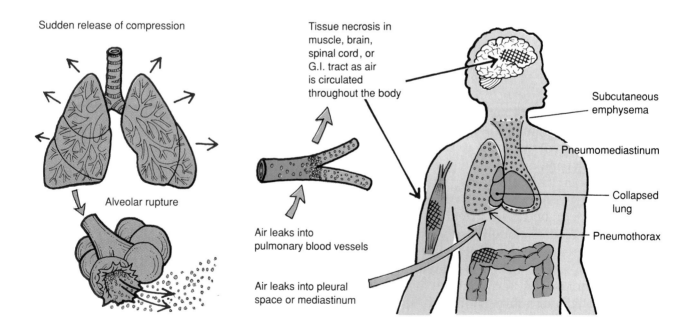

Sudden release of compression

Alveolar rupture

Tissue necrosis in muscle, brain, spinal cord, or G.I. tract as air is circulated throughout the body

Air leaks into pulmonary blood vessels

Air leaks into pleural space or mediastinum

Subcutaneous emphysema

Pneumomediastinum

Collapsed lung

Pneumothorax

FIGURE 43–4   Air embolism occurs as air in the lungs rapidly expands when compression on the chest is suddenly released. The resulting outward pressure can rupture alveoli and bronchioles and create the conditions shown here.

Decompression Sickness (The Bends)

Decompression sickness (the bends) also results from too rapid an ascent from a dive, although the mechanism of injury is different. In decompression sickness, bubbles of nitrogen form in the blood vessels and body tissues when the diver ascends rapidly. During the dive, nitrogen that is being breathed dissolves in the blood because it is under pressure. When the diver ascends rapidly, the external pressure is decreased, and the dissolved nitrogen forms small bubbles within the blood vessels. These bubbles of nitrogen cause the same problem that occurs in air embolism—blockage of blood vessels that deprives the affected parts of the body of their normal blood supply.

The signs and symptoms of decompression sickness may be similar to those of air embolism. The most striking symptom is severe abdominal and/or joint pain—so severe that the patient literally doubles up or "bends." Dive tables are available to show the proper rate of ascent from a dive, including the number and length of pauses that a diver should make on the way up from a deep, long dive. If these tables are followed, decompression sickness should not occur.

After a safe dive, decompression sickness can also occur from driving a car up a mountain or flying in an unpressurized airplane that climbs too rapidly to a great height. The problem is exactly the same as ascent from a deep dive: a sudden decrease of external pressure on the body and release of dissolved nitrogen from the blood that forms bubbles of nitrogen gas within the blood vessels. Some also claim that a hot shower or bath after a cold dive may bring on the bends.

Often it is difficult to distinguish between air embolism and decompression sickness. As a general rule, air embolism occurs immediately on return to the surface, whereas the symptoms of decompression sickness may not occur for several hours. The emergency treatment is the same for both: basic life support followed by recompression in a **recompression chamber.** In treating patients suspected of having air embolism or decompression sickness, you should follow these accepted treatment steps:

1. Remove the patient from the water. Try to keep the person calm.
2. Begin basic life support and administer oxygen.
3. Place the patient on his or her left side, with the head lower than the feet (the Trendelenberg position). This position will decrease the chance of an air embolism traveling to the brain.
4. Listen to the chest carefully for absent or decreased breath sounds that would indicate a pneumothorax.
5. Transport the patient promptly to the nearest recompression chamber (also called *hyperbaric oxygen chamber*) for treatment (Figure 43–5). Know the locations and means of access to the chambers in your area. Most of these can easily be reached by air transport, even if they are several miles from the incident. Transport the patient at or near sea level or in an aircraft pressurized to sea level atmosphere.
6. Continue to administer oxygen during transport to the chamber.

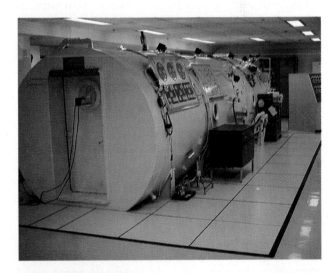

FIGURE 43–5

Treatment in a recompression chamber may be lifesaving for a patient with air embolism or decompression sickness.

7. If possible, obtain a history of the duration and depth of the dive. If facilities are available, the patient's scuba tank should be analyzed for the amount of air and other gases remaining in it.

8. Assess and monitor the victim's level of consciousness using the AVPU scale. This information will assist the personnel at the chamber in selecting the appropriate treatment program.

The aim of recompression treatment is to restore the body to a high-pressure environment so that the bubbles of gas (air or nitrogen) can be redissolved into the blood and the pressures inside and outside the lungs can be equalized. Once these pressures are equalized, gradual decompression can be accomplished under controlled conditions to prevent the bubbles from reforming.

Injury from decompression sickness is usually reversible with proper treatment. However, if the bubbles block critical blood vessels that supply the brain or spinal cord, permanent central nervous system injury may result. Therefore, the key in emergency management of these serious ascent problems is to first recognize that an emergency exists. You should begin basic life support, administer oxygen, and arrange for recompression as rapidly as possible.

OTHER WATER HAZARDS
· ·

Hypothermia may occur in patients who have been immersed in cold water. The progressive lowering of the body temperature makes it more difficult for these victims to help themselves. After removal from the water, the patient will continue to lose body heat. You must pay close attention to the body temperature of a person who is rescued from cold water. The same rules that are used for treating hypothermia caused by cold exposure apply to hypothermia from immersion in cold water: prevent further heat loss from contact with the ground, stretcher, or air and transport the patient promptly.

Breath-holding blackout sometimes occurs in shallow water. Swimmers who are trying to prolong their capacity to stay underwater breathe in and out rapidly and deeply prior to entering the water. This hyperventilation lowers the carbon dioxide level in the blood stream while increasing the oxygen level. Swimming underwater, the person consumes the oxygen but does not build up a high enough level of carbon dioxide, because so much of it has been blown off by hyperventilation. An elevated level of carbon dioxide in the blood is the strongest stimulus for breathing. Without this stimulus, the swimmer will not feel the need to breathe even though all of the oxygen in the lungs has been consumed. The person will then lose consciousness and may drown. The emergency treatment for a breath-holding blackout is the same as that for a drowning or near drowning.

Associated injuries may occur in the water. For example, contact with boat propellers, sharp rocks, water skis, or dangerous marine life can result in injury compounded by the problem of water immersion incidents. Remove the patient from the water (taking care to protect the spine from further injury) and give basic life support as needed. Apply dressings and splints if indicated, and monitor all patients closely for any signs of immersion or cold injury.

Child abuse may also occur in a water setting. You must be aware that a child involved in a drowning or near drowning may be the victim of child abuse. Although it may be difficult to prove, such incidents should be handled according to the applicable rules in suspected child abuse.

PREVENTION
· ·

Most immersion accidents are preventable when appropriate precautions are taken. Residential pools and other bodies of water should be surrounded by a fence that is at least 6 feet high with slats no farther apart than 3 inches. Fence gates should be self-closing with self-locking mechanisms. This is an appropriate precaution considering the number of children who drown in residential pools each year.

Additionally, 50 percent of teenage and adult drownings are associated with the use of alcohol. The public must be made aware of this association and the preventable nature of many of these problems. As a member of a health care profession, you should be involved in public education efforts that make people aware of the hazards of swimming pools and water recreation.

YOU ARE THE EMT

1. You have responded to a swimming pool diving accident. The victim's friends have pulled him to the surface, and he is floating face up when you arrive. He is unconscious but alive. Should you remove him from the pool or start ventilation in the water? Why will this patient need CPR? When will you start CPR?

2. How can hypothermia increase the chances of resuscitation after a near drowning?

3. Describe the diving reflex. What cardiac condition can it cause?

4. How does air embolism differ from the bends? What do these two problems have in common?

PSYCHOLOGICAL ASPECTS OF EMERGENCY CARE

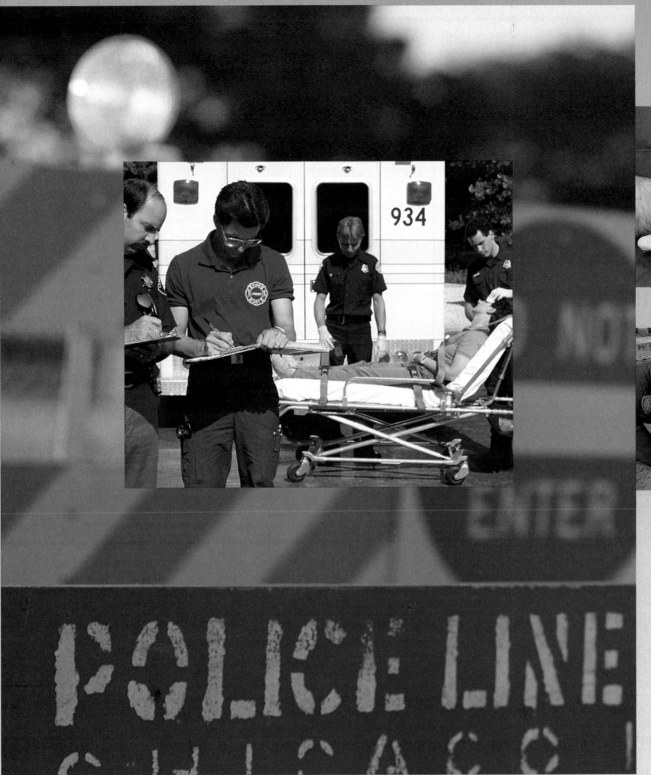

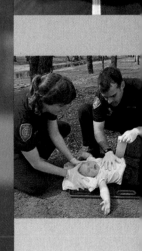

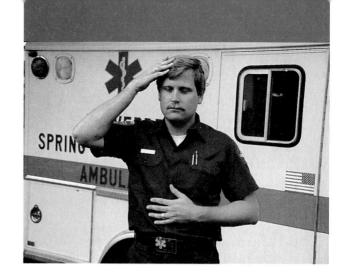

INTERACTING WITH PATIENTS

depression (de-presh'un) A mental state in which the patient has no interests, may not speak, or thinks of committing suicide.

disruptive behavior Behavior that causes a potential danger to the patient or to others, or causes a delay in treatment.

geriatric (jer"e-at'rik) Pertaining to the aged or elderly.

lucid (loo'sid) Alert, aware of surroundings, able to communicate.

malingering (mah-ling'gering) A condition in which a patient pretends to have an illness or injury.

mania (ma'ne-ah) A mental state in which the patient is hyperactive, ranging from mildly agitated to wildly uncontrollable.

organic brain syndrome A disease of the brain in which the patient's mental functioning is impaired, usually by old age or other disease; a cause of disruptive behavior.

paranoia (par"ah-noi'ah) A mental state in which the patient believes that others are talking about or plotting against him or her.

rational The ability to think and act clearly.

OVERVIEW

All emergency situations create stress in the patient, the patient's family, and the EMT who is called to the scene. The most important aspect of your initial assessment and treatment is your ability to communicate with the patient. The patient should understand who is carrying out the treatment, what is happening, and why it is happening. The patient must be able to trust you.

Sometimes, unfortunately, normal communication is not effective. When a patient displays disruptive behavior, special techniques are required before the person can be treated. In addition to understanding these techniques and knowing when they need to be applied, you should understand why they are needed—what causes disruptive behavior. Knowing some of the common causes will help you to manage the disruptive patient.

Chapter 44 begins by presenting the principles of effective communication with all patients. It then focuses on certain specific communications problems, such as communicating with the elderly, the child, hearing-impaired, blind, confused, and others with special problems. The last section of Chapter 44 discusses disruptive behavior—its causes and how it is managed.

GOALS

The goals of Chapter 44 are to
- become familiar with the principles of effective communication.
- identify specific communication problems and learn how to communicate with patients who have them.
- recognize the common causes of disruptive behavior and learn how to manage the disruptive patient.

PRINCIPLES OF EFFECTIVE COMMUNICATION

Effective communication will come more easily to you when you realize that the sick or injured patient is frightened and may misinterpret your gestures, body movements, and attitude. The following guidelines will help you to relate to a patient and keep the patient calm:

1. Make and keep eye contact with the patient at all times. Give the patient your undivided attention and let the patient know that he or she is your main—indeed, your only—interest. Look the patient "straight in the eye." This helps to establish rapport and to communicate your concern with the medical problem.
2. Tell the truth. Even if you have to say something very unpleasant, it is better than lying. Telling an untruth destroys the patient's trust in you and decreases your own confidence. You may not always tell the patient everything, but, in general, if the patient or family asks a specific question, answer truthfully. A straightforward question deserves a straightforward answer. If you do not know the answer to the patient's question, say so. To the questions, "Am I having a heart attack?" or "How long will I have to stay in the hospital?", "I don't know" is an adequate answer.
3. Communicate at a level that the patient can understand. Don't "talk up" or "talk down" or be patronizing in any way. Do not assume that an elderly person is deaf or otherwise unable to understand you. Never use "baby talk" with elderly people.

4. Be particularly careful about what you say to others. Although the patient who is ill or injured may have a heightened awareness of what people are saying, he or she may only hear part of your conversation and may seriously misinterpret, and remember for a long time, what you are saying to a co-worker or family member. Assume that the patient can hear every word you say, even if you are speaking to others.

5. Be aware of your body language. People may misinterpret gestures that you may make. Be particularly careful not to assume a threatening posture; instead, maintain yourself in a calm, professional stance. Nonverbal communication is extremely important in dealing with patients.

6. Always speak slowly, clearly, and distinctly.

7. Use a patient's proper name. Do not use terms such as "pops" or "lady" or "kid." Except with children, try to avoid using first names. Rather, use the patient's last name, preceded by the proper qualifier (Mr., Mrs., or Ms.).

8. If a patient is hearing impaired, speak clearly and face the person so that he or she can read your lips. Be careful not to shout at a hearing-impaired person. Shouting will not make it any easier for the patient to understand you, and shouting may frighten the person.

9. Allow time for the patient to answer or respond to your questions. Do not rush the patient unless there is immediate danger. Sick and injured people may not be thinking clearly and will need time to answer even simple questions.

10. Try to make the patient comfortable and relaxed. Is the patient more comfortable sitting or lying down? Is she cold or hot? Does she want a friend or relative to be with her?

SPECIFIC COMMUNICATION PROBLEMS
·······························

Elderly Patients

The **geriatric** population (people over age 65) is the fastest growing segment of the American population. By the year 2000, it is estimated that 13 percent of the U.S. population will be over 65 years old. The patient's actual age may not be the most important factor in making him or her "elderly," but rather the patient's functioning, mental state, and activity pattern usually determine the functional age. Most of these geriatric patients are **rational** (clear thinking) and can give a clear medical history. Most older patients are not senile or confused. However, some elderly patients are extremely difficult to communicate with; they may be hostile, unkempt, irritable, and/or confused. It takes great patience for you to deal with such a patient effectively and compassionately. If you pretend that the patient is your grandmother or grandfather, or indeed yourself when you reach that age, you will understand how important it is for you to have the necessary patience and persistence. Approach an elderly patient slowly and calmly, allowing plenty of time for the patient to respond to your questions. Be alert for signs of confusion, anxiety, or impaired hearing or vision. The patient should feel confident that you are in charge and that everything possible is being done for him or her.

Elderly patients often do not feel much pain. Do not be misled by an elderly person who, perhaps, has fainted, is dyspneic, but has no pain. Such a patient may very well have suffered a "silent" myocardial infarction. Even minor changes in an elderly person's breathing or mental state may signify major problems.

The elderly patient's spouse will also need attention. Seeing a person whom one has loved or been married to for many years taken away in an ambulance can be a particularly frightening and anxiety-producing experience. Take some time to speak with the patient's spouse or family, telling those who are close to the patient what is being done and why such action is being taken.

Pediatric Patients

Although all persons in an emergency situation experience some degree of fright, fear is probably most severe and most obvious in children. Assume that any child will be frightened about what is happening during a medical emergency. The child will be frightened by your uniform, your ambulance, and by the number of people who have suddenly gathered around. Even the child who says little is very much aware of all that is going on. Familiar objects and faces will help to reduce this fright. Letting the child keep a favorite toy, doll, or "security blanket" gives the child some sense of security and a lot of comfort. So does having a relative or friend nearby; however, this person must be emotionally stable. Sometimes adults become too upset by what has happened to the child to be of assistance, and their presence around the sick or injured child only makes things worse. Be careful about selecting the proper adult for this role.

Children can easily see through lies or deceptions, so you must always be honest with them. Constantly and repeatedly explain to the child what is happening and why certain procedures are taking place. If your treatment is going to hurt (such as applying a splint), explain this to the child ahead of time. You may tell the patient that it will not hurt for long and, most importantly, that it will help "make it better."

Respect a child's modesty. Little girls and boys are embarrassed if they have to undress or be undressed in front of strangers. When a wound or site of injury has to be exposed, you should try to do so out of sight of strangers. Again, it is extremely important to tell the child what you are doing and why you are doing it.

Your tone of voice is also important: it should be professional yet friendly. The child should feel reassured that you are there to help in every way possible. Maintaining eye contact with the child will let the child know that you are helping, and that you can be trusted.

Hearing-Impaired Patients

Hearing-impaired (deaf) patients are rarely ashamed or embarrassed by their deafness. They have learned to deal with it long ago. It is those around the deaf person—in this case, the emergency medical service personnel—who may have a problem dealing with a hearing-impaired person. You should first assume that a hearing-impaired person has normal intelligence and is able to understand what is going on, provided that you can successfully communicate with him or her. Most deaf people can read lips to some extent, so you should position yourself so that the patient can see your lips. Many hearing-impaired patients have hearing aids that may have been lost in an accident or fall, or that the confused, ill person forgot to put on. Look around the scene for the hearing aid; ask the patient or family whether the patient does, indeed, have a hearing aid. The following reminders will also help you communicate successfully with the hearing-impaired person:

1. Don't cover your mouth or mumble. Speak slowly, clearly, and distinctly.
2. Don't shout!
3. Know some of the simple phrases used in sign language, including those for "sick," "hurt," and "help" (Figure 44–1).
4. Have a clipboard handy to write down questions and for the patient to write down answers if necessary.
5. Write legibly and use short questions and answers. Remember that many hearing-impaired people can speak distinctly, although others cannot.

Blind Patients

Like hearing-impaired patients, blind patients have usually accepted their disability long ago and have learned to deal with it. Most blind people have also developed very sharp and acute senses of hearing and touch. Therefore, you should assume that a blind person has normal hearing and normal intelligence. Explain everything you are doing in great detail. Not all blind people are totally blind; many have some perception of light and dark, or can see shadows or movement. Be aware of your sudden movements; ask the person whether he or she can see at all. You should also keep in physical contact with the patient, holding your hand lightly on the patient's shoulder or arm. When it is time to move the blind patient—if the patient can walk—you should lead him or her with a hand on the patient's arm, taking care not to push. Transport any mobility aids (such as a cane) with the patient to the hospital.

A blind person may have a seeing eye dog.

A

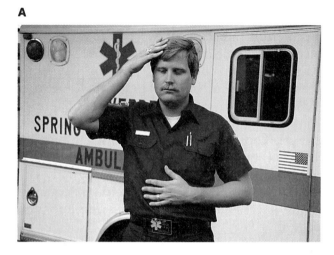

B

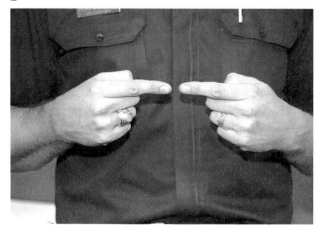

C

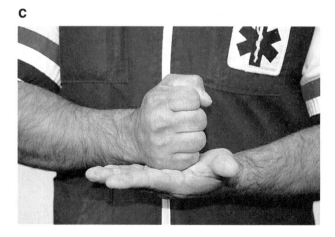

FIGURE 44–1

Some common hand sign language expressions to be used when communicating with hearing-impaired patients: (A) *sick*, (B) *hurt*, (C) *help*.

The dog can be identified by its special harness. Seeing eye dogs are trained not to leave their masters and not to respond to strangers. The blind patient who is conscious can tell you about the dog and give instructions for its care. Seeing eye dogs are often allowed into places where ordinary dogs are forbidden. If circumstances permit, bring the dog to the hospital with the patient. If the dog has to be left behind, you should make arrangements for its care.

Non-English-Speaking Patients

After the primary survey is completed and the patient's vital functions are stabilized, it is essential for you to obtain a medical history from the patient. This task is the responsibility of all medical personnel and cannot be omitted simply because the patient does not speak English. Many patients who do not speak English fluently will know certain important words or phrases.

Initially, you should determine how much English the patient can speak. If communication is impossible, seek out a family member or friend as an interpreter. Use short, simple questions and simple terms whenever possible. Be especially careful to avoid medical jargon. Questions can be supplemented with visual clues by using appropriate gestures and pointing to specific parts of the body. If you work in an area with a large non-English-speaking population, you should become familiar with their language, especially the common medical terms and phrases. You can carry cards that show the pronunciation of these terms.

Confused Patients

Patients may be confused for a variety of reasons. The stress of the emergency situation may be enough to confuse persons who ordinarily can function normally. Occasionally, illness or injury may cause confusion. Finally, some people appear constantly confused and cannot cope with normal daily routines, much less emergency situations. In communicating with a confused patient, you should assume that the confusion is only temporary and that the patient has normal intelligence. Speak slowly and distinctly, being certain that the patient understands what you are saying. Sometimes a confused patient's response time is quite long. This person needs and should be allowed plenty of time to respond to your questions and requests. Certain procedures may have to be explained more than once. It is important that you make every effort to communicate fully despite the patient's confused state. One final point to remember is that confusion may be a sign of significant injury or illness that will require medical care.

Mentally Retarded Patients

At times, severely mentally disturbed or retarded patients can be very difficult to communicate with. From the family, you should try to determine the patient's normal level of communication. The presence of a physical impairment does not necessarily mean that the patient cannot communicate. Even more important, most patients with physical impairments have normal intelligence and are able to understand the spoken word quite well.

When the patient is truly retarded, you should speak slowly, using short and simple words. As with the confused patient, the retarded patient sometimes needs to have sentences repeated more than once before he or she understands what is happening. These patients should be handled with an especially caring concern to minimize their fear and confusion.

DISRUPTIVE BEHAVIOR

Disruptive behavior is defined as behavior that presents a danger to the patient or others or causes a delay in treatment. The standard communication techniques outlined earlier in this chapter may be ineffective in altering disruptive behavior. Therefore, special techniques are required for dealing with such patients. Although there are many causes of disruptive behavior, it is important to remember that for some people it is simply a normal reaction to stress.

Possible Causes of Disruptive Behavior

Certain physical and medical conditions can result in disruptive behavior. One or more of these conditions may be present in an unruly patient.

Alcohol or drug abuse is discussed in Chapter 36. The presence of drug paraphernalia or an empty liquor bottle may point to the cause of disruptive behavior. Bear in mind that other causes of such behavior may be present in a patient who has been drinking or taking drugs. Be especially careful not to "write off" the unruly or abusive patient as "just another drunk."

Head injury may be a cause of disruptive behavior. The abnormal behavior may occur immediately after injury (from a concussion) or may be delayed for as long as two to three weeks after the injury (from a chronic subdural hematoma). When the family reports that the patient has had a significant change in personality, you must always consider the diagnosis of head injury.

Certain metabolic disorders can cause disruptive behavior. Both insulin shock and diabetic coma can result in abnormal patterns of behavior. Other endocrine disorders (especially thyroid disease) can produce wide ranges of abnormal behavior—from extreme agitation to marked lethargy. Attempt to determine whether the patient has a history of such a metabolic disorder. (Have similar reactions occurred before? Is the patient taking any prescribed medication?)

Neurological diseases may cause disruptive or irrational behavior. Many different terms are used to describe these diseases. The general descriptive term is **organic brain syndrome.** The vast majority of patients with organic brain syndrome are elderly and have experienced a gradual loss of function. Frequently, the first sign of organic brain syndrome is a change in personality. The family, and sometimes even the patient, will be aware of the personality change. Patients with organic brain syndrome are often disoriented. They do not know where they are; they may not know the date or they may not be able to answer a simple question such as "Who is the President of the United States?"

Many different forms of psychiatric illness also cause disruptive behavior. Psychiatric disorders may produce a wide range of behavioral problems, among them the following:

Paranoia   A patient may believe that people (including you) are plotting to hurt or kill him or her.

Mania   The patient may be severely agitated (manic)—moving around frantically and speaking rapidly but never finishing a sentence or a complete thought.

Depression   The patient may not want to do anything, even move, and will not cooperate or answer questions.

Suicidal act   The patient may be threatening to kill him- or herself or may have already made a suicide attempt.

These are just a few of the common presentations of psychiatric illness. Psychiatric patients may show great variations in their behavior over a short period of time. They often experience wide mood swings, appearing calm one minute and violent the next.

Management of the Disruptive Patient

Take the following steps in the management of any patient who is exhibiting disruptive behavior:

1. Assess the situation. Try to find out the cause of the patient's disruptive behavior. Unless the patient is in danger and must be moved immediately, you should spend some time assessing the situation. There frequently is no immediate need to hurry off to the hospital. Spending some extra time with the patient can often make the job of transporting him or her much easier. Look for a possible cause of a head injury or for drug or alcohol use. Try to obtain a history of the behavior. Did it come on suddenly or gradually? Does the patient have diabetes or other medical problems? Has he or she been ill recently? Does the patient have a history of similar previous behavior or psychiatric illness?

2. Protect the patient and yourself. Do not take your eyes off of the patient and be alert for any obviously aggressive behavior. Even small people can be dangerous if they are severely agitated. Never turn your back on the disturbed patient or leave him or her alone. If the patient has a knife or gun, stay clear: you do not want to become a casualty yourself. Do not attempt to deal with the disturbed, armed patient until he or she has been disarmed. Do not try to disarm the patient yourself. This is a job for the police.

3. Take charge. Establish yourself as the health care professional who is responsible for helping the patient. Act confidently and decisively. Your mood, your spoken and nonspoken communication to the patient, will go a long way toward beginning effective treatment.

4. Provide proper emergency medical care. If the patient has sustained an injury, self-inflicted or otherwise, carry out the appropriate emergency medical care as soon as it is safe for you to do so, and your own personal risk is minimal. Explain to the patient what you are doing to him or her.

5. Report the patient's behavior as accurately as possible. Is he **lucid** (alert and oriented and thinking clearly)? Calm or agitated? Frightened? Is there evidence of alcohol or drug use? Report these observations to medical control. Rarely will you be able to make a specific diagnosis. It is often difficult to distinguish between such diseases as organic brain syndrome and psychiatric illness. One important exception to this point is the diabetic patient in insulin shock. You must determine promptly whether the disruptive patient has diabetes or another metabolic disease that may be causing the abnormal behavior. These patients require prompt medical treatment.

6. Avoid expressing accusations and anger at a disruptive patient. These patients are frightened, and, to them, their fright is a real concern and has a real basis. Do not try to judge the patient's actions or lecture the person about substance abuse. Remember, this frightened patient is ill, and your re-

sponsibility is to provide emergency care and transport to a treatment facility.

7. Be careful about "labeling" a disturbed, disruptive patient. Do not use terms like "crazy" or "drunk," or, if the patient's symptoms seem minor, "a crock." Avoid labeling a patient as someone who is **malingering** (faking illness). That determination is often very difficult to make, even by experienced people. It is far better to be "taken in" by someone who fakes an illness than it is to deny treatment to someone who has a legitimate complaint but appears to be malingering. Assume that the patient's complaints are genuine. True malingering is rare.

There may be times when a patient simply cannot be approached; the person won't let anyone near and refuses to go to the hospital, despite all efforts to explain that you want to help, and that no one is going to hurt him or her. Sometimes family, neighbors, or friends will insist that a disturbed patient be taken to the hospital. You cannot do this unless you are ordered to by the police or another law enforcement agency. Furthermore, in most areas you cannot physically restrain a patient without police direction. Know your local laws regarding restraints. If you must restrain someone, get help. Frightened, agitated, disruptive pa-

tients may be capable of causing serious injury to you, to bystanders, or to themselves. When restraints are required, use soft, wide leather or cloth restraints, not police-type handcuffs (Figure 44–2).

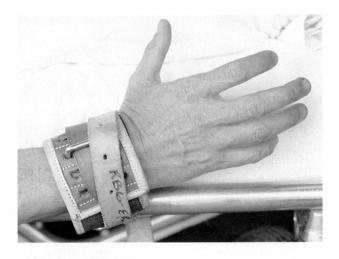

FIGURE 44–2

Soft, wide leather or padded cloth restraints—not police-type handcuffs—should be used when disruptive patients have to be restrained.

YOU ARE THE EMT

1. What is meant by the term *patronizing* a patient? Give an example of a patronizing statement and rewrite it so that it is no longer patronizing.
2. Your patient is a woman in her sixties who is deaf. She fainted while standing in line at the local supermarket. Write out 10 questions you would ask her. Keep the questions as short as possible and write them so that she can answer in one or two words.
3. Your patient is a 6-year-old boy who was struck by a car while chasing a ball into the street. He was not severely injured but has bleeding lacerations on his face and arms. You need to transport him, but his parents are not home. He is hysterical because of all the blood and because you have told him you have to take him to the hospital. How will you reassure him and how will you select someone from the neighborhood to ride in the ambulance if you feel that is necessary?
4. You have been called to treat a man who is exhibiting disruptive behavior. Identify three causes other than alcohol or drugs that might cause disruptive behavior and indicate how you might determine if this patient is suffering from any of these problems.

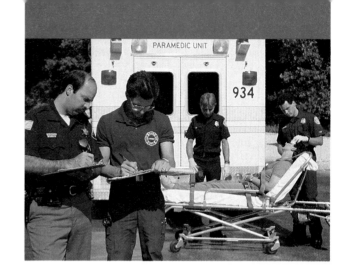

CHAPTER 45

CRISIS INTERVENTION

KEY TERMS

chain of evidence A protocol used by law enforcement agencies to collect and preserve evidence of a crime.

crisis A state of emotional confusion often caused by a sudden stressful situation, which the patient sees as causing a crucial turning point in his or her life.

Critical Incident Stress Debriefing (CISD) A program designed to help emergency medical personnel cope with the psychological reactions to stressful job-related incidents.

decapitation (de-kap″ĭ-ta′shun) Cutting off of the head.

decomposition (de″kom-po-zish′un) The gradual decaying of the body that follows death.

DNR (do not resuscitate) order A document by a patient or family that gives medical personnel permission not to attempt resuscitation in case of cardiac arrest.

dying declaration A statement made by someone who knows he or she is dying, which can be accepted as a legal document in a court; often a confession or revelation of a long-held secret.

exsanguinate (eks-sang′gwĭ-nāt) To bleed to death.

failure to thrive The failure of a child to grow and develop normally, frequently a sign of abuse.

lividity (lĭ-vid′ĭ-te) Discoloration of dependent body parts, by the gravitation of the blood.

rigor mortis (rig′or mor′tis) The stiffening of the entire body that follows death.

OVERVIEW

A crisis is a state of emotional confusion or turmoil that may develop suddenly or over a long period of time. It may be precipitated by a sudden, stressful situation that the patient sees as causing a crucial or critical turning point in his or her life. Any emergency medical situation, whether sickness or injury, may become a crisis in the patient's mind.

You may not think of a specific problem as a crisis, but if the patient thinks it is a crisis, you should manage it as a crisis.

Chapter 45 examines certain specific emergencies that are considered crisis events: sudden death; terminal illness; assault; rape; abuse of a child, elderly person or spouse; suicide; and SIDS (sudden infant death syndrome). Each crisis is discussed in terms of what you are likely to find when responding to such an emergency and how it should be managed. Throughout the chapter, the focus is on how you should be sympathetic to the patient and the problem while remaining objective and professional in your own behavior, and at all times being aware of steps for your own protection. The last section of Chapter 45 talks about the stress that crisis intervention puts on you, how to recognize and handle it; the chapter concludes by de-scribing the concept of Critical Incident Stress Debriefing (CISD).

GOALS

The goals of Chapter 45 are to
- learn how to face sudden and unexpected death.
- know how to provide care for the terminally ill patient and emotional support for the family.
- learn how to treat assaulted or abused patients of all ages and be aware of the additional responsibility of helping the police in these criminal cases.
- recognize the signs of child abuse and how to respond when faced with a possible child abuse case.
- realize that all suicide threats must be taken seriously, even after "arriving at the scene in time."
- learn how to cope with sudden infant death syndrome (SIDS).
- identify the signs and symptoms of chronic stress in an EMT, the sources of treatment, and the benefits of prompt treatment.
- understand the principles of Critical Incident Stress Debriefing (CISD).

SUDDEN DEATH CRISIS

Responding to a Sudden Death

Frequently, you are called to the scene of sudden and unexpected death. The causes of sudden death are many: trauma, myocardial infarction (heart attack), cerebrovascular acci-dent (stroke), sudden infant death syndrome (SIDS), suicide, and homicide are a few. Often, the patient will not have been previously ill or in any danger, and the death will come as a great shock to everyone.

As you arrive at the scene of sudden death, you must be prepared for a number of reactions from the patient's family and friends. A wide range of responses to sudden death can occur, especially from severely anxious and agitated family members. Remarks such as "He was never sick a day in his life" or "I warned him not to go out today" may be looked at as a family's way of coping with something that they do not understand.

Common, general emotional responses to sudden death include denial ("It can't be happening; I know he's going to be all right"); guilt ("It's my fault that I bought him that motorcycle" or "I knew I should have stayed home with her today"); obvious grief (hysterical sobbing, weeping, wringing of hands); and hostility and anger—to others, to the dead person, and to you ("Why did he have to go and do this?" or "If you had gotten here sooner, he wouldn't be dead," or "It's her fault; she drove him to it").

Sometimes the responses will come rapidly, one after another, and various people will demonstrate different types of responses. Occasionally, a person will withdraw and not show any response. This person might experience a delayed response, however, particularly if he or she appears unusually calm. Responses to sudden death are sometimes physical—that is, a person may feel faint, dizzy, or nauseated, and even have to vomit. The important thing to remember is that some type of emotional or physical response is a normal part of the grief that follows sudden and unexpected death.

Emergency medical personnel, including you and other EMTs, may experience some of these responses as well. You may feel helpless or frustrated because providing further medical care will not do any good. You may experience guilt ("Maybe if I had driven the ambulance faster. . ."), or anger ("What a stupid thing to do, driving his motorcycle into that truck. Now, I have to deal with his family"). You may even use avoidance or denial as a subconscious means of coping with these situations, such as wanting to leave the scene quickly, hoping that the memory will go away.

In an attempt to avoid the emotional impact of the situation, some EMTs may become "hyperclinical," discussing in great detail the medical and technical aspects of the problem with other medical personnel. A few may even

respond by making "sick jokes" about the situation or even about the people involved. Sometimes EMTs experience recurring memories of the tragic events surrounding sudden death and have nightmares or difficulty sleeping. All of these responses are normal and should lessen and end with time. You must acknowledge that these responses do accompany sudden death and be prepared to cope with them. The management of any of these responses that are long-lasting is discussed in more detail later in this chapter.

Management of Sudden Death

Only a licensed physician can legally pronounce a person dead—you, the EMT, cannot. The conclusive signs of death are **lividity, rigor mortis, decapitation,** or **decomposition** (see Chapter 5). If there is any doubt that the person is dead, you should initiate full resuscitation. Even if you are certain that the person is dead but the family feels "something has to be done," you should institute resuscitation. Understand that once you start resuscitation, you should not stop until a physician directs you to or the patient recovers.

When the person is obviously dead, you should turn your attention to the family and friends. Once again, you must be aware of and be prepared for the many and various responses these people may demonstrate. Keep the family informed of what is being done. Close relatives or friends may be allowed to see the body if they desire, unless there has been obvious mutilation. You should never raise false hopes. For example, if resuscitation is started on someone who is almost certainly dead, do not tell the family that everything is going to be all right; simply state that you are doing everything you can.

When you are confronted with a sudden death **crisis,** you should communicate with the family in the following manner:

- Answer questions as truthfully as possible. If you do not know the answer to a question, say so.
- Give straight answers to all questions. Don't hide unpleasant facts.

- Report all information that you know to be true.
- Don't guess about the unknown.
- Respect the family's need for sympathy. If family members want to be near the victim or want to be alone, try to follow their wishes.
- Do not try to argue with someone who is in a denial phase. Denial is sometimes a useful protective reaction to give someone time to adjust to what has happened.
- Maintain a professional attitude at all times. Control your own feelings, demonstrate caring and concern for the victim and the family, and go about your business calmly and efficiently. If anger is directed at you, do not take it personally; do not fight back. However, if you are in obvious danger, you should back away to avoid further confrontation. Wait for more help and allow time for the situation to calm down.

TERMINAL DISEASE CRISIS

Responding to Terminal Disease

When you are called to a scene where someone is dying after a long illness, you must also be prepared for the emotional and psychological responses of the patient and the patient's family. Although this type of call is not always as emotionally charged as the scene of a sudden and unexpected death, impending death from terminal disease can present you with a challenge.

Often the patient has been suffering from cancer or some other chronic, fatal disease. Usually the patient is elderly, although younger patients can also die from cancer or some congenital abnormality or defect. Usually, terminally ill patients know or strongly suspect that they are about to die. Most experience these four phases of emotional response to their impending death:

1. Denial: This is often the first response to the news of a fatal illness. Refusing to believe the doctors or assuming that "I'm going to beat this thing" is a common reaction.

2. Anger: This often follows denial. The patient wonders and asks, "Why is this happening to me?" "What have I done to deserve this?" or "Why did you have to tell me?" A dying patient often has a hostile, angry attitude to anyone around, and even to him- or herself.

3. Depression: Perhaps this is the most obvious and a very common response to the situation. The patient has no further interest in anything. The patient "turns his face to the wall" and refuses to participate in the activities of life.

4. Acceptance: Ultimately, resignation is the response of most terminally ill patients. They come to accept the condition and try to go on as best they can for as long as they can.

These four responses usually occur in the sequence listed above but may come in any order, and more than one response may occur at the same time. The family usually goes through the same responses of denial, anger, depression, and acceptance. Family responses may vary from extremely hostile and demanding ("Do something! He's going to die!") to so accepting that they do not want any efforts at all to change the inevitable ("Let her die in peace"). Remember that, to the family, the death of a loved one, even when it is expected, is always a major traumatic event, and may mean a radical change in life style, particularly when the dying person will leave behind a widow, a widower, or young children.

You may very well experience the same feelings of helplessness and inadequacy that accompany the sudden death crisis. The sadness of the situation may be overwhelming, particularly if the dying patient is a young person. Again, defense mechanisms may take over, and you may find yourself resenting being called to see a patient for whom little or nothing can be done.

Management of Terminal Disease

There may be little to do for the terminally ill patient other than to be certain that he or she is as comfortable as possible. Try to determine whether the patient and the family are aware that death is approaching and whether they are prepared for it. If death seems near, you should tell the family, pointing out the signs (hypotension, unconsciousness, bradycardia) that indicate the seriousness of the patient's condition. If you cannot determine the patient's status, you should tell the family so.

Do not separate the patient from the family. Keep familiar faces and voices around the patient and allow the family to be close in the last moments. Encourage the family and patient to talk about the imminent death if they wish and allow all to maintain their dignity. In general, the patient should not die alone if there are family or friends nearby. The family may or may not want to take the patient to the hospital. You should encourage transport to the hospital, but remember that a patient cannot be transported to a hospital against his or her will. If the family members strongly oppose transport, you should respect their wishes. If the patient is going to be transported to the hospital, you should let one or two family members ride along in the ambulance. If the patient is not going to be transported, you should contact medical control for further specific directions for his or her care.

A patient may have a living will. It is a legal document in most states with specific instructions that the patient does not want to be resuscitated—a **DNR (do not resuscitate) order**—or to be kept alive by mechanical life support systems. The patient's wishes expressed in a living will should be respected. On occasion, a serious conflict or problem with a living will may arise. A family member may disagree with the will's intent ("Grandpa was senile when he wrote that—we want you to give him mouth-to-mouth respiration"); or the will itself may not be available. In such situations, you should contact medical control for advice. Know what your local and state laws are, and what your system's prearranged protocol calls for to deal with a living will. In general, you will be directed to follow the patient's wishes.

If a cardiac arrest occurs, you should institute resuscitation efforts unless a specific state or local protocol directs otherwise. In general,

only a written order by a physician will permit an EMT *not* to resuscitate someone who has undergone a witnessed cardiac arrest. You should be in close touch with medical control when you are at the scene of an imminent death, particularly when there is a living will that specifically requests DNR. A properly organized EMS system will have a specific protocol in place to deal with this, as with other crises.

Let the patient make any statements desired. Sometimes a patient who knows he or she is dying may want to share some long-held secret or other important information. The laws in most states recognize that a statement by someone who knows he or she is dying may be accepted as a legal document, as a sworn statement in a court of law (a **dying declaration**). Listen to these statements carefully and write them down, word for word, because they may become very important to someone in the future.

To summarize: Make the dying patient as physically comfortable as possible. Address any of his or her wishes and concerns fully so that the patient's last minutes can be passed in peace and dignity.

ASSAULT CRISIS

Responding to Assault

Assault is, unfortunately, one of the more common crimes committed in America today. Violence, not only in the inner cities but all over the United States, is increasing in volume and severity. People frequently try to settle arguments with fists, knives, or guns. People in all walks of life are assaulted and injured each day in a great variety of ways. It is likely that, no matter where you are working, you will be called to assist someone who has been injured by assault. A person may have been robbed and beaten because he found himself in a dangerous part of town; a well-dressed woman may have had her expensive car stolen by a thief who jumped in through the unlocked door and threw her out onto the street; a college student may have been shot by a robber when he refused to give up his wallet; or a drug dealer may have been assaulted by a user. None of these people, even ones who could have avoided being hurt, wanted or expected to be assaulted; nobody wants to become a victim, regardless of his or her life style or economic level. Do not attempt to lecture or pass judgement on any assault victim.

In dealing with people injured in assaults, you may find yourself treating the perpetrator of the assault as well as the victim. Treat all injured patients in the same way. Your job is not to judge them, but to provide the necessary emergency care and leave the rest up to the police and the courts.

In criminal assault the police and other law enforcement agencies will become involved. Part of your responsibility, in addition to providing emergency care and transportation, is to cooperate with the law enforcement agencies (Figure 45–1). Many individuals who are responsible for a serious injury from criminal assault go free because there is not enough evidence to convict them of the crime. Sometimes critical evidence was present but was destroyed during the emergency care of the victim. Always bear in mind that in any criminal act, your personal testimony may be required in a court of law. That testimony may be an important factor in convicting a criminal or freeing an innocent person.

Assault victims may demonstrate any, or all, of several responses. The emotional damage done to a person who has been assaulted may be worse than the actual physical injuries that he or she suffers. No one believes that he or she personally will become a crime victim. Despite the wide publicity given to crimes of violence today, most of us believe "it can't happen to me." Therefore, the first reaction to a crime of violence is often disbelief. Be prepared for this response and help the victim accept the reality of the situation. Do not argue with the victim about the specific circumstances of the event. When questioned about specific details, always be truthful. Confirm or support only those facts of which you are certain.

In addition to disbelief, anger or outrage is a very common reaction of the victim. Sometimes this anger is directed at you; the police; the government; or anyone else, including the person who caused the injury. Allow the victim to talk as a way to "ventilate" some of this anger. Anger is part of the natural reaction to this particularly stressful situation. If it is directed at you, you must not take it personally. Remember, that anger can be "catching." Do nothing to further anger the victim. Do not add fuel to the fire.

FIGURE 45–1

When responding to an assault crisis, you must carry out the necessary emergency care, and assist law enforcement officers to maintain the chain of evidence.

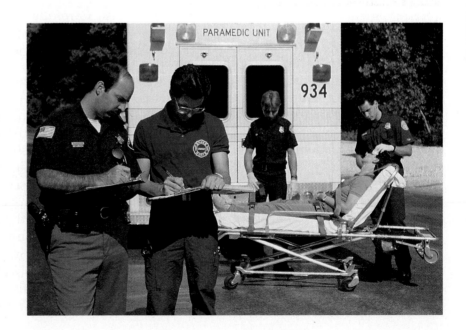

Withdrawal or depression is another common response. The victim may say little, appear not to care, or not want anyone near. This patient needs to be convinced that you are there to help. If you are able to calmly and professionally convey a genuine desire to provide care and support, you will often be successful in getting the victim to communicate. If you cannot obtain an accurate or complete history from the patient, you should obtain information about the event from relatives, friends, or witnesses.

Hysteria is another common reaction of a victim following assault. The patient may be screaming, crying, talking in unintelligible sentences, pacing, and refusing all attempts of help. Try to calm the patient and "talk the patient down," as when dealing with someone with a drug overdose (see Chapter 36). Often the right friend or family member can assist in calming the patient. You cannot forcibly restrain or transport anyone without a police order. Medical care cannot be forced on an adult patient who refuses treatment.

Guilt, the victim's feeling that somehow the victim is him- or herself responsible for what has happened, often occurs. You can best handle this situation by being professional. Never attempt to place blame, or judge the persons involved. A sympathetic, understanding manner on your part will help to start the patient's emotional recovery.

Management of an Assault Victim

The victim of an assault may have obvious injuries. Treat these using the standard emergency techniques. Gunshot wounds, particularly to the head or trunk, may be life-threatening, and you must evaluate, stabilize, and transport these patients rapidly. Patients who are not as seriously injured must be handled very carefully. Introduce yourself to the patient, explaining that you are there to help. Inform the victim of what you are doing and why. Stay calm, particularly if the patient is very upset. Maintain your professional manner. Listen to the victim. If the victim wants or does not want to talk, abide by his or her wishes. Above all, do not judge or lecture the victim, but let the patient know you are there to help. Conduct a thorough evaluation, stabilize all injuries and transport the patient promptly as you would with any other injured patient. Allow a friend or relative to accompany you in the ambulance if the patient so wishes.

If you are called to a scene of a crime and the crime is still in progress, stay out of the area until it is secured by law enforcement personnel. You are of no use to an assaulted person if you yourself become a victim.

Obtaining pertinent evidence is another important responsibility that you have in assault cases. Physical evidence of injury will be very critical to effective prosecution if legal remedies are sought. Although law enforcement agencies are ultimately responsible for collecting the physical evidence, you can be of significant assistance. You should maintain the **chain of evidence,** which means carrying out the following protocol:

1. Do not move or touch anything at the scene unless it is necessary to do so for medical reasons.
2. Avoid touching or disturbing any item that might have been used as a weapon (knife, gun, broken bottle, or other implement).
3. Note whether the patient's clothing has been torn, especially when it is necessary to cut away clothing to provide care for an injury.
4. Carefully note all injury sites.
5. Record a specific and complete list of injuries when more than one exists.

Your written record of observations and treatment may be used in court at some future date to document the extent of injuries. Therefore, you must carefully record all observations, the results of the patient examination, and a specific description of the treatment given at the scene. Record word for word, in quotation marks, any statements made by the patient. Months or years after the incident, a detailed, accurate written record will be of far greater value in court than vague recollections. You should always cooperate to the full extent with law enforcement officials at the scene. While your first priority is to provide medical care, you also have a responsibility to maintain the chain of evidence and to remain aware of the legal implications in any criminal action.

Rape Crisis

Rape is a particularly difficult form of assault to manage. Victims of rape require significant emotional support in addition to the kind of care that other assault victims receive. Male EMTs should obtain the assistance of a female EMT or police officer to assist in the care of a rape patient. Look for and carefully record any objective evidence of assault such as torn clothing, bruises (often about the head and face), and other injuries. Do not examine the patient's genitalia unless there is obvious bleeding that requires a sterile dressing.

Treat the female rape patient gently and professionally. Never criticize or condemn her, especially with comments such as "Don't you know that's a tough area?" or "What else could you expect, dressed like that?"

Rape victims will demonstrate the same variety of responses that other assault victims show. Most EMS systems have an established protocol for treating rape victims, which includes professional counseling as well as physician care. Use this service and consult medical control for advice on how best to manage these common reactions.

An established rape protocol includes directions about how to preserve the necessary evidence to prove that a rape took place. You must work closely with local law enforcement agencies to maintain the chain of evidence. Make sure that the rape victim does not bathe, urinate or douche before being examined at the hospital. If the vaginal area is not cleaned, the chances of recovering sperm are increased. The recovered sperm can be analyzed and used later as evidence of rape in a court of law.

All patients who have been raped or claim to have been raped should be evaluated by a physician in the emergency department. During transport, you should provide comfort and emotional support. If a friend or family member is nearby, have him or her accompany the victim in the ambulance.

Occasionally, you will be called to assist someone who has been the victim of a homosexual assault. Your approach to this person should be exactly the same as to any other victim of sexual assault. Do not try to judge or condemn the victim because of what you think may be his or her life style. In all cases of assault, you and all other health care professionals, run the danger of making it appear that the victim himself or herself is to blame. This attitude only increases the victim's feelings of guilt and helplessness and delays ultimate recovery.

ABUSE CRISIS

Abuse is another crisis that you, as an EMT, will encounter. Unlike assault, which is usually obvious, abuse may not be obvious at all. The victim may give no history of abuse and the injuries, at first glance, may appear to have resulted from an accidental injury. The exact incidence of abuse as a cause of injury is not known, but it is far more frequent than commonly thought. It is estimated that more than 1.5 million children, 1.8 million women, and over 1 million elderly people are the victims of abuse annually in the United States. Abuse is a crime. Thus, law enforcement agencies must and will become involved with the problem.

Abuse may take many forms—beatings, burns, neglect, or even attempted murder. Anyone may be the victim of abuse, although it is seen most often in children, women (often pregnant), and the elderly. It is particularly common in families and among people who live together. Abuse may even be "passed down" in a family from one generation to the next. People who cause abuse were often themselves abused as children.

The abused patient may have multiple bruises—evidence of beating, fractures, rope burns, or even cigarette burns. Or, the patient may show obvious signs of neglect such as dirty, unwashed clothes or lack of nourishment. The history often may be inconsistent with the victim's appearance ("Grandpa fell down the stairs"). The victim frequently will not tell you the truth about what happened, either. He or she may be too overwhelmed by the event or frightened of further abuse. A history of multiple calls to the same location for "falls" or other "accidents" should alert you to the possibility of abuse.

MANAGEMENT OF ABUSE

Regardless of the cause of abuse, your responsibilities are to provide proper emergency care, transport the patient to the hospital, and make sure the police can obtain the necessary evidence about the case. If the victim is unconscious, pay particular attention to maintaining the airway especially if the patient has been beaten about the head or face. Examine the patient carefully for rib fractures and blunt abdominal injuries. Dress and splint all wounds and limb injuries. Place the patient on a spine board. Transport the patient promptly. The patient may resist being transported to the emergency department, for a number of reasons. Remember that you cannot transport an adult patient against his or her will. However, when you suspect abuse, it is important to remove the patient from the environment. Persistent, gentle persuasion will usually allow you to convince the patient of the need for hospital evaluation.

Abused people will show the same kinds of emotional reactions as victims of assault. The same professional attitude on your part—concern for the victim and no attempt to judge or lecture—is a necessary part of your emergency care. The emotional scars of abuse, like assault, will remain long after the patient's injuries have healed. Assault or abuse victims will remember whether they were treated kindly, sympathetically, and compassionately by emergency service personnel.

Responding to Child Abuse

Child abuse was once believed to occur rarely and then only in lower-income families and broken homes. Now, estimates are that more than 10 percent of all pediatric patients seen in emergency rooms are victims of child abuse.

Child abuse is not always identified and reported for what it is. Although estimates of the incidence of child abuse in the United States run from 500,000 to 4 million per year, perhaps less than 10 percent of that number are actually reported or identified as such. Some 5,000 children die each year from child abuse. Child abuse is the only cause of death in children that has increased in incidence over the last 30 years.

Child abuse occurs at all social and economic levels and in various kinds of family structures. Child abuse may be caused by a parent; an older brother or sister; a baby-sitter; or an acquaintance of a parent, particularly a single parent. Some cases of child abuse are obvious, and some are not. Child abuse is often progressive; the child is abused with greater and greater severity over a period of time and ultimately can die from the injuries.

Child abuse is generally divided into four categories: physical abuse, emotional abuse, sexual abuse, and neglect. Physical abuse includes such actions as beating, burning (often with a lighted cigarette), and immersion in hot water. Sexual abuse (child molestation) can occur in boys and girls. Neglect (abandonment) may occur through inadequate provision of food or clothing. A combination of these abuses can prevent a child from gaining weight or growing properly, a condition described in medical terminology as the **failure to thrive.**

You should suspect child abuse if any of the following circumstances exist:

- If the history given does not fit the injury. For example, a fall from a chair will usually not be enough of an injury to cause a fracture of a femur in an otherwise normal child. Nor will that same "fall" produce multiple contusions on a child's body.
- If the history is vague or the person or persons who give the history say they didn't see the accident.
- If the child is obviously malnourished.
- If the child admits to having been beaten.
- If the child is withdrawn or refuses to tell what happened.

- If the child has multiple injuries that have occurred at different times, such as old bruises or healing burns in a child with a fresh injury (Figure 45–2).
- If the child has unusual wounds, such as cigarette burns, particularly about the genitalia.
- If you or one of your partners has been called to the same address before for injuries to the same child.

Management of Child Abuse

If you suspect child abuse, try to convince the parent (or whoever called the emergency medical service) that the child should be taken to the hospital. You can tell the parent or caretaker that a more thorough examination is necessary to provide better care for the child. You can suggest that the child may have a severe injury that can only be diagnosed in the hospital. However, you should never accuse anyone of child abuse. A calm and professional approach must be maintained at all times, although this is one time when doing so will be particularly difficult for you.

The first step in the treatment of child abuse is to remove the child from the environment that is producing the abuse. Therefore, with a case of suspected child abuse, you should transport the child to the hospital regardless of the apparent severity of the injuries. Hospital personnel can, if necessary, get a court order to admit the child. You cannot transport the child to a hospital against the wishes of the parent or legal guardian, regardless of how serious the injuries may be or how convinced you may be that the child is a victim of child abuse. If the parent or guardian refuses to allow transport of the child, you should stress the need for hospital evaluation for a potentially life-threatening injury. By emphasizing the need for X rays, "blood tests," and other hospital studies to rule out serious injury, an alert EMT can frequently convince a responsible adult to consent to transport. Certain x-ray findings, showing multiple fractures in different stages of healing, are characteristic of child abuse.

You are legally required to report all cases of suspected child abuse, whether the child was transported to the hospital or not, to the proper authorities. Any suspicion of abuse should always be reported to medical control. The law in every state requires all health care professionals to report suspected child abuse. The law also protects those who do report suspected child abuse from being sued by the person(s) whom they report. When the family refuses to allow you to transport the child to the hospital, the hospital personnel will contact the police or the local department of human services to investigate. Child abuse is a serious crime that could result in placement of the child in a foster home if the judge believes that child abuse has occurred. People convicted of child abuse face severe punishment.

Dealing with suspected child abuse can be a very difficult emotional experience for you. Perhaps the hardest part is keeping a calm, professional manner and avoiding judging or accusing anyone of child abuse. Such accusations must come from the law enforcement agencies and the courts.

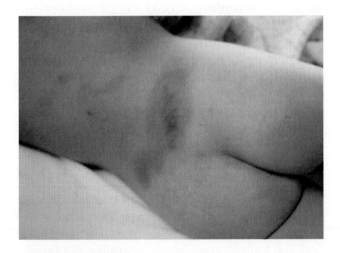

FIGURE 45–2

Old skin burns and multiple bruises that are apparent at the time of a fresh injury are signs that the patient may be an abused child.

Responding to a Suicide Attempt

Not all suicide attempts are fatal; nevertheless, suicide is a significant cause of death in the

United States. You may be called to the scene of a suicide attempt by a family member, a friend, or even by the patient. As with other crises, your first responsibility is to provide the necessary emergency care. In addition, you must deal with several special problems and considerations.

Some suicide attempts are serious—the patient would have succeeded except for some unforeseen event occurring. Others are gestures—a plea for help in which the patient did not actually intend to commit suicide. You will not be able to distinguish between a "gesture" for help and a serious suicide attempt that has failed. Therefore, you must assume that all suicide attempts are serious attempts. Someone who has tried suicide will try it again if given the chance. Do not provide that chance.

Most patients who attempt suicide have a severe psychiatric illness. Many are suffering from alcoholism or depression. Some people attempt suicide while under the influence of drugs. For many people, the underlying disease is treatable, and with proper treatment the patient will no longer be suicidal. However, until that treatment is carried out, you must assume that the patient remains suicidal and will try again. Even if the call for help has come from the patient himself, you should not assume the threat has passed and that he has given up on the idea of suicide. Once you have arrived at the scene of an attempted suicide, never turn away from the patient or leave the patient alone, even for a few seconds.

Management of Attempted Suicide

Patients may attempt suicide by ingesting poison, shooting themselves, jumping from a height, jumping in front of a speeding car or train, crashing their car at high speed, cutting their wrists or neck, or hanging, among other common methods. When you are called to the scene of a suicide attempt, find out how it was attempted. If the person swallowed a bottle of pills, examine the bottle. Most of the time, it will contain a narcotic, a sedative, or a tranquilizer that may have been prescribed by a physician or bought over the counter.

Be prepared to begin cardiopulmonary resuscitation, administer oxygen, and maintain the airway. The person may have serious injuries. For example, jumping from a height may have caused a spine fracture that will require moving the patient on a spine board. Splint obvious or suspected fractures, and dress obvious wounds.

Another problem occurs if the patient attempted suicide by more than one means—maybe swallowing a bottle of sedatives and then jumping out the window. Unconsciousness may be from a head injury or the sedatives or *both*. Patients who cut their wrists rarely **exsanguinate** (bleed to death) because the vessels involved are not that large. Often, however, they will have severely injured the median or ulnar nerves. And victims of self-inflicted gunshot wounds to the head may not have suffered fatal brain injury, but instead have sustained massive facial bleeding and airway obstruction.

Suicide by automobile is an increasing problem. One estimate is that 30 percent of all single car crashes are suicide attempts. The clues to a suicide attempt are a single car hitting an obstacle at high speed, absence of skid marks, and failure to wear a safety belt. Of course, these same findings could occur in someone who fell asleep at the wheel or suffered an AMI while driving. Your first priority in such a scene is to perform the proper emergency care procedures. If you do suspect that a vehicular crash was a suicide attempt, you must communicate your suspicions to medical control and to the hospital personnel.

The family of a suicide patient may need emotional support. Many ethnic groups consider suicide a sacrilege—something evil and against their religious beliefs. Be careful not to judge the victim, the family, or the victim's life style. A suicide attempt is often considered a "cry for help." You should reassure the family that suicide is not the fault of the family or friends.

SUDDEN INFANT DEATH SYNDROME (SIDS)

Sudden infant death syndrome (SIDS) is one of the most difficult crises you will ever be called on to manage. The death of a child, under any circumstances, is perhaps the greatest tragedy that can befall a family; parents never fully recover from the death of a child. SIDS occurs without warning in a healthy baby. The usual history is that the parents put the infant into the crib at night, and then find the baby unresponsive either later that night or the next morning. Approximately 7,000 infants, usually between the ages of 2 and 4 months of age, die each year this way.

If you are called to the scene of a SIDS crisis you will find very upset parents. However, you must focus on the infant. Often it is a good idea to begin resuscitation and transport the infant rapidly to the hospital, even if the infant appears to be dead. This response will assure the parents that everything possible has been done. However, if the baby is cold and stiff and has obviously been dead for several hours, resuscitation should not be undertaken. In that case, the family is usually aware that the baby is dead. However, if there is any doubt or the parents insist, you should go ahead with resuscitation efforts.

Be very careful not to raise the hopes of the parents; instead, keep them informed and reassured that everything possible is being done to revive the infant. It may be tempting to reassure the family that everything will be all right but if the infant is surely dead, then, sadly, everything will not be all right, and you cannot hide the eventual truth from the family. Therefore, any reassurance must be aimed at convincing the family that you are doing everything possible and that they will have to wait until hospital personnel can give a more definite statement. The parents usually want to ride in the ambulance with their baby, and they should be allowed to do so.

Sometimes you will not be sure whether the problem is SIDS or child abuse. There are several clues to distinguish these two prob-

lems. SIDS almost always occurs in infants between 2 and 4 months old, whereas child abuse can occur at any age. The characteristic feature of SIDS is that there are no marks on the infant, but an abused baby will usually have scars, bruises, or obvious deformities. A dead SIDS baby may have frothy sputum on the nose and mouth and dependent lividity (blood settling in the skin of the back or abdomen). In other words, the SIDS baby will show evidence of a quiet death, not a violent one. Any siblings are likely to be healthy appearing. An infant who has died from child abuse will look malnourished; so may the siblings. The typical history of SIDS is that the baby was perfectly healthy when put to bed. Your initial examination will support this: The baby looks like a normal, well-fed baby. On the other hand, the abused baby's family will often give a confused, unclear history that does not fit the infant's injuries or appearance.

Even if you are suspicious of child abuse, you should never accuse the parents. Instead, you need to extend to them sympathy for their tragedy and do all that is possible for the infant and the family. After bringing them to the hospital, however, you should report any suspicion of child abuse to the emergency department personnel. (SIDS and child abuse are also discussed in Chapter 38.)

THE EMT'S RESPONSE TO STRESS

In becoming an EMT, you have chosen a most stressful career. Life and death crises occur almost daily, and sometimes there is little you can do to alter the effects of serious illness or injury. Your work is fast paced and physically demanding; you work in a "pressure cooker." You may become emotionally involved with one or more of your patients and their problems. This is one of the more common difficulties in health care fields. It is natural and, of course, appropriate to care about the people you are helping. However, excessive emotional involvement will hinder your ability to carry out emergency care effectively and objectively.

At all times, you have to strive to keep a balance between sympathetic concern and emotional involvement.

Another problem that all EMTs and all EMS systems face following a life and death crisis is unfair and sometimes widely publicized criticism by a patient, the family, the community, the news media, or even by co-workers. It is very frustrating to be unable to reply to criticism that is based on inaccurate information or sensationalism.

The most difficult problem that will affect you is grief. Except in rare instances, repeated and prolonged contacts with grieving people will have an effect on you. Some of a family's grief will eventually rub off on you. The very nature of your responsibilities to the sick and injured prevents you from showing your true emotions; the "calm and professional manner" that you must maintain when you are handling a crisis prevents you from letting your own emotions of grief and sorrow show.

You are vulnerable to all the stresses that go with your profession. You must learn to recognize the symptoms of stress so that it does not interfere with your work or life away from work, including your family life. The signs and symptoms of chronic stress may not be obvious at first; they may be subtle and not present all of the time. The following may indicate a delayed grief reaction or the presence of excessive stress:

- An increase in stress-related physical complaints: headaches, gastrointestinal symptoms, and unexplained aches and pains.
- Anger and hostility—against your friends, the system, even patients.
- Feelings that life has lost its meaning; apathy, despair, or sadness; and lack of enthusiasm.
- Feelings characteristic of depression: chronic fatigue, difficulty sleeping, lack of concentration, loss of appetite, or even bouts of uncontrollable weeping.
- Periods of intense anxiety, even panic.
- Suicidal thoughts.
- Repeated thoughts about death, suffering, or pain.
- Nightmares.
- Alcohol and substance abuse.

- Flashbacks (vivid recollections) of severe accidents, tragedies, or incidents on the job.
- Loss of interest in family and in social activities.
- Desire to quit work.

Any of these symptoms may indicate chronic stress or delayed grieving. These symptoms are normal responses to the many daily stresses under which you work. You should recognize them as such and take steps to relieve their cause. Concerns should be discussed with co-workers, many of whom will have had similar experiences. Once you realize how common some of these symptoms are, such discussions may be enough to resolve the problem. However, persistent and severe symptoms may require professional guidance from a counselor within the EMS system, a physician, or a member of the clergy. Early recognition of chronic stress problems is most important, because a solution is much easier to achieve with early recognition. Persistent, untreated problems tend to get worse, making a solution much more difficult. Your EMS system should have a counseling program for this purpose. It should be confidential and easily available to anyone who needs it. Remember that the reaction to stress is normal, and common. With early recognition and counseling, you should be able to resume your normal functions and your normal efficiency and enthusiasm for your profession.

Critical Incident Stress Debriefing

After a particularly difficult incident, such as a mass casualty disaster, a particularly tragic death or group of deaths, an incident where you yourself narrowly escape death or serious injury, or any extraordinary situation, your reactions and those of other EMTs may be so severe that a special support service is needed. These special services are provided by the **Critical Incident Stress Debriefing (CISD)** program. This program provides a team of professionals, including EMTs, mental health specialists, and others with special training to handle the psychological reactions that commonly occur. A CISD program usually is started within 24 hours of the event and involves several steps to relieve the major stresses that you have undergone and prevent a major problem from occurring in the future. Most major EMS systems have a Critical Incident Stress Debriefing team, which can be activated rapidly as it is needed.

YOU ARE THE EMT

1. You are at the home of a terminally ill elderly woman. She is unconscious and is experiencing hypotension and bradycardia. Her husband wants to let her die in peace, in her own home. Her two daughters want their mother transported immediately. How will you proceed?

2. You are treating a woman who has been badly beaten by her husband or boyfriend—you are not sure what their relationship is. Prepare a written report of what you have observed. Include what is necessary to maintain the chain of evidence.

3. You suspect you are dealing with a serious child abuse case, and even though the toddler does not have life-threatening injuries, you want to transport him to the hospital. The parents "know you know" and are saying their child is fine and that you can go now. How can you convince them to let you transport the child?

4. You are called to assist a man who has been attacked by muggers, and resisted. In the course of the fighting, one of the muggers was hit in the head and now lies unconscious. The attack victim is alert and appears to have no injuries other than a bruised hand. What steps would you take, in what order, to carry out your mission of emergency care and transport?

5. Review the signs and symptoms of chronic stress. Choose one or two that you recognize as accompanying stressful situations in your life and describe how you know they relate to stress and what you do to relieve the problem.

PATIENT
HANDLING
AND
EXTRICATION

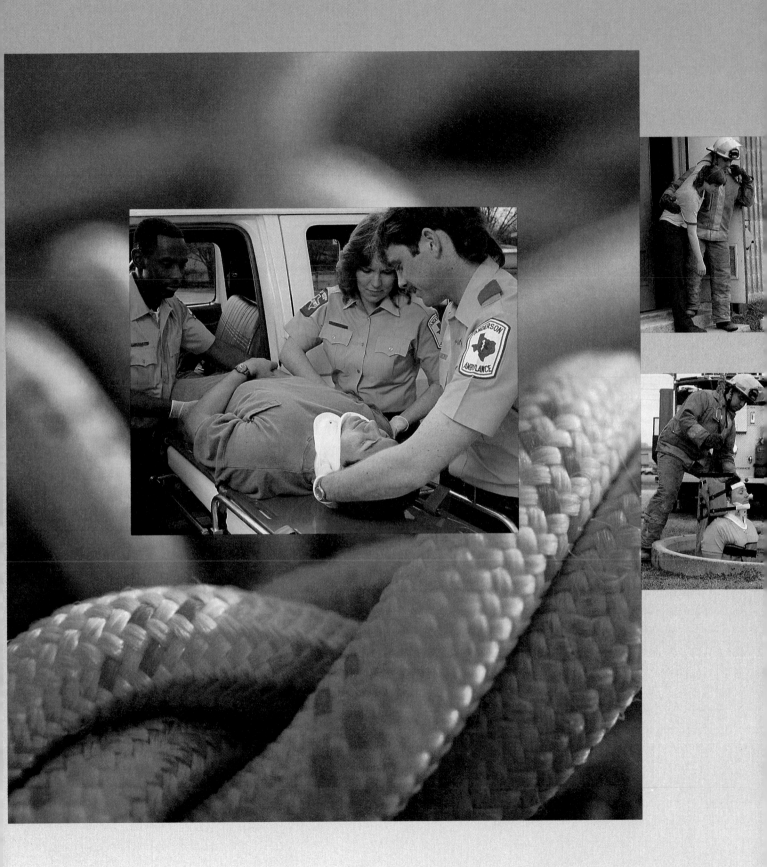

CHAPTER 46

PATIENT HANDLING AND TRIAGE

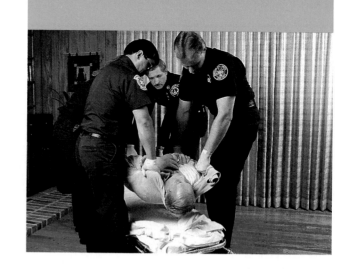

KEY TERMS

Critical Incident Stress Debriefing (CISD) A program designed to help emergency medical personnel cope with the psychological reactions to stressful job-related incidents.

disaster A human-caused or natural, sudden and serious disruption of life that causes or threatens injuries to a number of persons.

LAST An acronym for Locate, Access, Stabilize, and Transport; the four stages of the work phase of a disaster response.

Level One Trauma Center A medical center for severely injured patients.

packaging The positioning, covering, and securing of an ill or injured patient for transportation.

paraplegia (par"ah-ple'je-ah) Paralysis of the lower limbs.

quadriplegia (kwod"rĭ-ple'je-ah) Paralysis of all four limbs.

regionalized care Specific medical problems cared for at specialized centers.

START (Simple Triage And Rapid Treatment) A system of triage.

triage (tre-ahzh') Sorting. A technique of establishing treatment and transportation priorities in any event where the number of casualties is greater than the emergency facilities can handle.

OVERVIEW

The safe handling and extrication of patients, whether they are found on the street or highway, at home, or in the workplace, presents the EMT with a broad spectrum of challenges. The handling of patients falls into two general categories. The first is patients who are found in a readily accessible location. No matter how serious their injuries, they can be moved rather routinely from the home, building site, sidewalk, street, or wherever they are located. The second category is patients who must be extricated, or removed, from a location of difficult access, often with possible danger to the rescuer as well as to the patient. The patient's injuries may or may not be serious, but removing such patients from their precarious situations may require special techniques and tools of extrication (see Chapter 47).

Chapter 46 begins with the basics of handling patients with communicable diseases, violent patients, pediatric patients, geriatric patients, and handicapped patients. Then, the techniques of lifting and moving patients, transferring them to stretchers, and using specialized packaging techniques are described. The next section discusses ancillary patient-handling equipment, including spine boards and scoop stretchers. The last section of Chapter 46 concerns triage—the concept of sorting patients and allocating resources in a disaster.

GOALS

The goals of Chapter 46 are to

- understand the basics of patient handling and the specifics of handling patients with communicable diseases, violent patients, pediatric patients, geriatric patients, and handicapped patients.
- learn how to lift and move patients safely from one location to another.
- learn how to use a standard ambulance stretcher.
- become familiar with special patient packaging techniques and ancillary patient-handling equipment.
- understand the concept of triage and the duties of a triage officer.
- describe the components of the START triage system.

BASIC PATIENT HANDLING

After the safety of the patient and rescuer has been assured and the scene is "secured," your attention must be directed toward immediate life-threatening medical conditions. The patient's airway must be opened, breathing ensured, and major bleeding controlled. Although the procedures and protocols for the actual techniques of patient extrication and transfer have been relatively well defined (see Chapter 47), less attention has been paid to the medical aspects of vehicular space entrapment and extrication. In your zeal to free, treat, and transport the patient, do not forget the ABCs of basic life support once the safety of all concerned has been ensured. If advanced life support personnel are available, intravenous lines sometimes need to be placed prior to beginning extrication and transfer procedures. Carrying out emergency medical management procedures may be very difficult and sometimes impossible. In these situations you have to be creative in rendering emergency medical care, keeping in mind your duty to do no further harm.

After on-scene emergency medical care has been completed, the ill or injured patient must be transferred to a stretcher or other carrying device, positioned properly, covered as necessary, and securely strapped to the stretcher. This whole process is called **packaging** the patient. The stretcher or carrying device should be placed as close as possible to the patient before the transfer to minimize the distance the patient needs to be moved. Placing the patient on a long spine board or scoop stretcher will allow the easiest transfer to the ambulance stretcher, the emergency department stretcher, or an x-ray table, with minimal movement or risk of aggravating the patient's condition.

Except during the infrequent situations in which the life of the EMT or patient is in danger, movement of the ill or injured patient should be orderly, planned, and unhurried. This approach will protect the patient from further injury and reduce the risk of aggravating the original condition. For the most part, such movement will consist of transferring the patient from a bed, the floor, or the ground to an ambulance stretcher. The transfer should be carried out by at least two EMTs, with bystanders used for assistance only if absolutely necessary. These recruits must be instructed simply, but in detail, about their role before actual patient movement is carried out. Such movement involves lifting, lowering, pulling, and supporting both patient and equipment. If any of these tasks is conducted improperly, discomfort and additional injury may result to both the patient and rescuers.

One of the main goals in planning the transfer should be to eliminate or reduce the need for additional movement of the patient after the transfer is completed. The trauma patient should be placed on a long board or scoop stretcher with an antishock garment in place, ready to be applied (Figure 46–1).

The only time the patient should be moved prior to completion of the initial care, assessment, stabilization, and treatment is when the patient's or EMT's life is in immediate danger. This would be the case if the victim were in a burning building, toxic fumes were present, or

Transport any seriously injured patients on a spine board with an antishock garment in place ready for prompt application and inflation should the patient develop hypotension.

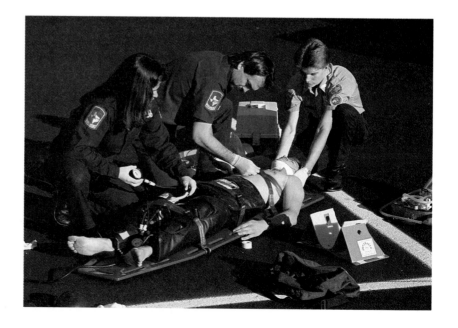

you were unable to administer the needed emergency medical care due to the location or position of the patient. The objective of every patient-handling situation is to ensure that the victim and the rescuer do not sustain additional injury during the rescue.

Patient packaging and handling are technical skills that are learned and perfected through practice and training. The only way you can be sure of using the best technique for a particular situation is to practice continually the various skills listed. After each patient transfer has been completed, you should evaluate the appropriateness of the actual techniques used as well as your technical skill in completing the techniques.

The overriding objective for each rescue/transfer is to complete it as safely and as efficiently as possible. As a rescuer, you must consider the use of your body and your skills. The outcome of a rescue is frequently determined by your ability to provide the needed care. Therefore, it is important for you to use good body mechanics; practice size-up, patient-packaging, and transportation skills; and understand safe versus risky patient transfer/transport techniques.

Handling Patients with Communicable Diseases

Health care workers are never immune from harm; selectively treating patients does not afford you any greater protection. When you are at the scene of an injury, there is always a threat to your personal safety; AIDS and hepatitis are common diseases. Therefore, you must take precautions at all times. Anything done infrequently is usually done poorly; tasks done often are usually done well. When there is any risk of contact with a patient's body fluids, use gloves, no matter how "inconvenient" it may seem. The basic universal precaution is to not expose your skin, eyes, or mucous membranes; therefore, always use gloves, goggles, and a mask when there is any risk of coming in contact with a patient's body fluids.

For emphasis and to dispel concerns due to lack of knowledge, some points in the handling of patients with communicable diseases previously covered in Chapter 35 are repeated here. Several guidelines apply when you care for potentially infected patients. The following steps should decrease the risk to you and to other patients you care for on subsequent rescue incidents:

- Use disposable, one-time-only equipment and supplies. Reusable equipment must be cleaned and disinfected after each use.
- Even though you wear gloves, thoroughly wash your hands after each patient contact. Friction and an antibacterial soap, such as a hexachlorophene soap, are excellent tools in decreasing the spread of germs.
- Dispose of all infected or contaminated items properly. Disposable items should be double-bagged and thrown away in an appropriate waste container. Wash reusable equipment, such as a bag-valve-mask, airway, scissors, splints, cervical collars, and cots, with a clean cloth and a disinfectant soap. Small equipment, such as the bag-valve itself, should be autoclaved. If mattresses or cots become contaminated, follow the washing with air/sun drying.
- Bathe yourself and launder all clothing after exposure to patients with a known communicable disease. At the end of each day, bathe all your body surface and change clothes even if exposure has not knowingly occurred. Wash clothing in hot, soapy water and dry it in a warm dryer. Wear a clean uniform each day.
- Maintain your own health at an optimum level, keeping immunizations up to date and participating regularly in an individualized exercise program.
- Handle contaminated needles with extreme care. Use specially designed disposal units for all sharp objects.
- Use a mechanical device whenever possible for respiratory assistance or resuscitation.

Whether or not you know in advance that a patient has a communicable disease, preventive universal precaution measures can, to a great extent, protect you and the ambulance from contamination. Precautions that you can take when transporting a patient known to have a communicable disease include the following:

1. Wear clean coveralls for the purpose of handling patients with known infections.
2. Wear a surgical mask and also place one on the patient.
3. Remove all but the needed basic equipment from the ambulance prior to the run.
4. Use disposable equipment whenever possible (for example, gloves and bed linen).
5. Isolate the patient by wrapping wounds in clean/sterile bandages and sheets.
6. On termination of the run, double-bag your coveralls and turn them in for decontamination. Clean and disinfect the ambulance. Shower immediately.

In view of the prevalence of some communicable diseases in the general population and in the patient groups often cared for by prehospital personnel, you must wear disposable gloves when there is a risk of coming in contact with the patient's body fluids and secretions, particularly blood, vomitus, and feces. Frequent handwashing should be a standard practice, particularly after you handle any patient or any equipment that has been used on or by a patient. All EMS systems should have medical policies and procedures relating to the protection of field personnel against disease. These should include recommended immunization levels, booster (reimmunization) intervals, postexposure precautions, and treatment recommendations for all EMTs who might have come in contact with an infected patient.

Handling Patients Who Are Violent

Rescue situations outside of a hospital environment contain many unforeseen possibilities that may endanger both the patient and you. You must be able to anticipate dealing with any situation and always be prepared for the violence. A patient who cannot be brought under control cannot be treated. An EMT who is injured cannot render treatment.

Not all violent patients are "drug crazed"; there are many reasons why a patient may be or become violent. Additionally, it is very difficult to determine the exact set of circumstances or combination of circumstances that caused the violence. Give special concern to patients with head injuries, alcoholic intoxication, and psychological problems as you determine your course of action. When such conditions are combined with physical injury, the potential for violence becomes even greater. If there is ever any question about your ability to bring a patient under control, send for help. In some instances a backup unit will suffice; in others, police agencies must be asked for help.

Handling Pediatric Patients

Children who require transport come in all sizes and shapes. Most are lighter than a typical adult, and most have smaller body parts. They are generally easier to move. Few are able to tell you much about how they feel or where they hurt, and most are usually frightened of strangers. Because of this fear, it is important to include parents in the care and transportation of children. The reassurance of a familiar face does wonders for increasing cooperation and safety when you deal with the pediatric patient. Sometimes the assessment routine must be changed slightly until you have gained the confidence of the child (Figure 46–2).

Because most transport equipment is designed for the adult-sized body, children need to be securely strapped on the stretcher and observed continuously, so that their safety is not compromised (Figure 46–3). Another important factor in handling children is the tendency for them to lose body heat rapidly due to their relatively larger body surface area. This means that the younger the child, the more rapidly you should cover the child as a protection against the elements. If it is extremely cold, putting a hat or cover on the child's head will help decrease loss of body heat.

Handling Geriatric Patients

The older patient often has special needs during transport. For example, many older

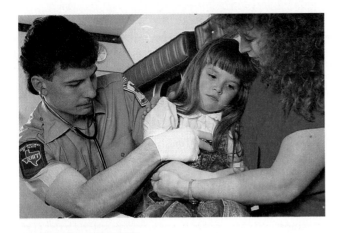

FIGURE 46–2

When you evaluate children, it is sometimes necessary to change the assessment routine because of the child's fear. Here the EMT is listening for breath sounds, leaving the child's shirt in place.

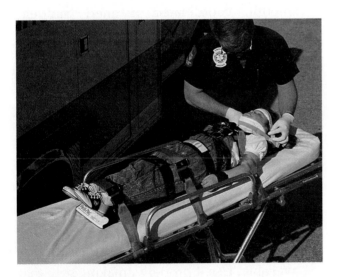

FIGURE 46–3

Children must be well secured to the stretcher designed to transport larger patients.

persons are very slow and deliberate in their movements. They may have decreased vision and hearing, along with slower general body movement. They are at greater risk for secondary injury. Older patients, especially women, frequently have osteoporosis, which causes their bones to be very brittle and easily fractured. You need to be aware of these limitations as you provide care and assistance. Also, you must remember to speak slowly, clearly, and directly to the older patient, carefully explaining everything that is being done. By maintaining a reassuring and calm attitude rather than one that is abrupt and impatient, you can care for the geriatric patient successfully.

Handling Handicapped Patients

Increasingly, more and more people with physical handicaps are living in the community. These people may be at increased risk for injury due to their decreased mobility. They must be handled with special care and all the protection available. Some may be at increased risk for pathologic fractures due to the handicap. The person who has muscle contractures or fused joints must be moved and stabilized in a position that suits and supports these deformities. This patient must be adequately restrained on the stretcher or in the wheelchair before being moved.

Patients with **quadriplegia** (paralysis of all four limbs) or **paraplegia** (paralysis of the lower limbs) have permanent paralysis and loss of feeling in the affected part of the body. These paralyzed limbs must be protected from injury and supported well during transfers. The paralyzed patient's wheelchair should be transported with the patient whenever possible.

Try to communicate using written messages, a word board, or signaling with pantomime with a patient who cannot speak or communicate normally. Talking slowly, simply, and directly toward this patient may also help. Handicapped patients deserve all the care and respect of any other injured patient, plus some special assistance. Deaf and non-English-speaking patients often have a relative or close friend who can act as an interpreter, using sign language or the patient's native tongue to communicate. Take special care to keep this individual near the patient at all times, and whenever possible, ask him or her to accompany the patient to the hospital.

LIFTING AND MOVING PATIENTS

Body Mechanics

Moving a patient from one location to another requires a definite plan. Just as you mentally organize for work each day, you need to have a strategy, thought out ahead of time, for packaging and transporting the patient. Part of the planning includes knowledge of your limitations and the availability of resources. Use assistive devices and equipment such as stretchers, blankets, straps, and splints, whenever possible. The rescue should be accomplished without undue risk or compromise to your health. Dead or injured EMTs cannot save lives. Among several elements you need to consider when you plan for the packaging and transfer of a patient are the following:

■ The patient's problem, including the actual and potential threats to the person's health and safety.

■ The environmental risks and limitations that may compromise the safety of the patient, you, or your fellow EMTs.

■ The availability of assistive equipment and/or emergency personnel at the scene.

■ Your own physical and technical capabilities and limitations, as well as those of your colleagues. If you have a weak or injured wrist, do not overstress the wrist and risk additional injury that could compromise the patient's safety.

When you actually perform a patient transfer, use the following principles of good lifting mechanics:

1. Only lift a patient whom you cannot roll, push, or pull.
2. Work with your limbs close to your body so that your center of gravity is not malaligned and your muscles are not overstressed.
3. Use the longest and strongest available muscle groups (biceps, quadriceps, and gluteals) to move patients. Maximum efficiency of contraction occurs when the muscle smoothly contracts at a moderate rate.

4. Flex your body at the knees and hips to keep your back straight when working below knuckle height. Try to avoid bending at the waist to lift.
5. Establish a firm support base by placing both feet flat on the ground, with one foot slightly in front of the other.
6. Distribute the patient's weight evenly over both of your feet.
7. Straighten your knees as you lift to help ensure that the major lifting forces will be provided by the thigh and buttocks muscles.
8. Hold your abdomen firm when you lift and tuck in the buttocks, keeping the shoulders aligned over the spine and pelvis.
9. Use pivoting movements rather than rotating or twisting actions when changing direction. Keep your shoulders square over your pelvis if possible.
10. Keep your head erect and move in a smooth, coordinated manner. Sudden, jerky movements tend to overstress muscles, resulting in injury.
11. Only lift weights you can comfortably handle. Weight maximums are individualized, based on age, sex, muscle mass, and condition.
12. Walk slowly, using coordinated movements. Steps should not be longer or wider than shoulder width when you carry a patient or stretcher.
13. Whenever possible, move forward rather than backward to facilitate normal balance and smoothness of movement.
14. Use assistive equipment whenever it is available. Use it properly, making sure that it is in good working order before you use it during a rescue.

The patient's transfer and transportation are not complete until the patient is safely delivered to the hospital. Restraining straps must be used and appropriately placed whenever you move the patient. All those helping to move the patient must know how the transfer is planned and what their specific duties are. When you help to lift and move a patient, a single leader should be designated to give commands and coordinate individual efforts. This coordination of movements will help to make patient transfer rapid and efficient.

After the patient is safely delivered to the emergency department, you must begin preparing for your next rescue effort. You should review the positive points that occurred during the transport. Then you should discuss adaptations or changes that would improve the management of the next patient. This review and evaluation process helps clarify procedures that need revision, identifies equipment that needs repair, and demonstrates skills that you need to review or acquire. Most important, a critical review assists in the development of more confident and better skilled EMTs.

Emergency One-Person Rescue Techniques

Only when prompt patient movement is necessary because of a life-threatening hazard and only one EMT is on the scene, should one-person rescue techniques for moving patients to a safe area be used. For example, you might have to act alone to remove a patient from a fire, a smoke-filled or contaminated area, or a building in danger of collapse. It must be emphasized that these are emergency transfer methods only. They are difficult and should not be used if there is time to obtain adequate assistance. You must also be aware that entrance to a hazardous environment such as a smoke-contaminated area requires protective equipment, including a self-contained breathing unit. EMTs should *not* attempt any hazardous environment rescue that poses a danger to themselves without proper training in the use of a self-contained breathing apparatus and protective equipment. Moreover, an incident scene is *not* the time or place for such training. The drag, carry, and lift techniques for one-person rescue are illustrated in Figures 46–4 through 46–10.

A

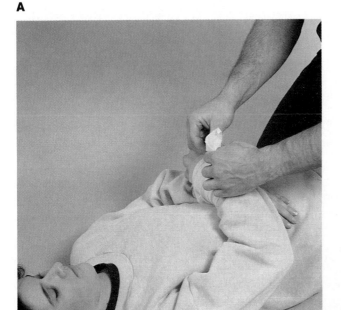

B

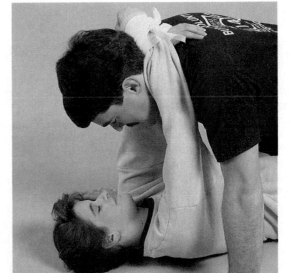

FIGURE 46–4　The firefighter's drag enables you to move a patient who is heavier than you are. (A) Tie the patient's wrists together with any available material: a cravat (a folded triangular bandage), gauze, belt, or necktie. (B) Next, get down on your hands and knees and straddle the patient. Put the patient's tied hands around your neck, straighten your arms, and drag the patient across the floor by crawling on your hands and knees.

FIGURE 46–5

The clothes drag. The rescuer must pull with the long axis of the patient's body. You can achieve the strongest pull using leg and back muscles and keeping your arms straight.

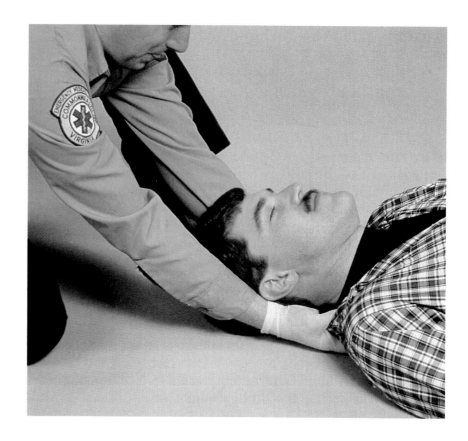

FIGURE 46–6

The blanket drag. The rescuer can reduce friction by using a blanket to drag the patient. The strongest pull is achieved using the leg and back muscles, keeping your arms straight. The blanket should encompass the body. It will provide some protection and support for the head, neck, and extremities.

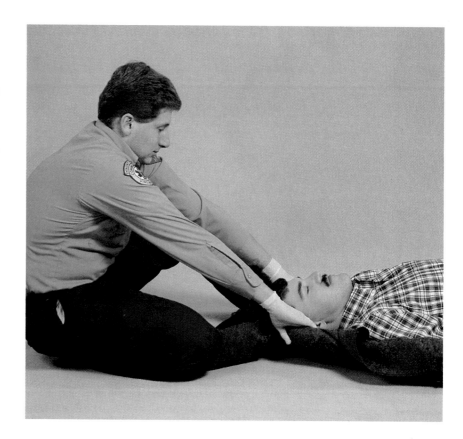

A

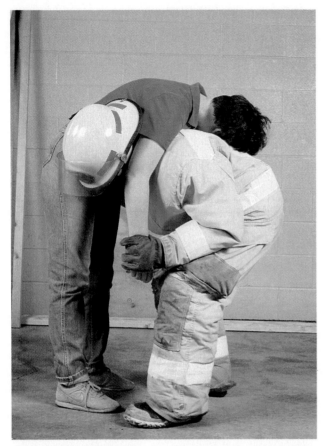

B

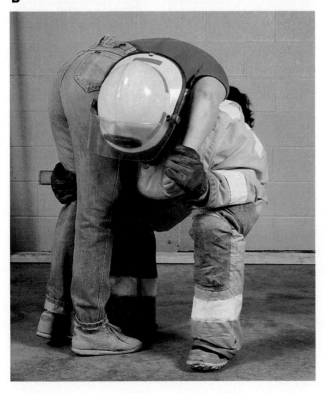

C

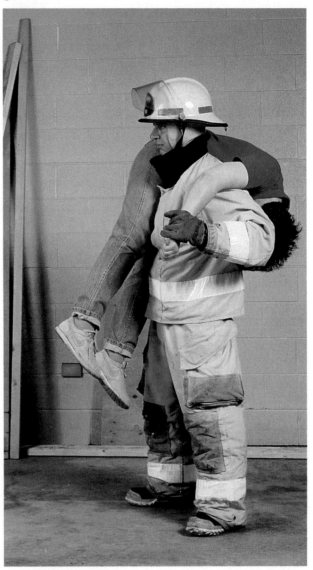

FIGURE 46–7

The firefighter's carry. (A) Balance and weight transfer are best achieved by drawing the patient's upper torso across the rescuer's shoulders. (B) At the same time, bend at the knees, to bring your hips under the patient's hips. (C) Lift with the legs, keeping your feet apart for stability. Be alert to loss of balance due to sudden weight shifts.

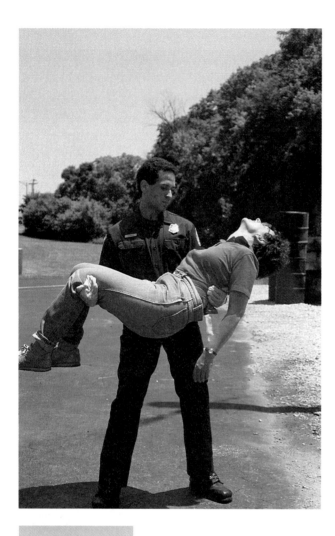

FIGURE 46–8

The front cradle. The rescuer bears considerable weight on his arms, shoulders, and back. The best balance and weight transfer is achieved by the rescuer bending at the hips and knees, using the legs for lifting. Leaning the patient's upper torso slightly back against the rescuer's arm may be helpful. Because the forward centered weight of the patient is in your arms, be careful to maintain your balance while moving with the patient.

A

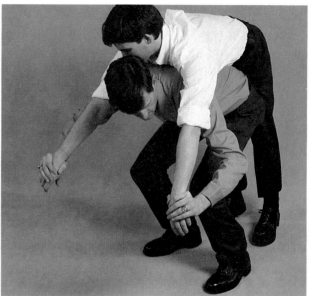

B

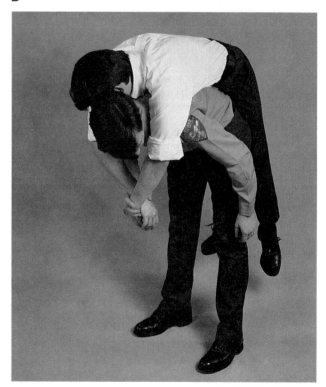

FIGURE 46–9

The pack strap. The rescuer bears the majority of the patient's weight along his spine, into his legs. (A) Weight transfer is best achieved by bending at your knees and hips and lifting with your legs. (B) Be alert to the position of the patient's legs to protect against tripping.

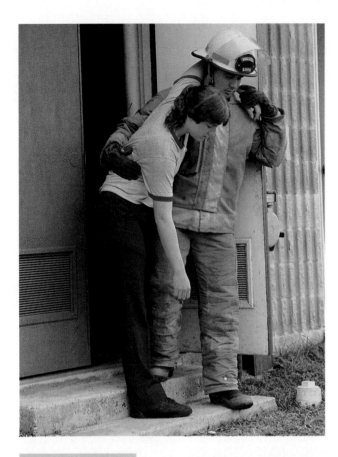

FIGURE 46-10

The one-person walking assist. The patient bears most of his or her own body weight. The rescuer supports a portion of the patient's weight only on demand. Be alert to the patient's loss of balance and subsequent sudden weight shift. Stand on the side opposite the injury.

A

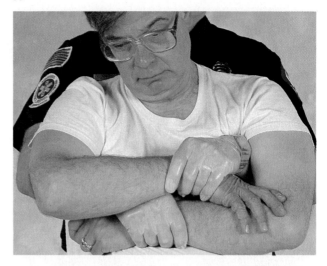

B

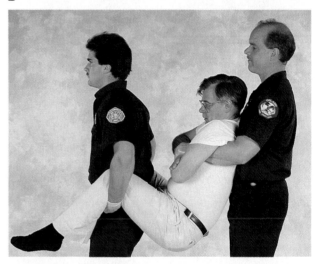

FIGURE 46-11

The extremity lift and carry. (A) Both rescuers must co-ordinate their movements through direct, verbal commands. The patient's hands should be crossed over his or her chest and grasped by the rescuer's arms coming through the axillae. (B) Balance and lifting are best achieved by the rescuers bending at their hips and knees, using their legs for lifting. The patient may experience a degree of discomfort in this position due to increased pressure against the thoracic cavity.

Emergency Two-Person Rescue Techniques

When two rescuers are available, both should work to remove the patient from danger using one of the techniques illustrated in Figures 46-11 through 46-13.

A

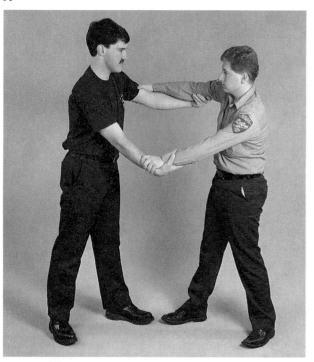

B

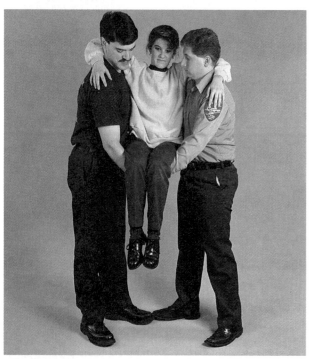

FIGURE 46–12

The seat (chair) lift and carry. (A) Two EMTs grasp each others' arms as illustrated. (B) Balance and lifting are accomplished by both rescuers bending at the hips and knees to use their legs for lifting.

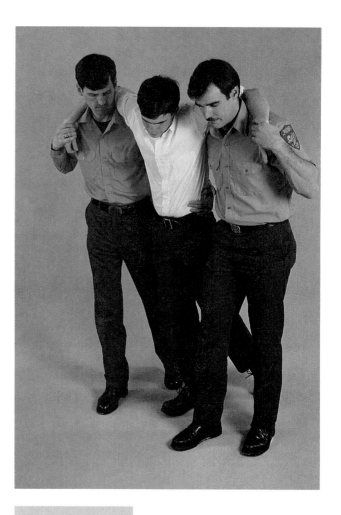

FIGURE 46–13

The two-person walking assist. The patient will bear a substantial portion of his or her own weight. The rescuers support a portion of the patient's weight on demand. The rescuers must be alert to the patient's loss of balance and sudden weight shift.

Patient Movement Under Stable Conditions

Figures 46–14 and 46–15 illustrate methods of moving patients when conditions are stable and adequate manpower can be recruited.

FIGURE 46–14

Log roll with no cervical injury. Coordination of movement during the log roll is achieved through direct, verbal commands. Positioning the hands on the far side of the patient increases leverage for the three rescuers. Weight control is best achieved through a smooth, coordinated pull using the rescuers' body weight and shoulder and back muscles to pull. The rescuers should concentrate their pull on the heavier portions of the patient's body.

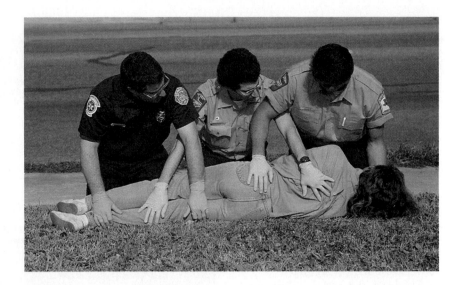

FIGURE 46–15

Log roll when cervical support is required. (A) In cases of suspected spine injuries, immediate gentle longitudinal support is applied to the cervical spine. (B) An extrication collar should be applied before the patient is moved. Cervical support must be maintained until the patient is secured on a spine board or equivalent, and the head and neck are stabilized and secured.
Continued

A

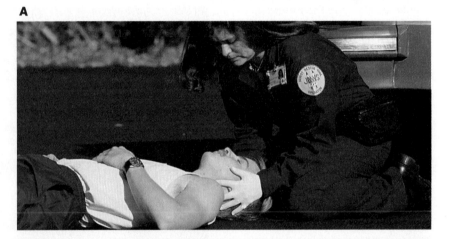

B

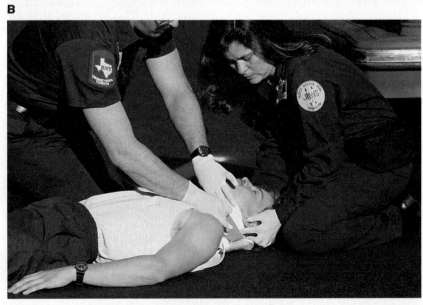

(C) The rescuer supporting the head and cervical spine is responsible for coordinating the log-roll procedure through direct, verbal commands. Positioning the hands on the far side of the patient increases leverage for the rescuers. Weight control is best achieved through a smooth, coordinated pull using the rescuers' body weight and shoulder and back muscles. The rescuers should concentrate pull on the heavier portions of the patient's body. The spine board is positioned as close as possible to the patient's body.(D) The patient is then slowly and gently rolled back onto the spine board and (E) secured.
(F) The head and neck are then secured to the spine board using foam blocks or a blanket roll. Straps may be placed over the forehead, but, to avoid airway management difficulties, should never be placed around the chin.

C

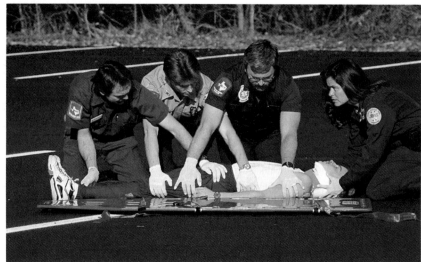

D

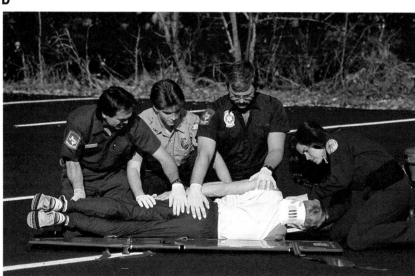

E

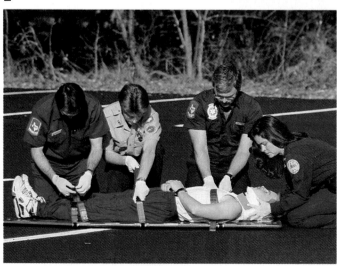

F

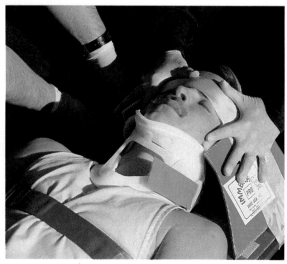

Stretchers

The standard ambulance stretcher has wheels and either a fixed or adjustable height. Attached handles are used for lifting and rolling. Side bars and restraint straps secure the patient. The stretcher should have a reasonably comfortable mattress. A good way to carry the short spine board is to place it beneath the mattress at the head of the stretcher. The board is then immediately available for extrication or for providing a firm surface on which to perform external cardiac compressions (when placed between the patient and the mattress). In medical emergencies such as angina or dyspnea, you generally will not have to remove the short board to allow the head of the stretcher to be elevated (Figure 46–16).

The techniques for transferring and lifting patients to the stretcher are illustrated in Figures 46–17 through 46–21. Figure 46–22 describes a chair-to-wheelchair transfer. The proper methods of lifting, moving, and loading stretchers are shown in Figures 46–23 through 46–27.

A

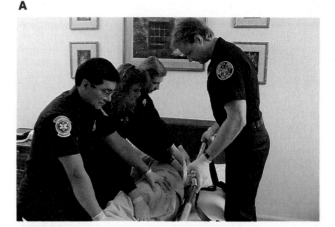

B

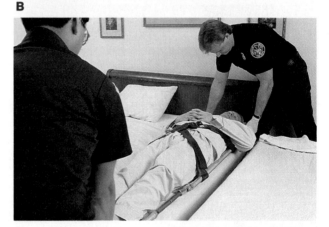

C

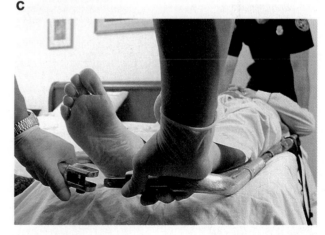

FIGURE 46–17

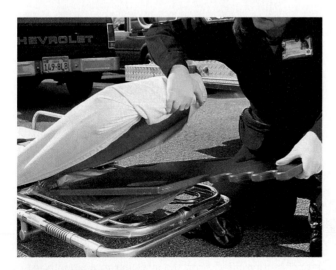

FIGURE 46–16

A short spine board should be placed beneath the mattress at the head of the stretcher to facilitate CPR.

Bed-to-stretcher transfers. (A) The patient is log-rolled onto the break-away stretcher. The stretcher is then positioned parallel to the bed and is locked or held in position. (B) The patient is then transferred from the bed onto the stretcher. (C) The break-away stretcher may then be removed if desired. The weight transfer is best achieved by the rescuers keeping their arms extended close to their bodies, heads up, and backs straight.

A

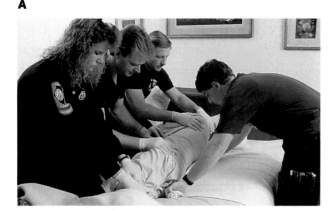

B

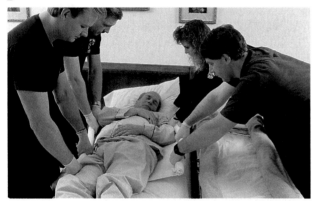

C

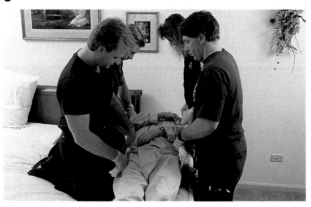

A

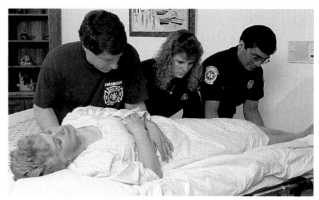

B

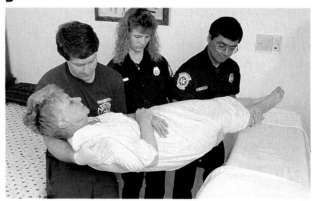

C

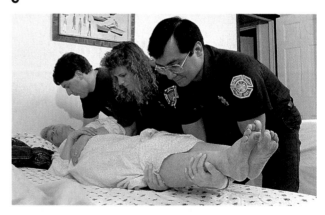

FIGURE 46–18

Bed-to-stretcher transfer using a drawsheet. (A) The patient is log-rolled onto a fan-folded draw sheet. (B) The stretcher is brought in parallel to the bed and secured. The patient is pulled gently to the edge of the bed. (C) The patient is then transferred to the stretcher. Weight transfer is best achieved by the rescuers using their shoulders, upper body weight, and back muscles to pull. The stretcher may roll if it is not secured during the patient transfer.

FIGURE 46–19

Stretcher-to-bed transfer using a three-person lift. (A) The stretcher is brought in parallel to the bed with the patient's feet facing toward the head of the bed. The stretcher should be secured to keep it from rolling. The patient is then lifted from the stretcher in a smooth, coordinated fashion. (B) The patient is slowly "walked around" into the appropriate position over the bed. (C) The patient is slowly and gently lowered into the bed.

A

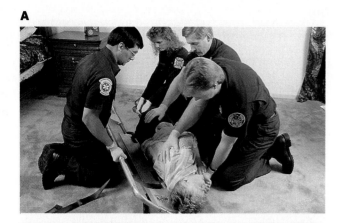

B

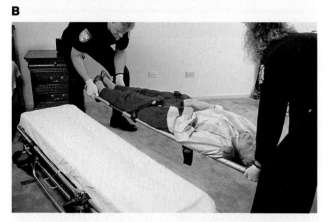

C

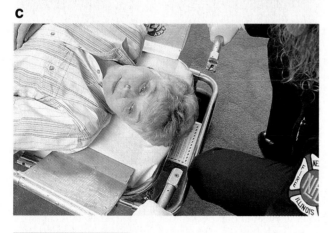

FIGURE 46–20

Floor-to-stretcher transfer. (A) The patient is log-rolled onto a long spine board or a scoop stretcher. (B) Then the patient is transferred to the stretcher. The best weight transfer is achieved by the rescuers bending at the hips and knees and using their legs to lift. (C) The scoop stretcher may then be removed if desired.

A

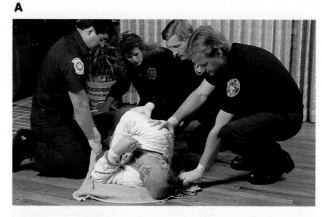

B

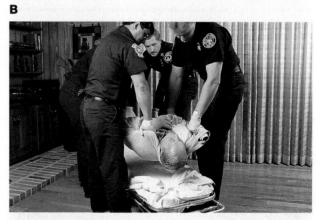

C

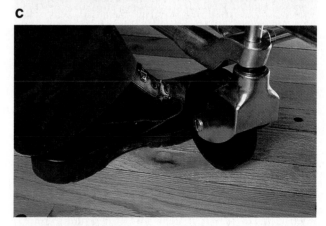

FIGURE 46–21

Floor-to-stretcher transfer using a blanket. (A) The patient is log-rolled onto a blanket. (B) Using the blanket, the rescuers gently lift the patient from the floor onto the stretcher. (C) The stretcher should be secured so that it does not roll during the transfer.

A

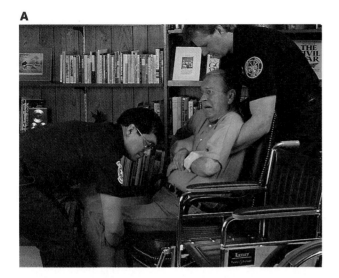

B

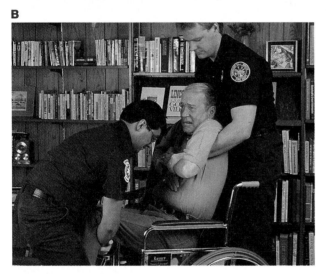

A

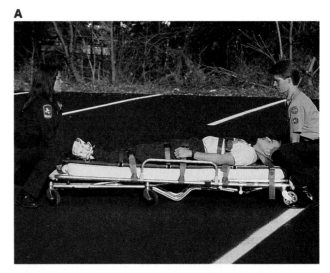

B

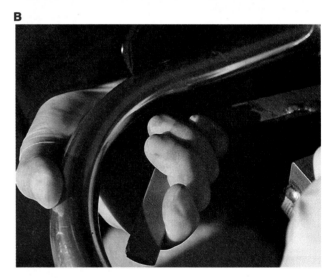

FIGURE 46-22

Chair-to-wheelchair transfer. (A) The EMT who is positioned behind the patient brings his arms through the patient's axillae and grasps the patient's crossed forearms. The second EMT grasps the patient's legs at the knees. (B) The patient is then gently lifted into the wheelchair, which must be secured to prevent it from rolling away. Transfers from a wheelchair to a chair or stretcher can be made in a similar fashion.

FIGURE 46-23

Raising the stretcher with a patient. (A) The rescuers must coordinate the lift with direct, verbal commands. Hips and knees should be bent and the arms held extended, with the back as straight as possible. (B) The release mechanism at the foot of the bed is activated.

(continued)

C

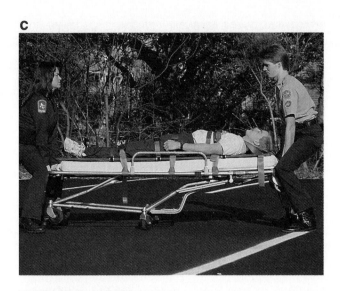

D

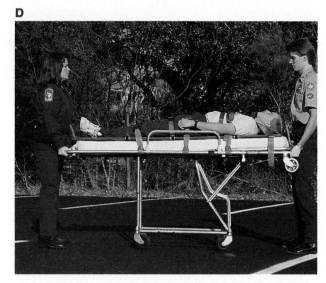

FIGURE 46–23

(continued)
(C) The lift should be a smooth straightening of the legs. (D) The rescuers may lift both ends or both sides of the stretcher simultaneously.

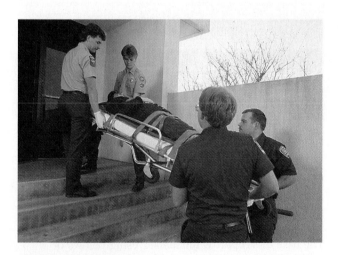

FIGURE 46–24

Ascending or descending stairs with a loaded stretcher. The rescuers must coordinate their moves with direct, verbal commands. The patient must be well secured with straps and other immobilizing devices. If the stretcher must be tipped on end, the patient's hips must be secured to keep him or her from slipping downward. The stretcher should be kept as level as possible. If there is a single rescuer on the lower end, he or she should be backed up by a watcher with a steadying hand.

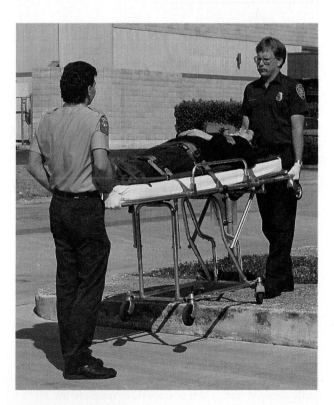

FIGURE 46–25

Moving the stretcher over obstacles. On firm surfaces, it is usually easiest to maneuver the stretcher in the elevated position. When an obstacle such as a curb or fire-hose is encountered, the stretcher should be lifted over the obstacle while keeping it as level as possible.

A

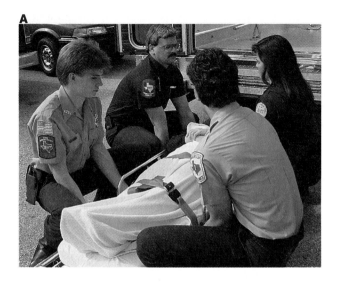

B

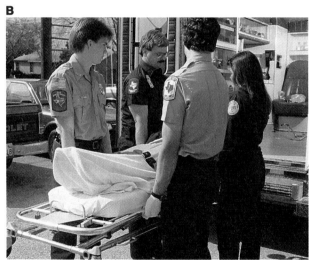

FIGURE 46–26

Loading a multi-level stretcher into the ambulance.
(A) The rescuers must coordinate their moves with direct, verbal commands. The stretcher must be locked into its lowest position. There must be an open pathway to the ambulance, and the ambulance doors must be secured in the open position. The rescuers should position themselves around the sides of the stretcher, with their feet sufficiently apart to give a stable base. (B) Bending at the hip and knees with their backs and arms straight, the rescuers smoothly complete the lift using the legs and then stop. On a second command, the stretcher is moved into the ambulance. If sufficient rescue personnel are available, it is best to have at least two rescuers on each side of the stretcher and another inside the ambulance to guide the stretcher into position.

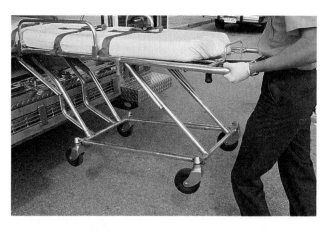

FIGURE 46–27

Loading a "Knockdown" stretcher into the ambulance. The stretcher is brought up to the rear entrance of the ambulance. When the wheels are in the ambulance, the stretcher is allowed to collapse as it is pushed into the patient compartment of the ambulance and secured. A second attendant should lift the undercarriage up to meet the bed frame.

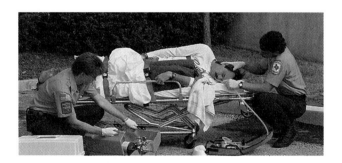

FIGURE 46–28

Packaging techniques for the unconscious patient, lateral position. The patient is placed on his or her side. The base of support is broadened using pillows or rolled blankets to support the flexed extremities, the head, and the back.

SPECIAL PATIENT-PACKAGING TECHNIQUES

Certain unusual circumstances will necessitate specialized packaging of the patient. Figures 46–28 through 46–32 illustrate some of these techniques.

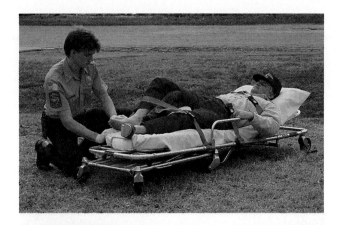

FIGURE 46–29

Packaging techniques for the patient with a dislocated hip. The patient is placed in a position of comfort, and pillows or rolled blankets are added as needed to support the injured extremity.

A

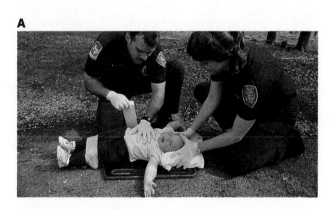

B

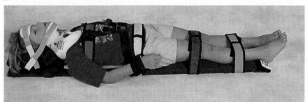

FIGURE 46–30

Packaging techniques for pediatric patients. (A) The standard ambulance stretcher and equipment are often not appropriately sized for children and must be adapted for the pediatric patient—for example, a short spine board can be used as a long board. (B) Equipment sized for pediatric patients should be used when available.

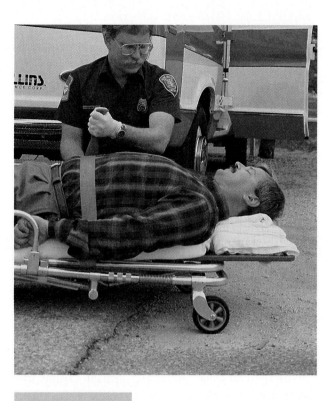

FIGURE 46–31

Packaging techniques for the extra-tall patient (or overhanging equipment). Extending the standard ambulance stretcher with a short spine board may prove effective for the extra-tall patient. Place the spine board at the head end of the stretcher to allow rear doors of the ambulance to close.

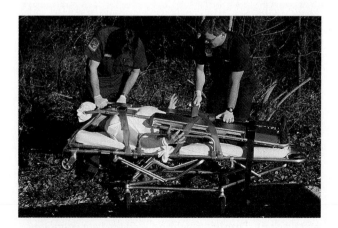

FIGURE 46–32

Packaging techniques for the combative patient. A scoop stretcher secured over the combative patient is one option to protect both the patient and the EMTs.

ANCILLARY PATIENT-HANDLING EQUIPMENT

Special skills are required to use the equipment described in this section. All of this equipment will be very useful to you in stabilizing and transporting patients. You must master the skills necessary for its use. A stair chair is illustrated in Figure 46–33. Figure 46–34 illustrates management of the wheelchair patient.

Another important piece of ancillary patient-handling equipment is the *split-frame* or *scoop stretcher* (known by names such as Robinson, Green, and Sarole). Although efficient, it requires both sides of the patient to be accessible. Unlike a long spine board, this stretcher cannot be slipped under the patient in the long axis of the body. Scoop stretchers are narrow, well constructed, compact for storage, and have excellent body support features; however, they are insufficient for standard spinal injury immobilization. Considerable practice is required

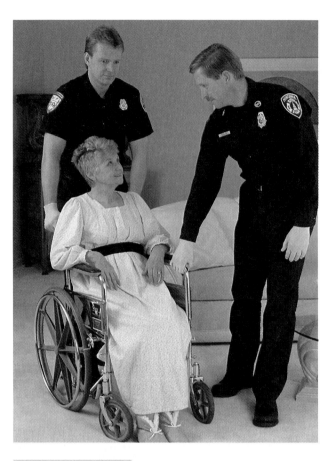

FIGURE 46–34

Wheelchairs, when available, provide easy management of the patient. The patient should be well secured in the wheelchair. At least two EMTs should manage the wheelchair patient—one in front and one behind. Movement should be as smooth as possible without sudden jerks or maneuvers.

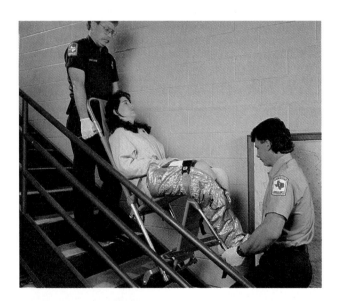

FIGURE 46–33

A stair chair. Sturdy straight-back chairs or a commercial stair chair may be used as an effective method of patient movement in a narrow corridor, small elevator, or a steep stairwell where other methods are not available. The patient must be *well secured* to the chair. The EMTs must communicate with each other and the patient continuously to coordinate movements.

to maintain proficiency in the use of scoop stretchers. You must be careful if you use a scoop stretcher in cold environments, because heat conduction from the body is significantly greater than on a regular stretcher because the patient's back is exposed.

"Scooping" a patient requires special attention to the closure area beneath the patient. The stretcher may trap clothing, skin, or other objects. As with the long spine board, complete, full body stabilization and securing of the patient are essential for good patient care. Scoop stretchers are illustrated in Figure 46–35.

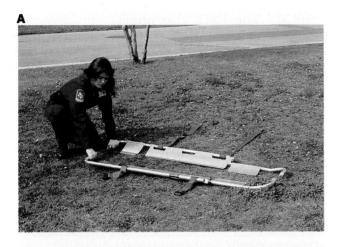
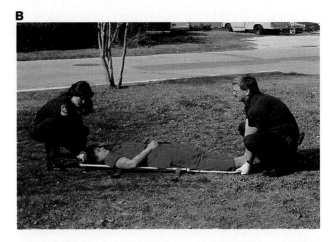
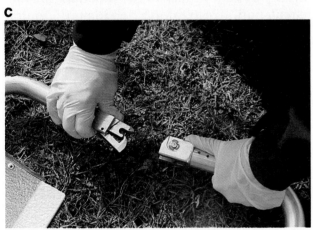
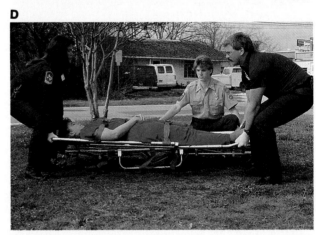

FIGURE 46–35 The split-frame or scoop stretcher. (A) To apply a scoop stretcher, it is first separated lengthwise. (B) The two halves are then slid under the patient from each side. Pinching of the patient or catching of clothing between the stretcher's halves may be prevented if the patient is gently lifted by his or her clothes as the halves are closed. (C) The locking brackets or knobs are latched and checked to make sure they are secure. (D) The patient is now loaded on the scoop stretcher and is ready to be transferred to the wheeled litter. Once the scoop stretcher is beneath the patient and he or she is secured by straps, the patient may be picked up without changing the body's position. The patient may be moved down narrow stairs without fear of slipping, even if the stretcher must be tipped sideways or tilted as much as 10 to 15 degrees. If the stretcher must be tipped on end, the patient's hips should be secured to prevent him or her from slipping downward.

TRIAGE

So far, this chapter has reviewed situations involving only one patient. You will frequently encounter situations in which there are two or more patients. The circumstances may range from an auto accident with two victims to a natural disaster such as a tornado with dozens of injured or dying patients. A disaster cannot be defined simply by the number of injured. A

disaster is a sudden and serious disruption of life caused by nature or humans that create or threaten to create injuries to a number of persons. It is best defined as any incident that will overload the capabilities and resources of the local medical community.

There are three phases of response to a disaster. The first is the *alarm phase,* which is concerned with the immediate activation of adequate and appropriate resources. The second phase of the response is the *work phase,* or implementation phase. It is subdivided into four overlapping steps, known by the acronym **LAST.**

1. Locate
2. Access
3. Stabilize
4. Transport

The final phase in response to a disaster is the *letdown phase.* After the work is completed, all personnel must recover from the stress of the disaster. The emotional impact on the health care providers may be immediate or delayed. **Critical Incident Stress Debriefing (CISD)** and counseling have been found to be useful methods for dealing with such stress.

In disaster situations, the concept of **triage** comes into play. Triage is a French word meaning to pick, sort, or choose. With multiple patients, it describes the process of sorting patients and allocating resources according to a system of priorities. Triage is a continuing process that is directed by the most highly trained medical individual at the scene of the incident or disaster.

Procedures for the Initial Triage Officer

The first EMT on the scene is responsible for beginning the triage process and contacting the dispatch center for additional equipment and personnel. This is the alarm phase of the response, which is concerned with activation of resources. It is better to overmobilize and later cancel responding units than to come up short-handed. This EMT then surveys the scene by making the first triage round and determining the number of victims who require priority medical treatment based on the familiar

"ABCs." The EMT also notifies the dispatch center of the number of victims so that area hospitals can be alerted. Having assumed the initial duties of the triage officer, this first EMT should not become involved in patient care but rather assign assistants to handle such duties.

Patients who are obviously dead or have such devastating injuries that they are unlikely to survive are bypassed during the initial round of triage. Although it seems cruel and uncaring, these patients must be left untended if there are limited personnel and resources to treat the people who can be saved. A trauma scoring system similar to the modified *CRAMS* (circulation, respiratory, abdomen, motor, speech) *scale* of Clemmer (Figure 46–36) can be

---

CRAMS Scale

Circulation
2—Normal cap. refill and BP > 100 mm Hg systolic
1—Delayed cap. refill or BP 85-99 mm Hg systolic
0—No cap. refill or BP < 85 mm Hg systolic

Respiration
2—Normal
1—Abnormal (labored, shallow, or rate > 35)
0—Absent

Abdomen
2—Abdomen and thorax not tender
1—Abdomen or thorax tender
0—Abdomen rigid, thorax flail, or deep penetrating
    injury to either chest or abdomen

Motor
2—Normal (obeys commands)
1—Responds only to pain—no posturing
0—Postures or no response

Speech
2—Normal (oriented)
1—Confused or inappropriate
0—No or unintelligible sounds

_____ Total CRAMS score (add the five areas)

Note: The CRAMS Score for trauma patients is determined by adding the scores from the five body areas. A score of 6 or less indicates a critically injured patient. (Clemmer, et al., *J. Trauma* 25(3): 188-191, Mar. 1985.)

FIGURE 46–36   CRAMS Scale.

used to determine the probability of survival. The cardinal rule of triage is to *do the greatest good for the greatest number*. Patients whose injuries are not an immediate threat to their airway, breathing, or circulation are also bypassed on the first round of triage.

Subsequent Triage Officer's Role

In the meantime, other rescuers should have arrived and will be unloading equipment and supplies and establishing a triage area. The triage officer will continue triage rounds in the triage area. As more experienced medical personnel arrive, the initial triage officer may relinquish his or her duties, after giving an oral briefing to the party assuming the duties of the triage officer. The briefing should be short and succinct. It must include the number of injured and a rough estimate of the severity of their injuries. The steps that have been taken regarding triage and treatment must be reported, and requests for additional personnel and supplies made. If any patients have been transported, the new triage officer must know their number, the severity of their injuries, and to what medical facilities they were transported.

During the second round of triage, those patients who require more definitive care for airway, breathing, and/or circulation problems are identified; preparations then are begun for priority transport. The second rule of triage is that *preservation of life takes precedence over preservation of limbs*. The third round of triage begins after immediate life-threatening conditions have been controlled. Secondary injuries such as spine injuries, major or open fractures, burns, and abdominal trauma are identified and stabilized. This round of triage is similar to the secondary assessment phase of the patient examination.

Triage rounds continue until all patients have been treated and transported. Patients must be evaluated during these continuing rounds of triage for any deterioration in their condition that might elevate their priority for treatment and transportation. The triage officer must maintain a record of all patients, their medical priority status, and to which medical facility they have been taken. The triage officer

should try to allocate patients, based on number and severity, among local medical facilities to minimize the overload on any one facility. These record keeping and allocation duties may be delegated, but the ultimate responsibility comes back to the triage officer. If the magnitude of the situation warrants, the triage officer may designate a communications officer to control and direct radio traffic to free the triage officer for other duties. In a major disaster, a medical triage officer may be responsible for patient care and an incident commander may be responsible for all support services.

Triage Priorities

A variety of systems are used to identify patients and treatment priorities in a disaster situation. You must become familiar with the system used in your locale. All the systems are based on the four following basic categories of patient treatment priority and injury severity. Patients with certain conditions or injuries are granted priority for treatment and transportation over others:

1. Highest priority: patients requiring immediate care and transportation. These patients must be treated first at the scene and then transported as soon as possible. They will have one or more of the following problems:

   - airway and breathing difficulties.
   - exsanguinating hemorrhage.
   - open chest or abdominal wounds.
   - severe head injuries or head injuries with decreasing levels of consciousness.
   - major or complicated burns.
   - tension pneumothorax.
   - pericardial tamponade.
   - impending shock.
   - complicating severe medical problems— poisonings, diabetes with complications, cardiac disease, pregnancy.

2. Intermediate priority: patients whose treatment and transportation can be delayed temporarily. These patients are likely to have injuries such as the following:

   - burns without complications.

- back injuries with or without spinal injuries.
- major, open, or multiple fractures.
- eye injuries.
- stable abdominal injuries.

3. Delayed or low priority ("the walking wounded"): patients whose treatment and transportation can be delayed until last. These patients will have fractures and sprains, lacerations, soft tissue injuries, and other lesser injuries.

4. Lowest priority: patients who are dead or are near death. These patients are already deceased or have such devastating injuries that they have little chance for survival. If resources are limited, these patients must be ignored to enable these resources to be used on "salvageable" patients.

The use of a priority system such as this will maximize the percentage of victims surviving the disaster.

The START System

The **START (Simple Triage and Rapid Treatment)** system is one method of triage that has proven to be very effective. It is based on three primary observations: breathing, circulation, and mental status (BCM).

In this system patients are tagged for easy recognition by other rescuers using one of a variety of methods. Colored surveyor's tape or colored paper tags are very effective (Figure 46–37). The four levels of triage are identified by color codes:

1. Priority one (red tag): Immediate care; life-threatening.
2. Priority two (yellow tag): Urgent care; can delay transport and treatment up to one hour.
3. Priority three (green tag): Delayed care; can delay transport and treatment up to three hours.
4. Priority four (black tag): No care required; patient is dead.

A

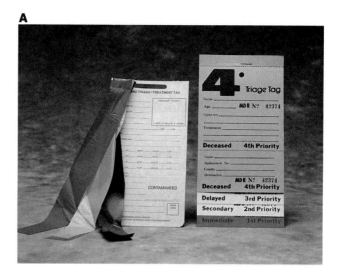

B

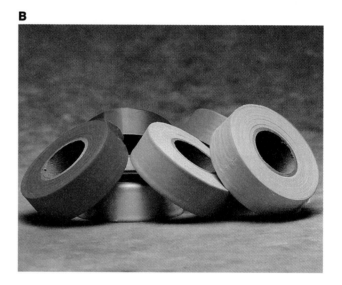

FIGURE 46–37

(A) Triage tags. (B) Triage tape.   *Continued*

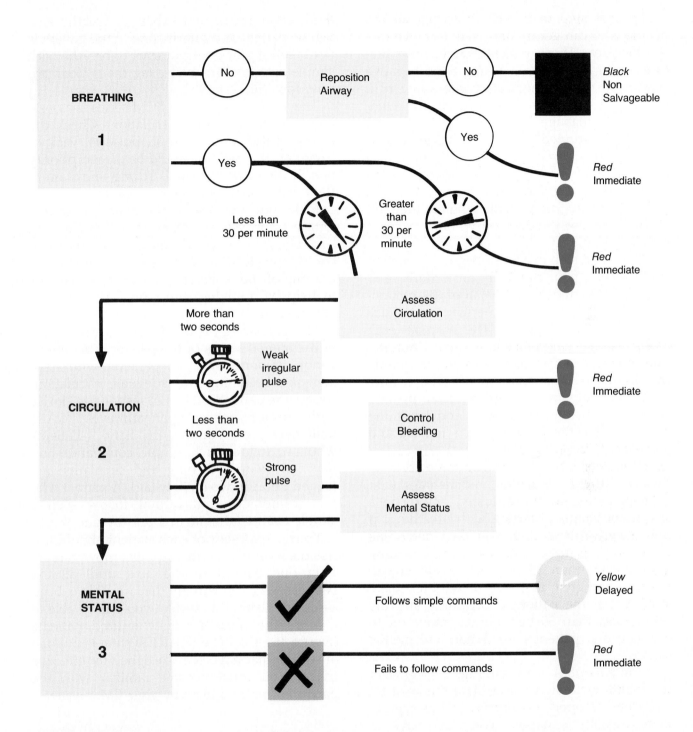

FIGURE 46–37 *Continued* (C) START algorithm.

The first step in START is to tell all the people who can get up and walk to move to a specific area. These patients rarely have life-threatening injuries and asking them to move away from the immediate rescue scene to a specific, designated safe area makes the situation more manageable. These patients (the "walking wounded") are then designated as priority three (green or delayed care). If a patient complains of pain on attempting to move to the designated area, do not force him or her to do so. The patients who are then left at the scene are the ones on whom you must now concentrate.

The second step in START begins by moving from where you stand in an orderly and systematic manner to assess all of the remaining victims. Stop at each person for a quick assessment and tagging. The stop at each patient should never take more than 1 minute. Your purpose at this point is to define and tag the priority one patients—those who require immediate attention. Examine each patient, correct life-threatening airway and breathing problems, tag the patient with a red tag and move on.

Patient evaluation is based on three observations: breathing, circulation, and mental status. Each patient must be evaluated quickly in a systematic manner starting with breathing. If the patient is breathing, you then determine the breathing rate. Patients with breathing rates greater than 30 per minute are tagged priority one (red tag) and need immediate attention. If the patient is breathing and the rate is less than 30 per minute, move on to evaluate that patient's circulation and mental status.

If the patient is not breathing, quickly clear the mouth of foreign matter. Use the head-tilt maneuver to open the airway. In this type of mass casualty situation, you may have to ignore the usual warnings about cervical spine injury when opening the airway. This mass casualty situation is the only time in emergency care when there may not be time to properly stabilize every injured patient's spine. Open the airway; position the patient to maintain the airway; and if the patient breathes, tag the patient priority one (red tag). If you are in

doubt about the patient's ability to breathe, also tag the patient as a priority one. If the patient is not breathing or does not start to breathe with simple airway maneuvers, tag the patient priority four (black tag).

The second step of the BCM series is assessment of the patient's circulation. Check the carotid pulse. If the carotid pulse is weak or irregular, the patient should be tagged priority one. If the carotid pulse is strong, move on to the third observation, mental status.

If the pulse is absent, the patient is tagged with a priority four. If the patient is bleeding severely, do not spend time yourself trying to control the bleeding. Get the patient to assist or ask one of the walking, priority-three patients to help by applying direct pressure over the bleeding site.

The last part of the BCM series is assessment of the mental status of the patient. This observation is done only on patients who have adequate breathing and adequate circulation. Assess the patient's ability to respond to simple verbal stimuli such as "open your eyes," "close your eyes," or "squeeze my hand." Patients who can follow such simple commands and have adequate breathing and circulation are tagged priority two (yellow tag). A patient who is unresponsive and cannot follow such a simple command is tagged priority one.

Your assessment of each patient should last less than 1 minute and you must move rapidly from one patient to the next until all the patients who remain in the area have been assessed. Using this system you will be able to identify the most seriously injured patients (Figure 46–37c). The START system is but one of several that have been designed for effective triage. You must become familiar with the particular method used by your EMS System.

Special Triage Situations

There is a separate category of triage for patients who have suffered radiation contamination and who are themselves carrying radiation particles. This category supersedes all others. Contaminated patients *must* be segregated immediately as an initial step. They must not be allowed to contaminate other patients, the EMTs, ambulances, or hospitals. A discussion of radiation injury management is found in Chapter 40.

In certain large metropolitan areas where regionalized care is provided, another concept of triage is used. Single patients with specific medical problems (burns, trauma, cardiac, or neonatal, for example) are "triaged" to specialized regional centers for treatment. Deciding whom to transport and to what treatment center is difficult and depends on many factors including, but not limited to

- the specific illness or injury.
- the severity of the illness or injury.
- the availability of local resources at the time of the event.
- local rules and protocols.

If you work in a region with specialized treatment centers you must know the specific triage protocols that apply.

Most major metropolitan areas have regional trauma care centers. Specific guidelines have been developed by the American College of Surgeons to define the **regionalized care** resources needed by a hospital to qualify for the care of the various levels of severity of injury. Severe, life-threatening injuries should be treated in facilities prepared to deal immediately and completely with the problem. Ideally, severely injured patients should be identified in the field and triaged to a designated **Level One Trauma Center.** However, in the field specific identification to discover which patients need to be transported is a difficult task. Various *trauma triage predictors* have been developed to aid field personnel in determining the need for transport to a trauma center. These predictors have three components:

- Physiological (blood pressure, pulse, respiratory rate, and level of consciousness).
- Anatomical (the number and location of wounds).
- Mechanism of injury (for example, missile wounds, falls from heights, and blunt injury secondary to automobile accidents).

When all three of these components are used together, one can reliably identify in the field a high percentage of those patients who should be transported to a level one trauma center. You should become very knowledgeable about all triage methods used by your EMS system to identify patients who should be transported to specialized treatment facilities.

As with other EMT skills, you must practice triage techniques to maintain your proficiency with them. Disaster drills should be run at least yearly, preferably in conjunction with local hospitals and other public safety and rescue units. Disaster plans must be developed and practiced in advance of need. The mass confusion of a disaster site is no time to experiment with organization.

YOU ARE THE EMT

1. In what ways is handling a geriatric patient the same as handling a pediatric patient? In what ways is it different?
2. What are some of the factors you must consider before attempting a one-person rescue?
3. Describe the differences between a standard stretcher and a scoop stretcher. Under what conditions are each best used?
4. Identify the resources available in your community that could be used in a disaster. Divide these resources into people and equipment who would respond to the scene and facilities that would receive the injured.
5. How would you use the START system to triage the victims of a tornado?

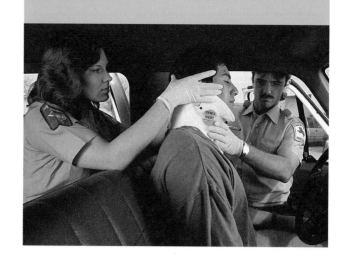

CHAPTER 47

EXTRICATION AND RESCUE

KEY TERMS

belay (bi-lā) A rescue line.

extrication (eks′trĭ-kay′shun) Removal from a difficult situation or position; often used to mean removal of a patient from a wrecked car or other place of entrapment.

incident command system An accepted local protocol of assigning responsibility in advance to manage medical emergencies and natural disasters.

LAST An acronym for Locate, Access, Stabilize, and Transport; the four stages of the work phase of a disaster response.

MEDEVAC A method of speeding lifesaving care to patients and of transporting patients with life-threatening injury or illness to treatment facilities using medically equipped helicopters.

packaging The positioning, covering, and securing of an ill or injured patient for transportation.

personal floatation device A life jacket used during water rescue.

rescue To free from a dangerous, destructive, or life-threatening situation by prompt vigorous action.

size up To gather facts quickly about a situation, analyze the problem, and decide how to handle it.

tempered glass A type of glass that shatters into small pieces when struck with a sharp, pointed object.

OVERVIEW

Rescue, by definition, means to free from the danger of death or destruction by prompt, vigorous action. One aspect of rescue is extrication, a method of freeing patients from an entrapment by means of force, ingenuity, or both. Extrication may range from simply opening a car door to gain access to the patient to a complex situation involving multiple patients such as a passenger train derailment or the collapse of a building. In between are many emergency situations—such as fires, cave-ins, water accidents, farm machine injuries, and snowmobiling accidents—that require the use of extrication skills.

Because of the specialized skills and equipment needed for complex extrication work, the EMT is not supposed to be an expert in every aspect of rescue and extrication; nor will this chapter attempt to cover the total field. Furthermore, in many areas of the country, the extrication phase of a rescue is under the control of specialized rescue units that are often attached to the local fire department.

Because extrication is often one of the early priorities and involves "hands on" exposure to victims, the EMT must be properly equipped and attired to avoid injury and illness.

Chapter 47 begins with an explanation of how rescue operations are classified. Then the eight principles of extrication are presented. Next, extrication techniques and tools are described, with a focus on vehicle entrapment, the most common extrication problem. Preparing the patient for transfer to an ambulance follows. The last section of Chapter 47 explores specialized rescue—which includes rescue in rough terrain, water, cold weather, and ice—and urban rescue.

GOALS

The goals of Chapter 47 are to
- see how rescue operations are classified.
- identify the nine principles of extrication.
- become familiar with commonly used extrication techniques and tools.
- learn how to prepare and package a patient for removal to an ambulance.
- know what is required for specialized rescue in rough terrain, water, cold weather, ice, and in an urban setting.
- be aware of and know how to avoid personal hazards.

CLASSIFICATION OF RESCUE OPERATIONS

Basic rescue involves the transfer of injured patients from uncomplicated motor vehicle accidents and from stable buildings. Basic rescue is the simplest to carry out and generally is handled with a minimum of equipment. For the most part, you will be involved in **rescue** and **extrication** activities that fall in this category of rescue.

Even if a rescue vehicle accompanies the ambulance on every accident run, basic rescue tools should be standard equipment on all ambulances, whether in rural, suburban, or urban service. Every EMT must be trained in the use of this extrication equipment. Multiple vehicle accidents requiring simultaneous patient access or delay of the rescue vehicle by traffic or a breakdown are sufficient reasons to require basic rescue equipment to be carried on all ambulances. The element of time is so critical in life-threatening situations that waiting for the arrival of basic extrication tools and equipment cannot be tolerated. But even in such situations, you must not attempt extrications beyond your training and expertise.

Medium rescue involves specialized equipment normally found on a rescue vehicle. Medium rescue implies the use of rigging, A-frames, and tripods for patient access. Medium rescue also involves the use of extrication tools for disentanglement of the patient.

Heavy rescue may include complicated rigging, patient handling under extremely difficult or adverse conditions, breaching of walls, disimpaction of vehicles, and all types of rescue involving buildings with major structural damage.

Incidents involving medium and heavy rescue usually involve the fire department rescue squad, and the fire department will receive the initial call. Under protocol in many areas of the country, the EMT uses light extrication skills and equipment to gain access to the patient to provide emergency medical care, while the rescue squad provides the extrication capabilities for disimpaction and disentanglement of the patient.[1]

In the work phase of a multiple casualty disaster you should follow the **LAST** (Locate, Access, Stabilize, and Transport) principle as described in Chapter 46. As many patients as possible should be located first. Because extrication of some may be quite difficult, consume much time, and require specialized equipment, the priorities of assessment, stabilization, and transport may need to be adjusted for certain patients. In such complex extrication operations the following priorities should be established:

1. Lightly pinned casualties—those who can be freed by lifting a beam or removing a small amount of debris—are extricated and stabilized first.
2. Those patients who are trapped in more difficult circumstances but who can still be rescued by use of the equipment at hand in a minimum amount of time are extricated next.
3. Those patients who require an extended time commitment for a difficult extraction are removed from entrapment next. Such rescue may involve cutting through floors, breaching walls, removing large amounts of debris, or cutting through an expanse of metal. An example would be removing a worker from under a large piece of machinery.
4. The bodies of those who have died are extricated last.

During all phases of rescue and extrication operations, your primary responsibilities are to provide emergency medical care to the patient and to prevent further injury to the patient or others. Although occasionally there are too few personnel to begin the routine of patient care immediately, this is the exception rather than the rule. Usually, far too many people are involved in the extrication process; some are of little use, and others may be dangerous to themselves and others when placed in such uncontrolled and anxiety-provoking situations.

The most evident problem in rescue situations involving several medical and rescue units is the lack of identifiable leadership at the scene and the accompanying disorganized provision of care. It is essential for one person to be in charge of the overall rescue operation. This person must be medically trained and qualified to judge the priorities of patient care. This person has to assume responsibility for the overall management of the extrication process,

---

[1] The textbook *Basic Rescue and Emergency Care* published by the American Academy of Orthopaedic Surgeons in 1990 provides a more complete and detailed description of the principles and techniques of all phases of rescue.

as well as the details of patient care. It is best to reach an agreement on the protocol of assigning this responsibility in advance through the development of an **incident command system** or as a part of the local disaster plan.

PRINCIPLES OF EXTRICATION

Although no two accident situations will be identical, the following basic principles of extrication apply to all rescue situations:

1. Evaluate (**size up**) the situation.
2. Locate all victims.
3. Provide for the safety of rescue personnel and the patient.
4. Secure the scene.
5. Gain access to the patient.
6. Provide emergency medical care (stabilize the patient).
7. Disentangle the patient.
8. Prepare the patient for transfer.
9. Transfer the patient.

Ingenuity, common sense, and a basic knowledge of mechanics will solve most extrication problems. All EMTs should enhance their basic training through additional workshops and courses, as well as with practice sessions on wrecked vehicles at the local junkyard.

Evaluation of the Situation (Size-up)

Size-up is a term used by firefighters that means to rapidly gather facts about the situation, analyze the problem, and decide how to handle it. Sizing up differs from triage in that it involves all aspects of the situation, including the type, severity, and location of the incident; the environmental conditions and hazards; the equipment and emergency personnel resources; and the number of victims and their medical conditions. All victims must be found and accounted for. Frequently, victims are thrown from vehicles and explosions and are missed due to darkness, uneven terrain, tall grass, shrubbery, or the wreckage. Selection of the extrication procedures is based on decisions made during size-up. Size-up must be a continuing evaluation of the situation throughout extrication, because new problems may arise that demand alterations in the extrication process.

A few of the frequently conflicting factors you must anticipate and evaluate during size-up are provided here in order to stimulate thought and discussion. The list is not complete, nor is it meant to serve as a checklist.

- Is the patient located in a building with stairwells that will require a special litter? Is there an elevator in the building? Will the ambulance stretcher fit in the elevator?
- Is there a fire involved? The presence of a fire complicates the extrication process by altering the available methods of patient removal and provision of emergency medical care.
- If a vehicle is involved, is it stable? All unstable vehicles must be stabilized before you attempt entry. This is one of the reasons why shoring blocks and ropes are standard ambulance equipment. Some services have installed towing hooks on their vehicles to provide a rapid method of securing an unstable vehicle.
- Is the vehicle right-side up, upside down, or lying on its side?
- Is the patient hanging from a seatbelt or lying crammed under the dash and up against the firewall?
- Are there objects protruding from the vehicle that must be removed before you can accomplish entry?
- Is the equipment necessary for extrication available on the ambulance? Will specialized equipment and personnel be required?
- Are all patients accounted for? A "head count" must be routine in the questioning of patients. Ideally, such questions should be directed at the least-injured patients. Witnesses should be questioned as to whether anyone left the scene or if passersby took any victims away.
- Are there hazards present—such as spilled gas, downed electrical wires, or hazardous materials—that could endanger the patient or the rescue personnel?

Safety of Rescue Personnel and the Patient

EMTs are frequently called on to undertake rescue and extrication activities at dangerous locations. A prime consideration for you should be avoiding personal injury and preventing further injury to the patient. To be successful in this endeavor, you must be properly prepared and equipped before the call comes in. Special equipment should be worn or be available for your protection.

Safety of Rescue Personnel

While on duty, all EMTs should wear sturdy shoes or workboots. Glass and sharp metal are frequently encountered at accident scenes. A rescuer with a lacerated foot only complicates the incident.

In cool environments, long underwear provides warmth even when it is wet or when you are perspiring. During the cooler months, you may be uncomfortable sitting around in "longies" waiting for a call, but at an accident scene, you can cool down very rapidly, especially if you have to stay in one position for an extended period during a prolonged extrication. A stocking cap or other hat will significantly decrease the loss of body heat. Hypothermia is as dangerous for the rescuer as for the patient.

It cannot be overemphasized that the use of latex or plastic disposable gloves *at all times* during patient contact will minimize the risk of contracting infectious diseases at the rescue site.

A pair of leather gloves should be worn over disposable gloves by all rescue personnel to protect their hands during the rescue and extrication process. Handling ropes, broken glass, hot or cold objects, or sharp metal can be dangerous to the unprotected rescuer. Chemical resistant gloves should also be available for handling toxic or corrosive materials that may be present.

A hard hat or protective helmet is very useful, both for identification of rescue personnel and personal safety (Figure 47–1). The hard hat is designed to protect against fixed objects, as well as light missiles such as falling rock or

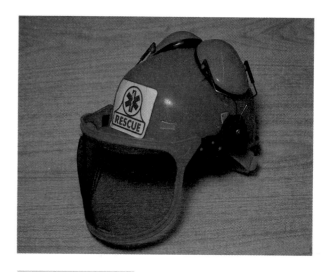

FIGURE 47–1

A hard hat is an essential piece of protective equipment during any rescue activity.

flying glass. Some services prefer the hard hat used by lumberjacks and tree trimmers, because it has a fine metal mesh face guard to protect the face from branches or small flying objects. Because the face mask is mesh rather than plexiglass, it does not fog up in cold weather and seems to provide good visibility in the rain. The helmet also has ear protectors that provide some protection from the high-decibel sound levels of portable power units that are used for the extrication equipment or machines found in a heavy industrial environment.

A hand-held strobe light may help EMTs keep track of each other in a crowd or in rural or wilderness locations (Figure 47–2). When working along the highway, you can hook these lights to your belts, or attach them to your upper arm to provide additional visibility to oncoming vehicles. Strobe lights are lightweight, quite durable, and readily visible at night at a distance of approximately 1 mile.

Safety of the Patient

While you are gaining access to the patient and during disentanglement, exercise great care to avoid further injury to the patient. This is the time when extrication tools and equipment are closest to the patient. You should cover the

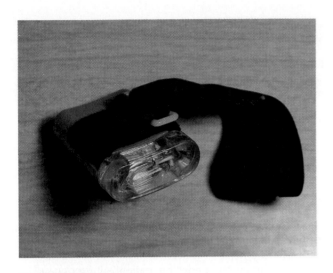

A durable lightweight strobe light provides increased visibility in many situations.

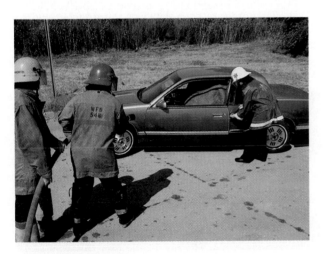

During extrication, always cover the patient with a heavy, nonflammable blanket to protect from further injury.

patient with a heavy, nonflammable blanket to protect against flying glass or other missiles (Figure 47–3). The EMT who is maintaining traction or providing other care during the extrication should be covered with a blanket as

well. A short spine board may also be used as a protective shield. Heat, noise, and force should be kept to the minimum required to extricate the patient safely.

Securing the Scene

One of the most common environmental hazards is spilled gasoline, which must be washed down at the scene of an incident. If gasoline or other flammable material is present, a fire crew with charged hoses should be standing by during the rescue and extrication process. You should make sure that your vehicle ignition is turned off and the key removed at any accident scene.

Hazardous materials, sometimes in tremendous quantities, are transported over our highways and railways each year. The release of these agents by an accident may endanger the lives of all those nearby. Vehicles transporting such material are usually marked with warning signs. When you respond to such incidents, your ability to identify the hazardous cargo from outside the danger zone may save your own life as well as the lives of other EMTs and rescue personnel (see Chapter 41). Carrying a pair of binoculars in the ambulance may allow you to observe the scene from a distance.

Downed electrical wires are another significant potential danger to you and your patient. The utility company must be notified of any downed or sagging wires at once. When informed that an accident involves a utility pole, the dispatcher should inquire about downed or dangling wires and notify the utility company if wires are damaged. Do *not* attempt to deal with downed power lines. You must also be extremely alert to the lethal potential of standing in water in the area of downed power lines.

Environmental hazards include adverse conditions such as collapsed buildings or mine shafts; temperature extremes with risk of hypothermia or hyperthermia; and dangerous locales, such as a freeway off-ramp at rush hour. Ingenuity and resourcefulness are required to handle such situations.

Poor visibility at the rescue scene can be a serious problem. It is impossible to work in the dark or with inadequate lighting. However, there is no excuse for inadequate lighting. Each ambulance must be equipped with sufficient stand-up flashlights, as well as sufficient flood-lights, to provide adequate lighting at a distance from the ambulance.

Finally, bystanders, relatives, and others can pose significant hazards to themselves and to the overall management of the incident. They must be controlled by the police or other personnel at the scene. Occasionally, a by-stander, particularly one with some medical credentials, may be difficult to manage. This situation is always challenging. All services are advised to have a protocol for dealing with this potential problem. Many states provide wallet-sized copies of licensure to physicians for use as identification, although, unfortunately, not all physicians are as well versed in field emergency medical care as is desirable. Communication between medical control and the physician at the scene may eliminate some of these problems. You may also find it helpful to assign the individual particular duties that provide minimal actual involvement in the rescue process, yet occupy the eager volunteer. This will reduce the potential of confrontation and tension that direct attention away from the primary goal of patient management.

Gaining Access to the Patient

Your means of gaining access to the patient depends on the type of incident—for example, the location and position of the vehicle, the damage to the vehicle, and the position of the patient. The means of gaining access to the patient must take into account the patient's injuries and their severity. You may have to change the chosen means of access during the course of the extrication as the nature or severity of the patient's injuries becomes more apparent.

Occasionally, it is necessary to extricate an injured patient from a threatening environment or to position the patient in an environment more conducive to performing CPR and other basic life support measures. The technique illustrated in Figure 47–4 will allow adequate manual immobilization of the injured spine, thorax, and extremities as long as a sufficient

FIGURE 47–4

Emergency patient removal. (A) With the patient seated, EMT A gets behind the patient and positions the head in a neutral, in-line position, with gentle longitudinal traction. (B) EMT B performs a rapid primary assessment. An extrication collar is applied to help stabilize the cervical spine. (C) Meanwhile, EMT C has placed a long spine board on the stretcher. With the door opened as wide as possible, the stretcher height is adjusted if necessary. (If there is a possibility that the pneumatic antishock trousers will be needed, they should be laid out on the spine board at this point so that the patient may be transferred directly from the car into the trousers.) (D) EMTs B and C then slide the spine board onto the car seat. The edge of the spine board should be just under the patient's buttocks and thigh. (E) EMT B stands as close to the rear of the door opening as possible, with arms extended and hands perpendicular to the arms. (F) EMT B reaches into the door opening and places one hand on each side of the patient's head, maintaining the neutral position and longitudinal traction on the cervical spine. (G) EMT A then moves into position alongside the patient, placing her arms under the patient's legs just above the knees. (H) While another rescuer stabilizes the stretcher and the spine board to prevent movement, EMT C places one hand in the patient's armpit.   (continued)

A

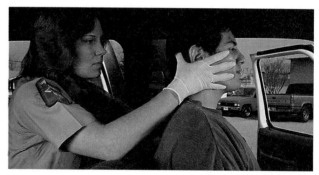

B

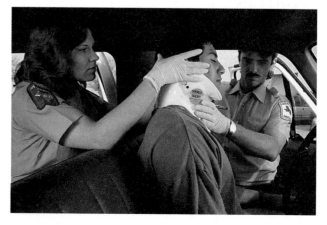

C

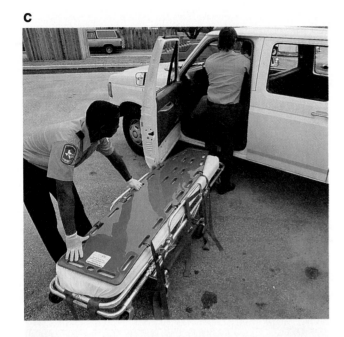

D

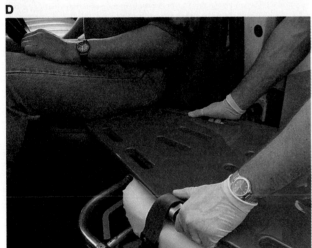

E

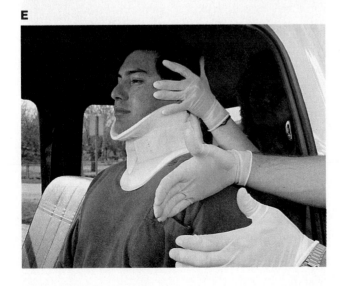

F

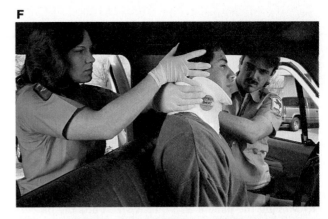

G

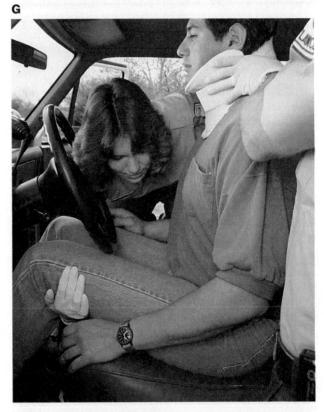

H

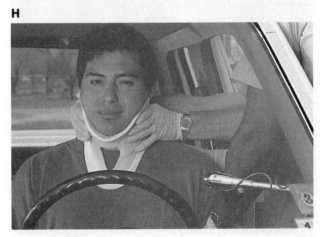

FIGURE 47–4

(continued) (I) EMT C places his other hand behind the patient's back to provide support in the mid-thorax. (It is best if EMT C can stand on the side of the stretcher opposite EMT B as illustrated. If there is inadequate room, EMT C may stand behind EMT B and reach between EMT B and the car to stabilize the mid-thorax.) (J) While EMT B maintains neutral, in-line traction, EMT A, controlling the patient's legs, and EMT C, controlling the patient's back, rotate the patient in a sitting position as a unit until lined up with the spine board. (K) Moving the patient as a unit, EMT A lifts the patient's legs, as EMTs B and C lower the patient onto the backboard, maintaining the sitting position. EMT B must continue to maintain neutral, in-line traction during this movement. (L) The patient is then gently slid up the spine board as a unit 6 to 12 inches at a time, as EMT B maintains neutral, in-line traction.

(M) The head and cervical spine are then stabilized with a blanket roll, foam blocks, or sandbags. (N) The patient is secured to the stretcher and may be moved to a less hazardous area where basic life support measures may begin. If the patient cannot be extricated through his or her door, he or she may be rotated out through the door on the opposite side. This will require that the spine board be placed across the seat. EMT B will also have to get inside the vehicle to maintain neutral, in-line traction on the patient's head and neck.

I

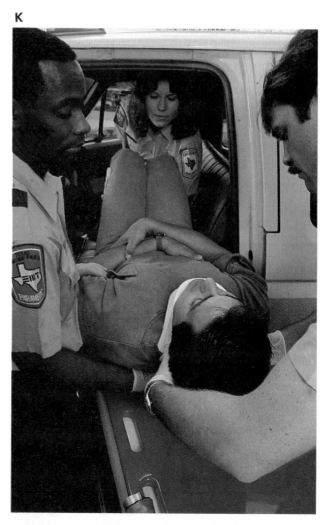

J

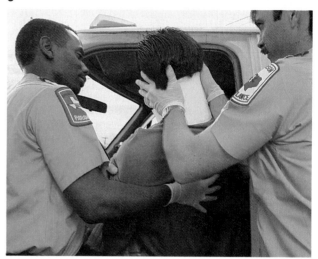

K

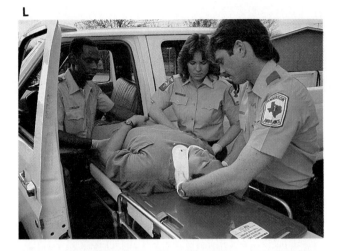

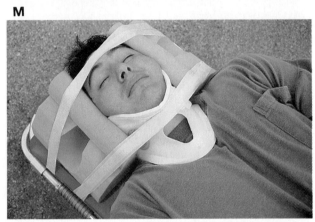

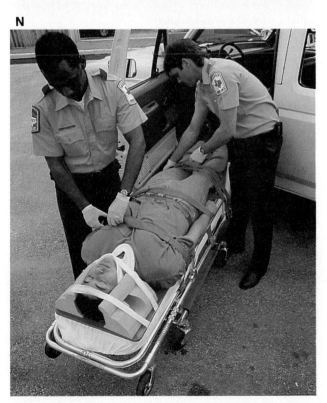

number of hands are available to support the injured body parts. The use of this technique is indicated only in those instances when there is a fire or high probability of fire; when the patient has rapidly deteriorating or absent vital signs, requiring the rapid initiation of resuscitation techniques such as airway management, ventilation, CPR, or the management of shock with pneumatic antishock trousers; or when the position of the vehicle poses a significant hazard to you or the patient. You should not use this technique if there is enough time to stabilize the patient with appropriate immobilization devices. There are two key elements to the successful use of this emergency extrication technique:

1. An adequate number of people must be available to stabilize all of the patient's injuries.
2. The lead EMT must coordinate the activities of all rescuers to ensure that the patient is moved as a unit.

Figure 47–5 illustrates the technique of rapidly removing a patient, if there is no danger of a cervical injury, using a special sling. Again, this procedure is for emergency removal only.

Providing Emergency Medical Care (Stabilization)

Providing emergency care is the same for the entrapped patient as for any other. However, often it needs to be divided into two phases: before and after disentanglement. Particularly when the extrication will be extended, it is essential to first perform an initial assessment, then stabilize the patient's vital functions, before the extrication process begins. Establish and maintain an airway, control bleeding, and support the cervical spine and any grossly unstable fractures before you begin the extrication. Monitor the vital functions during disentanglement. Once the patient is freed, remove him or her to a safe area, reassess the vital functions, perform a secondary survey, stabilize all injuries, and prepare for transport.

Remember that for cardiopulmonary resuscitation to be effective, the patient must be supine on a hard, flat surface. The patient

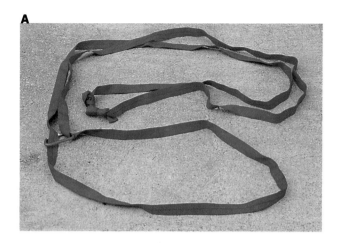

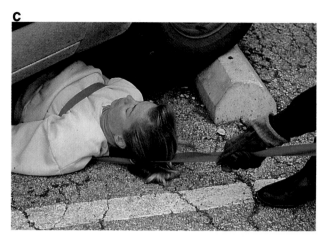

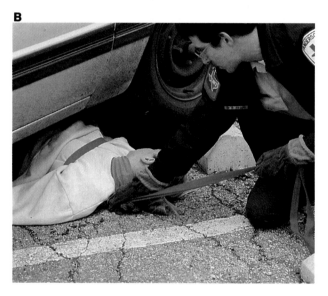

FIGURE 47–5

Emergency removal using a sling. (A) If there is no danger of a cervical injury and the patient must be moved rapidly from a danger area, drag the patient using a special sling consisting of an 8-foot loop of tubular nylon or a 1-inch rope with a metal ring sliding connector. (B) Do not use the traction loop without the sliding connector. Place the slide on the loop before the loop is spliced. Force the "slide" down between the shoulders at the base of the neck before traction is exerted on the loop. Take this precaution so that there is no danger of the loop pressing against the axillae of the patient and injuring the nerves and vessels to the arm. (C) Drag the patient from the area of danger.

should be placed on a long or short spine board and external cardiac compression begun as soon as the patient is removed from the entrapment. External cardiac compression is not effective when the patient is in a sitting position or on the soft seat of a vehicle.

Disentanglement of the Patient

Disentanglement of the patient requires medium to heavy extrication skills, which for the most part are beyond the scope of this text. The technique section of this chapter will show only some light extrication techniques for disentanglement of the patient.

Preparation of the Patient for Transfer

Preparing the patient for transfer means maintaining continued control of all life-threatening problems, dressing all wounds, splinting all suspected spinal injuries, and immobilizing all suspected fractures. The use of standard splints in confined areas is difficult and frequently impossible, but stabilization of the arms to the patient's trunk and of the legs to each other will often be adequate until the patient is positioned on a long spine board, which may serve as the ultimate splint for the whole body.

Packaging (preparing the patient for movement as a unit) is best accomplished by means of a spine board or a similar device. The boards are essential in moving patients with potential or actual spine injuries; they are helpful in other cases as well.

Transfer of the Patient

Transfer of the patient from the injury site to the ambulance is usually accomplished using a long spine board, or equivalent, as described later in this chapter.

EXTRICATION TECHNIQUES AND TOOLS

The most common extrication problem you will encounter is the entrapped patient following a motor vehicle accident. The basic principles, skills, and tools used in the extrication of a patient from an automobile may be used in many other rescue situations involving entrapped patients. Commonly used vehicle extrication equipment is illustrated in Figures 47–6 through 47–12.

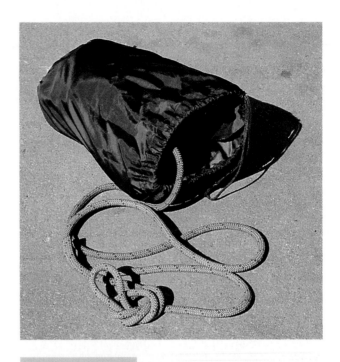

FIGURE 47–7

Rope for use in extrication should be a low-stretch, high-strength rope. It must be maintained in good condition. Carry each rope segment in a bag for easy deployment and storage. Do not use manila ropes for rescue, extrication, or stabilization. They lose up to 20% of their strength each time they get wet.

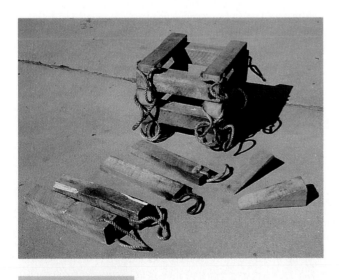

FIGURE 47–6

Shoring (cribbing) normally consists of pieces of unpainted wood, cut in standard, easy-to-carry lengths, with draw cord attached.

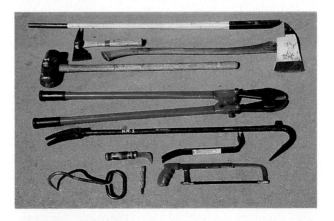

FIGURE 47–8

Hand tools. Carry light extrication tools on every ambulance. They allow prying of lightly damaged doors and sheet metal. They also may allow limited access to the patient through cutting of some sheet metal components on the vehicle or breakage of the glass.

A

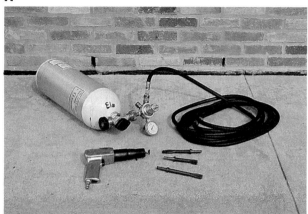

C

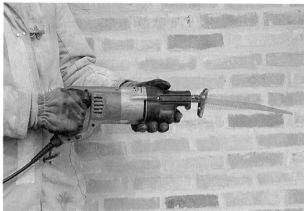

B

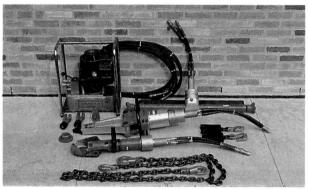

D

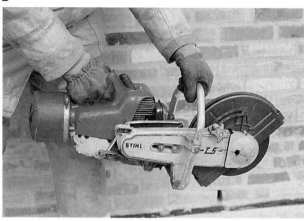

FIGURE 47–9

Cutting tools. (A) Use air chisels to cut sheet metal and supporting columns. They require an air compressor or a compressed air cylinder at the scene. (B) Hydraulic shears allow fast cuts of supporting columns using the hydraulic power from pumps that may be manually activated, or powered by a gasoline or electric motor. Use extreme caution to protect the patient and the rescuers from exposure to the hydraulic fluid, which is extremely corrosive. Wear goggles or a full face shield to protect the eyes whenever hydraulic equipment is being used. Wear gloves to protect the skin from exposure. Cover the patient with a protective blanket. (C) Use the electric saw-all to cut sheet metal and supporting columns. It requires an electric generator on the scene. There is a potential fire hazard from sparking. (D) High-speed saws, normally powered by a gasoline engine, are capable of cutting sheet metal and heavier supporting components. Consider the risk of fire and explosion from the sparks created when using this tool. (E) Cutting torches, usually oxygen/acetylene, allow you to cut through heavy metal components, including vehicle frames. In addition to the considerable risk of fire and explosion which you must consider, there is the potential for burning the patient from the heat generated during the cutting process. Use cutting torches only when no other alternative exists.

E

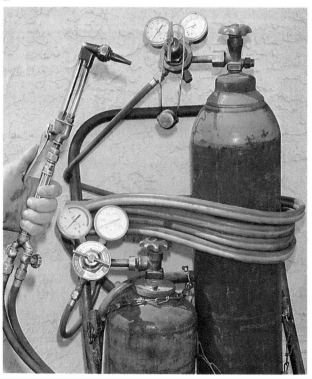

A

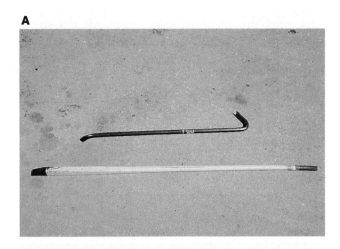

B

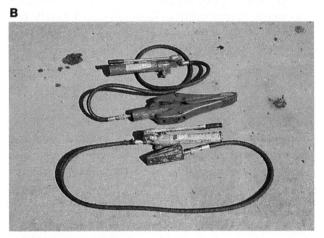

C

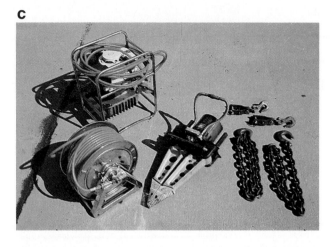

D

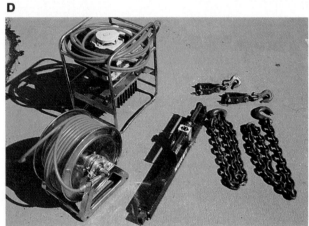

FIGURE 47–10

Spreading tools. (A) The pry bar and crowbar are hand tools commonly used to expose door-locking mechanisms and to bend sheet metal components. (B) Normally powered by hand pumps, Porta-power spreaders use hydraulic fluid as a power transfer medium to develop spreading forces in excess of 2,000 foot-pounds. As with all hydraulic equipment, exposure to the corrosive hydraulic fluid must be carefully avoided. (C) Hydraulic spreaders ("jaws") require manual, electric, or gasoline-powered hydraulic pumps to develop spreading forces from 10,000 to 16,000 foot-pounds. They may also be used for lifting. (D) Hydraulic rams require manual, electric, or gasoline-powered hydraulic pumps to develop spreading forces ranging from 8,000 to greater than 20,000 foot-pounds. They may also be used for lifting and pulling.

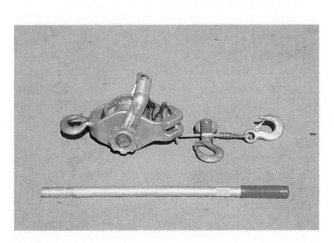

FIGURE 47–11

Pulling tools. A come-along is a manually powered tool with continuous pulling capability. It normally has a cable, a pulley, and a break-away handle. It requires chains or other devices to anchor it to the vehicle. Most will generate 4,000 lbs of pulling force. Hydraulic-powered rams and spreaders, normally used with chains for attachment, may also be used as tools for pulling, as demonstrated later in this chapter.

A

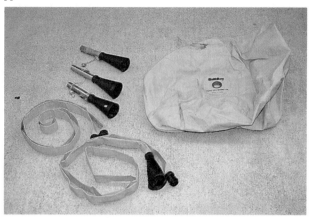

B

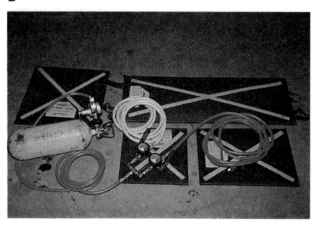

FIGURE 47–12

Lifting tools. (A) Low-pressure air bags are inflated with a compressor, compressed gas cylinders, or exhaust from a running vehicle. Regulate pressure to a maximum of 7 pounds per square inch (psi). They require a control valve for raising and lowering single bags. They have the capability to lift in the range of 4,000 to 20,000 lbs. (B) High-pressure air bags use a compressor or compressed gas cylinder regulated to a maximum of 110 psi to 135 psi. They require a control valve for raising or lowering. Single bags have lifting capabilities in the range of 2,000 to 150,000 lbs.

Passenger Vehicle Stabilization

Before extrication can begin, rescue personnel must stabilize the vehicle. The overall goal of stabilization is to broaden the vehicle's base of support and/or restrict the vehicle's movement. If the transmission has not already been put in

park and the ignition key removed, do so as soon as possible. The parking brake should also be set. Figure 47–13 illustrates the technique of vehicle stabilization.

Passenger Vehicle Extrication

Automobiles have a structural framework that gives strength, stability, and passenger protection. Rescuers may use the vehicle framework as anchors or push/lift points for extrication equipment.

The exterior "skin" of most passenger vehicles is made up of sheet metal and/or plastic or fiberglass components. Rescuers can easily cut through this skin with a variety of extrication tools, if necessary, to gain access to the patient. Figures 47–14 and 47–15 illustrate methods of opening a vehicle door to gain access to trapped victims.

If these relatively easy methods fail to gain rapid access to the patient, it may become necessary to break out a window to get at the door locks or to access the patient while heavier extrication equipment is used to disentangle the patient.

Automobiles usually use either **tempered glass,** which shatters into small pieces when struck with a sharp, pointed object, or a laminate of two pieces of glass with a binding layer of plastic between the glass sheets. Side and rear windows commonly have tempered glass, whereas the windshield is usually laminated. Figure 47–16 illustrates removal of tempered glass windows. Figure 47–17 shows how to remove the laminated glass of a windshield.

If the car is equipped with a safety air bag restraint device, special precautions may be necessary. The air bag is designed to deploy in certain frontal or near frontal crashes, but not in rear impacts, side impacts, or rollovers. It is possible, therefore, that you will be involved in rescue operations after crashes in which the air bag did not deploy. In some models, a late deployment of the air bag can be triggered if the positive battery terminal is disconnected first or if a jump start of the car is attempted or inadvertently caused while an EMT is securing an unstable car. The negative battery terminal should always be disconnected first.

A

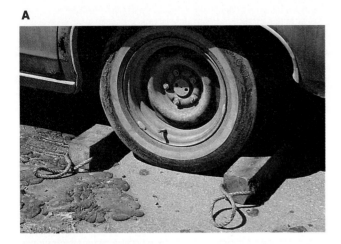

B

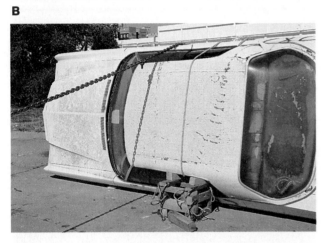

C

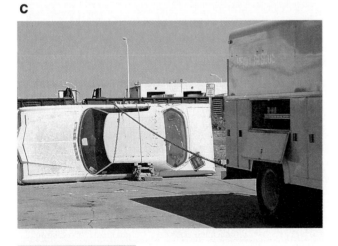

FIGURE 47–13

Vehicle stabilization. (A) If there is a danger of the vehicle rolling, place wooden cribbing to block the wheels. (B) Use wooden cribbing to extend the base of support of the vehicle if it is unstable or on uneven ground. Also, use cribbing to build a force point against which a ram or spreader may apply its force. (C) Use ropes, cables, and chains to restrict movement of the vehicle and broaden the base. Some services have special hooks attached to their rescue vehicles to allow rapid attachment of such stabilizers.

A

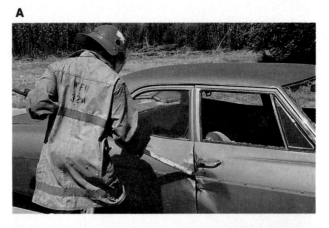

B

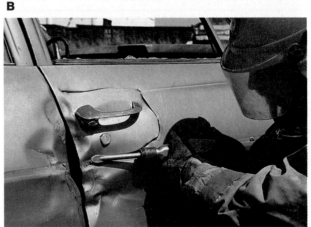

C

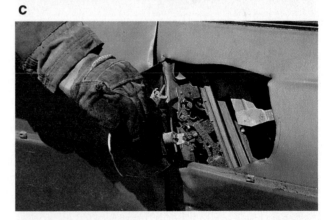

FIGURE 47–14

Opening a door with structural deformity. (A) If the door is lightly damaged and cannot be unlocked, a pry bar may be used to attempt to spring the door and unjam the lock bolt. (B) Another method is to insert a "can opener" or air chisel into the door and cut a flap of sheet metal around the door handle. (C) Turn the flap back to expose the lock. Strike the door jamb a heavy blow at the lock, relieving the tension on the tempered bolt and allowing the door to be opened.

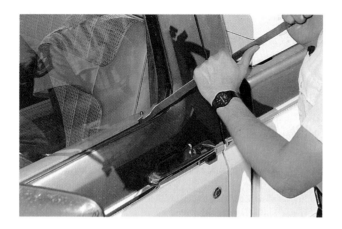

FIGURE 47–15

Opening a door with no structural damage. First, attempt to access and release the lock in order to activate the normal latch. The metal safety lock on newer cars may prevent the usual methods of opening doors. A thin metal strip with a slot in the end (thief's bar) is a handy tool for rapidly unlocking a door to access a patient. It is inserted between the window and the rubber seal of the door until it can be hooked on the lever controlling the lock bolt.

A

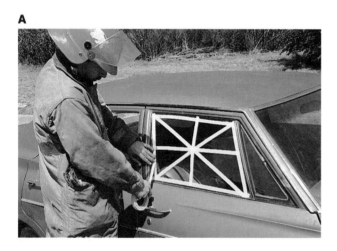

B

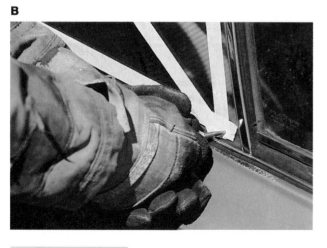

C

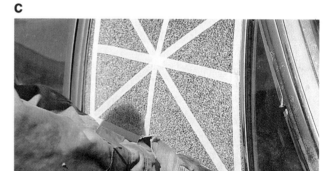

D

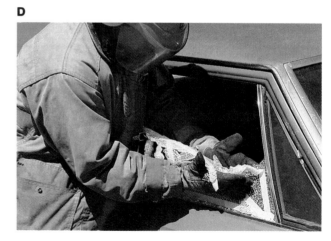

FIGURE 47–16

Removal of tempered glass. (A) Remove a tempered glass window by taping it with masking or adhesive tape to cut down on the risk of flying glass. (B) Apply a center punch to one corner. (C) Fire the center punch to shatter the glass. An alternate method is to strike the window a sharp blow with the point of a fire axe or head of a small hammer in one corner. (D) Remove the glass to allow access to the interior of the car. To avoid additional injuries from the glass, it is a good idea to place the removed glass out of the way under the vehicle.

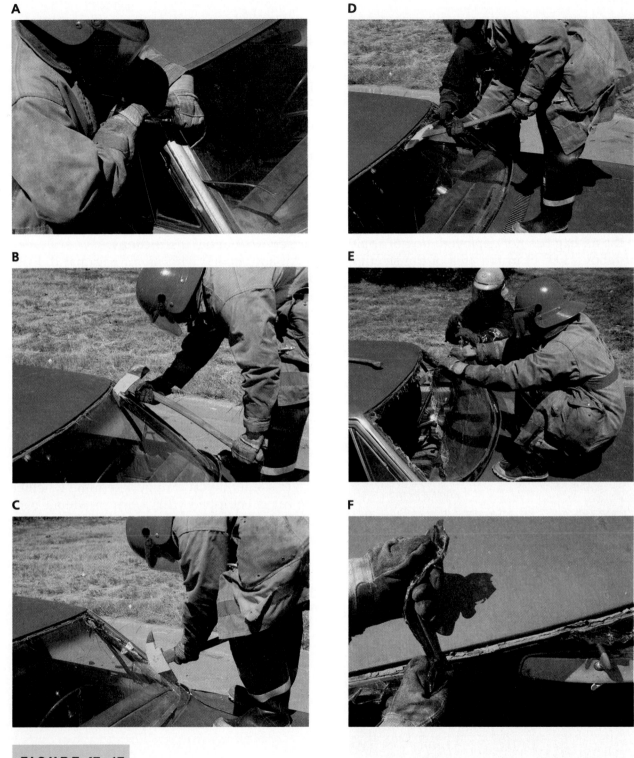

FIGURE 47–17

Removal of laminated glass. (A) Removal of the laminated glass of a windshield requires a different technique. First, remove all chrome trim strips. A baling hook will facilitate the removal. It is a good idea to kick the removed trim strips under the car to avoid additional injuries. (B) Make a hole in one of the upper corners of the windshield with the point of a fire axe. (C) Cut both sides of the windshield with a fire axe. (D) With another rescuer supporting the windshield, cut the upper edge with a fire axe. (E) Pull out and lift free the windshield. (F) Remove any remaining fragments of glass.

Some cars are equipped with an energy reserve feature that has the power to deploy the air bag for up to 20 minutes after the battery has been disconnected or the ignition turned off. The energy reserve and all air bag sensors can be disabled by disconnecting the air bag harness connector at the base of the steering column (Figure 47–18). If you cannot disconnect the harness connector, carry out your normal patient care and extrication operations, but do not place your body against or very close to the air bag module except for essential maneuvers.

If the air bag has not deployed, do not apply heat (above 300° F) in the area of the steering wheel hub. The air bag module is designed to self-deploy in the event of a fire. Applying heat

could activate the self-deployment feature. Do not cut or drill into the air bag module.

After deployment, the residue on and around the bag may contain a small amount of sodium hydroxide dust. Gloves and glasses should be worn to prevent any irritation to the skin or eyes. Do not allow any of this air bag residue to get into your eyes or the patient's eyes or wounds. In the unlikely event that the disk shaped canister in the module is ruptured, do not touch or ingest any exposed chemicals.

Before using a car with an air bag for training purposes, first deploy the bag according to the car service manual instructions.

An automobile with an air bag that did not deploy can be identified by several methods. Some models with driver-side air bags will have the words "Supplemental Inflatable Restraint" or "S.I.R." on the steering wheel hub (Figure 47–19). Otherwise, the driver-side air bag can usually be identified by the large size of the steering wheel hub, approximately 6 × 9 inches, which contains the bag. General Motors cars equipped with air bags have the number "3" in the seventh position of the VIN (vehicle identification number), which is visible through the bottom of the windshield on the driver's side. If you cannot determine whether the car is equipped with a driver-side air bag, take the same precautions as if it were equipped with an undeployed air bag.

If a door is sufficiently damaged so that it cannot be opened in the standard fashion or with a pry bar, hydraulic devices may be required. Figures 47–20 and 47–21 illustrate the use of hydraulic equipment to open a vehicle door.

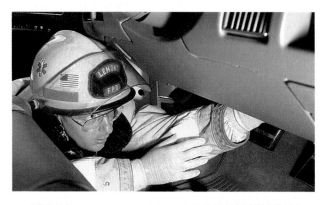

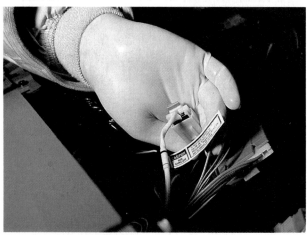

FIGURE 47–18

The energy reserve and all air bag sensors can be disabled by disconnecting the air bag harness at the base of the steering column.

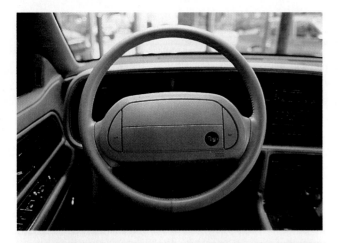

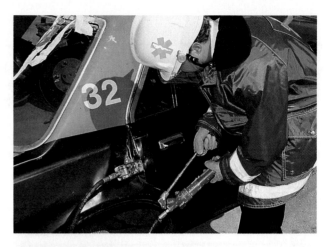

FIGURE 47–20

A Porta-power spreader may be used for doors with mild to moderate structural damage. Insert and pump up the spreader jaws between the door and frame to open the door by springing the lock bolt. Use caution with the longer spreader blades, as they may shatter if excessive force is generated.

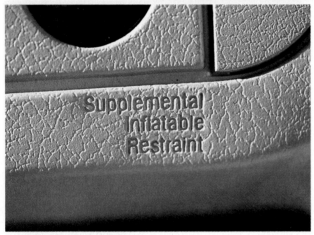

FIGURE 47–19

A car with an air bag that did not deploy can be identified by several methods. Some models with driver-side air bags will have the words "Supplemental Inflatable Restraint" or "S.I.R." on the steering wheel hub.

Sometimes it may be necessary to access the patient through the roof of the vehicle. Figures 47–22 and 47–23 illustrate vehicle access through the roof.

Sometimes the patient is trapped beneath the steering wheel. Figures 47–24 through 47–26 illustrate the techniques of pulling a steering wheel with a jack, a come-along, and a ram. Do not use these techniques to pull a tilt steering wheel or work with a front-wheel-drive vehicle, because a break may occur at the universal joint and force the steering column up into the patient.

Figure 47–27 shows how to remove a brake pedal that may be entrapping a patient's foot. The same technique can be used to free a patient caught between bars or to free a foot caught under a car (Figure 47–28). Figures 47–29 and 47–30 illustrate lifting equipment.

A

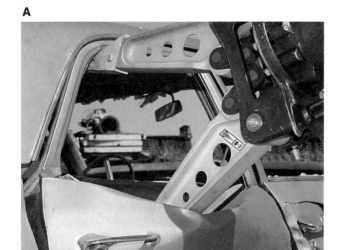

B

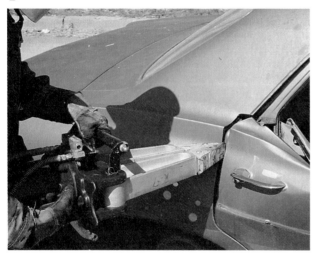

C

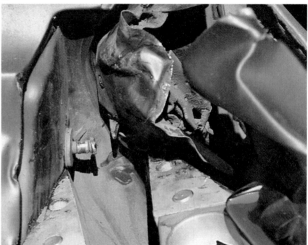

FIGURE 47–21

To open a door with major structural damage, the hydraulic spreader tool is frequently used.
(A) Develop an insertion point for the jaws between the door and the frame at about the level of the lock bolt. Develop this insertion point by placing the hydraulic spreader jaws between the roof and the door frame.
(B) Spread the jaws until the door is sufficiently deformed to allow the jaws to be reinserted at the level of the lock bolt. The porta-power spreader may also be used to develop this insertion point. (C) Insert the jaws at the level of the lock bolt and spread them until the lock mechanism has been popped free of the lock bolt. Open the door on its hinges.

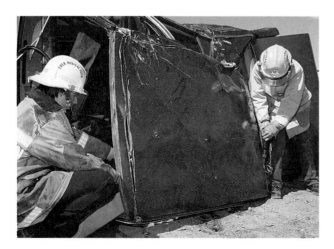

FIGURE 47–22

Rapid cutting of sheet metal is possible with a pneumatic air chisel. Replace the T-type chisel with the flat chisel to cut supporting members. Make the cuts in a "U" shape, and roll the roof back like a sardine can. If possible, cover, protect, and support the patient before cutting through the top.

A

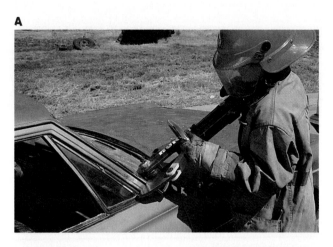

B

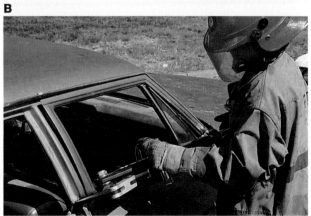

C

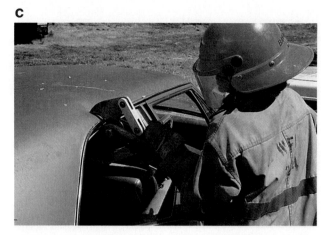

D

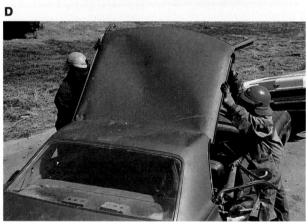

FIGURE 47–23

Sometimes it is necessary to completely remove the roof to access the patient. (A) Initially, remove the windshield, and roll down or remove the side windows. Then, use a hydraulic shear to cut the front pillars at their bases. (B) Cut the center door posts at their bases.

(C) Use the shears to cut the curve of the roof just in front of the rear pillars. If necessary, crease the roof with a sledge hammer along the line between the rearmost cuts. (D) Lift the roof from both sides and bend it backwards out of the way.

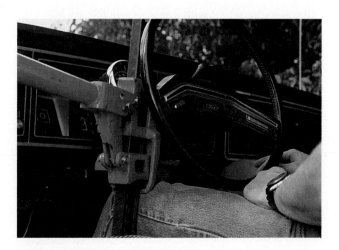

FIGURE 47–24

If a patient is trapped beneath the steering wheel, use a standard automotive jack between the floor and the steering wheel to free the patient.

A

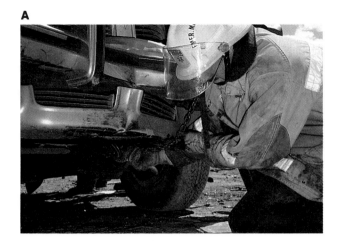

B

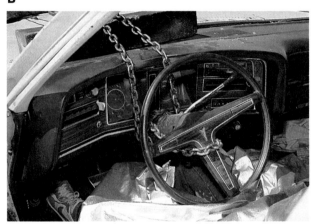

C

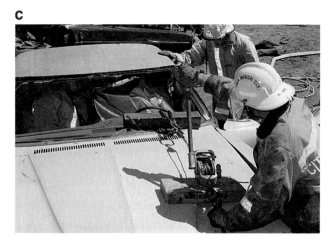

FIGURE 47-25

Pull a steering wheel away with a come-along. (A) A suitable anchor point is located on the vehicle, and the come-along is attached using chains or webbing.
(B) Keeping the patient covered and informed, the rescuer attaches a second chain to the steering wheel, positioned so that it will pull upward on the outer end of the steering wheel shaft. (C) Place the cribbing wherever the chains, come-along, and cable touch the vehicle. A stack of cribbing in front of the steering wheel provides excellent leverage.

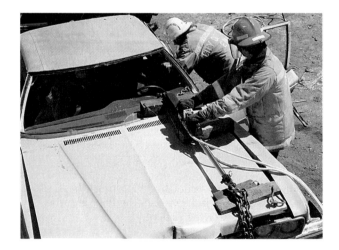

FIGURE 47-26

Pull a steering wheel with a ram. A suitable anchor point is located in line with the required direction of pull on the steering wheel. Secure the ram to the anchoring point using chains or webbing. Keep the patient covered and informed. Attach a second chain around the steering wheel as low as possible. Place cribbing at points where the chains and equipment contact the vehicle.

A

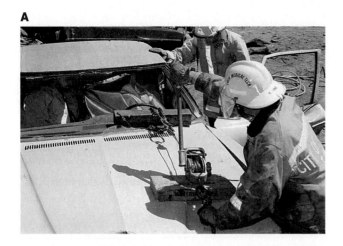

B

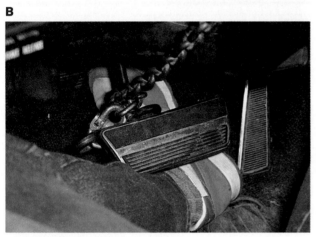

A

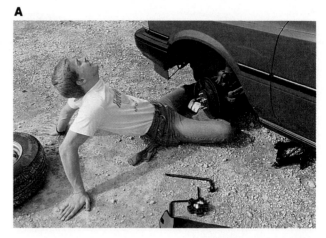

B

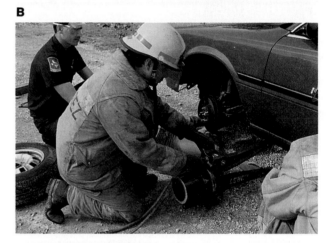

FIGURE 47–27

A brake pedal can be moved with a come-along and a deflector. (A) After locating an anchor point at the front of the vehicle, anchor the come-along with chains or webbing. Locate the pulley at an angle in the direction of pull, and anchor the pulley. (B) Using chains or webbing around the pedal, attach the loose end of the come-along to the cable hook. Utilize cribbing at all points of contact between the cable and the vehicle.

FIGURE 47–28

(A) To free an entrapped limb, (B) place the hydraulic spreader under the entrapping object, and expand the jaws until there is sufficient room to remove the entrapped body part.

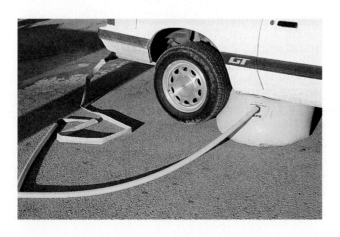

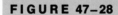

FIGURE 47–29

Lifting a vehicle with low-pressure air bags. The low-pressure air bags provide a wide base of support for lifting. Add additional puncture protection where necessary. Use box cribbing during the lift to protect the patient and the rescuers. Again, it is advisable to stabilize the vehicle to avoid slippage.

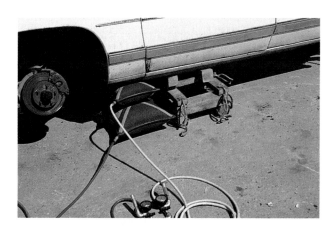

FIGURE 47-30

Lifting a vehicle with high-pressure air bags. High-pressure air bags provide a fairly wide base of support. Additional cribbing may be necessary to provide an adequate base for lifting. Once again, secure the vehicle to prevent rollover or slippage. Use wide box cribbing to maintain the position of the vehicle to prevent further injury to the patient or rescuer.

PREPARING AND "PACKAGING" THE PATIENT

Preparation for patient removal entails the basic elements previously described. Immobilization of fractures and the dressing of wounds should be balanced against the overall condition of the patient and the feasibility of carrying out such tasks in confined spaces. Do not remove a helmet in the field unless it is necessary to protect or preserve the airway or if you need to gain access to the skull. Stabilizing the legs to each other or the arms to the body will suffice if movement is gentle and planned. Some patients may have to be removed quickly because their general condition is deteriorating, and time will not permit meticulous splinting and dressing procedures. Clinical judgment must determine priorities in such cases.

Packaging the patient for removal to the ambulance is best accomplished by means of spine boards or similar devices. Such packaging will convert difficult situations to easier ones. The long spine board is essential in moving patients with potential or suspected

spine injuries. They are very helpful in other cases as well. Figure 47-31 illustrates packaging techniques using a spine board.

Clinical studies suggest that up to 25 percent of patients with neurological injuries secondary to cervical fractures become quadriplegic or have their injuries exacerbated during extrication, transport, and evaluation. This is presumably due to inadequate immobilization. New devices such as the noninvasive halo or appositional halo (Figure 47-32) may improve immobilization techniques.

SPECIALIZED RESCUE

In certain situations or disasters, specialized rescue teams are necessary. If the situation warrants and the dispatcher has not already done so, you must request a specialized rescue team. You then stand ready to provide all assistance necessary. Specialized rescue team members are trained in emergency medical care as well as in their rescue specialty. They are capable of providing basic emergency medical care to the patient.

Specialized rescue requires many skills not taught in the basic EMT training programs. A few general principles involving rough terrain and inaccessible areas, water rescue, snow and ice rescue, and urban rescue are all that will be covered here. Those who have an interest in specialized rescue are urged to contact the rescue team in their community. Most rescue services are anxious for additional volunteers and will assist in providing the additional training needed to become a member of the team.

Rescue in Rough Terrain and Inaccessible Areas

Rescue in rough terrain includes hilly or mountainous regions, flooded areas, or places where travel by road is impossible. Conditions may be aggravated by snow, ice, or rain. The main considerations in rough terrain rescue are locating the patient, providing emergency medical care as necessary, and using appropriate equipment to transport the patient to medical care.

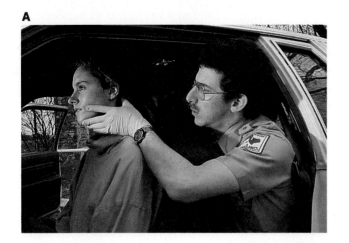

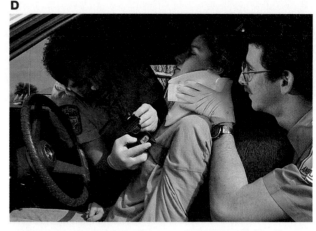

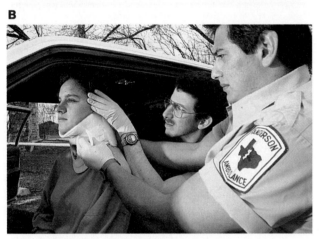

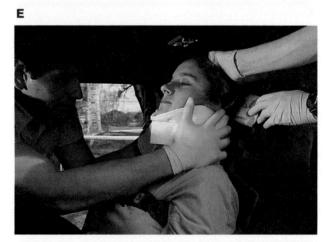

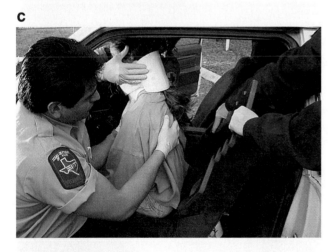

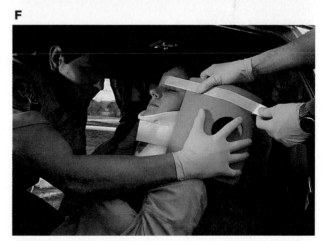

FIGURE 47–31

Packaging techniques using a spine board. (A) The short spine board (or equivalent) is used most frequently for stabilization of the sitting patient. The patient's head is supported by an EMT who applies neutral in-line traction. (B) A second EMT should stabilize the neck with a firm extrication collar. (C) Position the short board behind the patient while providing gentle support to the thoracic spine. (D) Secure the patient to the body of the board by the attached straps. There are several satisfactory methods for securing the straps. (E) Place an occipital pad behind the head to prevent hyperextension of the neck. Do not place this pad down in the curve of the neck, as it might increase neck extension in that position. (F) Secure the patient's head to the board with tape or Velcro straps. Do not use chin straps because of the danger of vomiting and difficulty with airway management.

G

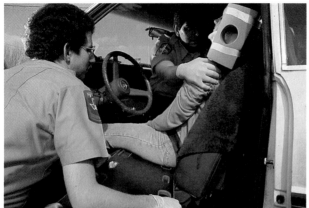

H

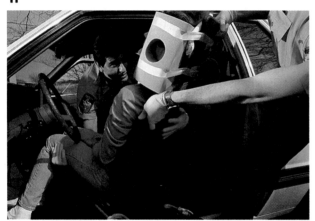

I

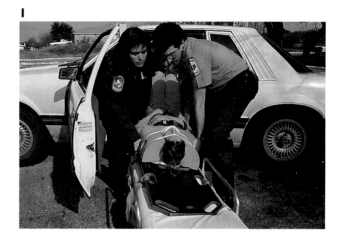

J

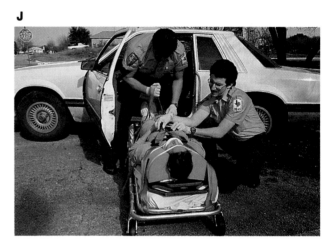

FIGURE 47–31

(continued) (G) Move the long spine board in under the patient's hips. (H) Rotate/lift the patient onto the long spine board. (I) Position and secure the patient on the long spine board. (J) Slide and secure the long board and patient onto the stretcher. If the patient's injuries demand, then position her on her side.

FIGURE 47–32

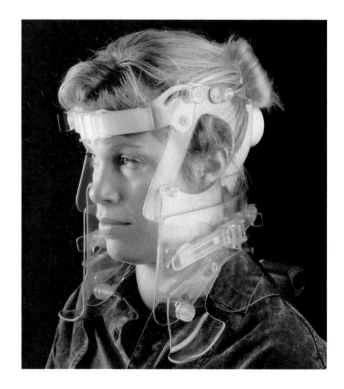

The halo spinal immobilization device.

Rough terrain rescues may involve such techniques as multiple-person stretcher passes up and over rough terrain, stream fording, or technical rock-climbing skills. Four-wheel-drive, high-clearance vehicles may be required to transport stretchers. Rescues in rough terrain often require great ingenuity to suspend or pad a stretcher so that the patient is provided a reasonably comfortable ride. Padding such as inflated inner tubes, 4- to 5-inch foam padding, or loosely rolled blankets may be used and is superior to "slinging" the stretcher on straps, which may allow excessive swaying and bouncing.

Helicopters are increasingly being used for quick patient evacuation from remote areas. Additionally, they are used to transport EMTs to the scene of an emergency in a remote area. If you are frequently faced with such situations, you should learn the various standard hand signals used for ground-to-air communication with the helicopter. As a rule, the crew of the helicopter is trained in emergency medical care, and you need to learn the techniques of boarding and off-loading helicopters. The methods of opening a landing area should also be learned. Chapter 48 contains more information regarding **MEDEVAC** helicopters and important guidelines for personal safety when MEDEVAC helicopters are in the vicinity.

Water Rescue

Water rescue involves rescue from a body of water, boats, marine structures, or areas flooded by excessive rain or by overflowing dams and reservoirs. The extent of your involvement in water rescue depends on the local protocol.

To be effective in water rescue, you must have a basic knowledge of water safety. All personnel involved in water rescue should be strong swimmers, preferably trained as water safety instructors or lifeguards. All water rescue personnel must wear an approved **personal flotation device** at all times. Never enter a boat without *wearing* (not carrying) an approved personal flotation device.

There is a great difference between simply wading out into a calm pond to rescue a person already hanging onto a flotation device and attempting to cross a river at flood crest to rescue a person off a bridge, pier, or rock. Likewise, the ocean front may create additional problems such as tides, large waves, and undercurrents. Personnel working in such dangerous areas should be attached to shore by a lifeline so they can be retrieved if necessary.

In water rescue situations, you must be alert to hypothermia in the patient as well as in yourself. Hypothermia may have some protective effect on the drowning victim, making delayed resuscitation possible. Chapter 42 contains additional information on hypothermia.

Cold Weather Rescue

Incidents involving snow and ice rescue are frequently encountered in association with recreational activities such as mountain climbing, technical ice and rock climbing, snowmobiling, ice fishing, cross-country and alpine skiing, snowshoeing, and skating. Incidents may also occur as a result of employment, particularly for workers such as snowplow drivers, farmers, mail carriers, and foresters.

The most common source of injury in the snowy or icy environment is the motor vehicle accident. Management of a motor vehicle accident is complicated by winter conditions. Your response time may frequently be longer in winter months because of additional clothing requirements, prolonged warm-up time for the response vehicle, and hazardous driving conditions. Frequently, the environment will be both cold and dark. There will be rapid cooling of the accident vehicle, because automobiles have exceptionally poor insulating qualities. This will result in rapid cooling of the occupants and a significant risk of hypothermia. Therefore, in addition to your usual concerns about the patient's airway, breathing, circulation, and the need for splinting of the injuries, there is the concern for hypothermia.

Splinting techniques may have to be modified under these circumstances. Specifically, if a pneumatic antishock garment is indicated, the protocol that calls for removing all clothing has to be modified. Opening the front crease of the pant legs with scissors, examining the leg, and then allowing the clothing to fall back over the leg to keep it warm is a reasonable alternative. Pneumatic antishock garments, when partially inflated, provide good insulation, minimizing further heat loss from the lower extremities and lower abdomen.

Anyone who as a child placed a moistened tongue against a very cold metal object will vividly recall the incident. Likewise, you must take care to avoid exposing your or the patient's skin to cold metal splints and stretchers, because the skin may freeze to the metal.

Use of inflatable splints must be carefully monitored. Warm air from your lungs will cool rapidly once the splint is applied, resulting in loss of pressure in the splint and loss of immobilization. This can be prevented by frequent observation of the splint as the air cools and further inflation becomes necessary. When the patient is placed in the warm ambulance, the splint may develop excessive pressure as the contained air warms. This can be prevented through close observation and releasing of the air from the splint as necessary.

Both the inflatable plastic splints and the newer vacuum splints have a significant potential for cracking as they are handled under frigid conditions. Some services do not use the inflatable plastic splints during the winter months to avoid this high complication rate. Pneumatic antishock garments do not seem to be as significantly affected by cold weather.

An effective splint for cold weather situations is the cardboard box splint (Figure 47–33). It is inexpensive and readily stored in quantity. It may be used once and discarded. Ski patrol units have found that nylon straps with Velcro® closures work well for securing these splints. Such straps are easily managed with mittens or gloves. The Velcro straps will not freeze together like metal buckles. The straps are easily exchanged for disposable ties before or during the patient's evacuation to the hospital.

In addition to the triangular bandage, the large safety pin or blanket pin is a versatile piece of equipment for winter management of extremity injuries, particularly of the upper extremity. They can be used to fashion a sling by simply pinning the arm of the outer garment

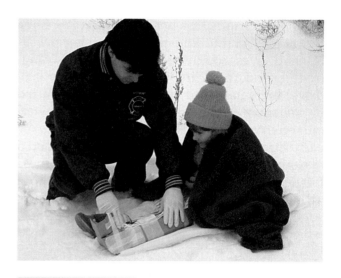

FIGURE 47–33

Cardboard box splints provide effective immobilization and are easy to work with in a cold environment.

to the chest of the garment (Figure 47–34). This provides secure immobilization of the upper extremity without sacrificing the warmth the garment provides. In addition, the extent to which the extremities can be examined at the scene depends to a considerable extent on the weather conditions and other circumstances.

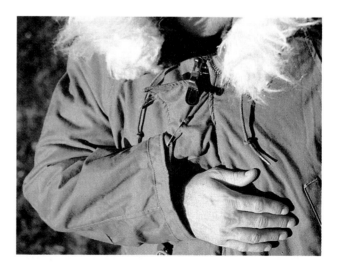

FIGURE 47–34

Preliminary immobilization of an injured upper extremity can be achieved with a large safety pin holding the injured arm against the chest wall.

Safety pin immobilization of one pant leg to the other, and the sleeves to the chest of the jacket, can provide good temporary immobilization until a warm, dry shelter can be reached, and more definitive secondary evaluation can be accomplished. Also, the patient's head should be covered, if at all possible, after you examine it. Fifteen percent of body heat can be dissipated through the exposed scalp.

Ice Rescue

As with all forms of technical rescue, ice rescue is not properly learned until it has been practiced. People who may be outstanding fire rescue or ambulance personnel may find themselves overwhelmed by the prospect of undertaking a difficult technical rescue. In areas where ponds, lakes, and rivers commonly freeze, practicing various ice rescue procedures is of great benefit.

The toughest problem in ice rescue is timing. The cold water begins to affect the victim immediately. Setting up equipment for a safe rescue is time-consuming. Only through careful preparation and prior planning can the necessary equipment and personnel be gathered and put into service in time to save a life. Preplanning should include the following:

- The community should know how to access the proper dispatch center.
- Dispatchers should alert, by protocol, those persons previously identified as having a specific role to play in the specialized rescue team (for example, scuba team, fire rescue, water rescue, drowning team). In areas where key personnel are not always on duty, locating them by beeper may be necessary.
- Required equipment should be stored and dispatched by protocol, unless countermanded by the on-scene commander. Such equipment includes the air supply truck, ladder truck, rescue boat, and special rescue gear, including waterproof rope, harnesses, slings, belaying equipment, throwing lines, line gun, and a personal flotation device for each individual at the scene.

Keeping the victim located is a prime concern. If possible, two observers should be situated a moderate distance apart from each other on the shore. They should keep constant visual contact with the victim or the victim's last visible location using a stationary reference point. Throwing a rope or flotation device to the victim will save the victim from having to waste energy swimming or treading water, and buy time to arrange a safe extrication.

Removing a victim over thin ice is a very dangerous procedure. It should only be accomplished by personnel who are prepared for immersion themselves—that is, they should be wearing wet or dry suits or "exposure suits" and flotation devices. They should be attached to shore with a lifeline. They may well use an inflatable rubber boat; the boat should be tethered ashore with a good rope.

Urban Rescue

For years technical rescue in an urban setting has been accomplished in admirable fashion by the local fire department. Rescue techniques using ladders and other equipment applicable to elevator shafts, building roofs, subway tunnels, and bridges have been developed. Recently, advances in the technology of mountaineering and technical climbing have fostered the production of new equipment that has been adapted to urban rescue. The use of figure-eight rapelling devices, the Russ Anderson "figure-eight with ears," belaying plates, bongs, shocks, nuts, and assorted mechanical jamming devices can all be of value in establishing **belays** (rescue lines) for rescuers and victims as well. Even if the fire department is going to use a direct ladder approach to a victim, the additional safety of a rope belay can be desirable when the belay is handled by well-trained personnel.

Experience must be gained in the use of such rescue techniques to recognize secure belaying points. A bong jammed under a door is only as strong as the door and door jamb. A sling around a pipe can be dangerous if the pipe is hot or rusty. Belaying to plumbing fixtures or furniture can lead to nasty surprises at the most inopportune times. Under all circumstances a secondary or backup belay point should be established. Before putting tension on a line, all

A

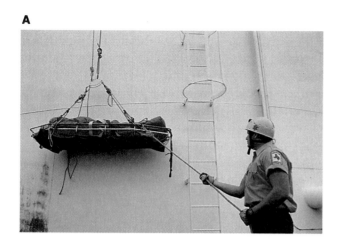

B

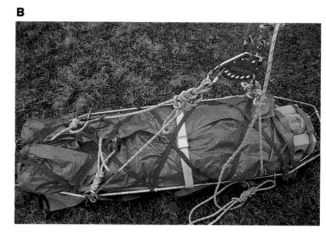

FIGURE 47-35

(A) Patients may be evacuated from a building using a Stokes stretcher or similar device. (B) The bridle can be used to elevate or lower the head of the stretcher.

A

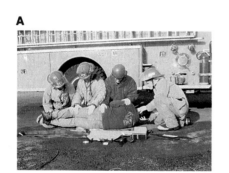

B

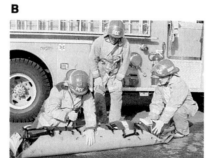

C

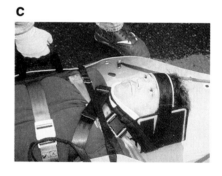

D

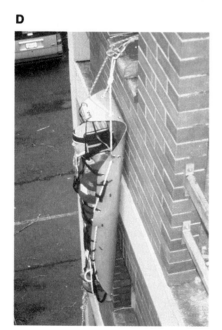

E

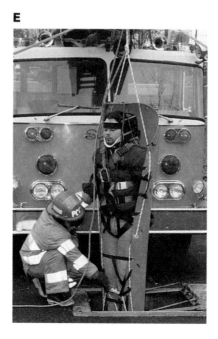

FIGURE 47-36

(A) An alternate method of vertical extrication using the SKED device. Place the patient in a spinal immobilization jacket or on a short board to prevent forced flexion of the cervical spine during the extrication. Log-roll the patient onto the SKED. (B) Secure the patient into the SKED. (C) Stabilize the head with foam blocks or a blanket roll. (D) With this kind of a protective packaging, the person can be lifted vertically without slipping out the bottom. (E) The packaged patient is compact enough to be removed through a standard manhole.

belay points should be inspected for security by a second team member.

All patients suspected of spinal injuries should be evacuated in a horizontal position in a Stokes stretcher or similar device. Patients with spinal injuries or major fractures may be evacuated from the upper levels of buildings that lack functioning elevators by a horizontal lowering in a Stokes stretcher, either in an elevator shaft or stairwell, or perhaps outside the building. The use of an adjustable bridle on the Stokes stretcher will allow some head-up positioning for head injuries, or head-down positioning for management of shock (Figure 47-35). Vertical evacuation (Figure 47-36) requires specialized packaging techniques to protect the injured spine.

Careful thought should go into the selection of the ropes used in rescue; some are now quite use-specific. Rope that does not soak up or retain water or increase in weight is now specifically manufactured for water rescue. Some synthetic ropes have a definite stretch factor that may be of value if it is required to withstand the shock of a fall. On the other hand, Dacron™ and some of the other synthetic ropes have very little stretch, which is much more suitable for tension lines. Obviously, it is very important to handle these ropes with care; they should be inspected and tested frequently and discarded when they begin to show signs of heavy use. Ridge or hose rollers should be employed where necessary to prevent ropes from fraying.

The use of rescue pulleys with carabiners and various belaying equipment can greatly facilitate and enhance the safety of technical urban rescue. Gasoline, electric, and hand-powered winches are also available to assist with long lifts.

Training for the techniques, skills, and activities involved in technical urban rescue can be accomplished in a variety of ways, but adequate basic training, frequent practice sessions, and scheduled retraining are mandatory for those planning to use technical urban rescue. The use of an "Outward Bound" type of program, which involves training in the use of climbing skills, becoming familiar with belaying techniques, and relying upon one's partner for security, has been found beneficial to many rescue services.

YOU ARE THE EMT

1. How does size-up differ from triage?
2. How does the glass in side and rear windows differ from the glass in windshields?
3. You have responded to an automobile accident in which two people have received injuries after their car skidded off the road and hit a telephone pole during a snowstorm. How will you combat hypothermia during treatment?
4. Describe four rescue situations in which a rope belay would be an essential piece of equipment. Specify the type of rope that should be used in each example.
5. How are hepatitis and HIV viruses spread? What is the easiest way to minimize your exposure? What do you do if you get inadvertently contaminated? Are your immunizations up to date?

SECTION 11

AMBULANCE
OPERATIONS

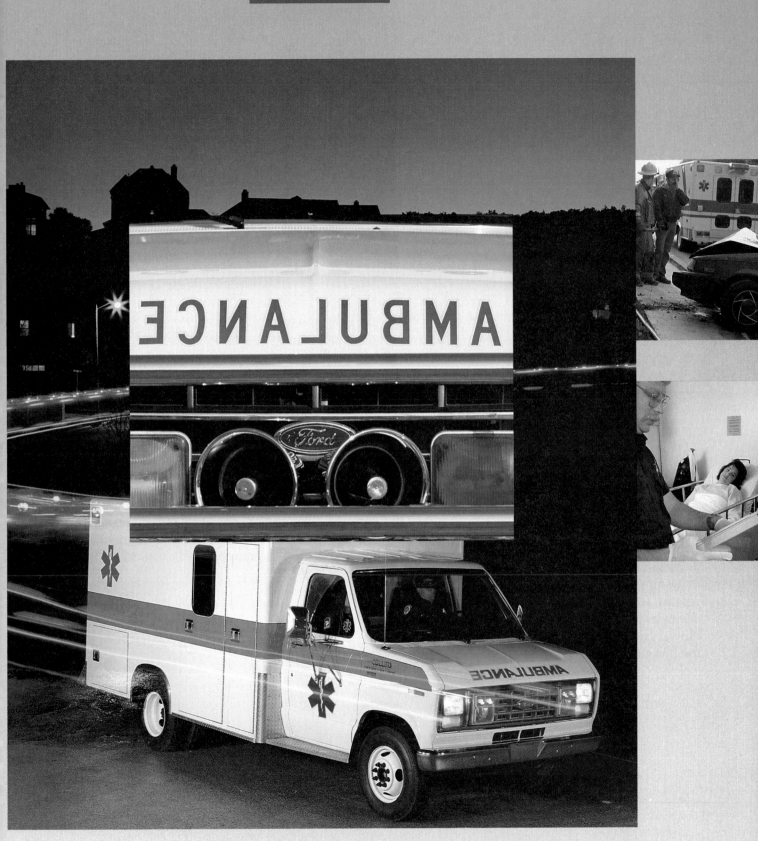

CHAPTER 48

THE MODERN EMERGENCY VEHICLE

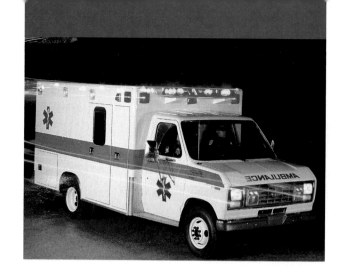

ambulance (am′bu-lans) Vehicle for emergency medical care.

chassis (shas′ē) The frame and working parts of a vehicle.

decontamination (de″kon-tam-ĭ-na′shun) The orderly process by which radiation or chemical hazards can be removed from clothing, equipment, vehicles, and personnel.

jump kit A lightweight, durable, waterproof kit used in the immediate care of the patient, usually by the EMT who initially leaves the vehicle while the EMT-driver parks the ambulance and secures the scene.

litter A type of stretcher for moving or carrying patients.

MEDEVAC A method of speeding lifesaving care to patients and of transporting patients with life-threatening injury or illness to treatment facilities using medically equipped helicopters.

Star of Life® Emblem that identifies true ambulances.

OVERVIEW

For many decades following the introduction of the first motor-driven ambulance in 1906, a hearse was the vehicle most frequently used as an ambulance because it could transport the patient in a recumbent position on a portable litter or stretcher. Few supplies were carried, and there was little space for the attendant in the back with the patient.

The hearse-ambulance has gone the way of its horse-drawn predecessor as better-equipped and better-designed emergency vehicles have become available. Ambulances are currently designed in accordance with government regulations (KKK specifications and ASTM standards) based on suggestions from the ambulance services and the EMTs who use them. One of the most significant developments in ambulance design has been the greater width, length, and height of the patient compartment.

Chapter 48 begins with an overview of ambulance design. This section discusses the definition of an ambulance, how a vehicle qualifies as an ambulance, standard external identification emblems and markings used on ambulances, and design specifications for an ambulance chassis and body. This section also describes ambulance acceleration capabilities and warning devices. The chapter then lists the various types of equipment and supplies that an ambulance should carry, including equipment and supplies for patient care and equipment for personal safety and extrication. The next section of Chapter 48 talks about the increasing role of air ambulances and the safety issues that are so important to their use.

GOALS

The goals of Chapter 48 are to

- become familiar with modern emergency vehicle design as it relates to national, state, and local standards.
- identify basic emergency vehicle equipment and supplies, including patient-care equipment and supplies, a jump kit, and equipment for personal safety and extrication.
- recognize the increasing role of air ambulances and learn how to approach a MEDEVAC helicopter safely and how to assist a MEDEVAC pilot in the sometimes difficult task of landing the aircraft.

EMERGENCY VEHICLE DESIGN

Manufacturers have enlarged and improved the **ambulance** in accordance with government-mandated design criteria and in response to the recommendations of those who use them—EMTs and other emergency personnel. Thus, more working space in the patient compartment, including room for at least two **litters,** and storage facilities for the essential equipment as recommended by the Committee on Trauma of the American College of Surgeons, are among the additions that have resulted in greater width, length, and height of the patient compartment. In a highly competitive and limited-output industry, these medically necessary improvements have added significantly to the cost of the modern ambulance.

Manufacturers have welcomed the consolidated recommendations of EMTs, ambulance operators, physicians, and automobile design engineers who, through the National Academy of Sciences-National Research Council (NAS-NRC) and the National Highway Traffic Safety Administration, have established national standards. In addition to bringing about greater uniformity of design and equipment, these standards have provided not only for the needs of today but also for adaptation for future medical advances without the necessity for radical changes in ambulance design.

Regardless of whether ambulances are used in urban or rural areas, they must be standardized to carry the essential recommended equipment. The need for equipment for the personal safety of the patient and EMTs, for extrication, and for road clearance is just as necessary in the city as in rural areas.

Continued research and development of vehicles with more sophisticated equipment for EMT-paramedics will undoubtedly continue, but the presently recommended standard ambulance can provide storage for all the supplies as well as the space necessary for basic and advanced life support at the scene and during transport.

NAS-NRC Definition of an Ambulance

The NAS-NRC defines an ambulance as a vehicle for emergency medical care, designed to provide a driver's compartment and a patient compartment that can accommodate two EMTs and two litter patients. The patients must be positioned so that at least one can be given intensive lifesaving care—cardiopulmonary resuscitation (CPR)—during transit. This vehicle must carry equipment and supplies to provide emergency medical care at the scene and during transport, to safeguard personnel and patients from hazardous conditions, and to carry out light extrication procedures. It must have two-way radio communication to enable the ambulance personnel to contact the dispatcher, the hospital, public safety authorities, and medical control. It must be designed and

constructed to afford maximal safety and comfort so that transportation does not aggravate the patient's injury or illness.

Restrictions on Designation as an Ambulance

Each state establishes its own standards for ambulance licensure. In most states, to qualify as an ambulance, a vehicle must meet all of the NAS-NRC requirements just stated. Unless it is fully equipped and staffed to serve as an ambulance, no vehicle employed to transport nonemergency patients (litter, wheelchair, or seated) will be licensed as an ambulance. Specially designed mobile intensive care units may be licensed as ambulances, depending on the state in which they are registered.

Federal specifications (KKK-A-1822C, 1990) have been developed and are used by most states as the basis for their ambulance licensure requirements. Pertinent portions of these recommended specifications are discussed in this chapter. These specifications are for the following three types of basic ambulance designs:

- Type I: conventional, truck cab-chassis with modular ambulance body that can be transferred to a newer chassis as needed (Figure 48–1a).
- Type II: standard van, forward-control integral cab-body ambulance (Figure 48–1b).
- Type III: specialty van, forward-control integral cab-body ambulance (Figure 48–1c).

External Identification

To ensure that the ambulance will be universally distinguished from all other vehicles, the exterior color should be basically white, in combination with an orange stripe and blue lettering and emblems. The materials used for the emblems and markings should be reflectorized. The **Star of Life**® emblem should be on the sides, rear, and roof of the vehicle (Figure 48–2). Local licensing authorities determine what emblems may be displayed on the side of a prehospital care ambulance, but there is no regulation for interhospital transport ambulances, and their emblems may look almost the

A

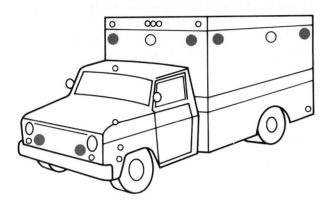

B

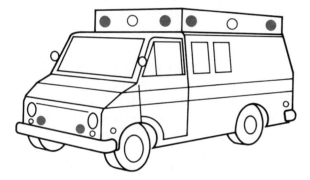

C

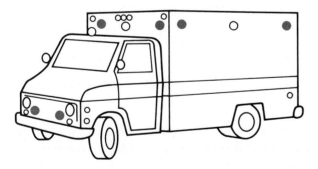

FIGURE 48-1

Three ambulance designs that meet federal specifications: (A) Type I, conventional truck cab-chassis with modular ambulance body; (B) Type II, standard van, forward-control integral cab-body ambulance; (C) Type III, specialty van, forward control integral cab-body ambulance.

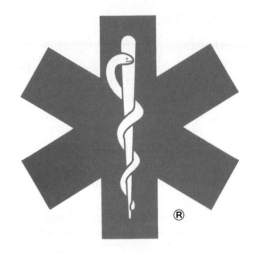

FIGURE 48-2

The Star of Life® emblem is displayed on the sides, rear, and roof of emergency vehicles that meet federal specifications as licensed ambulances.

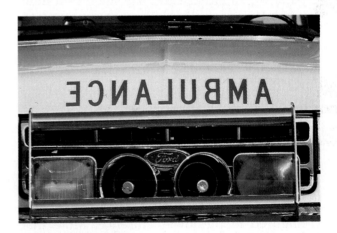

FIGURE 48-3

The word "ambulance" appears in mirror image letters on the front of the rescue vehicle.

same as the Star of Life. State and local regulations specify the numbers, type, colors, and locations of the warning lights. The siren should be capable of varying in pitch ("warbling") so that the drivers of other vehicles can recognize the sound. The word *ambulance* should be in mirror image letters on the front of the vehicle for easy identification by drivers ahead who see an ambulance approaching in their rear-view mirror (Figure 48-3).

Ambulance Chassis

The **chassis** should provide optimal smooth-riding qualities. It should have a road clearance of at least 6 inches when loaded and be able to ford water up to 12 inches deep. It must have a heavy-duty braking system and the highest-quality tires. A fuel range of at least 150 miles is suggested. Higher road clearance, dual rear wheels, and four-wheel-drive may be necessary where geographic location, climate, or frequent off-highway operations dictate. The ambulance body may be mounted on a passenger or truck chassis. Compliance should be made with general federal motor vehicle safety standards that are applicable to the chassis.

The overall length of the ambulance may vary according to whether the patient's and driver's compartments are constructed as a single unit or the driver's cab is mounted separately. In either case, the suggested minimum interior length of the patient compartment is 116 inches. The maximum overall length of the entire vehicle over the bumpers should not exceed 22 feet. The height at curbside should not exceed 110 inches, including roof-mounted equipment but excluding the flexible portion of radio antennas.

Keep in mind that many hospitals were designed long before the modern ambulance. Therefore, if a service frequently transports to a hospital with an entrance lower than 110 inches, it might want to obtain a vehicle configured to the lower entrance. More than one ambulance has lost its expensive roof-mounted equipment on a low overhang or garage door.

Ambulance Body

The body must be crashworthy and free of interior protrusions and unsecured objects that could be dangerous to you or your patient. It should be climate-controlled, insulated, and easily cleaned. It must be large enough to accommodate two litter patients, two EMTs, and all installed and portable equipment and supplies necessary for optimal patient care. There should be no windows except in the front, rear, and curbside doors of the patient compartment (additional windows take up necessary storage space). Direct access between the driver and passenger compartments is desirable. If there is a passageway, a door should be provided that can be locked from the driver's side. In either case, there should be a window or intercom between the driver's and patient's compartments. The driver should be shielded from the light in the rear compartment when driving at night.

There should be a clear space of 25 inches at the head and 15 inches at the foot of a standard 76-inch litter in the patient compartment. Inside width should provide for two 23-inch-wide litters, with sufficient space between them to permit you to kneel at the side of the primary patient and perform CPR. Thus, a 25-inch working area is required, part of which can be unobstructed space for the lower legs and feet of the EMT beneath the second litter or squad bench. The minimum acceptable ceiling height is 60 inches, with no protrusions over the aisle between the litters nor over the head and chest of either litter patient.

All equipment necessary for patient care in transit must be permanently installed, secured, or stored in cabinets inside the patient compartment. Once again, eliminating side windows and extra doors frees up more space for needed storage. All items must be adequately secured so that in the event of an accident, equipment and supplies will not become potentially harmful missiles.

Acceleration

The fully loaded ambulance should be capable of acceleration such that it is able to maintain its position in traffic on highways, as well as avoid hazardous situations in moving traffic. The criterion of acceleration is designed to ensure safety of the ambulance in traffic on interstate highways. Training in defensive driving, operational judgment, and a primary concern for the safety of the patient as well as the public will determine the manner in which the driver responsibly uses the ambulance's capabilities.

Warning Devices

A siren and a public address system should be mounted on each ambulance. They may be a combined system. A noise-canceling microphone, manual and automatic siren undulation, and yelp should be part of the system. Two speakers are desirable. An air horn is a useful additional warning and signaling device. Warning lights, including colors, are specified by state or local regulation.

EMERGENCY VEHICLE EQUIPMENT AND SUPPLIES

In order to estimate the space requirements for installed, portable, and stored equipment and supplies, as well as to house them for easy accessibility, ambulance designers must be familiar with the size, weight, shape, and power requirements for each item. No new equipment or supplies should be ordered by EMTs without consultation with the medical director of the ambulance service.

Many items offered for use by EMS systems have never been rigorously tested and evaluated for effectiveness under field conditions. Therefore, purchase of such items may turn out to be expensive or perhaps even dangerous mistakes. As a general rule of thumb, the more complex a piece of equipment, the more difficult it is to learn how to use it properly, especially under adverse field conditions, and the more likely the equipment is to malfunction during a medical emergency.

Equipment and supplies should be located according to the relative importance of the item and its frequency of use. Priority should be given to items necessary to cope with life-threatening conditions. Equipment and supplies necessary for airway care, artificial ventilation, and oxygenation must be within easy reach of the EMT positioned at the head of the primary litter. Equipment and supplies for cardiac resuscitation, control of external bleeding, and monitoring blood pressure must be easily available at the side of the litter.

To the greatest extent possible, equipment and supplies should be durable and standardized so that exchanges can be made between ambulances or between ambulances and emergency departments. Exchange is an important consideration for any ambulance service, because it decreases the delay in transfer of patients, prevents premature and possibly dangerous removal of required equipment from the patient, and decreases the time the EMTs and ambulance are detained at the hospital.

Storage cabinets and kits should open easily but must be fastened securely to keep them from opening during transit. The use of transparent construction materials for the fronts of cabinets and drawers allows rapid identification of their contents; otherwise, labeling of the contents on the cabinet fronts is recommended.

Equipment for Patient Care

Patient Transfer Litters Each ambulance should have a wheeled litter, a folding litter, and a collapsible chair device that enables you to carry a patient in stairways and other narrow spaces where a full-length litter cannot be used because of its size. The collapsible and folding litters may be combined as one unit. Litters must be easy to move, store, clean, and disinfect. The folding litter should keep the patient elevated above floor level when in the flat, extended position.

The wheeled litter should be adjustable in height and designed so that when secured in the lowest position, the top is between 11 and 15 inches above the floor of the ambulance. The head of the litter should be capable of being tilted upward to a 60-degree semisitting position, and the entire litter should be capable of being tilted into 10 degrees of the Trendelenburg position (head down) for airway care. So that patients can be full length in the supine, prone, or lateral position, litters must be at least 76 inches long and 23 inches wide. The frame or handles must be designed to permit up to four persons to carry the litter. Fasteners to secure the litter firmly to the floor or to the side of the vehicle during transport must be provided. The litter restraints should be capable of securing the litter to withstand a rollover of the ambulance. A minimum of two restraining devices must be provided to prevent the patient from falling off the sides or sliding off the end of the litter and to protect the upper and lower body.

Some ambulance services use an x-ray permeable, removable panel, such as the top of an emergency room cot or backboard, on top of the litter. This allows the patient to be moved easily through all the necessary diagnostic and treatment facilities, including surgery, without being removed from the panel until placed in a hospital bed (Figure 48–4). Such a panel decreases the discomfort for the patient during transfers, as well as the risk of further injury. The disadvantage of such a panel is that it prevents the patient from being placed in the semisitting position while the panel is in place on the litter.

Airways Oropharyngeal airways for adults, children, and infants must be carried. Nasal airways for adults and children should also be available.

Artificial Ventilation Devices Portable artificial ventilation devices that operate independently of a supply of oxygen must be provided.

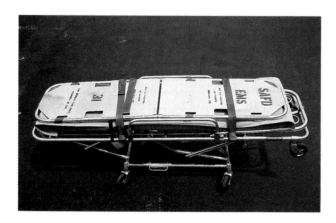

FIGURE 48–4

A wheeled ambulance litter with an x-ray permeable, removable panel from an emergency department cot or backboard placed on top. The patient can be moved easily from the ambulance to the emergency department to surgery without risk of further injury or discomfort.

Two units are desirable—one for use in the ambulance and the other for use outside the vehicle or as a spare. Portable artificial ventilation devices of the manually operated, self-filling, bag-valve-mask type that are capable of oxygen enrichment should also be carried. When attached to an oxygen supply, with the oxygen reservoir in place, the unit should be capable of supplying almost 100 percent oxygen to the patient. The unit must be easy to clean and **decontaminate.** The nonrebreathing valve must permit inhalation of oxygen during both artificial and spontaneous respirations. A pediatric-sized bag-valve-mask should also be carried.

Masks in a variety of sizes from infant to adult must be stocked. They should be transparent to permit the rapid recognition of color change in the patient and to detect vomiting or respiratory abnormalities. Adult and pediatric-sized bags should be used with the corresponding mask to deliver the proper volume of oxygen-enriched air to the patient.

Suction Equipment Portable and installed suction equipment is very important. The suction units must be powerful enough to provide an airflow of 30 liters per minute at the end of the suction tube and a vacuum of 300 mm Hg (mercury) when the tube is clamped. The suction force must be adjusted for use on children and infants. It should be fitted with large-bore, nonkinking suction tubing with a semirigid pharyngeal tip. There should be an additional set of semirigid suction tips. On the installed unit, the suction yoke, unbreakable collection bottle, water for rinsing the suction tips, and suction tubing must be readily accessible to the EMT at the head of the litter. The tubing must reach the patient's airway, regardless of the patient's position. All suction apparatus must be of the type that is easily cleaned and decontaminated.

Oxygen Inhalation Equipment An emergency vehicle must be equipped with two oxygen supply units—one portable and the other installed. The portable unit (300 liter capacity) should be located near a door for ready use outside the vehicle. It should be equipped with a yoke, pressure gauge, flowmeter (not gravity-dependent), delivery tubing, and oxygen mask. The unit must be capable of delivering oxygen at a flow rate of between 2 and 15 liters/minute (lpm). An extra portable 300 liter cylinder should be kept on the ambulance. Many services equip the backup cylinder with its own yoke, gauge, regulator, and tubing so that it can be used for a second patient in an emergency.

The installed oxygen unit must be supplied by at least 3,000 liters of oxygen, delivered by a two-stage regulator under pressure of 50 psi (pounds per square inch). The unit must be fitted with yokes, reducing valves, and flowmeters (not gravity-dependent). The flowmeters must be visible and accessible to an EMT seated at the head of the litter. The system must be capable of delivering oxygen at a flow rate of between 2 and 15 liters/minute. Delivery tubes must reach the face of the patient who is being transported in a horizontal position. They should connect readily to oxygen masks and to bag-valve mask ventilation devices. Oxygen masks (with and without bags) should be semiopen, valveless, transparent, and disposable. Masks should be available in sizes for adults, children, and infants. Nasal cannulae should also be available.

Ambulance services that frequently transport patients on runs lasting longer than 1 hour should consider using a disposable, single-use humidifier for the installed oxygen system. For runs of less than 1 hour, humidification is rarely indicated and may actually lead to an increased risk of infection in patients if the humidifiers are not scrupulously maintained.

Cardiac Compression Equipment A spine board, when placed under the patient on the litter, provides the necessary resistance for effective external chest compression. A tightly rolled sheet on the board will raise the patient's shoulders 3 to 4 inches above the level of the board and keep the head in a position of maximum backward tilt, while maintaining the shoulders and thorax in a straight position without manual support. If you suspect a neck injury, do not use such a roll for hyperextension of the neck.

Supplies for Patient Care

Basic Supplies Ambulances should carry the following basic supplies:

- A minimum of 2 pillows.
- A minimum of 2 pillow cases.
- A minimum of 2 spare sheets.
- 4 blankets.
- 4 towels.
- 6 disposable emesis bags or basins.
- 2 boxes of disposable tissue.
- 1 bedpan (optional).
- 1 urinal (optional).
- 2 disposable thermometers (optional).
- 4 sandbags.
- 1 blood pressure cuff.
- 1 stethoscope.
- 1 pair trauma shears.
- 1 package of disposable drinking cups.
- 1 unbreakable container of water.
- 1 package of wet wipes.
- 4 cold packs.
- 4 liters of irrigation fluid.
- 2 restraining devices.
- 1 package of plastic bags for waste or severed parts.
- disposable gloves.
- 1 Sharps container.
- 1 set of hearing protectors.
- 2 infection control kits (goggles, masks, and waterproof gowns).

Splinting Supplies The following supplies should be on hand for splinting fractures and dislocations:

- One lower extremity traction splint, with minimum 9-inch ring size and 43-inch length, with commercial limb-support slings, padded ankle hitch, traction strap with buckle, and a windlass. A telescoping splint may replace a rigid unit. A pediatric-sized splint should also be carried.
- Splints for the upper and lower extremities, such as uncomplicated inflatable, vacuum,

cardboard, plastic, wire-ladder, canvas-slotted, lace-on, or padded board. The number and types of splints should be determined by the local medical director or state law.

- Triangular bandages and conforming roller bandages for fractures of the shoulder and upper arm and for fixation of rigid splints when necessary.
- Short and long spine boards, cervical collars, and accessories for safe extrication, as well as splinting in case of suspected injuries of the spine.
- A pneumatic antishock garment with inflation equipment to be used for the splinting of severe pelvic and upper femur fractures as well as in the treatment of hemorrhagic shock.

Dressing Supplies Supplies to be carried for the dressing of open wounds and for application and padding of splints include the following:

- Sterile universal trauma dressing, approximately 10 × 36 inches, packaged folded to 9 × 10 inches.
- Self-adhering, soft roller bandages, 4 inches × 5 yards.
- Self-adhering, soft roller bandages, 2 inches × 5 yards.
- Sterile, nonporous, nonadherent dressing for occlusion of sucking chest wounds and eviscerations (aluminum foil sterilized in original package).
- Adhesive tape in several widths.
- Safety pins, large.
- Sterile dressings, gauze, 4 × 4 inches.
- Sterile dressings, laparotomy, 6 × 9 inches.

Childbirth Supplies A sterile obstetrical delivery (OB) pack must be carried. It should contain the following supplies:

- 1 pair surgical scissors.
- 3 cord clamps or umbilical tapes.
- 5 towels.
- 12 sponges, 4 × 4 inches.
- 4 pairs sterile surgical gloves.
- 1 baby blanket.
- 2 large plastic bags.
- 1 syringe, rubber-bulb type, for aspiration of baby's mouth and airway.

- 1 box sanitary napkins, individually wrapped and sterilized.

Each ambulance service must be able to obtain immediately, from a hospital or another source, a portable infant incubator that can either be fastened to the litter or stand alone for transporting newborn infants. The carrier should permit oxygen enrichment, humidification, control of body temperature, and accessibility to the baby's head for resuscitation. There must be artificial ventilation and sterile oropharyngeal suction equipment in appropriate sizes for this purpose.

Acute Poisoning Supplies Activated charcoal and syrup of ipecac in premeasured doses should be provided, as well as drinkable water and cups. A sufficient number of emesis basins or bags should be available. The phone number of the local poison control center should be prominently displayed on the "poisoning kit."

There should also be equipment and supplies for irrigation of the skin and eyes following exposure to toxic substances. A snakebite kit may be required by local protocol.

The Jump Kit The ambulance should have a **jump kit** that will be used by the EMT who initially leaves the vehicle to tend to the patient while the EMT-driver parks the ambulance and secures the scene as necessary. Such a kit must be light, durable, waterproof, quick to open, and easy to secure (Figure 48–5). It should also have the phone number of the local poison control center. The jump kit should contain the following supplies:

- Disposable gloves.
- Triangular bandages.
- Trauma shears.
- Adhesive tape in various widths.
- Universal trauma dressings.
- Self-adhering soft roller bandages, 4 inches × 5 yards and 2 inches × 5 yards.
- Oropharyngeal airways in adult, child, and infant sizes.
- Bag-valve-mask artificial respiration unit with masks for adults, children, and infants.
- Blood pressure cuff.
- Stethoscope.
- Penlight.

A typical jump kit. The kit must be light, durable, waterproof, quick to open, and easy to secure.

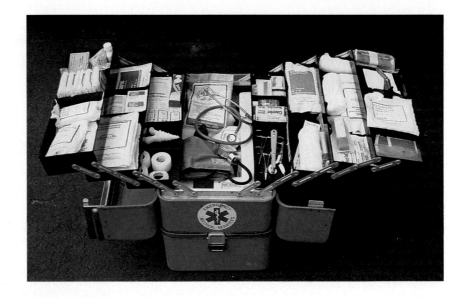

- Portable suction with pharyngeal tips.
- Sterile gauze pads, 4 × 4 inches.
- Sterile "lap" pads, 6 × 9 inches.
- Thermometer.
- Bandaids®.
- Sterile, nonporous, nonadherent dressing for occlusion of sucking chest wounds and eviscerations (aluminum foil sterilized in original package).

Equipment for Personal Safety

A weatherproof compartment that is accessible from outside the patient compartment should provide equipment to safeguard patients and EMTs, control traffic and bystanders, and illuminate work areas. These items include the following:

- Reflectorized or intermittently flashing warning devices (replacing the formerly recommended flares, which have caused fires at the accident scene).
- 2 high-intensity halogen 20,000 candle flashlights, battery powered, stand-up type.
- Fire extinguisher, type BC, dry powder, size 5.
- Hard hats with face shields or safety goggles.
- 2 portable floodlights (if not easily and quickly available from other primary response vehicles).

Extrication Equipment

A weatherproof compartment outside the patient compartment should contain equipment needed for simple, light extrication, even if an extrication and rescue unit is readily available. The following items should be available:

- Wrench, 12-inch, adjustable, open-end.
- Screwdriver, 12-inch, standard square bar.
- Screwdriver, 8-inch, Phillips head.
- Hacksaw with 12-inch carbide wire blades.
- Vise-grip® pliers, 10-inch.
- Hammer, 5 pound, with 15-inch handle.
- Fire ax, butt, 24-inch handle.
- Wrecking bar, 24-inch handle. (Hammer, ax, and wrecking bar may be one combination tool.)
- Crowbar, 51-inch, pinch point.
- Bolt cutter with 1 to 1-1/4 inch jaw opening.
- Shovel, folding, pointed blade.
- Tin snips, double action, 8-inch minimum.
- Gauntlets, reinforced, leather covering past mid-forearm (one pair per crew member).
- Rescue blanket.
- Ropes, 5,400 pound tensile strength in 50-foot lengths in protective bags.
- Mastic knife (able to cut seatbelt webbings).
- Bale hooks (2).
- Spring-load center punch.
- Pruning saw.
- Heavy duty 2 × 4 and 4 × 4 shoring (cribbing) blocks, various lengths.

Additional extrication equipment may be required based on the needs of the area serviced. This would be especially true if rescue and extrication services were not easily and immediately available, such as for a rural EMS agency without the support of a fire service.

AIR AMBULANCES

Air ambulances are not the modern medical development they may seem. In 1870, 36 years before the first use of a motor-driven land ambulance, 160 wounded soldiers and civilians were safely evacuated by hot air balloon during the Prussian siege of Paris.

You will be exposed to increasing use of air ambulances in the future. There are two basic types of air ambulances: fixed-wing and helicopters (rotary wing) (Figure 48–6). Fixed-wing aircraft are generally used for interhospital patient transfers over distances of greater than 100 miles; for shorter distances, rotary-wing aircraft are more efficient. Specially trained medical flight crews accompany these flights. Your involvement with fixed-wing aircraft transfers will probably be limited to providing ground transportation for the patient and medical flight crew between the hospital and the airport.

Rotary-wing aircraft are increasingly becoming an important tool in providing emergency medical care. For example, in many areas, it is an everyday occurrence to see a **MEDEVAC** helicopter land at an accident scene and transport the victims to a trauma facility far distant from the accident. MEDEVAC helicopters have the potential to speed the delivery of appropriate lifesaving care to a patient, as well as speed the delivery of the patient to a lifesaving treatment facility. In order to use them safely and effectively, you should be thoroughly familiar with the capabilities, protocols, and methods for accessing MEDEVAC helicopters available in your area. EMS crews should be cross-trained by local MEDEVAC crews in ground safety when working in and around rotary wing aircraft.

Medical experiences in Korea, Vietnam, and the Middle East proved that patient survival is

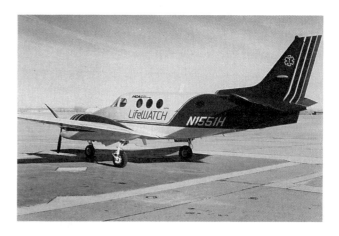

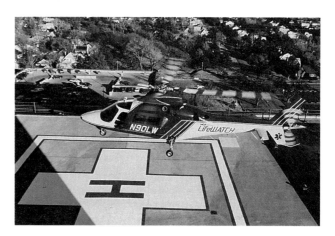

FIGURE 48–6

Air ambulances are playing an increasingly important role in the transportation of the sick and injured. The two basic types of air ambulances are (top) fixed-wing and (bottom) rotor-wing (helicopter) aircraft.

directly related to the time that elapses between injury and definitive treatment. The speed and versatility of helicopters in transporting injured military personnel to military medical facilities have been adapted to emergency medical care in the civilian conflict that may be referred to as "the war on trauma." Most of the helicopters used for emergency medical operations fly well in excess of 100 mph in a straight line, without road or traffic hazards. The patient can receive varying degrees of medical care during the flight, based on the capabilities of the aircraft and the MEDEVAC flight crew; the crew may include EMTs, paramedics, flight nurses, or physicians.

The types of helicopters used for MEDEVAC operations vary, but the dangers are the same. Helicopter safety is nothing more than good common sense, coupled with a constant awareness of the need for personal safety. If you become familiar with the way helicopters operate and if you follow the instructions of the pilots, you should minimize any dangers involved in being part of a MEDEVAC operation. The most important rule is to stay a safe distance from the aircraft or helicopter whenever it is on the ground and "hot" (the rotors are spinning). Remember, the tips of the rotor blades are traveling near the speed of sound.

When accompanying a flight crew member of the aircraft, either to go on the mission or to assist in the loading of a patient, you must follow the directions of the flight crew exactly. You should *never* attempt to open any aircraft door or move equipment unless instructed to do so by the flight crew member. Likewise, when directed to approach the aircraft, you should do so with extreme caution, paying constant attention to the hazards present.

Another important safety rule is never to approach the helicopter from the rear, even if it is not a hot load situation. The approach area is between nine and three o'clock as the pilot faces forward (Figure 48–7). The approach area has been strictly defined because of the hazard of the tail rotor. In addition, the pilot may need to swing the tail boom to a different direction for takeoff.

The tail rotor is a spinning blade that is sometimes almost impossible to see because of its excessive speed of rotation. All ground personnel must stay away from the tail rotor. If it is necessary to move from one side of the helicopter to the other, you should go around the front of the aircraft. Never duck under the

FIGURE 48–7

Always approach a helicopter from the front. The tail rotor moves so fast that it is sometimes impossible to see. The pilot cannot see the area behind the helicopter or any person who might be standing there.

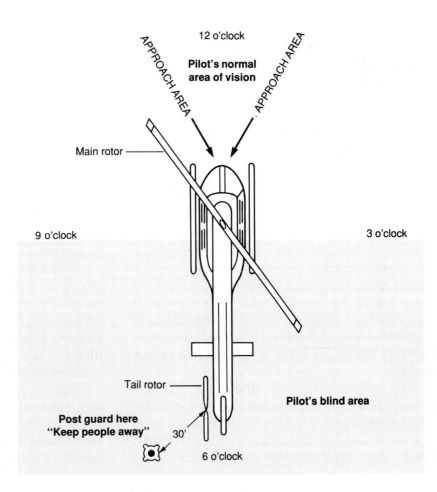

FIGURE 48–8

Always approach the front of a helicopter in a crouched position because the main rotor blade can dip
to as low as 4 feet off the ground.

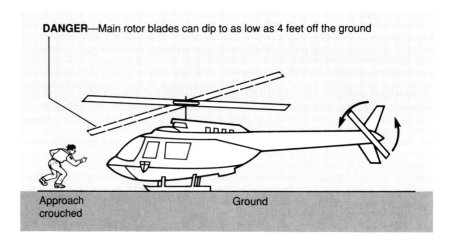

DANGER—Main rotor blades can dip to as low as 4 feet off the ground

Approach
crouched

Ground

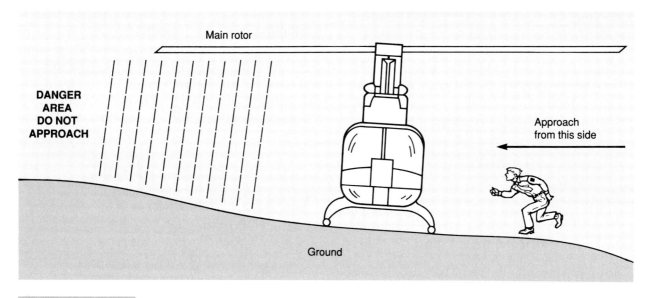

Main rotor

DANGER
AREA
DO NOT
APPROACH

Approach
from this side

Ground

FIGURE 48–9   Use extreme caution when approaching a helicopter that
is on an incline. The main rotor blade will be close to
the ground on the uphill side, so you must approach
from the downhill side.

body, the boom, or the rear section of the
helicopter. The pilot cannot see in these areas.
An unseen rescuer could very quickly experience a fatal injury and disable a helicopter by
being struck by the tail rotor. When enough
personnel are available, someone should stand
toward the rear of the aircraft, outside the arc of
the rotor blades, to warn spectators and others
away.

Another area of concern when approaching a
helicopter is the height of the main rotor blade.
Due to the flexibility of the blade, it may dip as
low as 4 feet off the ground (Figure 48–8).
When you approach the aircraft, walk in a

crouched position until at the helicopter. Wind
gusts influence the blade height without warning. Special care must be used when you carry
IVs and equipment under the blades. Air
turbulence created by the rotor blades can blow
off hats and loose equipment and cause them to
become a danger to the aircraft and personnel
in the area.

Keeping low is especially important if the air
ambulance is an increased capacity helicopter
that loads from the rear, such as the BK117.
After landing, the pilot locks the controls on
the ground, then goes to the rear rotor to route
boarders away from the blade.

If no other site is available and the helicopter must land on a grade, further caution must be exercised. The main rotor blade will be closer to the ground on the uphill side (Figure 48–9). Under these circumstances, the aircraft must be approached from the downhill side only. Do not move the patient to the helicopter until the helicopter crew has signaled that they are ready to receive you. A flight crew member will direct and assist you with loading the patient.

The following information is presented to minimize the dangers associated with landing sites. Although a helicopter can fly straight up and down, this is the most dangerous mode of operation. The safest and most effective way to land and take off is similar to that used by fixed-wing aircraft. Landing at a slight angle allows for safer operations. Takeoff is a reversal of this process, combining a gradual lift and forward motion to travel up and out on a slight angle.

Clearing a landing site is another important role that you can perform. You should look for loose debris, electric or telephone wires, poles, or any other obstacles that might interfere with the safe operation of the helicopter. If you note any obstacles, notify the pilot of them by radio or other signal. The pilot will usually "overfly" or make a reconnaissance of the landing site before final approach and landing to ensure that all potential dangers are identified. The pilot makes the final determination of the landing site. However, you should designate suggested landing sites. If they are appropriate, the pilot will use them. Variables such as temperature, winds, and helicopter payload play a part in the pilot's final selection of a landing site. Local protocols will determine whether flags, lights, or other signaling devices should be used to mark the proposed landing site.

Nighttime operations are considerably more hazardous than daytime, because obstacles are not as visible to the pilot. Frequently, the pilot will fly over the area with the helicopter's lights on, not only to show obstacles, but also to have the lights reveal the shadows of overhead wires; while the wires may not be visible, the changing shadows are often noted. Rescuers should not shine spotlights in the air to help the pilot. These lights may temporarily blind the pilot. Light beams should be directed toward the ground at the landing site. Even after the helicopter is on the ground, lights should not be aimed anywhere near it. Of course, smoking, open lights or flames, and flares are prohibited within 50 feet of the aircraft at all times.

EMTs are increasingly coming to recognize that MEDEVAC operations are a welcome and valuable tool in emergency medical care. These operations are most effectively used by those who have taken the time to familiarize themselves with locally available MEDEVAC services. For further information on the subject of air ambulances, refer to DOT publication HS805-703, *Air Ambulance Guidelines*, February 1981, and DOT publication HS806-841, Proceedings: National MEDEVAC Helicopter Conference.

YOU ARE THE EMT

1. What kind of litter is needed in order to place a patient in the Trendelenburg position? What are the advantages and disadvantages of an x-ray permeable, removable litter panel?
2. In addition to containing certain supplies, what else should characterize a jump kit?
3. What is more dangerous—the main rotor or the tail rotor of a helicopter? How do you avoid both of these dangers?
4. You are on the ground helping a MEDEVAC pilot land the helicopter at night. What should you do?

CHAPTER 49

EMERGENCY DRIVING AND VEHICLE OPERATIONS

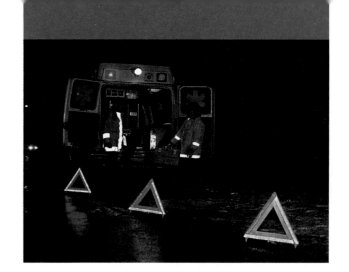

KEY TERMS

acceleration (ak-sel″er-a′shun) The process of increasing speed.

chassis set (shas′ē set) The transfer of the center of mass to various locations in a moving ambulance.

coefficient of friction A measure of the "grip" of the tire on the road surface.

footprint The area of contact between the ambulance tire and the road surface.

friction The rubbing of one body against another.

hydroplaning (hī″dro-pla′ ning) Driving on tires lifted from the road surface by a sheet of water.

OVERVIEW

Many patients have said that the most frightening part of the experience of being suddenly ill or injured was not the problem itself but the ambulance ride to the hospital. The terrifying effect of a fast, swaying ride with a siren blaring overhead is not very reassuring to an already upset patient. Although sometimes this kind of a ride is truly "lifesaving," usually excessive speed is unnecessary. What is necessary is that the patient be transported to a hospital safely in the shortest practical time. This takes common sense and defensive driving techniques on the part of the EMT, and speed should never be used to cover up a lack of these qualities.

Chapter 49 focuses on the techniques and judgment that an EMT has to learn in order to drive an emergency vehicle. The chapter begins with an explanation of why so many ambulance drivers are guilty of using excessive speed. The chapter next discusses emergency vehicle control and emergency vehicle operation. Both these topics are important factors in safe driving. The chapter then talks about the qualifications needed to drive an ambulance. Then the discussion focuses on emergency vehicles at the accident scene—where the ambulance should park and how the EMT should control traffic in the absence of police help. The chapter concludes with a discussion of ambulance maintenance.

GOALS

The goals of Chapter 49 are to

- identify four factors that contribute to the problem of excessive speed in driving the emergency vehicle.
- become familiar with emergency vehicle control, including steering techniques, chassis set, fender judgment, road position, controlled acceleration and braking, and special driving situations.
- become familiar with emergency vehicle operations, including right-of-way privileges, use of the siren, planning alternate routes, intersection hazards, and safe driving guidelines.
- describe the qualifications needed to be an emergency vehicle driver.
- learn where the ambulance should be parked and how traffic should be controlled at the scene.
- learn the procedures for inspecting the emergency vehicle after a daily shift change; after a run; and during periodic, scheduled maintenance checks.

THE PROBLEM OF EXCESSIVE SPEED

EMTs who operate an ambulance assume great responsibility. They must employ the knowledge they have gained through training and experience to get the patient to the hospital in a safe and efficient manner. Only in extreme life-and-death emergencies is speed an important factor. In most instances, if the patient is properly assessed and stabilized at the scene, speed during transport is unnecessary, undesirable, and dangerous. The emergency vehicle operator should *never* travel at a speed that is not prudently safe.

Unfortunately, use of excessive vehicle speed during emergency calls is not uncommon. Four factors that contribute to this problem have been identified. The first is lack of expertise on the part of the dispatcher. Dispatching is a job that requires a trained, experienced EMT. Only with a working knowledge of emergency calls can a dispatcher be in a position to help determine the urgency of the calls received. Dispatchers who are no more than switchboard operators cannot make such decisions properly. Even with EMT dispatchers, most services will respond to an incident with red lights and siren, mainly because it is very difficult to assess reliably the exact situation from an excited, distraught caller.

The second factor identified in the use of excessive speed is inadequate equipment in the ambulance. The EMT who does not have the equipment and supplies necessary to stabilize the patient may have little choice but to speed to the hospital to pass on the responsibility presented by the condition of the patient. The third factor is inadequate training of the EMT. The EMT who is inadequately trained or who lacks confidence in being able to care for the patient will tend to transport the patient rapidly to the hospital, in effect acting as a chauffeur rather than an EMT.

The fourth and final factor is inadequate driving ability. The emergency vehicle operator who has not received training in the safe operation of the ambulance will be unaware of the principles governing its proper use. This driver, lacking understanding of the added risks that excessive speed entails, may be inclined to select speed over safety.

EMERGENCY VEHICLE CONTROL

The ambulance driver has only two means of controlling the vehicle: changing its direction or changing its speed. To accomplish either maneuver safely means maintaining a continuous rolling contact between the bottom surface of the tires and the surface of the road. Two factors are involved in this contact: the **coefficient of friction** (a measure of the "grip" of the tire on the road surface) and the **foot-prints** of the ambulance's tires through which the grip is applied. An ambulance tire's typical footprint is approximately 8 inches long and as wide as the tire.

The coefficient of **friction** may vary widely on different parts of the same road, depending on the condition of its surface, its age, and the weather. The coefficient of friction also varies according to tread design and tire tread wear. A driver must constantly evaluate the road surface with regard to the frictional force the tires can apply to the road surface at a given speed before a skid will begin. This observation is especially important in cornering, where additional centrifugal force is acting on the vehicle.

Steering Techniques

The method of holding the steering wheel, its movement, and the timing of movements are all factors in steering technique. The steering wheel should be held with the hands at the nine o'clock and the three o'clock positions. These positions allow the wheel to be turned without removing either hand. In moving the steering wheel, one hand pulls while the other slides, paralleling the pulling hand's position on the wheel (Figure 49–1). When turning the vehicle, the hands should not pass the twelve o'clock or the six o'clock positions, because the hands will cross and become tangled. When these limits are reached, the opposite hand begins to grip the wheel, and the first hand slides. This technique will allow the wheel to be held firmly by at least one hand at all times.

Timing of steering wheel movement is proportional to the speed of the vehicle. All vehicles lag somewhat when responding to steering input. The faster a vehicle is traveling, the greater the lag becomes. The required steering input should anticipate the desired movement of the vehicle.

Chassis Set

Chassis set refers to the transfer of weight (center of mass) of the vehicle to different points on the chassis or frame. Basically, the weight of a vehicle is concentrated over one of three points on the chassis: in the front over the

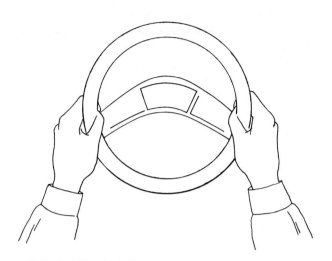

FIGURE 49–1

The hands of the driver should be at the 9 o'clock (left) and 3 o'clock (right) position on the steering wheel when driving straight ahead. A left turn is initiated by the left hand pulling the steering wheel in a counter-clockwise direction while the right hand slides along the wheel. The driver's hands should never cross.

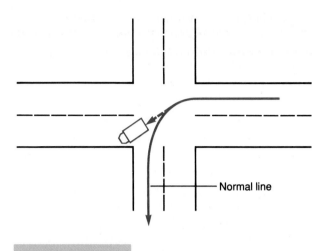

Normal line

FIGURE 49–2

When a vehicle accelerates, the front wheels lose some traction. The vehicle becomes harder to steer because it has a tendency to travel in a straight line as the center of mass moves toward the rear of the vehicle.

front wheels, in the rear over the rear wheels, or in the center between the front and rear wheels. The transfer of weight from one point to another is caused by **acceleration** or deceleration of the vehicle. When a vehicle accelerates, the weight is transferred to the rear; the front wheels lose some traction, which results in decreased ability to steer the vehicle—that is, the ambulance will have a tendency to travel in a straight line (Figure 49–2). When there is deceleration or braking, the opposite weight shift occurs and weight is transferred to the front of the vehicle; the rear end of the vehicle then tends to slide to the outside of a curve when cornering (Figure 49–3).

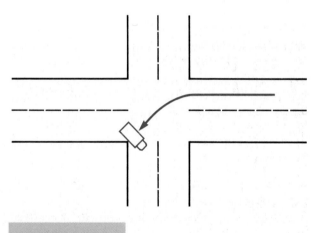

FIGURE 49–3

When a vehicle decelerates, the rear of the vehicle tends to slide to the outside of a curve when cornering.

Vehicle Size and Distance Judgment

Vehicle length and width are critical factors when maneuvering, driving, and parking an emergency vehicle. These factors are particularly important with types I and III vehicles, because they are wider than they appear to be from behind the steering wheel. Vehicle size and weight will greatly influence braking and stopping distances. It is essential to know the width and length of your vehicle for effective passing and parking. Accidents frequently occur when the emergency vehicle is backing up. The driver should always use a ground guide whenever backing the vehicle to avoid any unexpected surprises. Good peripheral vision and depth perception will help the driver to judge distances, but intensive training combined with experience are required for efficient and safe driving of all emergency vehicles.

Road Position and Cornering

Road position describes the position of the vehicle on the roadway relative to the inside or outside edge of the paved surface and the interaction of this position with cornering efficiency. Knowing the vehicle's present position as well as its projected position is necessary in order to achieve efficient cornering.

Efficient *cornering* means negotiating a curve at the optimum speed to achieve good road position as you exit the curve. The vehicle's position is projected so that its path will apex at the desired point in the curve. The apex of curve is the point at which the vehicle is closest to the inside edge of the roadway or traffic lane. The position of the apex depends on the desired road position at the exit point of the curve. An apex early in the curve will usually result in the vehicle's being forced toward the outside of the roadway when the vehicle exits the curve, whereas an apex late in the curve allows the vehicle to stay to the inside of the roadway, which helps keep the vehicle in the proper lane (Figure 49–4).

Controlled Acceleration

Controlled acceleration means the use of a controlled pressure on the accelerator and the use of acceleration to control the vehicle. Acceleration is most efficient when the vehicle is traveling in a straight line, because the force of acceleration is equally distributed to the rear wheels. Acceleration in a curve or during a turn results in a reduction of actual linear acceleration in the desired direction and an increase in acceleration to the outside of the curve. If the acceleration to the outside of the curve becomes excessive, the vehicle may drift out of control and into a skid or spin.

Controlled Braking

Controlled braking refers both to the use of the brakes to control the vehicle and the controlled

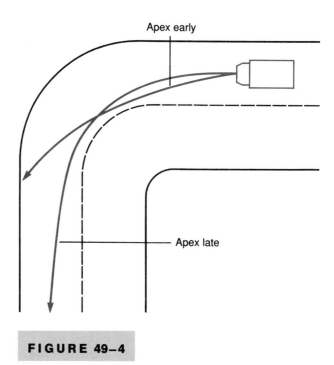

FIGURE 49–4

A vehicle will stay to the inside of the curve if the apex of the curve occurs late in the curve. An early apex will force the vehicle to the outside of the roadway.

application of pressure to the brake pedal. Brakes not only control the movement of the vehicle, causing it to slow or stop; they also aid in directional control. Braking while the vehicle is traveling in a straight line is the safest and most efficient method. Braking in a turn causes a loss of efficiency that may be barely noticeable at low speed but becomes more apparent with increased vehicle speed. Applying the brakes while cornering has little effect on slowing the vehicle and may actually cause a skid or spin. The proper method for use of the brake during a turn or in a curve is to gradually ease off brake pressure and increase accelerator pressure to maintain the speed of the vehicle.

Getting the feel for the proper brake pressure comes with experience and practice driving your assigned vehicle. You will experience a different braking action and feel with each vehicle. For example, brakes on Types I and III vehicles have a "heavier" feel than do the brakes of a Type II vehicle. Certain heavy vehicles use air brakes which have yet another feel. You must become familiar with each vehicle you drive and be sure you understand its particular braking characteristics and the best down shifting technique for that vehicle.

Special Driving Situations

Even the most conscientious driver occasionally will run into unexpected situations that may require special driving skills. Driving at a speed appropriate for the weather and road conditions will decrease the need to use these techniques.

Hydroplaning On a wet road, a tire tends to displace the water on the surface and make direct contact with the road. As the vehicle's speed increases above 30 miles per hour, the tire may be lifted off the road surface by water piling up under it; there is not enough time for the driver to slow down and force the water out from under the tire. This is known as **hydroplaning.** At higher speeds on wet roadways, the front wheels may thus be riding on a sheet of water, giving the driver no control over the vehicle. If hydroplaning occurs, the driver should gradually slow the vehicle without jamming on the brakes.

Water on the Roadway If at all possible, driving through large pools of water should be avoided. If it cannot be avoided, you should slow down and turn on the windshield wipers. After exiting the pool, you should lightly tap the brakes several times until they are dry. Once the brakes are dry, they will slow the vehicle without pulling it to one side or the other.

Decreased Visibility During periods of decreased visibility caused by fog, smog, snow, or heavy rain, common sense dictates that you slow down carefully after giving sufficient warning to following vehicles. At night, only low beams should be used to provide maximum visibility without reflection. You should use headlights during the day to increase your visibility to other drivers. You should also watch carefully for stopped or slow-moving cars.

Ice and Slippery Surfaces A light mist on an oily, dusty road can be just as slippery as a patch of ice. Good all-weather tires and an appropriate speed can help decrease traction problems significantly. Studded snow tires should be considered for vehicles frequently used in snow or icy conditions (where permitted by law).

You should be especially wary of bridges and overpasses when temperatures are close to freezing. These road surfaces will freeze much faster than surrounding road surfaces because they lack the warming effect of the underlying ground.

EMERGENCY VEHICLE OPERATION

Safe driving during transportation is an important phase of the emergency care of the sick and injured. It requires training and judgment in the operation of the emergency vehicle. There is an old cliche that applies very well to emergency driving: "Practice makes perfect." You can practice anytime, any place, and in any vehicle. No one is so proficient that additional practice will not be beneficial. And no one, EMTs included, can get too much practice.

The first rule in the safe operation of an emergency vehicle is that speed does not save lives. The second rule is that the driver and all passengers wear seat belts and shoulder restraints at all times. Other EMTs should wear them en route to the scene and when not actively engaged in direct patient care. Seat belts are without doubt the most important items of safety equipment on every ambulance.

You have to become familiar with the characteristics of your vehicle with regard to acceleration, cornering, swaying, and stopping. For example, disc booster brakes improve braking efficiency but increase the sway. You must also know exactly what the vehicle will do and how it will respond to steering, braking, and acceleration inputs under various conditions.

You should be constantly alert to changing weather, road, and driving conditions. Warnings of ice or hazardous conditions must be taken seriously. Whether en route to an emergency or returning to the hospital, you must modify your speed according to road conditions. Although you should follow specified routes for most runs, you should have alternate routes available for contingencies. During a major disaster, it is especially important that all public safety and emergency services be coordinated, with all vehicles following assigned routes. A driver who encounters unexpected traffic congestion should notify the dispatcher so that other emergency vehicles can be advised of the congestion and delays and select alternate routes.

In most instances, on a multilane highway, the ambulance should keep to the extreme left-hand (fast) lane. Use of this lane offers the least amount of traffic under most conditions and allows other motorists to move over in a normal right-hand manner.

You must always drive defensively. You should never rely on what another motorist will do unless a clear visual signal is received. Even then, you must be prepared to take defensive action in case of a misunderstanding, panic on the part of the other party, or careless driving.

Right-of-way Privilege

State laws vary regarding the right-of-way privileges of an ambulance. Some states allow an emergency vehicle to proceed through a red light or stop sign after stopping. Others allow emergency vehicles to proceed through a controlled intersection *with due regard* using flashing lights and siren. This means that the emergency vehicle must be driven with due regard for the safety of all persons using the highway. Failure to use due regard may expose your organization to a liability claim and expose you to punitive damages if you are found at fault.

The driver of an emergency vehicle must be familiar with the local right-of-way laws and should exercise these privileges only when it is absolutely necessary for the patient's well-being. The truth is, very few emergencies re-

quire extremely rapid transportation of the patient.

Use of the Siren

Probably the most overused piece of equipment on an ambulance is the siren. In general, the siren does not help the EMT driver. The automobile driver sitting in a closed car, proceeding at the speed limit, with the radio playing and the air conditioner or heater fan going full volume, cannot hear even a penetrating electronic siren until the ambulance is only a short distance away. If the radio is particularly loud, such a driver may not hear the siren at all.

The use of a police escort is an extremely dangerous practice. The motorist, hearing a siren and seeing a police car passing, may assume that the police car was the only emergency vehicle and may begin to proceed, causing an accident with the ambulance that is being escorted.

Planning Alternate Routes

The EMT who plans and executes the necessary moves in proper sequence will gain time. Becoming familiar with the various routes in the town or city will enable you to plan alternate ways to reach the destination. In fact, switching to alternate routes will save more time than increasing the speed of the ambulance. Knowing alternate routes around frequently opened bridges or blocked railroad crossings is especially important.

Intersection Hazards

The EMT driver often assumes that motorists and the public will do the "right thing" when an emergency vehicle is in the vicinity or is following a car. You should anticipate that motorists will pull to the nearest curb and stop or drive as close to the nearest curb as possible. However, the motorist might stop suddenly in front of the ambulance. If the ambulance is not under control, a serious accident could occur.

Intersection accidents are the most frequent and usually the most serious. Intersections abound with hazards for which you must be on the alert. If the call is so urgent that the ambulance cannot wait for red lights to change, you should still come to a momentary stop at the light and survey the intersection, looking for those drivers who will go around traffic and enter the intersection, usually at high speed.

Another serious hazard at the intersection is the motorist who times the traffic lights and arrives just as the lights are changing, thereby avoiding a stop. This person is often an experienced truck driver who is hauling a heavy load that makes a quick stop impossible. Such a driver will arrive at the intersection knowing that the traffic light is about to change and expect to go through. If your ambulance arrives at the same time, with the green light in your favor but about to change, and you are expecting to proceed through the intersection, the stage has been set for a serious accident.

Still another intersection hazard is created when the driver of one emergency vehicle follows another emergency vehicle through an intersection without assessing the situation carefully. A motorist who has yielded the right-of-way to the first vehicle may proceed into the intersection not expecting a second emergency vehicle close behind. You should never accept a police escort, and when following another emergency vehicle, you must exercise extreme caution. Use of a siren tone different from that of the first emergency vehicle may be useful in warning other drivers of the approach of a second unit.

The driver of an emergency vehicle must also be alert for other emergency vehicles that might be approaching an intersection with their sirens on and expecting to proceed through without yielding. An open window and a "tuned" ear can significantly reduce this risk. However, the most desirable siren practice is to respond with the windows up and the use of hearing protectors in conjunction with headset communication, taking care to stop and look at intersections.

Driving through an intersection when vision is obstructed, without stopping to make sure that the passage is clear, is equivalent to driving blindfolded. Even more likely than the

possibility of colliding with another vehicle is the possibility of striking a pedestrian who steps from behind an obstruction, such as a bus or truck.

Guidelines for Safe Driving

The following guidelines should help you operate the ambulance safely:

- At the time of dispatch, select the shortest and, normally, the least congested route to the scene.
- Avoid routes with heavy traffic congestion. Know alternate routes to each hospital destination during rush hours.
- Avoid one-way streets. They may become clogged by the sound of your siren. Do not try to go against the flow of traffic on a one-way street.
- When you approach the scene, be very careful and alert for pedestrians. Curiosity seekers rarely move out of the way.
- At the scene, park in a safe place. If you are parked facing into traffic, turn off your headlights as they may blind oncoming traffic. Do keep warning lights on, however, to alert oncoming motorists.
- When transporting the patient to the hospital, operate the ambulance within the stated speed limits for the area, except for the rare extreme emergency.
- Go with the flow of traffic.
- Use the siren as little as possible en route to the hospital. The patient is being cared for, and your duty as the driver is to reach the hospital safely. If you do have to use the siren, be sure to warn the patient before activating it.
- If it is necessary to use the siren, you should still travel at a speed that will enable you to be able to stop the ambulance safely at all times if other drivers do not give you the right-of-way.
- Never assume that warning lights and sirens will allow an ambulance to pass through a congested area.
- Always assume that other drivers will have their car windows rolled up, their radios

playing, conversation going on, and the heater or air conditioner fans going at full volume. They will not be looking for an ambulance and will not hear the siren, even though it is only a short distance away.

- Always drive defensively.
- Always maintain a safe following distance. Use the "four-second rule" of following at least four seconds behind another vehicle in the same lane.
- Try to maintain an open space in an adjacent lane as an escape route if the vehicle in front should stop suddenly.
- Except for freeway use, emergency lights should always be used with a siren.

EMERGENCY VEHICLE DRIVERS

Not all persons who drive an automobile are qualified to drive an emergency vehicle. Drivers should be screened carefully. The same requirements for a person who is to perform as an EMT hold true for an EMT who is assigned to emergency driving duties.

One of the basic requirements is that the driver be physically fit. Experience has shown that many accidents can be attributed to a physical impairment. You should not attempt to drive while taking medications such as cold remedies, analgesics, or tranquilizers that may induce sleep or slow reaction times. And of course, an EMT should never drive or provide medical care after drinking alcohol.

Another requirement is that the driver be emotionally fit. Emotions must be given much consideration. For example, the personality of an individual may change behind a steering wheel. Closely tied to emotional stability is the ability to operate under stress. You must be capable of acting properly under the stresses of emergency conditions. In addition to knowing exactly what to do, you must be able to do it under trying conditions.

The EMT who is serving as the driver must be aware of the important responsibilities of emergency driving and develop the proper attitude. Although an ambulance is usually granted right-of-way privileges, the laws are emphatic about the responsibility of the driver

who exercises those privileges. Any idea that an emergency vehicle driver can do no wrong must be abandoned. Being able to drive to one's destination without interruption (as granted in right-of-way privileges) and being permitted to move from one lane of traffic into the opposite lane are valuable, time saving privileges that must never be abused.

EMERGENCY VEHICLES AT THE ACCIDENT SCENE

Safe Parking

Emergency vehicles must be properly parked to maintain efficient traffic control and flow. The ambulance should not be parked beside the accident site, because it may block the movement of other emergency vehicles. The ambulance should instead pull ahead of the accident and park on the same side of the road. It is best to park uphill and/or upwind of the incident if smoke or hazardous material is present (Figure 49–5). If it becomes necessary to park on the backside of a hill or curve, and at all times after dark, you must put out warning devices (Figure 49–6). All emergency vehicles should park well away from any collapsing structures, fire, explosive hazards, or downed wires.

An overall guideline is to park your vehicle as close to the accident as the immediate need for emergency medical care and personal safety indicates. If possible, on approaching the scene, you should make a quick survey and choose the best place to park to unload equipment and to load patients. If necessary, the ambulance can be temporarily moved into a position to block traffic so that a patient can be moved safely and quickly. If this maneuver is required, it should be carried out as quickly as possible. Traffic should not be blocked any longer than is absolutely necessary. Of course, while traffic flow should continue with as little interruption as possible, the emergency medical care of the patient does take precedence over all else. Therefore, harassment by other motorists because traffic is obstructed should never affect the care the patient receives.

FIGURE 49–5

Park the ambulance uphill and/or upwind from smoke or hazardous substances such as gasoline.

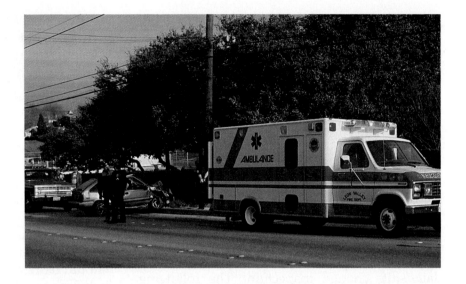

FIGURE 49–6

Place warning devices if it becomes necessary to park on the backside of a hill or drive.

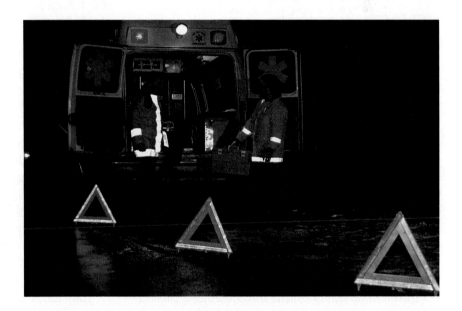

Traffic Control

Your first responsibility at an accident scene is to care for the patients. Only when all the patients have been treated and the emergency situation is under control should you be concerned with restoring the flow of traffic. If the police are delayed in arriving at the scene, you may then be required to take action.

The purpose of traffic control is to ensure an orderly traffic flow and prevent another accident. Under ordinary circumstances, traffic control is difficult. Under the conditions that exist at the scene of an accident or disaster, traffic control presents serious additional problems. Passing motorists often try to observe the scene as they drive by, paying little attention to the roadway in front of them. Some curiosity seekers may park and return on foot, creating still other hazards. As soon as possible, appropriate warning devices, such as reflectors, should be placed at a sufficient distance on both sides of the accident. Ordinarily, you will need to concern yourself with traffic control for only a short time until the police arrive. Remember, the main objectives in directing traffic are to forewarn other drivers, prevent additional accidents, and keep vehicles moving in an orderly fashion so that continued care of the injured is not interrupted.

EMERGENCY VEHICLE MAINTENANCE

You are responsible for the maintenance of the ambulance—it must be safe and available on a moment's notice. Routine inspections must be regularly scheduled, using a written checklist that documents needed repairs or replacement of equipment and supplies.

The first type of routine inspection is the daily/shift change inspection. The following items should be on the checklist.

- Chassis systems: brakes; battery(s); engine cooling system, including fluid levels, fan belts, and water hoses; all lights, interior and exterior; warning equipment and sirens; and power systems.
- Wheels and tires, including the spare: check inflation pressures and unusual wear or any damage.
- Doors for proper opening, closing, latching, and locking.
- Temperature control systems.
- Communications systems, vehicle and portable.
- Fuel tank: should be at least one-half full unless local circumstances demand larger reserves.
- Fluid levels: oil, coolant, transmission, power steering, power brakes, windshield washer.
- Test drive once daily to check brakes and handling.
- Check windows and mirrors for cleanliness and position; check wipers for proper functioning.
- Emergency medical supplies: oxygen, onboard and portable; jump kits; splints; backboards; OB pack; poison kit; and all other supplies.
- Housekeeping supplies.

- "Run sheets" and other report forms.
- 10 percent solution of chlorox in water should be used to clean the ambulance after any contamination.

The second type of inspection is the run inspection. After each trip, the interior of the ambulance should be cleaned and decontaminated as needed, in accordance with state and local health department regulations. Blood, vomitus, and other contaminants must be scrubbed from the floors, walls, and ceilings. The exterior of the vehicle should be cleaned as needed. Broken or damaged equipment should be replaced or repaired without delay. Supplies should be restocked as needed. If the fuel tank is below required reserves, the vehicle should be refueled. The oil level should be checked each time the vehicle is refueled.

The third type of inspection is carried out during prescheduled preventive maintenance checks of the emergency vehicle. Ambulance chassis and engine components are subjected to significantly greater stresses than the typical automobile or truck. For this reason, the manufacturer's recommendations for periodic preventive maintenance must be strictly followed, especially regarding lubrication, oil and filter changes, transmission and differential service, brakes, wheel alignment, wheel bearings, and steering components. Many services are now using a Hobbs or engine hour meter in addition to the odometer to help determine periodic maintenance requirements.

Just as is the case with emergency medical care report forms, local and individual differences affect inspection routines. Ambulance services should develop their own inspection forms for at least the inspection time intervals just listed. These forms should include those items listed for inspection. They should be used as a checklist so that nothing is overlooked or omitted. The forms should then be filed for inspection and legal documentation, and retained for a minimum of three years.

YOU ARE THE EMT

1. An EMT driver controls the vehicle by changing what two factors? What role does friction play in vehicle control?
2. Explain what happens when a vehicle hydroplanes. What corrective action should a driver take?
3. Give five examples of how you can drive defensively.
4. Research and report on the right-of-way privileges of ambulances in your state.

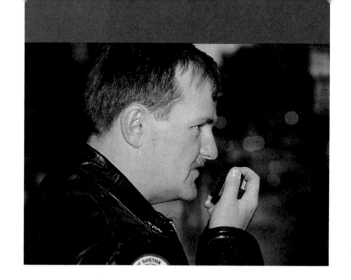

CHAPTER 50

COMMUNICATIONS

base station Any fixed radio hardware containing a transmitter and receiver. For EMS purposes, they will generally be within the class, land mobile service, as defined by the Federal Communications Commission (FCC).

carrier A basic radio signal (wave) generated by a transmitter without voice or other information imposed on it.

channel An assigned frequency or frequencies used to carry voice and/or data communications.

dedicated line A special telephone circuit used for specific point-to-point communications purposes such as remote control of a base station or alerting EMS crew quarters.

duplex The ability to transmit and receive traffic simultaneously on a particular channel.

hot line A dedicated telephone line between two specific points. It is always "open" or under the control of an individual at each end. The line is immediately available by lifting the receiver. Outside access cannot be obtained.

land mobile service Specified by the FCC; mobile communication service between a base station and mobile stations on land, or between two mobile stations on land.

scanner A radio receiver in which the frequency being received is automatically and instantaneously changed until a frequency carrying some message is detected. At that time, the receiver locks on to that frequency until the message is completed. The process is then repeated.

simplex Single-frequency operating capability; radio transmissions can occur in either direction but not simultaneously in both; one party transmits, and the other receives.

tone An audio signal or carrier wave of controlled amplitude and frequency that is used for equipment control purposes or to selectively signal a receiver, such as activating a pager.

UHF (ultrahigh frequency) Radio frequencies between 300 and 3,000 MHz. (A frequency of 800 MHz has better building and underground penetration than do frequencies below 300 MHz.)

VHF (very high frequency) Radio frequencies between 30 and 300 MHz. The VHF spectrum is further divided into "high" and "low" bands.

OVERVIEW

Radio and telephone communications are the framework that binds the components of an EMS system together. The communication system links one emergency health care provider with other members of the emergency health care team, thus permitting them to function effectively. It is imperative that all EMTs know the communication capabilities of their EMS delivery system. Especially important is knowing the equipment's limitations. EMTs must also become proficient in the effective and efficient use of the EMS communication system. They must be able to transmit concise, accurate reports relating to ambulance status, conditions at the emergency site, and the condition and treatment of the patient.

The chapter discusses the skills that an EMT has to possess in order to be an effective communicator. Next the chapter looks at the capabilities that an EMS communication system must offer and how patients access that system. The alert and dispatch phase is examined next. It emphasizes the crucial role of the dispatcher. The last section of Chapter 50 is about radio communications—the kinds of units used, the standard radio operating procedures, the medical communication capabilities possible, and the jurisdiction of the Federal Communications Commission over all radio communications.

GOALS

The goals of Chapter 50 are to
- identify the training and skills an EMT needs for effective communication.
- describe the capabilities of EMS communication systems and how patients access the EMS system.
- recognize the essential role of the dispatcher in the alert and dispatch phase of EMS communications.
- become familiar with radio communications, including the type of units, standard operating procedures, medical communication capabilities, and the role of the Federal Communications Commission.

THE EMT AS A COMMUNICATOR

Communications equipment, capabilities, and operating procedures vary among EMS systems, but all services rely on properly trained personnel to transmit concise, accurate reports. To achieve effective, efficient EMS communication, you must be well trained in the following communications elements:

- How to operate each piece of radio and telephone hardware.
- The appropriate voice communication procedures.
- The appropriate message to send and when to send it.
- The current status of EMS unit readiness.
- The relationships among EMS providers if a variety of providers or levels of service are available in the community.
- The relationship of the EMS system to the community's health care system and other public safety services.

As an EMT you must master many communications skills, including verbal communication, written reports, and radio skills. There are no substitutes for these skills. Efficiency and effectiveness in delivering patient care are directly related to how well you can communicate with the rest of the emergency medical care team. You must develop the following traits of a good communicator:

- Use of good judgment and common sense whenever you operate equipment and communicate with other EMS personnel.
- Ability to concentrate, listen, and follow instructions and protocols.
- Ability to speak intelligibly.
- Familiarity with all the communication tools available in the EMS system and how to use them. These include not only the radio and telephone, but also the vehicle lights, siren and PA system, hand signals, and written messages and reports.

Today, with the widespread public use of **scanners,** any EMS communication system can be readily evaluated. In fact, the community perception of the quality of the local EMS system may be greatly influenced by how efficiently and professionally its communications are conducted. That professionalism depends on your performance.

THE EMS COMMUNICATION SYSTEM

Communication Capabilities

The EMS communication system must be operational 24 hours a day and must provide the following capabilities:

- Public access for patient entry into the EMS system.
- Assignment and dispatch of the appropriate EMS unit, with assistance in routing it to the scene as necessary.
- Communications between EMS units at the scene.
- Communications between other public safety units involved in the incident (police, highway patrol, fire, civil preparedness, Red Cross, mutual assistance EMS units).
- Patient care communication between EMS field units and hospital emergency department personnel, including transmission of signs and symptoms, medical consultation, and medical control of treatment procedures at the scene.

The equipment and organization of EMS communication systems may vary significantly. But the key objective must be rapid mobilization and efficient coordination of EMS and public safety resources. Effective communication systems are configured to allow all local EMS services access to the system, as well as to provide compatible links to units from adjoining EMS services.

The heart of any EMS system is the communications control center (Figure 50-1). This may be a simple radio **base station** staffed by a single communications operator, or it may involve computers, sophisticated electronics, and a large staff of communication specialists. The control center's primary task is to monitor and coordinate the operation of the other communication components—base stations, repeaters, mobile units, hand-held portables, remote consoles, and telephone sets.

Patient Entry into the EMS System

The critical, though often overlooked, initial task of an EMS communication system is to promote rapid patient access to the EMS system. The telephone is the primary means of public access to the EMS system. Poorly publicized EMS numbers, with too many digits to remember in an emergency, have for years been a common problem throughout the country. This creates confusion for callers, unnecessary delays, relaying of messages among public

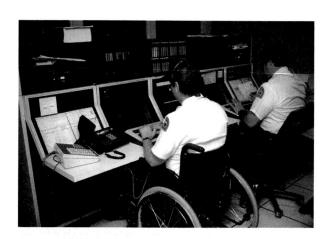

FIGURE 50-1

A communications control center.

safety agencies, and delays in response by the appropriate EMS unit. An effective public access mechanism should

- Be easily remembered and utilized by all citizens.
- Provide rapid, direct contact with the appropriate EMS dispatcher.
- Have sufficient telephone line capacity and staff to handle anticipated "peak" call volume.
- Offer reliable service with mechanisms to prevent calls from going unanswered, being lost, misunderstood, or left waiting unnecessarily.

In the past few years, there has been a significant increase in the use of the 911 universal emergency telephone number to access all public safety services, including EMS. The *Enhanced 911 System*, or *E911*, is the most technologically advanced version of this telephone service. It is available to all communities in which the local telephone companies have installed electronic switching equipment. The key technical features of E911 for improved public access include automatic number identification (ANI), automatic call location identification (ALI), and automatic ringback. These features allow public safety dispatch personnel to view a digital display of the telephone number and the street address from which the call is being made. In addition, if the caller hangs up, the E911 equipment can prevent disconnection of the call, and automatically "ring back" the number (Figure 50–2).

There is little debate that E911 is technically effective for public access. Everyone agrees that 911 is a number easily remembered and dialed in an emergency. It provides the necessary reliability and capacity for busy situations. One of the chief obstacles to implementing 911, in addition to the expense of special telephone switching equipment, is the agreement required among public safety agencies and community leaders to determine the location for the 911 communications control center and to designate the group responsible for managing the center. Such agreements for a centralized public safety communication system have not been easy to achieve. EMS providers may sometimes become unwilling participants in political con-

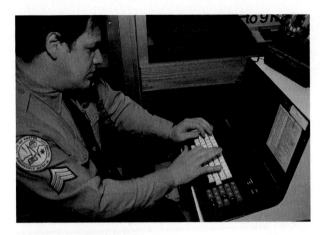

FIGURE 50–2

The 911 emergency telephone number and especially the Enhanced 911 system allow ready access of the patient to the EMS system.

troversies and interagency rivalries surrounding the planning of a centralized 911 system. By being well informed on the importance of easy, rapid public access for effective EMS and public safety services and on the capabilities of an E911 system, you may make a positive contribution to the planning and implementation of such a central communication system in your community.

Despite the capabilities of 911 and E911 systems, most EMS systems still rely on a single, seven-digit telephone number for public access. In some areas, several numbers may be required to summon a variety of EMS response units. In other areas, public access to EMS resources may be accomplished by other means. These include citizen band (CB) and other amateur radio networks (such as RACES and REACT), highway call boxes, and governmental or mutual-aid radio systems. Whatever the public access mechanism, the key elements of this initial phase of EMS communications are that the call be promptly received, properly triaged, and efficiently acted on by the EMS dispatcher.

ALERT AND DISPATCH PHASE

If the control center is the cornerstone of the EMS communication system, then the dispatcher is the key to the control center. The EMS communication system can perform only as well as the dispatcher performs. Thus, it is essential that the EMS dispatcher be trained to at least the EMT-basic level. This will help the dispatcher understand the medical functions of the EMS system, including the roles, responsibilities, and capabilities of the EMTs who render patient care. The dispatcher must also be thoroughly familiar with the capabilities and limitations of the mobile and portable radio units in the ambulances and other EMS response units.

In addition, the dispatcher must be aware of the level of training of the EMTs in each EMS response unit, as well as the medical equipment carried on board. In appropriate emergencies, the dispatcher must be able to provide effective emergency self-help advice to the caller. Although the specific role of the dispatcher may differ from one EMS system to another, each dispatcher must have a working knowledge of the operation and limitations of each piece of radio and telephone hardware in the control center, know the applicable Federal Communications Commission (FCC) rules regarding that center and its equipment, and understand the general operations, responsibilities, and interrelationships of the public safety service agencies in the area.

The alert and dispatch phase of EMS communications requires several important actions by the dispatcher. These include

- Properly screening and determining the priority of each call.
- Selecting and alerting the appropriate EMS response unit(s).
- Dispatching and directing the selected unit(s) to the correct incident location.
- Coordinating the response of the EMS unit(s) with that of other public safety services until the conclusion of the incident.

After receiving the original call for assistance, the dispatcher must attempt to assess its relative importance in order to initiate the appropriate EMS response. The dispatcher must elicit the exact location of the patient needing help, the nature and severity of the emergency, some description of the surrounding scene (number of patients in a multiple injury situation, special environmental hazards, and so on), and, if possible, additional information such as the telephone number from which the call is being made, the patient's age and name, and other information determined by local protocol. From this information, the dispatcher will assign the appropriate EMS unit to respond based on the following criteria:

- The dispatcher's perception of the severity of the problem.
- Proximity of EMS units to the scene (response time).
- Level of training (first responder, BLS, ALS) and experience of available EMS units.
- The need for additional response units (such as EMS, fire department, hazardous materials handling team, MEDEVAC helicopter, or additional police units).

Having made a decision, the dispatcher's next task is to alert and mobilize the appropriate unit(s). A variety of equipment may be used for the alerting function. The dispatch radio system may be used to alert those units already in service and monitoring the **channel.** Frequently, there will be a unit-specific **tone** generated to alert the selected unit of an incoming message. Special telephone circuits or **hot lines** may be used between the control center and the EMS crew station or "quarters." These circuits will ring without dialing whenever the dispatcher lifts the telephone handset. Another method is special tone-generating radio equipment that is activated by the dispatcher; it not only alerts the selected EMS crew, but also turns on the station lights and opens vehicle access doors at a distance of several miles from the communications center.

In EMS systems that rely on volunteer or part-time personnel not exclusively engaged in staffing EMS response units, paging is a common alerting system. *Paging* involves the use of a coded tone radio signal, and sometimes a voice message, transmitted to small individual radio receivers (beepers). The paging signals may be sent selectively to alert only certain individuals, or a blanket signal can be sent that activates all of the pagers of that service. Alerted personnel must then contact the dispatcher, by radio or telephone, to acknowledge the message and receive details on the assignment.

Once the selected units have been alerted, all units must be properly dispatched and routed to the incident. Every EMS system should use a standard dispatching procedure. The dispatcher's instructions to the alerted units should be given by a distinct voice protocol that includes the following details:

- The nature and severity of the injury, illness, or incident.
- The exact location of the incident.
- The number of patients.
- Responses by other public safety agencies.
- Special directions or advisories such as known adverse road or traffic conditions.
- The time at which the units are dispatched.

All radio communications during the dispatch, as well as other phases of operations, must be brief and easily understood. Although plain English transmissions are preferred, many locales find that prearranged "10 codes" enhance brevity and work well for routine communications requirements.

The dispatcher's job includes accurate tracking of EMS units and other public safety units throughout the incident. Personnel in responding units are responsible for keeping the dispatcher informed of their location and status.

An EMS system's dispatch protocol should designate the type of unit to respond to a particular situation. Many variations of such protocols are found. Based on the local situation, these may include the dispatch of a single emergency ambulance; a two-tiered response of basic life support (BLS) and advanced life support (ALS) units, with one unit providing transport capability; or a multitiered system in which first responders, such as fire or police units, are dispatched with BLS and/or ALS units to reduce response time. Dispatch protocols should be in effect before a call is prioritized. Whatever protocol is employed, the EMT dispatcher must maintain accurate status reports of all units being dispatched. To do so requires that the dispatcher concentrate, follow established procedures, and successfully employ any available status-keeping aids. These aids might range from a simple matrix board

with flags or lights to indicate a unit's status and location to a sophisticated *computer-aided dispatch (CAD)* display (Figure 50–3).

The aims of the EMT dispatcher's actions during the dispatch phase are to mobilize the appropriate resources quickly and to ensure the accurate exchange of information. The desired result is the shortest possible response time for the appropriate EMS unit. An effective EMS communication system will also mandate that its EMT dispatchers contribute their knowledge and training to the care being rendered. Instances of dispatchers providing emergency medical self-help information and advice to callers are increasing. In these medical self-help situations, the EMT-dispatcher gives callers information and instructions on effective actions to take for themselves or the patient until the EMS or first responder unit arrives. This self-help information may include

- How to administer cardiopulmonary resuscitation.
- How to control bleeding with direct pressure.
- How to perform the abdominal thrust maneuver on a choking victim.
- How to keep a victim of overexposure warm.
- How to cool off a heat stroke victim.
- How to prevent further injury to a victim with a neck injury or serious fractures.

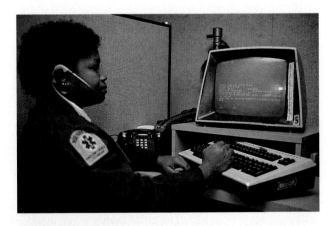

FIGURE 50–3

A sophisticated computer-aided dispatch (CAD) display.

This critical, medical self-help role of the EMT dispatcher may require calming a hysterical caller and remaining on the line for a considerable time, while simultaneously maintaining effective communication with EMS field units and other public safety agencies.

RADIO COMMUNICATIONS

Mobile and Portable EMS Communications

Every EMT who staffs an ambulance or other EMS response unit must be familiar with two-way radio communication. This means a thorough working knowledge of the vehicle's mobile radios and the hand-held portables. In addition, you must know when to use them and what to say when you are transmitting.

The EMT dispatcher usually communicates with field units by transmitting from a fixed radio base or repeater station controlled at the dispatch center (Figure 50–4). In a similar fashion, EMTs in an ambulance rely on their **land mobile service** and portable radios for communications. The portable radio is used to communicate with the dispatcher, hospital emergency department, medical control physician, or other EMS or public safety units at the scene. Portable radios are essential in helping coordinate EMS response at the scene of a multiple casualty incident. They are also effective in urban areas when you are searching for a patient in a multistory building; one EMT has to stay with the unit until directed to the proper location by the other EMT after the patient has been found.

Ambulances are usually equipped with an external public address system, which may be a component of the mobile radio. Similarly, the intercom between the cab and patient compartment may also be a component of the mobile radio. EMS systems may employ a variety of two-way radio hardware. Some operate **very high frequency (VHF)** equipment in the **simplex** (push-to-talk, release-to-listen) mode, while others conduct **duplex** (simultaneous talk-listen) on **ultrahigh frequencies (UHF)** ("MED" channels).

Some EMS radio systems are simply configured so that they require no off-site control links. Other systems rely on special telephone lines as control links for their remotely located base stations and antennae. Whatever equipment design is used, all EMS communications systems have some basic limitations. You must know the operational limitations of your communication equipment and understand how to cope effectively with and minimize them.

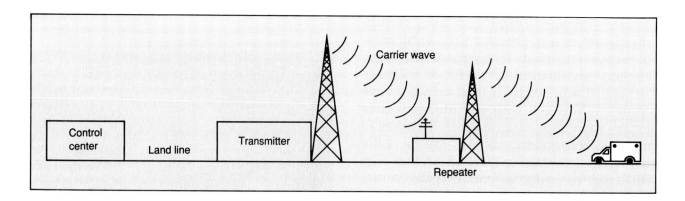

FIGURE 50–4   Two-way radio communication. The message is sent from the control center by a land line to the transmitter. The radio carrier wave is picked up by the repeater for rebroadcast to outlying units. Return radio traffic is picked up by the repeater and rebroadcast to the control center.

In any EMS radio system, the effectiveness and the extent of communication coverage are determined primarily by the "talk-back" capability of the weaker of either the mobile or portable units. Because the base and repeater stations normally have much greater power and higher antenna placement, their signal will generally be heard and understood at a much greater distance than the signal produced from a mobile unit. A portable or hand-held radio has an even shorter effective communication range, as it has the lowest power output and, frequently, the lowest antenna location. When you are on field assignment, realize that although you can clearly receive the dispatcher or hospital on your radios, you may not be heard or understood. Even small changes in the transmitting location of the portable or mobile unit can produce significant variations in the reception quality of the radio traffic.

You must also be aware that the efficiency of the radio system's equipment greatly influences the success of communications. The antenna of an ambulance radio that has been loosened by a hospital overhang or a damaged microphone often prevents high-quality communications. The field EMT and the EMT dispatcher are responsible for checking the condition and status of the communication equipment they will be using at the start of each shift and for correcting or replacing any deficiencies.

Standard Radio Operating Procedures

From the time you acknowledge receiving a call until completion of the run, you must use your radio communication system effectively. Frequently, you must demonstrate your communications skills. To help all EMTs, dispatchers, and others in the EMS system communicate properly, EMS system directors should establish a standard radio communications protocol. This protocol should include the appropriate format for transmitting messages, a definition of key communications words and key phrases, and procedures for troubleshooting common radio communications problems. For example, the "call-up" for establishing radio contact

between two units is made by transmitting the identification of the called unit first, followed by the identification of the unit calling, as in "Dispatch, this is Medic One." Using this format, the EMT initiating the call gives the radio transmitter a chance to turn on and generate a suitable **carrier** wave for the voice message. This procedure alerts the unit being called to listen for the identity of the transmitting unit and helps eliminate the caller's clipping the first part of the message by speaking too soon.

Standard radio operating procedures are designed to reduce the number of misunderstood messages, to keep transmissions as brief as possible (thus making more "air time" available), and to develop effective radio discipline for use in critical situations. In addition to learning standard message formats, you should practice these radio techniques:

- Always monitor the channel before transmitting to avoid interfering with another unit's radio traffic.
- Plan what you will say before pushing the transmit switch. This will help keep your transmissions brief and precise.
- Speak distinctly and directly into the microphone, but never shout. The microphone should be held about 2 inches from your mouth (Figure 50–5).
- Always acknowledge a transmission promptly. If you are otherwise occupied and cannot immediately take a long incoming message, simply acknowledge the call-up with "stand by."
- Use standard English language. Avoid slang phrases or complex codes.
- Speak at a moderate, understandable rate.
- Avoid showing negative emotions, such as anger or irritation, when transmitting. Your tone of voice should indicate courtesy, making it unnecessary to say "please" or "thank you," which wastes air time.

Becoming familiar with standard radio formats and techniques will help you perform your job more effectively through proper use of the EMS communication system. From acknowledgment of the dispatch call until you are

Hold a radio microphone about 2 inches from the mouth. Speak distinctly and directly; never shout.

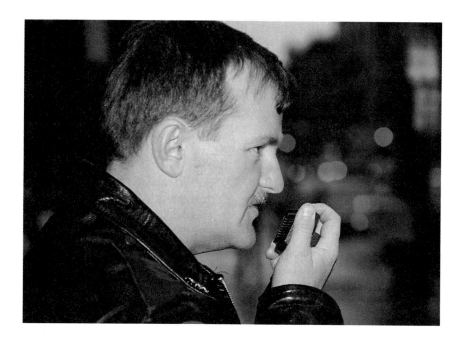

cleared from the medical emergency, the mobile radio communications capability of the EMS system will be in use at several key points. You must report at these intervals:

1. To acknowledge the dispatch information.
2. To estimate time of arrival (ETA) once you respond to the scene.
3. To announce unit's arrival on the scene.
4. To announce unit's departure from the scene and the destination hospital. (Include the number of patients transported if more than one.) Include the ETA.
5. To announce unit's arrival at the hospital or other facility.
6. To announce that unit is clear of the incident or hospital and is available for another assignment.
7. To announce unit's arrival back at quarters.

While en route to and from the scene, you should also report to the dispatcher special road conditions that might affect other responding units. You should report any unusual delays, such as road blockages or elevated bridges. At the scene, you may use the radio system to request additional EMS or other public safety assistance, and then help coordinate the response.

Medical Communication Capability

Every EMS system must have physician input and involvement. The physicians who provide medical consultation and control for you must be familiar with the EMS communication system and protocols (Figure 50–6). They must be readily available to communicate on the radio

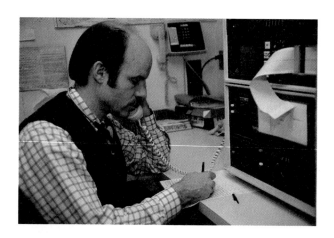

The physicians at the hospital must be familiar with the EMS communication system and protocols so they can provide medical consultation and control for EMTs in the field.

equipment installed at the hospital or on a mobile or portable unit. It is essential that the EMS director, medical control officers, and providers develop standard medical treatment and radio communications protocols for use by the physicians and EMTs in EMS field operations. Such protocols help to decrease misunderstandings between physician and EMTs regarding patient reports and orders.

Cellular telephones are an invaluable aid for physicians and scene commanders to confer with and talk to hospitals. Information can be gathered regarding hospital bed and physician availability, as well as conditions at the scene which may require the mobilization of specialized resources. Due to economic constraints, however, cellular telephones are not being widely used at the present time for routine communications by EMTs.

Ambulance-to-Hospital Communication

Field EMTs must have the capability of direct radio contact with hospital emergency department personnel. You can use your vehicle or portable radios to request physician consultation and to transmit the patient assessment report. The patient report should follow the classical medical case presentation and briefly include these elements:

1. Patient's age and sex (the patient's name should not be used over the radio because it is an invasion of one's privacy).
2. Patient's chief complaint or your perception of the problem and its severity.
3. Brief pertinent history of the patient's illness or injury, including medications, allergies, pertinent systemic problems such as diabetes, cardiac conditions, pregnancy.
4. Brief report of physical findings to include vital signs, level of consciousness, and general appearance and degree of distress.
5. Brief summary of emergency treatment administered to the patient and patient's response, if any.
6. Estimated time of arrival at the hospital.

When there are multiple patients at an incident, you should carefully identify each

patient with an appropriate number by using an established triage protocol. This will decrease confusion at the hospital.

Medical control communication must be conducted on radio channels that are relatively free of other radio traffic and interference. EMS systems may employ a variety of means for controlling access on the ambulance-to-hospital channels. In some cases, the ambulance dispatcher also monitors and assigns appropriate, clear medical control channels. Other systems rely on special communications operations, such as *CMEDS (centralized medical emergency dispatch) or resource coordination centers*, to monitor and allocate the medical control channels among EMS providers. Still others use a scanning capability built into their radio system, such as a *RTSS (radio-telephone switch station)* base and its associated mobiles. This unit automatically selects a clear channel from among several UHF frequencies. The ham radio network is also of great value, especially during natural disasters such as an earthquake.

When communication personnel regularly monitor channels and assign clear ones to EMS providers as needed, they use the "real-time" method of channel allocation. This method provides maximum flexibility for control and use of all EMS radio channels during busy radio traffic periods. An alternate method for allocating EMS radio channels may be used in some areas. This is the assignment of channels according to geographic sector. Only certain available channels are assigned to different providers in any one geographic area. Each channel is then designated for "primary," "secondary," or other use by the appropriate EMS providers. This allocation method severely restricts the flexibility for using the radio frequencies, but it may be satisfactorily used in areas that have several providers operating in adjacent service sectors with relatively low radio traffic demands.

Hospital-to-Hospital Communications

Most day-to-day hospital communications rely on the commercial telephone system. Regular telephones, and even **dedicated lines** or "hot lines," connect departments within the hospital or link closely related hospital facilities for a variety of everyday activities. In addition, hospitals are heavy users of paging systems to maintain contact with their own personnel within and outside the hospital's facilities.

In times of natural disasters, two-way radio communications may become important to the hospitals. During severe weather, or in incidents involving many sick or injured, the telephone network may fail or be overloaded with calls. Vital information may not be available to hospital personnel by routine means. In such situations, the EMS radio communications system may be used to send reports on bed availability, status of blood bank supplies, and other medical resource availability. Such interhospital communications should not interfere with EMS-to-hospital communications. EMS directors should make certain that their radio communication links among hospitals and the rest of the EMS system are tested regularly to ensure proper readiness.

The Federal Communications Commission (FCC)

All radio operations in the United States, including those used by EMS systems, are conducted according to regulations developed and enforced by the Federal Communications Commission. That agency also has jurisdiction over interstate and international telephone and telegraph services, which may occasionally involve EMS activity.

The FCC's main EMS-related responsibilities include

- Allocating specific radio frequencies for use by EMS providers. The "modern era" of EMS communication began in 1974, when the FCC created a block of 10 UHF "MED" channels to be used by EMS providers. These were added to several VHF frequencies that were previously available for EMS systems, but were often simultaneously used by interfering non-EMS activities.
- Licensing eligible individual base station operations and assigning appropriate radio call signs relating to those stations. An authoriz-

ing license is usually issued by the FCC to the operator for a five-year period, after which it must be renewed. Each FCC license is granted only for a specific operating group—for example, a specific base station control location on a specific **frequency** with specific antenna locations and for a specific number of associated mobile or portable units.

- Establishing licensing standards and operating specifications for radio equipment to be used by EMS providers. Before it can be licensed, a particular item of radio equipment must be submitted, by its manufacturer, to the FCC for type-acceptance based on the established operating specifications and regulations.
- Establishing limitations for transmitter power output. This principally involves base station hardware.
- Monitoring radio operations, including making spot field checks to help ensure compliance with FCC rules and regulations.
- Requiring that EMTs also be individually licensed before they are allowed to use prehospital care radio systems.

FCC rules and regulations can be purchased from the Government Printing Office in Washington, D.C. They are contained in many volumes of technical and legal language with only a very small section devoted to EMS communication issues (Part 90, subpart C). Most EMS systems have radio and telephone communication expertise available. Thus, EMTs need not read these government publications for appropriate guidance on technical issues; instead, they should rely on their EMS system supervisors.

One important element that the FCC has largely relegated to EMS system providers and directors is proper and effective communication planning and coordination. You should participate in this process at all available opportunities. You can contribute knowledge of how communications will assist in providing emergency medical care in the field, what interference problems have traditionally occurred on particular frequencies, where the "dead" spots are located, and what needs exist for radio communications with other public safety, rescue, or adjacent EMS organizations. Although there are many possible solutions for hardware and system design problems, the planning process must first define the needs for a particular communication system in the form of answers to the following questions: Who needs to talk to whom, from where, and when?

YOU ARE THE EMT

1. In addition to disagreeing over the location of a 911 communication control center, why do you think a lot of communities have not been able to implement an E911 system?

2. Why is it important that an EMS dispatcher have EMT training? What kind of problems could a dispatcher experience without such training?

3. You are a dispatcher and have received a call from a woman who says her 2-year-old is choking and turning blue. What information must you obtain from her? What advice will you give her?

4. Research and report on the radio communication protocol in your community's EMS system.

CHAPTER 51

RECORDS AND REPORTS

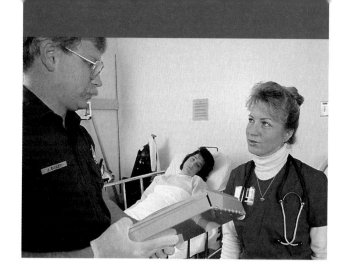

KEY TERMS

AVPU scale Level of consciousness scale.

P-Q-R-S-T A method used to describe the patterns and types of pain.

run report Verbal and narrative of events during a run.

street form A compact form, frequently printed on a 3 × 5 index card, that allows you to obtain and record the information needed to make a radio report to the emergency department. This information is also used to fill out the more detailed, permanent ambulance run record.

OVERVIEW

Paperwork is a pain. It is not the exciting, "save-a-life" part of the EMT's job that most people identify with. Nevertheless, it is a vital part of providing emergency medical care. Adequate reporting and development of accurate records ensure the continuity of patient care, guarantee proper transfer of responsibility, comply with the requirements of health departments and law enforcement agencies, and fulfill the EMT's administrative needs. Although these reporting and record keeping duties are essential for you, they must never come before patient care. With experience and alertness, you will soon learn to obtain most of the necessary information from simple observation, listening, and quick questioning while rendering emergency care to the patient.

Chapter 51 begins with an overview of the general information requirements of ambulance report forms. Then the chapter describes the general procedures for filling out the forms, usually a preliminary street form, followed by a permanent ambulance run report. Throughout the chapter, the importance of accurate record keeping is stressed—these records are often consulted long after the incident has occurred.

GOALS

The goals of Chapter 51 are to
- list the general information requirements of ambulance reports.
- describe the general procedures for record keeping, including how to fill out a preliminary street form and a permanent ambulance run report.

GENERAL INFORMATION REQUIREMENTS

Record keeping serves several important purposes. By describing the nature of the patient's injuries or illness at the scene and the initial treatment provided by you, ambulance report forms provide a mechanism for the efficient continuation of patient care. The forms should also be used in an ongoing program for evaluation of the quality of patient care. All records will be reviewed periodically by your system to ensure that trauma triage or other prehospital care criteria have been met. Additional data may be obtained from the forms to analyze causes, severity, and types of illness or injury requiring emergency medical care.

Records also provide administrative information for patient billing. In addition, they can be used to evaluate response times, equipment usage, and other areas of administrative responsibility.

The requirements on an ambulance report form are many and vary from jurisdiction to jurisdiction, mainly because so many agencies derive information from them. There is no universally accepted form and the following information is typically obtained:

Patient Information
- Patient's name, age, sex.
- Address.
- Nature of call.

- Mechanism of injury.
- Location of patient when first seen (specific details noted, especially if incident is a vehicular accident or criminal activity is suspected).
- Rescue and treatment measures by first responders.
- Signs and symptoms found during the primary and secondary surveys.
- Care and treatment given at site and during transport.
- Vital signs, patient condition, and changes in vital signs and condition during transport.
- Medications used by patient.
- Allergies.
- Hospital to which patient was taken.
- Disposition of patient's valuables.
- Signature of patient or relatives if medical care is refused.
- Procedures followed and disposition of body in the event of death.
- Dying statements.
- Circumstances involved if there are potential legal concerns such as homicide, suicide, or physical abuse.
- Statements made by patient or others that might serve as legal testimony.

Administrative Information

- Date of call.
- Time of call.
- Name and telephone number of caller.
- The location of the call.
- Time of dispatch.
- Time of arrival at scene.
- Time of leaving the scene.
- Time of arrival at hospital.
- Time of leaving hospital.
- Time of return to base.
- Patient's insurance information.
- Dispatching agency.
- Names of EMTs responding to call.
- The identity of the rescue units.
- The base hospital involved in the run.
- Type of run to scene, emergency/routine.
- Type of run to hospital, emergency/routine.

GENERAL PROCEDURES FOR RECORD KEEPING

Specific procedures for collecting, reporting, and recording the information for each run will vary from community to community. You must become familiar with local requirements, but general principles do apply.

Ambulance Street Forms

Initially, most EMTs make use of an ambulance **street form.** This is a compact form, sometimes printed on a 3 × 5 index card, that allows you to obtain and record the information needed to make a radio report to the emergency department (Figure 51–1). This information is also used to fill out the more detailed, permanent ambulance run record.

Reporting and record keeping begin with the dispatcher's notification of the need for the ambulance at the scene of an accident or illness. The first entry is the location to which the ambulance is being sent. En route to the scene, the dispatcher may provide additional information on the patient or situation. Report any unexpected delays in responding while you are en route to the scene to the dispatcher, especially traffic problems or road blockages that might affect other emergency vehicles. Notify the dispatcher of your arrival at the scene, the initial condition of the scene, and the need, if any, for additional units.

You will then record the number of patients, if more than one, and begin recording pertinent information for each patient, such as name, age, injuries, signs, symptoms, vital signs, medications, and allergies as the primary and secondary surveys are performed. Following treatment of the patient, the dispatcher should be notified that the ambulance is en route to a specific hospital. During transport, notify the emergency department of the condition of the patient if you have not already contacted the hospital. Report any significant change in the condition of the patient to the emergency

AMBULANCE STREET FORM

Run number _____ Name _____ Age ____ Sex ____ Date _____

COMPLAINT _____

_____

_____

ASSESSMENT _____

_____

_____

	BLOOD PRESSURE	PULSE	RESP.	NEUROLOGICAL			
Time ____	____ ____	____	____	Time			
Time ____	____ ____	____	____	Talks	yes/no	yes/no	yes/no
Time ____	____ ____	____	____	Follows commands	yes/no	yes/no	yes/no

SKIN
- normal ____   warm, dry ____
- pale ____   cold, clammy ____
- cyanotic ____   warm, moist ____
- flushed ____   cold, dry ____

BLOOD LOSS
- None ____
- Minor ____
- Moderate ____
- Severe ____

Pupil diameter	L R	L R	L R
	mm mm	mm mm	mm mm

SITES OF INJURY

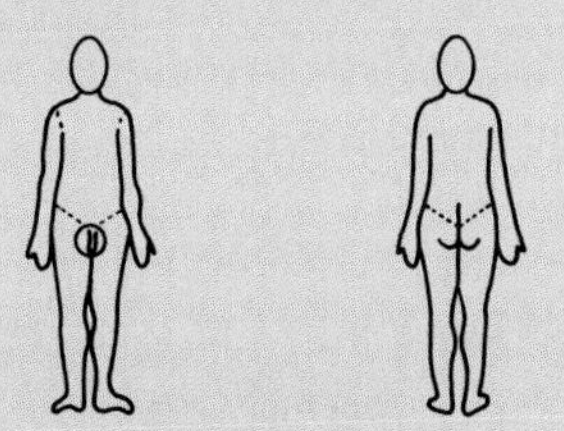

ANTERIOR   POSTERIOR

NEUROVASCULAR

	UPPER R or L		LOWER R or L	
Sensation				
Movement				
Pulse				
Capillary filling				
Time				

CHEST
- clear ____
- rales ____
- wheezes ____
- other ____

EMERGENCY MEDICAL CARE RENDERED

_____

_____

TIME
- Enroute _____
- Arrival _____
- Depart _____
- Hospital _____

CREW

_____

FIGURE 51–1 Ambulance street form. This is a preliminary report to record the information that will later be entered on a permanent ambulance run report.

department and record the change on the run report as well. During transport to the hospital, you may begin filling out the permanent run report if the patient is stable and does not require care or reassurance.

Run Reports

On arrival at the emergency department, you should give a verbal report to the physician or emergency department staff describing the patient's condition and the treatment given (Figure 51–2). Once your assistance in the emergency department is no longer needed, the permanent ambulance **run report** is completed (Figure 51–3). All parts of the report should be completed at this time and not left until later to be filled out. Appropriate copies of the permanent run report are left with the emergency department.

When you are completing the narrative portion of the run report, the following format will be helpful in organizing information. Each narrative report must include the following four basic components:

1. The patient's history.
2. The findings on physical examination.
3. Your working impression.

4. The treatment rendered.

The history section should contain information concerning the patient's chief complaint or problem. This includes a brief description of the patient's present illness or injury, including mechanism of injury, position found, significant environmental findings, and so on. The **P-Q-R-S-T** of pain should be used to describe the patient's pain:

P Provokes: What brought on the pain? What makes it better or worse?
Q Quality: Sharp, dull, achy, burning, etc.?
R Region: Where is the pain located?
S Severity: Mild, moderate, severe?
T Time: Onset, duration, recurrence?

The history section should also contain pertinent past medical history, including medications; allergies; and significant medical problems such as cardiac disease, diabetes, or pulmonary problems.

The next component of the narrative—findings on physical examination—contains information on the following:

1. Position in which the patient was found.
2. Respiratory status (airway; respiratory rate, rhythm, and effort).

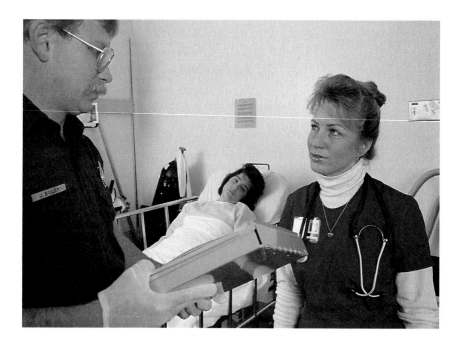

FIGURE 51–2

Upon arriving at the hospital, give a verbal report to emergency department personnel on the patient's condition and the treatment provided.

EMERGENCY MEDICAL SERVICE PATIENT FORM

_____ of _____

Date:_____
Unit No.:_____
Case No.:_____
Time:_____

Shift A B C D

Police/Sheriff:
on scene   requested

A Single Pt/Trans
B Multi Pt/Trans
C Multi Unit/Trans
D Aid Only/No Trans
E No Aid/No Trans
F Other _____

Location_____ Type of Call_____
Name_____ Age____ Sex M F DOB_____
Address_____ City_____ State_____ Zip_____
Responsible Adult_____ Relationship_____ Phone_____
EMT-P_____ Badge No._____ Pt's MD_____
EMT-P_____ Badge No._____ Extra Attn._____
Back-up EMS/Fire_____ Authorizing M.D._____

Chief Complaint:_____
Injury/Illness Description:_____

Remarks/Hx:_____

Medications:_____

Vital Signs Lying Sitting Standing   BP_____ Pulse_____ Resp_____ Temp_____

PATIENT STATUS	DRUGS	AID

PATIENT STATUS

Repeat VS
2   3
BP _____ _____
P _____ _____
R _____ _____

Skin
normal   cyanotic
pale   flushed
dry   moist

Respirations
normal   shallow
labored

Breath Sounds
left   right
normal   normal
decreased   decreased
rales   rales
wheezes   wheezes
absent   absent

Bleeding
none
min mod sev

Pain
none
min mod sev

Level of Consciousness
Initial
A—Alert
V—Responds to Verbal
P—Responds to Pain
U—Unresponsive
Repeat
A V P U

Pupils
left   right
size   size
● ● ●   ● ● ●
react   react
nr   nr

DRUGS

amt.   time   amt.   time

Atropine   Dextrose
1.____ ____:____   1.____ ____:____
2.____ ____:____   2.____ ____:____

Bicarb   Epinephrine
1.____ ____:____   1.____ ____:____
2.____ ____:____   2.____ ____:____
3.____ ____:____   3.____ ____:____

Bretylium   Lidocaine
1.____ ____:____   1.____ ____:____
2.____ ____:____   2.____ ____:____

Calcium   Oxygen
1.____ ____:____   nasal cannula
2.____ ____:____   face mask
                          L/min:____
Naloxone   bag-mask
1.____ ____:____   demand valve
2.____ ____:____

Other:_____

Allergies:_____

AID

Antishock pants
Bandaging
Burn kit
CPR
C-Collar
Defibrillate/Cardiovert
  Joules:_____
Dextrostix:_____mg%
Extrication/KED
EDA
ET:_____mm
EKG
  Rhythm:_____
Ice pack
OB kit
Oral/Nasal Airway
Spine board
Splinting
Suction

IV RL D5W
    gauge time
1.____ ____:____
2.____ ____:____

Response code to hospital:_____ Hospital:_____ Receiving M.D.:_____

I was offered aid by the City of _____ EMS, but chose not to accept emergency treatment and/or transportation.

Signature_____ Witness_____

FIGURE 51–3 Ambulance run report. This form is used by both EMTs and EMT-paramedics to document the four basic elements of prehospital care: patient identification and history, physical findings, the EMT's diagnostic impressions, and the treatment given.

3. Cardiac status (pulse rate and character; perfusion).
4. Level of consciousness—**AVPU scale.**

   A   Alert: oriented to time, person, place
   V   Verbal: responds to verbal stimuli
   P   Pain: responds to painful stimuli
   U   Unresponsive

5. Visual exam (wounds: location, type, severity; deformities: location, type, severity).
6. Secondary assessment findings (reported by body systems).

When you write the physical examination section, include significant negative findings—for example, "The abdomen nontender on palpation"—as well as the positive findings.

The third section of the narrative is *your* assessment of the clinical syndrome or medical problem that is present. This constitutes the field impression of the patient's condition on which you based your prehospital care. It should not, in any way, rule out or cause one to overlook other possibilities that may not be immediately apparent. The final diagnosis is made only after further evaluation and hospital care.

The final section is treatment. In this section you briefly describe what was done to the patient, such as splinting, oxygen administration, and so forth. Changes in the patient's condition as a result of treatment are also included in this section.

Accurate recording of information on the ambulance run report form, especially in the narrative section, will answer many questions that might arise at a later date. In addition, such information provides a useful tool in a program for evaluating the quality of patient care. Many EMS systems are developing computerized records and report forms to improve their accuracy and aid in the delivery of patient care and research in the field.

Ambulance records must be handled with care and stored in an appropriate manner once you complete them. They are confidential documents of significant potential legal consequence and must be treated as such.

Additional Records and Reports

In some instances, you may be required to file special reports with appropriate authorities. These may include incidents involving gunshot wounds; dog bites; certain infectious diseases; suspected physical, sexual, or substance abuse; and so on. You must be familiar with local requirements for reporting these incidents, because failure to report them may have legal ramifications.

YOU ARE THE EMT

1. What is the difference between an ambulance street form and an ambulance run report?
2. What kind of information on the street form can be transferred to the ambulance run report?
3. How can an EMS system use its ambulance run reports to review its performance and project future needs?
4. Research and report on the special reports that EMTs have to file in your community.

SECTION 12
....

....

SUPPLEMENTS

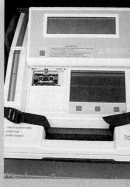

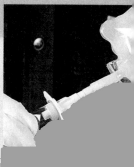

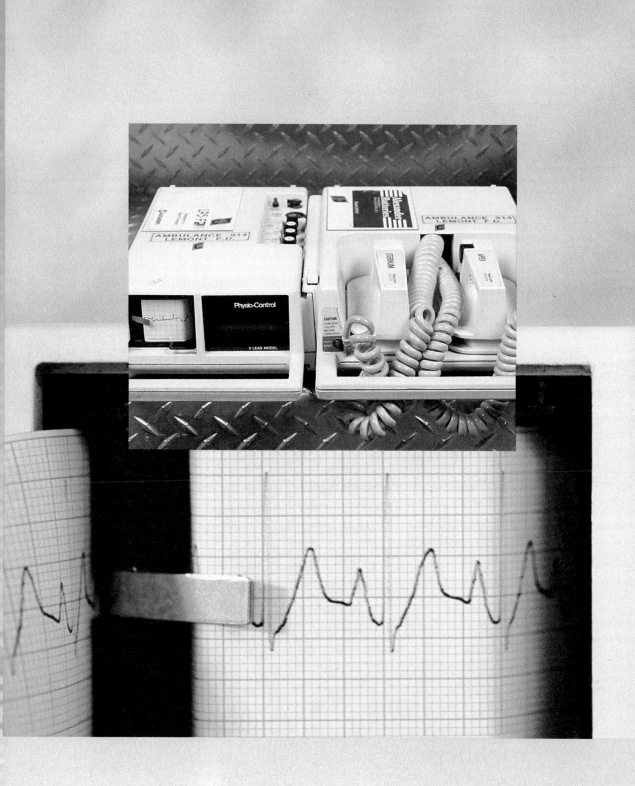

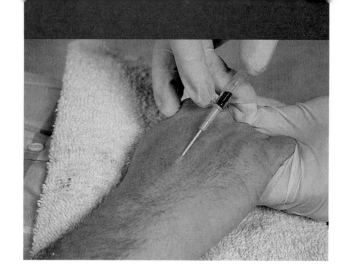

INTRAVENOUS THERAPY

KEY TERMS

air embolism (ār em′bo-lizm) A condition caused by a bubble of air in the blood stream.

catheter (kath′ĕ-ter) A hollow, cylindrical structure that can be inserted into the body to drain or deliver fluids.

circulating blood volume The amount of blood contained within the circulatory system (about 6 liters in the adult).

electrolyte (e-lek′tro-līt) Salts dissolved in body fluids and cells.

electrolyte solution Fluids used for intravenous infusion that contain electrolytes.

infiltration (in″fil-tra′shun) A condition in which the fluid for intravenous therapy enters the surrounding subcutaneous tissue instead of the vein.

infusion (in-fu′zhun) The introduction of fluid other than blood or blood products into the vascular system.

intravenous (in″trah-ve′nus) Within a vein.

transfusion The introduction of whole blood or blood products into the vascular system.

venipuncture (ven′ĭ-punk″tūr) The site on an extremity where the needle for intravenous fluid therapy is inserted into a vein.

OVERVIEW

Intravenous therapy may be an important procedure during the resuscitation of the patient who is suffering from volume depletion, burn injury, blood loss, heat illness, shock, electrolyte imbalance, and many other medical and surgical conditions. It is also important in providing an avenue of medication delivery in many medical situations such as cardiac arrest, seizure disorder, asthma attacks, and other assorted medical emergencies. As an EMT with specialized training you may be authorized to initiate intravenous therapy according to local medical director protocol in accordance with state and local ordinances and guidelines. Even if you do not initiate this invasive procedure, you may be responsible for monitoring intravenous therapy while transporting a patient to a treatment facility.

This therapeutic modality requires extensive training in its use as well as an ongoing program of retraining to maintain the necessary skills level. In addition, you must be aware of the indications for the use and maintenance of IV therapy as well as possible complications. Medical control and supervision, plus medical reviews, are mandatory when you perform invasive intravenous techniques.

Supplement A begins with a definition of intravenous fluid therapy and the terms related to its use. Then the equipment and supplies needed to provide IV therapy are listed. Next, the steps to start IV infusions are described, followed by a discussion of the importance of monitoring the patient and the IV. The last section of Supplement A discusses the possible complications of IV therapy.

GOALS

The goals of Supplement A are to
- define intravenous fluid therapy.
- identify the equipment and supplies needed to provide IV therapy.
- learn the steps to start an IV infusion.
- discuss the importance of monitoring the patient and the IV.
- recognize the possible complications of IV therapy.

PURPOSE OF IV THERAPY

Intravenous fluid therapy (IV therapy) is an intermediate or advanced EMT skill. The ability to use this skill is determined by state and local laws, ordinances, and standards of practice. Implementation of this level of care requires intensive training, clinical practice, and continuing education and skills practice. Additional requirements include mandatory medical control and medical quality assessment follow-up. As with any patient care procedure, meticulous documentation of indications for and patient response to the procedure are required. When the patient refuses intravenous therapy directed by medical director protocol, it too must be carefully documented. Additionally, you must document the physician's order for IV therapy. Ongoing medical quality control is necessary to ensure appropriate and efficient patient care.

Intravenous fluid therapy is not a difficult skill to learn, although once learned, continuous practice is necessary to maintain it. This skill should be learned in a well-controlled environment, but it generally will be practiced during stressful situations, under adverse environmental conditions and when time is a critical factor. In addition, potentially serious complications, of which you must be aware, can accompany the use of IV therapy.

You must understand the difference between *transfusion* and *infusion*. **Transfusion** is the introduction of whole blood or blood products into the vascular system. You will probably never institute a field transfusion. Because a patient may be receiving a transfusion during interhospital transfers, however, you must be familiar with the equipment and techniques used and the complications of transfusions.

Infusion is the introduction of fluid other than blood or blood products into the vascular system. You use this technique to establish and maintain direct access to the circulation or to provide fluids in order to maintain an adequate **circulating blood volume.** Fluids used for intravenous infusion are frequently referred to as **electrolyte solutions** because the chemical compounds they contain are **electrolytes.** A compound that, in solution, will conduct an electrical current is an electrolyte. The most common electrolyte solutions used are salt (sodium chloride) solutions. Other electrolytes in the body are potassium, calcium, magnesium, and chloride compounds. The most common solutions, their abbreviations, and components are listed in Table A–1.

Occasionally, you may use another group of solutions called plasma expanders or colloids. These include Dextran® (large molecules of dextrose that are not metabolized), albumin, and Plasmanate.® Although plasma expanders and electrolyte solutions may be used to replace up to two-thirds of the normal circulating blood volume, they have no oxygen-carrying capacity. They may enable the support of blood pressure but only hemoglobin carries oxygen to the tissues.

The appropriate fluid necessary for each patient situation will be determined by local medical control personnel or by written protocol.

EQUIPMENT AND SUPPLIES

The following equipment and supplies are needed in order to provide intravenous infusion therapy:

TABLE A–1   Common Intravenous Fluids

Solution	Abbreviation	Component Electrolytes
5% dextrose	D5W	5% dextrose
10% dextrose	D10W	10% dextrose
Normal saline	NS	0.9% sodium chloride (NaCl)
Half-normal saline	1/2NS	0.45% NaCl
Quarter-normal saline	1/4NS	0.2% NaCl
Lactated Ringer's	LR	NaCl, potassium chloride (KCl), calcium chloride (CaCl), sodium lactate

Note: All solutions may also be made containing dextrose, in which case they are abbreviated by adding D5 or D10 as a prefix. For example, Lactated Ringer's in 5% dextrose would be abbreviated D5LR.

- Appropriate fluid (in an unbreakable container).
- IV administration sets (tubing).
- IV needles, various sizes (catheter and/or butterfly).
- Prep swabs (povoiodine and/or alcohol).
- Tape.
- Constricting band (Penrose or IV tourniquet).
- Sterile pads (2 × 2 inch or 4 × 4 inch).
- Bandaids.
- Immobilization boards.
- Cot-mounted IV pole.
- Contaminated needle container.

Optional supplies may be added according to local preference:

- Transparent IV site dressing.
- Antiseptic ointment for dressing IV site.
- Tubes for the collection of blood samples.
- Syringes for the collection of blood samples.

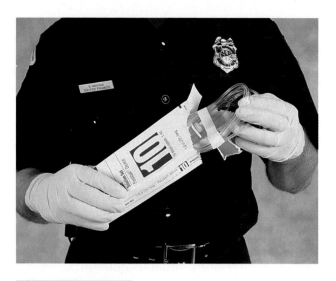

FIGURE A–1

An administration set for IV therapy.

PROCEDURE TO START IV INFUSION

As with any procedure that you perform, the patient must be prepared beforehand. You should explain to the patient that an IV is going to be started, that it is medically necessary to do so, and that there may be some temporary discomfort.

Step 1: Preparing the Solution

First select the solution—either ordered by medical control or appropriate for the particular situation—and check the labeling on the container to see that it is the correct solution. Checking includes making sure that the expiration date on the container has not been exceeded, that the sterile seals on the container are intact, and that the solution is clear, without cloudiness, color change, or precipitates (particles).

Next, select the administration set ordered by medical control or appropriate for the patient situation (Figure A–1). *Mini-drip sets* (with a needle in the drip chamber) are designed to keep an IV line open—that is, flowing with minimal volume infusion. These sets are generally used for medical type emergencies; they

are manufactured to deliver 60 drops/cc. They generally keep an IV open while infusing less than 0.5cc (30 drops) per minute. *Solution sets* are capable of providing much larger volumes in a shorter period of time. Designed without a needle in the drip chamber, they deliver 10 to 17 drops/cc. They are used for patients who require, or may require, large volumes of fluid to be infused over a short period of time, such as the adult trauma patient who is in hypovolemic shock. Special large bore trauma infusion tubing may enable the administration of up to one liter of fluid per minute. Also available are devices that, when applied to the IV solution bag, apply increased pressure to the bag and thus deliver a higher-volume flow rate through the tubing.

After selecting the appropriate administration set, you must ensure that the sterile seals are intact. Also inspect the set for cracks, discoloration, or holes. Move the flow control clamp to the desired position 6 to 8 inches from the drip chamber, and close it. Then remove the sterile seal from the end of the tubing closest to the drip chamber. After the sterile seal is removed from the fluid container, insert the tubing spike end into the fluid container with one quick twisting motion. Take care not to contaminate any of the sterile area.

While you are holding the fluid container higher than the drip chamber, squeeze the drip chamber and release it until the chamber is approximately half full (Figure A–2). Open the flow control and allow the fluid to flush all remaining air from the administration set. Although it may be necessary to loosen the sterile seal on the tubing to get the fluid to flow, it should not be removed. Be sure that there are no air bubbles in the administration tubing and that the drip chamber is still approximately half full. Place the tube near to where it will be applied. Next, lay out the three or four pieces of 1/2-inch tape that will be used to secure the needle or **catheter** in place, along with the dressing and antibiotic ointment if local practice requires. An arm board should be available to immobilize the IV site.

The IV needle or catheter to be used should be selected but not opened. EMTs generally use two types: the steel needle, or "butterfly," and the catheter over the needle (Figure A–3). In most situations, you will use the catheter over the needle type because it is easier to use and immobilize and less likely to injure the vein once in place.

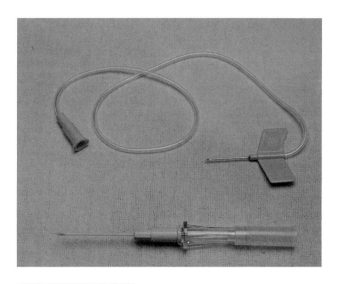

FIGURE A–3

The types of IV needle assemblies most commonly used to administer IV fluids in the prehospital setting: (top) butterfly; (bottom) catheter over the needle.

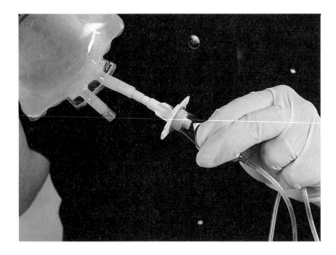

FIGURE A–2

Hold the fluid container higher than the drip chamber while squeezing and releasing the drip chamber until it is about half full.

Needles and catheters are sized by gauge—the smaller the gauge number (such as 14 or 16), the larger the internal diameter. The larger the internal diameter, the faster fluid can be infused. The size you use depends on the size of the vein, the amount or rate of administration desired, and how thick the solution is. Blood, for instance, requires 18 gauge or larger. Thus, you should use large-bore catheters (14, 16, or 18) for situations that may require large volume infusions, and small-bore catheters when the patient requires vascular access or an IV lifeline with minimal volume infusion.

Step 2: Selecting the Site

Talk to the patient. Explain the procedure and inquire about any known allergies. Inquire specifically about iodine and adhesive allergies as well as medication allergies. Explain to the patient about IV discomfort and the need to limit movement of the limb once the catheter is in place. Warn the patient not to manipulate the needle, catheter, or flow clamp. You should wear gloves and eye protection.

Next, select the site for the **venipuncture** (Figure A–4). When possible, an uninjured upper extremity should be used. You should try to use the most distal upper extremity site compatible with the gauge of catheter to be used. The veins in the antecubital fossa are the largest but should be used only as a last resort or when severe circulatory collapse exists. Veins over other joints should also be avoided if possible, because they tend to be close to arteries and also are difficult to immobilize. Avoid infected, injured, or irritated areas to minimize the chance of contamination and infection.

Place the constricting band about the extremity six to eight inches proximal to the selected site (Figure A–5). Apply the band tightly enough to restrict venous return but not arterial flow. Keep the extremity below the level of the heart and instruct the patient to clench and unclench the fist several times to enhance venous distension and to make the veins easier to detect. Once a straight, easily accessible vein is identified, palpate the vein to determine its location and degree of distension, and to be certain that the vein will not "roll away" from the needle.

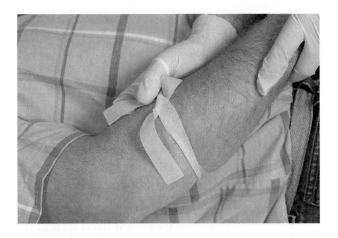

FIGURE A–5

Place a constricting band about the extremity, about six inches above the site for the venipuncture.

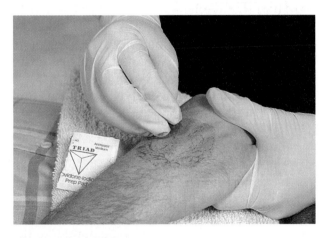

FIGURE A–6

The site of injection must be thoroughly disinfected.

Step 3: Preparation of the Site

Preparation of the site, the next step, is of utmost importance. The site must be thoroughly disinfected to prevent contaminants on the skin from being introduced directly into the bloodstream (Figure A–6). This step is particularly important in the undesirable environments in which you routinely work. Use a povoiodine swab for the initial cleansing. Begin to wipe over the selected site, then move in

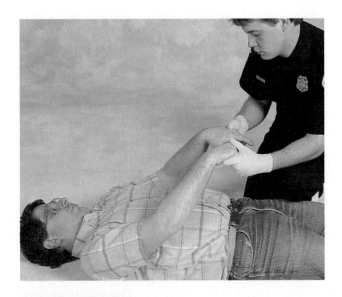

FIGURE A–4

Select the best site for the venipuncture.

ever-widening circles outward from the site. Then repeat the procedure using an alcohol swab to remove the povoiodine.

Step 4: Performing the Venipuncture

You should now be ready mentally and physically to perform the venipuncture. Be sure you are wearing gloves and eye protection, keep the extremity at the level of the heart or lower, and proceed in the following manner:

1. Remove the protective cap from the catheter/needle, being careful not to contaminate the needle and place the IV needle/catheter in your dominant hand.
2. With one finger of the other hand, apply light traction to the skin and vein, distal and slightly to the side of the site selected, to keep the vein from moving.
3. Hold the needle at a 30-degree angle, with the bevel facing up.
4. Firmly and quickly perforate the skin 2 to 5 mm distal to the intended point of entry into the vein (Figure A–7).
5. Then, firmly and quickly enter the vein from above or from the side. You should feel resistance, then a "pop" as the needle enters the vein. If the vein is successfully entered, there should be a "flash back" of blood at the needle hub (Figure A–8).
6. If you are unsuccessful (no flashback is seen), pull the needle back slightly and attempt to redirect the needle point into the vein again. If you are still unsuccessful, release the tourniquet, then withdraw the catheter/needle. Apply firm finger pressure over the puncture site for 1 minute.
7. Open a new catheter/needle and reattempt venipuncture at a point higher than the first attempt. If again unsuccessful, get someone else to start the IV or follow your local medical director protocol.
8. When you are using steel needles, carefully thread the needle up the vein. For a catheter over the needle, insert the needle approximately 2 to 3 mm past the entry point in the vein and carefully slide the catheter off the needle into the vein and remove the needle. *Important note:* If a

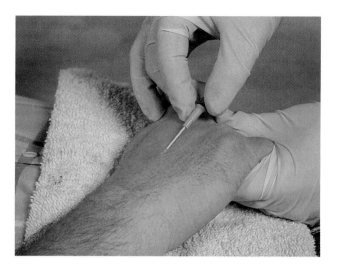

FIGURE A–7

Holding the needle at a 30-degree angle, quickly and firmly perforate the skin 2 to 5 mm distal to the vein.

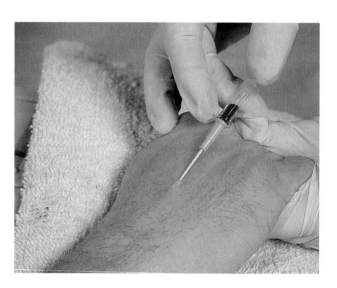

FIGURE A–8

When the vein has been entered, a small amount of blood will "flash back" at the needle hub.

problem should arise in threading a catheter off of a needle, do not pull the catheter back onto the needle. The end of the catheter might be sheared off by the needle point and cause a plastic catheter embolus which is a potentially serious complication for the patient.

9. If blood samples are to be taken, the syringe should be attached to the needle hub, the constricting band released, and the blood drawn up into the syringe.

10. To connect the tubing, remove the sterile seal on the free end of the administration set tubing and attach it firmly to the hub of the catheter, being careful not to contaminate any of the sterile areas (Figure A–9). To facilitate needle withdrawal and syringe or tubing attachment without unnecessary blood loss, place one finger over the vein just proximal to where the tip of the catheter can be seen or felt and apply gentle pressure. When the administration set tubing is attached, check to ensure that the constricting band has been removed.

11. Slowly open the flow control clamp to allow fluid to infuse. Make sure that fluid is flowing into the vein and not infusing into the surrounding tissue **(infiltration).** Infiltration is the leaking of IV fluid into the tissues around the IV site. It is evidenced by pain, swelling, and redness at the site, coolness to the touch, or fluid leaking from the infusion site. To confirm that the needle or catheter is inside the vein, place the fluid container below the level of the venipuncture site for a few seconds. If the needle or catheter is properly placed, blood will back up into the tubing of the administration set.

12. Unclamp the IV tubing and adjust the rate as described below. Reexamine the infusion site to rule out infiltration.

13. After you ensure that the IV is flowing smoothly, securely tape the catheter and tubing in place using an arm board if necessary (Figure A–10). When local guidelines dictate, antiseptic dressings may be used. They are applied as part of the securing process. Many localities now use a see-through dressing. Mark on the securing tape the catheter size, and date and time started. To ensure that the catheter stays in place, immobilize the extremity.

14. Record the treatment provided and the

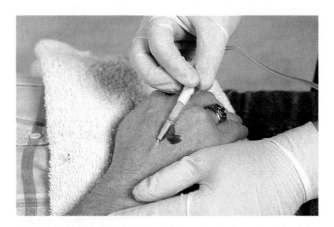

FIGURE A–9

Attach the tubing from the administration set firmly to the hub of the catheter.

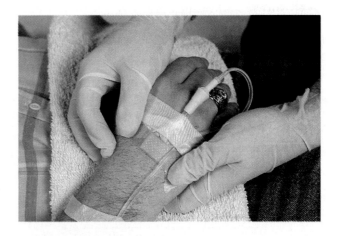

FIGURE A–10

Secure the catheter and tubing by tape, and immobilize the limb using an arm board.

physical results observed on the appropriate patient form.

15. When you use a butterfly needle, the steps are essentially the same as previously outlined; however, you must take greater care to ensure that the bevel of the needle that remains inside the vein is not manipulated or moved. This is necessary to minimize the possibility of cutting the vein.

MONITORING THE PATIENT AND THE IV

You must monitor the patient and the IV closely. The patient requires frequent monitoring of vital signs on a continuing basis to ensure that the appropriate rate of fluid administration is being maintained. In addition, the patient must be observed for signs of overhydration, such as distension of the neck veins, high blood pressure, rales in the chest, and dyspnea. If these signs appear, the flow rate must be decreased to the absolute minimum. The blood pressure should not be taken in the extremity in which the IV is running unless the other extremity is injured and unavailable.

In general, you will be given a specific order for a flow rate by medical control such as TKO (to keep open, the minimum flow rate), wide open (maximum or full flow), or a specific number of cubic centimeters per hour (cc/ hour). The flow rate in drops per minute is determined using the following formula:

$$\text{Flow rate in drops/min (abbreviated gtts/min)} = \frac{\text{cc/hr ordered} \times \text{drops/cc for drip chamber}}{\text{Time of infusion}}$$

As an example, assume you were ordered to infuse a fluid at 100 cc/hr using a drip chamber manufactured to produce 10 drops/cc; the flow rate in drops per minute would be:

$$17 \text{ drops (gtts)/min} = \frac{100 \text{ cc/hr} \times 10 \text{ drops (gtts)/cc}}{60 \text{ minutes}}$$

Check the IV periodically to ensure a proper flow rate. The flow rate must be checked each time the height of the fluid container changes in relation to the patient. If blood is "backflowing" into the tubing, the fluid container is too low in relation to the patient, and you should raise or gently compress it. If the IV stops running or the flow rate slows, check to see if the tubing has become kinked or compressed. Also, check the IV site to make sure that the catheter remains fixed in position, that the

extremity is not bent and impeding flow, and that the IV fluid is not infiltrating into the surrounding tissue. If infiltration is suspected, check the surrounding area for swelling and tenderness. If the IV is infiltrating, the flow must be stopped immediately and the IV discontinued.

If it becomes necessary to discontinue an IV due to infiltration or an IV malfunction, first close the flow control clamp and then gently remove the tape securing the catheter. Place a small, sterile dressing over the IV insertion site, firmly grasp the catheter hub, then quickly and smoothly withdraw the catheter. Maintain pressure over the venipuncture site until bleeding stops to prevent the formation of a hematoma. After the bleeding has been controlled, dress the site with a Bandaid.

When you are ordered to start a new IV, try to use another extremity. If the same extremity must be used, select a site proximal to the original site. You should never start an IV at a site distal to a recently discontinued infusion.

Should a fluid container begin to "run dry," exchange it for a full container before the drip chamber has emptied. Remove the old container from the tubing, taking care to prevent contamination of the tubing end. Insert the tubing end into the new container, as you did to prepare the IV initially, and partially refill the drip chamber.

COMPLICATIONS OF IV THERAPY

When you provide IV therapy, you must know how to manage the complications that may arise during or after therapy. Complications may be local, such as infiltration, or systemic, such as plastic catheter embolus. Certain complications may have grave consequences.

Local Complications

Some pain from the needle stick is to be expected. The pain may continue as the infusion begins, but it should subside rapidly. Continued pain or burning is probably a sign of infiltration or a local adverse reaction, and the IV should be discontinued. Cold IV solutions will feel cool as they enter an extremity. This also must be taken into consideration, especially in frigid weather.

The most common problem is hematoma formation at failed IV sites. Usually, pressure applied continuously for 3 to 5 minutes is sufficient to promote clotting and decrease hematoma formation.

Infection is another complication that may be caused by contaminants inadvertently introduced through the skin. Though not readily apparent at first, swelling, redness, and increased skin temperature at the site are possible indications of infection. The infected venipuncture site should be changed, preferably to another extremity.

Accidental arterial puncture may also occur, especially if venipuncture is performed over a joint. If bright, red, pulsatile arterial bleeding should occur through or around a catheter, withdraw the catheter immediately. Apply firm, direct pressure or a pressure dressing to the site for at least 10 minutes until the bleeding stops.

Other possible local complications include nerve damage, tissue slough, and thrombophlebitis. The latter is a late complication not ordinarily seen by EMTs initiating therapy.

Systemic Complications

Systemic complications tend to be more serious than the local complications. Some complications may result in circulatory collapse. You must be able to recognize these problems and be able to deal with them effectively.

Simple fainting may occur due to the emotional response of the patient to the venipuncture procedure. Supportive therapy may be required. All patients should be lying down when IV therapy is started. An **air embolism** may occur if air is allowed to leak into the IV line. In this case, the patient may rapidly lose consciousness and develop shock and cyanosis. The IV must be discontinued immediately and the patient transported as rapidly as possible in a head-down position. Give high flow oxygen and assist ventilation if necessary. Careful attention to the details of IV administration will minimize the chances of this potentially fatal complication.

Circulatory overload (the administration of an excessive amount of IV fluids) should be a rare occurrence when the patient and the IV have been properly monitored. Signs and symptoms of circulatory overload are the same as those of congestive heart failure (dyspnea, rales, and neck vein distension). Should a circulation overload occur, reduce the flow to the minimum rate and administer oxygen. Anaphylaxis is also rare. This condition usually occurs from medications added to the IV solution rather than from the solution itself. You must discontinue the infusion and begin treatment should anaphylaxis occur.

Environmental Complications

A final set of complications of IV therapy is related to the environment. In colder climates, the IV solutions may freeze in the tubing or container very rapidly. Under these circumstances, you may prefer to start the IV in the ambulance or in a heated building rather than in the field. During transport between the ambulance and a building, the fluid container should be protected from exposure to the cold. Another effect of cold can occur in the patient who is receiving a large volume of fluids for hypovolemic shock; if the fluids being administered have not been kept warm, it is possible that the patient's core temperature will drop, which could lead to hypothermia.

Safety cannot be overemphasized. The EMT who removes the needle safety cover is responsible for the needle and should ensure that it is properly disposed of in a sharps container after its purpose is fulfilled. Do *not* recap needles

(Figure A–11). If it must be recapped, place the safety cap on the ground or floor under your boot and slip the needle into the cap. The risk of AIDS following a needle stick contaminated from a high-risk patient is estimated at 0.5 percent; the risk of Hepatitis B is 10 to 20 times greater. There is no excuse for lack of proper precautions when handling needles. There are several new "self-recapping" or self-sheathing needles now on the market to satisfy the need to provide safer IV and injection devices.

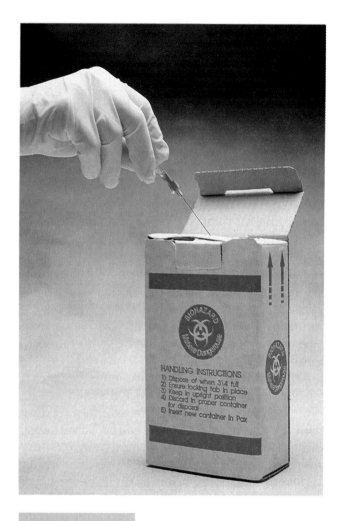

FIGURE A–11

Never recap a needle. Dispose of all needles in a sharps container.

YOU ARE THE EMT

1. How does an infusion differ from transfusion? Why must you be familiar with the equipment and techniques of transfusions even though you may never initiate one?

2. Describe the major difference between mini-drip sets and standard infusion sets. Give an example of a medical emergency that would require the use of each of these types of IV administration sets.

3. What signs should you look for while monitoring the patient on an IV? What should you do if any of these signs appears?

4. How do you check the flow rate of an IV? What would cause blood to "backflow" into the tubing?

5. The physician orders an IV at 2000 ml to be delivered over 10 hours. The administration set being used delivers 15 gtts/cc. Calculate the drops/minute to be given.

ADVANCED AIRWAY MANAGEMENT

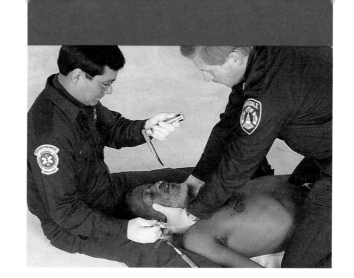

complication A difficult factor appearing unexpectedly.

contraindication A condition that renders a medical procedure, treatment, or medication undesirable.

endotracheal intubation (en"do-tra'ke-al in"tu-ba'shun) A method of intubation in which a tube is placed through a patient's mouth or nose and directly through the larynx between the vocal cords into the trachea for the purpose of opening and maintaining an airway.

esophageal gastric tube airway (EGTA) (ĕ-sof"ah-je'al gas'trik tūb ār'wa) An esophageal obturator airway with an added gastric decompression tube; it allows gas in the stomach to be vented to the outside, thereby decreasing gastric distension.

esophageal obturator airway (EOA) (ĕ-sof"ah-je'al ob'too-ra"tor ār'wa) A plastic, semi-rigid tube that can be inserted in the esophagus. The upper one-third, which has holes in it, lies at the level of the pharynx and provides free passage of oxygen-enriched air to the lungs.

intubation (in"tu-ba'shun) The placement of a tube in the airway to improve ventilation.

laryngoscope (lah-ring'go-skōp) An instrument used to give a direct view of the patient's vocal cords during endotracheal intubation.

Pharyngeotracheal Lumen Airway An airway management device designed to ventilate the lungs when placed in either the trachea or the esophagus.

stylet (sti'let) A plastic-coated wire that, when inserted into the endotracheal tube, adds rigidity to the tube.

vallecula (vah-lek'u-lah) The space between the base of the tongue and the epiglottis.

Advanced airway management means placing a tube into the airway to maintain an open airway, to prevent aspiration of foreign bodies and stomach contents, and to ensure an open channel for the delivery of oxygen-enriched air. Three types of devices are used in advanced airway management to achieve these objectives: the endotracheal tube, the esophageal obturator airway, and pharyngeotracheal airways. These devices require varying degrees of skill and instruction for proper insertion and use. Once you develop these skills, each device can be used to maintain and protect the patient's airway and provide effective ventilation.

Local ordinances and laws determine the level of EMT who may be authorized to use these advanced airways. Use of any of these devices requires consent of a medical director and adherence to written protocols.

Supplement B begins with a reminder of the importance of primary patient assessment and the need to establish and maintain an adequate airway. Then the chapter describes the three methods of advanced airway management and the contraindications and possible complications of each technique. A brief mention of end tidal carbon dioxide detection is included.

GOALS

The goals of Supplement B are to
- understand the importance of patient assessment.
- know how to perform advanced airway management using endotracheal intubation.
- know how to perform advanced airway management using an esophageal obturator airway.
- know how to perform advanced airway management using a pharyngeotracheal airway.

PATIENT ASSESSMENT

As always, the highest priority in the primary assessment of a patient must be the airway, breathing, and circulation. This rule applies to every patient. The obviously broken leg or amputated finger may be eye-catching, but the blocked airway must be cleared immediately or the patient will die. Always, you must first think A (airway), B (breathing), C (circulation). If a major problem is found in any of these areas during the primary survey, you must correct it immediately.

The most important skill you will employ is the ability to establish and maintain a clear airway. Most conscious patients are able to maintain an adequate airway. As long as the gag reflex is present, most patients can clear their own airway. Thus, in the management of the conscious patient, you may need only to provide oxygen and monitor the patient closely for any change. Semiconscious patients may require an oral or nasal airway and airway suctioning. However, those patients who cannot ventilate adequately, and those for whom the simpler, noninvasive airway management techniques described in Chapter 7 and 10 are found to be ineffective, will fare better with the advanced airway techniques described in this supplement.

ENDOTRACHEAL INTUBATION
· ·

The standard practice of advanced airway man agement is **endotracheal intubation**—the placement of a tube into the lower airway to protect and improve ventilation. Endotracheal intubation is a method of **intubation** in which an endotracheal tube (ETT) is placed through a patient's mouth or nose and directly through the larynx between the vocal cords into the trachea (Figure B–1). A **laryngoscope** is usually used to view the vocal cords as the tube passes through (Figure B–2), or the tube may be placed blindly through the cords using the sounds of labored respirations as a guide, or placed by feel through the vocal cords. After placement, a soft balloon cuff near the end of the tube is then inflated with 5 to 10 cc of air to seal the trachea and anchor the tube, so that air can be blown directly into the lungs.

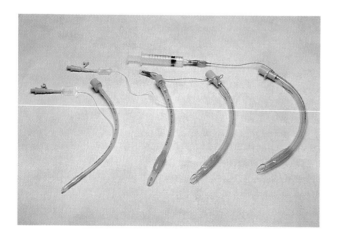

FIGURE B–1

Endotracheal tubes are available in several sizes. The inflatable balloon seals the airway when the tube is properly positioned.

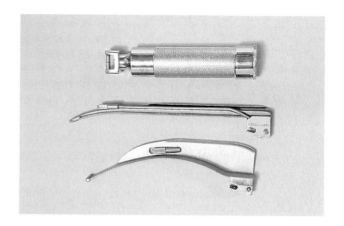

FIGURE B–2

Use a laryngoscope to insert the endotracheal tube. The detachable laryngoscope blades are straight or curved.

The advantages of endotracheal intubation are worth considering. The ETT completely controls and protects the airway and can be left in place for a long time if necessary. It prevents aspiration and gastric distension. It facilitates airway suctioning. The ETT enables the delivery of high volumes of oxygen at higher than normal pressures. Certain medications may be given down the tube. The ETT may also be placed around an esophageal obturator airway.

Endotracheal intubation is a difficult skill to master; it requires considerable practice and expert initial instruction. Direct visualization of the vocal cords is an important skill and observing the ETT passing through them ensures proper tube placement and minimizes laryngeal and tracheal damage. Esophageal intubation frequently occurs and must be immediately recognized and corrected. If intubation takes too long, the resulting delay in oxygenation may lead to brain damage. The maximum interruption of CPR ventilation should be no more than 30 seconds. Constant monitoring of lung sounds is needed to ensure that the tube stays in place and does not move during transfers and patient manipulations.

The endotracheal tube is available in many sizes from 2.5 mm to 9 mm inside diameter; a complete selection of tube sizes must be carried. Most adult males will need a 7.5 or 8 mm diameter tube, whereas most adult females will accept a 7 or 7.5 mm diameter tube. Thus 7.5 mm is a good emergency tube to use for all adults. For children, a rough guide for the appropriately sized tube is to select one equal in size to the diameter of the patient's little finger across the nailbed (Figure B–3). After selecting a tube of proper size, use a syringe to inflate the balloon to test for air leaks (Figure B–4). Pediatric ET tubes for children under 5 years of age (under 5 mm) do not have balloon cuffs. After testing, the balloon should be completely deflated, and the syringe left attached to the tube and filled with 10 cc of air.

A plastic-coated wire **stylet** (Figure B–5) may be inserted into the ETT. The stylet will give added rigidity to the tube, and it can be bent to maintain the desired curvature of the endotracheal tube during insertion. The tip of the stylet should be bent to form a gentle curve. It must not protrude from the end of the tube, because

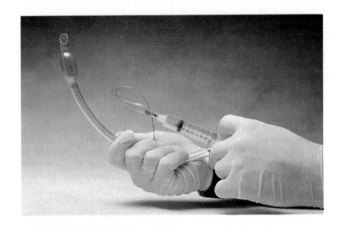

FIGURE B–4

Prior to placement, test the balloon of the ETT for air leaks.

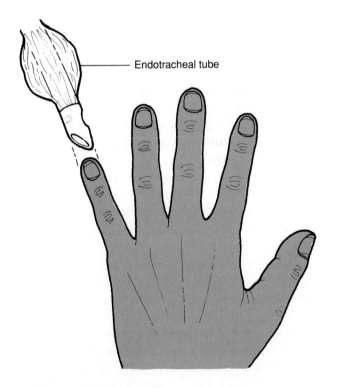

Endotracheal tube

FIGURE B–3

Use the diameter of the patient's little finger at the nailbed as a rough guide to ETT size selection for a child.

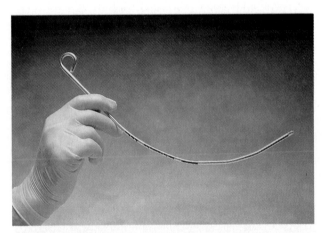

FIGURE B–5

Use a plastic-coated wire stylet to hold the best shape of the flexible ETT during intubation. The tip of the stylet should be bent and must never protrude from the end of the tube.

it could puncture or lacerate delicate airway tissues.

The laryngoscope is used to give you a direct view of the patient's vocal cords. The blade of the laryngoscope is detachable from the handle. Multiple blade sizes are available, all either curved or straight. Adequate lighting is essential for intubation. For this purpose, there is a light bulb near the tip of the blade. The light is activated by lifting the blade away from the handle until it locks at a right angle (Figure B–6). The light will not come on if the blade is not attached properly, if it is burned out, if it is loose, or if the batteries in the handle are dead. You must check your equipment daily to be certain that the light is working, especially before you try to intubate the patient.

Inserting the ETT

Use the following steps to insert an endotracheal tube:

1. Assemble equipment: proper ET tube, laryngoscope, syringe, stylet, suction apparatus, Magill forceps, suction tubes and tonsil sucker, lubricating gel, gloves, eye protection.
2. Check equipment: light, balloon cuff, syringe, suction apparatus, lubricate tube.
3. Hyperventilate the patient.
4. Position the patient's head and neck (hyperextended).
5. Clear the mouth of dentures, vomitus, or blood (use Magill forceps for objects).

6. Open the airway.
7. Gently position the laryngoscope.
8. Moving the mandible and tongue, expose the vocal cords (*Sellick's Maneuver*).
9. Slip the tubes through the cords.
10. Remove the laryngoscope and hold the tube.
11. Remove the stylet and hold the tube.
12. Inflate the cuff and ventilate the patient.
13. Check breath sounds; look for chest to rise.
14. Place the oral airway.
15. Secure the tube.
16. Continually monitor the tube and patient.
17. Suction as required (never for more than 10 seconds).

Once the equipment is ready, the patient should be positioned properly. To simplify intubation, the three parts of the airway (the mouth, pharynx, and trachea) should be positioned in a straight line. First, flex the neck on the chest to align the pharynx and trachea (Figure B–7a). Then extend the head on the neck, lining up the mouth and pharynx (Figure B–7b). These maneuvers cannot be used without special considerations if the patient is a trauma victim. Methods used for the trauma patient will be covered later.

Once you have aligned the airway, clear the mouth of any loose or obstructing materials. Remove dentures or partial plates. Use suction to remove vomitus, blood clots, or other material present in the upper airway. Special forceps, called Magill forceps, can be used to grasp objects obstructing the airway.

Just prior to intubation, the patient must be well oxygenated. Hyperventilate the patient for 2 to 3 minutes using the mouth-to-mask technique or preferably a bag-valve-mask with 100 percent supplemental oxygen at a rate of 20 to 30 breaths per minute. Next, grasp the laryngoscope handle in your left hand. Open the patient's mouth with the gloved fingers of your right hand by placing the right thumb on the lower first molar and hooking the index finger behind the thumb exerting force just behind the upper first molar. Place this blade in the right side of the patient's mouth, then move it to the center, gently pushing the tongue to the left. The final position of the blade will vary,

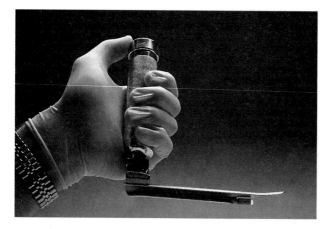

FIGURE B–6

Activate the light at the end of the laryngoscope blade by locking the blade at a right angle to the handle.

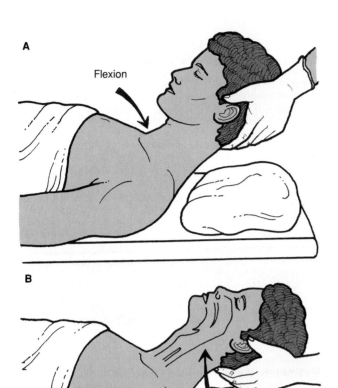

A

Flexion

B

Extension

FIGURE B–7

To facilitate placement of the endotracheal tube, align the pharynx with the trachea by (A) first flexing the neck on the chest and then (B) extending the head on the neck.

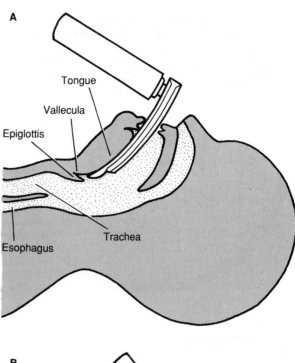

A

Tongue
Vallecula
Epiglottis
Esophagus
Trachea

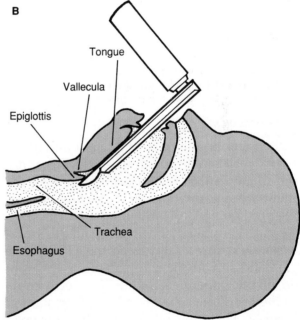

B

Tongue
Vallecula
Epiglottis
Esophagus
Trachea

FIGURE B–8

To visualize the vocal cords, (A) advance a curved blade along the base of the tongue until its tip rests at the vallecula; (B) advance a straight blade slightly farther to lift the epiglottis forward.

depending on whether it is curved or straight. A curved blade is advanced along the base of the tongue until its tip rests at the **vallecula**—the space between the base of the tongue and the epiglottis (Figure B–8a). A straight blade is advanced slightly farther, catching and pulling the epiglottis itself anteriorly (Figure B–8b). The laryngoscope must be lifted away from the posterior pharynx enough so the vocal cords can be visualized. The lifting force is directed straight up, parallel to the long axis of the laryngoscope handle. Neither type of blade is used as a lever against the upper teeth. This maneuver will break teeth and will not facilitate visualization of the vocal cords (Figure B–9).

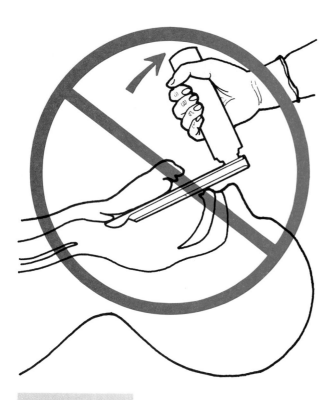

FIGURE B–9

The laryngoscope should never be pried or levered against the upper teeth. Achieve visualization of the vocal cords only by lifting the tongue forward.

Whenever possible, cricoid pressure should be applied by a second rescuer during endotracheal intubation. This further protects the patient from aspiration of stomach contents. Pressure should be maintained until the ETT tube cuff is inflated. With the patient's vocal cords now in direct view, hold the ETT in your right hand and advance the tube from the right side of the patient's mouth. The vocal cords and the tip of the tube must be kept in sight at all times. The tube should not be advanced down the center of the laryngoscope blade, because you will not be able to see its tip. The tip of the ETT must be observed as it passes through the vocal cords. Also, watch the uninflated balloon as it passes through the vocal cords. Then advance the ETT 1 inch beyond the upper edge of the balloon (Figure B–10). This should place the tip halfway between the *carina* and the vocal cords. Once the tube has been placed through the vocal cords into the trachea, remove the stylet.

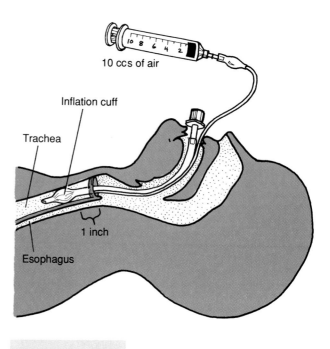

10 ccs of air

Inflation cuff

Trachea

1 inch

Esophagus

FIGURE B–10

When properly positioned, the upper edge of the balloon should lie approximately 1 inch below the level of the vocal cords.

Following the ETT placement, check for proper tube position by listening with a stethoscope over both lungs and the stomach while you ventilate the patient through the tube. Audible breath sounds should be heard over both right and left lung fields, in the axillae, and not in the stomach. The chest should rise symmetrically. If good breath sounds cannot be heard on both sides, the ETT should be pulled back approximately 1 inch and the position checked again by listening for bilateral breath sounds. Following the ETT placement verification, using the syringe, inflate the balloon with 5 to 10 cc of air—just enough to block the passage of air around the tube. The syringe must then be detached or the air in the balloon will empty back into it. After you inflate the balloon, recheck both lungs for breath sounds.

Even with the balloon inflated, the endotracheal tube can migrate in the trachea. Therefore, you must secure the ETT in the proper position. You should never let go of the tube until it has been secured in place with tape. Adhesive tape can be used to secure the tube to the patient's mouth or a 30-inch length of umbilical tape can be wrapped around the tube and then around the patient's head to maintain its proper position. Commercial products made of a plastic bite block and Velcro fasteners are also available to facilitate securing the ETT tube to the patient.

Once the properly placed ETT is secured, an oropharyngeal airway or a bite block should be placed between the patient's teeth to prevent the patient from biting on the tube (Figure B–11).

The placement of an endotracheal tube should be accomplished quickly and efficiently. No more than 30 seconds should be required to place the ETT in the proper position. If the ETT is not properly placed by then, it should be removed and positive pressure hyperventilation given for approximately 2 to 3 minutes before a second intubation attempt is made.

The most frequent error made during endotracheal intubation is to advance the tube too far, placing it in the right mainstem bronchus where it will ventilate only the right lung. Definitely audible breath sounds must be heard on both sides of the chest to confirm proper tube placement. If breath sounds are heard only on the right, the balloon should be deflated, the tube withdrawn about 1 inch, the

balloon reinflated, and both lungs rechecked for breath sounds.

The other common error occurs when intubation is forced without adequate visualization of the vocal cords. In this situation, the ETT usually ends up in the esophagus. In every patient, you must see the vocal cords and must watch the tip of the tube as it passes between them. A second EMT can make it easier to see the vocal cords by pushing on the cricoid cartilage using the Sellick's maneuver (Figure B–12). Although it may help to bring the vocal cords into view, this maneuver also may cause the patient to gag and vomit. As long as firm pressure is maintained on the cricoid cartilage, the esophagus will be blocked, thereby preventing regurgitation of food into the airway. Therefore, once pressure is applied to the cricoid cartilage, it must be maintained until the ETT is properly placed and the balloon is inflated.

Infrequently, the patient will regain a gag reflex or regain consciousness and not be able to tolerate the ETT. Field removal is not indicated unless the tube has moved to the esophagus or the patient will no longer permit the tube to remain in place. Before extubating the patient in these circumstances, suction should

FIGURE B–11

Once proper position of the ETT is assured, tape it in place. Insert an oropharyngeal airway to prevent biting of the ETT.

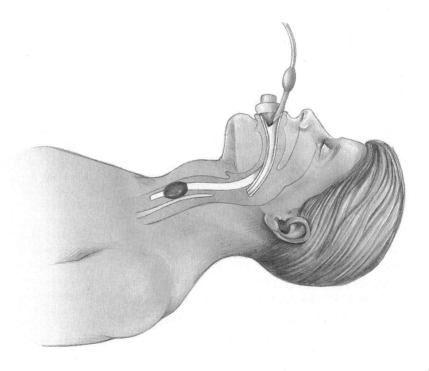

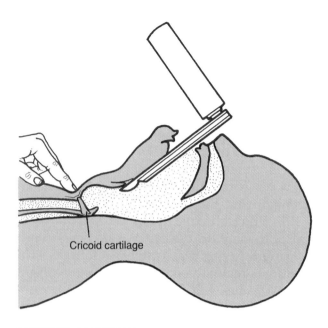

FIGURE B–12

Applying pressure on the cricoid cartilage will improve visualization of the vocal cords and block the esophagus.

be functioning and very close at hand. The recommended procedure is then to deflate the cuff and withdraw the tube as the patient inhales. Immediately suction if any vomiting occurs, assess the airway, and administer supplemental oxygen.

Cervical Trauma and Endotracheal Intubation

The endotracheal tube provides the best means of ventilation for the unconscious patient. Airway and breathing still have the highest priority. However, you must avoid further injury to a patient who may have a spinal injury. The patient in cardiac arrest that is not due to trauma should be intubated in the standard fashion just described, using laryngoscope, neck flexion, and head extension. The patient who is unconscious because of injury presents a more difficult situation. In such a patient, an alternative means of controlling the airway (the trauma chin-lift or trauma jaw-thrust maneuver, oropharyngeal airway, and bag-valve-mask) will usually suffice.

However, if you must intubate the unconscious trauma patient, a second EMT should kneel straddling the patient and hold the patient's head in a neutral in-line position during the intubation (Figure B–13). A third rescuer can improve visualization of the vocal cords by performing a Sellick's maneuver in the fashion described earlier. The major difficulty in the patient with a possible neck injury is lifting the mandible and tongue sufficiently to visualize the cords while maintaining vertebral alignment in a neutral position. For injured patients, some local medical directors may recommend the blind orotracheal technique of feeling the cords and then passing the ETT through the vocal cords by feel.

Complications of Endotracheal Intubation

As mentioned earlier, pushing the ETT too far through the vocal cords is the most common **complication** of its use. This causes the tube to pass into the right mainstem bronchus. In this position it will ventilate only the right lung.

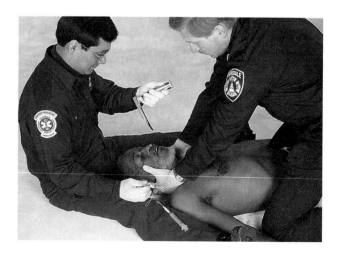

FIGURE B–13

If you suspect spinal injury, modify the endotracheal intubation technique. One EMT must straddle the patient and hold the neck in a neutral position. The Sellick's maneuver will improve the chances of successful intubation.

Even when placed properly, the ETT will migrate if not secured. You must never let go of the tube until it is adequately taped in place. Even then, the tube placement must be monitored continuously.

A second complication occurs when the endotracheal tube is placed without seeing the vocal cords. Usually, the ETT goes into the esophagus. In this position it will rapidly inflate the stomach and will not ventilate the lungs at all. Therefore, it is essential to watch the ETT as it passes through the vocal cords and check breath sounds in four locations as well as observing the rise and fall of the chest during the assisted ventilatory cycle.

A third complication of using the ETT is aggravation of a spinal injury. Whenever there is concern about a neck injury, you must intubate without moving the patient's neck from the neutral in-line position.

A fourth complication occurs when *too* much time is spent placing the tube. You should never spend more than 30 seconds trying to intubate. If it takes longer than this, you should stop and ventilate the patient with 100 percent oxygen for at least 2 to 3 minutes before trying again. If after two tries at intubation the tube cannot be passed, then an alternative ventilation technique should be used or another qualified rescuer should try.

Finally, the laryngoscope and the tip of the ETT can injure the airway and teeth. If the laryngoscope blade is used as a lever, teeth can be broken easily. If the tube is blindly pushed forward without watching the vocal cords, it can lacerate the pharynx. The advantages and disadvantages of endotracheal intubation are listed in Table B–1.

Carbon Dioxide Detection for Proper ETT Placement

The FEF® end tidal carbon dioxide detector is a plastic disposable indicator that helps you to verify proper placement of an ETT in the trachea simply by color change (Figure B–14). The color may vary with expiration and inspiration as the CO_2 levels rise and fall in the airway. The device is placed over the end of the

TABLE B–1	Endotracheal Intubation
Advantages	**Disadvantages**
Definitive airway	If placed in esophagus and not recognized, the patient gets no air
Easy to ventilate	
Prevents aspiration	
Can be left in for long time	Neck manipulation in patient with possible neck injury
Easy to maintain good seal	
Some cardiac medications can be administered through ETT	Requires frequent practice to maintain skill
Can suction lungs through ETT	

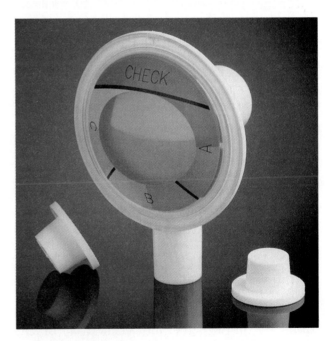

FIGURE B–14

The end tidal carbon dioxide detector.

ETT where the inspiratory and expiratory gases can pass through it. The chemically treated paper changes from purple to yellow in the presence of CO_2. If the ETT is properly placed in the trachea, and if carbon dioxide is being produced by bodily metabolism during CPR, then the device will indicate proper placement. Several studies are ongoing to determine the role of this device in demonstrating proper ETT placement. Consult your local medical director for more information on this potentially useful device.

THE ESOPHAGEAL OBTURATOR AIRWAY (EOA) AND THE ESOPHAGEAL GASTRIC TUBE AIRWAY (EGTA)

Advanced airway management can also be achieved by using an **esophageal obturator airway (EOA)** or its more modern form, the **esophageal gastric tube airway (EGTA).** The EOA has been used since 1973 to facilitate airway management in cardiopulmonary resuscitation. There is no doubt that a properly placed endotracheal tube provides the most effective possible delivery of oxygen to the lungs, but some studies have shown that the EOA, when properly used, may be as effective as endotracheal intubation in the short term when combined with the use of demand valve oxygen. Less practice and skill are required to insert the EOA, because you do not have to use a laryngoscope to visualize the vocal cords during intubation.

The EOA airway is a plastic, semirigid tube 34 cm long and 13 mm in diameter (Figure B–15). The lower end is smooth, rounded, and closed. The EGTA's esophageal tube differs because it has a valve designed to permit a tube to be passed through it and into the stomach to allow decompression and suctioning of the stomach (Figure B–16). The upper one-third of both is designed to function as an airway; it has 16 holes in its wall at the junction of the middle and upper thirds. When properly placed, these holes will lie at the level of the pharynx and provide free passage of oxygen-enriched air to the lungs. The lower two-thirds of the EOA or the EGTA should lie in the esophagus. The balloon surrounding the end of the tube is normally inflated to block the esophagus and

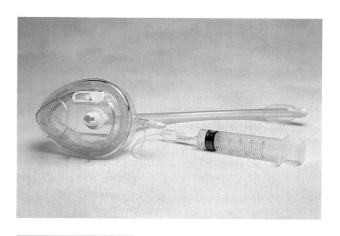

FIGURE B–15

The assembled esophageal obturator airway.

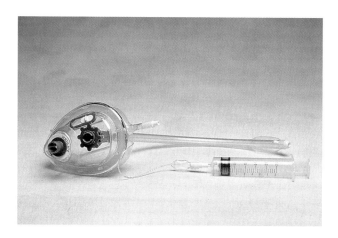

FIGURE B–16

An esophageal gastric tube airway. The gastric decompression tube allows the stomach to be vented of excessive air.

prevent the regurgitation of stomach contents into the airway.

The face mask that comes with the EOA or EGTA is designed to fit snugly about the patient's nose and mouth and must provide a tight seal. Oxygen-enriched air given through the 15-mm standard opening in the tube passes to the face mask and then passes through the upper portion of the airway and into the lungs through the side holes in the esophageal tube, because the esophagus is blocked by the inflated balloon and the obturator (Figure B–17). The oxygen inlet port for the EGTA is in the face mask, not the esophageal tube. This arrangement is believed to supply a greater volume flow of oxygen to the lungs than the EOA.

Inserting the EOA or EGTA

Use the following steps to insert an EOA or EGTA:

1. Assemble equipment:

   - EGTA or EOA
   - 30 cc syringe
   - Water soluble lubricant
   - Suction equipment
   - Oral airway
   - Oxygen delivery device
   - Gloves
   - Goggles

2. Check equipment.

3. Snap tube into lock at mask-tube connection.
4. Lubricate esophageal tube.
5. Position head, flexed slightly forward (except in a trauma patient where neutral in-line position must be maintained).
6. Hyperventilate the patient with 100 percent oxygen.
7. Open and clear the mouth.
8. Gently guide esophageal tube into place.
9. Inflate obturator balloon.
10. Place oropharyngeal airway.
11. Seal mask to face.
12. Ventilate the patient.
13. Check the chest for breath sounds.
14. Use oxygen-powered breathing device.
15. Maintain effective mask-face seal.

Always check first for proper function of the EOA/EGTA prior to insertion. Inflate the face mask with 20 to 30 cc of air. Then attach the 30-cc syringe filled with air to the valve supplying the obturator's balloon cuff. Inflate the balloon cuff with 20 cc of air and check for leaks. Then deflate the balloon and leave the syringe attached. Next, attach the mask to the

FIGURE B–17

When properly placed, the EOA will allow oxygen-enriched air to pass only from the side holes into the trachea.

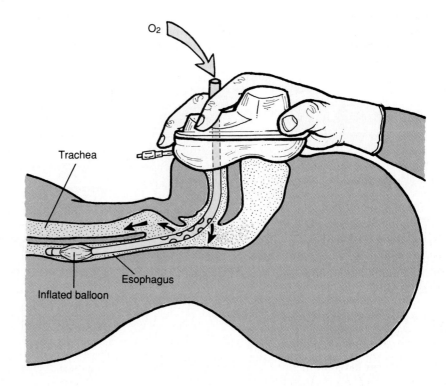

O₂

Trachea

Esophagus

Inflated balloon

tube. It is designed to lock into proper position with a definite snap. Lubricate the lower two-thirds of the tube well with a water-soluble gel. Before the EOA or EGTA is inserted, you must hyperventilate the patient for 2 to 3 minutes with a bag-valve-mask or pocket mask device with 100 percent oxygen.

The tube is designed to be placed with the head slightly flexed or in a neutral position. Flexion of the head on the trunk will decrease the risk of inserting the tube incorrectly into the larynx and trachea because it brings the opening of the esophagus into a more exposed position. In a patient who is not suspected of having sustained a neck injury, the head should be flexed slightly forward. In the unconscious trauma patient, the head must be secured in an in-line neutral position by one EMT while a second EMT opens the patient's airway and performs the EOA/EGTA insertion.

Open the patient's airway and prepare for intubation by grasping the tongue and mandible between your gloved thumb and index finger and lifting them forward with the left hand (Figure B–18). Grasp the EOA with the

mask attached with your right hand and insert it along the tongue and against the posterior wall of the pharynx in the midline (Figure B–19a). You do not have to use great force to insert the EOA/EGTA. Only light to moderate pressure is needed. The EOA/EGTA is inserted until the mask makes good contact with the face and the bite block lies at the level of the incisor teeth (Figure B–19b).

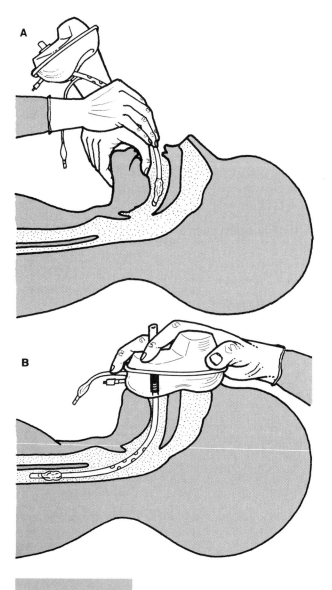

FIGURE B–18

With the head flexed on the trunk, grasp the mandible and lift forward in preparation for EOA insertion.

FIGURE B–19

(A) The EOA is inserted along the tongue (B) until the face mask makes good contact with the face. Only moderate pressure should be required to insert the EOA.

Using both hands, hold the face mask firmly against the face and check the EOA/EGTA for proper placement. Give mouth-to-mask or bag-valve-mask ventilation, while a second EMT listens for breath sounds over both lung fields with a stethoscope. If the EOA/EGTA is in the esophagus, breath sounds should be heard over both lung fields. If it has been placed in the trachea, no breath sounds will be heard. If it has been placed in the right mainstem bronchus, breath sounds will be heard only on the *left* side. If there is uncertainty about its position, remove the EOA/EGTA and ventilate the patient before you make another attempt to place the EOA/EGTA properly. If good breath sounds are heard over both lung fields, inflate the esophageal balloon with 20 to 30 cc of air and remove the syringe to keep the balloon inflated (Figure B–20).

With the tube in proper position, the mask still must be held firmly against the patient's face. Stay at the head of the patient and use the index finger and thumb to hold the mask to the face and the other three fingers to hold the mandible against the mask. If there is no concern about neck injury, you can extend the head to further open the airway. Then attach the opening in the face mask to a manual oxygen-powered positive pressure device for ventilation. This device provides the necessary volume and pressure of oxygen for effective ventilation with an EOA/EGTA. These levels cannot be achieved with a bag-valve-mask system.

Removing the EOA/EGTA

The EOA/EGTA is used only for short-term airway management. It should be removed only when the unconscious patient awakens and is able to protect the airway or when endotracheal intubation has been performed over the EOA/EGTA. There is a very high risk of vomiting and/or regurgitation of gastric contents when the balloon is deflated and the EOA/EGTA is removed. Therefore, the conscious patient should be turned onto his or her side and suction should be available prior to removal unless an ETT has been placed and properly inflated. Once ready, the EOA/EGTA is easily removed by fully deflating the balloon and sliding it out.

If long-term airway management is required in the hospital, the EOA/EGTA should be replaced by an endotracheal tube. In this circumstance, the EOA/EGTA must be left in place until the ETT is securely and properly placed.

Contraindications to the Use of an EOA/EGTA

Under the following circumstances, the EOA/EGTA is **contraindicated** (should not be used):

- On patients who are awake. EOA/EGTA placement will cause vomiting and aspiration of vomitus. The EOA/EGTA should be used only in deeply unconscious patients, usually after an ETT has failed.
- On small children. The EOA/EGTA should not be used for children under 16 years of age. Because there is only one size of EOA/EGTA, it is too large for children and it does not work effectively.
- On patients with known esophageal disease.

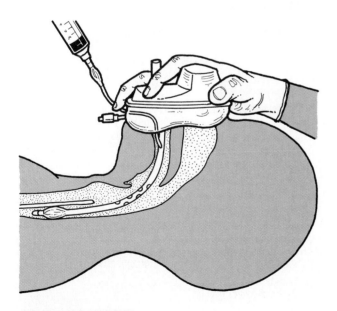

FIGURE B–20

Once properly placed, the esophageal obturator balloon is inflated with 20 cc of air, and a secure fit of the face mask is maintained manually.

The EOA/EGTA may cause serious problems for a patient with esophageal cancer or esophageal varices. If a patient has swallowed a caustic agent such as lye, the EOA/EGTA may perforate the injured esophagus.

■ On patients with significant upper airway bleeding. Blood from the nose or mouth will pass directly into the lungs once the esophageal balloon is inflated. If the patient accumulates some blood, mucus, or saliva in the upper airway once an EOA/EGTA is in place, it must be cleared by suctioning under the transparent mask.

Complications of Using the EOA/EGTA

The most common complication of using the EOA/EGTA is accidental placement into the trachea rather than the esophagus. Once the EOA/EGTA is placed, you must listen carefully for breath sounds with the stethoscope over both the right and left chest. Improper position of the EOA/EGTA is confirmed by the absence of breath sounds on one (usually the right) or both sides. In this instance, you must remove and replace the tube promptly. Tracheal intubation is more likely to occur if the head is extended on the neck. The head should be flexed or held in a neutral in-line position when you insert the EOA/EGTA. An excessive curvature to the EOA/EGTA will also increase the likelihood of entering the trachea. Excessive curving of the tube results from storing the EOA/EGTA in too small a plastic bag, where it stays bent for some time prior to use; it can also become kinked. The EOA/EGTA should always be stored in its original packaging to prevent this problem.

Esophageal rupture or tear can also result from the use of this device. The EOA/EGTA should never be inserted roughly or with excessive force. Although the balloon will hold up to 35 cc of air, 20 to 30 cc is usually sufficient to block the esophagus, and this smaller volume of air is less likely to injure the esophagus. Furthermore, the EOA/EGTA should not be stored in a cold ambulance or kept in a cold environment, as it will become stiff and be more likely to injure the esophagus when inserted.

The third complication is inadequate ventilation, despite proper placement of the airway. A major cause of this problem is persistent leakage of air around the face mask. A firm seal of the mask against the face must be maintained at all times during the use of the EOA/EGTA. It has an inflatable, balloon-like seal around the edge of the mask to provide a leakproof contact to the contours of the face. This balloon should contain just enough air to allow the finger, when pressed against it, to make contact with the edge of the underlying plastic mask. Another cause of inadequate ventilation is the delivery of an inadequate volume of air to the airway using a bag-valve-mask delivery system. The proper delivery system is an oxygen-powered positive pressure device.

The advantages and disadvantages of the EOA/EGTA are listed in Table B–2.

TABLE B–2 EOA/EGTA Airway	
Advantages	**Disadvantages**
Rapid, blind insertion	Requires good mask seal
Can be placed with minimal neck movement	Requires frequent practice
Can be used in all types of arrests	Blood and vomitus may be forced into lungs
Prevents gastric distension	Patients do *not* tolerate it well
Prevents gastric regurgitation	Laceration of esophagus
Permits easy ETT placement over it	

PHARYNGEOTRACHEAL AIRWAYS

Pharyngeotracheal airways have been designed to provide lung ventilation when placed either in the trachea or the esophagus. Several such devices are available. The **Pharyngeotracheal Lumen Airway** (PtL®) will be described here. It consists of two tubes, two balloon cuffs, a bite block, and a neck retaining strap (Figure B–21). The long, clear #3 tube contains a stylet and a low pressure balloon cuff near its tip. This #3 tube is left plugged by the stylet if it is placed in the esophagus, and the stylet is removed if the tube winds up in the trachea. In both cases, the balloon cuff prevents gastric contents from entering the lungs when it is inflated. This #3 tube passes through the larger diameter green #2 tube. This tube has a large balloon cuff designed to seal off the oropharynx not only to allow ventilation gas to pass through it into the trachea (should the #3 tube be placed in the esophagus), but also to prevent blood and debris from entering the airway from above. This balloon cuff essentially functions as the mask seal. The #1 tube is connected to the balloon cuffs to facilitate simultaneous inflation of these important airway seals.

This device is designed to be inserted blindly into the oropharynx and esophagus by those who have received training and are authorized to use it. The PtL airway is similar to the EGTA except it is designed to function like an ET tube if, when it is blindly inserted, it happens to go into the trachea (Figure B–22), or like an EGTA if its long tube goes into the esophagus (Figure B–23). However, in the latter case, maintaining a constant face mask seal is not necessary, because it forms an inflated cuff seal in the oropharynx and the trachea may be ventilated via a tube rather than a mask.

Inserting the Pharyngeotracheal Lumen Airway

The steps involved in the insertion of the PtL airway are listed here. The basic concept is to intubate the patient blindly and inflate the balloon cuffs. Then ventilation is attempted via the green (#2) tube. If no breath sounds are

The Pharyngeotracheal Airway consists of two tubes, two balloon cuffs, a bite block, and a neck retaining strap.

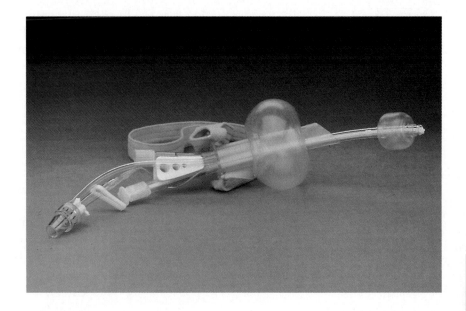

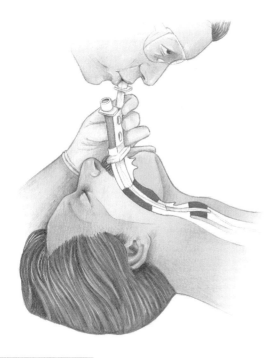

When the PtL airway is placed in the trachea, it can function as an endotracheal tube.

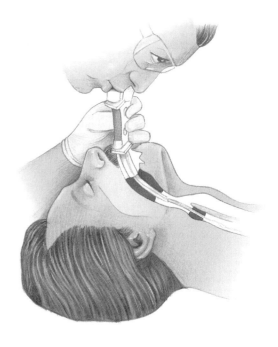

When the PtL airway is placed in the esophagus, it can function as an esophageal obturator airway. A constant face mask seal is not necessary because the inflated cuff seals the oropharynx.

heard, the #3 tube should be used as an ETT to ventilate the patient.

Begin the procedure by preparing and checking the materials while the patient is being hyperventilated with 100 percent oxygen. Lubricate the long clear #3 tube with a water soluble lubricant.

Inserting a PtL

Use the following steps to insert a PtL:

1. Assemble the equipment.

  - PtL
  - Water soluble lubricant
  - Suction equipment
  - Oxygen delivery device
  - Gloves
  - Goggles

2. Check all equipment.
3. Lubricate PtL #3 long tube.
4. Position head, in extension (except for trauma patient where neutral in-line position must be maintained).
5. Hyperventilate the patient with 100 percent oxygen.
6. Open and clear the mouth.
7. Lift the mandible and tongue away from the posterior pharynx.
8. Gently guide the PtL along the base of the tongue and into the airway until the teeth are against the teeth strap.
9. Inflate balloon cuffs with tube #1 (be sure to close the white cap).
10. Attempt to ventilate (mouth to tube) the patient through the short, green #2 tube.
11. Check the patient's chest for breath sounds.

12. If #3 is not in trachea, ventilate patient using #2.
13. If #3 is in trachea, remove stylet and ventilate with tube #3.
14. Check the patient's chest for breath sounds.
15. Ventilate with oxygen using the demand valve.
16. If ventilating via tube #2, consider ETT with tube #3 occluding the esophagus during the procedure.

First, open the patient's mouth and clear it of foreign objects, including vomitus, dentures, and blood clots. If the patient is not a trauma patient, open the airway via hyperextension. For a trauma patient, a second rescuer must maintain the neck in a neutral in-line position while the intubation proceeds. Insert your thumb deep into the patient's mouth, grasping the tongue and lower jaw between your thumb and index finger and lift them directly away from the posterior pharynx.

Hold the PtL so that it curves in the same direction as the natural curvature of the pharynx. Insert the tip into the mouth and advance it carefully along the tongue until the teeth strap touches the patient's teeth. The PtL should not be forced; if resistance is met, pull back and redirect it. When the PtL is at the proper depth, place the neck strap over the patient's head and tighten it with the Velcro closures on both sides.

Immediately inflate both cuffs simultaneously via tube #1 with a sustained breath into the inflation valve. Then, be sure to close the white cap. Once the cuffs are inflated and the little pilot balloon is tense, immediately blow forcefully into the #2 short, green tube. Observe and listen to the chest. If the chest rises and breath sounds are heard, the long, clear #3 tube is in the esophagus and ventilation is being achieved as with an EOA. When this is the case, continue to ventilate through the #2 green tube. If the chest does not rise, and breath sounds are not heard, you can assume that the long, clear #3 tube is in the trachea. In this case, remove the stylet from the long, clear #3 tube and ventilate the patient through it. Again listen to the lungs on both sides anteriorly, and in both axillae. Also listen over the stomach to verify the position and that effective ventilation is occurring. Once you are certain, connect the PtL to an oxygen powered ventilation device. Continuously monitor the patient. Occasionally, the balloon cuffs leak. This must be watched carefully. Use inlet tube #1 to keep the balloon cuffs properly inflated. The balloon cuffs are easily torn by jagged, broken teeth, dentures, and bones; thus special care must be exercised especially in the event of facial trauma.

Removal of the PtL airway is easily accomplished. If the ventilation is via the short, green #2 tube (with the long, clear #3 tube being essentially an esophageal obturator), then the patient should either undergo endotracheal intubation (if in deep coma) over the #3 tube, or be extubated if the patient will no longer tolerate the tube. Remember, the patient will vomit when the #3 tube is removed from the esophagus. Suction must be at hand and the patient must be turned on the side to facilitate keeping the airway clear of emesis. Simply deflate the balloon cuffs and gently remove the tube.

This is a single use item and must be discarded after use. It should *not* be cleaned and reused.

Contraindications to Use of the PtL

The PtL is contraindicated in conscious or semiconscious patients with a gag reflex. It should not be used in children under the age of 14 years or adults under 5 feet tall. Of course, like the EOA/EGTA, it should not be used in patients who are known to have suffered caustic ingestion and those who have known esophageal disease.

Advantages and Disadvantages of the PtL

Table B–3 lists the advantages and disadvantages of the PtL airway.

TABLE B-3 PtL Airway	
Advantages	**Disadvantages**
Difficult to place improperly	Loses effectiveness (cuff malfunction)
No mask seal necessary	Requires deeply comatose patient
Requires minimal skill and practice to maintain	Requires constant balloon observation
Easily used in spine injury patients	Cannot be used on patients under 5 feet tall
May be inserted blindly	Requires great care in listening for breath sounds
Protects the airway from upper airway secretions	

SUMMARY

While several advanced airway devices have been discussed in this supplement, it must be emphasized that application of these techniques requires not only advanced skills, but also medical control and direction overseeing their use. The medical director is responsible for ensuring that these procedures, which involve greater risk, also are more diligently applied for proper quality assurance and risk management.

The EMT who performs advanced airway techniques is responsible for documenting the placement. This documentation must include the following information as a minimum:

- The indication for the intubation.
- The device and size used for the intubation.
- Any injury or untoward occurrence involved with the intubation.
- An explicit statement of exactly what signs were observed to demonstrate that the intubation was successfully accomplished.

With the use of any of these airway devices, the patient may regain consciousness while intubated. Such patients will invariably gag, choke, and grasp at the device in an attempt to remove it. Often this results in injury to the airway. Therefore, it is of paramount importance to restrain the patients' hands immediately. A patient with an EOA/EGTA should be turned to the side and prepared for immediate removal of the device (suction and additional help should be available). A patient with an ETT in place should be restrained while you calmly explain that a plastic tube has been inserted to help with breathing. Advise the patient that the tube prevents him or her from talking and encourage the patient to relax and not fight against the tube. American Heart Association guidelines have assigned EOA, EGTA, Combitube, and PtL as interventions that are acceptable and possibly helpful. The preferred method of airway control is the ETT.

YOU ARE THE EMT

1. What is the difference between an endotracheal tube, a pharnygeotracheal airway, and an esophageal obturator airway?
2. When should an EOA/EGTA *not be* used?
3. What must you do to prepare a patient before you insert an ETT? What should you do after it is inserted?
4. Why is an EOA or an EGTA useful only for short-term airway management?
5. What would you do if the unconscious patient regained consciousness with an EOA or an EGTA in place?

DEFIBRILLATION BY EMTs

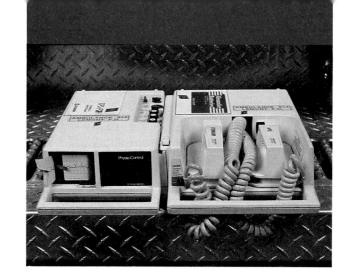

KEY TERMS

agonal rhythm (ag'o-nal rith'im) A cardiac rhythm that shows a flat line with a weak QRS complex less than once every 5 to 10 seconds; it may be observed early in asystole.

artifacts Extra or extraneous ECG signals.

asystole (ah"sis'to-le) Complete absence of heart activity.

automated external defibrillator (AED) Equipment that analyzes the electrical activity of the patient's heart and, under the right conditions, delivers an electrical charge to restore the heartbeat.

countershock The electrical charge generated and delivered by a defibrillator.

defibrillation (de-fib"rĭ-la'shun) Delivery of an electric current through a person's chest wall and heart for the purpose of ending ventricular fibrillation.

defibrillators (de-fib"rĭ-la'tors) Portable battery-powered devices that are used to record cardiac rhythm and to generate and deliver an electrical charge to patients with ventricular fibrillation.

depolarization (de-po"lar-i-za'shun) One of two electrical processes involving the heart, during which the electrical charges on the surface of the muscle cell change from positive to negative.

interference (in"ter-fēr'ens) Stray or undesirable signals on the ECG tracing.

joule (jōōl) A measure of the electrical current delivered by defibrillators.

normal sinus rhythm The coordinated pumping contractions of a healthy normal heart.

premature ventricular contraction (PVC) A type of abnormal heartbeat.

repolarization (re-po"lar-ĭ-za'shun) One of two electrical processes of the heart, during which the electrical charges on the surface of the muscle cell change from negative to positive.

ventricular fibrillation (VF) (ven-trik'u-lar fi-brĭ-la'shun) A continuous, uncoordinated quivering of the cardiac muscle.

ventricular tachycardia (VT) (ven-trik'u-lar tak"e-kar'de-ah) A very rapid heart rate.

Defibrillation can be a lifesaving measure in the treatment of sudden cardiac arrest. Great skill is needed to apply this technique, and training over and above basic EMT training is required. Once trained, you must frequently review your skills and update your knowledge in this area. An essential component of an effective prehospital defibrillation program is strict medical control with constant supervision of the performance of the EMT. In such a setting, the effectiveness of an EMS system can be expanded to provide an even more valuable service to the community.

Automated external defibrillation is described in Chapter 8 and will only be mentioned occasionally in this supplement. Supplement C first describes the role of the EMT in defibrillation. The principles of defibrillation are discussed next—how the heart's electrical system operates, how cardiac arrhythmias are detected, and how to recognize ventricular fibrillation using the electrocardiogram. Supplement C goes on to describe manual defibrillation equipment and gives a detailed explanation of how it is used. Some of the problems you may encounter during defibrillation are then presented, followed by guidelines for maintaining the defibrillation equipment. The last section talks about the requirements and local variations in defibrillator training programs.

GOALS

The goals of Supplement C are to

- understand the EMT's involvement in defibrillation programs, when the EMT should use defibrillation, and the difference between manual and automated defibrillators.
- understand the principles of defibrillation, including the heart's electrical system, cardiac arrhythmias, and the basic electrocardiogram.
- become familiar with defibrillation equipment.
- learn the steps of defibrillation.
- recognize the problems that may occur during defibrillation.
- realize the importance of maintaining defibrillation equipment.
- distinguish between the essential requirements and local variations in defibrillator programs.

DEFINITION OF TERMS

Defibrillation is the delivery of an electric current through a person's chest wall and heart for the purpose of ending a lethal cardiac arrhythmia called **ventricular fibrillation (VF).** This therapy is also used to treat another lethal cardiac arrhythmia called *pulseless* **ventricular tachycardia (VT)** which is present when the heart's ventricles are beating too fast to effec-tively circulate the blood. Portable battery-powered devices called **defibrillators** are used to record the cardiac rhythm and to generate and deliver the electrical charge (a **countershock**). An EMT-defibrillation (EMT-D) program is one in which fully trained EMTs undergo further training and are then certified to perform defibrillation on people in cardiac arrest due to ventricular fibrillation. In a *manual* EMT-defibrillation program, the EMT must learn to recognize VF when it is displayed on the screen of the monitor/defibrillator, and then to charge and deliver the electrical countershock with a manual defibrillator. In an automated defibrillation program, EMTs attach and operate **automated external defibrillators (AEDs)** that use internal computer circuitry to detect and recognize VF or pulseless ventricular tachycardia. These *automated* defibrillators then proceed to charge and deliver the countershock (fully automatic defibrillators), or they advise the EMT that a countershock is needed (semiautomatic, or shock-advisory defibrillators).

THE EMT AND DEFIBRILLATION

In the past, and still today in many programs, defibrillation is a special skill level over and above the basic EMT training. Its legal requirements are very state-specific but no requirements exist in a significant number of states since the popularization of Automated External Defibrillator programs. The following features have been found common to most successful prehospital defibrillation programs:

■ Basic certification as an EMT by those who provide this skill.
■ A medical director who assumes responsibility for all prehospital medical care.
■ Patient care protocols in the form of standing orders, developed and authorized by the medical director and accepted by the medical community.
■ A state-EMS authorized defibrillation training program that includes written and practical testing initially.
■ A continuing education program that includes regular review of theory and practical defibrillation skills.
■ Defibrillators capable of electrocardiographic recording.
■ Written reports documenting all EMT cardiac patient encounters.
■ Satisfactory performance by the EMT to the level of training and within the guidelines provided by the medical director and confirmed by medical review of every patient.

Rationale for Early Defibrillation by the EMT

The leading cause of death in this country is heart-related disease. More than 350,000 people die suddenly of cardiac arrest each year. More than three-quarters of them die outside of the hospital. Many die unexpectedly in their homes. Research in prehospital treatment for sudden death has identified several factors commonly associated with successful resuscitation and subsequent survival. Among them are the following:

■ The collapse is observed by a witness who begins CPR.
■ The 911 EMS System is accessed and activated to enable its response to the patient's side in less than 4 to 6 minutes of arrest.
■ The electrical rhythm of the patient's heart is ventricular fibrillation.
■ CPR is begun early, within 4 to 6 minutes of the collapse.
■ Defibrillation is performed within 8 minutes of the cardiac arrest.
■ Advanced life support (either from paramedics or at the hospital emergency department) is available within 20 minutes of the arrest to provide further treatment for the patient.

Equipping the EMT with a defibrillator is an extension of the proven concept that early defibrillation improves the chances that a patient will survive a cardiac arrest.

Manual Versus Automated Defibrillation by EMTs

Only one major difference exists between manual and automated defibrillation by EMTs. Manual defibrillators require that you recognize shockable and unshockable cardiac rhythms; automatic and semiautomatic (automated) defibrillators recognize shockable rhythms for you and preclude the ability to shock an unshockable rhythm. In practice, this means that for automatic and semiautomatic defibrillator programs, the content of the initial training and the continuing education review sessions are simpler and much less time-consuming. Automated external defibrillator (AED) programs are also less expensive. Clinical studies have shown that skilled EMTs are equally successful at saving lives, whether those EMTs use manual or automated defibrillators. The final choice between manual and automated defibrillators will be determined by the economic considerations and by the EMS medical director. Both automated and manual defibrillators require close case-by-case medical review of EMT field performance.

THE PRINCIPLES OF DEFIBRILLATION

The Electrical System of the Heart

A network of specialized tissue, capable of conducting electrical current, runs throughout the heart muscle. The flow of electrical current through this network causes smooth, coordinated contractions of the heart. These contractions produce the pumping action of the heart (Figure C–1).

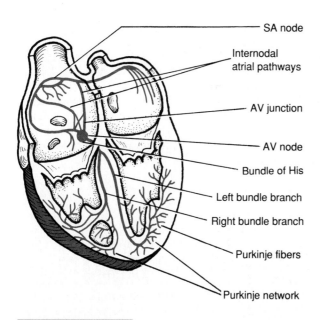

SA node

Internodal atrial pathways

AV junction

AV node

Bundle of His

Left bundle branch

Right bundle branch

Purkinje fibers

Purkinje network

FIGURE C–1

The electrical conduction system of the heart.

If part of the cardiac muscle becomes oxygen deficient, or is injured or dies, the electrical system becomes disturbed, and the heart may not continue to beat properly. The patient may not have an adequate blood pressure and thus may lose consciousness. Sometimes the injured area of the heart becomes irritable and begins to fire off uncoordinated electrical impulses. These impulses can initiate abnormal beats called **premature ventricular contractions (PVCs).** If several PVCs occur close together, they produce a rhythm called ventricular tachycardia (VT). The patient may still have a palpable pulse with ventricular tachycardia. If VT does not spontaneously convert to a normal rhythm, it rapidly degenerates into ventricular fibrillation. The heart in VT continues to beat faster until its oxygen supply is exhausted. At that point, tissue injury begins and the electrical impulses become completely uncoordinated and begin to fire off randomly. Effective pumping of the heart ceases. The heart muscle quivers ineffectively in the chest. This state is called ventricular fibrillation (VF). It is believed that 95 percent of VF is preceded by VT. The heart will continue to be in VF for several minutes until it runs out of energy and all detectable electrical activity in the heart muscle ceases. This final rhythm of complete electrical inactivity is called **asystole** (Figure C–2).

If a defibrillator can be applied to the patient and an electrical shock given to the heart during the time of ventricular fibrillation, there is a good possibility of restoring a more normal electrical activity. The countershock is believed to depolarize all of the cardiac muscle and conducting tissues instantaneously, essentially resetting the electrical energies to the depolarized state. Then, with enough energy, the patient's heart can begin its normal conduction and contractions without having to contend with randomly generated electrical impulses. If successful, the pumping action of the heart will resume, perfusion of the cardiac muscle will be restored, pumping will deliver blood at a sufficient pressure to cause the pulse to return (Figure C–3), and the patient will be resuscitated.

A Ventricular tachycardia

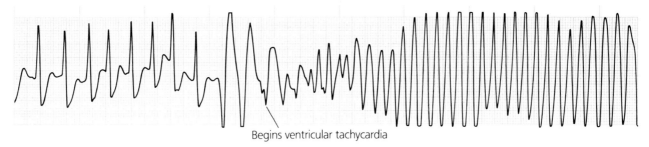

Begins ventricular tachycardia

B Ventricular fibrillation

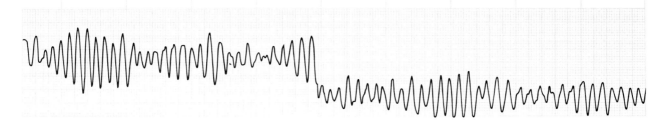

C Asystole

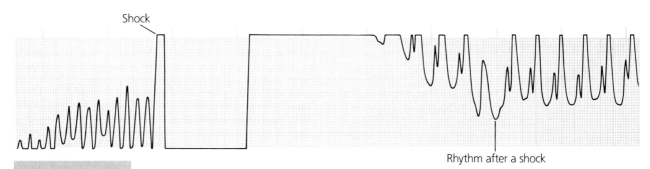

FIGURE C–2

Rhythms of the dying heart. Heart attack produces abnormal cardiac rhythms that can be analyzed on the ECG monitor. (A) Early cardiac disturbance is ventricular tachycardia. (B) Ventricular tachycardia often is followed promptly by ventricular fibrillation, a sign of ineffective cardiac function. (C) If untreated, asystole, or cardiac standstill will occur.

Shock

Rhythm after a shock

FIGURE C–3

If an electrical shock is applied to the heart during the time of ventricular fibrillation, normal electrical activity can be restored and effective cardiac contractions can resume.

Detecting Cardiac Arrhythmias

This discussion of the electrocardiogram and the visual detection of lethal cardiac rhythms are essential for programs that choose to use manual defibrillators. EMTs in programs that use automatic or semiautomatic external defibrillators may not have to learn to recognize the various lethal cardiac rhythms but should be familiar with the basic principles of the ECG.

The Electrocardiogram

An electrocardiogram (ECG or EKG) is a recording of the electrical current that flows through the heart (Figure C–4) as it is detected from the surface of the chest. Manual portable defibrillators display the electrocardiogram on a cathode ray monitor screen and should have the capability to print out the screen display on a paper strip chart.

Each mechanical contraction of the heart is associated with two electrical processes. The first is **depolarization,** during which the electrical charges on the surface of the muscle cell change from positive to negative. The second is **repolarization,** during which the heart returns to its resting state, and the positive charge is restored to the surface.

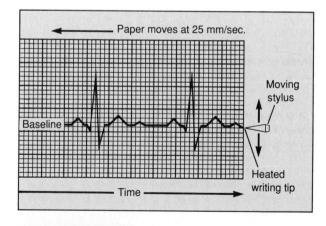

FIGURE C–4

The normal electrocardiogram recorded on a continuously moving strip of paper.

The body acts as a conductor of electrical current. Any two points on the body may be connected with electrical "leads" to record the electrical activity of the heart. The tracing produced by the electrical activity of the heart, as it depolarizes and repolarizes, forms a series of waves and complexes that are separated by regularly occurring intervals on the screen of the ECG monitor. The waves or deflections of the ECG are called the *P wave,* the *QRS complex,* and the *T wave.* Depolarization of the atria produces the P wave. Depolarization of the ventricles and repolarization of the atria produces the QRS complex; this is when the main mechanical contraction of the heart occurs. When the ventricles repolarize, the T wave is formed.

The *PR interval*—from the beginning of the P wave to the beginning of the QRS complex—records the time it takes for the heart's electrical impulse to go from the atria to the ventricles. The QRS complex, during which the ventricles are rapidly depolarized, should be narrow, no broader than 0.12 seconds, or three of the 1 mm boxes on the ECG paper strip.

When the heart is working normally, the heart's pacemaker is high in the atria at the *sinus node,* and there is a smooth flow of electricity through the heart, which depolarizes the muscle and produces a coordinated pumping contraction called **normal sinus rhythm.** The electrocardiogram of normal sinus rhythm looks like the drawing in Figure C–5.

Visual Recognition of Ventricular Fibrillation

During a cardiac arrest, EMTs who are trained to operate a manual defibrillator must perform a challenging task. They must view the squiggly line moving across a small monitor screen and decide whether the electrical activity of the heart is normal or if ventricular fibrillation is present. Research and clinical experience have clearly shown that the treatment of choice for VF is defibrillation via countershock. For most situations, therefore, you must be able to identify only two rhythms: VF or not-VF. You

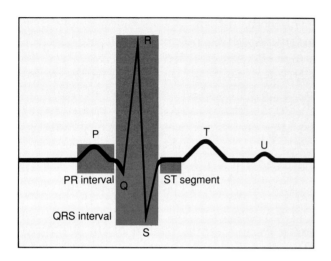

The components of a normal cardiac rhythm.

should look at three features of the electrical signal to detect ventricular fibrillation:

- *Overall pattern* The overall pattern should be irregularly shaped, chaotic, and lack any regular repeating features. Narrow (less than 3 boxes wide) QRS complexes are never present with VF.
- *Height* The electrical signal varies in height. As the energy of the heart decreases, the height or amplitude usually decreases from coarse VF to fine VF.
- *Rate* The distance between the erratic peaks of the VF signal varies greatly and is always irregular.

As shown in Figure C–6, ventricular fibrillation can vary from coarse to fine, but the three features of irregularity in pattern, height, and rate are always present. In addition, the patient in VF is always pulseless.

Visual Recognition of Other Rhythms

There are only four other rhythms that an EMT using a manual defibrillator needs to know: normal sinus rhythm, ventricular tachycardia, asystole and agonal rhythm. Normal sinus rhythm has already been described. Ventricular tachycardia is the rhythm produced when the

pacemaker for the heart is located somewhere in the ventricles. Beats that originate in the ventricles are broad, slurred, and slightly distorted. They are fast, between 140 to 200 beats per minute. When many of them occur one after another, they can produce a rhythm with the characteristics of consistent height and regular rate. Therefore, because there is a regularly shaped pattern, with little variation in signal height and rate, you can quickly conclude that this is a nonventricular fibrillation pattern (Figure C–7).

You should check the patient for a pulse whenever this rhythm is detected. Ventricular tachycardia must be carefully monitored, because it can deteriorate rapidly into ventricular fibrillation, often in seconds. If the patient is unconscious, no carotid pulse is present, and VT is present, countershock is indicated. This practice, however, should be covered by the local medical director's protocol.

Asystole is a rhythm that looks like a flat line and indicates no electrical activity in the heart (Figure C–8). **Agonal rhythm** must also be recognized. This rhythm shows a flat line with a weak QRS complex less than once every 5 to 10 seconds and may be observed just before asystole. Defibrillation has no effect on asystole or an agonal rhythm. In some programs, however, EMTs are instructed to shock a patient with asystole because of a small possibility that the heart does have some undetected ventricular fibrillation remaining and may respond to the shock. Other systems require the EMT to check other leads on the monitor/defibrillator to see whether asystole is present there also. This may also be accomplished by moving the paddles to other positions on the chest to verify asystole. Again, local medical director protocols must be followed in these instances.

DEFIBRILLATION EQUIPMENT
· ·

Portable Defibrillators

A number of companies manufacture portable defibrillators specifically designed for prehos-

A Coarse ventricular fibrillation

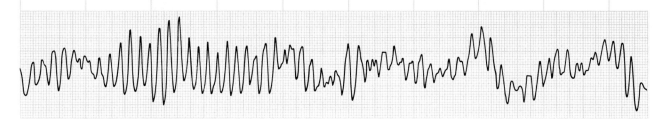

B Fine ventricular fibrillation

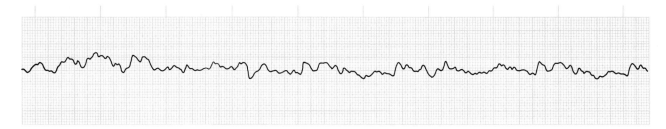

FIGURE C–6   Ventricular fibrillation is irregular, chaotic, and lacks regular, repeating features. The signal may vary in height and width. (A) Coarse, ventricular fibrillation and (B) fine ventricular fibrillation.

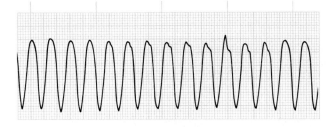
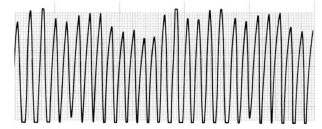

FIGURE C–7   Two examples of ventricular tachycardia. Note the regular pattern with little variation in height and rate.

pital use. These devices should have the following features:

- *Rechargeable power source.* The defibrillator must have a portable energy supply, usually rechargeable nickel-cadmium batteries.
- *Portability.* The defibrillator should be lightweight (less than 30 pounds) and designed for easy carrying.
- *Construction for prehospital care.* The defibrillators should be environmentally sealed for all weather conditions and be resistant to rough usage.
- *Event recording.* Defibrillators used in the prehospital setting must be capable of recording the cardiac rhythm on a strip chart for documentation.

Manual Defibrillators

Manual defibrillators (Figure C–9) must accurately record the patient's rhythm and then

A Asystole

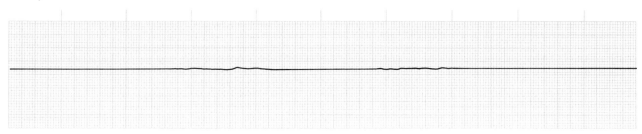

B Asystole with p waves present

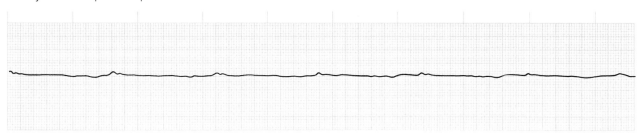

FIGURE C–8   (A) Asystole indicates no electrical activity of the ventricles of the heart. (B) On occasion, P waves indicating some residual electrical activity in the atria may persist with asystole.

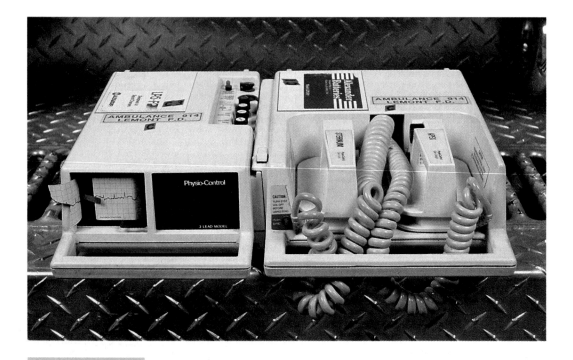

FIGURE C–9   A typical manual defibrillator.

display the rhythm in a clear, easy-to-see manner in all lighting conditions. This allows the EMT to interpret the patient's rhythm for the presence or absence of ventricular fibrillation.

The rhythm can be recorded in two ways: through standard cardiac monitor electrodes that are attached to the patient's chest or through the two paddles of the defibrillator. To lower the electrical resistance between the patient's skin and the defibrillator paddles, a special gel is applied or special conductive defibrillator pads are placed on the patient.

Rhythm assessment through the handheld defibrillator paddles is difficult, because **artifacts** on the ECG tracing frequently occur from motion of the paddles and the monitor cables. You must be especially careful not to interpret that artifact as VF; some programs allow rhythm interpretation by the EMT only through the small monitor electrodes directly attached to the patient. State and local protocols must be followed in this area of rhythm interpretation in the field. The R2® and Cardiotronix Systems involve a closed pad system similar to the automated external defibrillator wherein the pads serve both a monitoring and shock-delivering function.

Most manual defibrillators may simultaneously display the rhythm on a paper rhythm strip and on a cardiac monitor screen. Both of these methods are useful. The paper rhythm strip provides a physical copy of the rhythm for immediate review at the scene and for later review after use of the defibrillator. The cardiac monitor screen allows long periods of monitoring, without an accumulation of large amounts of ECG recording paper.

If the rhythm is ventricular fibrillation, you must press the "charge" switch on the defibrillator or on the paddle handles to allow the power source to charge the capacitors. It is a common practice to have the strip chart recorder record the rhythm for 6 seconds prior to the shock and for 6 seconds after the shock has been delivered to document the event. You deliver the electrical countershock across the chest by pressing appropriate "discharge" or "shock" buttons on each paddle simultaneously. When using handheld paddles, it is

recommended that the paddles be pressed onto the chest with at least 25 pounds of force.

Automatic and semiautomatic defibrillators can also be configured by a given EMS system to function as manual defibrillators. These instruments are attached to the patient's chest with two large adhesive pads precoated with an electrode gel held onto the patient by a special "diphoretic adhesive," as described in Chapter 9. These pads serve a dual function—to pick up the EKG signal from the heart and also to deliver the countershock. The energy levels and the electrical characteristics of the countershocks are virtually identical to the countershocks delivered by manual defibrillators.

Energy Levels of Defibrillators

The electrical current delivered by defibrillators is measured in units called **joules** or *watt-seconds*. Manual defibrillators can deliver countershocks measuring from 10 to 360 joules. You should use the energy level determined by local standing orders by your medical director. In most programs the first shock is 200 joules, the second shock is 200 to 300 joules, and the third and subsequent shocks are at the full 360-joule level. Automated and semiautomated defibrillators are preset to medical director-dictated energy levels.

PREHOSPITAL DEFIBRILLATION BY EMTs

Standing Orders Versus Telemetry

Standing orders are a direct order from the program medical director to perform certain tasks for a patient under a specific set of circumstances (Figure C–10). Virtually all programs use standing orders rather than telemetric transmission of an ECG recording to a base station physician. This is because speed is so important during a cardiac arrest, and because telemetry frequently causes long decision-making delays. Also, telemetry is expensive and does not function reliably in many locations.

SAMPLE STANDING ORDERS FOR PATIENT TREATMENT FOR EMTs CERTIFIED IN MANUAL, AUTOMATIC, OR SEMI-AUTOMATIC DEFIBRILLATION

Purpose: The purpose of these orders is to provide prompt defibrillation for patients who have confirmed circulatory arrest due to ventricular fibrillation.

Authorization: In the event of a cardiac arrest, the medical director authorizes you to perform the following:

1. Immediately upon arrival, verify circulatory and respiratory arrest by the absence of consciousness, normal respirations, and carotid pulses.

2. Initiate CPR and the defibrillation protocol.

3. Assessment. Assess the rhythm for the presence of ventricular fibrillation:

(1) Turn defibrillator POWER on.
(2) Turn recorder on.
(3) Begin verbal report.
(4) Attach monitor leads or defibrillator pads.

Manual Defibrillators
(1) Gel defibrillation paddles.
(2) Charge to 200 joules.
(3) Start paper chart recorder.
(4) Place paddles against the chest.
(5) Inspect the rhythm.

Automatic Defibrillators
(1) Clear the patient.
(2) Switch to AUTO MODE.
(3) Count to 15 seconds.

Semi-Automatic Defibrillators
(1) Clear the patient.
(2) Press the ANALYZE switch.
(3) Count to 15 seconds.

4. Treatment. Treat ventricular fibrillation with a maximum of three countershocks. When VF is persistent, deliver up to three shocks without pausing for CPR between shocks, as outlined below:

Manual Defibrillators
(1) Deliver shock #1.
(2) Leave paddles on the chest.
(3) Recharge to 200 J.
(4) Clear the patient.
(5) Reassess the rhythm.

(6) Deliver countershock #2.
(7) Leave paddles on the chest.
(8) Recharge to 200 J.
(9) Clear the patient.
(10) Reassess the rhythm.
(11) Deliver countershock #3.

Automatic Defibrillators
(1) Allow the device to continue to assess and treat for up to 3 shocks in a row.
(2) Whenever a 15-second assessment period occurs without a shock, switch to MANUAL MODE, and resume CPR for 15 to 30 seconds.
(3) Switch back to AUTO MODE, and allow the device to assess and treat until a total of 3 shocks have been delivered.

Semi-Automatic Defibrillators
(1) Push the "shock" switch when the message screen displays "shock advised."
(2) Repeat "analyze," and repeat "shock" each time the message screen displays "shock advised" until a total of 3 shocks in a row have been delivered.
(3) Whenever the "shock not advised" message appears, resume CPR for 15 seconds.

5. Manual Defibrillators Only. The rhythm assessment reveals asystole.

(1) Resume CPR.
(2) Check lead connections to the patient.
(3) Check lead connections to the monitor/defibrillator.
(4) Check calibrations.
(5) Verify that lead selector switch is in the lead II position, *not* the paddles position.
(6) Check for possible hidden VF by assessing the rhythm for 5 seconds in lead I, and then 5 seconds in lead III.
(7) Follow *treatment* orders if VF is observed in any lead.

(*Note:* The details of standing orders may differ from program to program. These sample standing orders are for an EMT-D program that uses only 200-joule shocks, allows a total of three shocks for persistent VF, and does not permit shocks for asystole.)

FIGURE C–10 Sample standing orders for patient treatment of EMTs certified in manual, automated or semiautomated defibrillation.

When performing defibrillation, you must follow standing orders precisely. You will be acting under the authority of the medical director's medical license. When you successfully complete your training course, you will receive an authorization to function. This authorization from the medical director legally permits you to use the defibrillator in certain situations and in a prescribed manner, which are exactly defined in standing orders.

The Steps of Defibrillation

Defibrillation should not be thought of as simply the proper operation of the defibrillator. The steps of defibrillation are best understood as parts of three cycles. These cycles are similar for both manual and automated defibrillators.

Step 1. Assessment Cycle First, it must be ascertained that the patient is in cardiopulmonary arrest. The ABCs must be performed. Then the defibrillator must be properly attached to the patient who is in cardiac arrest, and the initial heart rhythm should be recorded. Assess the rhythm as it is displayed on the monitor screen and the paper rhythm strip to decide whether VF is present. CPR must cease while the monitor defibrillator is being used to assess the cardiac rhythm.

During an assessment cycle, you should follow these steps:

1. Attach monitor leads or defibrillatory pads to the patient's chest.
2. Discontinue CPR.
3. Clear all personnel from contact with the patient.
4. Make a visual inspection of the rhythm.

Step 2. Treatment Cycle Once the assessment has occurred and it is decided that VF is present, the capacitors of the defibrillator must be charged to the selected appropriate energy level. This level is 2 joules per kilogram in the pediatric age group, with maximums being the adult energies. The adult energies range from 200J to 360J. You should ensure that the patient is not lying in a pool of water or in an explosive environment. Having made sure that no one, including yourself, is touching the patient, deliver the countershock. All EMTs must recognize the sudden movement of the patient that indicates a countershock has been delivered.

When using a manual defibrillator, follow these steps composing the treatment cycle:

1. Apply gel to the paddles.
2. Select the energy level (as determined by standing order or directed by medical control).
3. Charge the defibrillator.
4. Apply the defibrillator paddles to the chest in the proper position (Figure C–11).
5. Recheck that no personnel are touching the patient and say "clear" to warn other rescuers to avoid any further contact.
6. Press the shock delivery controls.
7. Visually recognize that a shock has been delivered.
8. Check for the return of a spontaneous pulse and check the cardiac rhythm.

Step 3: CPR Cycle The importance of CPR must never be forgotten. CPR must be continued at all times, except during the assessment

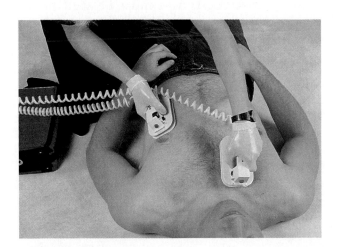

FIGURE C–11

The defibrillator paddles or monitor electrodes are positioned on the anterior chest wall, one to the right of the sternum at the level of the angle of Louis and the second over the apex of the heart.

and the defibrillation cycles. CPR is administered right up to the moment the assessment cycle begins, and it is resumed immediately after the treatment cycle ends. In some programs the medical director will require CPR cycles for a specified period prior to the assessment cycle and also between the treatment cycles. A CPR cycle begins and ends with a pulse check of the patient—if a pulse is present, the blood pressure is measured to see if the pulse is adequate. If a pulse is absent, the CPR cycles resume until the next treatment or assessment cycles begin.

You should therefore follow these steps of the CPR cycle:

1. Administer proper CPR.
2. Perform CPR for the specified time.
3. Stop CPR for 5 seconds to conduct a pulse check.
4. Restart CPR if the pulse is absent or follow the defibrillation cycle, depending on the patient's condition.

Successful Defibrillation

With the return of vital signs, the blood pressure should be monitored and respirations assisted as needed. You must be vigilant for relapse, because up to 25 percent of those patients defibrillated will refibrillate.

TROUBLESHOOTING
· ·

You must learn to recognize the most common problems that can occur while attempting to treat patients in cardiac arrest with a defibrillator. Each of these problems should trigger a mental checklist of possible causes and possible solutions.

Manual Defibrillators

Excessive Artifact Manual defibrillation is impossible when excessive artifact obscures the patient's rhythm on the monitor screen (Figure C–12). This prevents you from analyzing the rhythm and identifying VF. It must be removed. There are several causes of excessive

artifact, but probably the most common cause is unsnapped monitor leads; this produces a straight line tracing. You should quickly check to see whether the leads are snapped to the adhesive patches.

Cable movement is another problem that can be caused by the following:

- *Patient movement during transport.* The rhythm should never be analyzed during transport. The rescue vehicle should be brought to a complete stop to analyze the rhythm and to defibrillate.
- *Agonal respirations or muscle tremor.* Patients who are dying often have agonal respirations (irregular gasps) or have involuntary muscular twitching. Sometimes the rhythm can be properly assessed between agonal respirations. Otherwise, you must continue CPR until the agonal respirations cease.
- *Continued chest compressions or ventilations.* All contact with the patient must cease while the rhythm is being assessed.

Poor contact between adhesive monitor patches and the patient's skin is yet another problem. The first response should always be to push firmly against the monitor patches to see whether proper contact can be established. Other common causes include

- *Hairy chest.* A small safety razor should be carried to quickly shave a small area of the chest. This should not require an excessive amount of time.
- *Sweaty or wet chest.* Patients with severe chest pain who are in cardiac arrest are often covered with perspiration. They may also be wet from rain or from immersion. Alcohol swabs, 4 × 4 gauze, and a small towel to dry off the patient's chest should be available.
- *Small, bony or irregular chest.* The monitor leads should be quickly repositioned on the arms or another portion of the chest.
- *Dry or defective monitor patches.* The monitor patches can become outdated. They should be replaced. If some dryness is detected, a small amount of the electrode gel can be applied under the patches.

Excessive 60-Cycle Interference Sixty-cycle **interference** is usually due to electrical

FIGURE   C–12

(A) Faulty lead attachment or (B) patient muscle tremors may produce an artifact—an extraneous mechanical or electrical interference with ECG signal.

A Faulty lead attachment

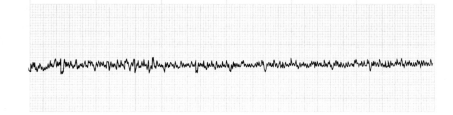

B Muscle tremors

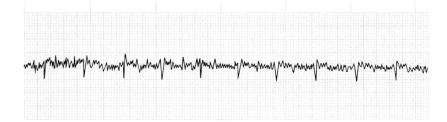

FIGURE   C–13

Sixty-cycle interference is usually due to electrical appliances operating in the vicinity of the ECG.

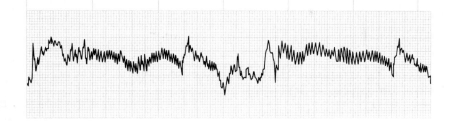

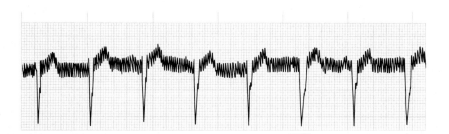

appliances in the vicinity such as electric blankets, televisions, fluorescent lights, clocks, and radios (Figure C–13). Nearby appliances should be unplugged, or the patient should be moved to a different location.

Equipment Problems Manual defibrillators contain a number of warning signals to indicate low batteries, end of tape cassettes, aborted charges, or other equipment failure. Also, several components of manual defibrillators will occasionally produce problems such as blown fuses, paper recorders that do not run, defective ECG paper stylus, and prolonged charge times. You should become thoroughly familiar with the operating manual of the defibrillator so you can quickly recognize these problems and respond correctly. One or more fully charged spare batteries should always be close at hand.

Automated Defibrillators

Inadequate Contact Between the Skin and the Pads Poor skin contact will not allow the automated defibrillators to interpret the cardiac signals properly. Use the following guidelines to ensure that proper contact is made between the skin and pads:

1. Firmly press the defibrillator pads against the chest.
2. Recheck all cable, pad, and device connections.
3. Consider whether the patient's chest has excessive hair or is too wet, sweaty, or irregularly shaped for proper contact. Respond to these problems as outlined for manual defibrillators.

Failure to Deliver Defibrillatory Shock When VF Exists Some of the reasons for this failure include the following:

1. Insufficient time to allow capacitors to charge.
2. Not pressing the defibrillator buttons simultaneously.
3. Leaving the defibrillator in the "Synchronizer" mode.
4. Equipment problems—usually inadequately charged batteries or batteries that have spontaneously discharged.

MAINTENANCE OF DEFIBRILLATION EQUIPMENT

The entire mechanical integrity of a defibrillator should be checked regularly, following a standard checklist. Manufacturers' recommenda-

tions will help determine the items in this checklist. Figure C–14 presents a sample checklist. Several areas need particular attention, as described here.

Battery Care and Maintenance

The charging and care of batteries is the most demanding feature of equipment maintenance. All defibrillators for prehospital use have rechargeable power sources: lead-acid, nickel-cadmium, or lithium batteries. Nickel-cadmium batteries require regular charge and discharge cycles to maintain optimal performance. Lead-acid batteries must be checked regularly, although their general maintenance is simpler than maintenance of nickel-cadmium batteries. Lithium batteries require no maintenance and

---

SAMPLE CHECKLIST FOR EQUIPMENT INSPECTIONS

1. Inspect for general mechanical integrity.
2. Check patient monitor leads and cables.
3. Check quality of monitor display.
4. Check all visual and audio indicator signals.
5. Check calibration setting.
6. Run the paper ECG drive and check quality of tracing.
7. Run the tape recorder and check that voice and rhythm are recorded.
8. Check defibrillator cords and the paddle surfaces. Clean if necessary.
9. Make sure batteries are adequately charged.
10. Charge defibrillator and discharge into test load to verify proper energy output.
11. Note time to charge to recommended energy level and compare with manufacturer's recommendations.
12. Check presence and condition of accessories and supplies:
    (1) tape cassette
    (2) ECG paper
    (3) defibrillatory pads
    (4) disposable monitor leads
    (5) electrode gel, paste, or disposable pads
    (6) safety razor blade
    (7) towel, alcohol swabs

FIGURE   C–14

Sample checklist for equipment inspections.

have an extremely long shelf life. They are used as a backup power source for emergencies, rather than as a primary power source. You must become thoroughly familiar with the manufacturer's recommendations for battery maintenance of the particular defibrillator used.

Defibrillator

The ability of the defibrillator to charge its capacitors and deliver a standard energy level must be checked regularly. Most manufacturers provide a method to measure defibrillator output. The defibrillator is charged to the specified level and then discharged against resistive test plates. Output indicators compare the selected charge level with the actual delivered charge. This procedure can identify problems with the batteries, the capacitor, or the general circuitry. This calibration procedure should be accomplished every six months.

ECG Monitor Screen/ECG Paper Recorder

The entire circuit, from the interface with the patient to the display on the monitor screen and ECG paper recorder, must be checked every shift. Monitor leads should be attached either to simulators that many manufacturers provide or to a volunteer. The paper supply must also be checked, and a spare roll must always be available on the rescue vehicle. The monitor display should be clear and easily seen, and the paper should run smoothly with a clear tracing produced by the stylus. Calibrations on some defibrillators need to be checked.

EMT-D PROGRAM REQUIREMENTS AND LOCAL VARIATIONS

Essential Requirements

The essential requirements for an EMT-defibrillation program that were presented earlier must be met by every program. This is true regardless of setting, population, or type or brand of defibrillator. It must be reemphasized that the purchase of automated or semiautomated external defibrillators does not eliminate any of these requirements. Use of automated defibrillators in a program changes only the final "decision maker" at the time of shock delivery; the content and complexity of the initial training and continuing education, in addition to all other requirements, remain the same.

Local Variations

A number of features of defibrillation programs do vary locally, however, based on the directives of the states' EMS offices and the local medical directors. Once the essential requirements have been met, local medical directors and state EMS offices have the option to establish local variations that, in their medical judgment, are best for their particular program. Examples of standing orders that demonstrate some of these local variations were presented in Figure C–10. Several others are discussed here.

Initial Training If a program selects manual defibrillators, EMTs must learn to recognize lethal cardiac rhythms and which rhythms are treated with a defibrillator. As stated previously, this is the cardinal distinction between a manual program and an automated program. The initial training for automated programs is consequently simpler and takes between 4 and 8 hours. Initial classes for manual programs range from 16 to 40 hours, depending primarily on the amount of rhythm recognition that is taught. Some program medical directors require only that the EMT distinguish between ventricular fibrillation and nonventricular fibrillation; other medical directors believe more advanced rhythm recognition is necessary.

Continuing Education The frequency of continuing education can vary from once a month to once every 6 months. The maximum time between reviews should be 90 days. The content of continuing education must emphasize the practical skills of proper attachment of the defibrillators, proper operation of the device, and close adherence to the standing orders. Rhythm recognition is an important component of these continuing education programs.

Electrical Countershocks The 1992 American Heart Association recommendations for the initial treatment of persistent ventricular fibrillation or pulseless ventricular tachycardia include the following:

1. ABC: determine cardiac arrest.
2. Apply countershock of 200 joules.
3. If VT or VF persists, countershock with 200-300 joules.
4. If VT or VF persists, countershock with 360 joules.
5. Initiate endotracheal intubation and intravenous therapy.
6. Apply additional countershocks of 360 joules.

Defibrillation programs should keep within these general guidelines and permit at least three countershocks for persistent VF, at the highest energy level. Many programs will not have paramedic backup, and consequently intubation and intravenous medications will not be available. In these systems, medical directors should issue standing orders that permit more than three countershocks for persistent ventricular fibrillation. Also, conditions for transport and medical control contact should be specified as dictated by local conditions and the medical director.

Stacked Shocks Properly performed CPR must be continued throughout the care of a person in cardiac arrest; it is stopped only during rhythm assessment and the actual delivery of the countershock. A prescribed period of CPR is not necessary prior to the first shock. Instead, CPR should be performed only for the length of time that it takes to attach the monitor leads, gel the defibrillator paddles, and charge the defibrillator. CPR is then stopped, the rhythm is assessed by the EMT, and the shock is delivered, if appropriate.

A number of protocols "stack" the second and sometimes the third countershocks, a procedure called *stacked shocks*. CPR is not resumed immediately after the first shock. Instead, the EMT continues the delivery of one or more shocks if VF persists without an intervening pulse check. With semiautomatic defibrillators, the "analyze" and the "shock" switches are pressed after each shock, without resumption of CPR. Similarly, when using manual defibrillators, do not remove the defibrillator paddles from the chest but treat persistent VF with continued shocks without interposed periods of CPR. Other programs may decide to provide a 15- to 30-second period of CPR after each shock. Local medical director protocols should prevail.

Shocking Asystole There is clinical evidence to suggest that in up to 5 percent of initial asystole findings, ventricular fibrillation may actually be present. To avoid the possibility of failure to shock occult ventricular fibrillation, some medical directors permit their EMTs to deliver a countershock during asystole. Others recommend checking the analyzed rhythm by moving the paddles to different positions on the chest. As a result, some successful conversions of "asystole" to an effective cardiac rhythm have been reported. Countershocks during asystole should be permitted only after you have verified that there is no alternative explanation for the apparent asystole, such as inadequate batteries, incorrect calibrations, or improper monitor connections. Automatic and semiautomatic defibrillators will not deliver a shock during asystole.

YOU ARE THE EMT

1. What factors must be present in order for defibrillation to be successful in reversing sudden death?

2. What three features are always present in an electrocardiogram showing ventricular fibrillation?

3. Why can't you use a defibrillator for nonventricular fibrillation? Why do some doctors instruct EMTs to use paddles on a patient with asystole?

4. You are unable to identify VF in your patient because of excessive artifact. You have checked the monitor leads and find they have not unsnapped. What other problems could be causing excessive artifact, and how should you deal with such problems?

GLOSSARY

. . . .

abandonment Failure of the EMT to continue emergency medical treatment.

abdomen (ab′do-men) The more inferior of the two major body cavities, lying between the thorax and the pelvis and containing the major organs of digestion and excretion.

abdominal catastrophe (ab-dom′ĭ-nal ka-tas′trafē) An inexact term to describe the most sudden and severe form of an acute abdomen.

abdominal cavity The cavity between the diaphragm and the pelvis that contains all the abdominal organs.

abdominal evisceration (ab-dom′ĭ-nal e-vis″er-a′shun) Injury in which abdominal organs are exposed.

abdominal quadrants (ab-dom′ĭ-nal kwod′rants) Four equal parts into which the abdomen is divided; they are separated by two imaginary lines that intersect at right angles at the umbilicus. The quadrants are the right upper, right lower, left upper, and left lower quadrants.

abdominal thrust maneuver A method of dislodging food or other material from the throat of a choking victim.

abduction (ab-duk′shun) Motion of a limb away from the midline.

abortion (ah-bor′shun) Miscarriage.

abrasion (ah-bra′zhun) Loss of skin as a result of a body part being rubbed or scraped across a rough or hard surface.

abruptio placentae (ab-rup′she-o pla-cen′tae) Early separation of the placenta from the wall of the uterus.

abscess (ab′ses) A localized collection of pus in a cavity formed by the disintegration of tissues.

absorption (ab-sorp′shun) A process of decontamination whereby the material is removed, usually from equipment, by special filters or materials designed to absorb the contaminants.

abuse A cause of injury that can take the form of beatings, burns, rape, attempted murder, and so on.

. . . .

Pronunciation Key
    ′ = primary stress
    ″ = secondary stress

acceleration (ak-sel″er-a′shun) The process of increasing speed.

acetabulum (as″ĕ-tab′u-lum) The socket portion of the hip joint, into which the femoral head fits.

acetone (as′ĕ-tōn) A colorless liquid found in small quantities in normal urine and in larger amounts in diabetic urine.

Achilles tendon (ah-kil′ēz ten′don) The tendon joining the muscles in the calf of the leg to the bone of the heel.

acid (as′id) Any compound of an electronegative element with one or more electropositive hydrogen ions. Acids can cause severe burns.

acidosis (as″ĭ-do′sis) A pathological condition resulting from the accumulation of acids in the body.

A/C joint *See* acromioclavicular joint.

acquired immunodeficiency syndrome (AIDS) A fatal disease first noted in 1978 and caused by a virus. Blood, semen, vaginal secretions, bone, and breast milk have been implicated in the transmission of this disease.

acromioclavicular (A/C) joint (ah-kro″me-o-klah-vik′u-lar joint) Joint at the top of the shoulder, formed by bony projections of the scapula and clavicle.

acromion process (ah-kro′me-on pros′es) Lateral extension of the spine of the scapula; the highest point of the shoulder.

A/C separation A dislocation of the acromioclavicular joint; shoulder separation.

activated charcoal Powdered charcoal that has been treated to increase its powers of adsorption; used as a general-purpose antidote.

actual consent Consent given by a person that authorizes the EMT to provide care or transportation.

acute A loss of volume taking place over 10 minutes or less.

acute abdomen A condition of sudden onset within the abdomen demanding immediate medical treatment.

acute cholecystitis (ah-kūt ko″le-sis-ti′tis) Inflammation of the gallbladder.

acute epiglottitis (ah-kūt ep″i-glot-ti′tis) A bacterial infection of the epiglottis. In children it can cause swelling severe enough to cause airway obstruction.

acute myocardial infarction (AMI) (ah-kūt mi″o-kar′de-al in-fark′shun) Heart attack; specifically, death of the heart muscle from obstruction of its blood flow.

acute pulmonary edema (ah-kūt pul′mo-ner″e•ĕ-de′mah) Severe fluid buildup in the lungs that usually occurs following acute myocardial infarction.

acute symptom A symptom of sudden onset.

acute urinary retention A condition common in the older male, often in conjunction with enlargement of the prostate gland, in which the urethral outlet of the bladder is obstructed and the patient is unable to void.

Adam's apple (ad′amz app′l) The firm prominence (more prominent in men than women) in the upper part of the larynx formed by the thyroid cartilage.

addiction (ah-dik′shun) A state characterized by an overwhelming desire or need (compulsion) to continue the use of a drug or agent and to obtain it by any means, with a tendency to increase the dosage.

adduction (ah-duk′shun) Motion of a limb toward the midline.

administration set Equipment used for intravenous fluid therapy; consists of a fluid container that holds the solution, tubing, and a drip chamber. *Minidrip sets* flow with minimum volume infusion; they are designed to keep an IV line open. *Solution sets* deliver large volumes of fluid to be infused over a short period of time.

adrenal glands (ah-dre′nal glandz) Glands that secrete hormones that control salt levels in the blood and some sexual function.

adult onset diabetes Milder form of diabetes mellitus that affects adults. Insulin is produced, but at a lower, insufficient level. Many of these patients can control their diabetes by diet alone or with pills that stimulate the pancreas.

advanced life support (ALS) Emergency lifesaving procedures, performed by trained professionals, including the use of advanced procedures such as cardiac monitoring, defibrillation, intravenous drugs and advanced airway management devices.

afterbirth (placenta) A special organ of pregnancy attached to the wall of the uterus through which the fetus receives its nourishment and gets rid of waste products.

agonal respiration (ag′o-nal res″pī-ra′shun) An irregular, gasping respiration, sometimes heard in dying patients.

agonal rhythm A cardiac rhythm that shows a flat line with a weak QRS complex less than once every 5-10 seconds and may be observed early in asystole.

AIDS *See* Acquired Immunodeficiency Syndrome (AIDS).

air ambulance An ambulance that is also an aircraft (a helicopter or fixed-wing aircraft).

airborne transmission A method of disease transmission in which the infective organism is introduced into the air by coughing or sneezing; droplets of mucus that carry bacteria or other organisms are then inhaled by another person.

air embolism (ār em′bo-lizm) A condition caused by a bubble of air in the blood stream.

air hunger A distressing dyspnea occurring in paroxysms; found in diabetic coma.

air splint A precontoured, inflatable plastic type of soft splint. After application, it is inflated by mouth, *never* with a pump.

airway Route for the passage of air into and out of the lungs; describing the upper airway, or air passages above the larynx: the nose, mouth, and throat.

alcohol A liquid obtained by fermentation of carbohydrates with yeast.

alcoholic hallucinations (al″ko-hol′ik hah-lu″sī-na-shuns) The awareness or perception of fantastic figures, often walking on the wall or appearing as if to attack the patient; the hallucinations are a manifestation of the alcoholic withdrawal syndrome.

alcoholism Addiction to alcohol; overuse that affects the individual's health and social and economic functioning.

alkali (al′kah-li) Any compound of an electropositive element with an electronegative hydroxyl ion or similar ion. Alkalis can cause severe burns.

alkaline Having a pH above the normal level of 7.45.

alkalosis (al″kah-lo′sis) A condition in which excessive breathing, such as from hyperventilating, "blows off" too much carbon dioxide. The patient experiences shortness of breath. This response is common in psychological stress.

allergen (al′er-jen) A substance causing an allergic reaction.

alopecia (al″o-pe′she-ah) Loss of hair.

alpha radiation A form of ionizing radiation that poses little danger; these rays are easily stopped by paper, a few inches of air, or light clothing.

alveoli (al-ve′o-li) The air sacs of the lungs in which the exchange of oxygen and carbon dioxide takes place.

ambient temperature (am′be-ent tem′per-ah-tūr) The temperature of the environment that is surrounding the body.

ambulance (am′byu-lens) Vehicle for emergency medical care.

ambulance run report A permanent run report filled out by the EMT after the patient has been delivered to the emergency department.

ambulance street form A compact form, frequently printed on a 3 × 5 card, that allows the EMT to record the information needed to make a radio report to the emergency department.

American Standard System Safety system for large cylinders of gas in which gas outlet valves are threaded to accept matching regulator valves so that a regulator cannot be attached to a wrong supply tank.

amino acids (ah-me′no as′idz) Organic compounds that form the chief structure of proteins.

aminophylline (ah-me″no-fil′in) A smooth muscle relaxant occurring as white or slightly yellowish granules or powder.

amnesia (am-ne′ze-ah) Lack or loss of memory; inability to remember past experiences.

amniotic fluid (am″ne-ot′ik floo′id) A liquid that surrounds the fetus in the uterus and protects it from injury.

amniotic sac The fluid-filled cavity that grows around the developing fetus, inside the uterus.

anoxic (ah-nok′sik) Characterized by a total lack of oxygen.

amphetamine (am-fet′ah-min) A stimulant that is taken to produce a general mood elevation, improve task performance, suppress appetite, or prevent sleepiness; common forms are "speed," "uppers," or "Bennies."

amputation (am″pu-ta′shun) Removal of a body part.

anabolism (ah-nab′o-lizm) The building of body tissue from simpler substances.

anal (a′nal) The lower end of the alimentary canal.

anaphylactic shock (an″ah-fĭ-lak′tik shok) Severe shock caused by an allergic reaction.

anaphylaxis (an″ah-fĭ-lak′sis) An unusual or exaggerated allergic reaction of the organism to foreign protein or other substances.

anatomic position (an″ah-tom′ik po-zish′un) A point of reference with the patient standing, facing the examiner, arms at the sides, with palms forward.

anesthesia (an″es-the′ze-ah) The loss of sensation from injury or from the administration of drugs.

anesthetic (an″es-thet′ik) Without feeling.

aneurysm (an′u-rizm) A swelling or enlargement of a part of an artery, resulting from weakening of the arterial wall.

angina *See* angina pectoris.

angina pectoris (an-ji′nah pek-to′ris) Chest pain from heart disease that is brought on by excitement or exertion and relieved by rest and nitroglycerin tablets.

angioplasty (an′je-o-plas″te) Dilatation of a blood vessel by means of a balloon catheter inserted through the skin and through the lumen of the vessel to the site of the narrowing, where the balloon is inflated to flatten plaque against the artery wall.

angle of Louis A bony prominence on the breast bone, just inferior to the junction of the clavicle and sternum and just opposite the second intercostal space.

angulation (ang″gu-la′shun) Departure from a straight line, as in a broken bone.

anisocoria (an-i″so-ko′re-ah) Unequal size of the pupils of the eyes.

ankle joint A hinge joint that allows flexion and extension of the foot on the leg.

anorexia (an″o-rek′se-ah) Lack or loss of appetite for food.

anorexia nervosa (an″o-rek′se-ah ner-vo′sa) A condition more common in young females in which the patient eats less and less food and may become seriously emaciated and malnourished. It is a manifestation of a severe underlying psychological disorder.

anoxia (ah-nok′se-ah) A lack of oxygen.

antecubital fossa (an″te-kyu′bĭ-tal fos′ah) The depression in the anterior region of the elbow.

anterior Situated in front of or in the forward part of the body.

anterior superior iliac spines The hard bony prominences at the front on each side of the lower abdomen just below the plane of the umbilicus; they form the anterior ends of the iliac crest.

anterior surface The front surface of the body, facing the examiner.

antibiotic (an″tĭ-bi-ot′ik) A chemical substance produced by a microorganism, which has the capacity to kill other microorganisms.

antidote (an′tĭ-dōt) A specific substance to neutralize or counteract a poison.

antihistamine (an″tĭ-his′tah-mēn) A drug that counteracts the effects of histamine and relieves the symptoms of an allergic reaction.

antivenin (an″tĭ-ven′in) A substance produced to counteract the effect of an animal or insect venom.

anus (a′nus) The distal or terminal ending of the alimentary canal.

aorta (a-or′tah) The major artery leaving the left side of the heart that carries freshly oxygenated blood to the body.

aortic valve (a-or′tik valv) A valve that guards the aortic opening in the left ventricle of the heart and prevents backflow into the left ventricle.

aortocoronary bypass (ay-or′to-kor′ə-na-rē bi′pas) An operation to bypass damaged coronary arteries to the heart; a vein from the leg or an artificial vessel is sewn directly from the aorta to a coronary artery beyond the point of obstruction.

Apgar score A measure of a baby's condition at birth.

aphasia (ah-fa′ze-ah) Loss of speech.

aphasic (ah-fa′zik) Unable to speak.

apneic (ap′ne-ik) Having no spontaneous breathing.

appendicitis (ah-pen″dĭ-si′tis) Inflammation of the appendix.

appendix (ah-pen′diks) A small tubular structure that is attached to the lower border of the cecum in the lower right quadrant of the abdomen.

aqueous humor (a′kwe-us hu′mor) The watery translucent content of the anterior and posterior chambers around the iris of the eye.

arachnoid (ah-rak′noid) Middle layer of the three layers of tissue that envelop the brain and spinal cord; lies between the dura mater and the pia mater.

arch of aorta Paired vessels arching from the ventral to the dorsal aorta through the branchial arches of fishes and amniote embryos.

arm Part of the upper extremity that extends from the shoulder to the elbow.

arrhythmia (ah-rith′me-ah) An irregular or abnormal heart rhythm.

arterial pressure (ar-te′re-al presh′ar) The pressure of the blood that flows through the artery.

arterial pressure points Points where an artery passes over a bony prominence or lies close to the skin.

arterial rupture Rupture of a cerebral artery.

arteriole (ar-te′re-ōl) Small branch of an artery, especially one just proximal to a capillary.

arteriosclerosis (ar-te″re-o-sklĕ-ro′sis) A disease characterized by a thickening and destruction of the arterial walls, caused by fatty deposits within them; the arteries lose the ability to dilate and carry oxygen-enriched blood.

artery (pl. arteries) A vessel through which blood passes away from the heart to the various parts of the body.

articular cartilage A thin layer of cartilage, covering the articular surface of bones in synovial joints.

articulation Joint; the juncture where two bones come in contact.

artifacts Extra or extraneous ECG signals.

artificial airway A device that is inserted through the nose or mouth to allow passage of air and oxygen to the lungs.

artificial circulation A means of providing circulation by external chest compression.

artificial respiration *See* artificial ventilation.

artificial ventilation (ar″ti-fish′al ven″tĭ-la′shun) Opening the airway and restoring breathing by mouth-to-mouth or mouth-to-nose ventilation and by the use of mechanical devices.

ascending colon Part of the colon that lies in the vertical position on the right side of the abdomen, extending up to the lower border of the liver.

ascent injuries Injuries in ascent from a dive, especially air embolism and decompression sickness.

aspiration (as″pĭ-ra′shun) Taking foreign matter such as vomitus into the lungs during inhalation.

asthma (az′mah) A disease of the lungs in which muscle spasms in the small air passageways and the production of a large amount of mucus result in airway obstruction.

asystole (ah-sis′to-le) Complete absence of heart activity.

ataxia Muscular incoordination.

atom (at′om) The smallest particle of an element that can enter into a chemical reaction.

atrial fibrillation (a′tre-al fi-brĭ-la′shun) Disorganized, ineffective quivering of the atria, causing an irregular, often rapid, ventricular heart rate.

atrial flutter Beating of the atria up to a rate of 300/minute, not associated with equal beating of the ventricles.

atrium (a′tre-um) Either of the two upper chambers of the heart.

auditory nerves (aw′di-to″re nervz) Nerves transmitting hearing sensations to the brain.

aura (aw-rah) A subjective sensation or phenomenon that precedes and marks the onset of a seizure.

auscultate (aws′kul-tāt) To listen.

auscultation (aws″kul-ta′shun) Listening to sounds within the organs, usually with a stethoscope; a method of taking a patient's blood pressure.

autoimmune A condition in which the body literally destroys its own tissues because it becomes allergic to them.

automated external defibrillator (aw″to-mat′ed eks-ter′nal de-fib′ri-la″tor) Equipment that analyzes the electrical activity of the patient's heart and, under the right conditions, delivers an electrical charge to restore the heartbeat.

autonomic nervous system (aw″to-nom′ik ner′vus sis′tem) (involuntary) That part of the nervous system that regulates functions, such as digestion and sweating, that are not controlled by a voluntary act of conscious will.

AVPU scale Level of consciousness scale.

avulse (ah-vuls′) To pull or tear away.

avulsion (ah-vul′shun) An injury in which a piece of skin is either torn completely loose from all of its attachments or is left hanging as a flap.

axilla (ak-sil′ah) The armpit.

back blows Sharp blows delivered with your hand over the patient's spine between the scapulae to relieve upper airway obstruction.

backdraft An explosion of gases in the smoldering phase of a fire.

bacterial (bak-te′re-al) Of or relating to bacteria.

bacterial meningitis (bak-te′re-al men″in-ji′tis) A form of meningitis that carries the risk of transmission.

bacterium (bak-te′re-um) Microorganism that causes infection.

bad trip An unpleasant or frightening hallucination caused by drugs.

bag of waters The amniotic sac.

bag-valve-mask resuscitators Equipment for supplying supplemental oxygen; consists of an inflatable, deflat-

bag, a face mask, and a valve that connects the face mask and bag and attaches to the oxygen supply.

bag-valve-mask system Method of delivering air with more than 90 percent oxygen; *see also* bag-valve-mask resuscitators.

ball-and-socket joint A joint that allows internal and external rotation as well as bending.

balloon angioplasty *See* angioplasty.

barbiturate (bar″bi-tūr′at) A drug that depresses the nervous system; it can alter the state of consciousness so that the individual may appear drowsy or peaceful. On the street, barbiturates are commonly known as "Goof Balls."

barrier device A protective item, such as gloves or a mask, that provides a relatively effective barrier to patient secretions and limits intimate patient contact during basic life support or mouth-to-mouth resuscitation.

basal skull fracture Fracture of the base of the skull; cerebrospinal fluid may leak from the ear, nose, or scalp laceration, or there may be hemorrhage from the ear without apparent cause.

base The nonacid part of any salt that combines with acids to form salts; an alkali.

base station Any fixed radio hardware containing a transmitter and receiver. For EMS purposes, they will generally be within the class, land mobile service, as defined by the Federal Communications Commission (FCC).

basic life support (BLS) Simple emergency lifesaving procedures which can aid a person in respiratory or circulatory failure.

basic rescue Rescue operation that involves the transfer of injured patients from uncomplicated motor vehicle accidents or stable buildings using a minimum of equipment.

basilar artery (bas′ĭ-lar ar′ter-e) Artery formed by two vertebral arteries that unite at the base of the brain; the basilar artery has connections that link with the two carotid arteries at the base of the brain to form a circle of vessels around the brain stem.

bee sting kit Kit with medications for the patient who has severe allergic reactions to bee stings.

belay (bi-lā′) A rescue line.

bends Decompression sickness; bubbles of nitrogen that form in the blood vessels when a diver ascends too rapidly.

benign (be-nīn′) Nonmalignant.

benzodiazepine A nonbarbiturate depressant drug.

beta cells of the islets of Langerhans Specialized cells in the pancreas that produce insulin.

beta particles Negatively charged electrons that are given off by the nuclei of radioactive material at fairly high energy levels.

beta radiation A form of ionizing radiation that can penetrate to a greater depth than alpha rays but that are effectively stopped by clothing, glass, or thin metal shielding.

biceps muscle (bi′seps mus′el) Large muscle that covers the front of the humerus.

bile (bīl) A fluid secreted by the liver and transmitted to the small intestine through the bile ducts. It is required for normal fat digestion.

bile ducts (bīl dukts) Ducts that convey bile between the liver and the intestines.

biliary tract (bil′e-a-re trakt) A ductal system through which bile passes from the liver into the intestines.

birth The act or process of being born; separation of the infant from the mother's body.

birth canal The vagina and the lower part of the uterus.

bite An injury caused by the teeth of an animal; the relation of the upper and lower teeth when in contact.

bite block Block to put in the patient's mouth to prevent biting of the tongue.

black widow spider A poisonous spider; the female is black with an hourglass-shaped red mark on the underside of the abdomen.

bladder A musculomembranous sac for collecting and storing urine.

blanched Paleness of skin.

blanket drag A method by which one EMT encloses a patient in a blanket and drags the patient to safety.

blood A complex, thick, red fluid composed of plasma, red blood cells (erythrocytes), white blood cells (leukocytes), and platelets.

blood-glucose self-monitoring units A method by which diabetics measure the amount of sugar in their blood. A drop of blood from the fingertip or ear lobe is placed on a strip of chemically treated paper. The color the paper turns is compared with a color chart. The readings are in milligrams per deciliter of blood.

blood pressure The pressure of the blood against the walls of the arteries.

blood volume The amount of blood within the circulatory system.

bloody show The appearance of a small blood and mucus plug from a pregnant woman's vagina, often signaling the beginning of labor.

blowout fracture Fracture of the orbit (eye socket) or of the bones that support the floor of the orbit.

blunt (closed) abdominal injuries Injuries to the abdomen caused by a blunt object like a steering wheel; the skin remains intact.

blunt injury (blunt in′ju-re) Injury in which the force of impact is concentrated over a large area of contact; the force of impact does not break the skin but damages the tissues and organs below the skin.

blunt trauma (blunt traw'mah) Injury in which the force of impact is concentrated on a large area of contact between the wounding object and the body; the force of impact is transmitted through the skin, not breaking the skin, but damaging the tissues and organs below the skin.

body (of the sternum) One of three parts of the sternum; (of the vertebra) the front part of a vertebra; a round solid block of bone.

body substance isolation (BSI) (bod'e sub'stans i"so-la'shun) The procedure of using barriers for self-protection when you handle blood and body fluids.

bone The hard form of connective tissue that makes up the skeleton.

bone marrow The central portion of all bones that produces red blood cells.

bony arch The back part of each vertebra; together, the bony arches form a tunnel that runs the length of the spine and protects the spinal cord.

bony rib cage Twelve pairs of ribs that extend from their respective thoracic vertebrae around to the front to create the walls of the chest.

borderline diabetes Jargon used to characterize the patient whose random blood sugar may be elevated or in whose urine sugar may be detected. It does not indicate the presence of the disease.

botulism (boch'oo-lizm) The most severe form of food poisoning; usually results from eating improperly canned food that contains bacterial toxins.

Bourdon gauge flowmeter A pressure gauge on a medical compressed gas cylinder calibrated to record flow rate.

brachial artery (bra'ke-al ar'ter-e) Artery on the inside of the arm between the elbow and the shoulder; used in taking blood pressure and for checking the pulse in infants.

brachial plexus (bra'ke-al plek'sus) A network of nerves originating from branches of the spinal nerves; located in the neck and the axilla.

bradycardia (brad"e-kar'de-ah) Slow but regular heart rhythm.

brain Controlling organ of the body; center of consciousness; functions include perception, control of reactions to the environment, emotional responses, and judgment.

brain stem Area of the brain between the spinal cord and cerebrum, surrounded by the cerebellum; controls functions necessary for life, such as respiration.

breath-holding blackout Loss of consciousness due to decreased stimulus for breathing.

breech presentation A delivery in which the baby's buttocks or feet appear first rather than the head.

bridge The proximal one-third of the nose that is formed by bone. The rest of the nose is made of cartilage.

bronchi (brong'ki) The two main branches of the trachea that lead into the right and left lungs. Within the lungs they branch into smaller airways. Three major bronchi form in the right lung. Two major bronchi form in the left lung.

bronchiole (brong'ke-ol) One of the finer subdivisions of the bronchi, less than 1 millimeter in diameter, having smooth muscle and elastic fibers in its walls.

bronchitis (brong-ki'tis) Irritation of the major lung passageways, either from infectious disease or irritants such as smoke.

brow One of two soft areas on a baby's head, located near the front.

brown recluse spider (brown rek-lüs spi'der) A poisonous spider with a violin-shaped mark on the head and thorax.

buccal vestibule (buk'al ves'ti-būl) The gum/cheek pouch.

bulb syringe (bulb si-rinj) A rubber or plastic device of defined capacity (60 cc) used for gentle suction and irrigation in neonates and small infants.

bulimia (bu-lim'e-ah) A condition in which the patient significantly overeats and then induces vomiting in an effort not to gain weight from the extra food. The condition is a manifestation of a severe underlying psychological disorder.

bulky hand dressing Dressing and splint for hand injuries.

burn A lesion caused by heat exposure or exposure to chemicals or electricity.

burp Regurgitation.

butterfly A steel needle that is used for intravenous fluid therapy.

caffeine (kah-fēn') A mild stimulant found in coffee and cola drinks.

calcaneus (Os calcis) (kal-ka'ne-us) The heel bone.

calcium (kal'se-um) An element found in nearly all organized tissues, especially bone.

cancer (kan'ser) A condition in which tissue develops a malignant neoplasm.

cannula A tube for insertion into a duct or cavity.

capillary perfusion (kap'ĭ-lar"e per-fu'zhun) The process whereby oxygen and nutrients are brought to every cell, and waste and carbon dioxide are removed.

capillary refill The ability of the circulatory system to restore blood to the capillary blood vessels after it has been squeezed out by the examiner.

capillary vessel (kap'ĭ-lar"e ves'el) Any one of the tiny vessels that connect the arterioles and venules at the cellular level, forming a network in all parts of the body.

carbohydrate (kar"bo-hi'drāt) Compound derived from alcohols. The starches, sugars, and cellulose, are examples.

carbon dioxide (kar'bon di-ok'sīd) An odorless, colorless gas, CO_2, resulting from the oxidation of carbon. It is formed in the tissues and eliminated by the lungs.

carbon dioxide drive The stimulus to breathing caused by the carbon dioxide level in the arterial blood; regulation of rate and depth of breathing by the carbon dioxide level.

carbon dioxide narcosis (kar'bon di-ok'sīd nar-ko'sis) A condition characterized by a chronically high blood level of carbon dioxide in which the respiratory center no longer responds to high blood levels of carbon dioxide.

carbon monoxide (kar'bon mon-ok'sīd) Colorless, poisonous gas, CO, formed by burning carbons or organic fuels with a scanty supply of oxygen; it causes asphyxiation by combining irreversibly with the blood hemoglobin.

cardiac arrest (kar'de-ak ah-rest) A sudden ceasing of heart function.

cardiac muscle (kar'de-ak mus'el) The muscle of the heart.

cardiac output (kar'de-ak owt'poot) The effective volume of blood expelled by either ventricle of the heart per unit of time.

cardiac pacemaker Device that imposes a regular rhythm on the heart by delivering an electrical impulse through wires sewn into the heart muscle.

cardiac tamponade (kar'de-ak tam"pon-ād') A condition in which the sac around the heart fills with blood.

cardiogenic shock (kar"de-o-jen'ik shok) Shock resulting from inadequate functioning of the heart.

cardiopulmonary resuscitation (CPR) The artificial establishment of circulation of the blood and movement of air into and out of the lungs in a pulseless, nonbreathing patient.

cardiovascular collapse *See* cardiac arrest.

cardiovascular (circulatory) system (kar"de-o-vas'ku-lar [ser'ku-lah-to"re] sis'tem) A complex arrangement of connected tubes that include arteries, arterioles, capillaries, venules, and veins; the heart pumps blood through this system.

carina (kah-ri'nah) A keel-shaped anatomical part, ridge, or process.

carotid artery (kah-rot'id ar'ter-e) The principal artery of the neck. It runs upward in the neck and divides into the external and internal carotid arteries to supply the face, head, and brain. It can be palpated on either side of the neck.

carotid artery pulse (kah-rot'id ar'ter-e puls) A pulse that can be felt at the upper portion of the neck where the carotid artery on each side of the neck is close to the skin.

carpal bones (kar'pal bōnz) The eight bones in the wrist.

carpometacarpal (kar"po-met"ah-kar'pal) The joint between the wrist bones and the metacarpals.

carpometacarpal joint (kar"po-met'ah-kar'pal joint) The joint between the wrist and the metacarpal bones.

carrier An animal or a person who may transmit an infectious disease but does not display any symptoms of it; base radio signal (wave) generated by a transmitter without voice or other information imposed on it.

cartilage (kar'ti-lij) A form of connective tissue containing a tough, elastic substance; found in joints, at the developing ends of bones, and in some specific areas such as the nose and ear.

case law Law established by judicial decision in particular cases.

cataract (kat'ah-rakt) Opacity developing over the lens of the eye, so that vision is impaired.

catheter (kath'ĕ-ter) A hollow, cylindrical structure that can be inserted into the body to drain or deliver fluids.

catheterization (kath"ĕ-ter-i-za'shun) A procedure in which a tube is inserted directly into the bladder to remove urine when a patient is unable to void.

catheter over the needle The most popular type of needle used with intravenous therapy.

catheter through the needle A type of needle used with intravenous therapy.

cecum (se'kum) The first part of the large intestine, into which the ileum opens.

cell A small mass of protoplasm (living matter) bounded by a membrane; the smallest unit of living matter that can function independently.

cellulitis (sel"u-li'tis) A spreading redness and inflammation under the skin, the result of infection.

Celsius (sel'se-us) Designation of temperature on a thermometer on which 0 degrees is the freezing point and 100 degrees is the boiling point of water; same as centigrade.

centigrade (sen'tĭ-grād) Designation of temperature on a thermometer on which 0 degrees is the freezing point and 100 degrees is the boiling point of water; same as Celsius.

centralized medical emergency dispatch (CMED) A special communications operation that monitors and allocates medical control channels among EMS providers.

central nervous system (CNS) The brain and spinal cord.

cerebellum (ser"ĕ-bel'um) One of three major subdivisions of the brain, sometimes called the "little brain"; coordinates the various activities of the brain, particularly body movements.

cerebral (ser'ĕ-bral) Pertaining to the brain.

cerebral arteries Arteries that supply blood to the brain.

cerebral concussion (ser'ĕ-bral kon-kush'un) A jarring injury of the brain resulting in disturbance of brain function. No permanent physical damage occurs to the brain tissue.

cerebral contusion Bruising of the brain tissue from a blow to the head that can cause bleeding, swelling, and brain damage.

cerebral edema (ser'ĕ-bral ĕ-de'mah) Swelling of the brain.

cerebral embolism Obstruction of a cerebral artery by a clot that formed elsewhere in the body and traveled to the brain.

cerebral hematoma A hematoma, or collection of blood, inside the brain tissue itself.

cerebrospinal fluid Fluid that fills the spaces between the arachnoid and the pia mater. The brain and spinal cord essentially float in this fluid.

cerebrovascular accident (CVA) (ser"ĕ-bro-vas'ku-lar ak'sĭ-dent) Stroke; a sudden lessening or loss of consciousness, sensation, and voluntary movement caused by rupture or obstruction of an artery in the brain.

cerebrovascular disease (ser"ĕ-bro-vas'ku-lar dĭ-zēz') Arteriosclerosis involving the vessels of the brain.

cerebrum (ser'ĕ-brum) The largest of the three subdivisions of the brain, sometimes called the "gray matter"; it is made up of several lobes that control movement, hearing, balance, speech, visual perception, emotions, and personality.

certification Formal notice of certain privileges and abilities after completion of certain training and testing.

cervical collar (ser'vĭ-kal kol'ler) A neck brace that partially stabilizes the neck following injury.

cervical spine That portion of the spinal column consisting of the seven vertebrae that lie in the neck.

cervical vertebrae (ser'vĭ-kal ver'tĕ-bre) The first seven vertebrae of the spinal column that lie in the neck.

cervix (ser'viks) The opening or mouth of the uterus.

chain of evidence A protocol used by law enforcement agencies to collect and preserve evidence of a crime.

channel An assigned frequency or frequencies used to carry voice and/or data communications.

chassis The frame and working parts of a vehicle.

chassis set (shas'ē set) The transfer of the center of mass to various locations in a moving ambulance.

chemical burn A burn that results from any toxic substance that contacts the body.

chemical pneumonia (kem'ĭ-kal nu-mo'ne-ah) Pneumonia caused by the aspiration of petroleum products or acid gastric juice into the lungs.

CHEMTREC (Chemical Transportation Emergency Center) A service organized by the chemical industry to assist emergency personnel in identifying and handling hazardous material spills.

chest-thrust maneuver A series of manual thrusts to the chest to relieve upper airway obstruction.

chief complaint The first words out of a patient's mouth in response to a general question such as "What's wrong?" or "What happened?"

child abuse The deliberate, intentional injury of a child physically and/or emotionally.

child molestation (chīld mo-les-ta'shun) Sexual abuse of children.

chin-lift maneuver *See* head-tilt/chin-lift maneuver.

cholesterol (ko-les'ter-ol) A fatlike substance found in animal fats and oils that is deposited on the inner walls of some people's arteries; the buildup of these deposits narrows the arteries and limits their ability to dilate, the disease process called arteriosclerosis.

choroid (koh'roid) The brown vascular coat covering the posterior half of the eyeball.

chronic bronchitis (kron'ik brong-ki'tis) Chronic irritation of the trachea and bronchi, with attacks of coughing and changes in the lung tissue.

chronic obstructive pulmonary (lung) disease (COPD) A slow process of dilation and disruption of the airways and alveoli, caused by chronic bronchial obstruction.

chronic symptoms Symptoms that are slowly progressive.

circulating blood volume The amount of blood contained within the circulatory system (about 6 liters in the adult).

circulatory overload The administration of an excessive amount of IV fluids.

circulatory system A complex arrangement of connected tubes that include arteries, arterioles, capillaries, venules, and veins; the heart pumps blood through this system.

cirrhosis (sir-ro'sis) A disease of the liver marked by progressive destruction of liver cells often causing jaundice.

clavicle (klav'ĭ-k'l) The collarbone. It is attached medially to the sternum and laterally to the scapula.

clinical (klin'e-k'l) Pertaining to or founded on actual observation and treatment of patients.

clinical sign A physical finding that can be elicited or viewed by the physician or EMT.

clonic muscular activity (klon′ik mus′ku-lar ak-tiv′ĭ-te) Spasms that occur during a generalized epileptic seizure.

closed (blunt) abdominal injury Any injury of the abdomen caused by a nonpenetrating instrument or force in which the skin remains intact.

closed chest injuries Injuries to the chest in which the skin has not been broken.

closed fracture A fracture in which the bone ends have not penetrated the skin and no wound exists near the fracture site.

closed wound Injury in which soft tissue damage occurs beneath the skin, but in which there is no break in the surface of the skin.

clothes drag A method by which one EMT can drag a patient to safety by grasping the patient's clothes.

Clostridium (klo-strid′e-um) A spore-forming bacteria.

CMED See centralized medical emergency dispatch.

CO₂ Carbon dioxide.

coagulation (ko-ag″u-la′shun) The process of blood clot formation; blood clotting.

cocaine (ko′kān) A powerful stimulant that induces an extreme state of euphoria. Legitimately, it is a potent local anesthetic. On the street, it is commonly known as "coke."

coccyx (kok′siks) The tailbone; the small bone below the sacrum formed by the final three to four vertebrae.

codeine (ko′dēn) A narcotic drug; a depressant.

coefficient of friction A measure of the "grip" of the tire on the road surface.

coffee ground vomitus Vomitus consisting of dark-colored matter, usually digested blood.

colic (kol′ik) Acute cramping abdominal pain.

colitis (ko-li′tis) Inflammation of the colon.

collateral circulation The ability of secondary blood vessels to replace or compensate for circulation lost by a damaged or blocked vessel.

Colles' fracture (kol′ēz frak′chur) Fracture of the distal radius, producing the silver-fork deformity in which the injured wrist assumes a curvature similar to the side view of a dinner fork.

colloids (kol′oidz) Fluids used for intravenous infusion that include Dextran® (large molecules of dextrose that are not metabolized) and Plasmanate®.

colon (ko′lon) The part of the large intestine that extends from the ileocecal valve to the rectum.

coma (ko′mah) A state of unconsciousness from which the patient cannot be aroused.

comatose (ko′mah-tōs) In a coma.

comminuted fracture (kom′ĭ-nūt′ed frak′chur) A fracture in which the bone is broken into more than two fragments.

communicable (kŏ-mu′nĭ-kah-b′l) (contagious) Capable of transmitting disease.

communicable (contagious, infectious) disease A disease that can be transmitted from one person to another.

complex partial seizure (kom′pleks pär-shel se′zhur) A partial epileptic seizure in which consciousness may be clouded, or the patient may display automatic behavior such as chewing, fumbling with clothes, or walking aimlessly.

complication A difficult factor appearing unexpectedly.

compound (open) fracture Any fracture in which the overlying skin has been damaged.

compression dressing (kom-presh′un dres′ing) A dressing by which pressure is applied to a limb to prevent edema or bleeding.

computer-aided dispatch (CAD) A sophisticated system that enables a dispatcher to input information from an emergency phone call into a computer terminal.

concussion (kon-kush′un) A temporary loss of some or all of the abilities of the brain to function without physical damage to the brain.

conduction (kon-duk′shun) The loss of heat by direct contact of a body part with a colder object.

conductor Any substance that allows an electrical current to flow through it.

condyles (kon′dīlz) Prominences at one or both ends of a bone.

congenital defect (kon-jen′ĭ-tal de′fekt) An imperfection, failure, or absence existing at and usually before birth.

congenital lesion (kon-jen′ĭ-tal le′zhun) A weakened portion of the arterial wall that has been present since birth.

congestive heart failure (CHF) (kon-jes′tiv hart fāl′yer) A disease in which the heart loses its ability to pump blood, usually as a result of damage to the heart muscle.

conjunctiva (kon″junk-ti′vah) The delicate membrane that lines the eyelids and covers the exposed surface of the eye.

conjunctivitis (kon-junk″tĭ-vi′tis) Inflammation of the conjunctiva.

connecting nerves Nerves that allow sensory and motor impulses to be transmitted from one nerve to another within the central nervous system.

consciousness (kon′shus-nes) The state of being conscious; responsiveness of the mind to the impressions made by the senses.

consent (kon-sent) To agree. See also actual consent; implied consent; informed consent.

constipation (kon″stĭ-pa′shun) Difficult, incomplete, or infrequent passage of stools, more common in older individuals who become less physically active.

contact transmission A method of disease transmission, either from direct physical contact between an individual and the infected person or from indirect physical contact between an individual and inanimate objects that may have infectious organisms on them.

contagious (communicable or infectious) disease (kon-ta′jus dī-zēz) A disease that can be transmitted from one person to another.

contamination The presence of infective organisms on or in objects such as dressings, water, food, or on the patient's body.

contraindication (kon″trah-in″dĭ-ka′shun) A condition that renders a medical procedure, treatment, or medication undesirable.

control console (kon-trōl kän′sōl) Typically, a desk-mounted, enclosed piece of equipment that contains the mechanical and electronic controls used to operate a radio base station.

controlled acceleration The use of a controlled pressure on the accelerator and the use of acceleration to control the vehicle.

controlled braking The use of the brakes to control the vehicle and the controlled application of pressure to the brake pedal.

contusion (kon-tu′zhun) A bruise.

convection (kon-vek′shun) The loss of heat through moving air, from the body to a colder environment.

convulsion (kon-vul′shun) A seizure.

convulsive seizure (kon-vul′siv se′zhur) A generalized epileptic seizure; also called a tonic-clonic seizure.

core temperature The temperature of the central part of the body, the heart, lungs, and vital organs.

cornea (kor′ne-ah) The transparent tissue layer in front of the pupil and iris of the eye.

cornering Negotiating a curve.

coronary arteries (kor′o-na-re ar′ter-ēz) Arteries of the heart.

coronary artery bypass graft (CABG) *See* aortocoronary bypass.

coroner (kor′o-ner) A public officer whose duty it is to inquire by an inquest into the cause of any death that there is reason to suppose may not be due to natural causes.

costal (kos′tal) Pertaining to the ribs.

costal arch The fused cartilages of the seventh to tenth ribs, forming the upper limit of the abdomen.

costovertebral angle (kos″to-ver′tĕ-bral ang′gl) Angle that is formed by the spine and the tenth rib. The kidneys lie beneath the back muscles in the costovertebral angle.

counteragent A drug or agent that opposes the effect of another drug or agent.

counterpressure Pressure countering the pressure that already exists.

countershock The electrical charge generated and delivered by a defibrillator.

countertraction Traction applied against a fixed point of the body.

coverage The geographic area in which reliable radio communications exist. Coverage is usually expressed as the radius in miles from a fixed base station.

CPR *See* cardiopulmonary resuscitation.

crack A form of cocaine.

cramp A painful spasm, usually of a muscle; a gripping pain in the abdominal area; colic.

crampon Spiked metal plate that attaches to boots or shoes in order to provide traction.

CRAMS scale A trauma scoring system (circulation, respiration, abdomen, motor, and speech) used to determine the probability of survival.

cranial nerves (kra′ne-al nervz) Twelve pairs of peripheral nerves that exit the brain through holes in the skull; they are specialized nerves that control specific functions in the head and face.

cranium (kra′ne-um) The area of the head above the ears and eyes; the skull. The cranium contains the brain.

crepitus (krep′ĭ-tus) A grating or grinding sensation generated when raw, fractured bone ends rub against each other.

crib death *See* sudden infant death syndrome (SIDS).

cricoid cartilage (kri′koid kar′tĭ-lij) A firm ridge of cartilage that forms the lower part of the larynx.

cricothyroid membrane (kri-ko-thi′roid mem′brān) A thin sheet of fascia that connects the thyroid and cricoid cartilages that make up the larynx.

crisis (kri′sis) A state of emotional confusion often caused by a sudden stressful situation, which the patient sees as causing a crucial turning point in his or her life.

critical burns The most serious burns. They include burns complicated by respiratory tract injury; third-degree burns involving critical areas or more than 10 percent of the body surface; second-degree burns involving more than 20 to 25 percent of the body surface; and any otherwise-moderate burn in an elderly or critically ill patient.

Critical Incident Stress Debriefing (CISD) (krit-i′kl in′sĭ-dent stres di-bref′ing) A program designed to help emergency medical personnel cope with the psychological reactions to stressful job-related incidents.

cross-finger technique A method of opening a patient's mouth; you cross your thumb under the index finger and brace both against the patient's lower and upper teeth. Then using your finger, pry open the jaws.

croup (krōōp) An infectious disease of the upper respiratory system that may cause partial airway obstruction and is characterized by a barking cough.

crowning The appearance of the baby's head at the cervix during labor.

crushing injury Injury resulting from the application of force to body tissue over a relatively long period of time. Crushing can cause soft tissue damage and cut off circulation.

curie (ku′re) A unit of measure of radiation from beta particles.

CVA *See* cerebrovascular accident.

cyanosis (si-ah-no′sis) Blue color of the skin resulting from poor oxygenation of the circulating blood.

cyanotic Having a bluish color.

cystitis (sis-ti′tis) Inflammation of the bladder.

decapitation (de-kap″ĭ-ta′shun) Cutting off of the head.

deceleration (de-sel″er-a′shun) Reduction in speed.

deciduous teeth (de-sid′u-us tēth) Baby teeth.

decompensated shock (de″kom-pen-sa′ted shok) Loss of ability to breathe due to insufficient circulation of blood.

decomposition (de″kom-po-zish′un) The gradual decaying of the body that follows death.

decompression sickness (the bends) (de″kom-presh′un sik′nes) A situation seen in divers in which gas, especially nitrogen, forms bubbles in blood vessels, obstructing them.

decongestants (de″kon-jes′tants) Drugs that reduce congestion or swelling of the mucous membranes.

decontamination (de″kon-tam-i-na′shun) The orderly process by which radiation or chemical hazards can be removed from clothing, equipment, vehicles, and personnel.

dedicated line A special telephone circuit used for specific point-to-point communications purposes, such as remote control of a base station or alerting EMS crew quarters.

deep Pertaining to or situated inside the body and away from the skin.

defibrillation (de′fib″rĭ-la′shun) Delivery of an electrical current through a person's chest wall and heart for the purpose of ending ventricular fibrillation.

defibrillator (de-fib″rĭ-la′tor) A portable battery-powered device that is used to record cardiac rhythm and to generate and deliver an electrical charge to patients with ventricular fibrillation.

deformity (de-for′mĭ-te) Distortion (twisting out of the natural shape) of a body part.

degeneration (de-jen″er-a′shun) Destruction of normal, health tissue from disease.

degenerative arthritis (de-jen′er-a-tiv ar-thritis) Deterioration of joints.

dehydration (de″hī-dray′shun) Loss of water from the tissues of the body.

deliberate abortion An abortion that is deliberately arranged. The abortion may be self-induced or performed in a hospital or clinic.

delirium (de-lēr′e-um) A mental disturbance marked by hallucination, cerebral excitement, and physical restlessness, usually lasting only a short time.

delirium tremens (DTs) (de-lēr′e-um trem′enz) A clinical withdrawal syndrome characterized by restlessness, fever, sweating, disorientation, agitation and convulsions seen in alcoholics who are acutely deprived of their source of supply.

dementia (de-men′she-ah) A severe emotionally disturbed state in which the patient acts irrationally.

dependency (de-pen′den-se) The total psychophysical state of an addict in which increasing doses of the drug are required to prevent the onset of abstinence symptoms.

dependent lividity (de-pen′dent lĭ-vid′ĭ-te) A sign of death; blood settling in the skin of a dependent body part, usually the back.

depolarization (de-po″lar-i-za′shun) Any of two electrical processes involving the heart, during which the electrical charges on the surface of the muscle cell change from positive to negative.

depressant (de-pres′ant) An agent that reduces functional activity.

depression (de-presh′un) A mental state whereby the patient has no interests, may not speak, or thinks of committing suicide.

dermis (der′mis) The inner layer of the skin, containing hair follicles, sweat glands, nerve endings, and blood vessels.

descending colon Part of the colon that lies on the left side of the abdomen, extending from a point below the stomach to the level of the iliac crest.

descent injury Compression problems caused by outside pressure on a diver's body.

diabetes (di″ah-be′tēz) A deficiency of insulin production marked by an inability of the body to metabolize sugar normally.

diabetes insipidus (di″ah-be′tēz in-sip′i-dus) A form of diabetes caused by a deficiency in the hormone which regulates urinary fluid reabsorption.

diabetes mellitus (di″ah-be′tēz mel′i-tus) A metabolic disorder in which the ability to metabolize carbohydrates is impaired, usually due to a lack of insulin.

diabetic (di″ah-bet′ik) One who has diabetes; pertaining to diabetes.

diabetic coma (di″ah-bet′ik ko′mah) Unconsciousness in uncontrolled diabetes caused by dehydration and acidosis.

diabetic ketoacidosis (di″ah-bet′ik ke″to-ah″sĭ-do′sis) A condition caused by excessive fluid and sugar loss in the kidneys and an excessive buildup in the bloodstream of acid metabolic products (ketones) caused by the body's use of substance other than sugar for energy.

diagnosis (di"ag-no′sis) Identifying a disease or injury from its signs and symptoms.

diaphoresis (di"ah-fo-re′sis) Perspiration; especially profuse sweating.

diaphragm (di-ah-fram) A muscular dome that forms the undersurface of the thorax, separating the chest from the abdominal cavity. Contraction of the diaphragm (and the chest wall muscles) brings air into the lungs. Relaxation allows air to be expelled from the lungs.

diarrhea (di"ah-re′ah) Abnormal frequency and liquidity of bowel movements.

diastole (di-as′to-le) The dilatation, or period dilatation, of the heart, especially of the ventricles.

diastolic blood pressure (di"ah-stol′ik blud presh′ur) The lower blood pressure noted during ventricular relaxation as the heart fills with blood.

Dieffenbachia (de′fen-bahk-e-ə) Dumbcane; a tropical American herb that when chewed causes the tongue to swell; the swelling may cause obstruction of the airway.

diffusion (dĭ-fu′zhun) The spontaneous movement of molecules or particles in solution.

digestion (di-jest′yun) The chemical conversion of food into simple sugars, fats, and proteins that can be absorbed into the body and used by cells for energy.

digestive system (di-jest′iv sis′tem) The gastrointestinal tract (stomach and intestines), mouth, salivary glands, pharynx, esophagus, liver, gallbladder, pancreas, rectum, and anus.

dilate (dī-layt) To swell, or become wide.

dilation (di-la′shun) Widening of a tubular structure such as a coronary artery.

dilation of the cervix A phase of labor just before delivery in which the cervix of the uterus opens so that the baby's head can pass through into the vagina.

dilution (di-lu′shun) A process of decontamination whereby the contamination is washed off with floods of water.

diphtheria (dif-the′re-ə) Acute bacterial infection of the throat, tonsils, nose, and sometimes skin, with local pain and swelling.

direct strike Lightning that hits a person directly, usually conducted through a metal object such as a golf club or umbrella.

disaster A human-caused or natural, sudden and serious disruption of life that causes or threatens injuries to a number of persons.

disentanglement Freeing; extricating.

dislocation (dis"lo-ka′shun) The disruption of a joint such that the bone ends are no longer in contact.

dispatcher One who transmits calls to service units, sending vehicles and EMTs on emergency assignments.

displaced fracture A fracture that produces deformity of the limb.

disruptive behavior Behavior that causes a danger to the patient or to others or causes a delay in treatment.

distal (dis′tal) Farther from any point of reference; opposed to proximal.

distension (dis-ten′shun) Bulging or swelling.

diverticulitis (di"ver-tik-u-li′tis) Inflammation of small pockets in the colon.

diving reflex Slowing of heart rate caused by submersion in cold water.

dizygotic twins (di"zi-got′ik twinz) Fraternal twins; they may be of the same sex or of different sexes.

DNR (do not resuscitate) order A document by a patient or family that gives medical personnel permission not to attempt resuscitation in case of cardiac arrest.

dorsal (dor′sal) Posterior, referring to the back or top.

dorsalis pedis artery (dor-sa′lis ped′is ar′ter-e) Artery on the anterior surface of the foot between the first and second metatarsals.

dorsal spine The 12 vertebrae that attach to the 12 ribs; the upper part of the back.

dorsiflex (dor′sĭ-fleks) To move a joint in the posterior direction.

"downer" A depressant.

dressing A bandage.

drowning Death from suffocation by submersion in water.

drug Any chemical or biological substance given to patients to aid in the diagnosis, treatment, or prevention of disease.

drug withdrawal A physical reaction characterized by anxiety, nausea, vomiting, convulsions, delirium, sweating, or cramps, that occurs when an addict is unable to get drugs.

duodenum (du"o-de′num) First or most proximal portion of the small intestine, passing from the stomach to the jejunum.

duplex The ability to transmit and receive traffic simultaneously on a particular channel.

dura mater (du′rah ma′ter) Outermost of the three layers of tissue that envelop the brain and spinal cord.

duty to respond The responsibility of an ambulance service attached to a government agency to respond to calls within its jurisdiction. A commercial or volunteer service is not so obligated unless such care is advertised or is a requirement of its licensure.

dying declaration A statement made by someone who knows he or she is dying, which can be accepted as a legal document in a court; often a confession or revelation of a long-held secret.

dysfunction (dis-funk′shun) Impaired or abnormal functioning.

dysphagia (dis-fa′je-ah) Difficulty in swallowing.

dysphasia (dis-fa′ze-ah) Difficulty in speaking.

dyspnea (disp′ne-ah) Difficult breathing.

dysuria (dis u′re-ah) Painful or difficult urination.

ear drum A thin, tense membrane forming the greater part of the outer wall of the middle ear and separating it from the outer ear canal.

ecchymosis (ek″ĭ-mo′sis) A small area of bleeding in the skin or mucous membrane; a bruise or "black and blue" mark.

eclampsia (ĕ-klamp′se-ah) A convulsive disorder of pregnancy associated with severe hypertension.

ecstasy A variation of an amphetamine compound and a legal drug until 1985, when its potential for abuse was determined to be higher than its medical benefit.

ectopic pregnancy (ek-top′ik preg′nan-se) A pregnancy where the fetus develops outside of the uterus, usually in a Fallopian tube.

edema fluid The presence of abnormally large amounts of fluid in the extracellular tissue spaces of the body, causing swelling of the affected area.

egg cell An ovum; a female gamete.

ejaculation (e-jak″u-la′shun) Act of expelling semen from the penis.

elbow joint The joint between the humerus and the radius and ulna.

electrical burns Burns caused by exposure to electric current.

electrical charge A definite quantity of electricity.

electrical shock The effects produced by the passage of an electric current through any part of the body.

electrocardiogram (ECG or EKG) (ĕ-lek″tro-kar′de-o-gram″) A recording of the electrical current that flows through the heart. The results are displayed on a paper strip or a display screen or (usually) both.

electrolytes (ĕ-lek′tro-lits) Salts dissolved in body fluids and cells.

electrolyte solutions Fluids used for intravenous infusion that contain electrolytes.

electron (e-lek′tron) A particle of an atom that has a negative charge.

embolism (em′bo-lizm) An embolus that causes an obstruction.

embolus (em′bo-lus) A blood clot or other substance that has formed in one blood vessel or the heart that breaks off and travels to another blood vessel, where it causes blockage.

emergency cardiac care (ECC) Subject addressed at na-

tional conferences at which techniques for providing ECC are reviewed and revised as necessary.

emergency delivery pack A kit kept on the emergency vehicle that contains supplies needed for an emergency delivery of a baby.

emergency medical identification card or tag Card carried or tag worn as a bracelet or necklace to warn of any serious medical problems the patient may have.

emergency medical services (EMS) The combined efforts of several professionals and agencies to provide prehospital emergency care to the sick and injured.

emergency medical technician (EMT) A member of a prehospital emergency medical system who is trained to provide basic life support.

emesis (em′ĕ-sis) Vomiting.

emetic (ĕ-met′ik) Medication to induce vomiting.

emphysema (em″fĭ-se′mah) Disease of the lungs in which there is extreme dilation and eventual destruction of pulmonary alveoli with poor exchange of oxygen and carbon dioxide. Also called chronic obstructive pulmonary disease (COPD).

EMS system *See* emergency medical services (EMS) system.

EMT-intermediate (EMT-D) program A training program in which fully trained EMTs undergo further instruction and are then certified to perform defibrillation on people in cardiac arrest.

EMT-intermediate (EMT-I) An EMT who has training in specific aspects of advanced life support such as intravenous therapy, cardiac defibrillation, or advanced airway management.

EMT-paramedic (EMT-P) An EMT who has received extensive training in advanced life support, including intravenous therapy, pharmacology, cardiac monitoring, defibrillation, advanced airway maintenance, including intubation and other advanced assessment and treatment skills.

endocarditis (en″do-kar-di′tis) Infection of the valves or the lining of the heart.

endocrine (en′do-krin) Those organs and structures whose function is to secrete into the blood or lymph a substance (hormone) that has a specific effect on another organ or part.

endocrine gland (en′do-krin gland) Gland that produces hormones that regulate specific bodily functions.

endometrium (en-do-me′tre-um) The lining of the uterus.

endotracheal intubation (en″do-tra′ke-al in′-tu-ba-shun) A method of intubation in which a tube is placed through a patient's mouth or nose and directly through the larynx between the vocal cords into the trachea for the purpose of opening and maintaining an airway.

endotracheal tube (ETT) (en"do-tra′ke-al toob) The tube that is placed in the airway during endotracheal intubation.

enhanced 911 system (E911) The most technologically advanced version of the 911 universal emergency telephone service; features include automatic number identification (ANI), automatic call location identification (ALI), and automatic ring-back.

envenomation (en-ven"o-ma′shun) The actual injecting of venom into a bite.

enzyme (en′zīm) A protein capable of producing or accelerating some change in a given substance.

ephedrine (ĕ-fed′rin) Almost colorless solid or white crystals or granules used to decongest the nasal mucosa.

epidermis (ep"ĭ-der′mis) The outer layer of skin, which is made up of cells that are sealed together to form a watertight protective covering for the body.

epididymis (ep"ĭ-did′ĭ-mis) The elongated cordlike structure along the posterior border of the testis, whose duct provides for storage, transit, and maturation of spermatozoa.

epididymitis Inflammation of epididymis.

epidural (ep"ĭ-du′ral) Superficial to the dura, deep to the skull.

epidural hematoma (ep"ĭ-du′ral hem"ah-to′mah) A hematoma, or collection of blood, outside the dura mater and under the skull.

epigastric (ep"ĭ-gas′trik) Relating to the epigastrium.

epigastrium (ep"ĭ-gas′tre-um) Upper-middle region of the abdomen.

epiglottis (ep"ĭ-glot′is) A thin, leaf-shaped valve that allows air to pass into the trachea but prevents food or liquid from entering.

epiglottitis (ep"ĭ-glot-ti′tis) An infectious disease in which the epiglottis becomes inflamed and enlarged and may cause upper respiratory obstruction.

epilepsy (ep′i-lep"se) A condition manifested by seizures that are caused by an abnormal focus of activity within the brain, producing severe motor responses or changes in consciousness.

epinephrine (ep"ĭ-nef′rin) A hormone used to stimulate the heart and the sympathetic nervous system.

epiphyseal fracture (ep"ĭ-fiz′e-al frak′chur) Injury to the growth plate of a long bone in children, which may lead to an arrest of bone growth if it is not properly treated.

epiphyseal plate (ep"ĭ-fiz′e-al plāt) A transverse cartilage plate near the end of a child's bone, responsible for growth in length of the bone.

epistaxis (ep"ĭ-stak′sis) Nosebleed; a hemorrhage from the nose.

erectile tissue (ĕ-rek′tīl tish′u) Tissue containing large vascular spaces that fill with blood on stimulation (a process called erection), as in the penis and clitoris.

erythematous (er"ĭ-them′ah-tus) Reddened.

erythrocyte (ĕ-rith′ro-sīt) A red blood cell.

esophageal gastric tube airway (EGTA) (ĕ-sof"ah-je′al gas′trik tūb ār′wa) An esophageal obturator airway with an added gastric decompression tube; it allows gas in the stomach to be vented to the outside, thereby decreasing gastric distension.

esophageal obturator airway (EOA) (ĕ-sof"ah-je′al ob′too-ra"tor ār′wa) A plastic, semirigid tube that can be inserted in the esophagus; the upper third, which has holes in it, lies at the level of the pharynx and provides free passage of oxygen-enriched air to the lungs.

esophageal reflux (heartburn) (ĕ-sof"ah-je′al re-fluks) A burning pain under the sternum caused by gastric juices that reflux into the lower esophagus and attack its lining.

esophageal varix (ĕ-sof"ah-je′al vār′iks) Dilated vein in the wall of the esophagus that develops in patients with liver disease. If such an enlarged vein ruptures, subsequent bleeding can be fatal.

esophagus (ĕ-sof′ah-gus) A collapsible tube about 10 inches long that extends from the pharynx to the stomach; contractions of the muscle in the wall of the esophagus propel food and liquids through it to the stomach.

ethics (eth′iks) The study of what is good and bad, and/or moral duty.

euphoria (u-fo′re-ah) A sense of well-being.

evaporation (e-vap"o-ra′shun) Conversion of water from a liquid to a gas.

Eve A variation of an amphetamine compound and a possible cause of deaths from cardiac arrhythmias.

evisceration (e-vis"er-a′shun) Disembowelment; the displacement of organs outside of the body.

excessive artifact (ek-ses′iv ar′tĭ-fakt) A problem that prevents the EMT-D from analyzing the rhythm on the monitor screen of a defibrillator.

excretion (eks-kre′shun) Eliminating material from the body.

exempt narcotic A drug that can be sold over the counter without a prescription.

expiration (eks"pĭ-ra′shun) Exhaling, breathing out or expelling air from the lungs.

exposure Potential for a fall.

exsanguinate (eks-sang′gwĭ-nāt) To bleed to death.

extend To straighten (a joint).

extension The straightening of a limb at a joint.

external auditory canal (eks-ter′nal aw′dĭ-to"re ka′nal) The ear canal.

external bleeding Hemorrhage that can be seen coming from a wound.

external chest compression A technique to produce artificial circulation by applying rhythmic pressure and relaxation to the lower half of the sternum, which has the effect of compressing the heart between the sternum and the spine.

external genitalia (eks-ter'nal jen"ĭ-ta'le-ah) The parts of the genitalia that are outside of the pelvis.

external maxillary artery Artery anterior to the angle of the mandible on the inner surface of the lower jaw that contributes much of the blood supply to the face.

extrasystole (eks"trah-sis'to-le) An irregular extra heartbeat.

extremities (eks-trem'ĭ-tēz) The arms and legs.

extrication (eks'trĭ-kay-shun) Removal from a difficult situation or position; often used to mean removal of a patient from a wrecked car or other place of entrapment.

eye The organ of vision.

face The front part of the head, including eyes, nose, cheeks, mouth, and forehead.

face mask A mask fitting to the face through which gas is delivered to the patient.

fahrenheit (F) designation of temperature on a thermometer on which 32 degrees is the freezing point and 212 degrees is the boiling point of water.

failure to thrive The failure of a child to grow and develop normally, frequently a sign of abuse.

faint Psychogenic shock; a temporary loss of consciousness, usually of brief duration and not serious.

Fallopian tubes (fal-lo'pe-an toobz) Long, slender tubes that extend from the uterus to the region of the ovary on the same side, and through which the ovum passes from ovary to uterus.

fall zone Area where you are most likely to encounter falling objects.

false motion Motion at a point in a limb where it usually does not occur; a positive indication of bone fracture.

fascia (fash'e-ah) A sheet or band of tough fibrous connective tissue. It lies deep under the skin and forms an outer layer for the muscles.

fat Adipose tissue; white or yellowish tissue that forms soft pads in the body and furnishes a reserve supply of energy.

fatty acid Any straight-chain monocarboxylic acid, especially those naturally occurring in fats.

febrile (feb'ril) Having fever.

febrile convulsion (feb'ril kon-vul'shun) A seizure, usually of short duration and not dangerous, that sometimes accompanies high fevers in children.

fecal (fe'kal) Pertaining to feces.

fecal impaction (fe'kal im-pak'shun) A collection of hardened feces in the bowel that produces an obstruction.

femoral artery (fem'or-al ar'ter-e) The principal artery of the thigh, a continuation of the external iliac artery.

It supplies blood to the lower abdominal wall, external genitalia, and legs. It can be palpated in the groin area.

femoral artery pulse (fem'or-al ar'ter-e puls) A pulse that can be felt in the groin where the femoral artery is close to the skin.

femoral condyles (fem'or-al kon'dīlz) Two surfaces at the distal end of the femur that articulate with the superior surfaces of the tibia.

femoral head The proximal end of the femur, articulating with the acetabulum.

femoral neck The heavy column of bone connecting the head and the shaft of the femur.

femoral nerve A major peripheral nerve, lying immediately lateral to the femoral artery in the groin.

femoral shaft The main part of the femur.

femoral vein A continuation of the popliteal vein that becomes the external iliac vein; the major vein draining the thigh.

femur (fe'mur) The thigh bone; it extends from the pelvis to the knee and is the longest and largest bone in the body.

fender judgment Knowing how much physical operating space a particular vehicle requires when traveling at a given speed.

fetal (fe'tal) Pertaining to the fetus.

fetal alcohol syndrome A condition of the children of alcoholic mothers characterized by growth retardation (low birth weight), failure to thrive, mental retardation, and a variety of specific congenital abnormalities.

fetus (fe'tus) A developing baby in the uterus.

fibrillation (fi-brĭ-la'shun) A form of arrhythmia characterized by completely disorganized, ineffective quivering of the heart muscle.

fibula (fib'u-lah) The outer and smaller of the two bones of the leg, extending from just below the knee and forming the lateral portion of the ankle joint.

finger probe A technique whereby the EMT probes a patient's mouth using the index finger as a hook in an attempt to dislodge a foreign body.

first aid Emergency care and treatment of an injured person before medical help can be secured.

first-degree burn Burn in which only the superficial part of the epidermis has been injured; an example is a sunburn.

first responder The first person present at the scene of sudden illness or injury.

first stage of labor The time from the beginning of contractions until the cervix is fully dilated.

flaccid (flak'sid) Soft and limp.

flaccid paralysis (flak'sid pah-ral'ĭ-sis) Paralysis in which the involved extremity or body part is limp.

flail chest (stove-in chest) A blunt chest injury in which three or more ribs are fractured in two or more places or in association with a sternal fracture so that a segment of chest wall is effectively detached from the rest of the thoracic cage.

flail segment That segment of the chest wall in a flail chest injury that lies between the rib fracture and moves paradoxically as the patient breathes.

flashover Violent reaction similar to an explosion; lightning current that travels over the surface of the person on its way to the ground.

flexion (flek′shun) Bending.

floating ribs The eleventh and twelfth ribs, which do not connect to the sternum.

flotation device A device that keeps one from sinking.

flowmeter A flow regulator attached to the pressure regulator on emergency medical equipment. It permits the regulated release of gas measured in liters per minute.

fontanelle (fon″tah-nel′) Soft area on a baby's head.

foot The distal portion of the lower extremity, on which one stands and walks.

foot drop Paralysis of the dorsiflexor muscles of the foot and ankle, so that the foot falls and the toes drag on the ground in walking.

footprint The area of contact between the ambulance tire and the road surface.

foramen magnum (fo-ra′men mag′num) A large opening in the base of the skull through which the brain connects to the spinal cord.

forearm The lower portion of the upper extremity, from the elbow to the wrist.

forehead The part of the face above the eyes.

foreskin The fold of skin covering the glans penis.

four-person log roll A method of placing a person on a carrying device, usually on a long spine board or a flat litter, by rolling the patient on one side and then back onto the litter.

fracture Any break in the continuity of a bone.

fracture-dislocation A two-fold injury in which the joint is dislocated and a part of the bone near the joint also fractures.

frequency An abnormally high number of voiding episodes during a 24-hour period; the number of repetitive cycles per second completed by a radio wave.

friction The rubbing of one body against another.

frontal (frun′tal) Of, relating to, or situated at the front; parallel to the main axis of the body and at right angles to the sagittal plane.

frontal region The forehead.

frostbite Damage to tissues as the result of exposure to low environmental temperatures.

frostnip A form of cold exposure that occurs after prolonged exposure to the cold. Freezing of the skin may be present, but freezing of the deeper tissues has not occurred.

fungal (fung′gal) Relating to a fungus, fungoril, fungous.

fungus A general term used to denote mushrooms, yeast, rust, molds, smuts, etc.

gallbladder (gawl′blad-der) A pear-shaped sac on the undersurface of the liver that collects bile from the liver and discharges it into the duodenum through the common bile duct.

gallstone A small hard concretion in the gallbladder or a bile duct, composed chiefly of cholesterol crystals.

gamma radiation A form of ionizing radiation that can penetrate through the human body; similar to X rays. Heavy shielding such as lead or concrete is necessary to protect against these rays.

gangrene (gang′grēn) Death of body tissues, usually the result of a loss of blood supply.

gastric distension (gas′trik dis-ten′shun) Inflation of the stomach caused when excessive pressures are used during artificial ventilation or when several breaths are administered quickly in succession.

gastric juice The digestive fluid secreted by glands of the stomach; it contains mainly hydrochloric acid, pepsin, and mucus.

gastric lavage (gas′trik lah-vahzh′) Flushing the stomach with fluids to remove ingested toxic substances.

gastritis (gas-tri′tis) Inflammation or irritation of the stomach lining.

gastroenteritis (gas″tro-en-ter-i′tis) A viral or bacterial infection of the lining of the stomach and/or the intestines.

gastrointestinal system The organs of the stomach and intestines involved in the digestion of food and excretion of the solid waste products of digestion.

Geiger counter (gi′ger kown′ter) An instrument used to measure the level of radioactivity in the environment; these instruments are usually designed to detect gamma radiation.

generalized seizure An epileptic seizure involving most of the brain; also called a convulsive or tonic-clonic seizure.

genitalia (jen″i-ta′le-ah) The male and female reproductive organs and the male urethra.

genital system (jen′i-tal sis′tem) The male and female reproductive systems.

genitourinary system (jen″i-to-u′rĭ-nar-e sis′tem) The organs of reproduction, together with the organs concerned in the production and excretion of urine.

geriatric (jer″e-at′rik) Pertaining to the aged or elderly.

geriatric patients Elderly patients.

German measles Viral illness with fever and rash; can cause birth defects in the fetus if contracted by the mother during the first three months of pregnancy.

germinal layer Layer of skin cells that constantly reproduce to replace outer cells that are being shed or rubbed off.

gestation period (jes-ta′shun pe′re-od) Period for the development of a baby; for humans this is 40 weeks.

Glasgow Coma Scale A rating system used to assess the patient's level of consciousness and the extent of loss of brain function.

glenohumeral joint (gle″no-hu′mer-al joint) The true shoulder joint.

glenoid fossa (gle′noid fos′ah) The recess in the scapula for the articulation of the humeral head laterally forming the glenohumeral joint.

globe The eyeball.

glucose (gloo′kōs) D-glucose or dextrose; one of the basic sugars.

glutethimide (gloo-teth′ĭ-mīd) A nonbarbiturate depressant drug.

gonorrhea Common venereal disease, a contagious infection of the genital mucous membrane.

"Good Samaritan" laws Laws that prevent an individual who voluntarily helps an injured or suddenly ill person from being legally liable for any errors of omissions in rendering good faith emergency.

gout (gowt) A hereditary form of arthritis, with excessive uric acid in the blood and recurrent painful attacks of arthritis in one joint.

governmental immunity The doctrine that government agencies are held to be immune from the legal consequences of their actions. Today, more than half of the states have abandoned the doctrine of governmental immunity.

great vessels The large vessels entering or leaving the heart, including the aorta, the pulmonary arteries and veins, and the venae cavae.

greater trochanter (grāt-er tro-kan′ter) A bony prominence on the lateral side of the thigh just below the hip joint to which several muscles are attached.

greenstick fracture An incomplete fracture that passes only partway through the shaft of a bone; occurs only in children.

guarding The involuntary protecting of the inflamed abdomen by abdominal wall muscular contraction.

gunshot wound A form of puncture wound; the amount of damage is directly proportional to the square of the velocity of the bullet.

hair follicles (hār fol′lĭ-k′lz) The small organs that produce hair; there is one for each hair, connected with a sebacous gland and a tiny muscle.

hallucinogen (hah-lu′sĭ-no-jen″) An agent that produces false perceptions in any one of the five senses.

hamstring muscles Two groups of muscles at the back of the knee.

hard hat A protective helmet worn during any rescue activity, both for the identification of rescue personnel and personal safety.

hard palate A bony plate forming the anterior part of the roof of the mouth.

hashish (hash-ēsh) Extracts of the stalks of *Cannabis indica*.

hay fever A common allergy problem caused by pollen in the air; symptoms include stuffy, runny nose, and sneezing.

hazardous material identification number A four-digit identification number displayed on a placard or orange panel on the ends of a tank, vehicle, or rail car transporting hazardous materials, as well as on the shipping paper of packaging of the material.

Hazmat Rule of Thumb A guide to how close you can come to a hazardous material spill before you know what the hazardous material is.

head-tilt/chin-lift maneuver Opening the airway by tilting the patient's head backward and lifting the chin forward, bringing the entire lower jaw with it.

head-tilt maneuver Opening the airway by tilting the patient's head backward as far as possible.

heart (hart) A hollow muscular organ that receives blood from the veins and propels it into the arteries.

heart attack *See* acute myocardial infarction (AMI).

heartburn (esophageal reflux) A burning pain under the sternum caused by gastric juices that reflux into the lower esophagus and attack its lining.

heart rate (pulse) The wave of pressure that is created by the heart contracting and forcing blood out the left ventricle and into the major arteries.

heat collapse (hēt kŏ-laps′) A mild form of shock that occurs when the body loses much water and electrolytes through very heavy sweating after exposure to heat; also called heat prostration or heat exhaustion.

heat cramps Painful muscle cramps associated with activity that occur in a warm or hot environment.

heat exhaustion A form of heat injury in which the body loses water and electrolytes from heavy sweating. (Also called heat collapse and heat prostration).

heat exposure A dose of excessive energy received by the human organism either locally or over its entire surface, for which its normal protective mechanisms are insufficient.

heat prostration *See* heat collapse.

heat stroke A life-threatening condition caused by exposure to excessive heat—natural or artificial—and marked by dry skin, dizziness, headache, nausea, and muscle cramps.

heavy rescue Rescue operations that involve the use of complicated rigging, patient handling under extremely difficult or adverse conditions, breaching of walls, disimpaction of vehicles, and all types of rescue involving buildings with major structural damage.

Heimlich (abdominal thrust) maneuver A series of 6 to 10 manual thrusts to the upper abdomen, just above the umbilicus and well below the xiphoid process, to relieve upper airway obstruction; the abdominal thrust maneuver.

hematemesis (hem″ah-tem′ĕ-sis) The vomiting of blood.

hematochezia (hem″ah-to-ke′ze-ah) The passage of bright red blood from the rectum.

hematoma (hem″ah-to′mah) A collection of blood contained within the body in tissue or in a cavity, occasionally palpable as a discrete mass.

hematuria (hem″ah-tu′re-ah) A discharge of blood in the urine.

hemiplegia (hem″e-ple′je-ah) Paralysis of one side (left or right) of the body.

hemithorax (hem″e-tho′raks) One side (half) of the chest.

hemoglobin (he′mo-glo″bin) The oxygen-carrying pigment of the red blood cells.

hemoptysis (he-mop′tĭ-sis) The expectoration of blood or blood-tinged sputum; the coughing up of blood.

hemorrhage (hem′or-ij) Bleeding.

hemorrhagic shock Shock resulting from blood loss.

hemorrhoid (hem′o-roid) Varicose dilation of a vein near the rectum.

hemothorax (he″mo-tho′raks) A collection of blood in the pleural cavity.

hepatitis (hep″ah-ti′tis) An infection of the liver caused by a virus that causes fever, loss of appetite, jaundice, and fatigue.

hepatitis A Type A (viral or infectious) hepatitis that is usually seen in children. It is a liver infection without serious consequences. Adults can be infected by their children or by ingestion of contaminated shellfish or water.

hepatitis B (serum hepatitis) Hepatitis caused by a virus that is spread through blood-to-blood contact (transfusion, needle stick), mucous membrane (saliva or sputum contact), or sexual contact. It is a serious disease with long-term side effects. Signs and symptoms are nausea, vomiting, fatigue, abdominal pain, and jaundice.

hernia The protrusion of a loop or knuckle of an organ or tissue through an abnormal body opening.

heroin (her′o-in) An opiate narcotic, often abused.

herpes (her′pēz) A spreading, recurrent skin eruption caused by infection from the herpes virus.

herpetic whitlow (her-pet′ik hwit′lo) A herpes virus infection of the finger.

hiccup (hik′up) A sudden inspiration of air that is rapidly checked by closure of the glottis, causing a characteristic sound.

hinge joint Joints that can bend and straighten but cannot rotate.

hip The joint where the femur articulates with the innominate bone.

hives (urticaria) (ur″tĭ-kār′e-ah) An allergic skin disorder marked by patches of swelling and intense itching; caused by contact with something to which the person is allergic.

HIV infection Infection of acquired immunodeficiency syndrome (AIDS).

hollow organs Tubes through which material passes, such as the stomach and intestines, ureters, and bladder.

hormone (hor′mōn) Chemical substance produced in the body by a gland that has special regulatory effects on the activity of another distant organ.

host The organism or individual attacked by the infecting agent.

hot line A dedicated telephone line between two specific points. It is always "open" or under the control of an individual at each end. The line is immediately available by lifting the receiver. Outside access cannot be obtained.

humeral condyles (hu′mer-al kon′dīlz) Bony prominences that form the medial and lateral borders of the upper surface of the elbow joint.

humerus (hu′mer-us) The supporting bone of the upper arm that articulates with the scapula to form the shoulder joint and with the ulna and radius to form the elbow joint.

humidification (hu-mid″ĭ-fi-kay′shun) Process of adding moisture during artificial ventilation to prevent pure oxygen from drying the patient's mucous membrane surfaces.

hydration (hi-dra′shun) The act of combining or causing to combine with water.

hydrocele A sac of water that is trapped about the testis or the spermatic cord.

hydrochloric acid (hi″dro-klor′ik as′id) A normal component of gastric juice.

hydrogen chloride (hi′dro-jen klo′rīd) hydrochloric acid.

hydrogen cyanide (hi′dro-jen si′ah-nīd) An extremely poisonous, colorless liquid or gas, HCN; inhalation can cause death within a minute.

hydroplaning (hi″dro-play′ning) Driving on tires lifted from the road surface by a sheet of water.

hyperbaric oxygen chamber A recompression chamber.

hypercapnia Excess of carbon dioxide in the blood.

hyperextension (hi″per-ek-sten′shun) Extreme extension or straightening of a limb or body part.

hyperflexion (hi″per-flek′shun) Forcible overflexion of a limb or part

hyperglycemia (hi″per-gli-se′me-ah) Abnormally increased glucose level in the blood; a factor in diabetic coma.

hypersensitive (hi″per-sen′sĭ-tiv) Allergic.

hypersensitive reaction Severe allergic reaction with

wheezing, cardiovascular collapse, and skin wheals (hives).

hypertension Abnormally and persistently high blood pressure.

hyperthermia (hi″per-ther′me-ah) A condition in which the internal body temperature increases above normal after prolonged exposure to heat.

hyperventilation (hi″per-ven″tĭ-la′shun) Rapid, deep breathing.

hyphema (hi-fe′me-ah) Bleeding into the anterior chamber of the eye, obscuring the iris.

hypnotic (hip-not′ik) Sleep inducing.

hypoglycemia (hi″po-gli-se′me-ah) Abnormally decreased glucose level in the blood.

hypotension (hi″po-ten′shun) Abnormally low blood pressure.

hypothermia (hi″po-ther′me-ah) A condition in which the internal body temperature falls below 95 degrees F after prolonged exposure to freezing or near-freezing temperatures.

hypovolemia (hi″po-vo-le′me-ah) A decrease in the volume of circulating blood or other body fluids.

hypovolemic shock Shock resulting from loss of body fluid or blood.

hypoxia (hi-pok′se-ah) A deficiency of oxygen reaching the tissues of the body.

hypoxic (hi-pok′sik) Oxygen-deficient.

hysteria (his″tēr′e-ah) A neurotic disturbance marked by excitement and self-consciousness, anxiety, symptoms of imaginary illness, and lack of emotional control.

idiopathic disease (id″e-o-path′ik dī-zēz) A disease of unknown cause.

ignite To catch on fire.

iliac arteries (il′e-ak ar′ter-ēz) Two branches of the aorta that carry blood to the lower extremities.

iliac crest The rim of the pelvic bone.

ileocecal valve (il″e-o-se′kal valv) Passage through which the contents of the small intestine empty into the large intestine. This valve allows passage of bowel contents in only one direction—into the colon.

ileum (il′e-um) The more distal portion of the small intestine between the jejunum and the colon.

ileus (il′e-us) Paralysis of bowel motility arising from any of a number of causes.

ilium (il′e-um) One of three bones (ilium, ischium, and pubis) that fuse to form the pelvic bones.

immersion foot (ĭ-mer′shun foot) A form of cold exposure that occurs when the feet suffer prolonged exposure to cold but not freezing water; also called trench foot.

immunity (ĭ-mu′nĭ″te) Exemptions granted by law to certain individuals or agencies freeing them from the burdens of compensating the injured or damaged individual.

immunization (im″u-ni-za′shun) The process by which resistance to an infectious disease is produced.

impaled foreign object (im-pay′eld for′en ob-jekt) An object such as a knife or splinter of wood or glass that penetrates the skin and remains in the body.

implied consent (im-plīd′ kon sent′) Consent that is given by the fact that the individual voluntarily entered a situation.

incident command system An accepted local protocol of assigning responsibility in advance to manage medical emergencies and natural disasters.

incomplete abortion Complication of abortion in which portions of the fetus or placenta are left in the uterus.

incontinence (in-kon′tĭ-nens) Involuntary emptying of bowels or bladder.

incubation period (in″ku-ba′shun pe′re-od) The time between exposure of the host to the infectious agent and the appearance of symptoms of that infection.

indirect contact Transmission of a communicable disease in which the person infected is not in direct contact with a host or carrier but touches some object that has been contaminated.

infarction (in-fark′shun) Death of tissue, usually caused by interruption of its blood supply.

infection (in-fek′shun) The invasion of a host or host tissue by organisms such as bacteria, viruses, or parasites.

infectious agent (in-fek′shus a′jent) The cause of an infectious disease, such as a virus, bacterium, or parasite.

infectious (communicable) diseases Diseases that can be transmitted from one person to another.

infectious disease Clinical disease resulting from an infection.

infectious hepatitis *See* hepatitis.

inferior (in-fēr′e-or) Referring to the lower portion of an organ or other structure.

inferior portion That portion of the body or body part that lies nearer to the feet than to the head.

inferior vena cava (in-fēr′e or ve′na ka′vah) One of the two largest veins in the body that carry blood from the lower extremities and the pelvic and abdominal organs into the heart.

infiltration (in″fil-tra′shun) A condition in which the fluid from intravenous therapy enters the surrounding subcutaneous tissue instead of the vein.

informed consent Consent given by a person who understands the nature and extent of any procedure before agreeing to it and who has sufficient mental and physical capacity to make such a judgment.

infusion (in-fu′zhun) The introduction of fluid other than blood or blood products into the vascular system.

ingestion (in-jes′chun) Swallowing; taking a substance by mouth.

inguinal hernia (ing′gwi-nal her′ne-ah) A common congenital defect in which a loop of intestine descends into the inguinal canal in the groin.

inguinal ligament (ing′gwi-nal lig′ah-ment) Tough, fibrous ligament that stretchs between the lateral edge of the pubic symphysis and the anterior superior iliac spine.

inhalant (in-ha′lant) A substance that is or may be taken into the body by way of the nose and trachea, or through the respiratory system.

inhalation (in″hah-la′shun) The drawing of air or other substances into the lungs.

inhalation injuries Injuries resulting from inhaling chemical fumes.

injection (in-jec′shun) Forcing a fluid into, as for medical purposes.

inoculation (ĭ-nok″u-la′shun) Introduction of a disease agent such as vaccine virus into a healthy person to produce a mild form of the disease followed by immunity.

insertion (in-ser′shun) Place of attachment of a muscle.

inspiration (in″spĭ-ra′shun) Inhaling; breathing in, or drawing air into the lungs.

institutional standards Specific rules and procedures of the ambulance service or organization with which the EMT is affiliated.

insulator (in′su-la″tor) Any substance that prevents an electrical current from flowing.

insulin (in′su-lin) A hormone produced by the pancreas that enables sugar in the blood to enter the cells of the body; insulin is used in the treatment and control of diabetes mellitus.

insulin-dependent diabetics Diabetics who must take one or more injections of insulin every day.

insulin shock Unconsciousness in a diabetic patient caused by hypoglycemia; often the result of extensive exercise or failure to eat after a routine dose of insulin.

Interagency Radiological Assistance Plan (IRAP) A national plan developed to provide professional guidance and assistance in the event of an accident involving radioactive materials.

intercostal (in″ter-kos′tal) Between the ribs.

intercourse (in′ter-kōrs) A sexual joining of two individuals during which seminal fluid, prostatic fluid, and sperm pass from the penis into the vagina during ejaculation.

interference (in″ter-fēr′ens) Stray or undesirable signals on the ECG tracing.

internal jugular vein (in-ter′nal jug′u-lar vān) Major vein draining the brain.

intertrochanteric fracture (in″ter-tro″kan-ter′ik frak′chur) A hip fracture

intervertebral disc (in″ter-ver′te-bral disk) A cushion between two vertebral bodies.

intestine (in-tes′tin) The part of the alimentary canal extending from the stomach to the anus.

intoxicated (in-toks′i-kay′ted) Affected by alcohol or another drug to the point of losing physical and mental control.

intraabdominal (in″trah-ab-dom′ĭ-nal) Within the abdomen.

intracerebral (in″trah-ser′ĕ-bral) Inside or within the brain.

intracerebral hematoma (in″trah-ser′ĕ-bral hem″ah-to′mah) A hematoma, or collection of blood, inside the brain tissue itself.

intracranial (in″trah-kra′ne-al) Within the skull.

intracranial pressure (in″trah-kra′ne-al presh′ur) Pressure from the brain swelling inside the rigid bony skull.

intramuscular Within the muscle.

intraperitoneal (in″trah-per′ĭ-to-ne′al) Within the peritoneal cavity.

intrathoracic (in″trah-tho-ras′ik) Within the chest.

intravascular (in″trah-vas′ku-lar) Within the vessel.

intravenous (in″trah-ve′nus) Within the vein.

intravenous fluid therapy (IV therapy) Infusion of fluid other than blood or blood products into the vascular system to establish and maintain access to the circulation or to provide fluids in order to maintain an adequate circulatory blood volume.

intravenous line A polyethylene catheter through which fluids are given directly into a vein.

intubation (in′tu-ba-shun) The placement of a tube in the airway to improve ventilation.

involuntary muscle Muscle that continues to contract, rhythmically, regardless of the conscious will of the individual.

involuntary (autonomic) nervous system That part of the nervous system that regulates functions not controlled by a voluntary act of conscious will, such as digestion or sweating.

ionizing radiation (i″on-īz-ing ra-de-a′shun) Nuclear radiation that has the capacity to alter body cells.

ipecac *See* syrup of ipecac.

iris (i′ris) The muscle and surrounding tissue behind the cornea that dilate and constrict the pupil, regulating the amount of light that enters the eye.

irrigation (ir″ĭ-ga′shun) Washing by a stream of water or other fluid.

ischemic (is-kem′ik) Lacking oxygen.

ischial tuberosities (is′ke-al too″bŏ-ros′i-tēz) The bony prominences felt in the middle of each buttock.

ischium (is′ke-um) One of three bones (ilium, ischium, and pubis) that fuse to form the pelvic bones. The two pelvic bones, together with the sacrum, form the pelvic ring.

islets of Langerhans (i′lets lahng′er-hanz) Glands scattered throughout the pancreas that produce insulin.

jaundice (jawn′dis) The deposition of bile pigment in the skin and mucous membrane resulting in a yellow appearance of the patient.

jaw-thrust maneuver Opening the airway by bringing the patient's jaw forward and pulling the lower lip down.

jejunum (jĕ-joo′num) That portion of the small intestine that extends from the duodenum to the ileum.

joint The place where two bones come in contact.

joint capsule (joint kap′sūl) A fibrous sac with synovial lining that encloses a joint.

joules (joolz) A measure of the electrical current delivered by defibrillators.

jugular notch The superior border of the sternum.

jump kit A lightweight, durable, waterproof kit used in the immediate care of the patient, usually by the EMT who initially leaves the vehicle while the EMT-driver parks the ambulance and secures the scene.

juvenile diabetics (joo′vĕ-nil di″ah-be′tiks) Children who have to take insulin every day.

ketoacidosis *See* diabetic ketoacidosis.

ketones Metabolic end products of the use of fat for routine energy needs.

kidneys The two retroperitoneal organs that excrete the end products of metabolism as urine and regulate the body's salt and water content.

kidney stone A stone that passes from the kidney into the ureter where it causes excruciating pain until it enters the bladder.

kinetic energy (kĭ-net′ik en′er-je) Energy associated with motion.

knee joint The articulation between the distal femur and the proximal tibia.

Kussmaul respiration Air hunger, manifested by deep sighing respirations.

labor The process by which the muscles of the uterus open the birth canal and push the baby down and through so that it can be born.

laceration (las″er-a′shun) A cut that may leave a smooth or jagged wound through the skin, subcutaneous tissues, muscles, and associated nerves and blood vessels.

lacrimal gland (lak′rĭ-mal gland) Tear duct.

lacrimal system (lak′rĭ-mal sis′tem) The tear glands and ducts of the eyes.

land mobile service Specified by the Federal Communications Commission (FCC); mobile communication service between a base station and mobile stations on land, or between two mobile stations on land.

large intestine (lärj in-tes′tin) The portion of the digestive tube that extends from the ileocecal valve to the anus. It is made up of the cecum, colon, and rectum.

laryngectomy (lar″in-jek′to-me) Surgical removal of the larynx.

laryngoscope (lah-ring′go-skōp) An instrument used to give a direct view of the patient's vocal cords during endotracheal intubation.

laryngospasm (lah-ring′go-spazm) A severe constriction of the vocal cords.

larynx (lar′niks) Voice box; a structure composed of thyroid cartilage on the top and cricoid cartilage on the bottom. It guards the entrance to the trachea and functions secondarily as the organ of voice.

laser (la′zer) A device that produces a beam of nonspreading, monochromatic, visible light. High energies are concentrated into a narrow beam.

LAST An acronym for locate, access, stabilize, and transport; the four stages of the work phase of a disaster response.

lateral (lat′er-al) Away from the midline of the body or a structure.

lateral malleolus (lat′er-al mah-le′o-lus) The bony prominence at the end of the fibula that, together with the medial malleolus, forms the socket of the ankle joint.

lateral structure Any part of the body that lies at some distance from the midline.

leg The lower extremity; specifically, the lower portion, from the knee to the ankle.

lens The transparent part of the eye through which images are focused on the retina.

letdown phase The period that follows the work phase, in which the EMT recovers from the disaster.

leukemia (loo-ke′me-ah) Cancer of the blood; characterized by an abnormal increase in the production of white blood cells and pathological changes in the bone marrow and other lymphoid tissue.

leukocyte (loo′ko-sīt) A white blood cell.

leukopenia (loo″ko-pe′ne-ah) Decrease in white blood cells.

levator palpebrae (le-va′tor pal′pĕ-brā) The muscle that lifts the upper eyelid.

level of consciousness The degree of alertness or awareness of the patient.

Level One Trauma Center A medical center for severely injured patients.

licensure Formal permission to perform certain acts.

ligament (lig′ah-ment) A band of the fibrous tissue that connect bones to bones. It supports and strengthens a joint.

limb presentation A delivery in which the baby's arm or leg appears first rather than the head.

lipid Fat.

lips Upper and lower fleshy margins of the mouth.

liter Base unit of capacity in the metric system.

litter A type of stretcher for moving or carrying patients.

liver A large solid organ that lies in the upper right quadrant. It produces bile, stores sugar for immediate use by the body, and chemically treats all products of absorption in the gastrointestinal tract.

liver mortis Discoloration appearing on dependent parts of the body after death, caused by pooling of the blood.

lividity (lĭ-vid'ĭ-te) Discoloration of dependent body parts by the gravitation of the blood.

living will A legal document with specific instructions stating whether the patient wants to be resuscitated or kept alive by mechanical life support systems.

lobe (lōb) The dependent fleshy portion of any structure such as the bottom of each ear.

lobulated (lob'u-lāt"ed) Consisting of lobes, as, for example, one of the surfaces of the placenta.

localized abdominal tenderness Tenderness in a specific part of the abdomen.

lower airway The larynx, the trachea, the major bronchi, and the other air passages within the lung.

lower urinary tract Bladder and urethra.

low volume (hypovolemic) shock Shock resulting from loss of body fluids or blood.

lucid (loo'sid) Alert, aware of surroundings, able to communicate.

lucid interval Time in which the patient seems normal between periods of unconsciousness.

lumbar spine (lum'bar spīn) The lower part of the back formed by the lowest five nonfused vertebrae.

lumbar vertebrae Vertebrae of the lumbar spine.

lumbosacral plexus (lum"bo-sa'kral plek'sus) A network of nerves originating from branches of the spinal nerves; the network is located in the lower extremity.

lumen (loo'men) The inside diameter of an artery or other hollow structure.

lungs The organs that aerate the blood; they occupy the lateral cavities of the chest and are separated from each other by the heart and mediastinal structures.

main bronchi (sing. main bronchus) (mān brong'ki) The two major branches of the trachea that lead into the left and right lungs.

malaria (mah-la're-ah) Parasitic tropical disease with cyclic fever, chills, and fatigue.

malingering (mah-ling'ger-ing) A condition in which a patient pretends to have an illness or injury.

malignant (mah-lig'nant) Cancerous.

malleolus (pl. malleoli) (mah-le'o-lus) The rounded projection on either side of the ankle joint.

mandible (man'di-b'l) The bone of the lower jaw.

mania (ma'ne-ah) A mental state in which the patient is hyperactive, ranging from mildly agitated to wildly uncontrollable.

manually controlled resuscitator (man'u-al-ē kon-trōld re-sus"ĭ-ta'tor) A resuscitator with manual control, used in ambulances.

manubrium (mah-nu'bre-um) One of three components (manubrium, body, and xiphoid process) of the sternum; the upper quarter of the sternum.

marijuana (mar"ĭ-hwah'nah) Extract from the plant top of the lowering hemp plant *Cannabus sativa* that when inhaled as smoke produces euphoria, relaxation, and drowsiness. It is often referred to as "pot."

mask and reservoir bag system A system of artificial ventilation in which the oxygen inflow fills a bag that is attached to a mask by a one-way valve.

mastoid process (mas'toid pros'es) A prominent, hard bony mass at the base of the skull behind the ear.

maturity onset diabetes *See* adult onset diabetes.

maxilla (pl. maxillae) (mak-sil'ah) The bone that forms the upper jaw on either side of the face; it contains the upper teeth, the orbit of the eye, the nasal cavity, and the palate.

measles Acute viral disease with fever, bronchitis, and red blotchy rash.

mechanism of injury Factors involved in producing the injury.

MEDEVAC A method of speeding lifesaving care to patients and of transporting patients with life-threatening injury or illness to treatment facilities using medically equipped helicopters.

medial (me'de-al) Pertaining to the middle; closer to the midline of the body or a structure.

medial malleolus (me'de-al mah-le'o-lus) The bony prominence at the end of the tibia that, together with the lateral malleolus, forms the socket of the ankle joint.

medial structure Any part of the body that lies close to the midline.

mediastinum (me"de-as-ti'num) The space between the lungs in which lie the heart, great vessels, esophagus, trachea, major bronchi, and many nerves.

medical disaster An incident that will overload the capabilities and resources of the local medical community.

medic-alert A bracelet, necklace, or card stating the patient's medical problems.

medical examiner A public officer who makes postmortem examinations of bodies to find the cause of death.

medicolegal (med″ĭ-ko-le′gal) Relating to both medicine and law.

medium rescue Rescue operations that involve specialized equipment normally found during a rescue.

melanin (mel′ah-nin) The pigment in the skin.

melena The passage of dark black stools that have the consistency of tar.

meninges (mě-nin′jēz) The three layers of tissue that envelop the brain and spinal cord: the dura mater, pia mater, and arachnoid.

meningitis (měn-in-ji′tis) An inflammation of the menigeal coverings of the brain; it can be caused by a virus or a bacterium.

meniscus (mě-nis′kus) A cushion of cartilage that fills up a space between bones and aids in the gliding motion of the joint.

menopause (men′o-pawz) Cessation of menstruation in the human female, occurring usually around the age of 50.

menstrual cycle The period of the regularly recurring changes in the uterus that result in blood and mucus being shed intermittently, usually every 28 days.

menstruation (men″stroo-a′shun) A periodic bleeding from the vagina that occurs at approximately four-week intervals, in which the lining of the uterus is shed.

meprobamate (mě-pro′bah-māt) A nonbarbiturate depressant drug.

mesentery (mes′en-ter″e) The delicate tissue formed by the peritoneum that suspends the organs within the abdomen and carries blood vessels and nerves to all these organs.

metabolic shock Shock caused by profound fluid losses from vomiting, diarrhea, or excess urination.

metabolism (mě-tab′o-lizm) The sum of all the physical and chemical processes of living organisms; the process by which energy is made available for the uses of the organism.

metacarpal bone (metacarpal) (met″ah-kar′pal bōn) Any of the five bones of the hand that extend from the wrist to the fingers.

metastasis (mě-tas′tah-sis) The transfer of a disease (usually a tumor) from one organ or part to another not directly connected with it.

metatarsal bones (metatarsals) The five long bones of the foot between the instep and the toes.

microcurie (mi″kro-ku′re) A finer subdivision of curie, a unit of measure of radiation from beta particles.

microwave A term applied to radio waves in the frequency range of 1,000 MHz and upward; the signals are generated by special equipment that depends on line-of-sight placement to operate properly.

middle ear The tympanic cavity with its ossicles.

midline The median line or median plane of the body.

midwife A woman who assists in childbirth.

mild diabetes *See* adult onset diabetes.

millicurie A finer subdivision of curie, a unit of measure of radiation from beta particles.

milliliter (mil′ĭ-le″ter) One-thousandth of a liter.

millimeters of mercury (mm Hg) (mil′ĭ-le″terz, mer′ku-re) Unit of pressure, used in measuring blood pressure.

milliroentgen (mil′ĭ-rent″gen) One-thousandth of a roentgen.

mineral A nonorganic substance usually occurring in the earth's crust.

mini-drip set A type of administration set for intravenous fluid therapy that is designed to keep an IV line open; it flows with minimal volume infusion.

minor burn Any third-degree burn that involves less than 2 percent of the body surface or a second-degree burn that involves less than 15 percent of the body surface.

minor's consent Consent given by person under legal age (usually 21).

miscarriage (abortion) (mis-kar′ij) Delivery of the fetus before 20 weeks gestation, for any reason.

mittelschmerz (mit′el-shmarts) Intermenstrual pain.

mobile relay station A fixed base station established for the automatic retransmission of mobile or portable radio communications.

mobile repeater station A mobile radio station in land mobile service that is authorized to automatically retransmit any radio traffic originated by a hand-held portable, by other mobiles, or by base stations.

mode of transmission The method of transfer of a communicable disease.

moderate burn Any burn that is less serious than a critical burn. These burns include third-degree burns that involve 2 to 10 percent of the body surface (excluding hands, feet, face, or genitalia); second-degree burns that involve 15 to 25 percent of the body surface; and first-degree burns that involve 50 to 75 percent of the body surface.

monitor A person who receives, and often records, radio messages without transmitting; to listen to radio messages without transmitting.

monitoring Checking constantly on physiological signs (cardiac, respiratory). *See also* monitor.

mononucleosis (mon″o-nu″kle-o′sis) Acute viral disease of the lumph nodes with fever and sore throat.

monoplegia (mon″o-ple′je-ah) Paralysis of one extremity.

monozygotic twins (mon″o-zi-got′ik twinz) Identical twins; they must both be of the same sex.

morphine (mor′fēn) A narcotic drug, a derivative of opium.

motor nerve A nerve that transmit impulses to muscles, causing them to move.

mouth The lips, cheeks, gums, teeth, and tongue.

mouth-to-mask ventilation A system of artificial ventilation in which the EMT ventilates the patient with supplemental oxygen through a mask while supplying air from his or her own lungs at the same time.

mouth-to-mouth ventilation Artificial ventilation in which the EMT's mouth makes a seal around the patient's mouth as the EMT exhales into the patient's mouth. The patient's nostrils are kept pinched together.

mouth-to-nose-and-mouth ventilation Artificial ventilation in which the EMT's mouth makes a seal around an infant's mouth and nose as the EMT exhales into both, simultaneously.

mouth-to-nose ventilation Artificial ventilation in which the EMT's lips makes a seal around the patient's nose as the EMT exhales into the patient's nose. The patient's mouth is kept closed, although sometimes the lips are spread apart during exhalation by the patient.

mouth-to-stoma ventilation Artificial ventilation for patients who, because of surgical removal of the larynx, have a tracheal stoma. The EMT blows into the tube. Usually the patient's mouth and nose are covered to prevent air from leaking up the trachea.

mucous membrane (mu′kus mem′brān) The lining of body cavities and passages that communicate directly or indirectly with the environment outside the body.

mucus (mu′kus) The opague, sticky secretion of the mucous membranes that lubricates the body openings.

multigravida (mul″tĭ-grav′ĭ-dah) A woman who has been pregnant more than one time.

multiplex (mul′tĭ-pleks) The ability to transmit simultaneously two or more different types of information in either or both directions over the same frequency.

mumps Acute viral disease with fever, swelling, and tenderness of the salivary glands.

muscle pull A stretched or torn muscle.

musculoskeletal (mus″ku-lo-skel′ĕ-tal) Pertaining to or composing the skeleton and the muscles, as the musculoskeletal system.

musculotendinous unit (mus″ku-lo-ten′dĭ-nus u′nit) The portion of fascia that extends beyond the muscle to attach to a bone; it crosses the joint and is responsible for movement of that joint.

mutation (mu-ta′shun) Altered heredity of offspring.

myocardial (mi″o-kar′de-al) Of the heart muscle.

myocardial contusion A bruise of the heart muscle.

myocardial infarction (mi″o-kar′de-al in-fark′shun) Heart attack; damage or death of an area of the heart muscle.

myocardium (mi″o-kar′de-um) The heart muscle.

narcosis (nar-ko′sis) Stupor or anesthesia produced by a narcotic drug.

narcotic (nar-kot′ik) An agent producing insensitivity or stupor.

narcotized (nar′ka-tīzd) A condition in which the respiratory center becomes depressed, with lower than normal activity; it is caused by high levels of carbon dioxide in the blood.

nasal Pertaining to the nose.

nasal bone One of the four major bones of the face.

nasal cannula (na′zal kan′u-lah) A tube for insertion into the nose; oxygen can be administered with it, through two small tubular prongs that fit into the nostrils.

nasal mucosa (na′zal mu-ko′sah) Membranes in the nasal passages that contain mucus-secreting glands.

nasal septum (na′zal sep′tum) The partition separating the two nostrils; composed of membrane, cartilage, and bone.

nasopharyngeal airway (na″zo-fah-rin′je-al ār′wa) An artificial airway placed in the nasal cavity.

nasopharynx (na″zo-far′inks) The part of the pharynx that lies above the level of the soft palate.

near drowning Survival, at least temporarily, after submersion in water.

neck of a bone The region below the head of the bone.

necrosis (nĕ-kro′sis) Destruction and death of tissue.

negligence (neg′li″jens) Failure to perform an important or necessary technique or performance of such a technique in a careless or unskilled manner so as to cause further injury.

neonate (ne′o-nāt) A newborn infant.

neoplasm (ne′o-plazm) Any new and abnormal growth such as a tumor.

nerve root The proximal (nearest) end of a spinal nerve.

nerves Branches from the spinal cord and brain; either sensory, motor, or a combination of both.

nervous system The brain, spinal cord, and nerves.

neurogenic shock (nu″ro-jen′ik shok) Circulatory failure caused by paralysis of the nerves that control the size of the blood vessels, seen in spinal cord injuries.

neurological (nu-ro-loj′ik-l) Relating to the branch of medical science that has to do with the nervous system and its disorders.

neuron (nu′ron) A nerve cell; the fundamental functional unit of nervous tissue.

neurosurgical (nu′ro-sur′ji-kl) Relating to surgery on any part of the nervous system.

neurotoxic (nu″ro-tok′sik) Poisonous to nerve tissue.

neutralize (nu'tral-īz) To render neutral; specifically, the chemical combination of hydrogen and hydroxyl ions to form water, thus rendering each ion harmless.

neutron The particle of an atom that has no electrical charge.

nicotine (nik'o-tēn) A mild stimulant that is present in tobacco that accounts for the addictive nature of cigarette smoking.

nitrogen (ni'tro-jen) A colorless, gaseous element; when released as bubbles of gas under conditions of reduced atmospheric pressure, it can cause serious sickness because of arterial embolization.

nitroglycerin (ni-tro-glis'er-in) A medicine used in treating angina pectoris; the medication relaxes vascular smooth muscle and increases blood flow and oxygen supply to the heart muscle.

nocturia (nok-tu're-ah) Excessive urination at night.

non-A, non-B hepatitis Viral hepatitis that is usually related to a transfusion or contaminated needle stick; the causative virus is unknown.

nonconductive Not transmitting an electrical current or any other source of energy.

nondisplaced fracture A fracture in which there is no deformity of the limb.

noninsulin-dependent diabetes The form of diabetes that can be managed without using insulin for control of blood sugar.

normal sinus rhythm The coordinated pumping contractions of a healthy, normal heart.

nose The part of the face that serves as an organ of smell; part of the respiratory system.

nostril One of the two external openings of the nose.

nuclear (nu'kle-ar) Relating to the atomic nucleus.

nutrients (nu'tre-ents) Substances that furnish nourishment to the body.

obesity (o-bēs'ĭ-te) Excessive body weight; an excessive amount of body fat.

obstetrical (ob-stet're-kal) Relating to childbirth.

occipital region (ok-sip'ĭ-tal re'jun) *See* occiput.

occiput (ok'sĭ-put) The most posterior (back) portion of the cranium (head).

occlude (ŏ-klood) To close or block.

occlusion (o-kloo'zhun) Blockage.

occlusive dressing (ŏ-kloo'siv dres'ing) A dressing or bandage that closes a wound and protects it from the air.

olecranon process (o-lek'rah-non pros'es) The superior tip of the ulna that forms most of the elbow joint where the ulna and radius articulate with the humerus.

open (penetrating) abdominal injury Any injury of the abdomen caused by a penetrating or piercing instru-

ment or force in which the skin is lacerated or perforated and the cavity itself opened to air.

open chest injuries Injuries to the chest in which the chest wall has been penetrated by some object such as a knife or bullet.

open fracture A fracture in which there is an external wound that communicates within the fracture site.

open wound Injury caused by a penetrating object that breaks the skin or the mucous membranes.

opium (o'pe-um) A bitter additive narcotic drug that consists of the dried juice of the opium poppy.

opium analgesic (o'pe-um an"al-je'zik) A pain medication that is a natural or synthetic derivative of opium from poppy seeds. These drugs include heroin, morphine, Demerol®, Dilaudid®, and Methadone®.

optic nerve (op'tik nerv) A cranial nerve that transmits visual sensations to the brain.

opportunistic infections Infections by organisms that do not commonly cause disease in humans.

oral content Contents of the mouth.

orbicularis oculi (or-bik'u-lar-is ok'u-li) The circular muscle around the eye whose contraction closes the eyelids.

orbit The eye socket.

orchitis (or-ki'tis) Inflammation of a testes.

organic brain syndrome A disease of the brain in which the patient's mental functioning is impaired, usually by old age or other disease; a cause of disruptive behavior.

organism An individual equipped to carry on the activities of life; a living being.

orifice An opening to the body (such as the mouth, nose, anus, or vagina).

origin The more fixed end or attachment of a muscle.

oropharyngeal Pertaining to the oropharynx, that division of the pharynx that lies between the soft palate and the upper edge of the epiglottis.

oropharyngeal airway (o"ro-fah-rin'je-al ār'wa) An artificial airway positioned in the mouth to prevent blockage of the upper airway by the tongue.

os calcis (calcaneus) The heel bone.

osteoporosis Reduction in the amount of bone mass, leading to fractures after minimal trauma.

ova (eggs) *See* ovum.

ovary Female gland that produces sex hormones and ova (eggs).

overdose An excessive dose of a drug.

ovum (o'vum) Female reproductive cell that, when fertilized by the sperm, develops a new member of the same species.

oxygen (O$_2$) (ok'sĭ-jen) A gas that is necessary for breathing and is found free in the air.

oxygenated (ok'sĭ-jĕ-nāt'ed) Supplied with oxygen.

oxygen exchange The process by which oxygen is provided to the blood, and carbon dioxide is taken from the blood to be expelled in the expired air.

pacemaker A device generally implanted under a heavy muscle or fold of skin that maintains a regular cardiac rhythm and rate by delivering an electrical impulse through wires that are in direct contact.

packaging The positioning, covering, and securing of an ill or injured patient for transportation.

pack years A measure of cigarette smoking: one package of cigarettes per day per year is a one-pack year.

paging A common alerting system that involves the use of a coded tone radio signal, and sometimes a voice message, transmitted to small individual radio receivers called "beepers."

palate (pal′āt) The roof of the mouth.

pallor (pal′or) Paleness; absence of skin color.

palmar (pal′mar) Pertaining to the palm.

palpate (pal′pāt) Feel; to examine by touch.

palpation (pal-pa′shun) Examination by touch.

pancreas (pan′kre-as) A large, elongated gland situated transversely behind the stomach, between the spleen and the duodenum; it is a major source of digestive enzymes and produces the hormone insulin, which regulates the metabolism of sugar.

pancreatic juice (pan″kre-at′ik joos) Juice secreted by the pancreas, which contains many enzymes acting in the digestion of fat, starch, and protein; pancreatic juice flows directly into the duodenum through the pancreatic ducts.

pancreatitis (pan″kre-ah-ti′tis) Inflammation of the pancreas.

paradoxical motion (par″ah-dok′se-kal mo-shun) The motion of the flail segment of a flail chest that is opposite to the normal chest wall movement.

paralysis (pah-ral′is-sis) The inability of a conscious patient to move voluntarily.

paramedic A trained professional EMT who provides sophisticated advanced life support in the field.

paranoia (par″ah-noi′ah) A mental state in which the patient believes that others are talking about or plotting against him or her.

paraplegia (par″ah-ple′je-ah) Paralysis of the lower limbs.

parasite An organism that lives within another living organism at whose expense it obtains some advantage.

parasitic (par-ah-sit′ik) Relating to parasites.

parasympathetic nervous system (par″ah-sim″pah-thet′ik ner′vus sis′tem) A part of the autonomic nervous system that causes blood vessels to dilate, slows the heart rate, and relaxes muscle sphincters.

parathyroid gland (par″ah-thi′roid gland) A gland that controls calcium levels in the blood, bone, and body fluids.

parietal (pah-rī′e-tal) Of or pertaining to the walls of a cavity; pertaining to or located near the parietal bone.

parietal peritoneum (pah-rī′e-tal per″i-to-ne′um) The portion of the peritoneum that lines the walls of the abdominal and pelvic cavities and the undersurface of the diaphragm.

parietal pleura (pah-ri′ĕ-tal ploor′ah) A smooth, glistening layer of tissue that lines the chest wall.

parietal region The more lateral portion of the cranium that lies between the temporal region and the occiput.

partial seizure An epileptic seizure involving a less extensive area of the brain than a generalized seizure.

patch A special connection between different communication systems—for example, the connection that allows a radio transmission to be carried over a telephone line.

patella (pah-tel′ah) The kneecap; a specialized bone that lies within the tendon of the quadriceps muscle.

pathogen Any disease-producing microorganism.

pathologic fracture (path″o-loj′ik frak′chur) A fracture that occurs from minimal force because the bone is weak or diseased.

pedal edema (ped′al ĕ-de′mah) Edema of the feet, usually seen in congestive heart failure.

pediatrics (pe″de-at′riks) Medical practice devoted to the care of children up to age 15.

pedicle (ped′ĭ-k′l) An elongated, somewhat slender anatomical structure resembling the stalk of a plant.

pelvic cavity (pel′vik kav′i-te) The space within the walls of the pelvis.

pelvic girdle The bony structure formed by the sacrum and the iliac bones that contain the abdominal and pelvic organs.

pelvic inflammatory disease (PID) (pel′vik in-flam′ah-to″re dĭ-zēz′) An infection in the Fallopian tube and the surrounding tissue of the pelvis.

pelvic outlet A layer of muscles that forms the inferior boundary of the pelvic cavity, with openings for the gastrointestinal tract, the female reproductive system, and the urinary tract.

pelvis A closed bony ring, consisting of the sacrum and two pelvic bones, that connects the trunk to the lower extremities.

penetrating (open) abdominal injury An injury in which a foreign body has entered the abdomen and opened the peritoneum-lined cavity to the outside.

penetrating chest injury Injury in which an object such as a knife or bullet has penetrated the chest wall.

penetrating injury Injury in which the force of impact is concentrated on a small point of contact between the skin and the wounding implement, creating an open wound.

penicillin (pen"ĭ-sil'in) An antibiotic extracted from culture of certain molds.

penis (pe'nis) The male organ of urinary excretion and copulation (sexual intercourse).

pentobarbital (pen"to-bar'bĭt-tal) A short- to intermediate-acting barbiturate occurring as a white, fine powder, used as a sedative.

pepsin (pep'sin) The only digestive enzyme produced in the stomach; it initiates the digestion of protein.

peptic ulcer (pep'tik ul'ser) Ulcer in the stomach or duodenum caused by the action of pepsin.

perforated tympanic membrane (per'fo-rāt"ed tim-pan'ik mem'brān) Ruptured eardrum.

perforating (through and through) wounds Wounds that traverse an entire limb to exit on the opposite side.

perforation (per"fo-ra'shun) A hole made through a part or substance.

perfusion (per-fu'zhun) The process whereby blood enters an organ or tissue through its arteries and leaves through the veins, providing tissue with nourishment and removing wastes.

pericardial sac (per"ĭ-kar'de-al sak) The sac that surrounds the heart and the root of the great vessels.

pericardial tamponade (per"ĭ-kar'de-al tam"pon-ād') Acute compression of the heart due to a buildup of fluid or blood in the pericardial sac.

pericardium (per"ĭ-kar'de-um) The fibrous sac that surrounds the heart.

perineum (per-i-ne'um) The space between the anus and the scrotum; the pelvic floor and associated structures.

periodic symptoms Symptoms that recur at intervals.

period of communicability The time during which an infectious agent may be transmitted to a host from another carrier.

peripheral nerve (pĕ-rif'er-al nerv) Nerve that carries electrical impulses to and from the cells in the brain.

peripheral nervous system The part of the nervous system that consists of 31 pairs of spinal nerves and 12 pairs of cranial nerves. These peripheral nerves may be sensory nerves or motor nerves.

peristalsis (per"ĭ-stal'sis) The wavelike movement by which the alimentary canal or other tubular organs propel their contents.

peristaltic contraction (per"i-stal'tik kon-trak'shun) The action of muscles to propel the contents of the intestines.

peritoneal cavity (per"ĭ-to-ne'al kav'ĭ-te) The abdominal cavity.

peritoneum (per"i-to-ne'um) The membrane lining the abdominal cavity (parietal peritoneum) and reflected inward over the abdominal organs (visceral peritoneum).

peritonitis (per"ĭ-to-ni'tis) Inflammation of the peritoneum.

peroneal nerve (per"o-ne'al nerv) A nerve lying below the head of the fibula that controls movement at the ankle and supplies sensation to the top of the foot.

personal flotation device A life jacket used during water rescue.

pH A scale used to represent acidity and alkalinity; a pH of 7 is neutral, one less than 7 shows increasing acidity (acidosis), and one greater than 7 shows increasing alkalinity (alkalosis).

phalanx (pl. phalanges) (fah'lanks) Any of the 14 bones that form the toes and fingers.

pharyngeal (fah-rin'je-al) Relating to the pharynx.

pharyngneal suctions tip (tonsil tip) Large-bore tip that fastens onto suction tubing used to suction the pharynx.

pharynx (far'inks) The throat; the cavity at the back of the nose and mouth.

phenobarbital (fe"no-bar'bĭ-tal) A barbiturate drug used as a sedative.

phlebitis (flĕ-bi'tis) Inflammation in the vein.

phosgene (fos'jen) A suffocating and highly poisonous war gas, carbonyl chloride, $COCl_2$.

phrenic nerve (fren'ik nerv) Nerve of the diaphragm.

physiologic (fiz"e-o-loj'ik) Characteristic of the state or functioning of the body or of a tissue or organ.

physiology (fiz"e-ol'o-je) A branch of biology that deals with the functions and actions of living matter and the physical and chemical factors involved.

pia mater (pi'ah ma'ter) Innermost of the three layers of tissue that envelop the brain and spinal cord.

pin-indexing safety attachment A safety system on a compressed gas cylinder that consists of a series of pins on the yoke that must be matched with the holes on the yoke attachment of the gas cylinder if a satisfactory connection is to be made.

"pink eye" (conjunctivitis) Inflammation of the conjunctiva of the eye.

pinna (pin'nah) The external part of the ear.

pit viper A poisonous snake with a triangular head, fangs, and a heat-sensitive pit between its nostril and eye.

placenta (plah-sen'tah) The afterbirth that grows during pregnancy, through which all the nutrients for the fetus pass during development.

placenta abruptio (plah-sen'tah ab-rup'she-o) Premature separation of the placenta from the wall of the uterus through which the baby receives its nourishment and gets rid of waste products. After the birth of the baby, the placenta is expelled through the birth canal.

placenta previa (plah-sen'tah pre'vi-ə) Development of

the placenta over the mouth of the uterus; severe hemorrhage results.

plasma (plaz′mah) A sticky, yellow component of blood that carries the blood cells and nutrients and transports cellular waste material to the organs of excretion.

plasma expander A fluid used for intravenous infusion; examples include Dextran® (large molecules of dextrose that are not metabolized) and Plasmanate®.

plastic catheter embolus A complication of intravenous fluid therapy in which the end of the catheter is sheared off by the needle point after venipuncture.

platelet Tiny disc-shaped element that is a component of blood; it is essential to the process of blood clot formation—the mechanism that stops bleeding.

plethoric (ple-thor′ik) Dark, reddish-purple skin color due to filling of all visible blood vessels.

pleura (ploor′ah) The serous membrane covering the lungs and lining the thoracic cavity, completely enclosing a potential space known as the pleural space.

pleural space (ploor′al spās) The potential space between the parietal pleura and the visceral pleura. It is described as "potential" because under normal conditions the lungs fill this space.

pleurisy (ploor′ĭ-se) Inflammation of the pleura.

pleuritic chest pain (ploo-rit′ik chest pān) Pain in the chest with respirations.

pleuritic pain (ploo-rit′ik pān) *See* pleuritic chest pain.

plexus (plek′sus) Complex nerve network.

pneumatic counterpressure device (nu-mat′ik kown′ter presh′ur dĕ-vīs) Large air splint for the lower half of the body to provide stability for severe pelvic, hip, and femoral fractures, and to combat shock.

pneumatic trouser *See* pneumatic counterpressure device.

pneumomediastinim (nu″mo-me″de-as-ti′num) The presence of air or gas in the mediastinum.

pneumonia (nu-mo′ne-ah) An infectious disease of the lung tissue.

pneumothorax (nu″mo-tho′raks) An accumulation of air or gas in the pleural cavity.

pocket mask Mask with an oxygen inlet that allows you to ventilate the patient with air from your own lungs while at the same time supplying supplemental oxygen.

point tenderness Tenderness at the site of injury or disease, which can be located by gently pressing with one finger.

poison Any substance that, when ingested, inhaled, or absorbed, or when applied to, infected into, or developed within the body, in relatively small amounts, by its chemical actions, may cause damage to structures or disturbance of function.

poliomyelitis (po″le-o-mi″ĕ-li′tis) Acute viral disease with fever, headache, gastrointestinal symptoms, stiff neck, and paralysis.

polydipsia (pol″e-dip′se-ah) Excessive thirst persisting for long periods of time.

polyuria (pol″e-u′re-ah) The passage of an unusually large volume of urine in a given period.

popliteal artery (pop-lit′e-al ar′ter-e) The continuation of the superficial femoral artery in the popliteal space (posterior surface of the knee).

posterior (pos-tēr′e-or) The back or dorsal surface of the body.

posterior spinous process That part of each vertebrae that can be palpated; it lies just under the skin in the midline of the back.

posterior surface The back surface of the body, away from the examiner.

posterior tibial artery (pos-tēr′e-or tib′e-al ar′ter-e) Artery just posterior to the medial malleolus; supplies blood to the foot.

postictal state (post″ik′tal stāt) Condition after an epileptic attack.

P-Q-R-S-T pain A method used to describe the patterns and types of pain.

precordial cardiac activity (pre-kor′de-al kar′de-ak ak′ti-vi-te) A transmitted impulse felt in the chest wall over the heart; it is not an arterial pulse and is therefore not reliable.

precordium (pre-kor′de-um) Chest wall over the heart.

pregnancy (preg′nan-se) Period during which a fertilized egg grows and develops in the uterus. Normal pregnancies come to completion at the end of nine months (40 weeks).

premature baby A baby who delivers before eight months gestation or who weighs less than 5-1/2 pounds at birth.

premature ventricular contractions (PVCs) A type of abnormal heartbeat.

presentation (pre″zen-ta′shun) The manner in which a baby is born; the part of the baby that appears first.

presenting part The part of the baby that is born first, usually the head.

pressure-compensated flowmeter A flowmeter with a float ball incorporated within a tapered calibrated tube. The float rises or falls according to the gas flow within the tube.

pressure point A point where a blood vessel runs near a bone; pressure can be applied to these points to stop bleeding.

pressure regulator A regulator attached to a medical gas cylinder in order to reduce pressure to suitable levels.

presumptive negligence Violation of a standard of emergency medical care imposed by statute, ordinances, administrative regulation, or case law.

priapism (pri′ah-pizm) A permanent and painful erection of the penis.

primary survey The process of finding and treating the most life-threatening emergencies first.

primigravida (pri″mĭ-grav′ĭ-dah) A woman who is pregnant for the first time.

PR interval From the beginning of the P wave to the beginning of the QRS complex.

PR level The time it take the electrical signal in the heart to travel from the atria to the ventricles, as measured by an electrocardiogram.

professional standard Published recommendation of organizations and societies involved in emergency medical care.

prolapse of the umbilical cord A delivery in which the umbilical cord appears before the baby; the baby's head compresses the cord during birth and cuts off all circulation to the baby.

prominence (prom′ĭ-nens) Projection, protrusion.

prostate gland (pros′tāt gland) A small gland that surrounds the male urethra where it emerges from the urinary bladder; it secretes a fluid that is part of the ejaculatory fluid.

prostatic hyertrophy (pros-tat′ik hi-per′tro-fe) Benign enlargement of the prostate gland.

prosthesis (pros-the′sis) An artificial substitute for a missing body part.

protection level A measure of the amount of protective equipment that someone must have to avoid injury during contact with a hazardous material.

protein (pro′tēn) One of a group of complex organic compounds, essential combinations of amino acids; principal constituent of the cell.

proton (pro′ton) The particle of an atom that has a positive electrical charge.

proximal (prok′sĭ-mal) Nearest; closer to any point of reference; opposed to distal.

psychiatric (si″ke-at′rik) Pertaining to psychiatry, that branch of medicine that deals with the study, treatment, and prevention of mental disorders.

psychogenic shock (si″ko-jen′ik shok) The common faint, caused by a temporary reduction in blood supply to the brain.

psychosis (si-ko′sis) A severely disturbed state of mind; a mental disorder characterized by defective or lost contact with reality.

ptyalin (ti′ah-lin) A digestive enzyme in saliva that converts starch to simple sugar.

pubic symphysis (symphysis pubis) (pu′bik sim′fĭ-sis) The firm fibrocartilaginous joint between the two pubic bones.

pubis (pu′bis) One of three bones (ilium, ischium, and pubis) that fuse to form the pelvic bones.

pulmonary (pul′mo-ner″e) Of the lung.

pulmonary abscess (pul′mo-ner″e ab′ses) An abscess that forms in damaged or diseased lung tissue.

pulmonary arteriole (pul′mo-ner″e ar-te′re-ol) A small arterial branch in the lungs.

pulmonary artery (pul′moner″e ar′ter-e) The major artery leading from the right ventricle of the heart to the lungs.

pulmonary capillary (pul′mon-ner″e kap′ĭ-lar″e) A capillary in the lungs that is located next to the alveoli (air sacs); here the exchange of oxygen and carbon dioxide takes place.

pulmonary circulation The circulation—sometimes called the lesser circulation—that carries unoxygenated blood from the right ventricle through the lungs and back to the left atrium; as it passes through the lungs, the blood gives up carbon dioxide and absorbs oxygen.

pulmonary contusion (pul′mo-ner″e kon-tu′zhun) A bruise of the lung.

pulmonary edema (pul′mo-ner″e ĕ-de′mah) Fluid building up in the lungs, a result of congestive heart failure.

pulmonary embolism (pul′mo-ner″e em′bo-lizm) The condition in which a blood clot breaks off from a large vein and travels to the lung.

pulmonary fibrosis (pul′mo-ner″e fi-bro′sis) Scarring of the lung.

pulmonary vein (pul′mo-ner″e vān) One of the four veins that return oxygenated blood from the lungs to the left atrium of the heart.

pulmonary venule (pul′mo-ner″e ven′ūl) A small vein in the lungs.

pulse The expansion and contraction of an artery, consistent with the beat of the heart, which may be felt with a finger.

pulseless electrical activity (PEA) The form of cardiac arrest in which the electrocardiogram displays an adequate heart rate and rhythm, but the heart is incapable of generating a palpable pulse and blood pressure in the circulation.

pulse point Point at which an artery lies close to the surface of the skin.

pulse rate The rate at which the heart is contracting. The normal pulse rate in an adult is 60 to 80 beats per minute; for a child the normal rate is 80 to 100 beats per minute.

pulse volume A rough indicator of the strength of the heart's contractions.

pump failure A condition that occurs when the heart fails to generate sufficient energy to move blood through the system.

puncture wound A wound resulting from a stab with a knife, ice pick, splinter, or any other pointed object or from a bullet.

pupil The circular opening in the middle of the iris of the eye.

purulent (pu'roo-lent) Consisting of or containing pus.

pus Liquid inflammation product made up of white cells and fluid.

P wave The wave on an electrocardiogram that represents depolorization of the atria.

pyloric stenosis (pi-lor'ik stĕ-no'sis) An obstruction of the outlet of the stomach, a congenital abnormal condition characterized by excessive growth of the pyloric muscle.

QRS complex The wave on an electrocardiogram that represents depolarization of the ventricles.

quadricep (kwod'rĭ-sep) The greater extensor muscle of the front of the thigh, divided into four parts.

quadriplegia (kowd"rĭ-ple"je-ah) Paralysis of all four limbs.

rabid An animal infected with rabies.

rabies(ra'bēz) An acute viral infection of the central nervous system, transmitted by the bite of a rabid animal.

"raccoon eyes" A sign of skull fracture in which ecchymosis develops under the eyes.

rad The unit of measurement for gamma and x-ray radiation.

radial artery (ra'de-al ar'ter-e) One of the major arteries of the arm; it can be palpated at the base of the thumb.

radial artery pulse A pulse that can be felt at the wrist, just at the base of the thumb, where the radial artery is close to the skin.

radial nerve Nerve carrying sensation to the greater portion of the back of the hand and controlling extension of the hand at the wrist.

radial nerve palsy An injury to the radial nerve in which the patient is unable to extend the wrist or fingers, producing "wrist drop."

radial styloid (ra'de-al sti'loid) Bony prominence felt on the lateral (thumb) side of the wrist.

radiant energy Any energy that is radiated from any source: electromagnetic waves, radio waves, visible light X rays, or nuclear radiation.

radiation The sending forth of light, short radio waves, ultraviolet waves, or X rays; the loss of heat through still air from the body to a colder environment.

Radiation Emergency Assistance REAC/TS A facility in Oak Ridge, Tennessee that serves as a worldwide hotline for the advice about and assistance following radiation accidents.

radioactivity The spontaneous release of energy by particles that make up atoms.

radio-telephone switch station (RTSS) Scanning capability built into a radio system that automatically selects a clear channel from among several VHF frequencies.

radium (ra'de-um) A radioactive element that is used in clinical therapy.

radius The bone on the thumb side of the forearm.

rale (rahl) Cracking, rattling breath sound that occurs in patients with fluid in the lungs.

rape Sexual intercourse without consent and chiefly by force or deception.

rational The ability to think and act clearly.

recessed (re-sest) In a hollow or cavity.

recompression (re"kom-presh'un) Restoration of pressure after the patient has been in a condition of greatly lowered pressure, as, for example, occurs from too rapid an ascent by a diver.

recompression chamber (re"kom-presh'un cham"ber) A single-person or multiperson capacity compressed air tank that is used by an experienced medical team to restore the body to a high-pressure environment.

record of live birth A recording of the birth of a live baby, with the exact time of birth.

recovery position Position used for a patient who is not a trauma victim prior to transport to facilitate spontaneous breathing.

rectosigmoid colon (rek"to-sig'moid ko'lon) Lower part of the large intestine that joins the rectum.

rectum (rek'tum) The lowermost end of the large intestine.

red blood cells Erythrocytes.

referred pain Pain felt in an area of the body other than where the cause of pain is located.

reflex (re'fleks) The sum total of any involuntary activity; *See also* reflex arc.

reflex arc The neutral arc used in a reflex action such as pulling the hand away from a hot stove; it involves sensory, short-circuiting internuncial, and motor nerves.

regionalized care Specific medical problems cared for at specialized centers.

regularity A characteristic of the pulse, occurring at constant intervals.

regulator A device that adjusts a condition to a certain standard.

regurgitation (re-gur"jĭ-ta'shun) A "burp" of air or fluid that is propelled as a result of the stomach being too full.

rehabilitation (re"hah-bil"ĭ-ta'shun) Restoration of the patient to self-sufficiency.

renal Pertaining to the kidney.

renal colic Excruciating pain caused by obstruction of the ureter by a kidney stone, as the ureter tries to pass the stone by peristalsis.

renal pelvis A cone-shaped collecting area that connects the ureter and the kidney.

repolarization (re-po″lar-ĭ-za′shun) One of two electrical processes of the heart, during which the electrical charges on the surface of the muscle cell change from negative to positive.

reproductive process (re″pro-duk′tiv pros′es) The process of conception, pregnancy, and birth.

reproductive system The anatomical system of a male or female body involved in reproduction.

rescue To free from a dangerous, destructive, or life-threatening situation by prompt vigorous action.

rescue vehicle A vehicle with equipment for providing rescue services; it should accompany the ambulance.

reservoir (rez′er-vwar) A place where infectious organisms live and multiply, such as stagnant water or a sewer.

resistance (re-zis′tans) The ability of an organism to remain unaffected by infectious agents.

resource coordination center Special communications operation that monitors and allocates medical control channels among EMS providers.

respiration (res″pĭ-ra′shun) Breathing.

respiratory center The area in the brain stem that senses the level of carbon dioxide and controls respiration.

respiratory distress Difficulty in breathing.

respiratory shock Shock caused by an insufficient amount of inspired oxygen.

respiratory system All the structures of the body that contribute to normal respiration or breathing.

respiratory tract The organs and structures of respiration, chiefly the nose, larynx, trachea, bronchi, and lungs.

resuscitation (re-sus″ĭ-ta′shun) Restoring to life or consciousness, using assisted breathing to restore ventilation and cardiac massage to restore circulation.

retina (ret′ĭ-nah) The light-sensitive area of the eye where images are projected; a layer of cells at the back of the eye that changes the light image into electrical impulses, which are carried by the optic nerve to the brain.

retinal detachment (ret′ĭ-nal de-tach′ment) A condition in which the retina is separated from its attachments at the back of the eye.

retrograde amnesia (ret′ro-grād am-ne′ze-ah) Inability to recall events that occurred before the actual onset of an event, such as a head injury.

retrolental fibroplasia (re″tro-len′tal fi″bro-play′se-ə) A disease of the eye in newborn infants in which an opaque fibrous membrane develops behind the lens of the eye; caused by high oxygen concentration.

retroperitoneal (re″tro-per″ĭ-to-ne′al) Behind the peritoneum.

retroperitoneal space (re″tro-per″ĭ-to-ne′al spās) The space between the abdominal cavity and the posterior abdominal wall, containing the kidneys, certain large vessels, and parts of the gastrointestinal tract.

rhonchi (rong′kī) Coarse breath sounds, seen in patients with chronic pulmonary disease.

ribs The paired arches of bone, 12 on either side, that extend from the thoracic vertebrae toward the anterior midline of the trunk.

rigid splints Splints made from firm material and applied to sides, front, and/or back of an injured extremity to prevent motion at the injury site.

rigor mortis (rig′or mor′tis) The stiffening of the entire body that follows death.

road position The position of the vehicle on the roadway relative to the inside or outside edge of the paved surface.

roentgen (rent′gen) The unit of measurement for gamma and x-ray radiation *See also* rad.

rotation (ro-ta′shun) A turning around on an axis; internal rotation: to the inside; external rotation: to the outside.

rubella (roo-bel′ah) German measles.

rubeola (roo-be′o-lah) Measles.

Rule of Nines A way to calculate the amount of body surface burned; the body is divided into sections each of which constitutes approximately 9 percent of the total body surface area.

rupture (rup′chur) A break or tear of an organ or tissue.

sacroiliac joint (sa″kro-il′e-ak joint) The joint formed by the articulation of the sacrum and ilium.

sacrum (sa′krum) One of three bones (sacrum and two pelvic bones) that make up the pelvic ring.

safe residual The point on the pressure gauge of a medical compressed gas cylinder at which the cylinder should be replaced with a new cylinder.

saliva (sah-li′vah) A secretion of water, protein, and salts into the mouth by salivary glands; makes food easier to chew and begins breaking starch down for digestion.

salivary gland Gland that produces saliva to keep the mouth and pharynx moist.

salmonella (sal″mo-nel′ah) A bacterium of the genus *Salmonella*.

salmonellosis Any disease caused by a salmonellal infection, which may be manifested as food poisoning with acute gastroenteritis, vomiting, and diarrhea.

SCBA *See* self-contained breathing apparatus (SCBA).

scalp The skin covering the cranium, usually bearing hair.

scanner A radio receiver in which the frequency being

received is automatically and instantaneously changed until a frequency carrying some message is detected. At that time, the receiver locks on to that frequency until the message is completed. The process is then repeated.

scapula The shoulder blade.

sciatic nerve The major nerve to the lower extremity.

sclera (skle′rah) The white portion of the eye; the tough outer coat of the eye that gives protection to the delicate, light-sensitive inner layer.

scleral icterus (skle′rahl ik′ter-us) Yellow color in the sclera of the eye, indicating jaundice.

scoop (split frame) stretcher Narrow stretcher that is first separated lengthwise, and then the two halves are slipped under the patient from each side. The halves are closed with locking brackets.

scrotum (skro′tum) A pouch of thickened skin hanging at the base of the penis, containing the testicles and their accessory ducts and vessels.

sebaceous gland (se-ba′shus gland) A gland that produces an oily substance called sebum, which discharges along the shafts of the hairs.

sebum (se′bum) Oily substance secreted by the sebaceous glands that seals the epidermal cells.

secondary survey The final step in the assessment process in which you carefully examine the patient from head to toe, looking for wounds and deformities and observing whether the patient feels pain or sensation.

second-degree burns Burns in which the epidermis and a varying extent of the dermis are burned; these burns are characterized by blister formation.

second stage of labor The time from the full dilation of the cervix until the baby is born.

sedative (sed′ah-tiv) A substance that allays activity and excitement.

seizure (se′zhur) Generalized, uncoordinated muscular activity usually associated with loss of consciousness; a convulsion.

self-contained breathing apparatus (SCBA) A respiratory aid that does not require outside air.

self-contained underwater breathing apparatus (SCUBA) A system that delivers air to the mouth and lungs at various atmospheric pressures, increasing with the depth of the dive.

Sellick's maneuver A technique whereby one EMT pushes on the cricoid cartilage to help a second EMT visualize the vocal cords during endotracheal intubation.

semen (se′men) Seminal fluid ejaculated from the penis and containing sperm.

semiconscious Partial consciousness.

seminal fluid (sem′i-nal floo′id) Semen.

seminal vesicles (sem′i-nal ves′i-k′lz) Storage sacs for sperm and seminal fluid, which empty into the urethra at the prostate.

senile dementia (se′nil de-men′she-ah) Loss of mental faculties occurring as a result of the aging process.

sensation (sen-sa′shun) A mental process, such as seeing, hearing, or smelling, due to immediate bodily stimulation.

sensitivity (sen″si-tiv′i-te) An overreaction or allergy to a substance.

sensory nerves (sen′so-re nervz) Nerves that carry sensations of touch, taste, heat, cold, pain, or other modalities.

sepsis (sep′sis) Blood poisoning; the presence in the blood or other tissues of harmful microorganisms or their poisons.

septic shock (sep′tik shok) Shock caused by infection that damages the walls of blood vessels.

septum (sep′tum) A dividing wall or membrane between body spaces or masses of soft tissue; a wall that divides the heart into the right and left sides.

serum hepatitis (se′rum hep″ah-ti′tis) Hepatitis B; hepatitis caused by a virus that is spread through blood-to-blood contact (transfusions, needle stick), mucous membrane (saliva or sputum contact), or sexual contact. It is a serious disease with long-term side effects.

sexual abuse Molestation or rape, often accompanied by physical abuse.

sexual intercourse (seks′u-al in′ter-kōrs) A sexual joining of two individuals during which seminal fluid, prostatic fluid, and sperm pass from the penis into the vagina during ejaculation.

shaft of a bone The long, straight, cylindrical midportion.

shock A condition of acute peripheral circulatory failure causing inadequate and progressively failing tissue perfusion.

shock position Position with the legs elevated and the knees straight so that blood drains from the enlarged vessels in the legs and returns to the heart for active circulation.

shoulder girdle The proximal portion of the upper extremity, made up of the clavicle, the scapula, and the humerus.

shoulder separation A/C Separation; a dislocation of the acromioclavicular joint.

side effect An effect of a drug other than the one for which it is given.

side flash Lightning that strikes near someone and "splashes" through the air to the person.

SIDS *See* sudden infant death syndrome (SIDS).

sign A condition that the EMT observes, such as bleeding or a contusion.

silver fork deformity Wrist injury from a fall on the

outstretched hand in which the injured wrist assumes a curvature similar to the profile of a dinner fork.

simple partial seizure A partial epileptic seizure in which the seizure activity is limited to one or more extremities or one side of the body.

simplex Single-frequency operating capability; radio transmissions can occur in either direction but not simultaneously in both; one party transmits, and the other receives.

sinusitis (si″nŭ-si′tis) Inflammation of a sinus.

sinus node Part of the electrical conduction system of the heart.

size up To gather facts quickly about a situation, analyze the problem, and decide how to handle it.

sixty-cycle interference A problem that prevents the EMT-D from analyzing the rhythm on the monitor screen of a manual defibrillator because of interference from electrical appliances in the vicinity.

skeletal muscle (skel′ĕ-tal mus′el) Striated muscles that are attached to bones and usually cross at least one joint.

skeleton (skel′ĕ-ton) The skeletal system; the supporting framework of the human body, composed of 206 bones.

skin The outer layer of the body, consisting of the dermis and epidermis and resting on subcutaneous tissue. It forms the largest organ of the body and serves to isolate the body from its environment, protect it from bacterial invasion, control temperature, retain fluids, and furnish information about the external environment to the brain through its nerve endings.

skull A collective term for the bones of the head.

sling A triangular bandage or material that is tied around the neck and is used to support the weight of the injured upper extremity.

small intestine The portion of the digestive tube between the stomach and the cecum, consisting of the duodenum, jejunum, and ileum.

smooth muscle Nonstriated, involuntary muscle; it constitutes the bulk of the gastrointestinal tract and is present in nearly every organ to regulate automatic activity.

soft palate (soft pal′at) A fold of mucous membrane and muscle that extends posteriorly into the throat. It is designed to hold food that is being chewed within the mouth and to initiate swallowing.

soft splint Air splint or splint made from soft material that provides gentle support.

solar burn Sunburn.

solar radiation Radiation from the sun.

solid organs Solid masses of tissue where much of the chemical work of the body takes place: the liver, spleen, pancreas, and kidneys.

solution sets A type of administration set for intrave-

nous fluid therapy that is designed for delivering large volumes of fluid to be infused over a short period of time.

somatic nervous system (so-mat′ik ner′vus sis′tem) Part of the nervous system that regulates functions over which there is voluntary control.

somnolent (som′no-lent) Sleepy.

source of infection The origin of the infection or infectious agent; such a source may be a person, object, or any substance carrying bacteria, viruses, or parasites.

sovereign immunity A doctrine in English common law, now abandoned, that individuals were deprived of a remedy when their injury or damage was caused by the negligence of the king or other members of the royal family.

Spanish Windlass A tourniquet consisting of a bandage tied around a body part and twisted.

spasm (spazm) A sudden, violent, involuntary contraction of a group of muscles.

"speed" Amphetamines.

sperm cell Male cell that fertilizes the ovum.

sphincter muscle (sfingk′ter mus′el) Circular muscles that encircle a duct, tube, or opening in such a way that their contraction constricts the opening.

sphygmomanometer (sfig″mo-mah-nom′ĕ-ter) An instrument used to measure blood pressure.

spinal canal A tunnel formed by the back part of each vertebra that encloses and protects the spinal cord.

spinal column The central supporting bony structure of the body.

spinal cord An extension of the brain, composed of virtually all the nerves carrying messages between the brain and the rest of the body. It lies inside of and is protected by the spinal canal.

spinal nerves Thirty one pairs of peripheral nerves that exit the spinal cord by passing between the vertebrae. They conduct sensory impulses from the skin and other organs to the spinal cord. They also conduct motor impulses from the spinal cord to the muscles that are present in that segment of the body.

spine A column of 33 vertebrae extending from the base of the skull to the tip of the coccyx.

spine board A wooden board primarily used for extrication and transportation of patients with actual or suspected spinal injuries; also serves as a litter.

spleen (splēn) A large glandlike organ in the upper left quadrant of the abdomen; its major function is the normal production and destruction of blood cells.

splint A rigid or flexible appliance used to protect and keep an injured part in place.

splinting Immobilizing an injured part by means of a device applying rigid support.

split-frame (scoop) stretcher Narrow stretcher that is first separated lengthwise, after which the two halves are slipped under the patient from each side. The halves are closed with locking brackets. These stretchers are not adequate for spinal immobilization.

spontaneous abortion (spon-ta′ne-us ah-bor′shun) An abortion that occurs for no known reason.

spontaneous pneumothorax (spon-ta′ne-us nu″mo-tho′raks) The presence of air in the chest cavity from the rupture of a congenitally weak area on the surface of the lungs.

sprain A joint injury in which some of the supporting ligaments are damaged.

sputum (spu′tum) Fluid that is coughed or spit up from the lungs.

squelch Several type of radio receiver circuits used for suppressing, though not eliminating, unwanted radio signals or radio noise.

stacked shocks Delivery of a second and sometimes a third countershock during defibrillation immediately after the first countershock has been delivered.

standard of care The manner in which an individual must act or behave when giving care.

standing orders A direct order from the program medical director to perform certain tasks for a patient under a specific set of circumstances.

staphylococcus An organism of the genus *Staphylococcus.*

Star of Life® Emblem that identifies true ambulances.

START (Simple Triage and Rapid Treatment) A system of triage.

state of consciousness The degree of consciousness.

status asthmaticus (sta′tus az-mat′ik-us) A severe episode of asthma that does not respond to typical therapeutic measures.

status epilepticus (sta′tus ep″ĭ-lep′tik-us) A series of rapidly repeated epileptic convulsions in one individual without any periods of consciousness between them.

sterilize (ster′ĭ-līz) To make sterile or free from bacterial contamination.

sternoclavicular joint (ster″no-klah-vik′u-lar joint) The joint formed by the articulation between the sternum and the clavicle.

sternocleidomastoid muscles (ster″no-kli″do-mas′toid mus′el) Muscles on either side of the neck that allow movement of the head.

sternum (ster′num) The breastbone.

stethoscope (steth′o-skōp) Instrument used in the determination of blood pressure and in the detection of heart, breath, and bowel sounds.

stimulant (stim′u-lant) Any agent producing excitation.

stimulus (pl. stimuli) (stim′u-lus) Something that rouses or attempts to rouse the patient to activity.

sting Injury caused by venom of a plant or animal.

Stoke's stretcher A basket stretcher shaped like an ob-

long plastic shell, useful in removing patients from heights or over difficult terrain or debris.

stoma (sto′mah) An opening or mouth.

stomach The expansion of the alimentary canal between the esophagus and the duodenum, which receives food, stores it, and provides for its movement into the small bowel.

stomach ulcers Lesions on the mucous surfaces of the stomach.

stool The fecal discharge from the bowels.

stove-in chest *See* flail chest.

straddle slide A method of placing a patient on a long spine board by straddling both board and patient and sliding the patient onto the board.

strain Muscle pull; a stretched, overexerted, or torn muscle.

strainer (strān′er) An obstruction that allows water to flow through, yet traps objects such as boats or people.

strangulation (strang″gu-la′shun) Arrest of the circulation in a part due to compression or entrapment; a situation causing death of tissue.

street drugs Drugs acquired "on the street" by addicts from pushers or other addicts, not prescribed by a physician.

street form A compact form, frequently printed on a 3 x 5-inch index card, that enables you to obtain and record the information needed to make a radio report to the emergency department. This information is also used to fill out the more detailed, permanent ambulance run record.

stress fracture One that occurs when the bone is subjected to frequent, repeated stress such as running or marching long distances.

stretcher A carrying device making it possible for two persons to lift and carry a patient who is lying down; used to transport patients to, from, and in an ambulance.

striated (stri′āt-ed) Marked by streaks or lines under the microscope.

striated muscle (stri′āt-ed mus′el) Muscle that has characteristic stripes, or striations, under the microscope; voluntary, skeletal muscle.

stride potential Lightning that strikes the ground near someone, travelling up one leg and down the other into the ground.

stridor (stri′dor) A harsh, high-pitched respiratory sound such as the inspiratory sound often heard in acute laryngeal obstruction.

strobe light Lightweight portable light that attaches to your arm or belt, enabling you to see other EMTs and enabling oncoming vehicles to see you.

stroke The loss of brain function, usually the result of a cerebrovascular accident.

stylet (sti′let) A plastic-coated wire that when inserted into the endotracheal tube, adds rigidity to the tube.

styloid processes (sti′loid pros es-ez) Bony prominences at the ends of the radius and ulna that form the socket for the wrist joint.

subarachnoid space (sub ah-rak noid spas) Space between the arachnoid and the pia mater.

subatomic particle A particle smaller than an atom.

subcutaneous (sub″ku-ta′ne-us) Under the skin.

subcutaneous emphysema (sub″ku-ta′ne-us em″ fi-se′mah) The presence of air in soft tissues, causing a very characteristic crackling sensation on palpation.

subcutaneously Under the skin.

subcutaneous tissue Tissue, largely fat, that lies directly under the dermis and serves as an insulator of the body.

subdiaphragmatic thrust (Heimlich) maneuver (sub″di-ah-frag-mat′ik thrust [him lik] mah-noo′ver) A series of manual thrusts to the upper abdomen just above the umbilicus and well below the xiphoid process to relieve upper airway obstruction; also called the abdominal thrust maneuver.

subdural (sub-du ral) Beneath the dura and outside the brain.

subdural hematoma (sub-du ral hem ah-to mah) A hematoma, or collection of blood, beneath the dura mater and outside the brain.

substance abuse The knowing misuse of any substance to produce some desired effect.

substernal (sub-ster nal) Under the breastbone.

subtrochanteric fracture (sub″tro-kan-ter′ik frak′chur) A fracture occurring below a trochanter.

sucking chest wound A open or penetrating chest wall wound through which air passes during inspiration and expiration.

suctioning (suk′shun-ing) Sucking out gas or fluid by mechanical means.

sudden infant death syndrome (SIDS) Death from unknown cause occurring during sleep in an otherwise healthy infant; also called crib death.

suffocate (suf′o-kayt) To stop breathing; to have one's breathing blocked; to suffer from lack of oxygen.

suicidal (soo′i-sīd-l) Describing a patient who may be threatening to kill himself.

suicide (soo′i-sīd) Self-inflicted death.

sunstroke *See* heat stroke.

superficial (soo″per-fish′al) Pertaining to or situated near the surface.

superficial temporal artery (soo″per-fish′al tem′po-ral ar′ter-e) An artery supplying the scalp, palpable just anterior to the ears at the temporomandibular joints.

superior (soo-pe′re-or) Situated above or directed upward.

superior portion That portion of the body or body part that lies nearer the head than the feet.

superior vena cava (soo-pe′re-or ven′ah ka′vah) One of the two largest veins in the body that carries blood from the upper extremities, head, neck, and chest into the heart.

supine (soo′pīn) Lying on the back or with the face upward.

supracondylar fracture (soo″prah-kon′di-lar frak′chur) Fracture of the distal end of the humerus in which the fracture line extends across the bone just above the condyles.

SURVIVE—study technique Composed of the following techniques: *s*kim, *u*nderline, *r*ead, *v*erbalize, *i*ntegrate, *v*ary, and *e*valuate.

sutured (su′churd) Describing a wound that was closed or repaired by stitching the opposing surfaces with a fibrous material.

swathe (swäth) A bandage that passes around the chest to secure an injured arm to the chest.

sweat glands The glands that secrete sweat.

swelling (swel′ing) An abnormal enlargement or increase in volume of a body part area not caused by proliferation of cells.

sympathetic nervous system A part of the autonomic nervous system that causes blood vessels to constrict, stimulates sweating, increases the heart rate, causes the sphincter muscles to constrict, and prepares the body to respond to stress.

symphysis (sim′fi-sis) An articulation in which the bony surfaces are connected by pads of fibrous cartilage without a synovial membrane.

symphysis pubis (pubic symphysis) (sim′fi-sis pu′bis) The firm fibrocartilaginous joint between the two pubic bones.

symptom (simp′tum) Something the patient tells you, such as "I feel dizzy."

syncope (sin′ ko-pe) Fainting.

synovial fluid (si-no′ve-al floo′id) Fluid produced by the synovium that nourishes and lubricates the articular cartilage of a joint.

synovium (si-no′ve-um) The inner surface of the joint capsule.

syphilis (sif′i-lis) Acute bacterial venereal disease with hard sores, secondary skin eruptions, and late complications of the heart and brain.

syringe (si-rinj) An instrument for injecting liquid into or withdrawing them from any vessel or cavity.

syrup of ipecac (sir′up, ip′ĕ-kak) Preparation of the dried root of a shrub found in Brazil and other parts of South America that can cause vomiting.

systemic (sis-tem′ik) Generalized throughout the body, such as fever, chills, and weakness.

systemic circulation Circulation, sometimes called the greater circulation, that carries oxygenated blood from the left ventricle of the heart throughout the body and back to the right atrium.

systemic hypothermia A systemic lowering of the body temperature below 95 degrees F.

systole (sis′to-le) The contraction, or period of contraction, of the heart, especially that of the ventricles.

systolic blood pressure The higher blood pressure noted at the moment of ventricular contraction of the heart.

systolic pressure *See* systolic blood pressure.

tachycardia (tak″e-kar′de-ah) Rapid but regular heart rhythm.

tachypnea (tak″ip-ne′ah) Excess, quick, shallow breathing.

talus (ta′lus) An ankle bone.

tarsal bones (tahr′sal bonz) Seven bones (the talus, calcaneus, and five other bones) that make up the rear portion of the foot.

tarsal plate (tahr′sal plat′) The firm framework of connective tissue that gives shape to the eyelids (upper and lower).

tear ducts Ducts located on the inner side of the eye along the upper and lower lids that drain the tears into the nose.

tear glands Lacrimal glands that produce tears that act to lubricate the eye and to flush out foreign material from the eye.

tears A fluid that acts as a lubricating substance to keep the eye from drying and flushes foreign material from the eye.

telemetric transmission Orders relayed from a program medical director to medical personnel in the field via radio transmission.

tempered glass A type of glass that shatters into small pieces when struck with a sharp, pointed object.

temples (temporal regions) The lateral portions of the cranium.

temporal (tem′po-ral) Pertaining to the lateral region of the head, above the zygomatic arch.

temporal artery The artery located on either side of the face that supplies blood to the scalp; it can be palpated just anterior to the ear at the temporomandibular joint.

temporal regions (temples) The lateral portions of the cranium.

temporomandibular joint (tem″po-ro-man-dib′u-lar joint) The joint formed by the articulation between the mandible and the cranium, just in front of the ear.

tenderness (ten′der-nes) Abnormal sensitivity to touch or pressure.

tendon (ten′dun) A tough, ropelike cord of fibrous tissue that attaches a skeletal muscle to a bone.

tension pneumothorax (ten′shun nu″mo-tho′raks) An accumulation of air or gas in the pleural cavity that progressively increases and causes a rise in intrathoracic pressure.

terminal disease Disease that is known to end in death.

testes (tes′tēz) Male reproductive glands.

testicles (tes′tĭ-k′lz) Male genital glands containing specialized cells that produce hormones and sperm.

tetanus (tet′ah-nus) An infectious disease in which a muscle spasm causes "lockjaw," arching of the back, and seizures.

tetanus prophylaxis (tet′ah-nus pro″fi-lak′sis) Treatment to prevent tetanus, a potentially fatal infectious disease characterized by extreme body rigidity and muscle spasms.

thebaine (the-ba′in) A crystalline, poisonous, and anodyne alkoloid from opium, having properties similar to those of strychnine.

thermal burn (ther′mal bern) A burn that is caused by heat.

third-degree burn Burns that extend through the dermis and into or beyond the subcutaneous fat.

third stage of labor The time from the birth of a baby until the delivery of the placenta.

Thomas (traction) splint Holds a lower extremity fracture or dislocation immobile and allows steady longitudinal pull on the extremity.

thoracic cage (tho-ras′ik kāj) The chest.

thoracic spine The 12 vertebrae that attached to the 12 ribs; the upper part of the back.

thoracic vertebrae The 12 vertebrae that lie between the cervical vertebrae and the lumbar vertebrae.

thorax (tho′raks) The chest; the upper part of the trunk between the neck and the abdomen.

thrombosis (throm-bo′sis) The formation of a blood clot in a blood vessel.

thrombus (throm′bus) The blood clot that forms in a vessel.

through and through (perforating) wounds Wounds that traverse an entire limb to exit on the opposite side.

thyroid cartilage (thi′roid kar′tĭ″lij) A firm prominence of cartilage that forms the upper part of the larynx; the Adam's apple.

thyroid gland A ductless gland lying on the upper part of the trachea; it produces the thyroid hormone thyroxin, which controls the general metabolism of the body.

tibia (tib′e-ah) The shin bone, the larger of the two bones of the leg.

tibial crest (tib′e-al krest) The lower end of the tibia from its point of insertion in the quadriceps tendon down to the ankle joint.

tibial plateau (tib′e-al plah-to′) The upper end of the tibia, which forms the interior surface of the knee joint.

tibial tuberosity A prominence on the tibia for the insertion of the quadriceps tendon.

tinnitus (tĭ-ni′tus) Ringing in the ear.

tolerance (tol′er-ans) The ability to endure large doses without ill effect, such as the ability to endure the continued or increasing use of a drug.

tone An audio signal or carrier wave of controlled amplitude and frequency that is used for equipment control purpose or to selectively signal a receiver, such as activating a pager.

tongue-jaw-lift maneuver A technique of opening the patient's mouth by grasping the tongue and lower jaw between the thumb and fingers and lifting them forward.

tonic-clonic seizure (ton′ik klon′ik se′zhur) A generalized epileptic seizure involving most of the brain; also called a convulsive seizure.

tonic-muscular contractions Sustained, rigid, muscular contractions that cause odd posturing of the body and occur during a generalized epileptic seizure.

tonsil tips (pharyngeal suction tips) Large-bore tips that fasten onto suction tubing used to suction the pharynx.

topographic anatomy (top″o-graf′ik ah-nat′o-me) The superficial landmarks of the body.

topography (to-pog′rah-fe) External features of the body.

torso (tor′so) The human trunk.

tourniquet (toor′nĭ-ket) An instrument for the compression of a blood vessel for the purpose of controlling the flow of blood.

toxic (tok′sik) Poisonous.

toxicity level (tok-sis′ĭ-te lev′el) A measure of the risk that anyone is subjected to by contact with a certain hazardous material.

toxin (tok′sin) A poison or harmful substance, produced by bacteria, animals or plants.

trachea (tra′ke-ah) The windpipe; the main trunk for air passing to and from the lungs.

tracheal stoma An opening in the neck that connects the trachea directly to the skin.

traction The act of exerting a pulling force on a structure.

traction splint Holds a lower extremity fracture or dislocation immobile and allows steady longitudinal pull on the extremity.

tragus (tra′gus) The small rounded fleshy protuberance immediately at the front of the ear canal.

tranquilizer (tran″kwĭ-līz′er) A drug that calms the patient without affecting the state of consciousness.

transfusion The introduction of whole blood or blood products into the vascular system.

transmission The manner by which an infection is spread: contact, airborne, by vehicles, or by vectors.

transverse colon The part of the colon that runs transversely across the upper part of the abdomen.

transverse presentation A delivery in which the baby is lying sideways inside the uterus.

trauma (traw′mah) A wound or injury.

trauma triage predictors (traw′mah tre-ahzh pri-dik-terz) The physiological, anatomical, and mechanism of injury indicators of the need to transport patients to a trauma center.

traumatic asphyxia (traw-mat′ik as-fik′se-ah) Impending or actual cessation of life as a result of sudden or severe compression of the thorax or upper abdomen, or both.

trench foot A form of cold exposure that occurs when the feet suffer prolonged exposure to cold but not freezing water; also called immersion foot.

Trendelenburg position The shock position, achieved by elevating the foot of the long spine board.

triage (tre-ahzh′) Sorting. A technique of establishing treatment and transportation priorities in any event where the number of casualties is greater than the emergency facilities can handle.

triceps muscle (tri′seps mus′el) The muscle in the back of the upper arm.

trimester (tri-mes′ter) A period of three months.

trochanters (tro-kan′terz) Prominences on a bone where tendons insert; specifically, two protuberances, greater and lesser, on the femur.

tuberculosis (TB) (too-ber″ku-lo′sis) A chronic bacterial disease that usually affects the lungs. Signs and symptoms are cough, fatigue, weight loss, chest pain, and coughing up of blood.

tuberosities (too″bĕ-ros′ĭ-tez) Prominences on a bone where tendons insert.

T wave The wave on an electrocardiogram that represents repolarization of the ventricles.

tympanic membrane (tim-pan′ik mem′brān) Eardrum.

type I diabetes The type of diabetic disease that usually starts in childhood and requires insulin for proper treatment and control.

type II diabetes The type of diabetic disease that usually starts in later life and is often treatable without the use of insulin.

UHF (ultrahigh frequency) Those radio frequencies between 300 and 3,000 MHz. (A frequency of 800 MHz has better building and underground penetration than do frequencies below 300 MHz.)

ulcer (ul′ser) A lesion on the surface of the skin or a mucous surface, caused by the superficial loss of tissue, usually with inflammation.

ulcerative colitis (ul′ser-a″tiv ko-li′tis) Chronic ulceration in the colon.

ulna (ul′nah) The inner and larger bone of the forearm, on the side opposite the thumb.

ulnar artery (ul′nah ar′ter-e) One of the major arteries of the arm; it can be palpated at the medial wrist at the base of the fifth finger.

ulnar styloid (ul′nar sti′loid) Bony prominence felt on the medial (little finger) side of the wrist.

ultraviolet light Those invisible rays of the spectrum that are beyond the violet rays.

umbilical cord (um-bil′ĭ-kal kord) The tissue connecting the placenta with the fetus.

umbilicus (um-bil′ĭ-kus) The navel; a small depression in the abdominal wall marking the point where the fetus was attached to the umbilical cord.

unconscious (un-kon′shus) Having lost consciousness.

unilateral On one side.

universal dressing Dressing made of thick, absorbent material, measuring 9 x 36 inches and packed folded into a compact size.

universal precautions (yü-ni-vər-səl pri-ko-shunz) Protective measures developed by the Centers for Disease Control (CDC) for use when dealing with objects that might accidentally puncture the skin of the health care worker.

"upper" A stimulant.

upper airway Air passage above the larynx: the nose, mouth, and throat.

uremia (u-re′me-ah) A toxic condition caused by waste products of metabolism accumulating in the blood as a result of failure of kidney function.

ureter (u-re′ter) A small, hollow tube that carries urine from the kidneys to the bladder.

urethra (u-re′thrah) The membranous canal conveying urine from the bladder to outside the body.

urethral discharge Any material that passes out of the male urethra other than urine or semen.

urinary bladder A musculomembranous sac for collecting and storing urine.

urinary system The organs that control the discharge of certain waste materials filtered from the blood and excreted as urine.

urine (u-rin) A fluid waste product of the body, excreted by the kidneys, passed through the ureters, stored in the bladder, and discharged through the urethra.

urticaria (ur″ti-kar′e-ah) Generalized itching, burning, and the development of multiple raised, reddened areas on the skin; hives.

uterus (u′ter-us) The womb.

vaccine (vak′sēn) A preparation of killed microorganisms or living organisms that is administered to produce or increase immunity to a disease.

vagina (vah-ji′nah) The birth canal.

vaginal discharge Blood discharge that occurs approximately once a month in healthy, nonpregnant women after puberty and before menopause.

vagus nerve (va′gus nerv) The tenth cranial nerve, which serves the larynx, lungs, heart, esophagus, stomach, and most of the abdominal viscera.

Valium® (val′e-um) A drug used as a tranquilizer and muscle relaxant.

vallecula (vah-lek′u-lah) The space between the base of the tongue and the epiglottis.

vascular (vas′ku-lar) Relating to or containing blood vessels.

vascular volume The capacity of the veins.

vas deferens (vas′def′er-ens) A spermatic duct of the testicles.

vector transmission A method of disease transmission in which the infective organism is transmitted to an individual by animals.

vehicle transmission A method of disease transmission in which the infective organism is introduced directly into the body through the ingestion of contaminated food or water or by the infusion of contaminated drugs, fluid, or blood.

vein (vān) A tubular vessel that carries blood from the capillaries and venules into the right atrium of the heart.

vena cava (ve′nah ka′vah) One of the two large veins conducting blood to the right upper chamber of the heart. Inferior vena cava: the venous trunk returning blood from the lower extremities and the pelvic and abdominal viscera. Superior vena cava: the venous trunk returning blood from the upper extremities and the head, neck, and chest.

venereal disease (ve-ne′re-al dĭ-zēz) A disease transmitted by sexual contact.

venipuncture (ven′i-punk″tūr) The site on an extremity where the needle for intravenous fluid therapy is inserted into a vein.

venom (ven′um) Poison secreted by animals and deposited in bite wounds.

venous pressure (ve′nus presh′ur) The pressure of blood that flows through the veins.

venous tourniquet A constricting band placed about and below the site of injection to block the flow of blood in the veins but not the arterial flow.

ventilation (ven″tĭ-la′shun) Exchange of air between the lungs and the air of the environment; breathing.

ventilator A device to aid breathing.

ventricle (ven′trĭ-k′l) Either of the two lower chambers of the heart.

ventricular extrasystoles Additional beats of the ventricle interspersed with the regular rhythm.

ventricular fibrillation (VF) A continuous, uncoordinated quivering of the cardiac muscle.

ventricular premature contractions *See* premature ventricular contractions.

ventricular tachycardia (VT) A very rapid heart rate.

Venturi mask (ven-tu(ə)r-ē mask) A breathing unit that provides a specific concentration of oxygen through a delivery tube connected to a standard face mask.

venule (ven′ūl) A small vein into which blood passes from the capillaries.

vertebra (ver′tĕ-brah) The 33 bones of the spinal column; there are 7 cervical, 12 thoracic, 5 lumbar, 5 sacral, and 4 coccygeal vertebrae.

vertebral arteries Two cerebral arteries that supply blood to the brain; they unite at the base of the brain to form the basiliar artery.

vertex presentation (ver′teks pre″zen-ta′shun) A normal delivery in which the baby's head appears first.

vertigo (ver′tĭ-go) Dizziness.

VHF (very high frequency) Those radio frequencies between 30 and 300 MHz. The VHF spectrum is further divided into "high" and "low" bands.

viral (vi′ral) Of or related to a group of pathogens not visible under a microscope and causing disease by intracellular invasion.

viral meningitis (vi′ral men″in-ji′tis) Meningitis, or inflammation of the meningeal coverings of the brain, caused by a virus; the viral form of meningitis is usually transmitted via food or water.

virulence (vir′u-lens) The degree to which an infectious organism survives after exposure to light and air; its strength.

virus (vi′rus) The specific agent of a type of infectious disease; specifically, a group of microbes that can pass through fine filters that bacteria cannot pass through. An incomplete organism, a virus cannot sustain life alone but is an obligate intracellular parasite that lives on the cells of the host or organism to which it is attached.

viscera (vis′er-ah) The internal organs of the body.

visceral peritoneum (vis′er-al per″i-to-ne′um) The portion of the peritoneum that covers the surface of all the abdominal organs.

visceral pleura (vis′er-al ploor′ah) Smooth, glistening tissue that covers the lungs.

vital signs Signs of life; pulse, respiration, blood pressure, and temperature.

vital statistics Age, sex, and kin of the patient.

vitamins Organic substances that occur in many foods and are necessary for normal metabolism in the body.

vitreous humor (vit′re-us hu′mor) Vitreous means glasslike; the translucent jellylike substance within the eye maintaining its pressure and form.

vocal cord (vo′kal kord) Either of two pairs of folds of mucous membranes that project into the cavity of the larynx and have free edges extending dorsoventrally toward the middle line.

voice box The larynx.

void To urinate.

voluntary muscle Muscle under direct voluntary control of the brain that can be contracted or relaxed at will; skeletal muscle.

voluntary nervous system *See* somatic nervous system.

vomiting (vom′it-ing) Disgorging the contents of the stomach through the mouth.

vomitus (vom′ĭ-tus) Vomited material.

vulva (vul′va) The external female genitalia.

watt-seconds A measure of the electrical current delivered by defibrillators.

wheal (hwel) A raised, whitish area on the skin resulting from an insect bite or allergic reaction.

wheeze (hwēz) A high-pitched, whistling breath sound, characteristically heard on expiration in patients with asthma.

whooping cough Acute bacterial disease with violent attacks of coughing and high-pitched whooping.

window phase of testing The time from exposure to a disease to the time lab tests note the presence of an antibody.

withdrawal Physical or psychological removal of oneself from a situation.

wrist Joint between the forearm and hand.

wrist drop Weakness in the wrist or fingers produced by injury of the radial nerve.

xiphoid process (zif′oid pros′es) One of three components (manubrium, body and xiphoid process) of the sternum; the narrow, cartilaginous lower tip of the sternum.

X ray An electromagnetic wave that penetrates various substances and can also affect a photographic plate; used in diagnosis and therapy.

zygoma (zi-go′mah) The quadrangular bone of the cheek, articulating with the frontal bone, the maxilla, the zygomatic process of the temporal bone, and the great wing of the sphenoid bone.

INDEX

. . . .